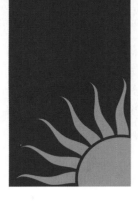

Cancer of the Skin

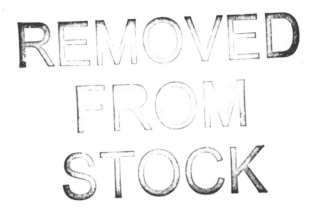

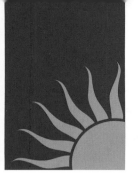

Cancer of the Skin

Edited by

Darrell S Rigel MD
Clinical Professor
Department of Dermatology
New York University School of Medicine
Adjunct Clinical Professor
Department of Dermatology
Mount Sinai School of Medicine
New York, NY, USA

Robert J Friedman MD MSc(Med)
Clinical Assistant Professor
Department of Dermatology
New York University School of Medicine
New York, NY, USA

Leonard M Dzubow MD
Clinical Professor of Dermatology
Department of Dermatology
University of Pennsylvania
Philadelphia, PA, USA

Douglas S Reintgen MD
Director
Lakeland Regional Cancer Center
Lakeland, FL, USA

Jean-Claude Bystryn MD
Professor of Dermatology
Department of Dermatology
New York University School of Medicine
New York, NY, USA

Robin Marks MB BS MPH FRACP FACD
Professor of Dermatology
Department of Dermatology
University of Melbourne
St Vincent's Hospital
Melbourne, Australia

ELSEVIER
SAUNDERS

Philadelphia   Edinburgh   London   New York   Oxford   St Louis   Sydney   Toronto   2005

ELSEVIER
SAUNDERS

An imprint of Elsevier Inc

ISBN 0 7216 0544 3

British Library Cataloguing in Publication Data
A catalogue record for this book is available from the British Library

Library of Congress Cataloging in Publication Data
A catalog record for this book is available from the Library of Congress

Notice
Medical knowledge is constantly changing. Standard safety precautions must be followed, but as new research and clinical experience broaden our knowledge, changes in treatment and drug therapy may become necessary or appropriate. Readers are advised to check the most current product information provided by the manufacturer of each drug to be administered to verify the recommended dose, the method and duration of administration, and contraindications. It is the responsibility of the practitioner, relying on experience and knowledge of the patient, to determine dosages and the best treatment for each individual patient. Neither the Publisher nor the editors or contributors assume any liability for any injury and/or damage to persons or property arising from this publication.
The Publisher

Printed in China

The
Publisher's
policy is to use
**paper manufactured
from sustainable forests**

Last digit is the print number : 9 8 7 6 5 4 3 2 1

Commissioning Editor: Sue Hodgson
Project Development Manager: Shuet-Kei Cheung
Project Manager: Glenys Norquay
Illustration Manager: Mick Ruddy
Design Manager: Andy Chapman
Illustrators: Mark Willey and Richard Prime

Contents

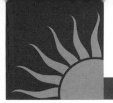

List of Contributors

Giuseppe Argenziano MD
Assistant Professor of Dermatology
Department of Dermatology
Second University of Naples
Naples, Italy

Shan R Baker MD FACS
Professor and Director
Center for Facial Cosmetic Surgery
University of Michigan
Livonia, MI, USA

Eric Berkowitz MD
Resident
Department of Dermatology
Mount Sinai Medical Center
New York, NY, USA

Brian Berman MD PhD
Professor of Dermatology and Internal Medicine
Department of Dermatology and Cutaneous Surgery
University of Miami School of Medicine
Miami, FL, USA

Jean L Bolognia MD
Professor of Dermatology
Department of Dermatology
Yale Medical School
New Haven, CT, USA

Thomas Brenn MD PhD
Instructor in Pathology
Harvard Medical School
Associate Pathologist
Brigham and Women's Hospital
Boston, MA, USA

Gregory M Bricca MD
Private Practice
Sacramento, CA, USA

David G Brodland MD
Assistant Clinical Professor
Departments of Dermatology and Otolaryngology
University of Pittsburgh Medical Center
Pittsburgh, PA, USA

Jean-Claude Bystryn MD
Professor of Dermatology
Department of Dermatology
New York University School of Medicine
New York, NY, USA

Jeffrey P Callen MD
Professor of Medicine (Dermatology)
Chief, Division of Dermatology
University of Louisville
Louisville, KY, USA

Leander Cannick MD
Medical University of South Carolina
Charleston, SC, USA

John A Carucci MD PhD
Chief, Mohs Micrographic and Dermatologic Surgery
Department of Dermatology
Weill Medical College of Cornell University
New York, NY, USA

J Christian Cather MD
Research Fellow
Texas Dermatology Associates
Dallas, Texas, USA

Jennifer Cather MD
Director of Clinical Research
Texas Dermatology Associates
Dallas, Texas, USA

Roger I Ceilley MD
Clinical Professor
Department of Dermatology
The University of Iowa
Iowa City, IA, USA

Lorenzo Cerroni MD
Professor of Dermatology
Department of Dermatology
Medical University of Graz,
Graz, Austria

Molly Chartier MD
University of Connecticut Health Center
Farmington, USA

Clay J Cockerell MD
Clinical Professor of Dermatology and Pathology
Director of Dermatopathology
University of Texas South Western Medical Center
Dallas, TX, USA

Jay S Cooper MD FACR FACRO
Professor of Radiation Oncology (Retired)
New York University Medical Center
New York, NY, USA

Michael Dans MD PhD
Resident Physician of Dermatology
Department of Dermatology
University of Pennsylvania Health System
Philadelphia, PA, USA

Vincent A DeLeo MD
Chairman
Department of Dermatology
St Luke's Roosevelt Hospital Center and Beth Israel
Medical Center
New York, NY, USA

James Q Del Rosso DO FAOCD
Clinical Assistant Professor
Department of Dermatology
University of Nevada School of Medicine
Las Vegas, NV, USA

Daihung V Do MD
Resident in Dermatology
Department of Dermatology
Tufts University School of Medicine
Boston, MA, USA

Marcia S Driscoll MD PharmD
Private Practice
Chevy Chase, MD, USA

Leonard M Dzubow MD
Clinical Professor of Dermatology
Department of Dermatology
University of Pennsylvania
Philadelphia, PA, USA

Melody J Eide MD
Fellow
Dermatoepidemiology Unit
Providence VA Medical Center
Providence, RI, USA

Steven S Fakharzadeh MD PhD
Assistant Professor of Dermatology
Department of Dermatology
University of Pennsylvania Health System
Philadelphia, PA, USA

Isaiah J Fidler DVM PhD
Chairman, Department of Cancer Biology
Professor of Cancer Biology
RE 'Bob' Smith Distinguished Chair in Cell Biology
The University of Texas MD Anderson Cancer Center
Houston, TX, USA

Robert J Friedman MD MSc
Clinical Assistant Professor
Department of Dermatology
New York University School of Medicine
New York, NY, USA

Alvin Friedman-Kien MD
Professor of Dermatology
Department of Dermatology
New York University School of Medicine
New York, NY, USA

Roy Geronemus MD
Director, Laser & Skin Surgery Center
of New York
Clinical Professor of Dermatology
New York University
New York, NY, USA

Glenn Goldman MD
Associate Professor of Dermatology
Director of Dermatologic Surgery
Division of Dermatology
University of Vermont
Burlington, VT, USA

Salvador González MD
Assistant Professor of Dermatology
Dermatology Department
Massachusetts General Hospital
Harvard Medical School, Boston;
Dermatology Service
Memorial Sloan-Kettering Cancer Center
New York, NY, USA

Marsha Gordon MD
Associate Clinical Professor
Department of Dermatology
Mount Sinai School of Medicine
New York, NY, USA

Annalisa Gorman MD
Dermatologic Surgery Fellow
Department of Dermatology
Oregon Health & Science University
Portland, OR, USA

Gloria F Graham MD
Associate Professor of Dermatology
Department of Dermatology
Wake Forest University School of Dermatology
Winston-Salem, NC, USA

Jane M Grant-Kels MD
Professor and Chair, Department of Dermatology
Director of Dermatopathology Laboratory
Assistant Dean of Clinical Affairs
University of Connecticut Health Center
Farmington, CT, USA

Caron M Grin MD
Professor of Dermatology
Director, Melanoma/Pigmented Lesion Clinic
University of Connecticut Health Center
Farmington, CT, USA

Karina Gritsenko BA
Department of Dermatology
The Mount Sinai School of Medicine
New York, NY, USA

David R Guillén MD
Clinical Assistant Professor
University of Texas Southwestern
Medical School
Dallas, TX, USA

Allan C Halpern MD MS
Chief of Dermatology Service
Memorial Sloan Kettering Cancer Center
New York, NY, USA

Edward R Heilman MD
Clinical Associate Professor of Dermatology and
Pathology
Department of Dermatology
SUNY Downstate Medical Center
Brooklyn, NY, USA

Carol L Huang MD
Clinical Assistant Attending
Dermatology Service
Memorial Sloan-Kettering Cancer Center
New York, NY, USA

Kenneth B Hymes MD
Associate Professor of Medicine
Department of Medicine (Hematology)
New York University Medical Center
New York, NY, USA

Stefania Jablonska MD
Professor of Dermatology
Department of Dermatology and Venereology
Warsaw School of Medicine
Warsaw, Poland

Laurie Jacobson MD
Attending Dermatologic Surgeon
Laser & Skin Surgery Center of New York
New York, NY, USA

James Jakub MD
Program Leader
Gastrointestinal Oncology Program
Lakeland Regional Cancer Center
Lakeland, FL, USA

Robert H Johr MD
Clinical Professor of Dermatology and Pediatrics
Director, Pigmented Lesion Clinic
University of Miami School of Medicine
Miami, FL, USA

Helmut Kerl MD
Professor of Dermatology
Chairman, Department of Dermatology
Medical University of Graz
Graz, Austria

John M Kirkwood MD
Professor and Vice Chairman for Clinical Research
Director of Melanoma Program
Hillman Cancer Research Pavilion
Pittsburgh, PA, USA

Niels Krejci-Papa MD
Assistant Professor of Dermatology
Department of Dermatology
Tufts University School of Medicine
Boston, MA, USA

Pearon G Lang MD
Professor of Dermatology, Pathology, Otolaryngology
and Communicative Sciences
Medical University of South Carolina
Charleston, SC, USA

Sancy A Leachman MD PhD
Huntsman Cancer Institute
University of Utah
Salt Lake City, UT, USA

Mark Lebwohl MD
Professor and Chairman
Department of Dermatology
The Mount Sinai School of Medicine
New York, NY, USA

Ken K Lee MD
Assistant Professor
Department of Dermatology, Surgery
Otolaryngology – Head and Neck Surgery
Oregon Health & Science University
Portland, OR, USA

Rebecca Lintner MD
Internal Medicine
New York University
New York, NY, USA

Katrina Lowstuter MS GCG
Huntsman Cancer Institute
University of Utah
Salt Lake City, UT, USA

John C Maize Sr MD
Clinical Professor of Dermatology and Chairman
Emeritus
Department of Dermatology
Medical University of South Carolina
Charleston, SC, USA

Slavomir Majewski MD
Professor of Dermatology
Department of Dermatology and Venereology
Warsaw School of Medicine
Warsaw, Poland

Ashfaq A Marghoob MD
Assistant Attending Physician
Memorial Sloan-Kettering Cancer Center
New York, NY, USA

Robin Marks MB BS MPH FRACP FACD
Professor of Dermatology
Department of Dermatology
University of Melbourne
St Vincent's Hospital
Melbourne, Australia

Phillip McKee MD FRCPath
Associate Professor of Pathology,
Harvard Medical School
Director, Division of Dermatopathology
Brigham and Women's Hospital
Boston, MA, USA

Martin Mihm MD
Clinical Professor of Pathology
Harvard Medical School
Senior Dermatopathologist
Chief, Vascular Malformation Clinic
Massachusetts General Hospital
Boston, MA, USA

Darren K Mollick MD
Clinical Assistant Professor of Dermatology
Department of Dermatology
SUNY Downstate Medical Center
Brooklyn, NY, USA

Colin A Morton MBChB FRCP MD
Consultant Dermatologist
Department of Dermatology
Falkirk Royal Infirmary
Falkirk, Scotland

Stergios J Moschos MD
Clinical Fellow in Hematology/Oncology
The Hillman Cancer Research Pavilion
University of Pittsburgh
Pittsburgh, PA, USA

Mark F Naylor MD
Associate Professor of Dermatology
Department of Dermatology
University of Oklahoma Health Sciences Center
Oklahoma City, OK, USA

Tri H Nguyen MD
Associate Professor of Dermatology and
Otolaryngology
Department of Dermatology
MD Anderson Cancer Center
University of Texas
Houston, TX, USA

George Niedt MD
Assistant Clinical Professor
Department of Dermatology
Columbia University in New York
New York, NY, USA

Agnieszka Niemeyer MD
San Bernadino, CA, USA

Margaret Oliviero ARNP
Nurse Practitioner
Skin and Cancer Associates
Plantation, FL, USA

Solange Pendas MD
Program Leader
Comprehensive Breast Cancer Program
Lakeland Regional Cancer Center
Lakeland, FL, USA

Andrew Pippas MD
Director
John B Amos Cancer Center
Columbus, GA, USA

David Polsky MD PhD
Associate Director, Pigmented Lesion Section
Department of Dermatology
New York University Medical Center
New York, NY, USA

Harold Rabinovitz MD
Voluntary Professor
Department of Dermatology
University of Miami School of Medicine
Miami, FL, USA

Babar Rao MD
Assistant Clinical Professor and Program Director
Division of Dermatology
Robert Wood Johnson Medical School
New Brunswick, NJ, USA

Douglas S Reintgen MD
Director
Lakeland Regional Cancer Center
Lakeland, FL, USA

Sandra R Reynolds MD
Assistant Professor
Department of Dermatology
New York University School of Medicine
New York, NY, USA

Darrell S Rigel MD
Clinical Professor
Department of Dermatology
New York University School of Medicine
Adjunct Clinical Professor
Department of Dermatology
Mount Sinai School of Medicine
New York, NY, USA

June K Robinson MD
Director
Division of Dermatology
Loyola University Medical Center
Maywood, IL, USA

Gary S Rogers MD
Director, Dermatologic Surgery and Oncology
Department of Dermatology
Tufts University School of Medicine
Boston, MA, USA

Les Rosen MD
Dermatopathologist
Ameripath, Fort Lauderdale;
Voluntary Associate Professor
University of Miami
Miami, FL, USA

Marti Jill Rothe MD
Associate Professor of Dermatology
Director of Phototherapy
University of Connecticut Health Center
Farmington, CT, USA

Thomas G Salopek MD FRCPC
Associate Professor of Medicine
University Dermatology Centre
University of Alberta
Edmonton, Canada

Julie V Schaffer MD
Dermatology Resident
Department of Dermatology
Yale University School of Medicine
New Haven, CT, USA

Noah Scheinfeld MD JD
Department of Dermatology
St Luke's Roosevelt Hospital Center
New York, NY, USA

Christopher M Scott MD
Resident in Dermatology
Department of Internal Medicine
The Brody School of Medicine at East Carolina
University
Greenville, NC, USA

William Slue Jr
Medical Photographer
William Slue Services, Inc
New Milford, NJ, USA

Arthur J Sober MD
Professor of Dermatology
Harvard Medical School
Associate Chief of Dermatology
Massachusetts General Hospital
Boston, MA, USA

Benjamin A Solky MD
Chief Resident for Education
Harvard Medical School Department of Dermatology
Massachusetts General Hospital
Boston, MA, USA

James M Spencer MD MS
Associate Professor and Vice Chairman
Department of Dermatology
Mount Sinai School of Medicine
New York, NY, USA

Neil A Swanson MD
Professor and Chair of Dermatology
Professor of Surgery, Otolaryngology, Head and Neck
Surgery
Department of Dermatology
Oregon Health & Science University
Portland, OR, USA

Gina Taylor MD
Clinical Assistant Instructor
Department of Dermatology
SUNY Downstate Medical Center
Brooklyn, NY, USA

Bruce H Thiers MD
Chief, Dermatology Service
Veterans Administration Medical Center
Professor of Dermatology
Medical University of South Carolina
Charleston, SC, USA

Abel Torres MD
Professor and Chief of Dermatology
Loma Linda University Faculty Medical Offices
Loma Linda, CA, USA

Hensin Tsao MD PhD
Assistant Professor of Dermatology
Wellman Center for Photomedicine
Department of Dermatology
Massachusetts General Hospital
Boston, MA, USA

Adriana M Villa MD
Clinical Research Fellow
Department of Dermatology and Cutaneous Surgery
University of Miami School of Medicine
Miami, FL, USA

Lisa M Wadge MS CGC
Licensed Genetic Counselor
Huntsman Cancer Institute
University of Utah
Salt Lake City, UT, USA

Steven Q Wang MD
Medical Resident
Department of Dermatology
University of Minnesota School of Medicine
Minneapolis, MN, USA

Martin A Weinstock MD PhD
Professor of Dermatology and Community Health
Brown University
Dermatoepidemiology Unit
Providence VA Medical Center
Providence, RI, USA

Jaeyoung Yoon MD PhD
Assistant Professor and Consultant
Department of Dermatology
Mayo Clinic
Rochester, USA

Iris Zalaudek MD
Assistant Professor
Department of Dermatology and Venereology
Medical University of Graz
Graz, Austria

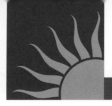

Acknowledgments

Because of the magnitude of the public health problem associated with cutaneous neoplasms, there are millions of people each year worldwide that are diagnosed with skin cancer. This text is dedicated to all who develop skin cancer and to those thousands who sadly succumb to its effects. In addition, we also dedicate this tome to those who are working tirelessly to hopefully provide the key to more effective diagnostic techniques and treatment modalities that will lower future morbidity and mortality from skin cancer.

A textbook of this magnitude could not be produced at the level that has been achieved without the help of many. I would like to thank my co-editors and academic collaborators over many years: Robert Friedman MD, Jean-Claude Bystryn MD, Leonard Dzubow MD, Robin Marks MD and Douglas Reintgen MD. Their incredibly detailed review significantly contributed to the successful outcome. The Editor Emeritus, Alfred W Kopf MD, who has been a life-long inspiration to those involved in the study of skin cancer, was always there for insight and guidance.

In addition, the efforts of the clinicians and researchers across multiple disciplines who generously provided their time and energy are reflected in the high quality of the chapters they wrote. They were particularly helpful in submitting their chapters in a very rapid timeframe so that the most recent up-to-date information could be provided. A special thanks to Clay Cockerell MD for his hard work above and beyond the "call of duty" in providing support for many of the chapters. Also, the New York University Department of Dermatology Skin and Cancer Photography Unit graciously supplied a number of clinical photos of many of the disorders presented in this textbook.

However, the successful culmination of a textbook depends on more than the editors and writers. We could not have reached the level of excellence that was achieved without the help of many others. My staff, Carol Gunther, Vanessa Sesclia, Elana Plemby and Jaquelyn Terhar, provided innumerable hours of coordination and logistics. The Elsevier team including Sue Hodgson, Shuet-Kei Cheung and Glenys Norquay were equally committed to a successful outcome.

Finally, I want to thank my wife Beth and children, Ethan, Adam and Ashlee for their love and encouragement and for allowing me all the time away from them while working on this textbook.

Darrell S Rigel MD

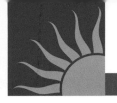

Foreword

It is now over one decade ago that several of the editors (Robert J Friedman, Darrell S Rigel and Alfred W Kopf) published the seminal comprehensive text entitled *Cancer of the Skin*. The current text is an update on the enormous progress that has been made on all levels, including clinical, therapeutic, epidemiologic, genetic and histopathologic, and on all levels of basic sciences with emphasis on neoplastic cellular biology.

Cancers of the skin in the United States of America have the highest incidence of malignancies of any organ system – and the incidence keeps rising inexorably. In addition to the over 1,200,000 non-malignant cancers of the skin anticipated in 2004, it is expected there will be over 55,000 new invasive melanomas diagnosed and almost 8000 deaths from melanomas. This translates to a lifetime risk of 1 in 57 for men and 1 in 81 for women!

A broad array of cancers of the skin is included in this comprehensive work. Special emphasis is placed on those cutaneous cancers that are particularly prevalent (e.g. basal-cell carcinoma) and those which are responsible for the highest number of fatalities (e.g. melanoma and squamous cell carcinoma).

In order to relay to the reader in the most vivid way, almost all of the photographs are published in full color. Every attempt has been made to provide clinical and histologic images of high quality.

Major emphasis in this text is on the diagnosis and management of cutaneous malignancies so that the reader is provided with the most advanced diagnostic and therapeutic measures available to date for each type of skin cancer. Thus, the editors and authors have made every effort to provide not only the commonly used therapeutic approaches, but also those modalities considered on the 'cutting edge' of our present therapeutic armamentaria.

The backbone of *Cancer of the Skin* is the remarkable productivity of the many authors who have been selected by the editors because of their interest and recognition of the specific malignant neoplasm dealt with in each of the chapters. Their broad experience in cutaneous oncology and the therapeutic guidelines they have documented are valuable assets to any individual involved in the multi-disciplinary needs of these patients. Thus, *Cancer of the Skin* serves as a valuable resource not only to physicians but also to all others who deal with the consequences of malignant tumors of the skin.

A major impetus to preventive methods and early detection of cancers of the skin is the establishment of The National Council on Skin Cancer Prevention, which is a coalition of organizations concerned about skin cancers. This Council was established by the Centers for Disease Control and Prevention at the request of the United States Congress. It is anticipated that the long-term effects of this Council may have a significant impact in reducing the incidence and, consequently, the mortality rates of cancers of the skin in our country.

It is our aspiration that you will find this comprehensive textbook a valuable summary of the current knowledge gleaned by the literally thousands of years of combined clinical and therapeutic experience coupled with extensive reviews of literature by the multiple authors who have so arduously presented in written and pictorial form the very best of what is known today.

Alfred W Kopf MD
Editor Emeritus
Clinical Professor of Dermatology
New York University School of Medicine

Preface

Skin cancer rates are rising dramatically. In the United States each year there are over 1 million newly diagnosed cases – more than all other cancers combined! One in five Americans will develop at least one skin cancer during their lifetime and similar rates are found in many other countries worldwide. This continued increase in skin cancer incidence is even more dramatic as it is occurring at a time when most other cancers are either stable or decreasing in rate.

The public health ramifications of these facts are profound. Skin cancer, once viewed as a relatively uncommon disease limited to dermatologists and surgeons, is now being seen on a daily basis by primary care physicians, oncologists and other health care professionals. The resulting need to educate all of these groups on recognizing and managing patients with this cancer is also increasing.

In addition, the advances that have occurred even in the past decade alone in our understanding of the basic biology, diagnosis, and treatment of skin cancer have been staggering. In sitting down to review the layout of this text, we were amazed at the multitude of new topics that had changed extensively or did not even exist for inclusion in our prior textbook 12 years ago. The advent of dermoscopy, confocal microscopy, computer-aided diagnosis, digital photographic documentation, topical immune response modulators, and advances in immunotherapy, lymph node biopsies, photoprotection agents and our understanding of the biologic basis of this cancer all demonstrate the dynamism of this field. Social issues that have arisen such as genetic testing and the deleterious effects of tanning salons also emphasize our need to understand this cancer within a broader context. All of these topics are covered in depth in this textbook to facilitate a wide-ranging understanding of skin neoplasms.

Primary prevention efforts are also becoming increasingly important. Skin cancer is one of the few cancers where we know the cause of the vast majority of neoplasms – excess ultraviolet exposure whether from the sun or artificial sources. Simple behavioral changes can lead to a significant decrease in a person's chance of developing skin cancer. An understanding of the mechanisms and risk factors of skin cancer are critical in counseling patients to facilitate prevention.

Skin cancer is also one of the most clear-cut cases of a disease where early detection and treatment are critical. Skin cancers treated early are virtually 100% curable with simple therapies, while lesions that are advanced often have no effective treatment available. Therefore, the need for medical practitioners to be able to recognize and treat skin cancer in its earliest phase cannot be overstated.

The changing demographics of skin cancer have also led to a need to focus prevention efforts on subsets of the population and to alter therapy for these groups. We have tried to meet this need through providing information on such topics as the management of melanoma in the pregnant patient.

To develop an inclusive understanding of skin cancer, one must remember that there are more than basal and squamous cell carcinoma and melanoma. This text has been designed to provide a comprehensive review of precursor lesions, other non-melanoma skin cancers and cutaneous neoplasms related to other disorders.

Cancer of the Skin has been designed to meet the aforementioned needs in a format that is conducive to effectively transmitting relevant data to the reader. Through the use of 100% color clinical images, photomicrographs and flow diagrams, information on diagnosing and treating skin cancer is portrayed in an easy-to-understand manner.

We hope that you will find *Cancer of the Skin* useful in the treatment of your patients with skin cancer and a help in reaching the goal that we all strive for – lowering the morbidity and mortality from this disease.

Darrell S Rigel MD
Robert J Friedman MD
Leonard M Dzubow MD
Douglas S Reintgen MD
Jean-Claude Bystryn MD
Robin Marks MD

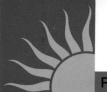

CHAPTER

1

The Biology of Skin Cancer Invasion and Metastasis

Isaiah J Fidler

Key points

- The major cause of death from skin cancer is due to metastases that are resistant to conventional therapies.
- Cancer of the skin consists of heterogeneous subpopulations of cells with different biological properties that include growth, angiogenesis, invasion, and metastasis.
- The process of metastasis is sequential and consists of many selective steps.
- To produce metastases, metastatic cells usurp homeostatic mechanisms representing a continuous 'cross-talk' of the 'seed and the soil'.
- Therapy of metastasis should be directed against the unique metastatic cells and the organ microenvironment of metastatic organs.

INTRODUCTION

Once a diagnosis of skin cancer is established, the urgent question is whether the cancer is localized to the skin or whether it has already spread to the regional lymph nodes and distant organs. The most fearsome aspect of cancer is metastasis, exemplified by the spread of cells from the primary neoplasm to distant organs where secondary growth occurs. This fear is well based. Despite great improvements in diagnosis, surgical techniques, general patient care, local and systemic adjuvant therapies, most deaths due to skin cancers are caused by the relentless growth of metastases that are resistant to conventional therapies. The production of metastasis varies among different types of skin cancers. Basal cell carcinomas rarely produce distant metastases. Squamous cell carcinomas metastasize infrequently. However, the high incidence of this tumor in the general population means that metastasis is a real clinical problem. Cutaneous melanomas metastasize more frequently than other skin cancers and are among the most malignant neoplasms in human beings.

In a large number of patients with melanoma and in some patients with squamous cell carcinomas, metastasis has occurred by the time the tumor is diagnosed. Metastases can be located in different organs and in different regions of the same organ. The organ micro-environment can modify the metastatic tumor cells' response to therapy and alter the effectiveness of anti-cancer agents in destroying the tumor cells without producing undesirable toxic effects. As is true for primary

neoplasms, the major obstacle to treating metastasis is the tumor cells' biological heterogeneity. By the time of diagnosis, cancers contain multiple cell populations with diverse characteristics of karyotype, growth rate, cell-surface properties, antigenicity, immunogenicity, marker enzymes, sensitivity to various cytotoxic drugs and ability to invade and produce metastasis.[1-4]

Understanding the mechanisms responsible for the development of biological heterogeneity in primary skin cancers and in metastases and the process by which tumor cells can invade local tissue and spread to distant organs must continue to be a primary goal of cancer research. Only from a better understanding will come improvements in the design of more effective therapy for malignant disease and in the way physicians deal with the problem of cancer metastasis. This chapter reviews some basic concepts of metastasis using melanoma as the primary example.

THE PROCESS OF CANCER METASTASIS

The process of cancer metastasis is dynamic, complex and consists of a large series of interrelated steps shown schematically in Figure 1.1. To produce a clinically relevant lesion, metastatic cells must survive all the steps of the process. If the disseminating tumor cell fails to complete any one of these steps, it will fail to produce a metastasis. The outcome of this process depends on both the intrinsic properties of the tumor cells and their interactions with host factors.[4,5]

The major steps in the formation of a metastasis are:

- After the initial transforming event, either unicellular or multicellular, growth of neoplastic cells must be progressive, with nutrients for the expanding tumor mass initially supplied by simple diffusion;

- extensive vascularization must occur if a tumor mass is to exceed 1–2 mm in diameter. The synthesis and secretion of proangiogenic angiogenesis factor probably plays a key role in establishing a neocapillary network from the surrounding host tissue;

- local invasion of the host stroma by some tumor cells could occur by several non-mutually exclusive mechanisms;

- thin-walled venules, like lymphatic channels, offer very little resistance to penetration by tumor cells and provide the most common pathways for tumor cell entry into the circulation. Although clinical observations

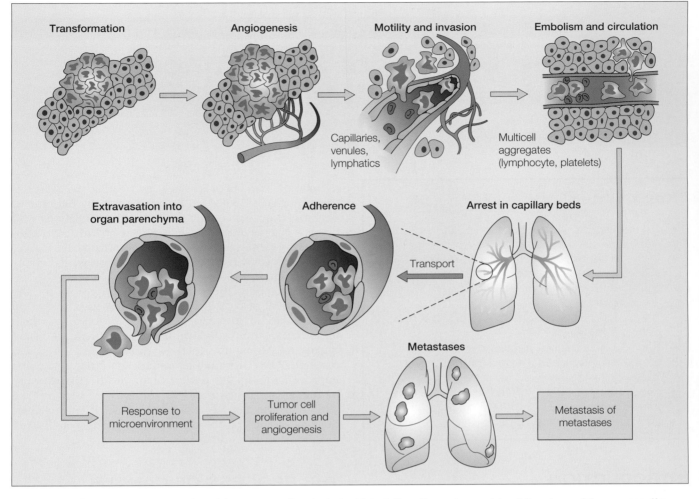

Figure 1.1 Schematic representation of the process of metastasis. Metastatic cells must complete all the steps of the process. If a disseminating tumor cell fails to survive any one of these steps, it will fail to produce a metastasis.

have suggested that carcinomas frequently metastasize and grow via the lymphatic system, whereas malignant tumors of mesenchymal origin more often spread by the hematogenous route, the presence of numerous venolymphatic anastomoses invalidates this concept;

- detachment and embolization of small tumor cell aggregates occurs next, the vast majority of circulating tumor cells being rapidly destroyed;

- once the tumor cells have survived the circulation, they must arrest in the capillary beds of organs, either by adhering to capillary endothelial cells or by adhering to subendothelial basement membrane, which may be exposed;

- extravasation occurs next, probably by the same mechanisms that influence initial invasion;

- proliferation within the organ parenchyma completes the metastatic process.

To continue growing, the micrometastases must develop a vascular network and continue to evade the host immune system. Moreover, the cells must invade, penetrate blood vessels and enter the circulation to produce additional metastases (Fig. 1.2).

The outcome of the metastatic process depends on multiple and complex interactions of metastatic cells with host homeostatic mechanisms.[2,5] Clinical observations of cancer patients and studies with experimental rodent tumors have concluded that certain tumors produce metastasis to specific organs independent of vascular anatomy, rate of blood flow and number of tumor cells delivered to each organ. The distribution and fate of hematogenously disseminated, radiolabeled melanoma cells in experimental animals conclusively demonstrated that tumor cells can reach the microvasculature of many organs, but growth in the organ parenchyma occurred in only specific organs.[1,2,6,7]

NEOVASCULARIZATION – ANGIOGENESIS

Oxygen can diffuse from capillaries for only 150–200 μm. When the distances of cells from a blood supply exceed this, cell death follows.[8,9] Thus, the expansion of tumor masses beyond 1 mm in diameter depends on neovascularization, i.e. angiogenesis.[8] The formation of new vasculature consists of multiple, interdependent steps. It begins with local degradation of the basement membrane surrounding capillaries, followed by invasion of the

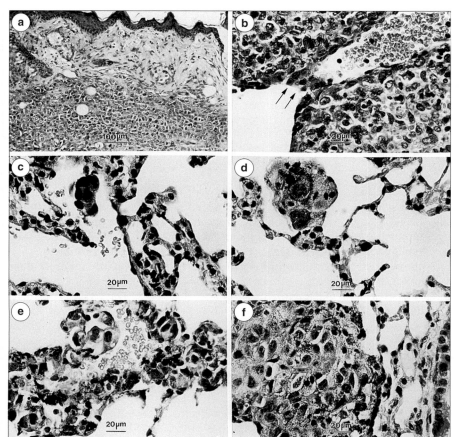

Figure 1.2 The pathogenesis of a mouse K-1735 melanoma metastasis: histologic studies. (a) Mouse K-1735 melanoma growing in the external ear of a syngeneic mouse. Note that tumor cells do not invade into cartilage. (b) Note the fibrous capsule surrounding the subcutaneous tumor, which is well vascularized. (c) Melanoma cell arrested in the microvasculature of the lung 1 day after intravenous injection. Proliferation of melanoma cells in lungs of mice (d) 10 and (e) 14 days after the tumor cells were injected intravenously. These are micrometastases. (f) 45 days after intravenous injection of K-1735 cells, large melanoma metastases replace normal lung parenchyma.

surrounding stroma and migration of endothelial cells in the direction of the angiogenic stimulus. Proliferation of endothelial cells occurs at the leading edge of the migrating column, and the endothelial cells begin to organize into three-dimensional structures to form new capillary tubes. Differences in cellular composition, vascular permeability, blood vessel stability and growth regulation distinguish vessels in neoplasms from those in normal tissue.[9–11]

The onset of angiogenesis involves a change in the local equilibrium between proangiogenic and antiangiogenic molecules.[3,4] Some of the common proangiogenic factors include bFGF which induces the proliferation of a variety of cells and has also been shown to stimulate endothelial cells to migrate, to increase production of proteases and to undergo morphogenesis.[12] Likewise, VEGF/VPF (vascular endothelial growth factor/vascular permeability factor) has been shown to induce the proliferation of endothelial cells, to increase vascular permeability, and to induce production of urokinase plasminogen activator by endothelial cells.[13] Additional proangiogenic factors include IL-8,[14] platelet-derived endothelial cell growth factor, which has been shown to stimulate endothelial cell DNA synthesis and to induce production of fibroblast growth factor (FGF), hepatocyte growth factor (HGF), or scatter factor, that increases endothelial cell migration, invasion, and the production of proteases, and platelet-derived growth factor (PDGF).[15]

The production of angiogenic molecules, e.g. VEGF, bFGF, and IL-8 by melanoma cells is regulated by complex interactions with keratinocytes in the skin.[16] Reports from our laboratory showed that IL-8 is an important molecule in melanoma growth and progression.

Constitutive expression of IL-8 directly correlated with the metastatic potential of human melanoma cells. Further, IL-8 induces proliferation, migration, and invasion of endothelial cells and, hence, neovascularization.[17] Several organ-derived cytokines (produced by inflammatory cells) are known to induce expression of IL-8 in normal and transformed cells.[16] Since IL-8 expression in melanocytes and melanoma cells can be induced by inflammatory signals, the question of whether specific organ microenvironments could influence the expression of IL-8 was analyzed. Melanoma cells were implanted into the subcutis, the spleen (to produce liver metastasis), and intravenously (to produce lung metastasis) of athymic nude mice. Subcutaneous tumors, lung lesions and liver lesions expressed high, intermediate and no IL-8, respectively, at both the mRNA and protein levels. Melanoma cells established from the tumors growing *in vivo* exhibited similar levels of IL-8 mRNA transcripts as continuously cultured cells, thus demonstrating that the differential expression of IL-8 was not due to the selection of a subpopulation of cells.[17]

IL-8 expression can be upregulated by co-culturing melanoma cells with keratinocytes (skin) and inhibited by co-culturing melanoma cells with hepatocytes (liver). The effects of two cytokines produced by keratinocytes (IL-1, IFN-β) and two cytokines produced by hepatocytes (TGF-α, TGF-β) on the regulation of IL-8 in human melanoma cells have also been investigated. IL-1 upregulated the expression of IL-8 in human melanoma cells at both the mRNA and protein levels in a dose- and time-dependent manner in the presence of *de novo* protein synthesis. IFN-β did not affect constitutive IL-8 mRNA and protein production in human melanoma cells, but it did block the induction of IL-8 by IL-1. TGF-β inhibited the expression of IL-8, while TGF-α had no effect on IL-8 expression.[18]

TUMOR CELL INVASION

To reach blood vessels or lymphatics, tumor cells must penetrate host stroma that includes basement membrane. The interaction with the basement membrane consists of attachment, matrix dissolution, motility and penetration.[19] At least three non-mutually excluding mechanisms can be involved in tumor cell invasion of tissues. First, mechanical pressure produced by rapidly proliferating neoplasms may force cords of tumor cells along tissue planes of least resistance.[19] Second, increased cell motility can contribute to tumor cell invasion. Most tumor cells possess the necessary cytoplasmic machinery for active locomotion and increased tumor cell motility is preceded by a loss of cell-to-cell cohesive forces. In epithelial cells, the loss of cell-to-cell contact is associated with downregulation of the expression of E-cadherin, a cell surface glycoprotein involved in calcium-dependent homotypic cell-to-cell cohesion. Reduced levels of E-cadherin are associated with a decrease in cellular/ tissue differentiation and increased grade in carcinomas.[20] Many differentiated carcinomas express higher levels of E-cadherin mRNA, as do adjacent normal epithelial cells, whereas poorly differentiated carcinomas do not. Mutations in the E-cadherin gene and abnormalities of α-catenin, which is an E-cadherin-associated protein, have been associated with the transition of cells from the noninvasive to the invasive phenotype.[21]

Third, invasive tumor cells secrete enzymes capable of degrading basement membranes, which constitute a barrier between epithelial cells and the stroma. Epithelial cells and stromal cells produce a complex mixture of collagens, proteoglycans, and other molecules, which contains ligands for adhesion receptors and is permeable to molecules but not to cells.[22]

To invade the basement membrane, a tumor cell must first attach to extracellular matrix (ECM) components by a receptor–ligand interaction. One group of such cell surface receptors are the integrins which specifically bind cells to laminin, collagen, or fibronectin.[23] Many integrins that bind to different components of the ECM are expressed on the surface of human carcinoma cells. Tumor progression has been associated with a gradual decrease of integrin expression suggesting that the loss of integrins, coupled with the loss of E-cadherin, may facilitate detachment from a primary neoplasm.

Subsequent to binding, tumor cells can degrade connective-tissue ECM and basement membrane components.[24] The production of enzymes such as type IV collagenase (gelatinase, matrix metalloproteinase) and heparinase in metastatic tumor cells correlates with invasive capacity of human carcinoma cells. Type IV collagenolytic metalloproteinases with apparent molecular masses of 98, 92, 80, 68, and 64-kDa have been detected in highly metastatic cells. Poorly metastatic cells, on the other hand, appear to secrete very low amounts of only the 92-kDa metalloproteinase.[25]

LYMPHATIC METASTASIS

Early clinical observations led to the impression that carcinomas spread mainly by the lymphatic route and mesenchymal tumors spread mainly by means of the bloodstream. It is now known, however, that the lymphatic and vascular systems have numerous connections and that disseminating tumor cells may pass from one system to the other.[26] For these reasons, the division of metastasis into lymphatic spread and hematogenous spread is arbitrary. During invasion, tumor cells can easily penetrate small lymphatic vessels and be passively transported in the lymph. Tumor emboli may be trapped in the first lymph node encountered on their route, or they may bypass regional draining lymph nodes to form distant nodal metastases ('skip metastasis'). Although this phenomenon was recognized in the late 1800s,[27] its implications for treatment were frequently ignored in the development of surgical approaches to treat cancers.[1]

Regional lymph nodes (RLN) in the area of a primary neoplasm may become enlarged as a result of hyperplasia or growth of tumor cells in the node. Although the use of morphologic criteria for assessing prognoses based on lymph node appearance is debatable, lymphocyte-depleted lymph nodes are believed to indicate a less favorable prognosis than those demonstrating reactive morphologic characteristics.[28] Hyperplastic responses could indicate reactivity to autochthonous tumors, and this could benefit the host.

Whether the RLN can retain tumor cells and serve as a temporary barrier for cell dissemination is controversial. In most experimental animal systems used to investigate this question, normal lymph nodes were subjected to a sudden challenge with a large number of tumor cells, a situation that may not be analogous to RLN at the early stages of cancer spread in humans, when small numbers of cancer cells continuously enter the lymphatics. This issue is important because of practical considerations for surgical management of such neoplasms as cutaneous melanoma. It raises the question: is elective prophylactic lymph node dissection appropriate for the treatment of micrometastases?

The biologic justification for elective lymph node dissection in patients with melanoma presumes that metastasis of some cutaneous melanomas occurs first in the RLN and that only at a later time do tumor cells gain access to the circulation to reach distant organs. If this is the case and RLN can act as a temporary barrier to the spread of cancer, removing the RLN with micrometastases could clearly increase the cure rate in subgroups of patients with melanoma. Some evidence exists that patients with melanomas of intermediate thickness (1–4 mm) do in fact have an improved survival rate subsequent to elective lymph node dissection. Similarly, some data suggest that an improved survival rate can be achieved for selected patients with head and neck cancers by elective lymph node dissection or local treatment with X-irradiation.[29]

Recent advances in mapping of the lymphatics draining cutaneous melanoma (by the use of dyes or radioactive tracers) have allowed surgeons to identify the lymph node draining the tumor site (i.e. the sentinel lymph node).[30] The presence of melanoma micrometastases in sentinel lymph nodes is correlated with poor prognosis and hence indicates wide field dissection. A series of more than 500 melanoma cases with longer than 4 years' median clinical follow-up concluded that absence of disease in sentinel lymph node correlates with increased disease-free status (in other nodes) and few or no skip metastases.[31,32] These data suggest that elective lymph node dissection when metastatic cells are present in sentinel lymph nodes may produce beneficial results in patients with melanoma.

HEMATOGENOUS METASTASIS

During blood-borne metastasis, tumor cells must survive transport in the circulation, adhere to small blood vessels or capillaries, and invade the vessel wall. The mere presence of tumor cells in the circulation does not in itself constitute metastasis, since most cells released into the bloodstream are eliminated rapidly.[1,6] Using radiolabeled tumor cells, we found that by 24 hrs after entry into the circulation, less than 1% of the cells are still viable and less than 0.1% of tumor cells placed into the circulation eventually survive to produce metastases.[6]

Although most tumor cells are destroyed in the bloodstream, it seems that the greater the number of cells released by a primary tumor, the greater the probability that some cells will survive to form metastases. The number of tumor emboli in the circulation appears to correlate well with the size and clinical duration of the primary tumor, and the development of necrotic and hemorrhagic areas in large tumors facilitates this process by providing tumor cells easy access to the circulation.[1] To a large degree, the rapid death of most circulating tumor cells is probably due to such simple mechanical factors as blood turbulence. Tumor cell survival can be increased by aggregation. Tumor cells can aggregate with each other or with host cells, such as platelets[33] and lymphocytes.[34]

Once metastatic cells reach the microcirculation, they interact with cells of the vascular endothelium. These interactions include non-specific mechanical lodgment of tumor cell emboli as well as formation of stable adhesions between tumor cells and small-vessel endothelial cells. The organ distribution of metastatic foci is believed to depend, in part, on the ability of blood-borne malignant cells to adhere to specific endothelium and produce endothelial cell retraction.[35]

The formation of fibrin clots at sites of tumor cell arrest in the microcirculation can result in blood vessel damage.[36] In some tumor systems, fibrin formation is not essential for tumor cell implantation or metastasis formation. The increased coagulability often observed in patients with cancer may be related to the high levels of thromboplastin found in certain tumors or to production of high levels of procoagulant-A activity, which can directly activate factor X in the clotting process. Since reduced blood flow could lead to increased trapping of circulating tumor cells and perhaps to their increased survival, the use of anticoagulants in the treatment or control of metastasis has been tried, albeit with limited success.

The adhesion of tumor cells to the vascular endothelium is regulated by mechanisms similar to those used by leukocytes. The initial attachment of leukocytes to vascular endothelial cells is regulated by the selectin family of adhesion molecules, which consists of three closely related cell surface molecules. E-selectin, which is expressed by endothelial cells, mediates initial attachment of lymphocytes (and tumor cells) by interaction with specific carbohydrate ligands that contain sialylated fucosylated lactosamines. The expression of mucin-type carbohydrates on the surface of human colon carcinoma has been correlated with their metastatic potential,[37] perhaps through differential interaction with E-selectins expressed on specific endothelial cells. The development of firm adhesion requires the interaction of other adhesion molecules, another selective process in metastasis. Several classes of cell-to-cell adhesion molecules regulate this adhesion. These include the hyaluronate receptor CD44 and its splice-variants,[38] the integrins $\alpha5\beta1$, $\alpha6\beta1$ and $\alpha6\beta4$, and the galactoside-binding galectin-3.[23] The arrest of tumor cells in capillary beds leads to the retraction of endothelial cells and the exposure of the tumor cells to the ECM. The adhesion of metastatic cells to components of the ECM, such as fibronectin, laminin and thrombospondin, facilitates metastasis to specific tissues, and peptides containing sequences of these components of the ECM can reduce formation of hematogenous metastases.[39]

Extravasation of arrested tumor cells is believed to operate by mechanisms similar to those responsible for local invasion. Tumor cells can grow and destroy the surrounding vessel, invade by penetrating the endothelial basement membrane, or they can follow migrating white blood cells.[40] The ability of malignant cells to extravasate into surrounding tissues of particular organs seems to arise, in part, from their selective adherence to and invasion of certain tissues.[41] Malignant cells frequently penetrate thin-walled capillaries but rarely invade arteries or arteriole walls, which are rich in elastin fibers. This resistance to invasion is not necessarily mediated by mechanical strength alone. Connective tissues have been shown to produce protease inhibitors, and these may block enzyme-dependent processes of invasion.

The invasion, survival and growth of malignant cells at particular secondary sites, also involve their responses to tissue or organ factors. Tumor cells can recognize tissue-specific motility factors that direct their movement and invasion.[42] After tumor cells invade organ parenchyma, they must also respond to organ-specific factors that influence their growth.[41]

METASTASIS FROM METASTASES

The tumor cells proliferating within metastases can invade host stroma, penetrate blood vessels, and enter the circulation to produce secondary metastases, the so-called 'metastasis of metastases'.[43,44] Hart and Fidler[45] used the preferential growth of B16 melanoma metastases in specific organs. Following the intravenous injection of B16 melanoma cells into syngeneic mice, tumor growths developed in the lungs and in fragments of lung or ovarian tissue implanted intramuscularly into the quadriceps femoris but not in renal tissue implanted as a control[45] (Fig. 1.3). Tumor growth in the specific

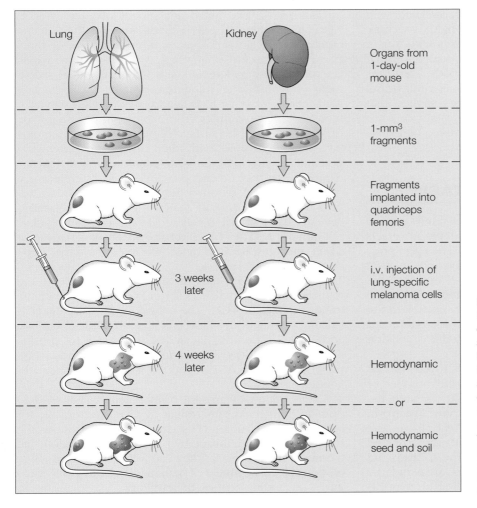

Lung

Kidney

Organs from 1-day-old mouse

1-mm³ fragments

Fragments implanted into quadriceps femoris

3 weeks later

i.v. injection of lung-specific melanoma cells

4 weeks later

Hemodynamic

— or —

Hemodynamic seed and soil

Figure 1.3 'Seed and soil' for metastasis. Design of the experiment that demonstrated that metastasis occurs to specific organs. Lungs and kidneys harvested from 1-day-old mice were cut into 1-mm fragments and implanted subcutaneously into the quadriceps femoris of syngeneic mice. Three weeks later, the mice were injected intravenously with B16 melanoma cells. Four weeks later, the mice were killed and autopsied. Metastatic lesions were found in the autochthcnous lungs and implanted lung fragments but not in the implanted kidney fragments serving as a trauma-organ-repair control.

transplanted organ could have been caused by the arrest and growth of tumor cells immediately following intravenous injection, i.e. 'initial metastases'. Alternatively, tumor cells injected intravenously could have been arrested in the lungs, where they developed; once metastases were established, tumor cells could enter the circulation to be arrested at other organs and produce 'secondary metastases'.[43] To distinguish between these possibilities, Nicolson and Fidler[44] performed several experiments: two weeks after normal, tumor-free mice were joined parabiotically to metastasis-bearing animals, there was no evidence of any tumor growth in the 'guest' animals. However, when the parabiont animals were allowed to survive for 4 weeks after separation from the metastasis-bearing animals, 40% developed lung metastases. Since the host mice did not have primary tumors at the time of parabiosis, the metastases in the guest mice could have only arisen as metastasis from metastases (Fig. 1.4).

THE BIOLOGIC HETEROGENEITY OF PRIMARY SKIN CANCERS AND THEIR METASTASES

From this discussion, it is clear that not all tumor cells in a primary neoplasm, nor those that enter the circulation can produce metastases. In fact, since less than 0.01% of

circulating cells are likely to produce a secondary growth, the development of metastases could represent the fortuitous survival of a few tumor cells or the selection from the parent tumor of a subpopulation of metastatic cells endowed with properties that enhance their survival.[46,47] Data generated by our research group and many others prove that neoplasms are biologically heterogeneous and that metastasis is indeed a selective process.

The first experimental proof of metastatic heterogeneity of neoplasms was provided by Fidler and Kripke in 1977[47] working with the murine B16 melanoma. Using the modified fluctuation assay of Luria and Delbruck,[48] we showed that different tumor cell clones, each derived from an individual cell isolated from the parent tumor, varied dramatically in their ability to produce pulmonary nodules after intravenous inoculation into syngeneic recipient mice (Fig. 1.5). Control subcloning procedures demonstrated that the observed diversity was not a consequence of the cloning procedure.[47] The finding that preexisting tumor cell subpopulations proliferating in the same tumor exhibit heterogeneous metastatic potential has since been confirmed in many laboratories with a wide range of experimental animal tumors of different histories and histologic origins.[2,49] In addition, studies using young nude mice as models for metastasis of human neoplasms have shown that several human tumor lines and freshly isolated tumors such as colon

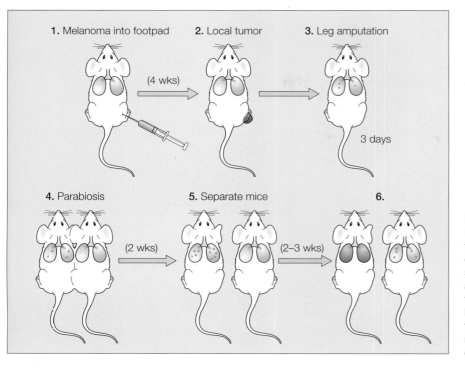

1. Melanoma into footpad   2. Local tumor   3. Leg amputation

(4 wks)

3 days

4. Parabiosis   5. Separate mice   6.

(2 wks)   (2–3 wks)

Figure 1.4 Metastasis of metastases. Design of the experiment that demonstrated that metastases metastasize. Melanoma cells were implanted into the footpads of syngeneic mice. The leg with tumor was amputated and the mice were parabiosed to normal syngeneic animals. Two weeks later, the mice were separated. The fact that the 'guest' mouse developed lung metastases proves that lung metastases can give rise to additional metastases.

carcinoma, renal carcinoma, and prostate cancer also contain subpopulations of cells with widely differing metastatic properties.[50]

We studied the biologic and metastatic heterogeneity in a mouse melanoma induced in C3H mice by chronic exposure to ultraviolet B radiation and painting with croton oil.[51] One mouse thus treated developed a melanoma designated by Kripke[51] as K-1735. The original K-1735 melanoma was established in culture and immediately cloned.[52] In an experiment similar in design to the one described for the B16 melanoma (Fig. 1.3), the clones differed greatly from each other and from the parent tumor in their ability to produce lung metastases. In addition to differences in number of metastases, we also found significant variability in the size and pigmentation of the metastases (Fig. 1.6). Metastases to the brain, heart, liver and skin were found as well; those growing in the brain were uniformly pigmented, whereas those growing in the lymph nodes, heart, liver, or skin generally had no pigment.

To determine whether the absence of metastasis production by some (but not all) clones of the K-1735 was a consequence of their immunologic rejection by the normal host,[53,54] we examined their metastatic behavior in young nude mice. In addition to the lack of a functional T-cell system, unstressed 3-week-old nude mice are also deficient in natural killer cell activity. In such recipients, the immunologic barrier to metastatic cells that also may be highly immunogenic is removed and they may thus successfully complete the process. This was true for cells of two clones that did not produce metastases in normal syngeneic mice but produced tumor foci in the young nude recipients. Most of the nonmetastatic clones were nonmetastatic in both normal syngeneic and in the nude recipients. Therefore, the clones' failure to metastasize in syngeneic mice probably was not caused by their immunologic rejection by the host but by their inability

to complete one or another step in the complex metastatic process.

ENHANCED METASTATIC POTENTIAL OF TUMOR CELLS HARVESTED FROM MELANOMA METASTASES

Our studies and most data reported by others have led us to conclude that metastasis is a highly selective process regulated by a number of as yet imperfectly understood mechanisms. This belief is contrary to the once widely accepted notion that neoplastic dissemination is the ultimate expression of cellular anarchy. In fact, suggesting that cancer metastasis is a selective process is a more optimistic view in terms of cancer therapy than one that postulates that tumor dissemination is an entirely random event. Belief that certain rules govern the spread of neoplastic disease implies that elucidation and understanding of these rules will lead to better therapeutic interventions.

We addressed the question of whether the cells that survive to form metastases possess a greater metastatic capacity than most cells in the parent neoplasm.[55] Some support for this possibility comes from the initial *in vivo* selection experiments of the highly metastatic B16-F10 cell line derived from the parent B16 melanoma[46] (Fig. 1.7). Comparable results have been obtained with the K-1735 tumor. When cells derived from the parent tumor were injected intramuscularly into the hind foot pads of syngeneic mice, the resulting skin tumors produced spontaneous pulmonary metastases. Four cell lines were established from four individual lung nodules harvested from four different mice. The finding that all the lines derived from metastatic deposits produced significantly more metastases than cells of the parent line

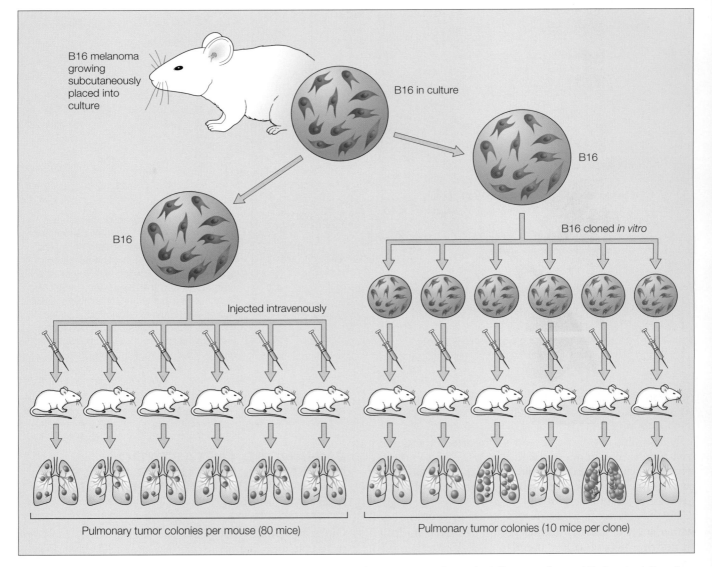

Figure 1.5 Design of the experiment demonstrating that tumors are heterogeneous for metastatic properties and that metastatic cells preexist within the primary neoplasm.

was good evidence for the hypothesis that metastasis is a selective process, that is, cells populating metastases have an increased metastatic capacity.[55]

Our studies demonstrate that the K-1735 melanoma is heterogeneous and contains both non-metastatic and metastatic cells. In contrast, individual metastases (spontaneous pulmonary metastases) are more uniform. This suggests that metastatic foci could develop by a clonal expansion of a few surviving metastatic cells. Moreover, it explains the observations showing that tumor cells in primary and metastatic lesions differ in their antigenic properties, biochemical characteristics and response to cytotoxic drugs.[4,56]

CLONAL ORIGIN OF CANCER METASTASES

Multiple metastases proliferating in a host, even in the same organ, often exhibit diverse biological characteristics of, for example, hormone receptors, antigenicity or immunogenicity, and response to various chemo-

therapeutic agents. This diversity may result from the nature of the pathogenesis of metastasis, the process of tumor evolution and progression, or both.

Pathologists have long been aware that neoplasms frequently exhibit different morphological appearances in different areas. For this reason, the malignant or benign nature of a tumor cannot be determined with confidence unless multiple sections obtained from all parts of the tumor are examined. The zonal differences in tumors are not restricted to morphology alone but include biological characteristics such as growth rates, sensitivity to cytotoxic drugs, antigenicity and pigmentation.[57] Since primary tumors are not uniform, it is possible that tumor cell aggregates entering the circulation from one zone of the tumor may be different from those entering from another zone. If an embolic aggregate originates from a primary tumor's homogeneous zone, regardless of whether only one cell or several cells survived to proliferate in distant organs, the resulting metastasis would be like a primary tumor of unicellular origin. If a mixed embolus derived from an area of zonal junctions enters the circulation, the unicellular or multicellular origin of the

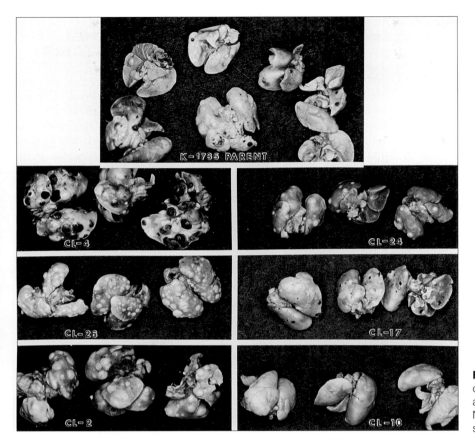

Figure 1.6 Lung metastases produced by cells from the parental K-1735 melanoma and various of its clonal subpopulations. Note the great variability in the number, size, and pigmentation of the metastases.

metastasis would depend on whether a single cell or multiple cells survived to proliferate. To determine whether individual metastases are clonal and whether different metastases can be produced by different progenitor cells, Talmadge *et al.*[58] performed a series of experiments using the fact that X-irradiation of tumor cells induces random chromosome breaks and rearrangements. Analyzing the karyotype composition of 21 individual melanoma lung metastases after cultivating cells from individual lesions, this research group found unique karyotypic patterns of abnormal, marker chromosomes in most of the lines established from metastases. This suggested that each metastasis originated from a single progenitor cell. Similar results have been obtained in other rodent tumor systems.[59] These studies reveal that the majority of metastases are of clonal origin. Moreover, variant clones with diverse phenotypes are formed, rapidly resulting in the generation of significant cellular diversity within individual metastases.[55]

Cancer metastases of a clonal origin can be produced by two different mechanisms, proliferation of a single cell or of many cells. In the case of the second possibility, the cell aggregate at the metastatic site must have a homogeneous composition. To determine which of these possibilities is responsible for the generation of clonal K-1735 melanoma metastases, we injected C3H mice intravenously with aggregates of K-1735 cells consisting of two distinct subpopulations.[7] Cells of line K-1735-M2 are highly metastatic and exhibit a stable normal karyotype. Cells of the X-met-21 line are also highly metastatic but exhibit a stable, submetacentric chromosomal marker. After mixed aggregates (>20 cells) of these two cell types were injected, individual lung metastases were recovered

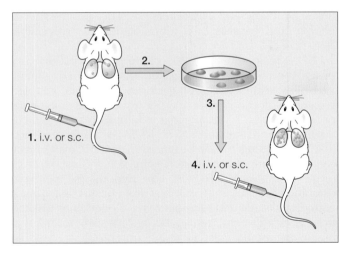

Figure 1.7 *In vivo* selection-enrichment for metastatic cells. Heterogeneous parental neoplasm cells are injected intravenously or subcutaneously (1). Metastases are harvested (2) and cells are grown in culture (3) The metastatic potential of the cells isolated from metastasis is determined subsequent to injection into mice (4).

and cultured, and each metastatic line was subjected to chromosome analysis. We reasoned that if an experimental metastasis originated from a single proliferating cell, all tumor cells within the metastatic focus should express either the K-1735-M2 or the X-met-21 chromosomal profile. This indeed was the case. Analysis of the distribution and fate of circulating tumor emboli has demonstrated that multicellular aggregates are more likely to give rise to a metastasis than a single-tumor-cell embolus. This is probably so because tumor cells not on the periphery of circulating emboli can be protected from destruction in the circulation, and a large aggregate of cells can more readily arrest in the capillary bed of an organ. Since the aggregates we injected were large, each containing more than 20 cells, the results suggest that the melanoma lung metastases resulted from the proliferation of a single viable cell within the embolus. Thus, regardless of whether an embolus is initially homogeneous or heterogeneous, metastases can be unicellular in origin.

Collectively, these observations indicate that different metastases arise from different progenitor cells and account for the well-documented differences in behavior of different metastases. Among individual metastases of proven clonal origins, however, heterogeneity can develop rapidly to create significant intralesional heterogeneity.

DEVELOPMENT OF BIOLOGICAL DIVERSITY WITHIN AND AMONG METASTASES

Clinical and histologic observations of neoplasms have suggested that tumors undergo a series of changes during the course of the disease. A tumor initially diagnosed as benign, for example, can evolve over a period of many months into a malignant tumor. This can best be demonstrated in the case of human cutaneous melanoma where the transformation of normal melanocytes and their conversion into metastatic cells has been studied in detail by Clark and coworkers.[60,61] This progression is gradual and consists of a series of discrete irreversible steps.[62]

To explain the process of tumor evolution and progression, Nowell[63] suggested that acquired genetic variability within developing clones of tumors, coupled with host selection pressures, can result in the emergence of new tumor cell variants that exhibit increasing growth autonomy or malignancy. Nowell's hypothesis[63] predicted that accelerating tumor progression toward malignancy can be accompanied by increasing genetic instability of the evolving cells. To test this hypothesis, we have examined the metastatic stability and rates of mutation of paired metastatic and non-metastatic cloned lines isolated from four different mouse neoplasms. We found that highly metastatic cells were phenotypically less stable than their nonmetastatic counterparts. Moreover, in highly metastatic clones, the rate of spontaneous mutation was found to be several-fold higher than in low-metastatic clones. These results are in accord with the hypothesis that tumor progression occurs as a result of acquired genetic alterations. Similar data have been reported for other neoplasms.[3,4] Evidence that genetic mechanisms can be responsible for tumor progression comes from mutagenesis experiments using nitrosoguanidine.

The finding that metastatic cells exhibit higher mutation rates than non-metastatic cells,[64] and that heterogeneity develops more rapidly in tumors containing few subpopulations of cells[65–67] suggest that accelerated tumor evolution and progression will result in the rapid development of biologic diversity in metastases, especially when such lesions are of clonal origin.

ROLE OF THE ORGAN MICROENVIRONMENT IN THE PATHOGENESIS OF METASTASIS

As stated above, the outcome of the metastatic process depends on multiple and complex interactions of metastatic cells with host homeostatic mechanisms. Clinical observations of cancer patients and studies with experimental rodent tumors have concluded that certain tumors produce metastasis to specific organs independent of vascular anatomy, rate of blood flow and number of tumor cells delivered to each organ. The distribution and fate of hematogenously disseminated, radiolabeled melanoma cells in experimental animals conclusively demonstrated that tumor cells can reach the microvasculature of many organs, but growth in the organ parenchyma occurred in only specific organs.[68–70] In 1889, Stephen Paget researched the mechanisms that regulate organ-specific metastasis, i.e. pattern of metastasis by different cancers. Paget questioned whether the organ distribution of metastases produced by different human neoplasms was due to chance and analyzed more than 700 autopsy records of women with breast cancer. His research documented a non-random pattern of visceral (and bone) metastasis. This finding suggested to Paget that the process was not due to chance but, rather, that certain tumor cells (the 'seed') had a specific affinity for the milieu of certain organs (the 'soil'). Metastases resulted only when the seed and soil were compatible.[27]

In 1928, J. Ewing challenged Paget's seed and soil theory and hypothesized that metastatic dissemination occurs by purely mechanical factors that are a result of the anatomical structure of the vascular system.[40] These explanations have been evoked separately or together to explain the metastatic site preference of certain types of neoplasms. In a review of clinical studies on site preferences of metastases produced by different human neoplasms, Sugarbaker concluded that common *regional* metastatic involvements could be attributed to anatomical or mechanical considerations, such as efferent venous circulation or lymphatic drainage to regional lymph nodes, but that metastasis in *distant* organs from numerous types of cancers were indeed site-specific.[71]

Experimental data supporting the 'seed and soil' hypothesis of Paget were derived from studies on the preferential invasion and growth of B16 melanoma metastases in specific organs[45] (Fig. 1.3). *In vitro* experiments demonstrating organ-selective adhesion, invasion, and growth as well as experiments with organ tissue-derived soluble growth factors indicate that soil factors can have profound effects on certain tumor cell subpopulations[56] also support Paget's hypothesis.

There is no question that the circulatory anatomy influences the dissemination of many malignant cells; however, it cannot, as Ewing proposed, fully explain the patterns of distribution of numerous tumors. Ethical considerations rule out the experimental analysis of cancer metastasis in patients as studied in laboratory animals, by which either Paget or Ewing might be proved correct. The introduction of peritoneovenous shunts for palliation of malignant ascites has, however, provided an opportunity to study some of the factors affecting metastatic spread in humans. Tarin and colleagues have described the outcome in patients with malignant ascites draining into the venous circulation, with the resulting entry of viable tumor cells into the jugular veins.[72] Good palliation with minimal complications was reported for 29 patients with different neoplasms. The autopsy findings in 15 patients substantiated the clinical observations that the shunts do not significantly increase the risk of metastasis. In fact, despite continuous entry of millions of tumor cells into the circulation, metastases in the lung (the first capillary bed encountered) were rare. These results provide compelling verification of the venerable 'seed and soil' hypothesis.[27]

An interesting demonstration for organ-specific metastasis comes from studies of experimental brain metastasis. Schackert and Fidler[73] described the development of a mouse model with which to study cerebral metastasis after injection of syngeneic tumor cells into the internal carotid artery.[73] A direct, intracranial injection of tumor cells was used to determine tumorigenicity. The injection of cells into the internal carotid artery of mice simulates the hematogenous spread of tumor emboli to the brain. Thus, this technique can examine the last steps of the metastatic process: release of tumor cells into the circulation, arrest of tumor cells in capillaries, penetration and extravasation of the tumor cells into the brain through the blood–brain barrier, and continuous growth of the cells in the tissue.

The two melanomas differed in patterns of brain metastasis: the K-1735 melanoma produced lesions only in the brain parenchyma, whereas the B16 melanoma produced only meningeal growths.[73] Similarly, different human melanomas[74] injected into the internal carotid artery of nude mice produce unique patterns of brain metastasis. These results demonstrate specificity for metastatic growth in different regions within a single organ. The results from site distribution analysis of radiolabeled murine melanoma cells injected into the internal carotid artery ruled out that the patterns of initial cell arrest in the microvasculature of the brain predicted the eventual sites of growth. Thus, an alternative explanation for the different sites of tumor growth involves interactions between the metastatic cells and the organ environment, possibly in terms of specific binding to endothelial cells and responses to local growth factors. In other words, organ-specific metastases are produced by tumor cells that are receptive to their new environment.

THE 'SEED AND SOIL' HYPOTHESIS – 2004

A current definition of the 'seed and soil' hypothesis consists of three principles. First, neoplasms are biologically heterogeneous and contain subpopulations of cells with different angiogenic, invasive, and metastatic properties. Second, the process of metastasis is selective for cells that succeed in invasion, embolization, survival in the circulation, arrest in a distant capillary bed, and

extravasation into and multiplication within the organ parenchyma. Although some of the steps in this process contain stochastic elements, as a whole, metastasis favors the survival and growth of a few subpopulations of cells that preexist within the parent neoplasm. Third, and perhaps the most important principle for the design of new cancer therapies, is that the outcome of metastasis depends on multiple interactions ('cross-talk') of metastatic cells with homeostatic mechanisms, which the tumor cells can usurp.[17] Therapy of metastasis, therefore, can be targeted not only against tumor cells but also against the homeostatic factors that promote tumor cell growth, survival, angiogenesis, invasion, and metastasis.

FUTURE OUTLOOK

The process of cancer metastasis is sequential, selective, and contains stochastic elements. The growth of metastases represents the endpoints of many lethal events that few tumor cells can survive (Fig. 1.8). Primary tumors contain multiple subpopulations of cells with heterogeneous metastatic properties and the outcome of metastasis depends on the interplay of tumor cells with various host factors. The findings that different metastases can originate from different progenitor cells account for the biological diversity that exists among various metastases. Even within a solitary metastasis of proven clonal origin, however, heterogeneity of various biologic characteristics can develop rapidly.

The pathogenesis of metastasis depends on multiple favorable interactions of metastatic cells with host homeostatic mechanisms. Interruption of one or more of these interactions can lead to the inhibition or eradication of cancer metastasis. For many years, all of

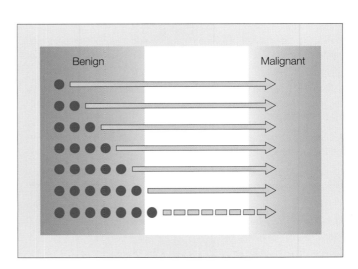
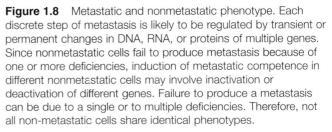

Figure 1.8 Metastatic and nonmetastatic phenotype. Each discrete step of metastasis is likely to be regulated by transient or permanent changes in DNA, RNA, or proteins of multiple genes. Since nonmetastatic cells fail to produce metastasis because of one or more deficiencies, induction of metastatic competence in different nonmetastatic cells may involve inactivation or deactivation of different genes. Failure to produce a metastasis can be due to a single or to multiple deficiencies. Therefore, not all non-metastatic cells share identical phenotypes.

our efforts to treat cancer have concentrated on the inhibition or destruction of tumor cells. Strategies both to treat tumor cells (e.g. chemotherapy and immunotherapy) and to modulate host microenvironment (e.g. tumor vas-culature) should provide additional approaches for cancer treatment. The recent advancements in our understanding of the biological basis of cancer metastasis present unprecedented possibilities for translating basic research to the clinical reality of cancer treatment.

ACKNOWLEDGMENT

This work was supported in part by Cancer Center Support Core Grant CA-16672 from the National Cancer Institute, National Institutes of Health.

REFERENCES

1 Weiss L. Principles of Metastasis. London: Academic Press; 1985.

2 Fidler IJ. Critical factors in the biology of human cancer metastasis: 28th GHA Clowes Memorial Award Lecture. Cancer Res 1990; 50:6130–6138.

3 Fidler IJ. Angiogenic heterogeneity: regulation of neoplastic angiogenesis by the organ microenvironment (editorial). J Natl Cancer Inst 2001a; 93:1040–1041.

4 Fidler IJ. 'Seed and soil' revisited: contribution of the organ microenvironment to cancer metastasis. In: Brodt P, ed. Surgical Oncology Clinics of NA: Cancer Metastasis: Biological and Clinical Aspects. Philadelphia: WB Saunders; 2001b:257.

5 Liotta LA, Kohn EC. The microenvironment of the tumor-host invasion field. Nature 2001:375–379.

6 Fidler IJ. Metastasis: quantitative analysis of distribution and fate of tumor emboli labeled with ^{125}I-5-iodo-2′-deoxyuridine. J Natl Cancer Inst 1970; 45:773–782.

7 Fidler IJ, Talmadge JE. Evidence that intravenously derived murine pulmonary metastases can originate from the expansion of a single tumor cell. Cancer Res 1986; 46:5167–5171.

8 Folkman J. How is blood vessel growth regulated in normal and neoplastic tissue? GHA Clowes Memorial Award Lecture. Cancer Res 1986; 46:467–473.

9 Folkman J. The role of angiogenesis in tumor growth. Semin Cancer Biol 1992; 3:65–71.

10 Liotta LA, Steeg PS, Stetler-Stevenson WG. Cancer metastasis and angiogenesis: an imbalance of positive and negative regulation. Cell 1991; 64:327–336.

11 Auerbach W, Auerbach R. Angiogenesis inhibition: a review. Pharm Ther 1994; 63:265–311.

12 Folkman J, Klagsburn M. Angiogenic factors. Science 1987; 235:444–447.

13 Dvorak HF, Brown LF, Detmar M, Dvorak AM. Vascular permeability factor/vascular endothelial growth factor, microvascular hyperpermeability, and angiogenesis. Am J Pathol 1995; 146:1029–1039.

14 Xu L, Xie K, Mukaida N, Matsushima K, Fidler IJ. Hypoxia-induced elevation in interleukin-8 expression by human ovarian carcinoma cells. Cancer Res 1999; 59:5822–5829.

15 Risau W, Drexler H, Mironov V, et al. Platelet-derived growth factor is angiogenic in vivo. Growth Factors 1992; 7:261–266.

16 Herlyn M. Human melanoma: development and progression. Cancer Metastasis Rev 1990; 9:101–129.

17 Gutman M, Singh RK, Xie K, Bucana CD, Fidler IJ. Regulation of IL-8 expression in human melanoma cells by the organ environment. Cancer Res 1995; 55:2470–2475.

18 Singh RK, Gutman M, Radinsky R, Bucana CD, Fidler IJ. Expression of interleukin 8 correlates with the metastatic potential of human melanoma cells in nude mice. Cancer Res 1994; 54:3242–3247.

19 Liotta LA. Tumor invasion and metastases – Role of the extracellular matrix: Rhoads Memorial Award Lecture. Cancer Res 1986; 46:1–7.

20 Kadowaki T, Shiozaki H, Inoue M, et al. E-cadherin and α-catenin expression in human esophageal cancer. Cancer Res 1994; 54:291–296.

21 Vermeulen SJ, Bruyneel EA, Bracke ME, et al. Transition from the noninvasive to the invasive phenotype and loss of α-catenin in human colon cancer cells. Cancer Res 1995; 55:4722–4728.

22 Sloane BF, Honn KV. Cysteine proteinase and metastasis. Cancer Metastasis Rev 1984; 3:249–265.

23 Ruoslahti E. Fibronectin and its α5β1 integrin receptor in malignancy. Inv Metastasis 1994–1995; 14:87–94.

24 Nakajima M, Irimura T, Nicolson GL. Heparanases and tumor metastasis. J Cell Biochem 1988; 36:157–164.

25 Morikawa K, Walker SM, Nakajima M, Pathak S, Jessup JM, Fidler IJ. The influence of organ environment on the growth, selection, and metastasis of human colon cancer cells in nude mice. Cancer Res 1988; 48:6863–6871.

26 Carr I. Lymphatic metastasis. Cancer Metastasis Rev 1983; 22:307–319.

27 Paget S. The distribution of secondary growths in cancer of the breast. Lancet 1889; 1:571–573.

28 Black MM, Freeman C, Mork T, Harvei S, Cutler SJ. Prognostic significance of microscopic structure of gastric carcinomas and their regional lymph nodes. Cancer 1971; 27:703–710.

29 Byers RM. Modified neck dissection: A study of 967 cases from 1970 to 1980. Am J Surg 1985; 150:414–421.

30 Cox CE, Pendas S, Cox JM, et al. Guidelines for sentinel node biopsy and lymphatic mapping of patients with breast cancer. Ann Surg 1998; 227:645–653.

31 Morton DL, Wen D-R, Wong JH, Cochran AJ. Technical details of intraoperative lymphatic mapping for early stage melanoma. Arch Surg 1992; 127:392–399.

32 Joseph E, Brobeil A, Glass F, et al. Results of complete lymph node dissection in 83 melanoma patients with positive sentinel nodes. Ann Surg Oncol 1998; 5:119–125.

33 Gasic GJ. Role of plasma, platelets and endothelial cells in tumor metastasis. Cancer Metastasis Rev 1984; 3:99–114.

34 Fidler IJ, Bucana C. Mechanism of tumor cell resistance to lysis by syngeneic lymphocytes. Cancer Res 1977; 37:3945–3956.

35 Nicolson GL. Metastatic tumor cell attachment and invasion assay utilizing vascular endothelial cell monolayer. J Histochem Cytochem 1982; 30:214–220.

36 Dvorak HF, Seneger DR, Dvorak AM. Fibrin as a component of the tumor stroma: Origins and biological significance. Cancer Metastasis Rev 1983; 2:41–75.

37 Mareel M, Vleminck K, Vermeulen S, Gao Y, Vakaet L Jr, Bracke M, van Roy F. Homotypic cell–cell adhesion molecules and tumor invasion. In: Graumann W, Drukker J (eds.) Progress in Histo- and Cytochemistry: Histochemistry of Receptors, Vol. 26. Stuttgart: Fischer Verlag; 1992:95–106.

38 Nesbit M, Herlyn M. Adhesion receptors in human melanoma progression. Inv Metastasis 1994–1995; 14:131–138.

39 Terranova VP, Hujanen ES, Martin GR. Basement membrane and the invasive activity of metastatic tumor cells. J Natl Cancer Inst 1986; 77:311–316.

40 Ewing J. Neoplastic diseases, 6th edn. Philadelphia: WB Saunders; 1928.

41 Nicolson GL, Dulski KM. Organ specificity of metastatic tumor colonization is related to organ-selective growth properties of malignant cells. Int J Cancer 1986; 38:289–294.

42 Pauli BU, Schwartz DE, Thonar EJM, Kuttner KE. Tumor invasion and host extracellular matrix. Cancer Metastasis Rev 1983; 2:129–153.

43 Sugarbaker EV, Cohen AM, Ketcham AS. Do metastases metastasize? Ann Surg 1971; 174:161–170.

44 Fidler IJ, Nicolson GL. Organ selectivity for implantation survival and growth of B16 melanoma variant tumor lines. J Natl Cancer Inst 1976; 57:1199–1202.

45 Hart IR, Fidler IJ. Role of organ selectivity in the determination of metastatic patterns of B16 melanoma. Cancer Res 1980; 40:2281–2287.

46 Fidler IJ. Selection of successive tumor lines for metastasis. Nature (New Biol) 1973; 242:148–149.

47 Fidler IJ, Kripke ML. Metastasis results from pre-existing variant cells within a malignant tumor. Science 1977; 197:893–895.

48 Luria SE, Delbruck M. Mutations of bacteria from virus sensitivity to virus resistant. Genetics 1943; 28:491–511.

49 Poste G, Fidler IJ. The pathogenesis of cancer metastasis. Nature 1979; 283 139–146.

50 Fidler IJ. Rationale and methods for the use of nude mice to study the biology and therapy of human cancer metastasis. Cancer Metastasis Rev 1986; 5:29–49.

51 Kripke ML. Speculation on the role of ultraviolet radiation in the development of malignant melanoma. J Natl Cancer Inst 1979; 63:541–545.

52 Fidler IJ, Gruys E, Cifone MA, Barnes Z, Bucana C. Demonstration of multiple phenotypic diversity in a murine melanoma of recent origin. J Natl Cancer Inst 1981; 67:947–956.

53 Kripke ML, Fidler IJ. Enhanced experimental metastasis of UV-induced fibrosarcomas in UV-irradiated syngeneic mice. Cancer Res 1980; 40:625–629.

54 Kripke ML. Immunologic mechanisms in UV radiation carcinogenesis. Adv Cancer Res 1981; 34:69–105.

55 Talmadge JE, Fidler IJ. Enhanced metastatic potential of tumor cells harvested from spontaneous metastases of heterogeneous murine tumors. J Natl Cancer Inst 1982; 69:975–980.

56 Fidler IJ .The pathogenesis of cancer metastasis: the 'seed and soil' revisited (Timeline). Nat Rev Cancer 2003; 3:453–458.

57 Fidler IJ, Poste G. The cellular heterogeneity of malignant neoplasms: Implications for adjuvant chemotherapy. Semin Oncol 1985; 12:207–221.

58 Talmadge JE, Wolman SR, Fidler IJ. Evidence for the clonal origin of spontaneous metastasis. Science 1982; 217:361–363.

59 Kerbel RS, Waghorne C, Man MS, Elliot B, Breitman ML. Alteration of the tumorigenic and metastatic properties of neoplastic cells is associated with the process of calcium phosphate-mediated DNA transfection. Proc Natl Acad Sci USA 1987; 84:1263–1267.

60 Clark WH, Elder DE, Guerry D, et al. A study of tumor progression: The precursor lesions of superficial spreading and nodular melanoma. Hum Pathol 1984; 15:1147–1162.

61 Clark WH, Elder DE, VanHorn M. The biologic forms of malignant melanoma. Hum Pathol 1986; 17:443–469.

62 Herlyn M, Clark WH, Rodeck U, et al. Biology of tumor progression in human melanocytes. Lab Invest 1987; 56:461–474.

63 Nowell PC. The clonal evolution of tumor cell populations. Science 1976; 194:23–28.

64 Cifone MA, Fidler IJ. Increasing metastatic potential is associated with increasing genetic instability of clones isolated from murine neoplasms. Proc Natl Acad Sci USA 1982; 78:6949–6952.

65 Poste G. Pathogenesis of metastatic disease: Implications for current therapy and for the development of new therapeutic strategies. Cancer Treat Rep 1986; 70:183–199.

66 Poste G, Doll J, Fidler IJ. Interactions among clonal subpopulations affect stability of the metastatic phenotype in polyclonal populations of B16 melanoma cells. Proc Natl Acad Sci USA 1981; 78:6226–6230.

67 Nicolson GL. Tumor cell instability, diversification, and progression to the metastatic phenotype: From oncogene to oncofetal expression. Cancer Res 1987; 47:1473–1487.

68 Hart IR. 'Seed and soil' revisited: Mechanisms of site-specific metastasis. Cancer Metastasis Rev 1982; 1:5–17.

69 Hart IR, Talmadge JE, Fidler IJ. Metastatic behavior of a murine reticulum cell sarcoma exhibiting organ-specific growth. Cancer Res 1981; 41:1281–1287.

70 Price JE, Aukerman SL, Fidler IJ. Evidence that the process of murine melanoma metastasis is sequential and selective and contains stochastic elements. Cancer Res 1986; 46:5172–5178.

71 Sugarbaker EV. Cancer metastasis: a product of tumor–host interactions. Curr Probl Cancer 1979; 3:1–59.

72 Tarin D, Price JE, Kettlewell MGW, et al. Mechanisms of human tumor metastasis studied in patients with peritoneovenous shunts. Cancer Res 1984; 44:3584–3592.

73 Schackert G, Fidler IJ. Site-specific metastasis of mouse melanomas and a fibrosarcoma in the brain or the meninges of syngeneic animals. Cancer Res 1988; 48:3478–3484.

74 Zhang R, Price JE, Fujimaki T, Bucana CD, Fidler IJ. Differential permeability of the blood–brain barrier in experimental brain metastases produced by human neoplasms implanted into nude mice. Am J Pathol 1992; 141:1115–1124.

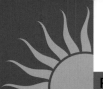

CHAPTER

2

Genetic Basis of Skin Cancer

Michael Dans and Steven S Fakharzadeh

Key points

- Specific genes implicated in causing each major form of skin cancer have been identified through genetic studies on hereditary and/or sporadic skin cancer. Their role in promoting cutaneous neoplasia is supported and confirmed by functional studies in animal model systems.
- Defects in the *CDKN2A* tumor suppressor locus are associated with both familial and sporadic cutaneous malignant melanoma and may cooperate with *RAS* or *RAF* proto-oncogene activation to promote tumor formation.
- Mutations resulting in *RAS* proto-oncogene activation may cooperate with inactivation of either *CDKN2A* or *p53* tumor suppressor genes in causing cutaneous squamous cell carcinoma.
- Defects in the *PTCH* gene have been implicated in both hereditary and sporadic basal cell carcinoma and mutations in genes encoding other components of the SHH signaling pathway have been associated with sporadic tumors. Defects in the *p53* tumor suppressor gene are common in basal cell carcinoma as well.
- Although significant advances have been made in identifying genes associated with skin cancers, additional yet to be identified genes likely contribute to the pathogenesis of each major form of skin cancer.

INTRODUCTION

Tumorigenesis is a multi-staged process deriving from a series of acquired, and in some cases inherited, genetic alterations.[1] Together, these aberrations create imbalances between critical cellular processes, such as cell cycle regulation/cell proliferation, cell death, and cell differentiation. Consequently, such imbalances permit clonal expansion of cells and ultimately tumor formation. Significant progress in delineating the genetic basis of skin cancers has been made in recent years. Specific genes implicated in causing cutaneous tumors when mutated have been identified through genetic studies of hereditary and/or sporadic skin cancer. In turn, functional studies in animal model systems support and confirm their role in cutaneous neoplasia.

Cancer genes fall into two general categories: proto-oncogenes and tumor suppressor genes. Proto-oncogenes, such as *RAS* and *RAF*, normally promote cell pro-

liferation or survival. However, upon mutation, proto-oncogenes may be activated (to become oncogenes), which allows them to bypass regulatory mechanisms that normally prevent their function in an uncontrolled manner. An activating mutation in just one allele typically is sufficient to contribute to tumorigenesis. In contrast, tumor suppressor genes, such as those encoded by the *CDKN2A* locus and the *p53* gene, normally inhibit cell cycle progression and proliferation. Characteristically, inactivation of both alleles of such genes, through mutation, deletion or silencing, is required to lose suppressor function and permit tumor formation.

This chapter reviews and summarizes the current understanding of the genetic basis of the three predominant forms of skin cancer, basal cell carcinoma, squamous cell carcinoma and melanoma.

BASAL CELL CARCINOMA

Hereditary basal cell carcinoma: Gorlin syndrome

Initial insights into the molecular pathogenesis of basal cell carcinoma (BCC) were derived from genetic analysis of families with Gorlin syndrome (basal cell nevus syndrome, nevoid basal cell carcinoma syndrome).[2,3] Affected individuals have normal-appearing skin early in life. However, during the course of their lifetime these patients develop BCCs, often numbering in the hundreds, in a generalized distribution. Palmoplantar pits and epidermal cysts represent other frequent cutaneous findings in these patients. In addition to BCC, affected individuals are predisposed to other tumors, including medulloblastoma, meningioma, rhabdomyosarcoma and ovarian tumors. Skeletal anomalies, such as odontogenic jaw cysts, bifid ribs, and tall stature may be observed, as well as craniofacial and brain defects, such as cleft palate, coarse facies, dysgenesis of the corpus callosum, mental retardation, and intracranial calcification.

Gorlin syndrome displays an autosomal dominant inheritance pattern. Linkage analysis of Gorlin syndrome families established a chromosomal locus for the disorder at 9q22.3.[4] Furthermore, both hereditary and sporadic BCCs commonly show deletion of this region.[4] Taken together, these observations suggested the presence of a tumor suppressor gene locus at chromosomal region 9q22.3. Subsequently, inactivating mutations in the human homolog of the Drosophila *patched* gene (*PTCH* in humans, *Ptc* in mice; italicized for gene, non-italicized for protein), which maps to this locus, were identified and implicated in causing Gorlin syndrome.[5,6]

Ptc function and the Shh signaling pathway

In vertebrate models the *Ptc* gene has been implicated in the development of a variety of structures, including neural tube, skeleton, limbs, craniofacial structures, skin and hair follicles. The *Ptc* gene effects its function through the Hedgehog (Hh) signaling pathway.[7] In vertebrates, there are three *Hh* homologs, *Sonic* (*Shh*), *Desert* (*Dhh*), and *Indian* (*Ihh*); of these *Shh* has been most extensively studied. Shh is a secreted factor that binds to the membrane-bound Ptc protein. Normally Ptc inhibits the capacity of Smoothened (Smo), a G-protein-coupled transmembrane receptor protein, to convey a signal to induce transcription of a variety of downstream target genes including pathway components, such as the *Ptc* and *Gli1* genes. Shh binding to Ptc relieves inhibition of Smo, enabling it to transduce its intracellular signal.

The *Gli* genes (*Gli1*, *Gli2*, and *Gli3*) are critical downstream effectors of Smo signaling once the Shh pathway has been activated.[8] The *Gli* genes encode a family of DNA-binding, zinc-finger transcription factors. An activation domain exists at the C-terminal of Gli1, which induces expression of downstream target genes in response to Shh signaling. In contrast, both Gli2 and Gli3 possess N-terminal repressor domains and C-terminal activator domains, and may display either transcriptional activator or repressor function. However, repression of *Shh*-responsive genes may be more pronounced through Gli3 than Gli2, and Gli2 may have more of a role as an activator of gene expression.

Activation of Shh signaling promotes cell proliferation, which may result in tumorigenesis if normal pathway controls are abrogated. Although the mechanisms mediating Shh-induced proliferation are not fully characterized, there is evidence suggesting that both Shh and Ptc may directly influence cell cycle progression.[7] Shh has been shown to antagonize function of the cyclin-dependent kinase (CDK) inhibitor p21[Cip1], which imposes restrictions upon cell cycle progression. Furthermore, Shh induces expression of D and E cyclins to promote progression through the G1 phase of the cell cycle and stimulate cell growth.[9] Conversely, Ptc was found to bind phosphorylated cyclin B1, thus altering its cellular distribution and imposing blockade of cell cycle progression in the G2 phase.[10] Thus, inactivation of the *Ptc* gene could lead to aberrant cell cycle progression both by mimicking constitutive Shh signaling and loss of Ptc inhibition of cyclin B1.

With knowledge of the molecular components of the SHH pathway, the role of *PTCH* as a tumor suppressor gene in Gorlin syndrome becomes apparent. Affected individuals have a germline defect in one allele of the *PTCH* gene. Mutation or deletion compromising the remaining normal *PTCH* allele in a given cell would lead to complete loss of PTCH function. In turn, this would result in constitutive activation of the SHH pathway, uninhibited SMO signaling (Fig. 2.1), unregulated cell proliferation and ultimately tumorigenesis.

SHH pathway gene defects in sporadic BCC

Evidence for *PTCH* inactivation in tumorigenesis in Gorlin syndrome led to speculation that *PTCH* gene defects may be involved in the pathogenesis of sporadic BCCs as well. Subsequent studies detected mutations in *PTCH* in 12–38% of sporadic BCCs examined.[11,12] Moreover, loss of DNA markers around the *PTCH* locus has been observed in roughly 40–67% of sporadic BCCs.[4,12,13] These findings indicate that *PTCH* gene defects are frequent in sporadic BCC and suggest that both hereditary and sporadic BCCs may develop through a common mechanism.

Further still, mutations in other components of the SHH pathway were speculated to result in BCC tumorigenesis. Dominant, activating mutations in *SMO* have been found in 6–20% of sporadic BCCs.[14,15] One example of an activating *SHH* mutation in BCC has been reported.[16] Additionally, there has been a report of mutation in the *PTCH2* gene, which shows strong homology to *PTCH* and is believed to be engaged in SHH signaling as well.[17] Thus, mutations in different components of the SHH pathway may deregulate signaling in a manner analogous to inactivation of *PTCH* and consequently lead to BCC tumorigenesis.

In addition, defects in the SHH signaling pathway may play a role in the pathogenesis of more benign forms of basaloid neoplasms. Some precedence for this derives from studies that implicate *PTCH* gene defects in sporadic trichoepitheliomas. Deletion of chromosomal region 9q22.3 was observed in about half of the samples examined in one study,[18] whereas specific mutations in the *PTCH* gene were identified in sporadic trichoepitheliomas in another report.[19] Sebaceous nevi are cutaneous congenital malformations that are susceptible to developing foci of basal cell carcinoma. Up to 40% of lesions in one study demonstrated loss of heterozygosity of at least one microsatellite marker at 9q22.3, suggesting a role for *PTCH* inactivation in the pathogenesis of sebaceous nevus.[20] Lastly, there is evidence for altered regulation of SHH signaling in basaloid follicular hamartoma (BFH). Increased levels of message for *PTCH* and other pathway target genes have been observed in BFH lesions.[21,22] However, lower levels and an altered distribution of transcripts for these genes were detected in BFH compared with BCC, suggesting that the magnitude and/or pattern of SHH signaling may influence skin tumor phenotype.

Experimental studies of Shh pathway genes in mouse models of BCC tumorigenesis

There is extensive experimental evidence from mouse models for a causative role for Shh pathway gene defects in BCC tumorigenesis. Results from such functional studies corroborate findings from genetic studies of hereditary and sporadic BCC identifying aberrations in these genes. Mice heterozygous for a *Ptc* null allele represent genetic murine equivalents of Gorlin syndrome patients. These mice spontaneously develop primordial follicular lesions resembling trichoblastoma,[23] and they develop tumors

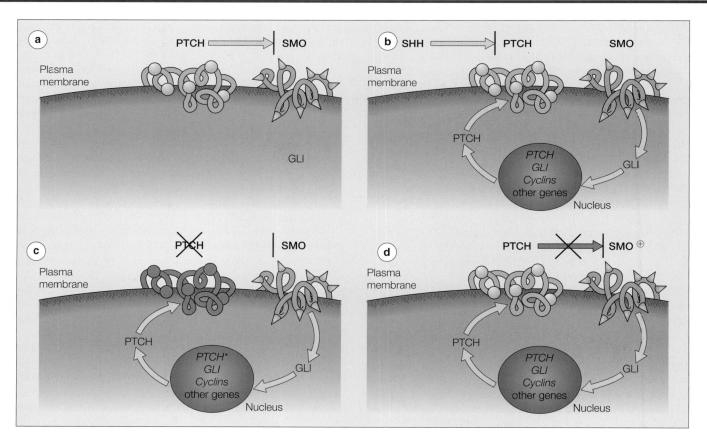

Figure 2.1 SHH signaling pathway. (a) PTCH normally inhibits SMO function. (b) SHH binding inactivates PTCH, allowing SMC to transmit its intracellular signal through GLI effectors. Transcription of a variety of downstream target genes, including pathway components, such as the *PTCH* and *GLI* genes, and genes that stimulate cell cycle progression and growth, is regulated by GLI transcription factors. Induction of PTCH expression reestablishes suppression of SMO as a negative feed back mechanism to prevent uncontrolled pathway activity. (c) If *PTCH* is inactivated by mutation and/or deletion (designated by *), SMO functions without inhibition and the pathway becomes constitutively active. Any PTCH produced from a mutant allele is non-functional and incapable of suppressing pathway signaling. (d) Activating *SMO* mutations (designated by ⊕), make its gene product unresponsive to PTCH suppression, allowing pathway signaling to proceed unopposed.

with features more similar to BCC in response to UV or ionizing radiation. These studies demonstrate that haplo-insufficiency of *Ptc*, as in Gorlin syndrome, increases susceptibility to basaloid neoplasia.

In addition, aberrant expression of other components of Shh pathway signaling to induce or mimic *Ptc* inactivation results in similar patterns of tumorigenesis in various mouse models. Transgenic mice that constitutively overexpress Shh in the skin, leading to inhibition of Ptc suppression of Smo, develop cutaneous tumors resembling BCC.[16] Similarly, primary human keratinocytes induced to overexpress SHH develop into BCC upon grafting onto immunodeficient mice.[24] Moreover, transgenic mice that overexpress an activated, mutant variant of human SMO which bypasses Ptc suppression, develop epidermal hyperplasia and down-growths of basaloid cells.[14,22] Similar findings have been observed in studies of downstream effectors of Shh signaling. Transgenic mice that target GLI1 expression to basal epidermis develop BCCs and trichoepitheliomas,[25] whereas transgenic mice that express Gli2 in the skin generate BCCs as well.[26] Taken together, these studies provide overwhelming experimental evidence that deregulation of the Shh pathway, through inactivation of *Ptc* or activation of pathway components either upstream or downstream of *Ptc*, plays a central role in mediating development of BCC as well as other related forms of basaloid neoplasia.

p53 mutations in basal cell carcinoma

The *p53* tumor suppressor gene is one of the most commonly mutated genes in human cancers. Given the frequency of *p53* defects in other cancers, a number of studies investigated BCCs for the presence of *p53* mutations. Approximately half of sporadic BCCs studied have been found to harbor *p53* mutations.[27–29] As for SCC, inactivating *p53* mutations observed in BCC typically display UV signature (C→T or CC→TT) features, implicating mutagenesis through solar irradiation.[29] Deletion of the *p53* locus, however, is an infrequent occurrence in BCC.[30]

After chromosomal aberrations at 9q and *PTCH* gene defects were identified in BCCs, studies were performed to determine whether both *p53* and 9q/*PTCH* defects are commonly observed in the same tumors. Of 18 tumors analyzed in one study, 11 (61%) BCCs demonstrated loss of 9q DNA markers and 11 (61%) carried *p53* mutations;

7 (39%) maintained alterations of both genes.[30] Similarly, 38% of early onset BCCs studied in another report showed mutations in both *PTCH* and *p53* genes, although this figure likely underestimates *PTCH* defects as allelic loss at 9q and was not assessed.[31] Yet another study reported both allelic loss of *PTCH* and *p53* mutations in 6 of 8 (75%) of sporadic BCCs.[32] Taken together, these findings indicate that defects in both *PTCH* and *p53* genes are frequently associated in BCC.

Alternative genes involved in the pathogenesis of BCC

Despite substantial evidence implicating *PTCH* or *SMO* mutations leading to deregulation of SHH signaling in BCC tumorigenesis, it is likely that defects in other genes may have similar consequences. Although mutations in *PTCH* or *SMO* have been observed in a high proportion of sporadic BCCs, as discussed above, mutations in neither gene have been identified in at least one third of sporadic BCCs. Although this, in part, may reflect limitations of the approaches used for mutation detection, a plausible alternative explanation for this observation is that defects in other genes may play a primary role in the pathogenesis of these BCCs. Mutations in other genes commonly associated with other forms of skin cancer, such as *RAS* and *CDKN2A* genes are rare in sporadic BCC.

Further evidence supporting alternative genes contributing to BCC neoplasia derive from genome-wide screenings for chromosomal aberrations in tumor-derived DNA. Comparative genomic hybridization studies revealed recurrent chromosomal losses at 9q including the region of the *PTCH* gene in a panel of BCCs, as expected, in one report.[33] However, recurrent chromosomal gains were observed at 5 loci. In particular, regional gains at 6p were detected in 47% of tumors studied, suggesting that a proto-oncogene localized to this region may become activated by virtue of its amplification and overexpression in a significant proportion of sporadic BCCs.

Similarly, additional genetic disorders, which, like Gorlin syndrome, predispose to multiple BCCs, yet are not attributable to mutations in *PTCH*, *SMO*, or other known components of SHH signaling have been defined. For example, linear unilateral basal cell nevus (LUBCN) is a rare disorder that predisposes to development of multiple BCCs, BFH, and comedonal and cystic lesions, in a limited unilateral distribution.[34] Although there is evidence for deregulation of SHH signaling in LUBCN lesions, underlying mutations in *PTCH* and *SMO* have been ruled out in at least one subject with this disorder (our unpublished observations). Bazex–Dupre–Christol syndrome is characterized by follicular atrophoderma, hypotyrichosis and development of multiple BCCs starting at an early age. This disorder displays an X-linked pattern of inheritance and linkage studies have identified a genetic locus for this disorder at Xq24–q27.[35] However, no known component of the SHH pathway maps to this region. Similarly, individuals with Rombo syndrome, another rare hereditary disorder, manifest a constellation of features including multiple BCCs, trichoepitheliomas,

vermiculate atrophoderma, milia, hypotrichosis, and peripheral vasodilation with cyanosis.[36] Neither a specific gene nor a genetic locus for this disorder has been identified as yet. Given that each of these disorders increase susceptibility to BCC, identifying the genes that cause them may provide further insight into mechanisms that contribute to tumorigenesis not only in these disorders, but potentially in sporadic BCCs as well.

Lastly, studies employing experimental animal models further suggest involvement of alternative genes in BCC neoplasia. The *Notch*1 gene is important in regulating normal development in a variety of tissues and altered Notch1 signaling has been implicated in tumorigenesis. Mice engineered to selectively inactivate the *Notch*1 gene in epidermis develop epidermal hyperplasia and skin tumors resembling BCC.[37] Moreover, tumors derived from these mice display increased and constitutive expression of *Gli*2. Therefore, in this model system, *Notch*1 displays tumor suppressor gene properties very much analogous to those of *Ptc*, whereby loss of function may lead to altered regulation of Shh signaling and BCC tumorigenesis. Although involvement of *NOTCH*1 in human BCC neoplasia has not yet been reported, it is conceivable that defects in the *NOTCH*1 gene or other genes engaged in *NOTCH*1 signaling may play a role in the pathogenesis of either sporadic or syndromic BCCs.

CUTANEOUS SQUAMOUS CELL CARCINOMA

In contrast to cutaneous malignant melanoma and basal cell carcinoma, cutaneous squamous cell carcinoma (SCC) is not specifically associated with a known hereditary syndrome or familial clustering. This absence of a hereditary syndrome that specifically increases susceptibility to SCC has made the identification of genes involved in SCC somewhat more complex. Most genetic analyses of cutaneous SCC have focused on oncogenes and tumor suppressor genes known to contribute to the development of other forms of cancers when altered. Studies have focused predominantly on *RAS* genes or the *CDKN2A* or *p53* tumor suppressor genes. A variety of mutation analysis studies on sporadic SCCs and functional studies forcing aberrant gene expression have provided considerable insight into the genetic basis of SCC.

RAS gene defects in SCC

Activating *RAS* mutations are among the most common genetic abnormalities in human cancers. This class of mutation promotes constitutive activation of molecular signaling pathways downstream of RAS, such as the MAPK-mediated signaling pathway, which in turn influences a variety of cellular processes such as cell proliferation.[38] Given the frequency of *RAS* mutations in other tumor types, a number of studies have examined sporadic SCCs for the presence of activating *RAS* mutations. Although the frequency of *RAS* mutations reported ranges widely, several studies indicate that *RAS* mutations are common in SCC. In one report, 46% of cutaneous SCCs examined harbored activating mutations substituting a valine for glycine at residue 12 of the *H-RAS* gene, while *K-RAS* mutations and *N-RAS* amplification events were less commonly observed.[39] Similarly, codon 12 *H-RAS* mutations were detected in 35% of SCCs screened in another study,[40] and activating *H-RAS* or *K-RAS* mutations were observed in 12% of SCCs and 16% of actinic keratoses (AKs) in an additional report.[41] Given that AKs represent precursor lesions to SCCs, these findings suggest that *RAS* mutation may represent an early event in SCC tumorigenesis. Taken together, these results indicate that mutations resulting in *RAS* gene activation may contribute to the development of a significant proportion of cutaneous SCCs.

CDKN2A gene defects in SCC

Chromosomal deletions or allelic losses are relatively common in SCC and may involve multiple chromosomes. In particular, deletions targeting chromosome 9p are frequent; DNA markers from this region are deleted in approximately 30–50% of SCCs.[42,43] Given that the *CDKN2A* locus maps to 9p21, studies to screen sporadic SCCs for mutations that disrupt p16^{INK4a}/p14^{ARF} function were performed. *CDKN2A* mutations were observed in 9–42% of cutaneous SCCs, demonstrating that inactivation of p16^{INK4a}/p14^{ARF} may occur commonly in SCC development.[43,44] In further support of this, Mortier *et al.*[45] observed loss of DNA markers flanking the *CDKN2A* locus in AKs as well as in SCCs. Deletion of the *CDKN2A* locus was detected in 21% of AKs compared with 46% of SCCs. Given the higher frequency of loss in SCCs, loss or inactivation of the *CDKN2A* locus may represent an important step in the progression of pre-malignant AK to malignant SCC.

p53 gene defects in SCC

The *p53* tumor suppressor gene represents yet another gene commonly altered in human cancers, and it has been studied extensively in cutaneous SCC. The product of the *p53* gene normally functions as a critical regulator of cell cycle progression and programmed cell death in response to insults that damage DNA, such as UV irradiation.[46] Induction of p53 expression occurs as a consequence of DNA strand breaks (Fig. 2.2). In turn, p53 stimulates expression of p21^{Cip1}, which imposes G1 blockade of cell cycle progression by binding to and inhibiting cyclin-dependent kinases (CDKs) 2 and 4. Inhibition of cell cycle progression allows for DNA repair before it is replicated in S phase to prevent retention of introduced mutations. Alternatively, if DNA damage is severe, cells undergo programmed cell death, mediated by p53 induction of BAX, which binds to BCL-2 and inhibits its anti-apoptotic activity. If the *p53* gene becomes inactivated through mutation or deletion, neither cell cycle blockade nor cell death would occur in response to DNA damage. Thus, mutations may not be repaired and consequently would be retained in genomic DNA. Damaged cells would persist and potentially undergo clonal expansion and tumorigenesis. Therefore, the *p53* gene serves as a 'guardian of the genome' and plays a central role as a tumor suppressor.

Substantial evidence implicates *p53* gene defects in SCC tumorigenesis. Although reported rates of *p53* mutations in SCC vary considerably, a number of studies observed *p53* gene defects to be common events in SCC. Mutations in *p53* were detected in 41%, 58% and 69% of SCC tumors in three independent studies.[27,47,48] These results support that compromise of p53 function may represent an important step in SCC tumorigenesis. Moreover, *p53* mutations have been found to be common in

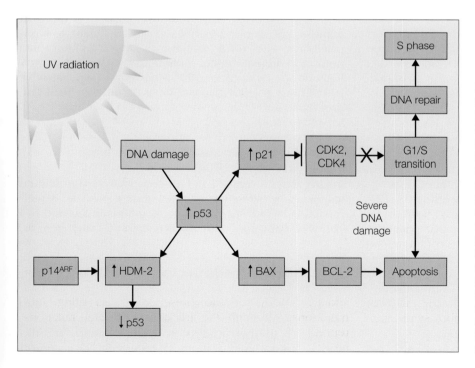

Figure 2.2 *p53* tumor suppressor gene function. Expression of p53 is induced by DNA damage incurred by insults such as UV irradiation. p53 induces expression of p21^{Cip1}, which blocks cell cycle transition from G1 to S phase by inhibiting CDK2 and CDK4. Cell cycle blockade allows for DNA repair before replication in S phase to prevent retention of mutations. If DNA damage is severe, cells undergo apoptosis mediated by p53-induced BAX. In addition, p53 induces HDM-2, which downregulates p53 to permit cell cycle progression when appropriate. p14^{ARF} inhibits HDM-2 to promote stabilization of p53. Inactivation of the *p53* gene through either mutation or deletion would eliminate p53-induced cell cycle blockade and cell death responses to DNA damage, and permit mutations to accumulate.

precursor lesions and early SCCs as well. Mutations in *p53* have been reported in approximately 50–60% of AKs[47,48] and 35% of *in situ* SCCs examined.[49] Further still, *p53* mutations have been observed in clonal expansions of keratinocytes in otherwise normal sun-exposed skin.[50,51] Moreover, mutations in the *p53* gene characteristically represent UV signature CC→TT or C→T tandem transition mutations at dipyrimidine sequences.[47] Taken together, these findings suggest that *p53* gene defects likely represent early events in squamous neoplasia that are induced by solar UV irradiation.

Experimental studies of *RAS*, *CDK* and *p53* genes in models of SCC tumorigenesis

Extensive studies in experimental model systems corroborate findings from genetic analysis of sporadic cutaneous SCC and implicate defects in *RAS*, *CDKN2A* and *p53* genes in the pathogenesis of SCC. Furthermore, these studies provide evidence that these genes may cooperate with each other to establish a molecular environment that facilitates SCC tumorigenesis.

Studies in mouse keratinocytes have demonstrated that Ras activation is an important early event in the stepwise development of SCC.[52] Primary murine keratinocytes that express oncogenic *v-ras*[Ha] have been found to develop into benign squamous papillomas upon grafting onto immunodeficient mice. Downstream effects of oncogenic Ras expression have been shown to be mediated by aberrant protein kinase C (PKC) signaling (upregulation of PKCα and inhibition of PKCδ), and is dependent on activation of the epidermal growth factor receptor (EGFR). However, Ras activation alone is insufficient to cause SCC, and additional genetic aberrations and alterations in gene expression are required for premalignant progression and malignant transformation resulting in unregulated cell proliferation.

Further insight into the consequences of RAS activation have been derived from models for human SCC development. Although similar findings have been observed in other cell types, recent studies showed that expression of an activated *H-RAS* gene in primary human keratinocytes induces growth arrest as a means of protecting against unregulated RAS activity.[53,54] Moreover, growth arrest appears to be mediated by RAS-induced expression of CDK inhibitors and suppression of CDK4 expression, leading to G1 blockade of cell cycle progression. However, when primary keratinocytes are forced to co-express activated RAS with either CDK4[53] or IκBα,[54] they produce tumors resembling invasive SCCs after grafting onto immunodeficient mice. IκBα is an inhibitor of NF-κB, a transcription factor that promotes proliferation and protects against apoptosis (programmed cell death) in many cell types yet paradoxically inhibits proliferation of primary keratinocytes.[55] Significantly, IκBα was shown to induce CDK4 expression in this model.[54] Therefore, either direct or induced expression of CDK4 may circumvent RAS-induced growth arrest and promote cell proliferation.

Despite its role in mediating growth arrest, activated RAS signaling must provide some alternative function to promote tumorigenesis given the frequent finding of RAS mutations in SCC. It has been recognized that activated RAS signaling may oppose apoptosis through multiple downstream pathways.[56,57] Although IκBα promotes cell proliferation by inducing CDK4 activation, a potential consequence of IκBα expression would be increased susceptibility to programmed cell death by antagonizing NF-κB function. However, studies by Dajee *et al.*[54] demonstrated that co-expressing RAS with IκBα in primary human keratinocytes countered the increased susceptibility to apoptosis imposed by blocking NF-κB. These studies, therefore, demonstrate that alterations in CDK4 and RAS pathways may cooperate to (1) bypass growth arrest to permit cell proliferation and (2) circumvent programmed cell death, respectively, to induce transformation of primary human keratinocytes and promote SCC tumorigenesis.

Similarly, experimental animal models support a role for p53 in SCC development. Mice completely deficient for p53 develop pre-malignant lesions resembling actinic keratoses and SCCs in response to UV irradiation.[58,59] Insights into early events that ultimately predispose to development of these lesions were derived from histologic examination of skin from normal and p53-deficient mice 24 hrs after irradiation.[60] Apoptotic keratinocytes ('sunburn cells') were evident in the epidermis of normal mice, but were not observed in the skin of p53 null mice. Thus, cells lacking p53 failed to undergo programmed cell death in response to UV irradiation, permitting them to accumulate mutations in their genomic DNA. Consequently, mutations occurring in proto-oncogenes and/ or tumor suppressor genes may facilitate clonal expansion and ultimately tumor formation. Therefore, this work establishes a clear role for p53 in protecting against early events that increase susceptibility to squamous neoplasia.

Furthermore, evidence supports that loss of p53-mediated cell cycle inhibition may be sufficient to overcome Ras-induced growth arrest in mouse models of SCC tumorigenesis. Primary murine keratinocytes that express oncogenic *v-ras*[Ha] and are deficient for p53 proliferate and form carcinomas upon grafting onto immunodeficient mice.[61] Similarly, primary mouse keratinocytes that lack p19[ARF] (the murine equivalent of p14[ARF]) are able to bypass Ras-induced growth arrest, proliferate and form tumors as well.[62] Given that p19[ARF] serves to stabilize p53, loss of p19[ARF] represents an alternative mechanism for impairing p53 function. Thus, elimination of p53-mediated cell cycle inhibition through either direct (p53 defect) or indirect (p19[ARF] defect) means circumvents Ras-induced growth arrest and stimulates proliferation. These studies provide experimental evidence showing that alterations in Ras and p53 pathways may cooperate to promote SCC tumorigenesis.

Alternative genetic loci in SCC

Despite advances in identifying genes that contribute to the pathogenesis of SCC, it is likely that additional genes contribute to this process as well. Evidence for this derives from identification of recurrent chromosomal aberrations through genome-wide analysis of SCC tumors.

Quinn *et al.* found that loss of DNA markers mapping to several chromosomes was common. In addition to loss of heterozygosity at 9p (41%), as discussed previously, frequent losses at 3p (23%), 13q (46%), 17p (33%), and 17q (33%) were observed.[42] Deletion of DNA markers at 17p, 17q and 13q were commonly observed in AKs as well, suggesting that loss of potential tumor suppressor genes that map to these regions may contribute to the pathogenesis of both AKs and SCCs.[63] While the p53 gene maps to 17p and may represent a target for deletion in some tumors, potential novel tumor suppressor genes may localize to other areas that are often deleted. More recent studies also found evidence for chromosomal losses at 13q, in addition to other regions of gain or loss, using the technique of comparative genomic hybridization.[64] Further studies evaluating larger numbers of tumors may permit more refined mapping and identification of a putative 13q tumor suppressor gene and possibly other genes that contribute to squamous neoplasia.

CUTANEOUS MALIGNANT MELANOMA

Familial melanoma: *CDKN2A* and *CDK4* gene defects

Although familial melanomas represent just 5–10% of all cases, genetic studies of families predisposed to developing cutaneous malignant melanoma (CMM) identified the first gene associated with this disease.[65] Early studies detected cytogenetic aberrations and deletion of DNA markers at the short arm of chromosome 9 in both primary CMMs and melanoma cell lines, and subsequent work localized a putative melanoma tumor suppressor gene to region 9p21.[66] Based on these early studies, linkage analysis was performed on several kindreds with a high incidence of CMM using markers derived 9p21 and established the presence of a genetic locus for familial melanoma in this region.[67] Subsequently, germline mutations were identified in the *CDKN2A* (p16^{INK4A}) gene in several affected members of families demonstrating linkage to the 9p21 chromosomal region.[68,69] Of those family members that inherit *CDKN2A* mutations, 55–100% ultimately develop CMM, indicating that *CDKN2A* mutations are highly penetrant.[70]

The *CDKN2A* gene encodes the p16^{INK4A} protein, which plays a key role in limiting cell cycle progression (Fig 2.3).[71,72] Advancement through the G1 phase of the cell cycle is dependent on a molecular complex formed by cyclin D1 and CDK4 (cyclin-dependent kinase 4). The CDK4 component of this complex phosphorylates the product of the retinoblastoma tumor suppressor gene (Rb), which then releases transcription factors of the E2F family. Once released by Rb, E2F transcription factors induce expression of genes necessary for exiting G1 and progression to the S phase of the cell cycle. To effect inhibition of cell cycle progression, p16^{INK4A} protein binds to CDK4 and inhibits its kinase activity. In turn, phosphorylation of Rb protein is impaired, hypophosphorylated Rb fails to release E2F transcription factors,

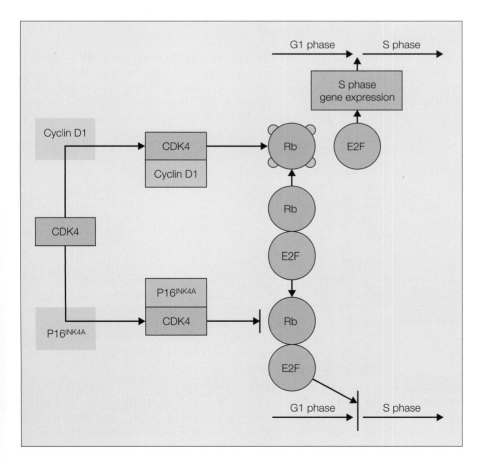

Figure 2.3 CDK4 and p16^{INK4A} regulation of the cell cycle. (Upper section) CDK4 and cyclin D1 form a complex that phosphorylates Rb through CDK4 kinase activity. Upon phosphorylation, Rb releases E2F transcription factors, which induce expression of genes required for exiting G1 and entering the S phase of the cell cycle. (Lower section) p16^{INK4A} binds CDK4, inhibits its kinase activity, and impairs phosphorylation of Rb. Hypophosphorylated Rb fails to release E2F transcription factors, preventing cell cycle progression to S phase.

and the cell cycle stalls in the G1 phase. Therefore, loss of p16^{INK4A} function by virtue of *CDKN2A* mutation and/or deletion would eliminate a critical inhibitor of cell cycle progression and suppressor of tumor development.

Most germline *CDKN2A* mutations in melanoma families appear to alter p16^{INK4A} protein in a manner that interferes with its binding to CDK4.[73] Abrogation of this interaction, in turn, would render p16^{INK4A} non-functional and negate its cell cycle regulatory and tumor suppressor activities. Similarly, defects in CDK4 that interfere with its binding to p16^{INK4A} would be predicted to yield the same result and lead to unregulated CDK4 activity. Thus, it is not surprising that melanoma families carrying germline mutations in the *CDK4* gene have been identified.[74] Notably, all *CDK4* mutations identified to date cause an amino acid substitution for the arginine at residue 24, which normally facilitates CDK4 interaction with p16^{INK4A}. Although *CDK4* mutations in melanoma families are rare, their identification further underscores that impairment of p16^{INK4A} interaction with CDK4 contributes to the pathogenesis of CMM.

Additional melanoma families showing linkage to chromosome 9p yet lacking mutations in p16^{INK4A} coding sequences have been identified, suggesting that an alternative melanoma susceptibility gene maps to this area. One candidate, p14^{ARF}, was recently shown to harbor germline mutations in some cases. The p14^{ARF} gene product is derived from the *CDKN2A* locus and shares sequences that encode p16^{INK4A}; however, it represents a completely distinct protein from p16^{INK4A}.[71,72] Alternative promoters initiate transcription of p16^{INK4A} and p14^{ARF} mRNA, and independent first exons, 1α and 1β, respectively, are incorporated into each transcript (Fig. 2.4). Alternative splicing allows for joining of both first exons with the same second and third exons. However, use of different translational reading frames (hence ARF for *a*lternative *r*eading *f*rame) in the latter exons gives rise to proteins with distinct amino acid sequences that share no homology.

Despite their derivation from a common locus, p16^{INK4A} and p14^{ARF} influence cell cycle progression through different mechanisms. Whereas p16^{INK4A} inhibits CDK4-mediated phosphorylation of Rb to block progression through the G1 phase of the cell cycle, p14^{ARF} promotes stabilization of p53 protein. Stabilization of p53 is mediated by p14^{ARF} binding to HDM2 (human homolog of murine Mdm2) and interfering with HDM2-directed ubiquitination and subsequent degradation of p53 (see Fig. 2.2). Thus, p16^{INK4A} and p14^{ARF} inhibit cell cycle progression through distinct, yet vital, alternative pathways.

Given that deletions of the *CDKN2A* locus commonly result in loss of expression of both p16^{INK4A} and p14^{ARF}, what, if any, role p14^{ARF} plays in tumor suppression independently of p16^{INK4A} was unclear. However, a number of recent reports directly associate germline defects in p14^{ARF} with increased predisposition to CMM. A deletion involving p14^{ARF} exon 1β which does not disrupt p16^{INK4A} coding sequences was identified in one melanoma family.[75] An individual with multiple CMMs was shown to harbor a germline 16 bp insertion into p14^{ARF} exon 1β sequences. This insertion causes a shift in translational reading frame and introduces a premature termination codon, which exclusively disrupts expression of p14^{ARF}.[76] Similarly, a germline mutation that alters the last nucleotide of exon 1β was detected in another melanoma family. This change interferes with normal mRNA splicing patterns resulting in complete loss of expression of p14^{ARF} transcripts from this allele.[77] Taken together, these examples demonstrate that germline defects specific to p14^{ARF} may cause increased susceptibility to CMM independently of p16^{INK4A} status.

CDKN2A and *CDK4* gene defects in melanoma cell lines and sporadic melanoma

In addition to their association with familial melanoma, *CDKN2A* gene defects have been detected in both cultured and uncultured cells derived from sporadic melanomas. *CDKN2A* inactivation, by virtue of deletion, mutation or transcriptional inhibition through promoter methylation,

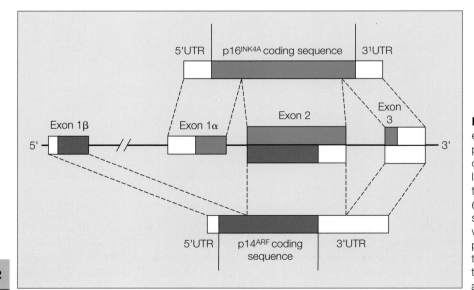

Figure 2.4 p16^{INK4A} and p14^{ARF} transcripts expressed from the *CDKN2A* locus. Both p16^{INK4A} and p14^{ARF} are expressed from overlapping sequences within the *CDKN2A* locus. Alternative promoters initiate transcription of independent first exons, 1α (p16^{INK4A}) and 1β (p14^{ARF}). Alternative splicing allows for joining of each first exon with the same second and third exons. The p16^{INK4A} and p14^{ARF} transcripts use different translational reading frames in exons 2 and 3 to give rise to proteins with distinct amino acid sequences that share no homology.

has been observed in nearly all melanoma cell lines.[78] In contrast, *CDKN2A* gene defects in uncultured melanomas are much less common. Data compiled from several studies revealed that approximately half of uncultured melanomas (54%) display loss of DNA markers in the region of the *CDKN2A* locus, whereas fewer either carry intragenic *CDKN2A* mutations (8%) or demonstrate *CDKN2A* inactivation through promoter methylation (6%).[79] Several factors may account for the discrepancy in frequency of *CDKN2A* aberrations between melanoma cell lines and uncultured melanomas. The presence of otherwise normal cells (e.g. stromal cells) in tumor samples may obscure detection of gene defects specific to melanoma cells and homozygous deletions may be difficult to detect. Furthermore, introduction of tumor cells into culture may select for cells that have acquired *CDKN2A* mutations. Nonetheless, these studies, when taken together, provide further support for alterations of the *CDKN2A* locus playing a role in the pathogenesis of CMM.

Similarly, examples of mutations in the *CDK4* gene have been identified in sporadic CMM. Two cases of sporadic CMM with mutations converting amino acid 24 of CDK4 from arginine to cysteine, which would interfere with p16^{INK4A} binding to CDK4, have been reported.[80] As with germline *CDK4* mutations in familial melanoma, however, *CDK4* mutations in sporadic melanoma are exceedingly rare.[81] In contrast, no mutations specific to exon 1β of p14^{ARF} resulting in its inactivation independently of p16^{INK4A} have been identified as of yet in CMM.[82]

Experimental studies of *CDKN2A* and *CDK4* genes in mouse models of CMM tumorigenesis

Functional studies using mouse models corroborate findings from mutation analysis of familial and sporadic CMM, and directly implicate genetic aberrations in *CDKN2A* and *CDK4* in causing CMM. Mice harboring a targeted deletion of the murine equivalent of the human *CDKN2A* locus that disrupts expression of both p16^{INK4A} and p19^{ARF} (the murine homolog of human p14^{ARF}), develop normally yet produce spontaneous tumors early in life and are highly susceptible to tumorigenesis in response to carcinogenic agents.[83] However, targeting expression of an activated variant of the *H-RAS* gene to melanocytes in *Cdkn2a*-deficient mice specifically induces melanoma.[84] This landmark study provides direct support for a causal relationship between gene defects at the *CDKN2A* locus and development of CMM in humans. Furthermore, this work directly implicates cooperation between *CDKN2A* and *RAS* genes in the pathogenesis of melanoma.

Similarly, mice that express activated *H-RAS* in melanocytes yet are deficient for either p16^{INK4A} or p19^{ARF} alone also develop melanoma. However, these mice develop tumors with a greater latency period compared with mice lacking both genes.[72] In addition, mutant mice that express a variant of Cdk4 that circumvents p16^{INK4A} binding and inhibition develop melanocytic tumors and invasive melanomas in response to treatment with topical carcinogens.[85] Thus, mouse models mimicking each class

of identified germline mutation in familial melanoma have been developed. Each faithfully recapitulated human susceptibility to melanoma and provides functional proof for defects in these genes causing melanoma.

Alternative genetic loci in CMM

In addition to *CDKN2A* and *CDK4* genes, there is substantial evidence that several other genes are likely to contribute to the pathogenesis of melanoma. Aberrations involving the *CDKN2A* locus have been documented in 25–40% of melanoma families.[65] Of those families that do not harbor *CDKN2A* defects, many show genetic linkage to markers on chromosome 9p nonetheless. One obvious candidate was the *CDKN2B* gene, which encodes p15, a cell cycle inhibitory protein similar to p16^{INK4A}. The *CDKN2B* gene lies in close proximity to the *CDKN2A* locus, and both are commonly deleted together in melanomas. However, mutation analysis failed to reveal any germline *CDKN2B* mutations in subjects from 154 families.[79] Additional evidence suggesting the presence of other CMM loci on chromosome 9p derives from studies demonstrating loss of DNA markers in regions distinct from the *CDKN2A* locus in sporadic melanoma.[86] However, no alternative tumor suppressor genes in these regions have been identified as of yet.

Similarly, linkage analysis of additional melanoma families, and loss of heterozygosity, cytogenetic, and comparative genomic hybridization studies in sporadic CMMs have defined several other genetic loci that may harbor genes that play some role in CMM development. Included among these are loci at chromosomes 1p, 3p, 6q, 6p, 10q, 11q and 17p.[87–90] Notably, a locus at 1p36 was the first to be identified by linkage analysis of families susceptible to CMM.[91] However, association of dysplastic nevi as a clinical feature of affected subjects may have clouded these studies and no subsequent studies have shown linkage of familial melanoma to 1p36.[71] Nonetheless, loss of DNA markers from the 1p36 region has been observed in sporadic CMMs, providing support for the presence of a putative melanoma-associated tumor suppressor gene in this region.[92] More recently, linkage analysis of 49 Australian melanoma families that lack *CDKN2A* or *CDK4* mutations revealed a novel susceptibility locus associated with early onset CMM at chromosomal region 1p22.[93] However, a specific familial melanoma candidate gene within this region has not been identified yet.

PTEN gene defects in CMM

DNA markers at chromosome 10q are frequently deleted in CMM, and recently defects in the *PTEN* gene, which maps to 10q23, have been detected. *PTEN* is a tumor suppressor gene that is commonly lost or mutated in a wide variety of cancers. Moreover, germline mutations in the *PTEN* gene cause Cowden's syndrome. Subjects with this disorder are prone to developing hamartomatous lesions and malignancies in several tissues, including skin, breast, thyroid and colon, although melanoma is not commonly associated with Cowden's syndrome.

PTEN protein functions as both a lipid and protein phosphatase, and may influence several cellular processes.[94] In particular, PTEN may exert control over cell cycle regulation by promoting p27 (another cyclin-dependent kinase inhibitor) suppression of the kinase activity of the cyclin E/CDK complex. In turn, this leads to hypophosphorylation of Rb protein, resulting in sequestration of E2F transcription factors and cell cycle arrest. Thus, in a manner analogous to p16[INK4A], loss of PTEN function would impair normal cell cycle regulation through mechanisms related to the Rb pathway.

Deletion and/or mutation of the *PTEN* gene in sporadic CMM has been examined in a number of studies. Although variable results have been reported, *PTEN* gene defects have been observed in approximately 30–50% of melanoma cell lines and approximately 5–20% of uncultured melanomas.[94] In addition, functional studies have demonstrated restoration of growth arrest in cultured melanoma cells upon re-introduction of a normal *PTEN* gene.[95] Taken together, these studies indicate that *PTEN* aberrations may contribute to the pathogenesis of some sporadic CMMs.

RAS and *RAF* gene defects in CMM

RAS family genes (*H-RAS*, *K-RAS* and *N-RAS*) encode membrane-associated GTPases that function downstream of cell surface receptors, such as tyrosine kinase receptors, G-protein-coupled receptors and integrin cell adhesion receptors. RAS proteins regulate signaling from the cell surface to the nucleus to alter patterns of gene expression and regulate cell proliferation and differentiation (Fig. 2.5).[38] *RAS* genes frequently become activated through mutation in human cancers, and may contribute to CMM development.[96] As discussed above, expression of activated RAS can cooperate with inactivation of the

Cdkn2a locus to promote progression of melanoma in a murine model.[84] These experimental studies correlate remarkably well with findings of *RAS* mutations in familial CMMs. Activating *N-RAS* mutations were detected in 95% (20 of 21) of primary hereditary melanomas from patients with germline *CDKN2A* mutations.[97] In contrast, *RAS* gene mutations are detected at a much lower frequency (4–31%) in uncultured sporadic melanomas and melanoma cell lines.[98,99] Nearly all represent activating mutations of *N-RAS* at codon 61, whereas only rare *H-RAS* mutations have been observed.[98]

The discrepancy between the high rate of *RAS* mutations in familial melanomas and the relative paucity of *RAS* mutations observed in sporadic CMMs, may be explained, in part, by the finding of *BRAF* mutations in a high proportion of sporadic CMMs.[100] RAF family proteins are serine/threonine kinases that function downstream of RAS proteins in the MAPK (mitogen-activated protein kinase) signal transduction pathway (Fig. 2.5).[38] RAF proteins localize to the plasma membrane through interaction with RAS proteins, and are activated by dimerization and phosphorylation. Activated RAF proteins then initiate a cascade of phosphorylation events to effect signal transduction. RAF proteins phosphorylate MEK1/2, which then phosphorylates ERK1/2. Various transcription factors are then phosphorylated by ERK1/2, allowing them to influence expression of a series of target genes. Because RAF proteins function immediately downstream of RAS, activating *RAF* mutations could have virtually the same influence on MAPK pathway activation as *RAS* mutations. Therefore, mutations in either *RAS* or *RAF* genes may be important in the pathogenesis of CMM.

Davies, *et al.*[100] reported that a remarkable 66% of melanoma samples screened carried *BRAF* mutations. All mutations documented occurred in the BRAF kinase domain, and 80% of these gave rise to the identical

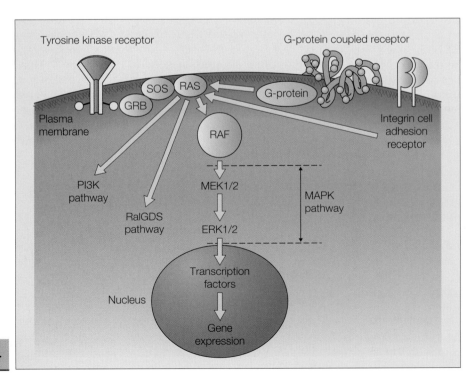

Figure 2.5 RAS/RAF signaling pathways. Normally, RAS may be activated through stimulation of cell surface tyrosine kinase receptors, G-protein-coupled receptors, or integrin cell adhesion receptors to trigger signal transduction through various effector pathways. RAF serine/threonine kinases function immediately downstream of RAS and activate the MAPK (mitogen-activated protein kinase) signaling pathway. Activating mutations in either *RAS* or *RAF* genes may bypass normal controls and lead to constitutive activity of this pathway.

valine to glutamic acid substitution at residue 599 (V599E). These mutations result in constitutive kinase activity, permitting BRAF to stimulate downstream signaling in the MAPK pathway independently of any requirement to interact with RAS or become phosphorylated itself. Notably, a single T→A change accounted for 92% of the V599E mutations observed. That this common mutation does not result from pyrimidine dimer formation (CC→TT or C→T) indicates that UV exposure is not a critical factor for inducing activating *BRAF* mutations in CMM development.

Given the high proportion of sporadic CMMs carrying *BRAF* mutations, melanoma families that did not show linkage to chromosome 9p were screened for germline *BRAF* mutations. However, none of 122 probands were shown to carry *BRAF* mutations, indicating that *BRAF* does not represent an alternative familial melanoma susceptibility gene.[101,102] In contrast, *BRAF* mutations appear to be common in benign melanocytic lesions. The identical V599E substitution mutation was observed in 82% of melanocytic nevi studied.[103] This finding suggests that activation of MAPK signaling may represent an important early event in melanocytic neoplasia. However, additional genetic aberrations, such as inactivation of the *CDKN2A* locus, would be required for development of CMM.

FUTURE OUTLOOK

Significant progress has been made in identifying oncogenes and tumor suppressor genes that, when activated or inactivated, respectively, cause CMM, SCC and BCC. Identification of such genes has permitted investigation of the molecular pathways they participate in and how mutations in different genes may interact or cooperate with each other to alter the balance between cell proliferation, cell death and differentiation in favor of tumorigenesis. However, our understanding of the genetic and molecular mechanisms underlying these cancers is far from complete.

There is substantial evidence indicating that additional genes may contribute to the development of CMM, SCC and BCC. The various screening studies discussed in this chapter have detected gene defects in only a portion of tumors examined. Although this, in part, may reflect limitations of techniques used to identify gene defects, it is likely that a number of cases derive from alterations in different genes. In addition, many tumor types carry recurrent, non-random genomic aberrations that may activate proto-oncogenes (through DNA amplification) or inactivate tumor suppressor genes (through gene deletion). Such aberrations frequently occur in regions distinct from sites of known cancer genes, indicating that they harbor novel genes that promote tumorigenesis.

Lastly, defects in alternative genes likely underlie various forms of hereditary skin cancer. Specific germline gene defects have not been identified in the majority of melanoma families and various genetic disorders that increase susceptibility to BCC appear to be unrelated to the *PTCH* gene.

In the course of future study, and with application of increasingly sophisticated technology, novel skin cancer genes will be identified. Further experimentation will elucidate the function of these genes, the consequences of altering them, and how they interact with other known cancer genes to promote tumorigenesis. As novel skin cancer genes are identified and studied, a more comprehensive understanding of the genetic and molecular basis of skin cancer will be achievable. Ultimately, this may permit development of novel therapies that target specific genes and the molecular pathways they participate in to treat skin cancer.

REFERENCES

1 Hanahan D, Weinberg RA. The hallmarks of cancer. Cell 2000; 100:57–70.

2 Gorlin RJ. Nevoid basal cell carcinoma syndrome. Derm Clin 1995; 13:113–125.

3 Kimonis VE, Goldstein AM, Pastakia B, et al. Clinical manifestations in 105 persons with nevoid basal cell carcinoma syndrome. Am J Med Genet 1997; 69:299–308.

4 Gailani MR, Bale SJ, Leffell DJ, et al. Developmental defects in Gorlin syndrome related to a putative tumor suppressor gene on chromosome 9. Cell 1992; 69:111–117.

5 Hahn H, Wicking C, Zaphiropoulous PG, et al. Mutations of the human homolog of Drosophila *patched* in the nevoid basal cell carcinoma syndrome. Cell 1996; 85:841–851.

6 Johnson RL, Rothman AL, Xie J, et al. Human homolog of *patched*, a candidate gene for the basal cell nevus syndrome. Science 1996; 272:1668–1671.

7 Wetmore C. Sonic hedgehog in normal and neoplastic proliferation: insight gained from human tumors and animal models. Curr Opin Genet Dev 2003; 13:34–42.

8 Ruiz i Altaba A, Sanchez P, Dahmane N. Gli and hedgehog in cancer: tumours, embryos and stem cells. Nat Rev Cancer 2002; 2:361–372.

9 Duman-Scheel M, Weng L, Xin S, et al. Hedgehog regulates cell growth and proliferation by inducing Cyclin D and Cyclin E. Nature 2002; 417:299–304.

10 Barnes EA, Kong M, Ollendorff V, et al. Patched1 interacts with cyclin B1 to regulate cell cycle progression. EMBO J 2001; 20:2214–2223.

11 Gailani MR, Stahle-Backdahl M, Leffell DJ, et al. The role of the human homologue of *Drosophila patched* in sporadic basal cell carcinomas. Nat Genet 1996; 14:78–81.

12 Aszterbaum M, Rothman A, Johnson RL, et al. Identification of mutations in the human *PATCHED* gene in sporadic basal cell carcinomas and in patients with the basal cell nevus syndrome. J Invest Derm 1998; 110:885–888.

13 Holmberg E, Rozell BL, Toftgard R. Differential allele loss on chromosome 9q22.3 in human non-melanoma skin cancer. Br J Cancer 1996; 74:246–250.

14 Xie J, Murone M, Luoh SM, et al. Activating *Smoothened* mutations in sporadic basal-cell carcinoma. Nature 1998; 391:90–92.

15 Lam CW, Xie J, To KF, et al. A frequent activated smoothened mutation in sporadic basal cell carcinomas. Oncogene 1999; 18:833–836.

16 Oro AE, Higgins KM, Hu Z, et al. Basal cell carcinomas in mice overexpressing sonic hedgehog. Science 1997; 276:817–821.

17 Smyth I, Narang MA, Evans T, et al. Isolation and characterization of human *patched 2 (PTCH2)*, a putative tumour suppressor gene in basal cell carcinoma and medulloblastoma on chromosome 1p32. Hum Mol Genet 1999; 8:291–297.

CHAPTER

3

The Biology of the Melanocyte

Julie V Schaffer and Jean L Bolognia

Key points

- The major determinant of human skin color and sensitivity to ultraviolet radiation (UVR) is the activity of melanocytes, i.e. the quantity and quality of pigment production, not the density of melanocytes.
- Melanocytes contain a unique lysosome-related intracytoplasmic organelle, the melanosome, which is the site of melanin biosynthesis.
- Compared with lightly pigmented skin, darkly pigmented skin has more numerous, larger melanosomes that contain more melanin; once transferred to keratinocytes, the melanosomes are singly dispersed and degraded more slowly.
- Tyrosinase is the key enzyme in the melanin biosynthetic pathway.
- Two major forms of melanin are produced by melanocytes: brown-black, photoprotective eumelanin and yellow-red, photolabile pheomelanin.
- In humans, binding of melanocyte-stimulating hormone (MSH) to the melanocortin-1 receptor (MC1R) stimulates eumelanogenesis, most notably as a protective response to UVR.
- Loss-of-function variants of the MC1R largely account for the red hair phenotype in humans, are associated with fair skin even in those without red hair, and confer a risk of melanoma and nonmelanoma skin cancer that appears to be independent of pigmentary phenotype.

INTRODUCTION

Pigmentation of the hair and skin is not only one of the most striking visible human traits, it also represents a major determinant of sensitivity to ultraviolet radiation (UVR) and risk of both melanoma and non-melanoma skin cancers (NMSC). An appreciation of the biology of the melanocyte is required in order to understand the physiology of normal constitutive and facultative pigmentation, as well as the biology of melanoma and the pathophysiology of disorders of pigmentation that predispose affected individuals to the development of skin cancer. A classic example of the latter is type 1 oculocutaneous albinism (OCA), a genodermatosis in which pigmentary dilution of the skin, hair and eyes due to absent or decreased tyrosinase activity results in a markedly increased risk of UVR-induced NMSC. With regard to melanoma, knowledge of melanosomal proteins such as tyrosinase, gp100/Pmel17 and MelanA/MART1 is critical

to the use of immunohistochemical methods of diagnosis, the understanding of immune responses such as melanoma-associated leukoderma, and the development of vaccine therapies. Furthermore, the elucidation of signaling pathways for proliferation and differentiation in normal melanocytes is fundamental to the understanding of melanoma tumorigenesis and progression.

Within the realm of physiologic pigmentation, the melanocyte melanocortin-1 receptor (MC1R), via interactions with α-melanocyte-stimulating hormone (α-MSH), plays a key role in the determination of skin type and hair color. Loss-of-function variants of the *MC1R* gene, which result in increased production of pheomelanin rather than eumelanin, have been shown to largely account for the red hair phenotype in humans and to have a strong association with fair skin and a decreased ability to tan even in individuals without red hair. Moreover, these *MC1R* variants also appear to confer a risk of melanoma and NMSC that is independent of pigmentary phenotype.[1]

This chapter is divided into three major sections:

- The structure and function of the melanocyte
- The structure and function of the melanosome
- Melanin biosynthesis and its regulation.

HISTORY

Although human epidermal melanocytes were first observed by Riehl in 1884, the cytologic basis of human pigment production was not yet known in the early twentieth century when Raper and others defined the metabolic pathway converting tyrosine to melanin in invertebrates. In 1917, research in human melanocyte biology began when Bloch developed a technique to stain pigment-producing cells by using dihydroxyphenylalanine (DOPA) as a substrate for melanin formation. Tyrosinase was identified in human melanocytes several decades later and in 1961, Seiji *et al.*[2] isolated and characterized the melanosome, the subcellular localization of melanin biosynthesis. Since that time, advances in molecular biology have facilitated the discovery of many genes, proteins and regulatory pathways important to melanogenesis.

STRUCTURE AND FUNCTION OF THE MELANOCYTE

Melanocytes are pigment-producing dendritic cells derived from the neural crest. During embryogenesis, pluripotent

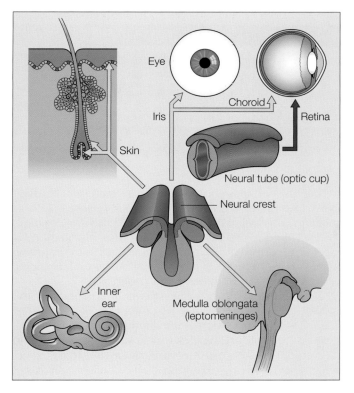

Figure 3.1 Migration of melanocytes from the neural crest. Melanocytes migrate to the uveal tract of the eye (iris and choroid), the cochlea of the inner ear, and the leptomeninges, as well as to the epidermis and the hair follicle. The retina actually represents an outpouching of the neural tube. (Adapted from Bolognia JL, *et al*. Dermatology. Philadelphia: Elsevier; 2003.)

neural crest cells develop into lineage-restricted melanocyte precursors (melanoblasts) as they migrate along the dorsolateral pathway between the somite and overlying ectoderm to the dermis, eventually reaching their final destinations in the epidermis and hair follicles. In addition, melanoblasts migrate to the uveal tract of the eye (choroid, ciliary body and iris), the inner ear (stria vascularis of the cochlea) and the leptomeninges (pia mater; Fig. 3.1). This distribution of melanocytes accounts for the melanocytosis and risk of developing melanoma in the eye (e.g. choroid) and leptomeninges that is seen in patients with nevus of Ota and the occurrence of neurocutaneous melanosis in patients with large posterior axial or multiple congenital melanocytic nevi.

The study of patients with and animal models of inherited pigmentary disorders has led to insights into critical signaling pathways in melanocyte development and homeostasis. The survival and migration of neural crest-derived cells during embryogenesis depend upon interactions between specific receptors on the cell surface and their extracellular ligands. For example, steel factor (stem cell factor (SCF), mast cell growth factor) binds to and activates the KIT transmembrane tyrosine kinase receptor on melanoblasts and melanocytes (Fig. 3.2). Heterozygous germline mutations in the *KIT* gene that result in receptors with decreased function cause human piebaldism, while mutations in either the *KIT* gene or the *steel* gene can lead to dominant white spotting in mice.[3] On the other hand, somatic *activating* mutations in the *KIT* gene are often found in adult human patients with

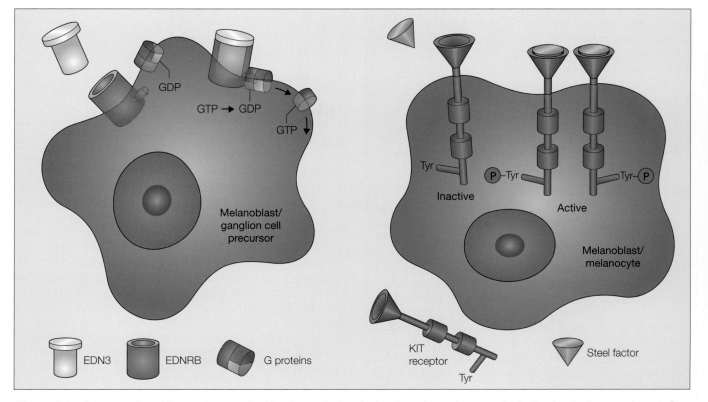

Figure 3.2 Receptor–ligand interactions required for the survival and migration of neural crest cells. In the developing neural crest, G protein-coupled endothelin B receptors (EDNRB) on melanoblast-ganglion cell precursors are activated by endothelin-3 (EDN3) (see also Fig. 3.16). In the mesenchyme and final destination sites, binding of steel factor to KIT tyrosine kinase receptors on melanoblasts and melanocytes induces activation via dimerization and autophosphorylation. (Adapted from Bolognia JL, *et al*. Dermatology. Philadelphia: Elsevier; 2003.)

mastocytosis/mast cell leukemia and gastrointestinal stromal tumors. The steel/KIT signaling pathway can stimulate melanocyte proliferation and dendricity in normal adult human skin, and has been shown to have a role in UVR-induced pigmentation.[4] In the developing neural crest, interactions also occur between endothelin-3 (EDN3) and the endothelin B receptors (EDNRB) found on melanoblast-ganglion cell precursors (Fig. 3.2). Mutations in both alleles of the *EDN3* gene or the *EDNRB* gene can produce a combination of Waardenburg syndrome (WS) and Hirschsprung disease (type IV WS).

Downstream of these receptor–ligand interactions, several transcription factors (i.e. proteins with the ability to bind to DNA and influence the activity of other genes) have important functions in melanocytes and their precursors. *M*icrophthalmia-associated *t*ranscription *f*actor (MITF), the earliest known marker of commitment to the melanocytic lineage, has been implicated as the 'master gene' for melanocyte survival as well as a key regulator of the promoters of the genes encoding tyrosinase and other major melanogenic proteins.[5] MITF activity is modulated both through a cAMP-dependent pathway of transcriptional upregulation (which can be induced by α-MSH, see below) and via *m*itogen-*a*ctivated *p*rotein *k*inase (MAPK)-dependent phosphorylation of MITF itself. The latter, which can be stimulated by the KIT signaling pathway, increases the intrinsic activity of MITF but also targets it to the proteasome for degradation. Heterozygous mutations in the *MITF* gene result in type II WS. Furthermore, MITF has recently been shown to mediate UVR-induced pigmentation and to promote viability of melanoma cells as well as melanocytes by up-regulating the expression of the anti-apoptotic protein Bcl2.[6] Other transcription factors expressed in melanocytes include paired box gene-3 (PAX3) and SRY box-containing gene 10 (SOX10), both with roles in regulating the expression of *MITF*. Heterozygous mutations in the *PAX3* gene or the *SOX10* gene can result in types I and III WS or type IV WS, respectively.[3]

As predicted by their migratory pathway, melanocytes are present throughout the dermis during intrauterine development. Dermal melanocytes first appear in the head and neck region, and begin to produce pigment at a gestational age of approximately 10 weeks. However, by the time of birth active dermal melanocytes have disappeared with the exception of three anatomic sites – the head and neck, the dorsal aspects of the distal extremities, and the presacral area.[7] Although a fraction of the 'lost' dermal melanocytes can be accounted for by migration to the epidermis, it is clear that cell death (presumably apoptotic) has also occurred. Of note, the three locations of persistent dermal melanocytes correspond to the most common locations for dermal melanocytosis and blue nevi, with the scalp representing a site of predilection for malignant blue nevi. Interestingly, hepatocyte growth factor (HGF), which binds and activates the MET tyrosine kinase receptor, has been shown to promote the survival, proliferation and differentiation of dermal melanocytes when it is overexpressed in transgenic mice, resulting in a 300-fold increase compared with normal mice in the number of active dermal melanocytes seen after birth. With autocrine HGF signaling in a similar transgenic mouse model, the development of cutaneous and metastatic melanomas was also observed.[8]

In the epidermis of the human fetus, melanocytes can be identified by immunohistochemical staining as early as 50 days' gestational age.[9] By the fourth month of gestation, melanin-containing melanosomes can be recognized within the epidermal melanocytes via electron microscopy. With the exception of benign and malignant neoplasms, melanocytes reside in the basal layer of the epidermis, accounting for approximately 10% of the cells in this location (Fig. 3.3). Although the cell bodies of melanocytes rest on the basal lamina, their dendrites reach keratinocytes as far away as the mid stratum spinosum. Each melanocyte supplies melanosomes to approximately 30–40 neighboring keratinocytes, an association referred to as the epidermal melanin unit.[10] As melanocytes represent intruders into the epidermis, they do not form desmosomal connections with surrounding keratinocytes.

The basal layer of the hair matrix and the outer root sheath of hair follicles are additional sites to which melanocytes migrate during development (Fig. 3.1).

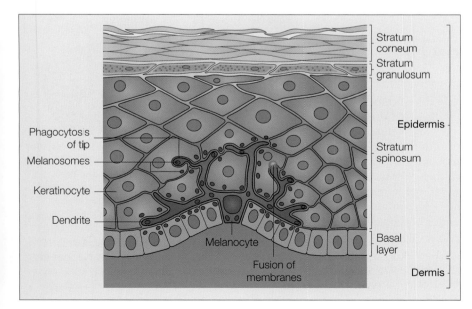

Phagocytosis of tip
Melanosomes
Keratinocyte
Dendrite
Melanocyte
Fusion of membranes

Stratum corneum
Stratum granulosum
Epidermis
Stratum spinosum
Basal layer
Dermis

Figure 3.3 A melanocyte residing in the basal layer of the epidermis. In normal skin, approximately every tenth cell in the basal layer is a melanocyte. Melanosomes are transferred from the dendrites of the melanocyte to approximately 30–40 neighboring keratinocytes, an association referred to as the epidermal melanin unit. (Adapted from Bolognia JL, et al. Dermatology. Philadelphia: Elsevier; 2003.)

While melanocytes in the matrices of pigmented anagen hairs actively produce melanin and are therefore easily recognized, those in the outer root sheath are usually amelanotic, less differentiated and more difficult to identify.[11] It has been suggested that melanocytes in the epidermis and the hair follicle represent two antigenically distinct populations,[12] explaining the preferential destruction of the former in vitiligo. Recently, a population of melanocyte stem cells was found to exist in the lower permanent portion of mouse hair follicles throughout the hair cycle, with activation at early anagen to supply progeny to the hair matrix.[13]

When DOPA-stained epidermal sheets from various anatomic sites are analyzed, regional differences are observed in the density of epidermal melanocytes, ranging from ~2000/mm^2 on the face and in the genital area to ~800/mm^2 on the trunk. However, despite the wide variation in pigmentation seen among humans, when the same anatomic site is examined there are no significant differences in melanocyte density between those with light and dark constitutive skin pigmentation. For example, a person who has extremely fair skin and an inability to tan has a density of epidermal melanocytes similar to that of a person whose natural skin color is dark brown to black. Even individuals with OCA type 1A, the most severe form of OCA, have a normal number of melanocytes. Nonetheless, melanocyte density does appear to decline with age, with a decrease by approximately 5–10% per decade during adulthood.[14]

The major determinant of human skin color is therefore not the density of melanocytes, but rather the activity of melanocytes.[15] In comparison with lightly pigmented skin, the melanocytes of darkly pigmented skin have increased dendricity and produce larger, more numerous melanosomes that are higher in melanin content. The quantity and quality of pigment production depend on constitutive (baseline, genetically programmed) and facultative (stimulated, e.g. by UVR) activity levels of the enzymes involved in melanin biosynthesis as well as the characteristics of individual melanosomes (e.g. diameter and ultrastructure). Interactions between the melanocyte MC1R and extracellular ligands such as α-MSH have important influences on both constitutive and facultative melanocytic activity (see below).

STRUCTURE AND FUNCTION OF THE MELANOSOME

Melanosomes are lysosome-related, membrane-bound intracytoplasmic organelles that specialize in the synthesis and storage of melanin.[16] Both melanocytes and retinal pigment epithelial cells produce melanosomes. However, while the latter cells retain the melanosomes within their own cytoplasm, the transfer of mature melanosomes to keratinocytes is an important function of epidermal and hair matrix melanocytes. By providing compartmentalization, melanosomes protect the remainder of the cell from reactive melanin precursors (e.g. phenols, quinones) that can oxidize lipid membranes; this is analogous to the protection conferred by sequestration of proteases and other degradative enzymes within lysosomes. Other features shared by melanosomes and lysosomes include

the potential to have a low intraluminal pH (although melanin production is optimal at a neutral pH), certain integral membrane proteins (e.g. lysosomal-associated membrane protein-1 (LAMP-1)) and resident hydrolases. However, melanosomes represent a distinct organelle lineage, separate from the conventional lysosomes that are also present within melanocytes. Melanosomes contain both specific matrix proteins that provide a striated scaffolding upon which melanin is deposited and enzymes that regulate melanin biosynthesis.

During their synthesis by ribosomes, proteins destined for melanosomes are targeted to the lumen of the rough endoplasmic reticulum (ER; Fig. 3.4) by an N-terminal signal sequence. In both normal melanocytes and melanoma cells, misfolded tyrosinase and aberrant *tyrosinase related protein 1* (TYRP1; see Fig. 3.10) produced from an alternate reading frame are 'sorted' via ER quality-control mechanisms for degradation in the cytosol by proteasomes (Fig. 3.4), resulting in the presentation of antigenic peptides to the immune system by MHC class I molecules. In amelanotic melanoma cell lines, wild-type tyrosinase is retained in the ER due to factors such as abnormal acidification of organelles and decreased expression of *TYRP1* (which facilitates tyrosinase processing in the ER), resulting in accelerated degradation of the enzyme and contributing to the dedifferentiated phenotype.[17]

The targeting of proteins to intracytoplasmic organelles versus the plasma membrane and the sorting of specific proteins to the correct type of organelle (e.g. melanosome versus lysosome) are complex processes. Most melanogenic enzymes are glycoproteins that must undergo post-translational modification (i.e. the attachment of sugars) in the ER and Golgi apparatus; they are then

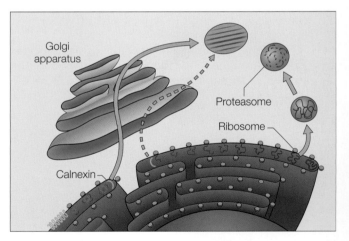

Figure 3.4 Synthesis and processing of glycoproteins destined for melanosomes. As they are synthesized by ribosomes, tyrosinase and other melanogenic enzymes are translocated into the lumen of the rough endoplasmic reticulum (ER), where co- and post-translational glycosylation begins and molecular chaperones (e.g. calnexin and calreticulin) bind the nascent glycoproteins and promote efficient folding. Properly folded proteins are exported from the ER to melanosomes via the Golgi apparatus (left), while misfolded proteins are targeted for degradation by the ubiquitin-dependent proteasome pathway (right). The latter process results in degradation of mutant tyrosinase in many patients with oculocutaneous albinism types 1A and 1B.

transferred from the *trans*-Golgi network (TGN) via clathrin-coated vesicles to join matrix proteins in endosomes or maturing melanosomes (Fig. 3.5).[18] This triaging from the TGN requires the equivalent of 'traffic police' within the cell, an example of which is the heterotetrameric adaptor protein-3 (AP-3). The binding of AP-3 to a di-leucine-based motif in the cytoplasmic domain of tyrosinase may facilitate this protein-sorting process. Mutations in the gene that encodes the β3A subunit of AP-3 can cause Hermansky–Pudlak syndrome, a disorder in which melanosomes and other intracytoplasmic organelles are defective and the resultant pigmentary dilution can increase the risk of NMSC (Fig. 3.6; Table 3.1).[19]

The progression of a melanosome from an organelle that lacks melanin to one that is fully melanized has been divided into four morphologic stages (Fig. 3.7). Cleavage and refolding of the matrix protein gp100/Pmel17 (the protein detected by the HMB45 immunohistochemical stain) accompanies the transition from a spherical, amorphous stage I melanosome (structurally similar to an early multivesicular endosome) to an elliptical, fibrillar, highly organized stage II melanosome.[20] At the same time, stabilization of melanogenic enzymes allows biosynthesis of melanin (eumelanin in particular) to begin. In the setting of pheomelanin rather than eumelanin

production (see below), pheomelanogenic melanosomes retain a spherical shape and an unstructured matrix with vesicular bodies.

As melanin is deposited within them, melanosomes migrate along microtubules from the cell body into the dendrites in preparation for transfer to neighboring keratinocytes (Fig. 3.8). Myosin Va is a dimeric molecular motor that captures the melanosomes when they reach the cell periphery, attaching them to the actin cytoskeleton beneath the plasma membrane.[18] Melanophilin links myosin Va with RAB27A, a GTPase that is present in mature melanosomes. Mutations in the *MYO5A*, *RAB27A* or *MLPH* genes cause different forms of Griscelli syndrome (Table 3.1), a disorder in which diffuse pigmentary dilution results from a lack of melanosome transfer to keratinocytes. In this condition, failure to securely attach the melanosomes to the actin cytoskeleton within the dendrites causes them to 'slip back' and accumulate in the center of the melanocyte, reminding us as do other disorders (e.g. hypopigmented mycosis fungoides) that normal cutaneous pigmentation depends on an orderly transfer of melanosomes from melanocytes to keratinocytes.

It is the activity of melanocytes, not their density, that determines skin color and sensitivity to UVR. The number and size of melanosomes produced, their degree of melanization, and the ability to transfer them efficiently to keratinocytes are all indicators of melanocyte activity. For example, stage II melanosomes predominate in lightly pigmented skin, whereas primarily stage IV melanosomes are seen in darkly pigmented skin (Table 3.2). Additional factors include the distribution and rate of degradation of the melanosomes after they are transferred to keratinocytes. The smaller melanosomes of lightly pigmented skin are clustered in groups of two to ten within secondary lysosomes, and are degraded by the time they reach the mid stratum spinosum. In contrast, the larger melanosomes found in darkly pigmented skin

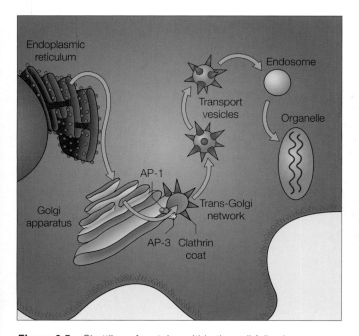

Figure 3.5 Shuttling of proteins within the cell following translation and post-translational processing. After modifications such as the attachment of sugar residues in the ER and Golgi apparatus, proteins must be triaged to the correct cellular location, either a specific organelle or the plasma membrane. Heterotetrameric adaptor proteins, AP-1 and AP-3, regulate this protein-sorting process. The latter binds to a di-leucine-based motif in the cytoplasmic tail of tyrosine, facilitating its transfer via clathrin-coated vesicles from the trans-Golgi network to maturing melanosomes. Mutations in the gene that encodes the β3A subunit of AP-3 can cause Hermansky–Pudlak syndrome. (Adapted from Bolognia JL, *et al*. Dermatology. Philadelphia: Elsevier; 2003.)

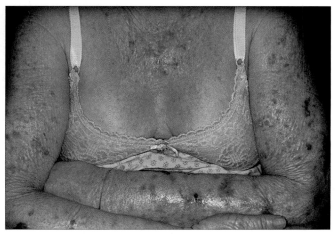

Figure 3.6 Diffuse pigmentary dilution in a patient with Hermansky–Pudlak syndrome. In addition to abnormal formation of melanosomes, defective protein trafficking results in a bleeding diathesis due to an absence of platelet dense granules. Note the development of multiple actinic keratoses and squamous cell carcinomas in sun-exposed areas.

Table 3.1 Disorders characterized by diffuse pigmentary dilution in which the genetic defect is known

Disorder	Gene	Protein	Clinical phenotype[a]	Pathogenesis
Oculocutaneous albinism (OCA)				
Type 1A	TYR	Tyrosinase	White hair, pink skin and gray eyes	Complete absence of tyrosinase activity and melanin production Retention of tyrosinase protein within the ER
Type 1B	TYR	Tyrosinase	Same as Type 1A at birth, but develop yellow to red hair with age ('yellow albinism')	Decreased tyrosinase activity; can produce pheomelanin Retention of tyrosinase protein within the ER Variant with temperature-sensitive tyrosinase – activity normal at 35°C, but diminished at 37°C
Type 2	P	P protein	Born with lightly pigmented hair (not white), skin and eyes Large, jagged lentigines Brown albinism in Africa	Transmembrane protein found in the ER as well as in melanosomes Possible functions include regulating organelle pH, facilitating vacuolar accumulation of glutathione, and processing/trafficking of tyrosinase
Type 3 (rufous/red)	TYRP1	Tyrosinase-related protein 1	Reddish hair and skin ('rufous')	TYRP1 stabilizes tyrosinase in mice and humans, and also functions as a DHICA oxidase in mice Retention within the ER and degradation of both mutant TYRP1 and tyrosinase
Type 4	MATP	Membrane-associated transporter protein	Similar to Type 2	Transmembrane transporter with a role in tyrosinase processing and intracellular trafficking to the melanosome
Hermansky-Pudlak syndrome (HPS)[b]				
1	HPS1	HPS1	Pigmentary dilution of hair, skin and eyes	Defective trafficking of organelle-specific proteins to melanosomes,
2	AP3B1	Adaptor protein 3, β3A subunit	Bleeding diathesis	lysosomes, and cytoplasmic granules (including platelet dense
3	HPS3	HPS3	Pulmonary fibrosis and	granules)
4	HPS4	HPS4	granulomatous colitis due to	Ru and ru2 proteins directly
5	HPS5	Ruby-eye 2 (ru2)	ceroid lipofuscin deposits	interact in a complex referred to
6	HPS6	Ruby-eye (ru)		as the biogenesis of lysosome-
7	DTNBP1	Dysbindin		related organelles complex 2
Chédiak–Higashi syndrome				
	CHS1 (LYST)	Lysosomal trafficking regulator	Mild pigmentary dilution Silvery hair Bleeding diathesis Neurologic abnormalities Recurrent infections Accelerated phase[c]	Abnormal vesicle trafficking results in giant organelles (e.g. melanosomes, neutrophil granules (lysosomes), platelet dense granules)
Griscelli syndrome				
1	MYO5A	Myosin Va	Mild pigmentary dilution Silvery hair Neurologic abnormalities	Defective attachment of organelles to the actin cytoskeleton; this normally occurs
2	RAB27A	RAB27A	Mild pigmentary dilution Silvery hair Recurrent infections Accelerated phase[c]	by linkage of myosin Va (via melanophilin) to RAB27A, a GTPase present in melanosomes Melanocytes are 'stuffed' with
3	MLPH	Melanophilin	Mild pigmentary dilution Silvery hair	melanosomes due to failure of transfer to keratinocytes

[a]All types of OCA and HPS result in an increased risk of ultraviolet-induced non-melanoma skin cancers, particularly squamous cell carcinoma.
[b]As there are ≥15 known loci for HPS-like phenotypes in mice, additional genes may be discovered in humans with this disorder.
[c]Characterized by pancytopenia and lymphohistiocytic infiltrates of the liver, spleen and lymph nodes.
ER, endoplasmic reticulum; DHICA, 5,6-dihydroxyindole-2-carboxylic acid.

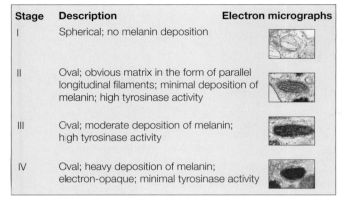

Stage	Description	Electron micrographs
I	Spherical; no melanin deposition	
II	Oval; obvious matrix in the form of parallel longitudinal filaments; minimal deposition of melanin; high tyrosinase activity	
III	Oval; moderate deposition of melanin; high tyrosinase activity	
IV	Oval; heavy deposition of melanin; electron-opaque; minimal tyrosinase activity	

Figure 3.7 Descriptions and electron photomicrographs of the four major stages of eumelanogenic melanosomes. (Reproduced with permission from Bolognia JL, *et al*. Dermatology. Philadelphia: Elsevier; 2003.)

Table 3.2 Variation in types of melanosomes within melanocytes and keratinocytes with level of cutaneous pigmentation

	Predominant melanosomal stages	
Pigmentation of skin	**Melanocytes**	**Keratinocytes**
Fair	II, III	Occasional III
Medium	II, III, IV	III, IV
Dark	IV > III	IV

(Courtesy of Ray Boissy PhD. Reproduced with permission from Bolognia JL, et al. Dermatology. Philadelphia: Elsevier; 2003.)

are singly dispersed and are degraded much more slowly, often remaining intact in the stratum corneum (Fig. 3.9).[15] Furthermore, mature eumelanogenic melanosomes form supranuclear melanin 'caps' that help shield the nuclei of keratinocytes from UVR.

MELANIN BIOSYNTHESIS AND ITS REGULATION

The functions of melanin in the skin and hair range from camouflage in animals to protection from UVR via photoabsorption and free-radical scavenging in humans. Melanin represents a group of complex polymeric pigments that exist in two basic forms in human skin, brown-black eumelanin and yellow-red pheomelanin. These types of melanin differ in their biochemical and photoprotective properties as well as the architecture of the melanosomes within which they are produced (see above). For example, the eumelanin found in elliptical, highly structured eumelanosomes is less soluble and has a higher molecular weight than the cysteine-rich pheomelanin found in spherical, unstructured pheomelanosomes. Moreover, pheomelanin is photolabile, generating oxidative stress and resulting in photosensitivity, whereas eumelanin may have some inherent cytotoxicity but confers substantial photoprotection.[21] This section begins with a review of the biosynthetic pathways for eumelanin and pheomelanin, and then examines the internal and external factors that influence the amount and type of melanin that is produced.

The melanin biosynthetic pathway

The amino acid tyrosine is the starting material for the production of both eumelanin and pheomelanin. Tyrosinase, the key enzyme in the melanin biosynthetic pathway, catalyzes the initial rate-limiting conversion of tyrosine to DOPA. It is also a copper-dependent enzyme with two copper-binding sites, which explains the diffuse pigmentary dilution seen in rare cases of copper deficiency and in patients with Menkes kinky hair syndrome. In addition to its essential role as a tyrosine hydroxylase, human tyrosinase has DOPA oxidase, 5,6-dihydroxyindole (DHI) oxidase, and perhaps 5,6-dihydroxyindole-2-carboxylic acid (DHICA) oxidase activities that regulate several other steps in the pathway (Fig. 3.10). The total

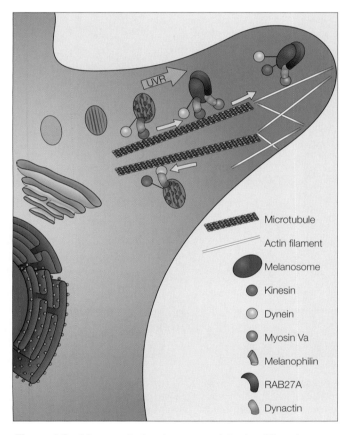

	Microtubule
	Actin filament
	Melanosome
	Kinesin
	Dynein
	Myosin Va
	Melanophilin
	RAB27A
	Dynactin

Figure 3.8 Movement of melanosomes into dendrites. As melanin is deposited within melanosomes, they migrate along microtubules from the cell body into dendrites in preparation for transfer to keratinocytes. Kinesin and dynein serve as molecular motors for microtubule-associated anterograde and retrograde melanosomal transport, respectively, and UVR results in augmented anterograde transport via increased kinesin and decreased dynein activity. Myosin Va, which is linked to the melanosomal RAB27A GTPase by melanophilin, captures mature melanosomes when they reach the cell periphery and attaches them to the actin cytoskeleton. (Adapted from Bolognia JL, *et al*. Dermatology. Philadelphia: Elsevier; 2003.)

35

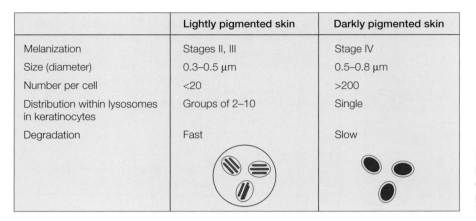

	Lightly pigmented skin	Darkly pigmented skin
Melanization	Stages II, III	Stage IV
Size (diameter)	0.3–0.5 μm	0.5–0.8 μm
Number per cell	<20	>200
Distribution within lysosomes in keratinocytes	Groups of 2–10	Single
Degradation	Fast	Slow

Figure 3.9 Differences between melanosomes in lightly pigmented and darkly pigmented skin. (Reproduced with permission from Bolognia JL, *et al*. Dermatology. Philadelphia: Elsevier; 2003.)

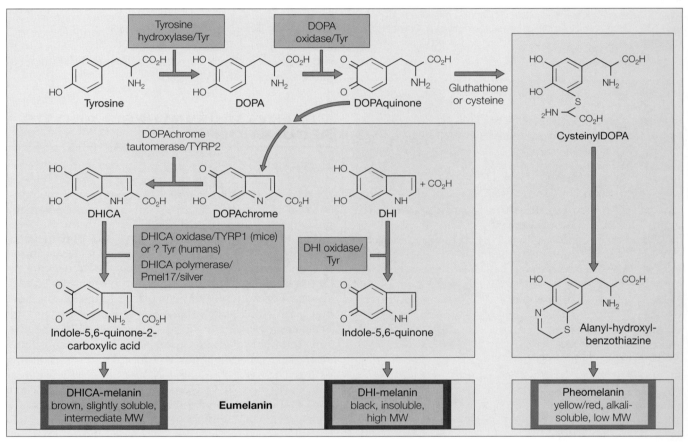

Figure 3.10 The melanin biosynthetic pathway. The pathway includes the sites of dysfunction in OCA1 (tyrosinase) and OCA3/rufous OCA (TRP1). The two major forms of melanin in the skin and hair are brown-black eumelanin and yellow-red pheomelanin. DHI, 5,6-dihydroxyindole; DHICA, 5,6-dihydroxyindole-2-carboxylic acid; DOPA, dihydroxyphenylalanine; MW, molecular weight; Tyr, tyrosine; TYRP, tyrosinase-related protein. (Courtesy of Dr Vincent Hearing.)

lack of melanin in the skin, hair and eyes of patients with OCA type 1A underscores the importance of tyrosinase in melanin biosynthesis. In this and other types of OCA (Table 3.1), the decreased production of photoprotective melanin results in increased susceptibility to the development of UVR-induced NMSC, in particular squamous cell carcinomas which can metastasize and lead to premature death, especially in those who reside in the tropics.

Once produced via tyrosinase activity, DOPA can spontaneously oxidize and cyclize to form melanin. However, although tyrosinase was initially thought to be the sole enzyme involved in melanin biosynthesis, by the late 1970s it became clear that there were additional regulators in the pathway. These include two tyrosine-related proteins (TYRPs) that have roles in eumelanogenesis, each a transmembrane protein with approximately 40% amino acid sequence homology with tyrosinase. The major function of TYRP1 is to stabilize tyrosinase; in mice Tyrp1 also acts as a DHICA oxidase, while in humans tyrosinase itself may have this catalytic capacity (Fig. 3.10).[22] Mutations in the *TYRP1* gene result in OCA type 3, which is typically associated with a 'rufous' phenotype of reddish-colored hair and skin.[3] TYRP2 serves as a DOPAchrome tautomerase, converting DOPAchrome to DHICA (Fig. 3.10). In the absence of

TYRP2, a carboxylic acid group is spontaneously lost and black, insoluble DHI-melanin that has cytotoxic effects as well as photoprotective properties is formed. With TYRP2 activity and the utilization of gp100/Pmel17 as a solid-phase substrate for polymerization, DHICA-melanin is produced. This brown, slightly soluble pigment provides photoprotection with minimal cytotoxicity.

The eumelanin and pheomelanin biosynthetic pathways diverge early on, following the formation of DOPAquinone (Fig. 3.10). At this point, the production of pheomelanin entails the addition of a cysteinyl group that accounts for its yellow-red color. Whereas eumelanin synthesis is associated with increased tyrosinase activity and involves additional melanogenic proteins such as TYRP1 and TYRP2, pheomelanin synthesis in murine melanocytes is associated with a reduction in tyrosinase and a marked reduction to absence of TYRP1, TYRP2, and the P protein (see below).[23] The formation of pheomelanin is therefore regarded as a default pathway.

The P protein, encoded at the *pink-eyed dilution* locus in mice, is a transmembrane protein with an important role in eumelanogenesis (Fig. 3.11),[24] although its exact function is not currently known. Mutations in the *P* gene in humans lead to OCA type 2 (Table 3.1).[25] Because its amino acid sequence is homologous to that of transmembrane transporters of small molecules and high concentrations of tyrosine can increase pigment production in *P*-null melanocytes, it was initially predicted that the P protein might serve to transport tyrosine across the melanosomal membrane. However, kinetic studies showed no difference between the melanosomes of wild-type and *P*-null melanocytes in the rate of tyrosine uptake. A second hypothesis is that the P protein regulates the pH of melanosomes and/or other organelles, potentially mediating neutralization of pH to optimize the activity and/or folding of tyrosinase.[26] The restoration of pigment production in *P*-null cells by vacuolar H+-ATPase inhibitors (e.g. bafilomycin A1) that are known to alkalinize (i.e. neutralize) organelles supports this theory. More recently, it was shown that the majority of the P protein in melanocytes is actually located in the ER rather than in melanosomes, and that abnormal processing and trafficking of tyrosinase occurs when the P protein is absent.[27] In addition, it was observed that the P protein facilitates vacuolar accumulation of glutathione, a major redox buffer that is required for the folding of cysteine-rich proteins such as tyrosinase. The P protein may thus regulate the processing of tyrosinase via control of glutathione. It has been speculated that the resistance of melanoma cells to chemotherapeutic agents detoxified by glutathione-dependent mechanisms (e.g. cisplatin and doxorubicin) could be related to decreased sequestration of glutathione due to a lack of P protein activity.

Melanogenesis-related proteins and other melanoma-associated antigens

A number of melanoma-associated antigens (MAA) have been identified and shown to induce both cytotoxic T-lymphocyte and antibody responses in melanoma patients, providing the basis for the development of vaccine therapies. There are two major types of MAA (Table 3.3):

(1) *melanocyte-differentiation antigens* and (2) *tumor/testis-specific antigens*.

The pathogenesis of melanoma-associated leukoderma (MAL) has important implications with regard to tumor immunity. Like vitiligo, it is associated with the presence of autoreactive T cells and antibodies directed against melanocyte-differentiation antigens (Fig. 3.12). The development of MAL can herald spontaneous disease regression in a small subset of patients with metastatic melanoma and is seen in responders to IL-2-based immunotherapy.[28]

The presence of melanocyte-differentiation antigens also serves as a diagnostic marker for melanoma. In addition to the use of immunohistochemical stains,

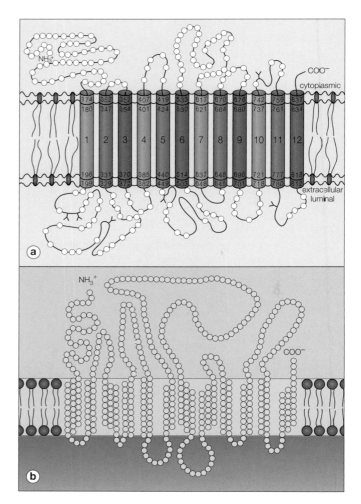

Figure 3.11 Proposed models for the arrangements of the P protein and membrane-associated transporter protein (MATP) within the lipid bilayer. (a) The P protein, which is defective in OCA type 2, has 12 putative transmembrane domains. (Reprinted with permission from Rinchik EM, *et al.* A gene for the mouse pink-eyed dilution locus and for human type II oculocutaneous albinism. Nature 1993; 361:72–76. Copyright © 1993 Macmillan Magazine Ltd.) (b) The membrane-associated transporter protein, which is defective in OCA type 4, also has 12 transmembrane domains. (Reproduced with permission of the University of Chicago from Newton JM, Cohen-Barak O, Hagiwara N, *et al.* Mutations in the human orthologue of the mouse underwhite gene (uw) underlie a new form of oculocutaneous albinism, OCA4. Am J Hum Genet 2001; 69:981–988. Copyright © 2001 American Society of Human Genetics.)

Table 3.3 Melanoma-associated antigens

Gene	Protein (immunohistochemical stain)	Functions
Melanocyte-differentiation antigens – melanogenesis-related proteins specific to melanocytes and melanoma cells		
TYR	Tyrosinase (T311)	Tyrosine hydroxylase, DOPA oxidase, DHI oxidase and, in humans, possibly DHICA oxidase
TYRP1	TYRP1/gp75 (MEL-5)	Stabilizes tyrosinase; in mice, also functions as DHICA oxidase
TYRP2	TYRP2/DCT	DOPAchrome tautomerase
P	P protein	Regulates organelle pH, glutathione accumulation, and/or processing/trafficking of tyrosinase
SILV	gp100/Pmel17/silver (HMB45)	Matrix protein; stabilizes melanogenic enzymes/intermediates and acts as a substrate for DHICA polymerization; marker for cellular activation
MART1	MelanA/MART1 (A103)	Membrane protein; may have a role in melanosome biogenesis
MC1R	MC1R	Stimulates eumelanin production, melanocyte proliferation, and dendricity
MITF	MITF	Regulates transcription of TYR, TYRP1, and TYRP2; also upregulates expression of the anti-apoptotic protein Bcl2
Tumor/testis-specific antigens[a] – proteins encoded by genes that are expressed in various tumors including melanomas, but are silent in normal adult tissues other than the testis		
MAGE1	MAGE1/MZ2-E	
MAGE3	MAGE3/MZ2-D	
BAGE	BAGE/Ba	
GAGE1/2	GAGE1/2/MZ2-F	
NY-ESO1	NY-ESO1	
Other types of tumor-specific antigens that result from mutated or aberrantly expressed genes Antigens that result from mutations (unique to each patient, with the exception of CDC27)		
MUM1–3	MUM1–3	
CDK4	Cyclin-dependent kinase 4	
CTNNB1	β-catenin	
MART2	MART2	
CDC27	CDC27	
Antigens that result from alternative transcription and/or splicing		
TYRP2	TYRP2-6b, TYRP2-INT2, others	
GNT-V	NA17-A (encoded by an intronic region in the N-acetylglucosaminyl-transferase V gene)	
Antigens reflecting selective overexpression in melanomas, other tumors, and leukemias of genes that are expressed at a low level in a variety of tissues		
PRAME	PRAME	
P15	p15	

[a]In general, lower immunogenicity than melanocyte-differentiation antigens.
TYRP, tyrosinase-related protein; MART, melanoma antigen recognized by T cells; MC1R, melanocortin-1 receptor; MITF, microphthalmia-associated transcription factor; MUM, melanoma-ubiquitously mutated; PRAME, preferentially expressed antigen in melanoma

reverse-transcriptase-polymerase chain reaction (PCR)-based assays have been developed to detect melanoma cells in tumor-draining lymph nodes (see Ch. 41) and in the circulation. However, it is important to be aware of the variable sensitivities and specificities of PCR-based tests, as well as other potential diagnostic pitfalls such as nodal nevi.

The regulation of melanin biosynthesis

The ratio of eumelanin to pheomelanin, as well as the total melanin content, is higher in skin types V to VI than in skin types I to II. Pheomelanin levels are greatest in 'fire' red hair, while eumelanin predominates in most

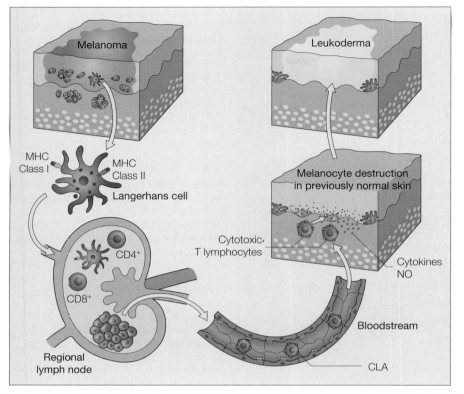

Figure 3.12 Model for the pathogenesis of melanoma-associated leukoderma. Sensitization to melanocyte-differentiation antigens expressed by melanoma cells can result in immunologic attack on normal melanocytes, producing vitiligo-like patches of depigmentation. CLA, cutaneous lymphocyte antigen; NO, nitric oxide.

human hair colors other than red.[29] The amount and type of melanin produced is determined by a complex interplay of the activity levels of the enzymes, transporters, and enzyme-stabilizing or structural proteins that are involved in melanogenesis. The factors known to influence the activity of these key proteins and control the eumelanin/pheomelanin switch include α-MSH, agouti signaling protein (ASIP), endothelin-1, basic fibroblast growth factor (bFGF), and UVR (Fig. 3.13).

The melanocortin peptides (including α-, β- and γ-MSH as well as adrenocorticotropic hormone (ACTH)), β-endorphin and β-lipotropic hormone are all cleavage products of a single precursor protein, proopiomelanocortin (POMC; Fig. 3.14). Although POMC-derived peptides were originally identified as pituitary hormones, POMC is also synthesized and differentially processed in the hypothalamus, other regions of the brain and a variety of peripheral tissues including the gastrointestinal tract, gonads and, of particular interest to us, the skin. In humans, α-MSH (the major type of MSH) and ACTH have similar potencies in activating the melanocyte MC1R,[30] and the relative contribution of centrally- and peripherally-derived forms of each to baseline melanogenesis *in vivo* has yet to be determined. Nevertheless, it is clear that centrally-produced melanocortins can dramatically influence cutaneous pigmentation, as evidenced by the generalized hyperpigmentation seen in disorders such as Addison's disease that are characterized by pituitary hypersecretion of ACTH and/or α-MSH.

Likewise, melanocortins produced peripherally by the skin can have a prominent role in promoting melanogenesis, most notably as a protective response to UVR. *POMC* is expressed by a variety of epidermal and dermal

cell types, including melanocytes, keratinocytes, fibroblasts, endothelial cells and antigen-presenting cells. Both UVR and the epidermally-derived, UVR-induced cytokine interleukin-1 (IL-1) stimulate increased synthesis and enzymatic processing of POMC by melanocytes and keratinocytes, providing autocrine as well as paracrine regulation of cutaneous pigmentation (Fig. 3.13).

In addition to their well-known roles in pigmentation and adrenocortical steroidogenesis, melanocortin peptides serve other important functions by binding to the various melanocortin receptors (MCRs) present in different tissues (Table 3.4). These biologic activities range from suppression of inflammation to regulation of body weight to stimulation of lipid production in sebaceous glands. A phenotype of severe early-onset obesity, adrenal insufficiency and red hair has been described in individuals with mutations in the *POMC* gene.[31] It is therefore not surprising that mutations in the genes that encode the receptors to which the POMC-derived peptides bind can produce similar clinical manifestations. For example, *MC4R* mutations result in morbid obesity, *MC2R* mutations cause adrenal insufficiency, and *MC1R* mutations are associated with red hair (see below).

To date, five MCRs (MC1R–MC5R) have been identified, each with distinctive tissue distribution, relative affinities for melanocortin ligands and physiologic roles (Table 3.4). The MCRs represent a subfamily of G protein-coupled receptors, all with seven transmembrane domains (Fig. 3.15) and signal transduction via an associated protein complex that binds guanosine triphosphate (GTP) and guanosine diphosphate (GDP). Upon ligand binding to a MCR, the α-subunit of the receptor-coupled stimulatory G protein ($G_s\alpha$) activates adenylate cyclase, which

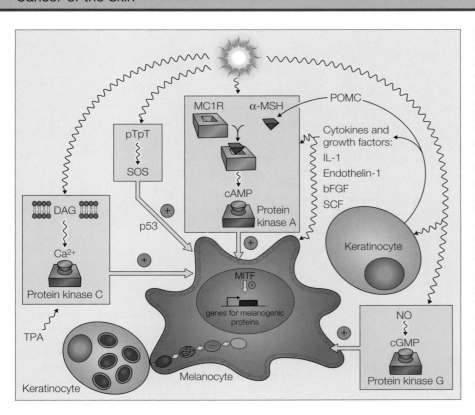

Figure 3.13 Mechanisms of UVR-induced melanogenesis. These include an increase in one or more of the following: (1) expression of POMC and its derivative peptides by keratinocytes, melanocytes and other cells in the skin; (2) the number of MC1R on melanocytes; (3) the release of diacylglycerol (DAG) from the plasma membrane, which activates protein kinase C; (4) the induction of an SOS response to UVR-induced DNA damage; (5) nitric oxide (NO) production, which activates the cGMP pathway; and (6) production of cytokines and growth factors by keratinocytes. As a result, there is enhanced transcription of the genes that encode MITF and melanogenic proteins including tyrosinase, TYRP1, TYRP2, gp100/Pmel17, and P. In addition, melanocyte dendricity and transfer of melanosomes to keratinocytes is stimulated via increased activity of RAC1 (involved in dendrite formation), ratio of kinesin to dynein, and expression of protease-activated receptor-2 (PAR2; involved in melanosome transfer). TPA, tetradecanoyl phorbol acetate. (Adapted from Bolognia JL, et al. Dermatology. Philadelphia: Elsevier; 2003.)

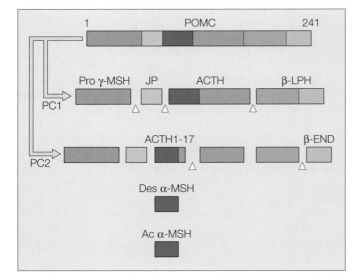

Figure 3.14 Post-translational processing of the proopiomelanocortin (POMC) precursor protein. Ac, acetylated; ACTH, adrenocorticotropic hormone; Des, desacetyl; END, endorphin; JP, joining peptide; LPH, lipotropic hormone; MSH, melanocyte-stimulating hormone; PC, prohormone-converting enzyme. (Adapted from Bolognia JL, et al. Dermatology. Philadelphia: Elsevier; 2003.)

Table 3.4 Melanocortin receptors

Receptor	Distribution		Ligands
	Major	Minor	
MC1R[a]	Melanocytes	Keratinocytes, fibroblasts, endothelial cells, antigen-presenting cells	α-MSH, ACTH > β-MSH
MC2R	Adrenal cortex	Adipocytes	ACTH
MC3R[b]	Brain	Gut, placenta	α-, β-, γ-MSH, ACTH
MC4R[b]	Brain		α-, β-MSH, ACTH
MC5R	Peripheral tissues	Fibroblasts, adipocytes, sebaceous glands	α-, β-MSH, ACTH

[a]Agouti protein (mouse) and agouti signaling protein (human) are the major antagonistic ligands.
[b]Agouti-related protein is the major antagonistic ligand.
(Reproduced with permission from Bolognia JL, et al. Dermatology. Philadelphia: Elsevier; 2003.)

increases production of the second messenger cyclic adenosine monophosphate (cAMP; Fig. 3.16).[32]

The key MCR in the skin, the MC1R, is found on many types of cells, including keratinocytes, fibroblasts, endothelial cells and antigen-presenting cells; however, melanocytes clearly have the highest MC1R density.[33] Melanocyte *MC1R* expression has a central role in the induction of photoprotective melanization in response to UV exposure, and is stimulated by α-MSH, ACTH, UVR and a variety of UVR-induced, keratinocyte-derived cytokines and growth factors such as IL-1, endothelin-1 and bFGF (Fig. 3.13). When the melanocyte MC1R is activated by ligand binding, elevated intracellular cAMP results in melanocyte proliferation, increased dendricity,

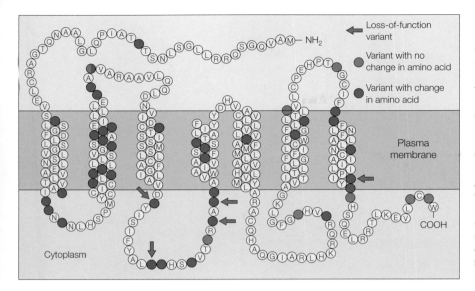

Figure 3.15 Melanocortin-1 receptor (MC1R) within the plasma membrane of a melanocyte. The red dots indicate the locations of amino acid changes (compared to the wild type) in MC1R variants that have been reported. Some of the variants are due to partial or complete loss-of-function mutations (i.e. the generation of cAMP in response to α-MSH binding is impaired), whereas others have no effect on function. Loss-of-function variants, e.g. Arg151Cys, Arg160His, and Asp294His, are associated with red hair, fair skin and increased risk of melanoma and non-melanoma skin cancers. The tan dots represent synonymous variants where there is no change in amino acid sequence. (Adapted from Bolognia JL, *et al.* Dermatology. Philadelphia: Elsevier; 2003.)

and stimulation of the expression and activity of tyrosinase and other melanogenic proteins, which leads to eumelanin production.[34] If the MC1R receptor is dysfunctional and ligand binding fails to induce cAMP production, pheomelanogenesis is favored (Fig. 3.17).

Although human pigmentation is genetically complex, thus far *MC1R* is the only gene that has been shown to play a major role in physiologic variation of hair and skin color.[35] The *MC1R* gene is highly polymorphic, with approximately 50% of individuals in white populations carrying at least one of more than 50 variant alleles reported to date (Fig. 3.15). Homozygous or compound heterozygous loss-of-function *MC1R* mutations (i.e. resulting in impaired cAMP generation in response to α-MSH) have been shown to largely account for the red hair phenotype in humans, which approximates an autosomal recessive trait and increases the risk of developing melanoma over 4-fold.[36] In addition, these loss-of-function *MC1R* mutations have a strong association with fair skin, a decreased ability to tan, and freckling, resulting in a significant heterozygote effect in individuals without red hair.

Moreover, loss-of-function *MC1R* mutations also confer a significantly increased risk of melanoma (approximately doubled for each variant allele carried) and NMSC (2–3-fold increase with two variant alleles) that is independent of pigmentary phenotype.[1] In the setting of familial melanoma, *MC1R* genotype modifies melanoma risk in individuals carrying mutations in the cyclin-dependent kinase inhibitor gene *CDKN2A*, with the presence of a variant *MC1R* allele significantly increasing raw penetrance (from 50 to 80%) and decreasing mean age of onset (from 58 years to 37 years; Fig. 3.18).[37] It was recently demonstrated that loss-of-function *MC1R* mutations markedly increase the sensitivity of melanocytes to the cytotoxic effects of UVR and, in melanoma cells, reduce α-MSH-induced effects such as suppression of proliferation and decreased binding to fibronectin.[38] The *MC1R* genotype may thus serve as a marker of susceptibility to skin cancer beyond its visible effects on pigmentary phenotype.

The switch between eumelanin and pheomelanin synthesis is regulated not only by the binding of melanocortin ligands that activate the MC1R, but also by a physiologic antagonist known as the agouti protein.[39] The latter is a soluble paracrine factor synthesized by dermal papilla cells within the hair follicle that acts as a competitive inhibitor of α-MSH binding to the MC1R and also reduces basal MC1R activity in the absence of α-MSH, likely by functioning as an inverse agonist or effecting MC1R desensitization. Binding of agouti protein to the MC1R thus blocks eumelanin production and induces pheomelanin synthesis (Fig. 3.17). The term 'agouti' refers to the presence of a subapical band of yellow pheomelanic pigment in an otherwise black eumelanic hair shaft; this pattern results from transient 'turning on' of agouti protein production during the mid phase of the hair growth cycle, and is seen in mice, dogs and foxes (Fig. 3.19). In mice with a dominant mutation at the *agouti* locus, excessive synthesis of agouti protein throughout the body results in a uniformly yellow coat and obesity, the latter caused by antagonism of the hypothalamic MC4R.

The human orthologue of the agouti protein (ASIP) is expressed in the skin, adipose tissue and pancreas. ASIP can antagonize all five MCRs, with most potent inhibition of MC1R and MC4R.[40] Recently, a polymorphism in the 3′ untranslated region of the *ASIP* gene was found to be significantly associated with dark hair and brown eyes in a large cohort of white Americans.[41] Destabilization of *ASIP* mRNA was proposed as a possible mechanism for the bias toward eumelanogenesis seen in individuals with the polymorphism. To date, over-production of ASIP leading to pheomelanogenesis and/or obesity has not been observed in humans. However, polymorphisms in the promoter and coding regions of the gene for agouti-related protein (*AGRP*), a MC3R and MC4R antagonist that is expressed in the hypothalamus, have been associated with human obesity.

In addition to signaling via the MC1R, pigment production can be enhanced by exposure of melanocytes to agents that increase cytoplasmic levels of cAMP, such

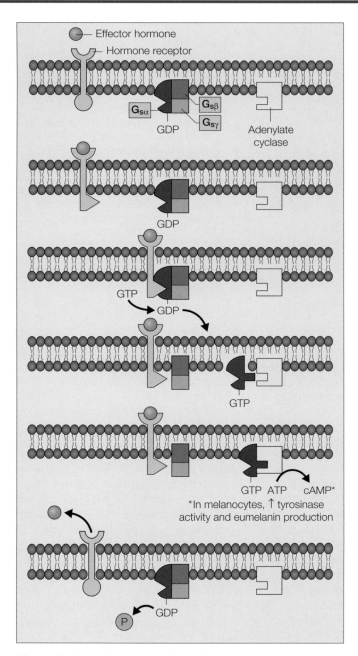

Figure 3.16 Activation of a G protein-coupled receptor such as the melanocortin-1 receptor (MC1R). Binding of a ligand to the receptor results in activation of adenylate cyclase via the α-subunit of the receptor-coupled stimulatory G protein ($G_{s\alpha}$). This produces an elevation in the intracellular concentration of cyclic adenosine monophosphate (cAMP), which, in the case of the MC1R, leads to an increase in tyrosinase activity and eumelanin production. GDP, guanosine diphosphate; GTP, guanosine triphosphate; P, phosphate group; ATP, adenosine triphosphate. (Adapted from Alberts et al.[32])

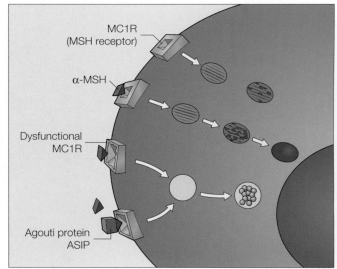

Figure 3.17 Interaction of α-melanocyte stimulating hormone (α-MSH) and agouti signaling protein (ASIP) with the melanocortin-1 receptor (MC1R). There is some baseline activity of the MC1R; this is enhanced by α-MSH-binding, resulting in increased eumelanogenesis. Dysfunction of the MC1R (as in the case of humans with red hair) or binding of ASIP, a physiologic antagonist, leads to pheomelanogenesis.

production of MITF (see above) in turn results in up-regulation of *TYR, TYRP1* and *TYRP2* gene expression.

Ultraviolet radiation

Stimulation of melanogenesis by UVR (i.e. tanning) is a well-known phenomenon (Fig. 3.13). Considering that the MCIR plays a central role in the process, it is not surprising that it closely resembles the pigmentary response of melanocytes to α-MSH.[23] Following either a single erythemal exposure or several suberythemal exposures to UVR, an increase in the size, dendricity and number of active melanocytes as well as enhanced tyrosinase function and melanin production can be observed.[42] Repeated exposures to UVR lead to increased formation of stage IV melanosomes and their efficient transfer to keratinocytes, while treatment with psoralens plus UVA (PUVA) also leads to an alteration in the size and aggregation pattern of melanosomes, which become larger and singly dispersed (i.e. similar to those found in darkly pigmented skin; Fig. 3.9). Chronically sun-exposed sites (e.g. the outer upper arm) have an up to two-fold higher density of melanocytes than adjacent sun-protected sites (e.g. the inner upper arm).[14] As melanocytes normally have a low mitotic rate, it is not clear whether the increased number of pigment-producing melanocytes results from a higher mitotic rate or an activation of 'dormant' melanocytes or melanocyte precursors. Recently, UVR exposure was shown to induce KIT+ melanocyte precursors in mouse epidermal sheets to proliferate and differentiate into mature melanocytes.[43]

In human skin, the pigmentary response to UVR has two phases. *Immediate pigmentary darkening* occurs

as isobutylmethylxanthine (Figs 3.13 and 3.16). The activation of protein kinase A (PKA) by cAMP leads to the phosphorylation of many substrates, one of which is the *cAMP responsive element binding* protein (CREB), a transcription factor that regulates the expression of multiple genes, including those with pivotal roles in melanogenesis (Fig. 3.20).[34] For example, CREB binds and activates the *MITF* promoter, and increased

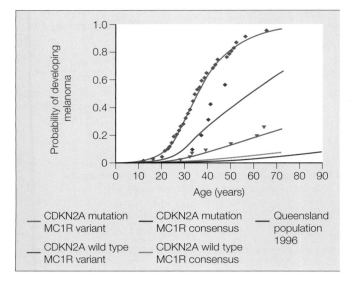

Figure 3.18 Modification of melanoma risk by the presence of a variant *MC1R* allele in individuals carrying mutations in the cyclin-dependent kinase inhibitor gene *CDKN2A*. (Reproduced by kind permission of the University of Chicago. Box NF, Duffy DL, Chen W, et al. MC1R genotype modifies risk of melanoma in families segregating CDKN2A mutations. Am J Hum Genet 2001; 69:765–773. Copyright © 2001 American Society of Human Genetics.)

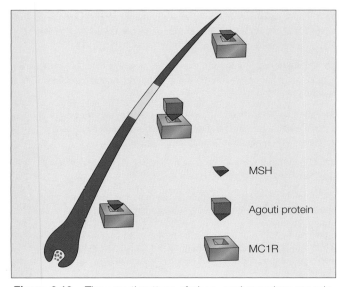

Figure 3.19 The agouti pattern of pheo- and eumelanogenesis. Transient 'turning on' of agouti protein production during the mid phase of hair growth results in a subapical band of yellow pheomelanic pigment in an otherwise black eumelanic hair shaft, as seen in mice, dogs and foxes.

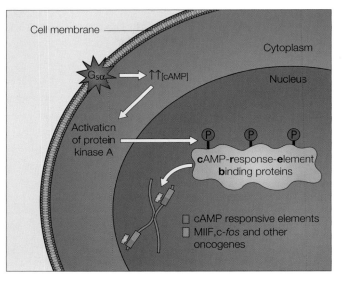

Figure 3.20 The cAMP cascade. In McCune–Albright syndrome (polyostotic fibrous dysplasia), post-zygotic activating mutations in the gene encoding $G_{s\alpha}$ permanently 'turn on' the cAMP signaling cascade, and segmental café-au-lait macules result from the increased melanogenic enzyme activity and eumelanin production. (Adapted from Bolognia JL, *et al.* Dermatology. Philadelphia: Elsevier; 2003.)

within minutes of exposure to UVA radiation and fades over 6–8 hrs. Most prominent in darkly pigmented skin, it is thought to result from photo-oxidation of pre-existing melanin or melanin precursors. The second phase, *delayed tanning*, is clinically apparent within 48–72 hrs of exposure to UVA and/or UVB radiation and represents *de novo* melanogenesis via an increase in tyrosinase activity. Of note, oxygen dependence is a feature particular to UVA-induced erythema and pigment production, explaining the lack of tanning over dorsal pressure points in those who use UVA tanning 'beds'.

Melanin defends the skin from UVR-induced damage not only by absorbing and scattering incident light, but also by scavenging reactive oxygen species. However, paradoxically, pheomelanin itself is photolabile, generating free radicals and oxidative stress upon UVR exposure. Individuals with increased pheomelanin production due to the presence of two *MC1R* variant alleles have significantly steeper dose-response curves for UVB radiation-induced erythema than those with one or no variant allele. In addition, the presence of certain pheomelanin derivatives in the hair has been shown to serve as a marker for individuals with extremely low minimal erythemal dose values.[29] The level of photoprotection thus depends both on the total content of melanin and the eumelanin:pheomelanin ratio. Although constitutive pigmentation has been estimated to provide the equivalent of a sun protection factor (SPF) of 10–15 in individuals with dark brown to black skin, with five times more UVR reaching the papillary dermis of Caucasian than black skin,[15,21] the 'induced' SPF provided by a tan is only 2–3 in those with skin types II–IV.[44]

FUTURE OUTLOOK

Overwhelming epidemiologic evidence implicates solar radiation as a major cause of skin cancer in humans. The photoprotective or photosensitizing properties of melanin pigment itself, which are largely determined by the functional status of the MC1R, represent critical factors in the development of both cutaneous melanoma and NMSC. In the future, characterization of the chemical nature of the melanin produced as well as the status of the *MC1R* gene, which appear to have effects on susceptibility to tumor development beyond the visible phenotype, may provide a more accurate method for assessment of an individual's risk for skin cancer.

REFERENCES

1 Sturm RA. Skin colour and cancer – MClR, the genetic link. Melanoma Res 2002; 12:405–416.

2 Seiji M, Fitzpatrick TB, Birbeck MSC. The melanosome: a distinctive subcellular particle of mammalian melanocytes and the site of melanogenesis. J Invest Dermatol 1961; 36:243–252.

3 Bolognia JL. Molecular advances in disorders of pigmentation. Adv Dermatol 1999; 15:341–365.

4 Hachiya A, Kobayashi A, Ohuchi A, et al. The paracrine role of stem cell factor/c-kit signaling in the activation of human melanocytes in ultraviolet-B-induced pigmentation. J Invest Dermatol 2001; 116:578–586.

5 Goding CR. Mitf from neural crest to melanoma: signal transduction and transcription in the melanocyte lineage. Genes Devel 2000; 14:1712–1728.

6 McGill GG, Horstmann M, Widlund HR, et al. Bcl2 regulation by the melanocyte master regulator Mitf modulates lineage survival and melanoma cell viability. Cell 2002; 109:707–718.

7 Zimmerman AA, Becker SW Jr. Precursors of epidermal melanocytes in the Negro fetus. In: Cordon M, ed. Pigment Cell Biology. New York, NY: Academic Press; 1959:159–170.

8 Kunisada T, Yamazaka H, Hayashi S. Ligands for receptor tyrosine kinases expressed in the skin as environmental factors for melanocyte development. J Invest Dermatol Symp Proc 2001; 6:6–9.

9 Holbrook KA, Underwood RA, Vogel AM, et al. The appearance, density and distribution of melanocytes in human embryonic and fetal skin revealed by the anti-melanoma monoclonal antibody, HMB-45. Anat Embryol 1989; 180:443–455.

10 Jimbow K, Quevedo WC Jr, Fitzpatrick TB, et al. Some aspects of melanin biology: 1950–1975. J Invest Dermatol 1976; 67:72–89.

11 Horikawa T, Norris DA, Johnson TW, et al. DOPA-negative melanocytes in the outer root sheath of human hair follicles express premelanosomal antigens but not a melanosomal antigen or the melanosome-associated glycoproteins tyrosinase, TRP-1, and TRP-2. J Invest Dermatol 1996; 106:28–35.

12 Tobin DJ, Bystryn JC. Different populations of melanocytes are present in hair follicles and epidermis. Pigment Cell Res 1996; 9:304–310.

13 Nishimura EK, Jordan SA, Oshima H, et al. Dominant role of the niche in melanocyte stem-cell fate determination. Nature 2002; 416:854–860.

14 Gilchrest BA, Blog FB, Szabo G. Effects of aging and chronic sun exposure on melanocytes in human skin. J Invest Dermatol 1979; 73:41–43.

15 Bolognia JL, Pawelek JM. Biology of hypopigmentation. J Am Acad Dermatol 1988; 19:217–255.

16 Orlow SJ. Melanosomes are specialized members of the lysosomal lineage of organelles. J Invest Dermatol 1995; 105:3–7.

17 Watabe H, Valencia JC, Yasumoto KI, et al. Regulation of tyrosinase processing and trafficking by organellar pH and by proteasome activity. J Biol Chem 2004; 279:7971–7981.

18 Marks MS, Seabra MC. The melanosome: membrane dynamics in black and white. Nat Rev Mol Cell Biol 2001; 2:1–11.

19 Angelica EC Dell, Shotelersuk V, Aguilar RC, et al. Altered trafficking of lysosomal proteins in Hermansky-Pudlak syndrome due to mutations in the beta 3A subunit of the AP-3 adaptor. Mol Cell 1999; 3:11–21.

20 Kushimoto T, Basrur V, Valencia J, et al. A model for melanosome biogenesis based on the purification and analysis of early melanosomes. Proc Natl Acad Sci USA 2001; 98:10698–10703.

21 Ortonne J-P. Photoprotective properties of skin melanin. Br J Dermatol 2002; 146:7–10.

22 Olivares C, Jiminez-Cervantes C, Lozano JA. The 5,6-dihydroxyindole-2-carboxylic acid (DHICA) oxidase activity of human tyrosinase. Biochem J 2001; 354:131–139.

23 Hearing VJ. Biochemical control of melanogenesis and melanosomal organization. J Invest Dermatol Symp Proc 1999; 4:24–28.

24 Newton JM, Cohen-Barak O, Hagiwara N, et al. Mutations in the human orthologue of the mouse underwhite gene (uw) underlie a new form of oculocutaneous albinism, OCA4. Am J Hum Genet 2001; 69:981–988.

25 Rinchik EM, Bultman SJ, Horsthemke B, et al. A gene for the mouse pink-eyed dilution locus and for human type II oculocutaneous albinism. Nature 1993; 361:72–76.

26 Ancans J, Tobin DJ, Hoogduijn MJ, et al. Melanosomal pH controls rate of melanogenesis, eumelanin/phaeomelanin ratio and melanosome maturation in melanocytes and melanoma cells. Exp Cell Res 2001; 268:26–35.

27 Chen K, Manga P, Orlow SJ. Pink-eyed dilution protein controls the processing of tyrosinase. Mol Biol Cell 2002; 13:1953–1964.

28 Rosenberg SA, White DE. Vitiligo in patients with melanomas: normal tissue antigens can be targets for cancer immunotherapy. J Immunother Emphasis Tumor Immunol 1996; 19:81–84.

29 Prota G. Melanins, melanogenesis and melanocytes: looking at their functional significance from the chemist's viewpoint. Pigment Cell Res 2000; 13:283–293.

30 Abdel-Malek Z, Swope VB, Suzuki I, et al. Mitogenic and melanogenic stimulation of normal human melanocytes by melanotropic peptides. Proc Natl Acad Sci USA 1995; 92:1789–1793.

31 Krude H, Biebermann H, Luck W, et al. Severe early-onset obesity, adrenal insufficiency and red hair pigmentation caused by POMC mutations in humans. Nat Genet 1998; 19:155–157.

32 Alberts B, Johnson A, Lewis J, et al. Molecular biology of the cell, 3rd edn. New York, NY: Garland; 1994.

33 Luger TA, Scholzen T, Grabbe S. The role of alpha-melanocyte stimulating hormone in cutaneous biology. J Invest Dermatol Symp Proc 1997; 2:87–93.

34 Busca R, Ballotti R. Cyclic AMP as key messenger in the regulation of skin pigmentation. Pigment Cell Res 2000; 13:60–69.

35 Sturm RA, Teasdale RD, Box NF. Human pigmentation genes: identification, structure and consequences of polymorphic variation. Gene 2001; 277:49–62.

36 Schaffer JV, Bolognia JL. The melanocortin-1 receptor: red hair and beyond. Arch Derm 2001; 137:1477–1485.

37 Box NF, Duffy DL, Chen W, et al. MC1R genotype modifies risk of melanoma in families segregating CDKN2A mutations. Am J Hum Genet 2001; 69:765–773.

38 Robinson SJ, Healy E. Human melanocortin 1 receptor (MC1R) gene variants alter melanoma cell growth and adhesion to extracellular matrix. Oncogene 2002; 21:8037–8046.

39 Lu D, Willard D, Patel IR, et al. Agouti protein is an antagonist of the melanocyte-stimulating hormone receptor. Nature 1994; 371:799–802.

40 Voisey J. Van Daal A. Agouti: from mouse to man, from skin to fat. Pigment Cell Res 2002; 15:10–18.

41 Kanetsky PA, Swoyer J, Panossian S, et al. A polymorphism in the agouti signaling protein gene is associated with human pigmentation. Am J Hum Genet 2002; 70:770–775.

42 An HT, Yoo J, Lee MK, et al. Single dose radiation is more effective for the UV-induced activation and proliferation of melanocytes than fractionated dose radiation. Photodermatol Photoimmunol Photomed 2001; 17:266–271.

43 Kawaguchi Y, Mori N, Nakayama A. Kit+ melanocytes seem to contribute to melanocyte proliferation after UV exposure as precursor cells. J Invest Dermatol 2001; 116:920–925.

44 Sheehan JM, Cragg N, Chadwick CA, et al. Repeated ultraviolet exposure affords the same protection against DNA photodamage and erythema in human skin types II and IV but is associated with faster DNA repair in skin type IV. J Invest Dermatol 2002; 118:825–829.

CHAPTER
4

Epidemiology of Skin Cancer

Melody J Eide and Martin A Weinstock

Key points

- Melanoma is 20 times more common today than 60 years ago.
- Melanoma incidence has leveled off in young men, but continues to increase in young women; it is increasing faster at older ages for both men and women.
- Overall melanoma mortality is increasing in the US, but is declining in younger generations.
- Keratinocyte carcinoma (basal and squamous cell carcinoma) is the most common malignancy in the US and it is estimated that over 1 million cases were diagnosed in 2004.

INTRODUCTION

Skin cancer is the most common malignancy in the US[1] and in many other nations worldwide, and consequently has substantial public health significance. Malignant melanoma (MM), keratinocyte carcinoma (KC), including basal cell carcinoma (BCC) and squamous cell carcinoma (SCC), and other cutaneous malignancies such as cutaneous lymphoma have increased in incidence over the last several decades. Dermatoepidemiology may be seen as the bridge between skin disease and its burden and relationship to society. Monitoring trends in disease, identifying risk factors for disease, and modifying these risks to reduce disease impact are a few of the many critical roles served by epidemiology. This chapter will discuss key issues in the descriptive, analytic, and interventional aspects of the dermatoepidemiology of cutaneous malignancies.

HISTORY

Epidemiology has a rich history in relation to skin diseases. Percival Pott's suspicion of the association between soot and scrotal cancer in British chimney sweeps in the eighteenth century eventually led to recognition of this occupational risk.[2] In 1956, it was HO Lancaster's classic report of the distribution of melanoma mortality that was pivotal in the recognition of the role of sun exposure in melanoma etiology.[3] Today, cancer registries of countries worldwide routinely include melanoma, and sometimes, other cutaneous malignancies. In the US, the longest record of melanoma incidence is provided by the Connecticut Tumor Registry. The Connecticut Tumor

Registry has kept a record of malignant melanoma diagnosed since 1935 and continues to be an important source of information on melanoma incidence today.[4] In 1973, the National Cancer Institute (NCI) initiated a system of population-based registries to track most cancers, including melanoma. The Surveillance, Epidemiology and End Results (SEER) program is the broadest system of cancer registration in the US. Originally, SEER included information representing ~10% of the US utilizing nine population-based cancer registries: the metropolitan areas of Atlanta, Detroit, San Francisco and Seattle, and the states of Connecticut (CT), Iowa, New Mexico, Utah and Hawaii. The registry has expanded over the years and now includes approximately 14% of the US population.[5]

DESCRIPTIVE EPIDEMIOLOGY

Melanomas

Melanoma incidence

Melanoma incidence has increased rapidly over the past 65 years. Between 1935 and 1939, the incidence of melanoma in CT was 1.0 per 100,000 (age-standardized, 1970).[6] In 1996, incidence rate of melanoma had increased to 20.3 per 100,000 (age-standardized, 1970)[4] (Fig. 4.1). Similar trends have been noted in the SEER registry. In 1973 the melanoma incidence rate was 6.8 per 100,000, but by 1999, this rate had climbed to 17.4 per 100,000.[5] It is estimated that in the US in 2004, there were 55,100 new cases of melanoma diagnosed and an additional 40,780 cases of melanoma *in situ*.[1] The increase in invasive melanoma incidence was 6.1% per year between 1973 and 1981 and 2.8% per year between 1981 and 1999 (based on rates age-adjusted to 2000 US standard population).[5] In the US in 2004, it is estimated that melanoma will be the fifth most common cancer (other than keratinocyte carcinoma) diagnosed in men, behind prostate, lung, colon and urinary bladder. In women, it is estimated to be the seventh most common cancer, behind breast, lung, colon, uterine, ovarian, and Non-Hodgkin lymphoma.[1] Melanoma is the fourth most common cancer (other than keratinocyte carcinoma) in Australia, New Zealand and Sweden, the tenth most common in Scandinavia and the eighteenth most common cancer in most of the UK (England, Scotland and Wales).[7–9]

Studies continue to examine incidence and mortality trends to further determine the contribution of increasing age or birth cohort. Birth cohort refers to all individuals born within a specific time period and who subsequently

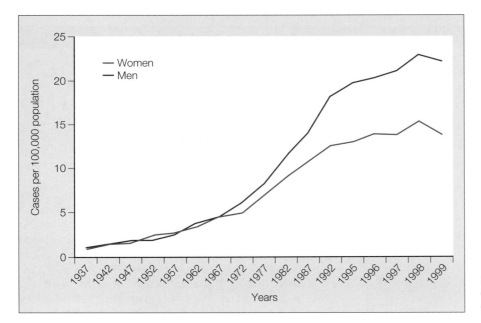

Figure 4.1 Melanoma incidence in Connecticut, 1937–1999. *Source*: Connecticut Tumor Registry.

may share similar early exposures and experiences. There have been attempts to distinguish a 'cohort' from a 'period' effect. The period effect is a concept which implies that time trends are influenced by more recent exposures or events, such as changes in diagnostic criteria or cancer screening. With a period effect, an increase in a given year (or other time period) is noted similarly in all age groups. Melanoma incidence, however, has generally been found to follow cohort patterns of changes. For example, assume incidence started to increase. With a cohort effect, this change would be noted first among more recent birth cohorts (younger people) and would not be observed in prior birth-cohorts (older people). A change in middle-age incidence first would be noted when these more recent birth cohort populations reached middle age.

It has been suggested that a 'leveling off' of the melanoma incidence is occurring in many countries. In the US, more recent generations of men have similar incidence rates compared with prior generations, even though these rates are still increasing in these older generations of men. However, incidence appears to be increasing in more recent generations of women. This is consistent with a cohort effect (Figs 4.2 and 4.3).[10] Incidence also appears to have leveled off in Australia, especially in younger cohorts born after 1960, supportive of a birth cohort effect.[10a] Incidence appears to even have fallen significantly in the last 20 years in young women (age groups 15–34 and 35–49) in New South Wales (annual per cent change −3% and −0.9%, respectively).[11] Trends in melanoma incidence in Europe (1953–1997) show a flattening of incidence rates in younger age groups in Scandinavian countries, whose rates are expected to remain stable or decrease further in the future, though these trends in incidence were less distinct in young people in other areas of northern and western Europe.[12]

The stabilization of melanoma incidence in recent cohorts may be related to the educational programs implemented in the last 30 years although this is not clear. Regardless of the apparent recent trend toward stabilization in the US and several other countries, the incidence rate of melanoma has increased faster than the mortality rate. Improved surveillance may have increased detection and resulted in the potential surgical removal of earlier 'cancers' that may never have progressed to become lesions of clinical significance, or may have increased removal of potentially fatal lesions at a curable point in their evolution, or a combination of both.

Because the frequency of skin cancer is significantly lower in non-white populations, epidemiological information is more limited. SEER provides detailed estimates of incidence by race only for blacks.[13] In 1999, SEER data showed an incidence rate in blacks of 1.2 per 100,000. Overall incidence rates are low in Hispanic, Asian/Pacific Islander and Black populations. The trend from 1992–1999 demonstrates an estimated annual percent increase in melanoma incidence as follows: Hispanic 4.0%; Black 4.9%; and Asian/Pacific Islander 3.0%. However, it is noted that these estimated increases are significantly different from zero only in the Hispanic population (Fig. 4.4).[5]

SEER incidence data indicate that melanoma incidence in the US trends upward with age, peaking between 80–84 years of age at a rate of 55.9 cases per 100,000 (Fig. 4.5). Similar age-trends have been seen in other countries, including Australia, Italy and the Netherlands.[14,15]

In the US, melanoma is more common in men than in women. In 1973, the incidence rates were 7.3 per 100,000 in men and 6.4 per 100,000 in women. In 1999, the incidence rate had risen in men and women respectively to 21.7 and 14.2 cases per 100,000 (Fig. 4.6). Gender differences have been noted in other countries, including Australia, where in 1999, incidence in males was 49 cases per 100,000 population while the female incidence was 34 cases per 100,000 (Fig. 4.7).[8] These gender differences appear to vary with age as well. In SEER registrants under age 40, melanoma incidence is higher in women while, after age 40, men have higher incidence rates.[5] Between 1995 and 1999 in the US, the

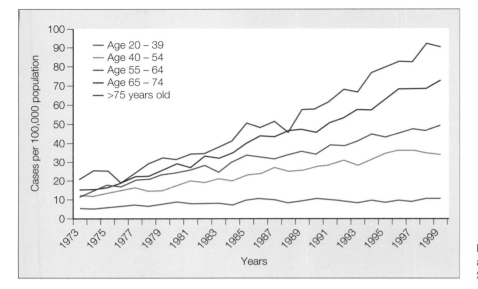

Figure 4.2 Incidence of melanoma by age in males, USA, 1973–1999. *Source*: SEER Registry.

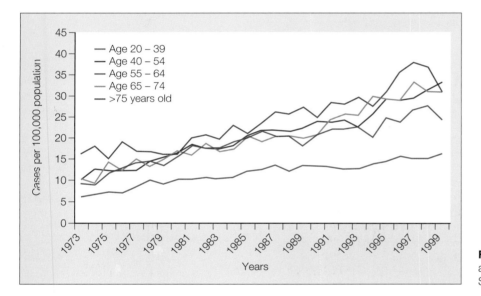

Figure 4.3 Incidence of melanoma by age in females, USA, 1973–1999. *Source*: SEER Registry.

incidence in males over age 65 was 77 per 100,000 while the incidence in females was 33 per 100,000.[5]

Incidence rates vary substantially, worldwide (Table 4.1). New Zealand and Australia have some of the highest rates. In Queensland, Australia, the incidence rate is three times that of the US.[16] These high rates have led to a large public health and economic burden which have motivated extensive and successful public health campaigns. Incidence in European nations ranges from 1.4–2.0 cases per 100,000 in Vila Nova de Gaia Portugal to 14.3–16.1 per 100,000 in Norway. In Africa and Central and South America, incidence is low. In Asia, it is remarkably low, with less than one case per 100,000 throughout the area. An exception is Israel, where the incidence varies with ancestry and place of birth. It is quite high in Israeli Jews, and those born in Israel have a higher incidence than Jews born outside the country.[16]

Trends in international incidence suggest that melanoma is continuing to increase.[17] Between the mid-1960s to the mid-1980s, the average annual percentage increase in melanoma incidence generally ranged from 3–6%, with the highest rate of increase noted in white residents of Hawaii, who had an over 9% increase.[17] Kricker and Armstrong examined international data for trends in age-specific rates, and found that incidence rates have stabilized or begun to fall in young people (less than age 55) in some populations including Denmark, Canada, the US, Australia, New Zealand, Norway and the UK, but are continuing to rise in other countries such as Poland, Spain and Yugoslavia.[17] There is evidence suggesting a latitudinal effect world wide in melanoma incidence, with generally higher incidence reported nearer the equator. In New Zealand data from 1968 to 1989, a latitudinal trend from north to south existed for each gender and across time. New Zealanders living in the northern region of the country may have at least 37% higher incidence than those living in the South.[18] There is a higher incidence in Scandinavian compared with Mediterranean countries, which is attributable to gradients in sun sensitivity in these populations.[16]

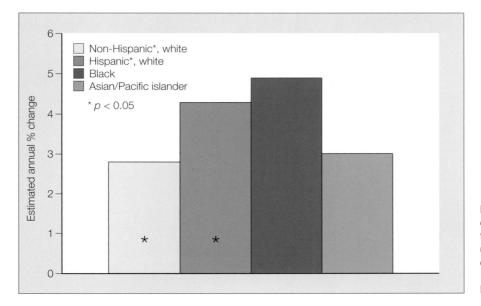

Figure 4.4 Estimated annual percentage change (%) in age-adjusted SEER incidence from 1992–1999 by race/ethnicity, USA. (*Source*: Ries LAG, Eisner MP, Kosary CL, et al. (eds) SEER Cancer Statistics Review, 1973–1999, Table XVI-9. Bethesda: National Cancer Institute; 2002.)

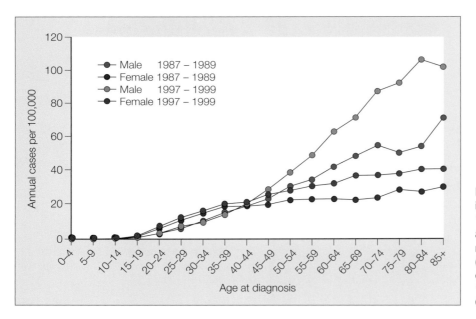

Figure 4.5 Melanoma of the skin, SEER incidence by age and sex, Whites 1987–1989 vs 1997–1999. Rates are age-adjusted to the 2000 US standard million population by 5-year age groups. (From: Ries LAG, Eisner MP, Kosary CL, et al. (eds) SEER Cancer Statistics Review, 1973–1999. Bethesda, MD: National Cancer Institute; 2002.)

Melanoma mortality

Nearly 75% of skin cancer deaths in the US are attributable to melanoma.[19] Melanoma mortality has increased substantially in the US over the last 30 years, although it is now stabilizing. Mortality increased 4.3% annually in the white population between 1973 and 1977, 1.5% annually between 1977 and 1990 and increased 0.2% per year between 1990 and 1999.[5] In 1999, according to the Centers for Disease Control, 7215 people died of melanoma in the US.[20] It was estimated that in 2003, 7600 Americans would die of this cancer.[1]

A recent analysis of World Health Organization (WHO) Cancer Mortality Data Bank data (examining Australia, Canada, Czechoslovakia, France, Italy, Japan, UK, the US and a combined Denmark, Finland, Sweden and Norway) examined mortality rates and recent trends from 1960 to 1994. In 1960, some of the lowest mortality rates for the 30–59 age group were seen in France, Italy

and Czechoslovakia (less than 0.5 deaths per 100,000 (world standard population)). However, over the last 30 years, the highest rates of increase in mortality were found in these same three countries, with death rates increasing annually by 9–16%. Age adjusted mortality in Japan remained low (less than one death per 100,000 in all age groups) over the entire time period.[21]

There are marked differences in mortality with increasing age in the US. The mortality rate in 1999 for men and women younger than age 65 was 1.9 and 1.0 deaths per 100,000, respectively. However for those ages 65 and older, the mortality rate for men was 18.0 per 100,000 and 7.6 per 100,000 in women. The highest mortality is seen in men over age 85: 28.8 per 100,000.[5]

There is also a higher mortality rate in men compared to women of the same age in the US.[5] In men, melanoma mortality increased 2.5% yearly between 1973 and 1987 and 0.7% from 1987 and 1999. In women, mortality rose

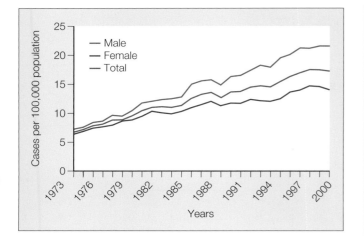

Figure 4.6 Age-adjusted incidence of melanoma in the US, 1973–1999. Age standardized to 2000 US census. *Source*: SEER Registry.

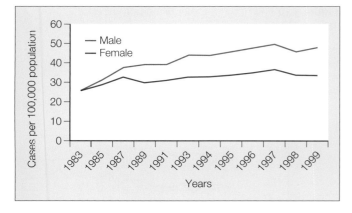

Figure 4.7 Age-adjusted incidence of melanoma in Australia, 1983–2000. Age standardized to 1991 Australian population. *Source*: National Health Priority Areas: Cancer Indicators, http://www.aihw.gov/au/hhpa/cancer (accessed 5 September 2003), Australian Institute of Health and Welfare, 2003.

Table 4.1 Age-standardized incidence of melanoma in selected countries of the world

Country	Incidence rate[a] per 100,000	
	Male	Female
Columbia, Cali	2.5	2.7
Canada	8.5	7.5
United States, SEER White	15.4	11.6
United States, SEER Black	1.0	0.5
India, Mumbai (Bombay)	0.3	0.2
Israel, Jews	11.7	11.3
Israel, Non-Jews	1.0	0.9
Japan, Hiroshima	0.4	0.5
China, Beijing	0.3	0.2
Czech Republic	8.1	7.9
Denmark	10.5	13.4
Finland	8.0	6.7
Germany, Saarland	6.3	6.1
The Netherlands	8.0	10.9
Poland, Warsaw City	4.1	4.1
Spain, Murcia	4.1	5.4
Sweden	11.8	11.9
UK, England	5.8	7.4
UK, Scotland	7.1	9.9
Australia, New South Wales	36.9	25.9
Australia, Queensland	51.1	38.1
New Zealand	32.8	30.6

[a]*Age standardized at world population.*
Source: Cancer Incidence in Five Continents, Vol. III. Lyon: IARC Scientific Publications; No 155, 2002

2.4% annually from 1973 to 1981, however in recent years (1981–1999) it has decreased by 0.1% annually[5] (Fig. 4.8). It was estimated that there would be approximately 1900 more deaths in men than women in the US in 2004.[1] The mortality rate in Australia is also higher for men than women (Fig. 4.9).

The age-adjusted death rate from melanoma in 1999 was 3.0 per 100,000 for the white population and 0.4 per 100,000 in the black population. Between 1973 through 1999, the mortality rate was unchanged in black women, while in black men there was actually a slight decrease.[5] In this time interval, however, the overall change in melanoma mortality amongst blacks was not significantly different from zero.[5] The 5-year relative survival rate of melanoma is lower in blacks compared with whites (all stages: 66% vs 90%).[1] Examination of stage of diagnosis reveals that a higher percentage of blacks diagnosed with melanoma between 1992 and 1998, had regional or distant disease-stage than the

white population. However, a survival rate inequality is also seen in localized disease.[1]

The mortality rate appears to be stabilizing in portions of the world, including the US, Australia and parts of Europe. Mortality has demonstrated a cohort effect, although unlike incidence, US mortality has declined in more recent birth cohorts. Death certificate or histopathology criteria changes are not felt to have a significant impact on this trend.[22] The stabilization of melanoma mortality in more recent cohorts may be the result of a combination of a slower increase in melanoma incidence and a lower case-fatality, presumably due at least in part to earlier detection. Age-specific mortality rates are displayed in Figures 4.10 and 4.11.

Cohort analysis of WHO mortality data have demonstrated several different patterns. In Australia, the US and the Scandinavian countries, there appears to be an increasing mortality rate for the generation born prior to 1940, followed by a decrease in mortality in younger cohorts. In the UK and Canada, the rates increase in the generation born between 1920 and 1950, with a stabilization in more recent cohorts In France, Czechoslovakia and Italy, there has been a steep

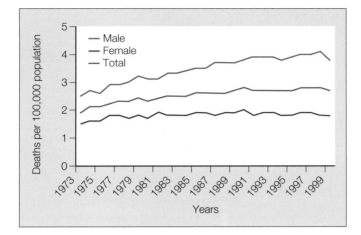

Figure 4.8 Age-adjusted melanoma mortality in the US, 1973–1999. Age standardized to 2000 US census. *Source*: SEER CanQues Results, http://canques.seer.cancer.gov (accessed 22 February, 2003).

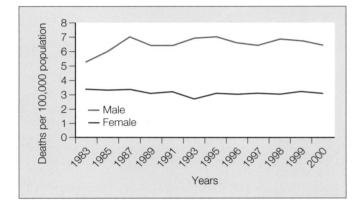

Figure 4.9 Age-adjusted melanoma mortality, Australia, 1983–2000. Age standardized to 1991 Australian population. *Source*: National Health Priority Areas: Cancer Indicators, http://www.aihw.gov.au/hhpa/cancer (accessed 5 September, 2003), Australian Institute of Health and Welfare, 2003.

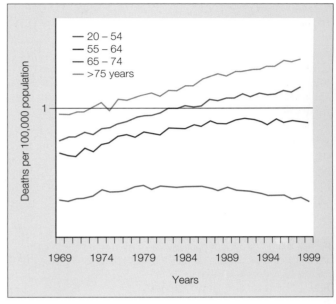

Figure 4.10 Trends in melanoma mortality in males, USA, 1969–1999. *Source*: SEER Registry.

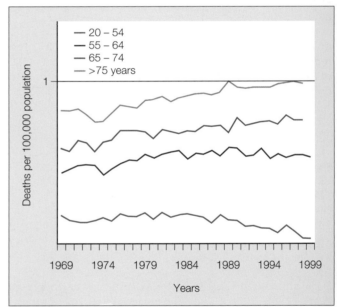

Figure 4.11 Trends in melanoma mortality in females, USA, 1969–1999. *Source*: SEER Registry.

increase in melanoma mortality that appears linear with little change in trend.[21] In Sweden, mortality has plateaued in men in the last 10–15 years and slightly decreased in women (−2.3%). Mortality has decreased in women among all age groups, but in men only for those younger than age 60, and analysis of trends has been suggestive of a period effect.[23]

Economic impact of melanoma

As the incidence of melanoma increases, the social and economic impact grows. With a mean age of diagnosis at 55, melanoma affects a younger population than many other cancers.[24] This occurrence of disease during an individual's 'working years' can have significant economic impact as well as social impact. Treatment costs also are substantial. It has been estimated that in 1997 the cumulative cost of treating newly diagnosed melanoma patients in the US was over US$560 million. Treatment of advanced disease is more expensive and it is estimated that treating a stage III or stage IV patient is almost 40 times the cost of treating someone with stage

I disease.[25] The increasing use of sentinel lymph node biopsies and chemotherapeutic agents such as adjuvant interferon in localized disease may further increase these costs. Physician skin examinations as a screening tool in high risk populations have been estimated in the US to have a cost-effectiveness ratio of US$29,170 per year of life saved.[26] Follow-up recommendations have been suggested that emphasize optimal patient care and resource allotment for melanoma patients.[27] The cost of follow-up in a German cohort per detected first recurrence for patients with a Breslow thickness less than 0.75 mm is €35,900 but dropping to €5704 when Breslow depth was greater than 4 mm.[28]

Cutaneous malignancies other than melanoma

Keratinocyte carcinoma (KC) includes both basal cell (BCC) and squamous cell carcinoma (SCC).[29,30] The term 'non-melanoma skin cancer' (NMSC) is commonly used to refer to KC, but also includes other cutaneous malignancies The fundamental problem with the term NMSC is that it defines our most common malignancy by what it is *not*, thereby impeding its proper study and demeaning its significance. The use of the more specific term of keratinocyte carcinoma may facilitate proper investigation of other cutaneous malignancies, including cutaneous lymphoma, Merkel cell carcinoma, Paget's disease, angiosarcomas, malignant histiocytomas, and many other cutaneous malignancies, each of which have different origins, pathological features, clinical and epidemiologic characteristics and prognosis.

Keratinocyte carcinomas

It is estimated that in 2004 there will be over 1 million cases of keratinocyte carcinoma (BCC and SCC) diagnosed in the US alone.[1] However, it should be noted that there are limited data sources available on keratinocyte carcinoma because they are not routinely included in cancer registries in the US or many other countries,[31] and thus precise incidence rates are typically unavailable (Table 4.2 and Fig. 4.12). In the few registries that include KC, there is concern that, because of their high incidence, generally excellent prognosis and potential for outpatient treatment without histologic evaluation, these cancers may be subject to significant under-registration.

Other sources have been used to evaluate the occurrence of KC including using information from large pre-paid health maintenance organizations (HMOs) and self-report surveys. Regardless of data source, there are several complicating factors. Some investigators choose to enumerate KC by individual person while others prefer counting all incident cancers as unique measures, regardless of multiplicity in a single person. The former method is the one most accepted by the scientific community and utilized in this chapter. However, when counting only first cancer, the observation interval may vary significantly between reports. For example, a report based on a 6-month interval will tend to yield higher incidence estimates than a report based on a 5-year interval because there will be fewer tumors uncounted among those who have many occurrences of KC in the 5 years. Furthermore, sometimes SCC and BCC are considered and studied together, despite the clinical and epidemiological differences. Hence, reports of incidence rates must be carefully scrutinized.

Squamous cell carcinoma incidence

The incidence of SCC has been rising worldwide over the last several decades at an estimated 3–10% per year.[6,32] It was estimated that in 1994 there were between 135,000 and 250,000 cases of SCC diagnosed in the US.[33] SCC incidence is generally higher in men.[34] The incidence rate of squamous cell carcinoma in Rochester, MN in 1992 was estimated in men and women

Table 4.2 Incidence rate of keratinocyte carcinoma

Location	Standard population	Year of study	Incidence rate of SCC per 100,000		Incidence rate of BCC per 100,000	
			Male	Female	Male	Female
Australia, Nambour[a]	World	1985–1992	600	298	2074	1579
Western Australia, Geraldton[b]	Crude	1987–1992	775	501	7067	3379
Switzerland, Canton of Vaud[c]	World	1991–1992	29	18	69	62
United States, New Hampshire[d]	US, 1970	1993–1994	97	32	310	166
Finland[e]	World	1991–1995	7	4	49	45
Australia[f]	World	1995	419	228	955	629
United States, Arizona[g]	US, 1970	1996	271	112	936	497

[a]Green A, Battistutta D, Hart V, Leslie D, Weedon D. Skin cancer in a subtropical Australian population: incidence and lack of assocation with occupation. The Nambour Study Group. Am J Epidemiol. 1996;144(11):1034–1040.
[b]English DR, Kricker A, Heenan PJ, Randell PL, Winter MG, Armstrong BK. Incidence of non-melanocytic skin cancer in Geraldton, Western Australia. Int J Cancer. 1997;73:629–633.
[c]Levi F, Franceschi S, Te VC, Randimbison L, La Vecchia C. Trends of skin cancer in Canton of Vaud, 1976–92. Br J Cancer. 1995;72(4):1047–1053.
[d]Karagas MR, Greenberg ER, Spencer SK, Stukel TA, Mott LA. Increase in incidence rates of basal cell and squamous cell skin cancer in New Hampshire, USA. Int J Cancer. 1999;81:555–559.
[e]Hannuksela-Svahn A, Pukkala E, Karvonen J. Basal cell skin carcinoma and other nonmelanoma skin cancers in Finland from 1956 through 1995. Arch Dermatol. 1999;135:781–786.
[f]Staples M, Marks R, Giles G. Trends in the incidence of non-melanocytic skin cancer (NMSC) treated in Australia 1985–1995: Are primary prevention programs starting to have an effect? Int J Cancer. 1998;78:144–148.
[g]Harris RB, Griffith K, Moon TE. Trends in incidence of nonmelanoma skin cancers in southeastern Arizona, 1985–1996. J Am Acad Dermatol. 2001;45(4):528–536

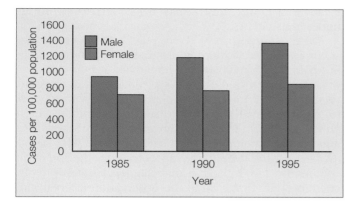

Figure 4.12 Age-adjusted incidence of non-melanoma skin cancer, Australia 1985–1995. Age standardized to World Standard Population. *Source*: National Health Priority Areas: Cancer Indicators, http://www.aihw.gov/au/hhpa/cancer (accessed 5 September, 2003), Australian Institute of Health and Welfare, 2003.

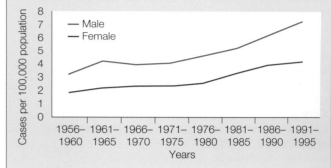

Figure 4.13 Age-adjusted incidence of squamous cell carcinoma, Finland, 1956–1995. Age standardized to World Standard Population. *Source*: Hannuksela-Svahn A, Pukkala E, et al. (1999) Basal cell skin carcinoma and other nonmelanoma skin cancers in Finland from 1956 through 1995. Arch Dermatol 135:781–786. Copyright © 1999 American Medical Association. All rights reserved.

respectively at 161.1 and 99.7 cases per 100,000 (age-standardized, 1990 US population), more than doubling compared with 1984.[35] The incidence of SCC in Finland was estimated in 1991–1995 for men and women, respectively at 7.2 and 4.2 cases per 100,000 (World Standard Population)[36] (Fig. 4.13). The majority of SCC occurs on the head, neck and upper extremities. In darker-skinned populations, the etiology of SCC may be unrelated to sun exposure, but may be associated with chronic irritation or injury while there is evidence to suggest that sun exposure is related to SCC development in lighter-skinned populations.[6]

The geographic distribution of SCC has been examined and in the US there appears to be a higher incidence with lower latitudes, with an approximate doubling when compared with northern areas.[2] A similar trend has been seen in Australia. Incidence rates in migrants to Australia have shown that the odds of developing SCC were lower among migrants than among persons born in Australia, with a trend of declining risk with more recent immigration (shorter lengths of time in the country).[34] The incidence rate has also been shown to increase with decreasing latitude in Norway.[37] However, this gradient may not be true in all of Europe.[16]

Trends in squamous cell carcinoma do not appear to be consistent across populations. In the US, no significant change in incidence was seen in southeastern Arizona from 1985 to 1996, however, incidence more than doubled in New Hampshire between 1978 and 1994.[38,39] Internationally, in South Wales, no significant difference was also seen in the standardized incidence rate from 1988 to 1998,[40] but the trend in Finland between 1956 and 1995 suggests a steady increase in squamous cell carcinoma incidence.[41] In Singapore, SCC incidence rates have decreased by 0.9% per year for both genders between 1968 and 1997.[42] There are several possible reasons for these ambiguities. Squamous cell carcinoma incidence may be affected by diagnostic accuracy (i.e. misclassification of actinic keratoses and SCC *in situ*) or changes in histologic criteria. Furthermore, some physicians may treat squamous cell carcinoma without histologic confirmation of the diagnosis.

Squamous cell carcinoma mortality
Inaccuracies in death certificate information limit direct epidemiological study. The age-adjusted mortality rate (1970 US standard) was calculated for confirmed cases of squamous cell carcinoma in Rhode Island (0.26 per 100,000), but the data to perform this calculation is unavailable in most locations.[43] Men have higher death rates from squamous cell carcinoma than women, a finding which is further amplified with age-adjustment. The age adjusted mortality rate ratio for men compared with women has been estimated to be roughly 3.9. Squamous cell carcinoma mortality is higher in whites and with increasing age. Case-fatality also appears to be higher in certain locations, including the ear, lip and genitalia.[43] While melanoma among whites is responsible for 90% of skin cancer deaths before 50 years of age, in adults over 85 years of age, the majority of skin cancer deaths are attributable to squamous cell carcinoma.[19] Between 1969 and 1988, there was a consistent decrease in the skin cancer mortality rate in the US, with an overall percent decline between 17 and 38%.[44] From 1988 to 2000, the mortality rate from SCC appears to have decreased even further, an additional 19% (unpublished data, Lewis and Weinstock), likely due in part to earlier detection, treatment or both.

Basal cell carcinoma incidence
Basal cell carcinoma is the most common skin cancer and is three to five times more common than squamous cell carcinoma in many Caucasian populations.[40] Men generally have higher rates of BCC than women, with a ratio of 1.3 to 1.9 in North America.[2] Like SCC, BCC commonly occurs on the head and neck[38] in both genders. However, women are more likely to have a greater frequency of BCC on the lower extremities than men, who have more ear lesions and this difference may be due to fashion differences, including clothing and hairstyle. Changes have been noted in the anatomic site over the last 20 years with larger increase in lesions located in anatomic sites other than head, including the trunk and limbs.[38]

The incidence of basal cell carcinoma is increasing. In the last 30 years, incidence rates have been estimated to have risen between 20 to 80%.[6] Basal cell carcinoma was estimated in Finland to have doubled from the late 1960s until the early 1990s, with an incidence in 1991–1995 of 49 and 45 cases per 100,000 in men and women respectively (age-standardized, World Standard Population)[36] (Fig. 4.14). In South Wales, the age-standardized rate for BCC in 1998 was 114.2 cases per 100,000 (World Standard Population), an increase of nearly 50% since 1988.[40] The incidence rate of BCC from the Neuchatel Cancer Registry in 1998 were 78 per 100,000 in men and 56 per 100,000 in women (age-adjusted, World Standard Population), doubling over a 20-year period.[45]

Basal cell carcinoma mortality

The mortality of basal cell carcinoma is lower and the mean age at time of death is higher than with squamous cell carcinoma. It has been suggested that squamous cell carcinoma is 12 times more likely to be fatal than basal cell carcinoma. The age-adjusted mortality rate for basal cell carcinoma has been estimated at 0.12 per 100,000.[43] More recent estimates suggest that between 1988 and 2000 mortality from BCC may have dropped further to 0.05 per 100,000 (Lewis and Weinstock, unpublished data). Higher mortality is seen with increasing age, male gender and in the white population. Age-adjusted rate ratios, which correct for the higher proportion of elderly females, suggested that mortality among men may be over twice that of women.[43]

Economic and social impact

It is difficult to determine the cost of the individual types of cutaneous malignancies. However, it has been estimated that the US spends more than US$2 billion each year treating cutaneous malignancies other than melanoma.[46] Recent estimates suggest that from 1992 to 1995 treatment of all cancers cost Medicare, the health insurance program for Americans over age 65, 13 billion dollars, and 4.5% of this cost is attributable to KC.[47] In this same time period, analysis of data from the Medicare Current Beneficiary Study provided an estimate for the cost of NMSC care for the entire US population (all ages) of US$650 million per year.[48] In the US, it has been estimated that the cost of treating a 1.5 cm facial skin tumor ranged from lesion destruction (electrodesiccation and curettage) with costs of approximately US$700 or outpatient Mohs micrographic surgery with costs of approximately US$1243 dollars (US$836–2940) to upwards of US$4500, with radiation therapy.[32] If these costs are applied to numbers of basal cell and squamous cell carcinoma from the last US national survey (1977–1978, at which time there were estimated to be approximately 500,000 cases of BCC and 100,000 cases of SCC annually, and assuming no recurrence, the minimum cost of treatment would have been US$350 million to treat BCC and US$70 million for SCC. It should also be noted that treatment costs do not include pathology fees and other diagnostic costs.

It is more difficult to quantify the morbidity impact associated with cutaneous malignancies. We have recently investigated factors, including patient and health system delay, associated with keratinocyte carcinoma morbidity, using the size of defect from Mohs micrographic surgery as proxy for size of malignancy. After controlling for anatomic site, histologic subtype, age and gender, we found that delay from first examination by a physician until having Mohs Micrographic Surgery (MMS) resulted in larger surgical defects. In fact, the lesions appeared to double in size in patients who had more than 1 year delay between first examination and MMS. Examination of contributors to delay from physician evaluation until MMS of more than 1 year included initial misdiagnosis, initial provider treatment and number of prior surgical treatments. Our preliminary findings suggest that attention to the process of care delivery for KC may have greater impact on morbidity than efforts at earlier detection by the public (Eide and Weinstock, unpublished data). Similar findings were noted in a recent doctoral dissertation.[49]

Disability and disfigurement may result from these malignancies and their treatment, with resultant economic and psychosocial implications. A recent study done in the UK investigated the handicap imposed by basal cell carcinoma and their treatment as measured by the UK Sickness Impact Profile and Dermatology Life Quality Index at baseline, 1 week and 3 months post-treatment. The study showed very little disability from BCCs, though there was an increase in disability score immediately post-treatment, which was presumed due to pain and minor sleep disturbances. No relationship was found between the quality of life scores and size of lesion.[50]

Other cancers of the skin

The epidemiology of other cutaneous malignancies is often obtained from defined populations or using cumulative cases from large registries such as the SEER registry.[51,52]

Cutaneous T-cell lymphoma

Incidence of cutaneous T-cell lymphoma (CTCL) in the US has been estimated at between 0.4–0.9 cases per 100,000 population.[51,52] Approximately 5% of these cases are classified as Sézary's syndrome. The incidence rate

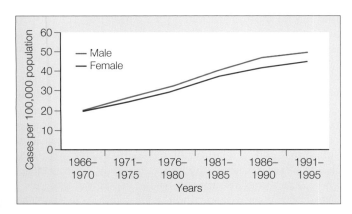

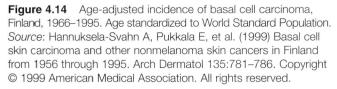

Figure 4.14 Age-adjusted incidence of basal cell carcinoma, Finland, 1966–1995. Age standardized to World Standard Population. *Source*: Hannuksela-Svahn A, Pukkala E, et al. (1999) Basal cell skin carcinoma and other nonmelanoma skin cancers in Finland from 1956 through 1995. Arch Dermatol 135:781–786. Copyright © 1999 American Medical Association. All rights reserved.

based on data from the SEER registry between 1973–1992 is 0.36 cases per 100,000.[53] SEER registry data from 1973 to 1984 reveals a three-fold increase in reported CTCL incidence.[52] However, the incidence rates for CTCL after 1984 have remained fairly constant.[53] Incidence of CTCL is higher with increasing age, male gender and in the black population. The etiology of CTCL remains unclear.[52,53]

The mortality rate for CTCL has decreased more than 20% since the early 1980s. This decline was seen regardless of gender or race. The age-adjusted estimated mortality from 1991 SEER registry data was 0.055 cases per 100,000. We have evidence, however, that this mortality rate substantially underestimates the true rate.[54] Higher CTCL mortality is seen in older adults, males, and in the black population.[53] In the US, between 1973 and 1992, the relative survival in CTCL patients was approximately 77% at 5 years and 69% at 10 years.[54]

Merkel cell carcinoma

Merkel cell carcinoma (MCC) was first reported in 1978. The SEER registry added MCC to its list of surveillance cancers in 1986 and between 1986 and 1994, only 425 people with MCC were reported to SEER.[55] Of these cases, 97% were white. The age-adjusted incidence per 100,000 is subsequently 0.23 in whites and 0.01 in blacks. The age-adjusted annual incidence of MCC is 0.35 per 100,000 in men and 0.15 per 100,000 in women. There is a higher incidence of MCC after approximately age 50. An increase in incidence has been noted in patients with other neoplasms and in organ transplant recipients.[55]

Kaposi's sarcoma

There are several types of Kaposi's sarcoma (KS): epidemic or HIV-associated, iatrogenic or transplant-associated, endemic African and classical. KS was a rare tumor among Western populations prior to 1981, occurring in only 0.02–0.06 per 100,000 people per year. It was classically seen in people of Mediterranean or Ashkenazi descent, often between the ages 40–70, and almost 10 times more often in men than women. With the arrival of acquired immunodeficiency syndrome (AIDS), incidence of KS increased dramatically. In the early years of the epidemic, it is estimated that between 15–25% of men affected with human immunodeficiency virus (HIV) in the US were diagnosed with KS. The endemic African type of KS occurs in blacks in equatorial Africa, such as Uganda where it accounts for between 3–9% of malignancies. The endemic type is seen in middle-aged adults and children, again more often in males than females. The immunosuppressive therapies necessary for organ-transplant success are responsible for the final type, iatrogenic. Recent reviews of iatrogenic KS note that incidence is approximately 80 to 500 times that of the non-immunosuppressed population, and that it is seen in transplant patients of all ages, though two to three times more frequently in males than females.[56,57]

ANALYTIC EPIDEMIOLOGY

Skin cancer has many causes. In 2002, ultraviolet light was added to the list of carcinogens reported in the Tenth Report on Carcinogens released by the National Institute of Environmental Health Sciences because of its association with cutaneous malignancies.[58] Size, type and multiplicity of nevi, personal and family history of melanoma, and early, intense and intermittent exposure are important risk factors for melanoma. Other risk factors include eye color, hair color, facultative skin color, and ethnicity. Immunosuppression and photochemotherapy also appear to have a role.[59] Many of these potential etiological factors have been identified through analytical epidemiology.

Both case–control and cohort investigations have led to improved knowledge about the etiology of melanoma. Cohort study design was used to identify the increased risk of melanoma in those who have a family history of the disease as well as the suggested association between dysplastic nevi and melanoma. Cohort studies have also been used to quantify these associations.[2] Studies of twins have also contributed. In the Finnish Twin Cohort, almost 26,000 twins were linked prospectively to the Finnish Cancer Registry and followed for 22 years. The incidence of cutaneous malignancies in this cohort reflected that of the general population. There were no twin pairs in which both of the twins developed melanoma, and only one pair in which both developed SCC.[60]

In a recently published case–case study, researchers examined melanoma patients in Queensland, Australia to explore their hypothesis that melanomas in different anatomic locations may arise through different causal pathways. Patient with lentigo maligna melanoma and melanomas on the head and neck were significantly more likely to have more solar keratoses and significantly fewer nevi than those patients who had melanoma on the trunk. This study was supportive of a divergent pathway for melanoma induction. It suggested that people who have a low tendency to develop nevi require more sunlight exposure to induce melanoma as opposed to those people with multiple nevi.[30]

Case–control studies have made major contributions to our knowledge of skin cancer. Case–control studies helped establish the link between melanoma and several factors: severe sunburns, extent of youth sun exposure and intense intermittent sun exposure.[2] In a case–control study conducted in Belgium, France and Germany, findings supported that ultraviolet exposure in childhood and adulthood were both associated with an increased risk of melanoma, and an interaction between early and later life exposure further magnified the risk.[61]

Other risk factors for keratinocyte carcinoma have also recently surfaced using the analytic type of study design, such as the association of cigarette smoking and basal cell carcinoma.[62] Ultraviolet exposure is a major contributor to the risk of developing basal cell and squamous cell carcinoma of the skin. People with evidence of solar damage including elastosis, telangiectasia and solar keratosis appear to be at higher risk. In a case–control study of squamous cell carcinoma in Australia, the relationship of sun exposure was investigated through the Geraldton Skin Cancer Prevention Survey. A large positive relationship with squamous cell carcinoma was seen with hours of bright sunlight accumulated over the course of a lifetime. Also, a strong association was noted for sunlight exposure with the specific anatomic site of the carcinoma, and this site-specific exposure risk was greater for exposure early in life. There was also a significant association between the number of blistering sunburns of the anatomic site with SCC. Investigators found little evidence that use of sunscreen or hats was associated with SCC risk in this study.[34]

Genetic factors play a role in the development of these cancers. Individuals with xeroderma pigmentosa have a significantly higher incidence of melanoma, basal cell carcinoma and squamous cell carcinoma. Familial risk for squamous cell carcinoma was recently examined using the national Swedish Family Cancer database from 1961 to 1998. Evidence of family clustering was found, with a standardized incidence ratio of 2.72 for invasive squamous cell carcinoma in offspring of parents with skin cancer. No correlation of squamous cell carcinoma was found between spouses suggesting that heritable factors may be more significant than adult environmental exposure.[9] Other potential genetic risk factors include racial origin, skin type, eye and hair color. Specific genes that have been linked to skin cancer include *CDKN2* and *MC1R* for melanoma, *p53* for squamous cell carcinoma and *PTCH* for basal cell carcinoma.[63–65]

INTERVENTIONAL EPIDEMIOLOGY

In a clinical trial, the investigator manipulates and allocates the exposure of subjects. Interventional studies provide the potential for a higher degree of validity of the findings of these types of studies and, potentially, for a more definitive result. The goals of interventional epidemiology include establishing reliable evidence on which public health policy and resources can be focused. Drawbacks of clinical trials include expense, ethical concerns related to exposure (or non-exposure) to the intervention, and feasibility of application.[66] To date, interventional epidemiologic design has played a more limited role in the study of cutaneous malignancies.

Trial evidence suggests that sunscreen use is important in skin cancer prevention.[6] Recently published data from the Nambour Trial, in which patients were randomly assigned to one of four treatment groups, including daily sunscreen use vs discretionary use (or beta carotene vs placebo tablets), investigators found a significant association with regular sunscreen use. Comparing 1994 with 1992, the estimated increase in the number of solar keratoses (SK) in the regular sunscreen users was 20% compared with an increase of 57% in the control group, which is the equivalent of one additional SK per person over time.[67] The Nambour Skin Cancer Prevention Trial also investigated the effectiveness of daily sunscreen use on the reduction of basal cell carcinoma and squamous cell carcinoma incidence. Daily sunscreen use had no effect on overall risk of basal cell carcinoma. However, an effect of daily sunscreen application did seem to decrease squamous cell carcinoma incidence.[68]

Sunscreen use and the development of melanocytic nevi has also been investigated in a randomized controlled trial. In British Columbia, white school children were randomly assigned to a group that was given a supply of sunscreen and application instruction, or to a control group that received neither advice nor sunscreen.

Children in the sunscreen group developed significantly fewer new nevi than the control group children, a difference in median count of 4 nevi.[69]

Clinical trials of this sort can provide additional evidence to support or to help reject suggested associations that arise from descriptive and analytic epidemiology reports. For example, findings from the Nutritional Prevention of Cancer Trial, a multi-center, randomized clinical trial of selenium supplementation in areas of the Southeastern US, were consistent with no association between selenium and melanoma, contradicting the previous associations from analytical studies that led the authors to investigate this area.[70]

Public health promotion and interventions

With the rise in skin cancer incidence, interest has increased in developing effective public health strategies to combat the disease. These strategies focus in either preventing the development of skin cancer through risk factor modification (primary prevention) or in improved disease surveillance and earlier detection of disease (secondary prevention).

Primary prevention efforts focus mainly on reducing ultraviolet exposure, a modifiable risk factor for melanoma and KC. The US Department of Health and Human Services in its Healthy People 2010 recommendations identified specific goals for reducing the risk of skin cancer. Measures identified are: sun avoidance between 10.00 hrs and 16.00 hrs, use of sun-protective clothing, use of sunscreen with a sun-protective factor (SPF) of at least 15 and avoidance of artificial ultraviolet exposure sources, like tanning beds. The goal of Healthy People 2010 is for 75% of the US population to use at least one of these sun-protective measures.[71] The American Cancer Society has followed the lead of the Australian public health authorities in publicizing the slogan, 'Slip! Slop! Slap!' This slogan encourages and reminds the public to 'slip' on a shirt, 'slop' on some sunscreen and 'slap' on a hat, for safety when outdoors in the sun.

Secondary prevention through improved and earlier detection is also encouraged. The prognosis of melanoma is closely associated with tumor thickness, and hence, detection of disease at a thinner stage should, in theory, result in an improved outcome.[10] Early detection campaigns often seek to educate health care providers and the general public on skin evaluation techniques and the appearance of suspicious lesions.[72] Both primary and secondary prevention of skin cancer are discussed in further detail in Chapter 7.

Public health interventions are often intensive and expensive. Because of resources necessary for such campaigns, measuring the impact and efficacy of promotion components is essential. Traditional programs are being improved and alternative behavior change methods are continuously being investigated. Some investigators have chosen to focus on raising awareness of the role of sun damage in aging (appearance-based as opposed to emphasizing cancer-risk), in an attempt to engage younger audiences earlier, but ultimately in an attempt to decrease cutaneous malignancies.[73] While there are numerous benefits of health promotion interventions, they also bring with them resultant costs. A cost effectiveness analysis of an Italian public education campaign for early diagnosis of melanoma was evaluated in terms of additional costs per year of life-year saved (LYS). The total cost from the educational campaign as well as the additional costs from resultant medical care (minus 'costs saved' estimated as the projected cost of treatment for stage II and stage III disease for patients healed after surgical excision for Stage I) was estimated at between L817 million to L905 million (US$519,400 to 575,300). Overall LYS was quantified by comparing the survival curves by thickness, with the LYS result from the curve of the thickness of that class and the mean of the curve below it. The estimated cost of the educational campaign per LYS was L5.28 million (US$3360).[74]

FUTURE OUTLOOK

For the past several decades, we have been able to measure melanoma incidence and mortality, and the picture has been clear and concerning: a meteoric rise in both incidence and mortality. The future situation will be more complex due to several factors, some artifactual and some real.

There may be pressures to shift diagnostic criteria for skin cancers. Pathologists' fear of legal liability may cause an artifactual increase in incidence (particularly for melanoma because of its relatively high case fatality) although there is no evidence that this is occurring to a significant degree at present. If this were to occur, the result would likely resemble a 'period' (as opposed to 'cohort') effect of increasing incidence, but have no impact on mortality.

The impact of the various diagnostic categories including dysplastic nevi, atypical nevi, Clark's nevi, lentigo maligna, and others that have been used for melanocytic dysplasias may also affect melanoma incidence, although no such effect has been documented to date. This may serve to artifactually decrease incidence due to the availability and frequent use of these alternate diagnostic categories for equivocal lesions, which are common. One might assume that the result would be a 'period effect' decrease, but since these equivocal lesions appear to be more common at younger adult ages, it may mimic a cohort effect.

Publicity around skin cancer issues has increased in recent years, and this may be causing more people to present to their physician with concern about a skin lesion, which may lead to more skin cancer diagnosis, and again leading to an artifactual increase in skin cancer incidence. In the US in recent years there appears to have been a substantial increase in visits to dermatologists for concern about skin cancer that could have some association.

Finally, changes in the healthcare system in the future will have an uncertain effect on the degree of under registration of skin cancer in established registries. For the past 30 years there has been a cycle of health system changes in the locus of skin cancer diagnosis followed by some cancer registry attempts to capture cases that might otherwise be missed due to these changes. Registries have varied in their efforts and success.

Beyond the above effects, future skin cancer rates are likely to show real impacts of several trends. First, access to sites of natural intense ultraviolet exposure may have reached a plateau in light-skinned populations worldwide, although this is uncertain. There may even be a decreasing trend among some segments of youth more enamored with video games than stickball. In either case the resulting trends in population-based incidence may not be manifest for quite some time for melanoma and BCC because of the long lag time between exposure and the cancer diagnosis. For SCC, the effect on incidence would become more rapidly apparent, although measures of SCC incidence are much less commonly available than those of melanoma incidence and the diagnostic issues for SCC are more problematic and not as well studied.

The most important issues for anticipating future trends in melanoma, SCC, and BCC are the impacts of technologic changes and of public health campaigns and awareness around skin cancer issues. One technology now in widespread use is the tanning lamp, particularly as used in commercial tanning facilities.[75,76] This allows a substantially higher ultraviolet exposure to the skin than was previously the case, and epidemiologic evidence has linked such exposures to skin cancers.[77,78] The industry that has grown around the commercialization of this practice has substantial resources and a financial interest in encouraging ultraviolet exposures in tanning parlors. The consequences for skin cancer of tanning parlors will unfold over the coming decades.

Sunscreens can reduce the risk of at least some of the adverse consequences of excessive exposure to ultraviolet radiation with appropriate application before the exposure. However, there is evidence that their use is often inadequate, so their exact impact on future skin cancer rates cannot yet be determined.[79]

Finally, the widespread campaigns aimed at skin cancer prevention do seem to be associated with improved prognosis and perhaps reduced incidence. It is clear that properly constructed campaigns can have an effect on sun-related behavior,[80] and can be associated with effects observable at the population level.[81]

The net result of these conflicting trends is uncertain. Hopefully, the effects of the above and yet heretofore undetermined factors will lead to our nearing a peak in skin cancer incidence and mortality and to decreasing rates in the future.

REFERENCES

1 Jemal A, Murray T, Samuels A, Ghafoor A, Ward E, Thun M. Cancer statistics, 2004. CA Cancer J Clin 2004, January; 54:8–29.

2 Weinstock MA. Ultraviolet radiation and skin cancer: Epidemiologic data from the USA and Canada. In: Young AR, Bjorn LO, Moan J, Nultsch W, eds. Environmental UV Photobiology. New York, NY: Plenum Press; 1993:295–344.

3 Lancaster HO. Some geographical aspects of the mortality from melanoma in Europeans. Med J Aust 1956; 1:1082–1087.

4 The Connecticut Tumor Registry. Hartford: State of Connecticut Department of Public Health, July 2001.

5 Ries LAG, Eisner MP, Kosary CL, et al. SEER Cancer Statistics Review, 1973–1999. Bethesda: National Cancer Institute; 2002.

6 Mikkilineni R, Weinstock MA. Epidemiology. In: Sober AJ, Haluska FG, eds. Atlas of Clinical Oncology: Skin Cancer. London: BC Decker, Inc; 2001:1–15.

7 Marks R. Epidemiology of melanoma. Clin Exp Dermatol 2000; 25:459–463.

8 Australian Institute of Health and Welfare. National Health Priority Areas: Cancer Indicators. http://www.aihw.gov/au/hhpa/cancer (accessed 5 September 2003).

9 Hemminki K, Zhang H, Czene K. Familiar invasive and in situ squamous cell carcinoma. Br J Cancer 2003; 88:1375–1380.

10 Weinstock MA. Skin Cancer I: Melanoma and nevi. In: Williams HC, Strachan DP, eds. The Challenge of Dermato-Epidemiology. Boca Raton, Florida: CRC Press; 1997:191–207.

10a Giles GG, Armstrong BK, Burton RC, Staples MP, Thursfield VJ. Has mortality from melanoma stopped rising in Australia? Analysis of trends between 1931 and 1934. BMJ 1996; 312:1121–1125.

11 Marrett LD, Nguyen HL, Armstrong BK. Trends in the incidence of cutaneous malignant melanoma in New South Wales, 1983–96. Int J Cancer 2001; 92:457–462.

12 de Vries E, Bray FI, Coebergh JWW, Parkin DM. Changing epidemiology of malignant cutaneous melanoma in Europe 1953–1997: Rising trends in incidence and mortality but recent stabilizations in western Europe and decreases in Scandinavia. Int J Cancer 2003; 107:119–126.

13 SEER. White, Black, Hispanic, and Asian/Pacific Islander, 1996. http://www.seer.cancer.gov (accessed 28 November 2003).

14 Boi S, Cristofolini M, Micciolo R, Palma PD. Epidemiology of Skin Tumors: Data from the Cutaneous Cancer Registry in Trentino, Italy: http://www.springerlink.com/app/home/content (accessed 19 August 2003).

15 de Vries E, Schouten LJ, Visser O, Eggermont AMM, Coebergh JWW. Rising trends in the incidence of and mortality from cutaneous melanoma in the Netherlands: a Northwest to Southeast gradient? Eur J Cancer 2002; 39:1439–1446.

16 Parkin DM, Whelan SL, Ferlay J, Teppo L, Thomas DB. Cancer Incidence in Five Continents, Vol. VIII. Lyon, France: IARC Scientific Publications; 2003.

17 Kricker A, Armstrong BK. International trends in skin cancer. Cancer Forum 1996; 20:192–195.

18 Bulliard J-L, Cox B, Elwood M. Latitude gradients in melanoma incidence and mortality in the non-Maori population of New Zealand. Cancer Causes Control 1994; 5(3):234–240.

19 Weinstock MA. Death from skin cancer among the elderly: epidemiologic patterns. Arch Dermatol 1997; 133:1207–1209.

20 CDC Wonder. Centers for Disease Control: http://wonder.cdc.gov/wonder (accessed 26 March 2003).

21 Severi G, Giles GG, Robertson C, Boyle P, Autier P. Mortality from cutaneous melanoma: evidence for contrasting trends between populations. Br J Dermatol 2000; 82(11):1887–1891.

22 van der Esch P, Muir CS, Nectoux J. Temporal change in diagnostic criteria as a cause of the increase of malignant melanoma over time is unlikely. Int J Cancer 1991; 47:483–490.

23 Cohn-Cedermark G, Mansson-Brahme E, Rutqvist LE, et al. Trends in mortality from malignant melanoma in Sweden, 1970–1996. Cancer 2000; 89:348–355.

24 Garbe C, McLeod GRC, Buettner PG. Time trends of cutaneous melanoma in Queensland, Australia and Central Europe. Cancer 2000; 89(6):1269–1278.

25 Tsao H, Rogers GS, Sober AJ. An estimate of the annual direct cost of treating cutaneous melanoma. J Am Acad Dermatol 1998; 38(5):669–680.

26 Freedberg KA, Geller AC, Lew RA, Koh HK. Screening for malignant melanoma: A cost-effectiveness analysis. J Am Acad Derm 1999; 41(5):738–745.

27 Sober AJ, Chuang T-Y, Duvic M, et al. Guidelines of care for primary cutaneous melanoma. J Am Acad Derm 2001; 45(4):579–586.

28 Hofmann U, Szedlak M, Rittgen W, Jung EG, Schadendorf D. Primary staging and follow-up in melanoma patients – monocenter evaluation of methods, costs and patient survival. Br J Cancer 2002; 87:151–157.

29 Weinstock MA, Bingham SF, Cole GW, et al. Reliability of counting actinic keratoses before and after brief consensus discussion. Arch Derm 2001; 137:1055–1058.

30 Whiteman DC, Watt P, Purdie DM, Hughes MC, Hayward NK. Green A. Melanocytic nevi, solar keratoses and divergent causal pathways to cutaneous melanoma. J Natl Cancer Inst 2003; 95(11):806–812.

31 Cancer Incidence in Five Continents, Vol. VII. Lyon: International Agency for Research on Cancer (IARC); 1997.

32 Cook J, Zitelli JA. Mohs micrographic surgery: a cost analysis. J Am Acad Derm 1998; 39:698–703.

33 Miller DL, Weinstock MA. Nonmelanoma skin cancer in the USA: Incidence. J Am Acad Dermatol 1994; 30(5):774–778.

34 English DR, Armstrong BK, Kricker A, Winter MG, Heenan PJ, Randell PL. Demographic characteristics, pigmentary and cutaneous risk factors for squamous cell carcinoma of the skin: a case-control study. Int J Cancer 1998; 76:628–634.

35 Gray DT, Suman VJ, Su WPD, et al. Trends in the population-based incidence of squamous cell carcinoma of the skin first diagnosed between 1984 and 1992. Arch Derm 1997; 133(6):735–740.

36 Hannuksela-Svahn A, Pukkala E, Karvonen J. Basal cell skin carcinoma and other non melanoma skin cancers in Finland from 1956 through 1995. Arch Derm 1999; 135:781–786.

37 Moan J, Dahlback A. The relationship between skin cancers, solar radiation and ozone depletion. Br J Cancer 1992; 65(6):916–921.

38 Karagas MR, Greenberg ER, Spencer SK, Stukel TA, Mott LA. Increase in incidence rates of basal cell and squamous cell skin cancer in New Hampshire, USA. Int J Cancer 1999; 81:555–559.

39 Harris RB, Griffith K, Moon TE. Trends in incidence of nonmelanoma skin cancers in southeastern Arizona, 1985–1996. J Am Acad Derm 2001; 45(4):528–536.

40 Holme SA, Malinovszky K, Robert DL. Changing trends in non-melanoma skin cancer in South Wales, 1988–98. Br J Dermatol 2000; 143:1224–1229.

41 Hannuksela-Svahn A, Pukkala E, Karvonen J. Basal cell skin carcinoma and other nonmelanoma skin cancers in Finland from 1956 through 1995. Arch Derm 1999; 135:781–786.

42 Koh D, Wang H, Lee J, et al. Basal cell carcinoma, squamous cell carcinoma and melanoma of the skin: analysis of the Singapore Cancer Registry data 1968–97. Br J Dermatol 2003; 148:1161–1166.

43 Weinstock MA, Bogaars HA, Ashley M, Litle V, Bilodeau E, Kimmel S. Non-melanoma skin cancer mortality. Archives of Dermatology 1991; 127:1194–1197.

44 Weinstock MA. Non-melanoma skin cancer mortality in the USA, 1969–1988. Arch Derm 1993; 129:1286–1290.

45 Levi F, Erler G, Te V-C, Randimbison L, La Vecchia C. Trends in skin cancer in Neuchatel, 1976–98. Tumori 2001; 87(5):288–289.

46 Chuang T-Y. Skin Cancer II: Nonmelanoma skin cancer. In: Williams HC, Strachan DP, eds. The Challenge of Dermato-Epidemiology. Boca Raton, Florida: CRC Press; 1997:209–222.

47 Housman TS, Feldman SR, Williford PM, et al. Skin cancer is among the most costly of all cancers to treat for the Medicare population. J Am Acad Dermatol March 2003; 48(3):425–429.

48 Chen GJ, Fleischer AB, Smith ED, et al. Cost of nonmelanoma skin cancer treatment in the United States. Derm Surg 2001; 27(12):1035.

49 Bandaranayake DM. Why do some non-melanocytic skin cancers reach an advanced stage before they are treated? The effect of delay and predictors of delay in presentation, referral and treatment of NMSC. Doctor of Philosophy dissertation, University of Newcastle, Newcastle, Australia 2002.

50 Blackford S, Roberts D, Salek MS, Finlay A. Basal cell carcinomas cause little handicap. Qual Life Res 1996; 5(2):191–194.

51 Chuang T-Y, Su WPD, Sigfrid AM. Incidence of cutaneous T cell lymphoma and other rare skin cancers in a defined population. J Am Acad Dermatol August 1990; 23(2):254–256.

52 Weinstock MA, Horm JW. Mycosis fungoides in the United States. JAMA 1988; 260(1):42–46.

53 Weinstock MA, Gardstein B. Twenty-year trends in the reported incidence of mycosis fungoides and associated mortality. Am J Public Health 1999; 89(8):1240–1244.

54 Weinstock MA, Reynes JF. The changing survival of patients with mycosis fungoides. CA Cancer J Clin 1999; 85(1):208–212.

55 Miller RW, Rabkin CS. Merkel cell carcinoma and melanoma: etiological similarities and differences. Cancer Epidemiology, Biomarkers and Prevention 1999; 8:153–158.

56 Aboulafia DM. Kaposi's sarcoma. Clin Dermatol 2001; 19:269–283.

57 Euvrard S, Kanitakis J, Claudy A. Skin cancers after organ transplantation. N Engl J Med 2003; 348:1681–1691.

58 Twonbly R. New carcinogen list includes estrogen, UV radiation. J Natl Cancer Inst 2003; 95(3):185–186.

59 Weinstock MA. Issues in the epidemiology of melanoma. Hematol/Oncol Clin North Am 1998; 12(4):681–698.

60 Milan T, Verkasalo PK, Kaprio J, Koskenvuo M, Pukkala E. Malignant skin cancers in the Finnish Twin Cohort: a population-based study, 1976–1997. Br J Dermatol 2002; 147:509–512.

61 Autier P, Dore J-F. Influence of sun exposure during childhood and during adulthood on melanoma risk. Int J Cancer 1998; 77:533–537.

62 Boyd AS, Shyr Y, King LE. Basal cell carcinoma in young women: an evaluation of the association of tanning bed use and smoking. J Am Acad Dermatol 2002; 46(5):706–709.

63 de Gruijl FR, van Kranen HJ, Mullenders LHF. UV-induced DNA damage, repair, mutations, and oncogenic pathways in skin cancer. J Photochem Photobiol 2001; 63:19–27.

64 Bataille V. Genetic epidemiology of melanoma. Eur J Cancer 2003; 39(10):1341–1347.

65 Giglia-Mari G, Sarasin A. P53 mutations in human skin cancers. Hum Mutat 2003; 21:217–228.

66 Hennekens CH, Buring JE. Epidemiology in Medicine, 1st edn. Philadelphia, PA: Lippincott Williams & Wilkins; 1987.

67 Darlington S, Williams G, Neale R, Frost C, Green A. A randomized controlled trial to assess sunscreen application and beta carotene supplementation in the prevention of solar keratoses. Arch Derm 2003; 139:451–455.

68 Green A, Williams G, Neale R, et al. Daily sunscreen application and beta carotene supplementation in prevention of basal-cell and squamous-cell carcinomas of the skin: a randomised controlled trial. Lancet 1999; 354:723–729.

69 Gallagner RP, Rivers JK, Lee TK, et al. Broad-spectrum sunscreen use and the development of new nevi in white children. JAMA 2000; 283(22):2955–2960.

70 Duffield-Lillico AJ, Reid ME, Turnbull BW, et al. Baseline characteristics and the effect of selenium supplementation on cancer incidence in a randomized clinical trial: a summary report of the Nutritional Prevention of Cancer Trial. Biomarkers and Prevention 2002; 11:630–639.

71 US Department of Health and Human Services. Health People 2010. Washington, DC: US Department of Health and Human Services; 2000.

72 Jones LME, Weinstock MA. Ultraviolet light. In: Colditz GA, Hunter D, eds. Cancer Prevention: The Causes and Prevention of Cancer, Vol 1. Dordrecht, Netherlands: Kluwer; 2000:111–122.

73 Mahler HIM, Kulik JA, Gibbons FX, Gerrard M, Harrell J. Effects of appearance-based interventions on sun protection intentions and self-reported behaviors. Health Psych 2003; 22(2):199–209.

74 Garattini L, Cainelli T, Tribbia G, Scopelliti D. Economic evaluation of an educational campaign for early diagnosis of cutaneous melanoma. Pharmaco Economics 1996; 9(2):146–155.

75 Cokkinides VE, Weinstock MA, O'Connell MC, Thun M. Use of indoor tanning sunlamps by US youth, ages 11–18 years, and by their parent or guardian caregivers: prevalence and correlates. Pediatrics 2002; 109(6):1124–1130.

76 Demko CA, Borawski EA, Debanne SM, Cooper KD, Stange KC. Use of indoor tanning facilities by white adolescents in the USA. Arch Pediatr Adolesc Med 2003; 157:854–860.

77 Swerdlow AJ, Weinstock MA. Do tanning lamps cause melanoma? An epidemiologic assessment. J Am Acad Derm 1998; 38(1):89–98.

78 Karagas MR, Stannard VA, Mott LA, et al. Use of tanning devices and risk of basal cell and squamous cell skin cancers. J Natl Cancer Inst 2002; 94(3):224–226.

79 Davis KJ, Cokkinides VE, Weinstock MA, O'Connell MC, Wingo PA. Summer sunburn and sun exposure among US youths ages 11 to 18: national prevalence and associated factors. Pediatrics 2002; 110(1):27–35.

80 Dietrich AJ, Olson AL, Sox CH, Tosteson TD, Grant-Petersson J. Persistent increase in children's sun protection in a randomized controlled community trial. Prev Med 2000; 31:569–574.

81 Staples M, Marks R, Giles G. Trends in the incidence of non-melanocytic skin cancer (NMSC) treated in Australia 1985–1995: Are primary prevention programs starting to have an effect? Int J Cancer 1998; 78:144–148.

CHAPTER
5

Etiological Factors in Skin Cancers: Environmental and Biological

Noah Scheinfeld and Vincent A DeLeo

Key points

- The cause of the vast majority of basal cell cancer, squamous cell cancer and melanoma is exposure to ultraviolet radiation.
- Less frequent causes of cutaneous cancer include viruses, ionizing radiation, chemical agents, heat and trauma.
- Cutaneous carcinogenesis is a multistage process involving initiation, promotion, conversion and progression – all of which can result from interaction of skin with ultraviolet radiation.
- Further research is necessary to understand the mechanisms involved in the development of skin cancer, particularly in the case of basal cell carcinoma and melanoma.

INTRODUCTION

The etiological factors that underlie the development of skin cancer are multiple and interrelated. Both endogenous factors (e.g. genes) and exogenous factors (e.g. ultraviolet radiation) are involved. The interaction of these factors is complex and they usually act synergistically in the multistage process of carcinogenesis, which includes tumor initiation, promotion, premalignant progression and malignant conversion of normal skin cells into skin cancers.

A variety of exogenous factors have been related to the development of skin cancer. By far the most important of these is ultraviolet radiation from sunlight. Other exogenous factors include: (1) ionizing radiation, (2) human papilloma virus, (3) chemical carcinogens that include industrial oils and hydrocarbons (e.g. coal, petroleum products), dyes, solvents and arsenic and pesticides, (4) chronic irritation and (5) hyperthermia (Table 5.1).

These exogenous factors and other endogenous factors affect DNA function and replication, cell membrane, immune function, enzymatic activity and overall cellular function. The exact mechanisms by which these etiologic factors induce changes in cellular function are an ongoing area of intense investigation.

As would be expected, different types of skin cancer are induced by different exogenous and endogenous factors. Most research has focused on squamous cell carcinoma (SCC), since only that skin cancer can be

reliably reproduced in animal models. This chapter will therefore focus on the environmental and biological factors that underlie SCC. Some mention will be made however concerning research on the causation of basal cell carcinoma (BCC) and malignant melanoma (MM).

HISTORY

The role of exogenous substances in the development of cancer has been a subject of investigation for almost three centuries. Interestingly, one of the earliest published observations dealt with chemical induction of SCC when in the 1750s, Percival Potts demonstrated that occupational exposures can result in cancers and specifically showed that chimney sweeps developed skin cancer of the scrotum from soot. By 1934, the link between ionizing radiation and SCC was already suspected when the International Congress of Radiology, a commission to assess the occurrence of cancers among medical users of radioactive chemicals, was created. In 1945, Harold Blum published work documenting a dose response relationship for the induction of skin tumors in mice by ultraviolet radiation and he demonstrated that ultraviolet B radiation was the causative portion of the solar spectrum.

Epidemiology

The vast majority of all skin cancers are thought to be caused by exposure to ultraviolet radiation. Thus, unsurprisingly, the incidence of BCC and SCC is highest among fair-skinned Caucasians who live close to the equator or in tropical regions. Being born into such regions confers a greater risk of developing skin cancer than emigrating to such regions. In this regard, blond or red hair and a pale complexion are major risk factors. As one might expect Australia, where fair-skinned people live closest to the equator, leads the world in the incidence of skin cancers.

There is also epidemiological evidence for involvement of chemical exposure in certain occupations, in increasing the risk of developing skin cancer. This includes occupations that involve work with oils, solvents and tars.[1] In this occupational context, it is interesting that conflicting evidence exists on whether airline personnel (ultraviolet exposure)[2] and those working in atomic laboratories (ionizing radiation) have an increased risk of skin cancer.[3,4]

Table 5.1 Etiologic factors in the development of skin cancers
Endogenous
Genes
Exogenous
Ultraviolet radiation
Ionizing radiation
Viruses
Chemicals
Industrial oils and hydrocarbons
Dyes
Solvents
Arsenic
Pesticides
Tobacco
Chronic irritation
Hyperthermia

Table 5.2 Stages of carcinogenesis
Initiation – induction
Promotion
Premalignant conversion
Malignant progression

Biochemistry of the induction, promotion and conversion of skin cancer

The biochemistry of the development of SCC has been extensively investigated in murine skin. The classic mouse model for the study of skin cancer has been used for decades to study the mechanism of development of SCC. From these studies, a multistage model of carcinogenesis has been developed. This multistage model of carcinogenesis, developed in skin, has been found to be relevant to development of most cancer regardless of tissue of origin.

The classic model involves four stages: initiation/induction, promotion, pre-malignant progression and malignant conversion (Table 5.2).

Initiation results when an exogenous agent causes genetic damage and results in mutations, which alter cellular proliferative controls and/or the machinery of differentiation. *Promotion* involves the expansion of the initiated cell population or clone and is thought to be due to epigenetic effects. *Progression* and *conversion* are marked by cells with a high level of genetic instability, chromosomal abnormalities, surface substance expression and oncogene activity. An in-depth discussion of the biochemistry behind the initiation/induction, promotion and conversion of skin cancer can be found in Chapter 1.

As an example of this complexity of the process of carcinogenesis a brief discussion of the role of soluble mediators is instructive. The regulation of these mediators by which cells and tissues communicate with each other locally and systemically occurs throughout the multistage process. For example, although TGFβ inhibits growth of normal epithelial cells, it is paradoxically overexpressed in many epithelial cancers. It has been postulated that TGFβ acts as a tumor suppressor at the early stages of carcinogenesis, but over-expression of TGFβ at late stages of carcinogenesis may be a critical factor for tumor invasion and metastasis.[5] Prostaglandins formed along a dysregulated cyclooxygenase (COX) pathway have been shown to mediate tumor promotion in animal experiments and may play a role, in addition, in other processes involved in tumor growth such as angiogenesis, metastasis and immunosuppression.[6] FasL-mediated apoptosis is important for skin homeostasis, suggesting that the dysregulation of Fas–FasL interactions may be central to the development of skin cancer.[7] Finally, PDGF, a major factor activated in wound healing, may play an important role as an endogenous promoter in epithelial tumor formation.[8]

Ultraviolet radiation

Ultraviolet radiation, visible light, infrared radiation, gamma rays, and X-rays are all parts of the electromagnetic spectrum. Visible, ultraviolet, and infrared radiation is incapable of causing ionization of molecules and is therefore referred to as non-ionizing. Such radiation travels as three-dimensional waves in a vacuum and acts as discrete 'packets' of energy or photons when interacting with matter. In order for such radiation to have an effect in biologic systems, it must be absorbed by the molecules of such systems. The energy of a photon of non-ionizing radiation defines its ability to interact with a given molecule. Energy of a photon varies inversely with its wavelength. Radiation by convention is described in terms of wavelength and the nanometer is the measure commonly used.

The effects of non-ionizing radiations on human cells rely on complex cellular interactions. Specifically, once the radiation is absorbed the molecule is raised to an excited state. In an effort to dissipate the absorbed energy and return to the ground or resting state the energy can be converted to chemical change which in turn results in biologic alterations.

Exposure to ultraviolet radiation is the most common etiological factor in the development of skin cancer. Persons who live close to the equator have a 2.4-fold higher incidence of SCC as contrasted to persons living in higher latitudes. Persons who are born in Australia, where ultraviolet exposure is great have higher rates of cancer than those who emigrate there suggesting that early exposure may be more damaging.

Ultraviolet-B (UVB) (290–320 nm), ultraviolet-A (UVA) (320–400 nm) (UVA1 340–400 and UVA2 320 nm–340 nm) and ultraviolet-C (UVC) (200–290 nm) radiation can induce DNA damage as well as a myriad of effects on other cellular structures and function. This damage results in SCC, BCC and MM. At the present time UVC does not reach the earth's surface since it is absorbed by the ozone layer and is therefore not important in inducing skin cancer from sunlight (Table 5.3).

UVB causes mutations and immunosuppressive effects that are essential to photo-carcinogenesis. UVB induced DNA damage leads to modifications in oncogene and tumor suppressor gene expression, which is probably the most important event in initiation of skin tumors.

The immunomodulatory effects of UVB occur through: (1) the induction of apoptosis, (2) the expression of cell-

Table 5.3 Non-ionizing radiation	
UVC	<290 nm
UVB	290–320 nm
UVA	320–400 nm
UVA2	320–340 nm
UVA1	340–400 nm
Visible	400–700 nm
Infra-red	>700 nm

surface receptors and (3) the production of soluble mediators.

UVB effects are primarily limited to the epidermis and involve disruption of cellular DNA. The type of mutation that ultraviolet B (UVB) causes is very specific. When ultraviolet radiation strikes the skin, it is absorbed by pyrimidine bases in DNA and induces the formation of cis-syn diastereomers of cyclobutane-type pyrimidine dimers and pyrimidine (6–4) pyrimidone lesions and alkali-able Dewar valence isomers.[9] These photoproducts result in the covalent association of adjacent pyrimidines and usually occur in areas of consecutive pyrimidine residues, which are preferential areas for mutation.[10] Cyclobutane dimers occur one third as commonly as (6–4) pyrimidone lesions[11] but the quantities and placements of such mutations vary based on the nucleotides flanking the mutations.[12]

The formation of these thymidine dimers and 6–4 photoproducts is the primary event in the induction of most skin cancers and represent the beginning of the initiation stage of carcinogenesis. This is true of SCC and likely important in BCC as well. Their role in the induction of MM is not documented, but may also play an important role.

Unrepaired or incorrectly repaired pyrimidine dimers lead to mutations that are very specific to UVB. In such mutations, cytosine (C) is changed to thymine (T), often when two cytosines are adjacent or a C is adjacent to a T. These specific types of mutations, that is C to T or CC to TT transitions, are referred to as the 'signature' or 'fingerprint' of the effect of UVB on DNA.

In addition to the direct results of UVB on DNA, many of the effects of UVB involve the production of reactive oxygen species (ROS). The absorbing molecule or chromophore for these reactions is unknown. The reactive species induced include hydrogen peroxide, superoxide anions and singlet oxygens. These induce single strand breaks in DNA,[9,10] purine base modifications[11] and alkali-labile sites.[12] Breakage effects have been found in cells from skin cancer-prone patients with the disorders dysplastic nevus syndrome and basal cell nevus syndrome.[13]

UVB induces immunosuppression in skin by affecting many cells and tissue functions including decreasing the number of Langerhans cells in the epidermis and modifying their antigen-presenting cell capacity.[14] One study has noted that systemic effect of UVB radiation can interfere with natural host control mechanisms and result in cancers at distant sites.[15]

Other reported effects of UVB radiation in skin include alteration of a number of systems, which may play a role in the promotion stage of carcinogenesis. These include UVB stimulation of production of both phospholipase A (1 or 2) and lysophospholipase which has profound effects on UVB-induced inflammation and control of cell growth in human skin.[16]

UVB used therapeutically has a low risk of producing cutaneous cancers, with the possible exception of those on male genital skin. In a study of 85 patients with psoriasis who received UVB for at most 25 years, Larko and Swanbeck did not demonstrate an increased risk for SCC and BCC in treated patients compared with controls.[17] Other studies have replicated these findings.

While most studies show that the primary part of the solar spectrum responsible for the development of SCC and BCC is UVB, UVA is also carcinogenic, but not as efficient, probably by orders of magnitude. UVA is important however since it makes up 90–95% of the ultraviolet radiation reaching human skin.

UVB and UVA radiation both exert immunomodulatory effects, which result from different photobiological mechanisms. UVA radiation affects both epidermal and dermal chromophores.[18] UVA induces persistent genomic instability in human keratinocytes through an oxidative stress mechanism.[19] Unlike UVB, UVA-mediated damage can occur indirectly through UV radiation absorption by non-DNA endogenous sensitizers, generating reactive oxygen species (ROS). ROS can cause DNA damage, breaks and, ultimately, mutations. The major UVA-induced ROS produced in DNA is 8-hydroxyguanine, which appears to be highly mutagenic.

In addition to DNA effects UVA induces phospholipase activation[20] and stimulates arachidonic acid release and cyclooxygenase activity in mammalian cells in culture.[21] UVA also induces protein kinase C activity.[22] UVA radiation transiently disrupts gap junctional communication in human keratinocytes.[23]

Experimental models have shown that UVA1 exposure induces SCC largely without the characteristic *p53* point mutations (see below). Both UVB and UVA radiation can give rise to ROS-related point mutations (e.g. G to T). Both result in genetic changes (e.g. frame-shifts) that may not be seen as normally initiated by ultraviolet radiation.

Photosensitizers can play an important role in UVA's carcinogenesis. The therapeutic combination of oral psoralen and UVA (PUVA) appears to be particularly capable of inducing skin cancers. PUVA appears to be a carcinogen by itself for SCC with a linear increase in tumor risk but this is not as true for BCC development.[24] Prior therapy with methotrexate might be a risk factor for skin cancer in PUVA-treated patients.[25]

The exposure to UVA may not be blocked by normal sun protection steps like sunscreen usage, which may be inadequate to shield persons from its effects. UVA also penetrates window glass so that exposure to UVA, but not UVB can occur in automobiles and inside home or workplace when near windows. UVA and UVB exposure can also come from sources other then sunlight such as sunlamps commonly used in tanning salons. In addition, a recent study demonstrated that summer clothing proved surprisingly ineffective as a barrier to UVA radiation, and that such clothing permitted a larger percent transmission of UVA than UVB.

UV induced mutations

The role of UVA and UVB in carcinogenesis is related in large part to their effect on the tumor suppressor gene *p53*. *p53* is the most commonly mutated tumor suppressor gene. *p53*'s role in the development of SCC is believed to be central. Mutated *p53* is present in more than 50% of breast, lung and colon cancers and is found in more than 90% of SCCs and in most BCCs. *p53* mutations are also found in most actinic keratoses. Mutations in the PTCH gene appears to also be important in the development of BCC and interestingly, BCCs have been reported with defects in both *p53* and PTCH.[26]

Over 90% of SCCs and more than 50% of BCCs contain UV-like mutations in the *p53* tumor suppressor gene. The function of *p53* in normal skin is indicated by the observation that inactivating *p53* in mouse skin reduces the appearance of sunburn cells, apoptotic keratinocytes generated by UV overexposure.[27] The apoptosis that *p53* induces helps to weed out precancerous cells. When *p53* does not function, a sunburn cell can lead to an actinic keratosis among the *p53*-mutated cells, suggesting that sunlight has a dual function: as tumor initiator and as tumor promoter. That is, UV drives a clonal selection process in favor of pre-cancerous and cancerous cells.[28] Studies have demonstrated that UVB can induce mutations in *p53* in mice transplanted with human skin that result in actinic keratoses and SCCs.[29]

MM risk appears associated with more intense, intermittent exposure to sunlight. The effects of ultraviolet radiation on melanocytes are complex. Its effects on *p53* in melanocytes are less dramatic then in keratinocytes. Tyrosinase and TRP1, which are involved in melanin synthesis, have also been implicated as downstream effectors of *p53*. Tyrosinase can be induced after UV radiation in a *p53*-dependent manner.

UV also stimulates production of growth factors in skin cells. How these factors result in MM has yet to be defined. Experimental studies with a fish model suggest that UVA may play a more significant role but the relationship of this model to humans should be severely scrutinized.[30]

Ionizing radiation

Ionizing radiation has electromagnetic forms (X-rays and gamma rays) and particulate forms (electrons, protons, alpha particles, and neutrons). X-rays, gamma rays and electrons are classified as sparsely ionizing, whereas alpha particles (such as those associated with radon) and neutrons are densely ionizing. Ionizing radiation can produce ionizations in target molecules, such as DNA, directly or indirectly by interactions with water molecules that result in the ROS formation. Because ionizing events from sparsely ionizing radiation exposures produce mostly ROS and are sparsely distributed, damage to DNA and other targets from such radiation is principally a result of indirect mechanisms mediated by ROSs. Densely ionizing radiation more commonly exerts direct effects and actual physical damage to DNA.

The incidence of skin cancers as related to ionizing radiation seems related and proportional to the total dose of radiation. Individual fractionated doses of more than 12–15 Gy are generally thought to be necessary to induce tumor formation. Most SCC and BCC that occur after exposure to ionizing radiation have a latency of several months to several decades with most cases occurring 20 years after initial exposure. One case was noted to appear 70 years after radiation treatment for tinea capitis.

Ionizing radiation most commonly induces BCC. Its role in the induction of SCC is controversial. These effects have been studied in mice.[31] One study noted that therapeutic radiation is associated with BCC but not with SCC.[32] Another study found increased risk of SCC and BCC from radiotherapy, especially in individuals prone to sunburn with sun exposure (facial areas in which acne was treated with radiation).[26]

Certain clinical situations have been well described with BCC after treatment with ionizing radiation. In a study of 2224 children given X-ray therapy for tinea capitis compared to a control group of 1380 tinea capitis patients given only topical medications, the relative risk (RR) for BCC of the head and neck among irradiated Caucasians was 3.6.[33] Specifically, treatment of tinea capitis with radiation has been linked to the development of multiple BCC.[34] In another study in mouse skin, radiation can act as a weak initiator of SCCs and induce BCCs.[35]

Portwine stains treated with radiation and argon lasers have developed BCC.[36] Multiple synchronous pigmented BCCs have been reported following radiotherapy for Hodgkin's disease.[37] Skin cancers have also been reported after accidental exposure to ionizing radiation.[36]

Recent studies suggest that ionizing radiation does not increase the risk of MM,[38] however there are case reports which dispute this. One report noted two patients with MM occurring within a previously irradiated area suggesting that genetic mutations (based on associated family history) probably underlie its etiology.[39] Another study showed that radiation technologists who started working before the 1950s had increased risk for developing MM.[40]

Basal cell nevus syndrome (Gorlin syndrome, BCNS) is an autosomal dominant disorder in which patients are abnormally susceptible to developing BCC after exposure to ionizing radiation. Affected persons usually have a defect in the PTCH gene. The effects of ionizing radiation on this gene have been studied,[41] but the mechanisms underlying the abnormal radio-susceptibility of cells in patients with BCNS has not been well characterized. One report noted an increase in the number of nucleoli in fibroblast cells from three patients with BCNS after ionizing radiation treatment concomitant with the increase of ribonucleoprotein immunoreactive aggregates within the nucleus. These changes were thought to be related to alterations in RNA synthesis metabolism.[42]

Viruses

To date, 86 distinct HPV types have been identified and fully sequenced, and more than 130 putative novel sequences have been partly characterized. All identified types appear to be strictly epitheliotropic, and the full vegetative viral lifecycle of HPV is precisely linked to keratinocyte differentiation.

The mechanism of HPV induction of SCC is best defined in anogenital cancers. Epidemiological and experimental studies now overwhelmingly implicate HPV as the causal agent in cervical cancer. Viral E6 and E7 proteins have been confirmed as cellular immortalizing agents that interfere with functions of the *p53* and retinoblastoma tumor suppressor proteins, respectively. Evidence for the involvement of specific HPV types in SCC originated from studies of patients suffering from the rare hereditary disease epidermodysplasia verruciformis (EV) and from patients who have had organ transplants and utilized immunosuppressive medications. In affected patients the role HPV exerts appears to be synergistic, that is, interactions of the virus and ultraviolet radiation with host cells lead to a multitude of changes that eventuate in SCC. This process has been shown to involve host cytokines and cellular proteins including *p53* and the pro-apoptotic protein Bak.

The role of viruses in skin cancer in otherwise healthy patients has yet to be defined. Specifically, the evidence for human papillomaviruses (HPV) role in carcinogenesis is considerably less convincing for non-anogenital skin cancers than for anogenital cancers. Interestingly, HPV DNA has been frequently detected in apparently normal skin, hair follicles and benign hyperproliferative dermatoses. Data on skin cancers from immunocompetent individuals have tended to report a lower prevalence of HPV DNA than in those from compromised individuals, ranging from 0 to 55% for SCC and 31–43.5% for BCC.

Epidermodysplasia verruciformis (EV)

EV is a rare genodermatosis caused by nonsense mutations in the genes EVER1 and EVER2 located at chromosome 17q25. The gene products of EVER1 and EVER2 have features of integral membrane proteins and are localized in the endoplasmic reticulum. The clinical picture of EV results from an abnormal susceptibility to infection with specific HPV types. These types include HPV 5, 8, 9, 12, 14, 15, 17, 19–25, 36–38, 47 and 49. SCCs occur on sun-exposed sites in 30–60% of EV patients, and over 90% contain mostly HPV5 and occasionally HPV8, 14, 17, 20 or 47. These HPV types occur with increased copy numbers in episomal rather than integrated forms.

Clinical pathological observations have repeatedly underlined the strict requirement for ultraviolet radiation (UVR) in EV carcinogenesis. This synergistic effect of virus and ultraviolet radiation has recently been underscored by the finding of *p53* mutations in over 60% of EV SCCs and up to 40% of pre-malignant lesions. The situation in EV tumors thus clearly differs from cervical cancer, in which *p53* is predominantly wild type as its function is undermined by E6 in a focused fashion. In EV it has been shown that the E6 contributes to tumor progression by degradation of the ultraviolet-induced protein, Bak. Diseases related to EV are covered in further depth in Chapter 12.

Transplant patients and warts

Fundamental to understanding the role of HPV in cancer has been the study of immunologically suppressed patients, especially those who have received organ transplants. The incidence of warts and SCC which arise on sun-exposed sites is greatly increased (up to 100-fold) in transplant patients. Transplant skin cancers are predominantly SCCs, with a reversal of the BCC to SCC ratio of approximately 3:1 seen in the general population, and tumors at times may be multiple and highly aggressive. Such tumors tend to recur and metastasize more often then in healthy controls.

Interestingly, SCCs in transplant patients usually show many clinical and histopathological features that are similar to transplant warts. Moreover, warts in transplant patients can demonstrate significant dysplasia. Skin cancers are the most common malignancies seen in transplant patients and they are independently associated with the presence of viral warts.

HPV DNA is found in approximately 70–90% of transplant-associated SCCs. Tumors from transplant recipients contain HPV strains that occur in common benign cutaneous lesions (HPV types 1 and 2), epidermodysplasia verruciformis (HPV 5), oncogenic (HPV types 16 and 18) and nononcogenic (HPV types 6 and 11). Sometimes, several HPV strains are detected within a single tumor. Persistent infection with either or both oncogenic and non-oncogenic HPV strains appears to be carcinogenic.

Interactions with *p53* may be involved in promotion of cancer by HPV. There is a consensus *p53*-binding motif in the upstream regulatory region of HPV77, a cutaneous HPV type first identified in a transplant patient. SCC physiological activation of *p53* by UVR leads to the stimulation of HPV77 promoter activity.[43]

There is conflicting evidence in the literature concerning a common *p53* polymorphism which has an arginine substitution for proline at codon 72. These two forms of the gene results in electrophoretically distinct forms of the protein. The two polymorphic alleles of *p53* have distinct biochemical and functional properties, including their ability to signal apoptosis following DNA damage. Preliminary studies suggest that the arginine form was preferentially degraded by E6 proteins from both high- and low-risk mucosal HPV types.

E7, as stated previously, interferes with the function of the retinoblastoma gene (RB). Its gene product is a negative regulator of growth and a positive affector of differentiation. Hypophosphorylated RB is active and binds and inactivates the function of transcription factors such as E2F. E7 binds and sequesters RB leaving factors such as E2F to activate the protooncogenes *myc*, *myb* and *fos*. The latter's gene products promote proliferation. The foregoing observations aside, the exact mechanism by which E7 induces its carcinogenic effects especially in concert E6, remain to be defined.

The risk of developing skin cancer in transplant patients is linked to the level of immunosuppression. A retrospective study showed that kidney-transplant recipients who were receiving prednisolone, azathioprine, and cyclosporine had a risk of SCC that was three times as high as the risk among those receiving prednisolone and azathioprine alone. In a related fashion, in patients with skin cancer type IV hypersensitivity responses to recall antigens was lower then in normal controls. These

70 Copcu E, Aktas A, Sisman N, Oztan Y. Thirty-one cases of Marjolin's ulcer. Clin Exp Derm 2003; 28(2):138–141.

71 Kurdina MI, Denisov LE, Vinogradova NN. Groups at high risk for skin cancer. Vopr Onkol 1994; 40:216–220.

72 Sehgal VN, Reddy BS, Koranne RV, et al. Squamous cell carcinoma complicating chronic discoid lupus erythematosus (CDLE). J Dermatol 1983; 10:81–84.

73 Camisa C. Squamous cell carcinoma arising in acne conglobata. Cutis 1984; 33:185–187.

74 Gooptu C, Marks N, Thomas J, James MP. Squamous cell carcinoma associated with lupus vulgaris. Clin Exp Dermatol 1988; 23:99–102.

General reference:

Miller SJ, Maloney ME (eds). Cutaneous oncology: pathophysiology, diagnosis and management. Malden: Blackwell Science 1998.

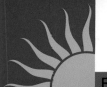

CHAPTER
6

Current Concepts in Sunscreens and Usage

Mark F Naylor and Darrell S Rigel

Key points

- Studies have demonstrated that the correct usage of sunscreens can lower subsequent risk for actinic keratoses, squamous cell carcinoma and nevi.
- Prospective studies are needed to better assess the magnitude of the protection provided.
- The combination of regularly using sunscreen, using protective clothing and avoiding mid-day sun appears to lower subsequent skin cancer risk.
- Clinical recommendations for regular sunscreen usage continue to be appropriate.

INTRODUCTION

Sunscreens are topical preparations that attenuate ultraviolet (UV) incident to the skin. Most commercial preparations try to maintain transparency in the visible ranges since an invisible preparation is more acceptable to the public. An ideal sunscreen should be cheap, easy to apply in a uniform layer that is sufficiently effective, be invisible on the skin, stop 100% of incident UV and the wearer should be unaware that it is present. Unfortunately, no such sunscreens exist. Even if ideal sunscreens existed, they would not be 100% effective because sunscreens are rarely, if ever, applied perfectly.

Sunscreens only attenuate sunlight and never completely eliminate it. The word 'block' implies that all of the harmful effects are being completely blocked leading to a false sense of security. Since real sunscreens never do this, the word 'block' should be completely eliminated from the lexicon used to describe them, particularly from sunscreen labels and advertising.

All of the preparations currently available are approximations that fall short of the mark of the 'ideal' sunscreen. However, even in their currently available forms, they are very useful pharmacological agents for attenuating the short and long-term effects of sunlight if used appropriately.

SPF, which stands for *Sun Protection Factor*, is a measure of a sunscreen's ability to prevent the development of one of the consequences of massive UV over-exposure, erythema. If a fair-skinned individual would normally sunburn in 10 min of exposure to noon sun, with an SPF 15 sunscreen properly applied, he would get the same sunburn in 150 min, or 2.5 hrs. In sunscreens, SPF measures their ability to attenuate UVB, the major contributor to sun-induced erythema.

'Sunscreening agent' is the term used in Medline to describe the individual active ingredients in sunscreens. The term 'sunscreen' is generally used to describe the mixture of several ingredients in an appropriate base, e.g. a usable product that can actually be applied to skin. For greater clarity, these conventions will be used throughout this chapter.

MECHANISMS OF ACTION

Sunscreening agents work primarily through two mechanisms: (1) scattering and reflection of UV energy and (2) absorption of UV energy. Many sunscreen preparations contain ingredients that work through both mechanisms.

Scattering and reflection

Submicroscopic particles of zinc oxide and titanium dioxide are the prototypical agents that work primarily by scattering and reflection. In this process, UV energy bounces off the sunscreen particulates and back into the environment (Fig. 6.1).

The manufacturing process in a particulate sunscreen is very important. Particle size is a critical determinant of its sunscreening characteristics. Small particle size is also important to minimize visibility. However, formulation chemists have generally found it impossible to produce a pure particulate sunscreen with an SPF >15 without some noticeable whitening effect (which many sunscreen users find objectionable). Tinting the sunscreen can help with this problem, but this makes assumptions about the skin color of the user. Frequently, particulate sunscreens are formulated in combination with the so-called chemical sunscreening agents, which are molecules (as opposed to submicroscopic particles) that act primarily by absorption of UV. This is usually done to get the SPF high enough for a satisfactory preparation without a significant whitening effect.

Coating the particles is a manufacturing process that is used to reduce free radical formation, an undesirable characteristic of particulate sunscreens. Particulate sunscreens also absorb some of the UV energy and their behavior is to some extent like a so-called chemical sunscreening agent that acts primarily by absorption of UV. Table 6.1 summarizes sunscreening agents used commonly in the US.

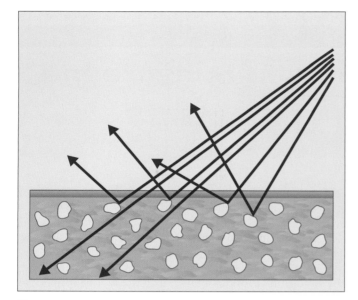

Figure 6.1 Attenuation of ultraviolet (UV) by scattering and reflection. Most of the incident UV is reflected and scattered back into the environment.

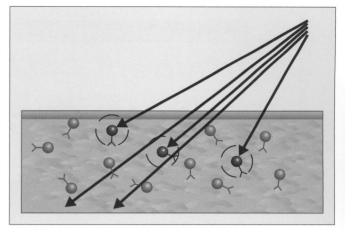

Figure 6.2 Attenuation of ultraviolet (UV) by absorption. Sunscreen molecules absorb UV energy in their electron structure and re-radiate the energy as less energetic radiation, usually infrared (heat).

Table 6.1 Commonly used sunscreening agents in the US
Chemical agents (UV absorbing molecules)
Benzophenones
Benzophenone
Oxybenzone
Cinnamates
Octyl methoxycinnamate
Cinoxate
Salicylates
Homosalicylate
Octyl salicylate
Other
Avobenzone
Octocrylene
Mexoryl SX
Physical agents (UV reflecting microscopic particles)
Titanium dioxide
Zinc oxide

Table 6.2 Current common sunscreening agents and their UV protective wavelengths

Sunscreening agent	Range of protection (nm)	Maximal effect of protection (nm)
PABA and PABA esters		
PABA	260–313	283
Padimate O	290–315	311
Padimate A	290–315	309
Glycerol aminobenzoate	260–313	297
Cinnamates		
Octyl methoxycinnamate	280–310	311
Cinoxate	270–328	290
Salicylates		
Homosalicylate	290–315	306
Octyl salicylate	260–310	307
Triethanolamine salicylate	269–320	298
Octocrylene	287–323	303
Etocrylene	296–383	303
Benzophenones		
Oxybenzone	270–350	290,325
Dioxybenzone	206–380	284,327
Sulisobenzone	250–380	286,324
Menthylanthranilate	200–380	336
Dibenzoylmethanes		
Tert-butylmethoxy-dibenzoylmethane (Parsol)	310–400	358
4-isopropyldibenzoyl-methane (Eusolex)	310–400	345
Mexoryl SX	295–390	338

Absorption

Sunscreening agents that primarily act through absorption of UV energy have been termed 'chemical' sunscreening agents to distinguish them from particulate sunscreening agents that act primarily by scattering and reflecting UV energy. Chemical sunscreening agents are individual molecules that absorb UV energy into their electron structures and re-radiate the energy at different (less dangerous) wavelengths, principally as infrared or heat energy (Fig. 6.2).

There are several classes of sunscreening agents available in the US that have different spectral absorption characteristics as summarized in Table 6.2. Usually these are blended together in various concentrations to try and achieve something closer to the ideal absorption profile (100% of all incident UV) than is achievable with each individual agent. The exact formulation of most successful sunscreens is a proprietary secret.

Para-amino benzoic acid (PABA) was introduced in the US in the early 1970s. One of the major characteristics of PABA that made it so effective as a sunscreening agent was its ability to bind to epidermal cells. This made PABA-based sunscreens fairly water and perspiration resistant, but also made them prone to staining. PABA attenuates UV radiation most effectively in the UVB range (290–320 nm). Although it was originally one of the most commonly used commercial sunscreening agents, because of problems with staining and with allergic contact sensitization it has largely been replaced by other agents or its derivatives, the PABA esters.

The PABA esters, Padimate A, Padimate O and Glyceryl PABA have the absorption characteristics of PABA but have the additional advantage of only rarely staining. Therefore, most current PABA containing sunscreens use the PABA esters.

However, PABA has a major disadvantage compared with other sunscreen components. There is a much higher presence of contact and photocontact allergy to PABA than to other sunscreening agents.[1] Among PABA-based chemicals, Padimate A is often chosen for use in sunscreen compounds due to the PABA esters' lower allergic incidence. However, sunscreens with PABA esters may contain up to 0.2–4.5% PABA. This may account for the many allergic reactions seen with these agents. For all of the above reasons, most new formulations do not include PABA or its derivatives.

Benzophenones are the second most commonly found component of sunscreens. Although their primary protective range is found in the UVA range (320–400 nm), a secondary protective band is noted in the UVB zone. Benzophenones were originally used alone as a PABA free sunscreen alternative, but are now combined with other sunscreening agents to provide broad-spectrum coverage.

The most commonly used benzophenone agents are oxybenzone and dioxybenzone. These ingredients are much less allergenic than PABA and do not stain. However, the benzophenones are less water resistant than PABA. Therefore, the bases that are used in benzophenone containing sunscreens must be thicker and less cosmetically acceptable.

Cinnamates, a derivative of cinnamon, also make good sunscreening agents. Their products are chemically related to balsam of Peru, tolu balsam, coca leaves, cinnamic aldehyde, and cinnamic oil. Therefore, persons with sensitivity to these items may cross-react to sunscreens containing cinnamates. The most commonly used cinnamates are octyl methoxycinnamate and cinoxate. Cinnamates are non-staining but also have poor water resistant qualities. Therefore, cinnamate products may require more frequent re-application and/or special substantive bases.

Salicylates are among the original sunscreen chemicals. Homomenthyl salicylate absorbs primarily in the UVB range and is typically added to other components to increase SPF. Octyl and triethanolamine salicylates are also used. They may cause photocontact dermatitis more frequently than homomenthyl salicylate and are therefore used less frequently.

Anthranilates, such as menthylanthranilate, provide low-level, yet broad-spectrum coverage, and are commonly added to sunscreens to augment protection.

Recent concerns over the effects of UVA radiation on the skin have demonstrated the need for better UVA protection in sunscreens. The newest ingredients that have shown to have the best UVA protection are the dibenzoylmethanes. Because they offer less protection from UVB, they must be used in combination with other ingredients. Tert-butylmethoxydibenzoylmethane (Avobenzone, Parsol 1789) is approved for use in the US. Its range of coverage is 310–400 nm with peak effectiveness at 358 nm. A second member of this family, Isopropyldibenzoylmethane (Eusolex 8020) has been used in Europe for several years. Because of the high incidence of contact dermatitis reactions associated with its use, it has not been approved for incorporation into sunscreens in the US.

Sunscreen bases are quite important to the success of a preparation. For example, the base can significantly affect the measured SPF. No matter how closely a laboratory preparation of sunscreening agents begins to approximate the ideal absorption profile (100% of all UV wavelengths), it can be quite difficult to reproduce this in something that can be applied to the skin. The base must perfectly disperse the active agents, and spread easily and uniformly so it will not produce thin areas that reduce effectiveness. The base is important for other critical characteristics such as substantivity (the ability to maintain SPF value over time) (Fig. 6.3), water resistance, and perhaps most importantly, its cosmetic properties, a set of factors which are critical to the acceptability of the preparation to the consumer.

SPECTRAL COVERAGE ISSUES

UVC radiation (260–290 nm) does not penetrate to the earth's surface in measurable amounts, so sunscreens do

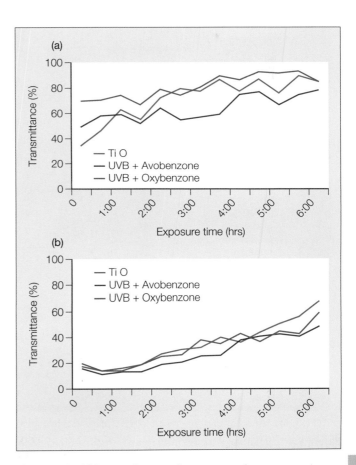

Figure 6.3 UV transmittance of sunscreen after exposure to sunlight over time: (a) UVA, (b) UVB.[76]

not need to cover these wavelengths. Only a small amount of UVB penetrates to the surface, although this energy is responsible for the majority of the biological effect of UV on human skin. Quantitatively, 4% of the total UV energy reaching the earth at sea level is UVB and 96% is UVA (Figs 6.4 and 6.5). The realization that most of the erythema provoking ability in natural sunlight came primarily from the UVB energy plus the demonstration that UVB could reproduce many of the pathologic changes observed with solar exposure led to an assumption early in the twentieth century that UVB was the only hazardous wavelength in sunlight.

For some time it was therefore believed that solar UVA did not contribute to the harmful effects of sunlight. UVB does contribute more to the harmful effect of sunlight including photoaging,[2–4] immunosuppression,[5,6] mutations, chromosome damage[7] and the generation of reactive oxygen species.[8–11] However, studies have now shown that UVA can contribute significantly to these harmful effects, including photoaging,[3,4,12,13] the production of reactive oxygen species,[14–16] chromosome damage,[7] immunosuppression[17] and carcinogenesis.[18–21] This is especially true of high intensity UVA sources such as those used in tanning beds, which typically produce several times the UVA energy output of sunlight and may be more carcinogenic than natural sunlight.[22] The realization that UVA can contribute to skin damage and cancer formation has ultimately led to a consensus opinion that sunscreens should include UVA in their spectral coverage. This has led to a concept that sunscreens should have broad-spectrum coverage, which should mean meaningful coverage of most of the UVA spectrum from 320 to 400 nm as well as UVB coverage.

Most commercially available sunscreens in the US do a good job covering UVB wavelengths, which remains a critical role for a sunscreen. Where sunscreens in the US have lagged behind other developed countries is in the coverage of UVA wavelengths and in the appropriate labeling of UVA coverage so that consumers can make informed choices.

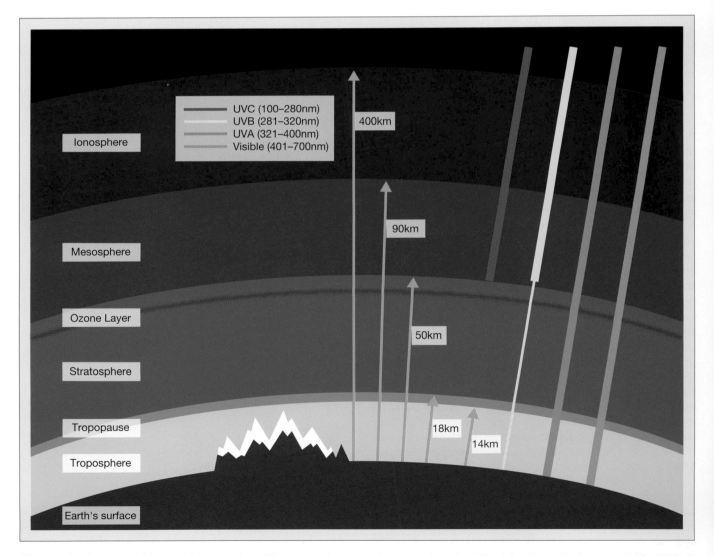

Figure 6.4 Structure of the earth's atmosphere. The troposphere contains approximately 10% of the atmospheric ozone, while 90% resides in a very thin layer just inside the outer reaches of the stratosphere and is commonly known as the ozone layer. Much of the natural resistance of the earth's atmosphere to penetration by harmful UV comes from this layer, which substantially attenuates UVC and UVB wavelengths.

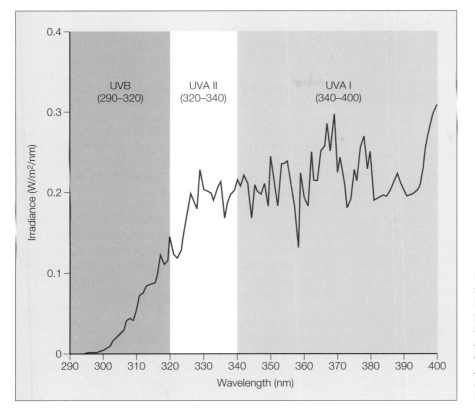

Figure 6.5 UV irradiance at earth's surface. All of the UVC and most of the UVB is filtered out by the atmosphere, particularly the stratospheric ozone layer. Sunscreens therefore do not need to cover against UVC since this does not reach the earth's surface for practical purposes. About 4% of the total UV energy that reaches the earth's surface at sea level is UVB and the rest is UVA (UVA I + UVA II).

Problems implementing new labeling requirements in the US stem from several sources. One is that the federal agency tasked with regulating sunscreens, the FDA, has other priorities that have in the past and continue to, usurp much of the needed effort and resources. Another related issue is the expense and difficulty of getting new sunscreen ingredients approved for use in the US that has made it difficult for manufacturers to produce new sunscreening agents that can meet standards for good, broad spectral coverage. Finally, a lack of consensus in the US on how American sunscreens should be tested and labeled for UVA protection has paralyzed further progress with regard to this issue.

A conference in 1999 organized by the American Academy of Dermatology between representatives from industry, academia and the FDA resulted in some guidelines to help initiate UVA labeling in the US.[23] Unfortunately, this effort and others have so far failed to produce a definite plan of action to test and label the efficacy of UVA protection in American sunscreens.

The best additives available in the US that contribute substantially to UVA protection are: (1) avobenzone (Parsol 1789), (2) zinc oxide and (3) titanium dioxide. While these ingredients can provide substantial UVA coverage, how they are formulated can markedly affect the result both in terms of SPF and spectral coverage. Unfortunately, at the present time, a claim of broad-spectrum coverage is no guarantee of good UVA coverage, as it has no specifically defined meaning. Until more reliable UVA protection labeling is approved by the FDA, consumers should use sunscreens that include one or more of the above ingredients and/or with companies that are known for better quality products. At the present time, the operative phrase is still *caveat emptor* (buyer beware) in the US with regard to UVA coverage.

CUTANEOUS REACTIONS TO SUNSCREENS

Many types of sunscreen reactions have been reported. People will often complain of a reaction to a specific sunscreen and will not subsequently use the product. These reactions include:

- allergic contact dermatitis
- photoallergic contact dermatitis
- irritant dermatitis
- acne
- aesthetic issues.

Because sunscreens are applied topically to the skin frequently and in relatively high concentrations (up to 26%), contact sensitization can occur. Since the active agents in sunscreens absorb radiation, they also have the potential to cause photosensitization. Both types of reactions can occur from not only the sunscreening agents themselves, but also from components of the vehicles. The most common offending agents in vehicles and preservatives can be found in Table 6.3.

The most common sunscreening agent causing allergic reactions is PABA. It has been estimated that 3–7% of the US population is PABA sensitive.[24] Both contact and

Table 6.3 Vehicles and preservatives that can cause contact or photocontact dermatitis

Avocado oil
t-Butyl alcohol
Methyl parabens
Phenyl dimethicone
Solvent red 1
Solvent red 3
Triethanolamine stearate
Benzyl alcohol
Cetylstearyl alcohol
Sorbitan sesquiolate
Imidazolidinyl urea (Germall 115)
Methylisothiazolin one/methylchloroisothiazolin one (Kathon CG)
Glyceryl monostearate
6-Acetoxy-2,4-dimethyl-m-dioxane
Carbowaxes
Ethyl alcohol
Glycerol
Isopropyl alcohol
Isopropyl myristate
Petrolatum
Stearyl alcohol

photoallergic reactions have been reported. Benzophenone sensitization has been estimated at 1–2%. Other sun-screening agents also can cause contact reactions.

By far the most common sunscreen reaction is due to 'sensitive' skin. It is estimated that up to one in three persons using sunscreens will at some time complain about sunscreens irritating their skin. Complaints include subjective signs such as stinging, burning and itching, as well as objective findings such as urticaria, and comedogenicity. The most effective method for alleviating these findings is to choose an alternative sunscreen from a different chemical family or with a different base.

True sunscreen reactions need to be both patch and photopatch tested to determine whether the reaction is allergic or light related. Use of too low a concentration of the testing materials may result in a false negative finding.

STUDIES RELATING SUNSCREEN USAGE TO SKIN CANCER PROTECTION

Numerous studies have been performed using conventional sunscreens to determine performance with regard to important long-term outcome measures such as photoaging and cancer. Sunscreen studies can be divided broadly into two categories: retrospective studies and intervention trials. These two types of studies tell us distinctly different things about sunscreens.

Under ideal circumstances, retrospective studies can tell us about what the actual effects of sunscreens were in the hands of the population under study over the period of time they were using them. Since the investigator collecting the data had no opportunity to instruct the subjects under study in the proper use of sunscreens at the time they were using them, retrospective studies are a measure of the effects of the untrained behavior of the population under study. This necessarily includes the inappropriate as well as the appropriate uses of sunscreen. As such, retrospective studies are a measure of how undirected sunscreen use in the hands of the general public is actually working. They can provide in effect, a benchmark of whether sunscreens work well in the hands of real people, influenced by the culture and mass media rather than physicians directing a study. However, in practice, retrospective studies are typically affected by a number of methodological problems which limits our ability to draw reliable conclusions from them.

Interventional trials, on the other hand, are a measure of what sunscreens can do under favorable circumstances, when the physician directing the trial has a chance to set the ground rules for behavior and sunscreen use, and has the opportunity to monitor and reinforce behavior during the study. In other words, interventional, prospective trials tell us what sunscreens can do under favorable conditions, while retrospective trials tell us the effects they actually have under less favorable, real world conditions, including contributions from both inappropriate and appropriate uses of sunscreens. This distinction is important to keep in mind when evaluating the results of sunscreen studies.

RETROSPECTIVE STUDIES

Table 6.4 summarizes the results of the major retrospective studies in this area.[25–38] As might be expected in retrospective trials, sunscreens do not always perform as hoped, probably in part due to methodological flaws, and in part because they are not used in the way dermatologists would intend for them to be used.

Most of the existing studies relating sunscreen usage to skin cancer prevention are retrospective and suffer from a number of methodological flaws including:

- *Recall bias* – In retrospective studies, data is collected about prior usage. Since sunscreen usage is generally deemed to be a 'healthy behavior,' persons may be more likely to report a greater use. In addition, parents may be more likely to say that they applied sunscreen to their children than may have been the case.

- *Interval bias* – These studies typically look at one interval in time. However, no data is collected or evaluated regarding behaviors of the subjects from during other periods of their lives. Given a latency in the clinical appearance of skin cancer from the time of initial UV insult, the assumption that only the behaviors that occurred in the study period influenced skin cancer development is flawed.

Table 6.4 Studies evaluating protective effects of sunscreens on melanoma

Study	Interval of sunscreen use examined	Findings
Klepp 1979[25]	1974–75	Increased MM in users
Graham 1985[26]	1974–80	n.s.
Herzfeld 1993[27]	1977–79	n.s.
Beitner 1990[28]	1978–83	Increased MM in a subset of users
Green 1986[29]	1979–80	Protective for MM
Holman 1986[30]	1980–82	n.s.
Osterlind 1988[31]	1981–85	n.s.
Holly 1995[32]	1981–86	Protective for MM
Westerdahl 1995[33]	1988–90	Increased MM in users
Rodenas 1996[34]	1989–93	Protective for MM
Autier 1995[35]	1991–92	Increased MM in users
Espinosa 1999[36]	1994–97	Protective for MM
Naldi 2000[37]	1994–98	n.s.
Westerdahl 2000[38]	1995–97	Increased MM in a subset of users

n.s., not significant

- *Lack of statistical power* – Many of the studies lack statistical power due to the low numbers of subjects involved and fail to show a protective effect that might actually exist.

- *Surrogate endpoints* – Many of the studies use endpoints that correlate with melanoma risk such as sunburning or number of nevi rather than using a direct measurement of melanoma incidence.

- *Lack of multivariate analysis* – Data on other factors (i.e. sun avoidance, seeking shade, etc.) as well as clothing usage needs to be evaluated in a careful multivariate analysis to determine which factors were directly protective and which might just be correlates. For example, in some of the studies, data on the use of protective clothing is collected, but the actual type of clothing worn is not defined. The SPF of a dry, white, cotton T-shirt is approximately six, wet approximately three.[39] Multivariate analysis might also demonstrate that fair skinned persons with high constitutional risk factors for skin cancer development might also be more likely to be 'high' sunscreen users rather than sunscreen use itself being the source of the problem. Finally and most importantly, those defined in these studies to be 'high' sunscreen users may have simply been those who received the highest dose of UV exposure due to a combination of inadequate sunscreen use and more time spent outdoors.

- *Sunscreen usage needs to be better defined* – Sunscreen use means different things to different persons and the definitions used in these studies were blurred. Studies show that far less sunscreen is

used than is recommended.[40] Frequency of application and time of application (whether applied before exposure or after exposure has begun)[41] need to be determined when data is collected to critically assess the impact of sunscreen on melanoma prevention.

Many existing retrospective studies evaluating sunscreen efficacy exhibit some or all of the above problems. These methodological issues may help to explain the markedly disparate conclusions reached in such studies. A recent meta-analysis of existing retroactive studies demonstrated no significant protective effect of sunscreen usage in the development of melanoma but also no increased risk for developing melanoma either.[42] Because no net detrimental effect on cancer rates attributable to sunscreen users has been convincingly shown in the majority of these studies, the use of sunscreens, especially in conjunction with other sun protective measures, continues to be recommended.

The most important endpoint for determining the effectiveness of public policies regarding sun protection is the melanoma incidence rate of a population. In Australia, where 74% of the population regularly uses sunscreen,[43] melanoma incidence and mortality rates are beginning to fall. Since sunscreens are the most commonly used method of sun protection in Australia, it is clear that sunscreens are a major factor in this outcome. Melanoma rates are also falling among Hawaiian Caucasians, a group that has among the highest *per capita* use of sunscreen in the US.[44] Until we have prospective data to show the effect of sunscreens on melanoma risk more directly, this is some of the best evidence of their effect on preventing melanoma in large populations of individuals.

INTERVENTIONAL TRIALS

Interventional trials are a measure of what sunscreens can do when used appropriately. In prospective interventional trials, physician investigators initially instruct study subjects in appropriate use of the agent. There are further opportunities during the study to monitor behavior and reinforce or change it as appropriate. This leads to much greater conformity with how the physician thinks the agent should be used. It is not surprising that sunscreens have faired much better in interventional trials than in the retrospective studies in which appropriate use of the agents may be partially or completely obscured by inappropriate use. The most important endpoint to consider in such studies, at least from a medical and social viewpoint are sun-induced neoplasms.

There are only four interventional trials in the literature that used actual sun-induced neoplasms as primary study endpoints. The first two of these were relatively short-term studies using actinic keratoses (AKs) as the primary outcome variable.[45,46] Since these first two studies were published, there has been one interventional study in nevi development in children[47] and one somewhat longer-term study in adults in which cutaneous squamous cell carcinoma was the primary outcome measure.[48]

The American AK study was carried out over a four year period in Lubbock, Texas and initially enrolled 53 people who had one or more AKs in the past or at study enrollment.[45] Each subject was followed for a minimum of 2 years from the time of enrollment, and the study was placebo-controlled. This showed that almost immediately the two groups diverged in terms of the numbers of new AKs that were forming over time. This implied that there was very little latency in the development of these lesions (AKs) and that they respond to UV reductions rather quickly. This study did not reveal much about the effect of sunscreens on skin cancer, since there were roughly equal numbers of cancers in both the placebo and treatment groups. The advantage of this study was that it was done over more than 1 year; the main limitation with this effort was that the number of subjects was small.

The Australian AK study was carried out over one summer in a much larger group of people (588 individuals).[46] In this prospective placebo-controlled trial, the AKs were not treated. This study showed a significant percentage of AKs disappearing during the study, suggesting that these lesions may have been dependent on the promoting influence of the sun. Another distinct possibility was that the immune system, which was held at bay by continued solar suppression, was unleashed by the protective effect of the sunscreen, allowing the immune response to eradicate many of the lesions. These potential explanations are not mutually exclusive and either or both could have contributed to this result.

Individuals in the sunscreen treated group experienced a significant reduction both in the number of countable lesions and in the number of new lesions, confirming the American study result. The advantage of this study was primarily that it included a relatively large number of subjects, and its main limitation was that the observations were made over a relatively short (6 months) period.

These two studies remained the only hard evidence for the positive effects of sunscreens until the next two sunscreen studies were published at the end of the twentieth century.[47,48] Both of these first two studies confirmed that appropriate use of these agents can have a significant beneficial effect on a skin-cancer related end point, namely development of AKs.[45,46] In spite of different study designs, this effect accrued fairly rapidly. However, due to the relatively short period of time covered by these early studies, nothing was learned about the eventual impact on skin cancer *per se* as an endpoint. This question was later addressed in a longitudinal study by Green *et al.*, which at the time of this writing is still underway.[48]

In 1992, Green *et al.* began a longitudinal study related to sun effects in the town of Nambor, Australia.[49] This study had the ambitious aim of including most of the residents of the town. This trial was interesting in that the authors did not believe it was ethical to use a placebo control, so what is actually being compared is active intervention to encourage daily use of an SPF 17 sunscreen vs background *ad lib* use of sunscreens by the population. This design obviously makes it more difficult to see differences than would a placebo control, but in spite of this handicap, the study demonstrated a significant difference developing between the two groups with regard to squamous cell carcinoma by 1999.[48] What was also interesting is that so far, a difference has not been detected between the two groups with regard to basal cell carcinomas, which probably says more about the differences in the biology of carcinogenesis between these two sun-induced tumor types (particularly biological differences in latency) than anything about the efficacy of sunscreens in preventing basal cell carcinoma. It seems reasonable to anticipate that if the study goes on long enough, that a difference may eventually be seen between the two groups with regard to basal cell carcinoma as well.

The biological endpoint that we are most interested in is melanoma. Unfortunately, although practical designs to study this endpoint exist, so far there has been no real interest in supporting such a prospective study. Until governmental agencies consider this a worthy effort and fund the studies that have been put forward, interventional studies to test the effects of sunscreen on melanoma development will have to depend on surrogate endpoints.

The only prospective, interventional study in this category is the Vancouver Mole study, a 2-year effort that compared sunscreen to placebo in school children living in Vancouver, British Columbia.[47] This study showed a significant reduction in nevi formation over the two years of the study in the sunscreen group compared to placebo. This report is significant because the process of nevus formation is probably similar to the process of melanoma development, differing more in degree than in kind.

As a group, what these prospective studies reveal is that sunscreens, when used appropriately, can produce significant improvements in the long-term consequences of sun exposure. Although many retrospective studies suffer from serious methodological defects as has been pointed out, this may not completely explain the poor showing of sunscreens, especially in certain populations. One explanation for a poor effect of sunscreens on cancer rates is that some populations may not be applying these agents very effectively, or worse, may be using sunscreens primarily as tanning aids. Using sunscreens to allow an individual to spend more time in the sun is a behavior that may counteract and even reverse the beneficial effects of a sunscreen due to excessive dosing with UV. Clearly, there is still much work that must be done to change how the public views sun exposure and how this affects their use of sunscreens.

Future trials

In order to better assess protective effects on skin cancer risk, more studies, both prospective and retrospective should be undertaken. However, there are significant problems that must be overcome. The prevalence of skin cancer in the population is relatively low. In order to have a study with adequate statistical power a large number of subjects are needed. In addition, studies have to take into consideration that there may be a 10–50 year latency period between the time that sun exposure initially occurs and the time that skin cancer appears clinically. Therefore, a follow up period of at least 10 years would be needed if a study uses children or young adults of average risk.

Also, the difficulties of obtaining accurate sun exposure and sunscreen usage history for the period prior to the studies' inception must be overcome to minimize the effects of earlier behaviors. Finally, any placebo-controlled interventional study will need to overcome the ethical dilemma of depriving a subject of the use of sunscreen when strong inferential data already suggests that sunscreens protect from skin cancer when used appropriately.

OTHER FACTORS

Vitamin D levels: do sunscreens create problems?

One source of vitamin D is skin synthesis from sun exposure. In the skin, 7-dehydrocholesterol is converted to a precursor (pre-vitamin D) which then undergoes a temperature-dependent molecular rearrangement that results in the production of vitamin D_3.[50] Vitamin D is then hydroxylated at the 25 position in the liver and at the 1 position in the kidney, producing the most physiologically active metabolite, 1,25-hydroxyvitamin D_2. Vitamin D is essential for calcium absorption from the gastrointestinal track, bone formation and calcium homeostasis.

Sunscreens, because they specifically absorb the UVB energy that most efficiently forms pre-vitamin D, have the potential to cause deficiencies of vitamin D, an idea that seemed to be supported by a few early case reports.[51,52] However, the bulk of the evidence does not support the notion that this is a common problem, no matter how plausible it may seem, probably because the primary source of vitamin D in Western societies is diet. Although lack of vitamin D can lead to bone disease and related problems, one prospective study specifically excluded the development of osteoporosis in sunscreen users followed over a 2-year period, suggesting that this is, at most, a rare event.[53]

In addition, Vitamin D sufficiency was tracked in at least two of the prospective sunscreen trials, and in neither was vitamin D deficiency a problem.[54] Other prospective studies designed to evaluate this issue also have not found a problem with vitamin D deficiency in sunscreen treated subjects.[55] Even a study of subjects with xeroderma pigmentosum, who use the most aggressive sun protection measures, confirmed the absence of vitamin D deficiency.[56]

Since sunlight is a known carcinogen and diet is the primary source of vitamin D, there seems little justification for calls to intentionally expose large portions of the population to the sun or artificial UV sources solely for the purpose of supplementing vitamin D. Vitamin D sufficiency is rarely a problem in individuals eating a well-balanced diet. If supraphysiological levels are eventually found to be of value in suppressing the incidence of certain cancers, dietary supplementation will be the safe and logical way to obtain high levels of vitamin D.

Recently there has been speculation that higher levels of vitamin D might have efficacy in reducing the incidence of certain cancers, although this has not yet been demonstrated in clinical trials. Speculation about the potential impact of supraphysiological levels of vitamin D has raised the possibility that sun protection, and specifically the use of sunscreens, may have adverse consequences by preventing a putative beneficial effect on cancer. While all of this is obviously speculative, the psychological impact of this hypothesis has been felt. Pronouncements coming from certain scientists may be negatively affecting the attitudes of the general public towards the whole issue of sun exposure. Caution should be used in interpreting these assertions. It seems likely that there are motives beyond reducing cancer risk, since if this were simply an issue of how to supplement vitamin D, responsible scientists would be advocating the safer alternative of oral supplementation, which will not make melanoma an any worse problem than it already is.

SPF: how high is enough?

American dermatologists have tended to support the trend for higher SPF values in sunscreen preparations. One reason for this is that keeping the overall SPF high (>30) usually has the effect of boosting UVA coverage when sunscreens are formulated with sunscreening agents currently available in the US. Another added benefit of higher sunscreen SPFs is that it makes them more difficult to use as tanning aids. However, there are other reasons that sunscreens with higher SPF values may be of benefit.

Federal regulators in the US may have founded their decisions on SPF in the past on incorrect assumptions. One assumption was that prevention of erythema meant that no meaningful harmful effects from sun exposure were occurring. This is clearly not the case, as shown by many studies that demonstrate almost all of the harmful effects of ultraviolet exposure can occur at suberythemal exposures.[12,57–67] Moreover, studies done directly in humans demonstrate that in situations of equal suppression of erythema, sunscreens with higher SPF prevent more of these suberythemal effects.[68] Since such effects are important for the development of long-term consequences such as photoaging and cancer, these studies imply that sunscreens with SPFs over 30 might be superior if used over long periods of time.

A second assumption is that SPF values, measured under controlled laboratory conditions with subjects using ideal applications of sunscreen, predict what will happen with consumers. There is good evidence that this assumption is incorrect. For example at least two studies have confirmed that most people who use sunscreen apply between 25–50% of the amount required to achieve the rated SPF.[69–71] Furthermore, other studies have established that most people do not apply sunscreens uniformly or as often as would be required to continue to achieve the rated SPF value.[72]

Because of such real world considerations, it is distinctly possible that SPFs above 30 may substantially outperform sunscreens of 30 or less, especially over the time of a human lifespan. Others who have looked at this issue outside commercial laboratory testing have also concluded that SPFs above 30 have merit.[73] Until prospective interventional trials are done in humans that specifically compare SPF values varying from 15 to >50, it is difficult to agree with the conclusion that SPF values >30 are of no benefit. Since sunscreens in the SPF 30–50 range have proved over time to be safe, the current recommendation for at least an SPF 30 certainly seems justified.

One issue that is frequently ignored when public health policy for sunscreen potency is considered, is whom are we trying to help? Another way of looking at this is whom are such policies going to exclude or hurt, particularly if such policies are going to limit the availability of sunscreens with adequate SPF? It is no wonder then, that when considering public health issues such as limiting improvements in commercial sunscreens such as higher SPFs, dermatologists have as a group tended to be against such ideas.

RECOMMENDATIONS FOR SUNSCREEN PHOTOPROTECTION

Sunscreens are an important part of our armamentarium for preventing skin cancer. The National Health Interview Survey data shows that it is the most common sun protection method employed by Americans compared with protective clothing and sun avoidance.

This use of sunscreen as the primary method of UV protection is both positive and negative. It is good that people are interested in using any sun protection method. Sunscreen is the least intrusive on lifestyles since it can be added to anyone's routine with very little change required in terms of sun exposure behavior. This is also good if it produces a reduction in overall UV exposure. It would be even better if sunscreen were used as part of an overall package of exposure reduction which included some changes in behavior and protective clothing.

Unfortunately, available evidence suggests that there may be a significant number of individuals who are misusing sunscreens to actually absorb even more UV than they otherwise would. Those who intentionally seek the sun for cosmetic tanning and misuse sunscreens as tanning aids (such that they absorb the same or even larger amounts of UV) may ultimately accrue skin cancers at an accelerated rate compared with the rest of the population and may further drive up skin cancer statistics.

As the American Academy of Dermatology has advocated for some time, it is important to use sunscreens as part of a total UV exposure reduction program with the intention of reducing as low as is reasonable the individual's exposure to ultraviolet, consistent with a healthy, active lifestyle.

In practice, this means three things. First, it is best to avoid direct exposure to mid-day sun whenever possible.

Ideally this means trying to schedule outdoor activities early or late in the day to avoid as much as possible being outdoors in direct sunlight between 1000 hrs and 1600 hrs. Second, clothing such as long-sleeved shirts, trousers and hats should be used as much as possible to limit direct exposure of skin to UV. Finally, when all other measures fail, sunscreens should be used as the 'fail-safe' method and applied to all skin exposed skin that cannot be covered with clothing, such as the face, hands and forearms.

Sunscreens should be applied as a daily routine instead of on an 'as needed' basis since anecdotal experience suggests that considerably more than half of the time it will be forgotten when it should have been used. It has also been demonstrated that these unprotected episodes can almost completely defeat a sun protection program.[74,75] Additionally, the effectiveness of the sunscreen begins to degrade after 2 hrs and therefore it needs to be reapplied after that interval of exposure has occurred.[76]

FUTURE SUNCREENING AGENTS

Some novel sunscreen additives have been proposed in the past few years although so far few of these have made their way into mainstream formulations that are readily available to the general public. These include antioxidants and DNA repair enzymes. While such additives may be able to effectively enhance the potency of sunscreens for preventing harmful effects from sunlight, it is important to realize that no additive is going to replace the need for good, broad-spectrum UV coverage. The task for sunscreen manufacturers will be to add such additives to their products without significant sacrifices in SPF or the broad-spectrum coverage required for a good sunscreen.

Adding potent antioxidants to sunscreens is based on the idea that both UVB and UVA generate damage to the skin as a result of the generation of oxygen radicals and related molecular species that can produce damage to DNA and other important cellular macromolecules. Logically, adding antioxidants to sunscreens as long as it can be done without significant sacrifices to the UV attenuating properties may produce a sunscreen with improved ability to prevent the harmful effects of sunlight.

The addition of DNA repair enzymes to sunscreens is an interesting idea that is being considered for commercial sunscreen products. UVB produces DNA damage through several mechanisms. The best understood mechanism involves the formation of 6–4 photoproducts and cyclobutane dimers in DNA strands. Low levels of this type of damage can usually be repaired via the excision repair mechanism in mammalian cells to restore normal cellular function. The concept of enhancing the efficacy of sunscreens with DNA repair enzymes is to enhance the process of repairing this type of damage caused by the UV that gets past the sunscreening agents and thus, to enhance the ability of the sunscreen to protect against the harmful effects of sunlight. If this could be accomplished without sacrificing the sunscreen's primary function of preventing the formation of the dimers in the first place, this approach might be effective. Most of the published work along these lines has been done with the addition of bacteriophage DNA repair enzyme, T4 endonuclease.[77]

Although these agents are based on logical concepts, it is important to remember that there are no studies that demonstrate the superiority of sunscreens containing such additives to conventional sunscreens for the purpose of ameliorating the most important long-term consequences of sun exposure such as photoaging and cancer.

FUTURE OUTLOOK

The usage of sunscreens has grown dramatically worldwide over the past decade. Current data suggests that a regimen of sun protection that includes protective clothing, avoiding midday sun, and regular use of broad-spectrum high SPF sunscreen (such as practiced in Australia[43]) appears to be reducing melanoma incidence rates. This is the current recommendation of the American Academy of Dermatology and it is also the recommendation that is best supported by existing data.

Except for total sun avoidance, sunscreens in conjunction with other protective measures remain the best method of protection from UV induced damage to the skin. Hopefully, we will have even more definitive answers to questions related to the effectiveness of sunscreens for reducing melanoma and non-melanoma skin cancer risk as better sunscreen components are developed and as studies are performed in the future that avoid some of the methodological problems in prior efforts.

REFERENCES

1 Mackie BS, Mackie LE. The PABA story. Australas J Derm 1999; 40:51–53.

2 Brenneisen P, Sies H, Scharffetter-Kochanek K. Ultraviolet-B irradiation and matrix metalloproteinases: from induction via signaling to initial events. Ann N Y Acad Sci 2002; 973:31–43.

3 Harrison JA, Walker SL, Plastow SR, et al. Sunscreens with low sun protection factor inhibit ultraviolet B and A photoaging in the skin of the hairless albino mouse. Photodermatol Photoimmunol Photomed 1991; 8:12–20.

4 Kligman LH, Akin FJ, Kligman AM. The contributions of UVA and UVB to connective tissue damage in hairless mice. J Invest Derm 1985; 84:272–276.

5 Garssen J, Vandebriel RJ, Loveren H van. Molecular aspects of UVB-induced immunosuppression. Arch Toxicol Suppl 1997; 19:97–109.

6 Whitmore SE, Morison WL. Prevention of UVB-induced immunosuppression in humans by a high sun protection factor sunscreen. Arch Derm 1995; 131:1128–1133.

7 Emri G, Wenczl E, Erp P Van, et al. Low doses of UVB or UVA induce chromosomal aberrations in cultured human skin cells. J Invest Derm 2000; 115:435–440.

8 Deliconstantinos G, Villiotou V, Stavrides JC. Increase of particulate nitric oxide synthase activity and peroxynitrite synthesis in UVB-irradiated keratinocyte membranes. Biochem J 1996; 320:997–1003.

9 Heck DE, Vetrano AM, Mariano TM, Laskin JD. UVB light stimulates production of reactive oxygen species: unexpected role for catalase. J Biol Chem 2003; 278:22432–22436.

10 Rosen JE, Prahalad AK, Williams GM. 8-Oxodeoxyguanosine formation in the DNA of cultured cells after exposure to H_2O_2 alone or with UVB or UVA irradiation [published erratum appears in Photochem Photobiol 1996 Sep;64(3):611] Photochem Photobiol 1996; 64:117–122.

11 Cejkova J, Stipek S, Crkovska J, Ardan T, Midelfart A. Reactive oxygen species (ROS)-generating oxidases in the normal rabbit cornea and their involvement in the corneal damage evoked by UVB rays. Histol Histopathol 2001; 16:523–533.

12 Lowe NJ, Meyers DP, Wieder JM, et al. Low doses of repetitive ultraviolet A induce morphologic changes in human skin. J Invest Derm 1995; 105:739–743.

13 Bernerd F, Asselineau D. UVA exposure of human skin reconstructed in vitro induces apoptosis of dermal fibroblasts: subsequent connective tissue repair and implications in photoaging. Cell Death Differ 1998; 5:792–802.

14 Berneburg M, Grether-Beck S, Kurten V, et al. Singlet oxygen mediates the UVA-induced generation of the photoaging-associated mitochondrial common deletion. J Biol Chem 1999; 274:15345–15349.

15 Linetsky M, Ortwerth BJ. Quantitation of the reactive oxygen species generated by the UVA irradiation of ascorbic acid-glycated lens proteins. Photochem Photobiol 1996; 63:649–655.

16 Wamer WG, Wei RR. In vitro photooxidation of nucleic acids by ultraviolet A radiation. Photochem Photobiol 1997; 65:560–563.

17 Reeve VE, Bosnic M, Boehm-Wilcox C, Ley RD. Differential protection by two sunscreens from UV radiation-induced immunosuppression. J Invest Derm 1991; 97:624–628.

18 Laat A de, Leun JC van der, Gruijl FR de. Carcinogenesis induced by UVA (365-nm) radiation: the dose-time dependence of tumor formation in hairless mice. Carcinogenesis 1997; 18:1013–1020.

19 de Gruijl FR. Photocarcinogenesis: UVA vs UVB radiation. Skin Pharmacol Appl Skin Physiol 2002; 15:316–320.

20 de Gruijl FR. Photocarcinogenesis: UVA vs UVB. Methods Enzymol 2000; 319:359–366.

21 Kranen HJ van, Laat A de, Ven J van de, et al. Low incidence of p53 mutations in UVA (365-nm)-induced skin tumors in hairless mice. Cancer Res 1997; 57:1238–1240.

22 Moseley H, Davidson M, Ferguson J. A hazard assessment of artificial tanning units. Photodermatol Photoimmunol Photomed 1998; 14:79–87.

23 Lim HW, Naylor M, Honigsmann H, et al. American Academy of Dermatology Consensus Conference on UVA protection of sunscreens: summary and recommendations. Washington, DC. J Am Acad Derm 2001; 44:505–508.

24 Darvay A, White IR, Rycroft RJ, et al. Photoallergic contact dermatitis is uncommon. Br J Derm 2001; 145:597–601.

25 Klepp O, Magnus K. Some environmental and bodily characteristics of melanoma patients. A case-control study. Int J Cancer 1979; 23:482–486.

26 Graham S, Marshall J, Haugney B, et al. An inquiry into the epidemiology of melanoma. Am J Epidemiol 1985; 122:606–619.

27 Herzfeld PM, Fitzgerald EF, Hwang SA, Stark A. A case-control study of malignant melanoma of the trunk among white males in upstate New York. Cancer Detect Prev 1993; 17:601–608.

28 Beitner H, Norell SE, Ringborg U, Wennersten G, Mattson B. Malignant melanoma: aetiological importance of individual pigmentation and sun exposure. Br J Cancer 1990; 122.43–51.

29 Green A, Bain C, McLennan R, Siskind V. Risk factors for cutaneous melanoma in Queensland. Recent Results Cancer Res 1986; 102:76–97.

30 Holman CD, Armstrong BK, Heenan PJ. Relationship of cutaneous malignant melanoma to individual sunlight-exposure habits. J Natl Cancer Inst 1986; 76:403–414.

31 Osterlind A, Tucker M, Stone B, Jensen O. The Danish case-control study of cutaneous malignant melanoma. II. Importance of UV-light exposure. Int J Cancer 1988; 42:319–324.

32 Holly EA, Aston DA, Cress RD, Ahn DK, Kristiansen JJ. Cutaneous melanoma in women. I. Exposure to sunlight, ability to tan, and other risk factors related to ultraviolet light. Am J Epidemiol 1995; 141:923–933.

33 Westerdahl J, Olsson H, Masback A, Ingvar C, Jonsson N. Is the use of sunscreens a risk factor for malignant melanoma? Melanoma Res 1995; 5:59–65.

34 Rodenas JM, Delgado-Rodriguez M, Herranz MT, Tercedor J, Serrano S. Sun exposure, pigmentary traits, and risk of cutaneous malignant melanoma: a case-control study in a Mediterranean population. Cancer Causes Control 1996; 7:275–283.

35 Autier P, Dore JF, Schifflers E, et al. Melanoma and use of sunscreens: an EORTC case-control study in Germany, Belgium and France. EORTC Melanoma Coop Group Int J Cancer 1995; 61:749–755.

36 Espinosa Arranz J, Sanchez Hernandez JJ, Bravo Fernandez P, et al. Cutaneous malignant melanoma and sun exposure in Spain. Melanoma Res 1999; 9:199–205.

37 Naldi L, Lorenzo Imberti G, Parazzini F, Gallus S, Vecchia C La. Pigmentary traits, modalities of sun reaction, history of sunburns, and melanocytic nevi as risk factors for cutaneous malignant melanoma in the Italian population: results of a collaborative case-control study. Cancer 2000; 88:2703–2710.

38 Westerdahl J, Ingvar C, Masback A, Olsson H. Sunscreen use and malignant melanoma. Int J Cancer 2000; 87:145–150.

39 Menter JM, Hollins TD, Sayre RM, et al. Protection against UV photocarcinogenesis by fabric materials. J Amer Acad Derm 1994; 31:711–716.

40 Stokes R, Diffey B. How well are sunscreen users protected? Photodermatol Photoimmunol Photomed 1997; 13:186–188.

41 Pruim B, Green A. Photobiological aspects of sunscreen re-application. Australas J Derm 1999; 40:14–18.

42 Huncharek M, Kupelnick B. Use of topical sunscreens and the risk of malignant melanoma: a meta-analysis of 9067 patients from 11 case-control studies. Am J Public Health 2002; 92:1173–1177.

43 Martin RH. Relationship between risk factors, knowledge and preventive behaviour relevant to skin cancer in general practice patients in south Australia. Br J Gen Pract 1995; 45:365–367.

44 Chuang TY, Charles J, Reizner GT, Elpern DJ, Farmer ER. Melanoma in Kauai, Hawaii, 1981–1990: the significance of in situ melanoma and the incidence trend. Int J Derm 1999; 38:101–107.

45 Naylor MF, Boyd A, Smith DW, Cameron GS, Hubbard D. Neldner KH. High sun protection factor (SPF) sunscreens in the suppression of actinic neoplasia. Arch Derm 1995; 131:170–175.

46 Thompson SC, Jolley D, Marks R. Reduction of solar keratoses by regular sunscreen use. N Engl J Med 1993; 329:1147–1151.

47 Gallagher RP, Rivers JK, Lee TK, et al. Broad-spectrum sunscreen use and the development of new nevi in white children: A randomized controlled trial. JAMA 2000; 283:2955–2960.

48 Green A, Williams G, Neale R, et al. Daily sunscreen application and betacarotene supplementation in prevention of basal-cell and squamous-cell carcinomas of the skin: a randomised controlled trial. Lancet 1999; 354:723–729.

49 Green A, Battistutta D, Hart V, et al. The Nambour Skin Cancer and Actinic Eye Disease Prevention Trial: design and baseline characteristics of participants. Control Clin Trials 1994; 15:512–522.

50 Holick MF, MacLaughlin JA, Clark MB, et al. Photosynthesis of previtamin D_3 in human skin and the physiologic consequences. Science 1980; 210:203–205.

51 Matsuoka LY, Ide L, Wortsman J, MacLaughlin JA, Holick MF. Sunscreens suppress cutaneous vitamin D_3 synthesis. J Clin Endocrinol Metab 1987; 64:1165–1168.

52 Matsuoka LY, Wortsman J, Hanifan N, Holick MF. Chronic sunscreen use decreases circulating concentrations of 25-hydroxyvitamin D. Arch Derm 1988; 124:1802–1804.

53 Farrerons J, Barnadas M, Lopez-Navidad A, et al. Sunscreen and risk of osteoporosis in the elderly: a two-year follow-up. Dermatology 2001; 202:27–30.

54 Marks R, Foley PA, Jolley D, et al. The effect of regular sunscreen use on vitamin D levels in an Australian population. Results of a randomized controlled trial. Arch Derm 1995; 131:415–421.

55 Farrerons J, Barnadas M, Rodriguez J, et al. Clinically prescribed sunscreen (sun protection factor 15) does not decrease serum vitamin D concentration sufficiently either to induce changes in parathyroid function or in metabolic markers. Br J Derm 1998; 139:422–427.

56 Sollitto RB, Kraemer KH, DiGiovanna JJ. Normal vitamin D levels can be maintained despite rigorous photoprotection: six years' experience with xeroderma pigmentosum. J Amer Acad Derm 1997; 37:942–947.

57 Bestak R, Barnetson RS, Nearn MR, Halliday GM. Sunscreen protection of contact hypersensitivity responses from chronic solar-simulated ultraviolet irradiation correlates with the absorption spectrum of the sunscreen. J Invest Derm 1995; 105:345–351.

58 Chouinard N, Therrien JP, Mitchell DL, et al. Repeated exposures of human skin equivalent to low doses of ultraviolet-B radiation lead to changes in cellular functions and accumulation of cyclobutane pyrimidine dimers. Biochem Cell Biol 2001; 79:507–515.

59 Bissett DL, Majeti S, Fu JJ, McBride JF, Wyder WE. Protective effect of topically applied conjugated hexadienes against ultraviolet radiation-induced chronic skin damage in the hairless mouse. Photodermatol Photoimmunol Photomed 1990; 7:63–67.

60 el-Ghorr AA, Norval M, Lappin MB, Crosby JC. The effect of chronic low-dose UVB radiation on Langerhans cells, sunburn cells, urocanic acid isomers, contact hypersensitivity and serum immunoglobulins in mice. Photochem Photobiol 1995; 62:326–332.

61 Gallagher CH, Canfield PJ, Greenoak GE, Reeve VE. Characterization and histogenesis of tumors in the hairless mouse produced by low-dosage incremental ultraviolet radiation. J Invest Derm 1984; 83:169–174.

62 Gange RW, Parrish JA. Recovery of skin from a single suberythemal dose of ultraviolet radiation. J Invest Derm 1983; 81:78–82.

63 Harber LC, Kochevar IE. Pyrimidine dimer formation and repair in human skin. Cancer Res 1980; 40:3181–3185.

64 Hofmann-Wellenhof R, Wolf P, Smolle J, et al. Influence of UVB therapy on dermoscopic features of acquired melanocytic nevi. J Am Acad Derm 1997; 37:559–563.

65 Lavker RM, Gerberick GF, Veres D, Irwin CJ, Kaidbey KH. Cumulative effects from repeated exposure to suberythemal doses of UVB and UVA in human skin. J Amer Acad Derm 1995; 32:53–62.

66 Weelden H van, Putte SC van der, Toonstra J, Leun JC van der. UVA-induced tumours in pigmented hairless mice and the carcinogenic risks of tanning with UVA. Arch Derm Res 1990; 282:289–294.

67 Wulf HC, Poulsen T, Brodthagen H, Hou-Jensen K. Sunscreens for delay of ultraviolet induction of skin tumors. J Amer Acad Derm 1982; 7:194–202.

68 Kaidbey KH. The photoprotective potential of the new superpotent sunscreens. J Amer Acad Derm 1990; 22:449–452.

69 Wulf HC, Stender IM, Lock-Andersen J. Sunscreens used at the beach do not protect against erythema: a new definition of SPF is proposed. Photodermatol Photoimmunol Photomed 1997; 13:129–132.

70 Stenberg C, Larko O. Sunscreen application and its importance for the sun protection factor. Arch Derm 1985; 121:1400–1402.

71 Azurdia RM, Pagliaro JA, Diffey BL, Rhodes LE. Sunscreen application by photosensitive patients is inadequate for protection. Br J Derm 1999; 140:255–258.

72 Azurdia RM, Pagliaro JA, Rhodes LE. Sunscreen application technique in photosensitive patients: a quantitative assessment of the effect of education. Photodermatol Photoimmunol Photomed 2000; 16:53–56.

73 Poon TS, Barnetson RS. The importance of using broad spectrum SPF 30+ sunscreens in tropical and subtropical climates. Photodermatol Photoimmunol Photomed 2002; 18:175–178.

74 Phillips TJ, Bhawan J, Yaar M, et al. Effect of daily versus intermittent sunscreen application on solar simulated UV radiation-induced skin response in humans. J Am Acad Derm 2000; 43:610–618.

75 Al Mahroos M, Yaar M, Phillips TJ, Bhawan J, Gilchrest BA. Effect of sunscreen application on UV-induced thymine dimers. Arch Derm 2002; 138:1480–1485.

76 Rigel D, Chen T, Appa Y. Sunscreens and UV protection. Washington, DC: Presented at American Academy of Dermatology Annual Meeting; 2001.

77 Wolf P, Cox P, Yarosh DB, Kripke ML. Sunscreens and T4N5 liposomes differ in their ability to protect against ultraviolet-induced sunburn cell formation, alterations of dendritic epidermal cells, and local suppression of contact hypersensitivity. J Invest Derm 1995; 104:287–292.

CHAPTER

7

The Importance of Primary and Secondary Prevention Programs for Skin Cancer

June K Robinson

Key points

- As the US population of adults 65 and older increases by an estimated 20% in the next decade, the number of people developing new skin cancers, or dying from them, will rise.
- Skin Self Examination (SSE) may achieve some reduction in the deaths from melanoma and reduce the physical and emotional burden of disease from both NMSC and CM.
- Having a partner enhances SSE performance.
- The role of adults in adolescent health and disease prevention has been suggested as being even more influential than school curricula.
- Parents may re-frame the sun-protection health promotion message with their children to, 'Daily sun protection now means fewer or no painful burns. Tanning now means loss of the skin's health and beauty; you may get wrinkles in your 20s'.

INTRODUCTION

Skin cancer, the most common malignancy in the US, is an important public health concern with an incidence rate that will continue to increase in the next decade. As the US population of adults 65 and older increases by an estimated 20% in the next decade, the incidence of and mortality from skin cancer will rise.[1] For those at risk to develop skin cancer, early detection by skin self-examination (SSE) is recommended to decrease mortality and the physical and emotional burden of the disease.[2]

While secondary prevention with early detection is the most effective strategy for those who sustained unprotected sun exposure in youth, primary prevention by effective sun protection throughout life for those at risk to develop skin cancer may reduce the incidence of skin cancer. Concentrated, intermittent sun exposure has been shown to increase the risk of melanoma and basal cell carcinoma (BCC) development, and childhood and adolescence exposure to ultraviolet radiation have been identified as key periods for the induction of melanoma and non-melanoma skin cancer (NMSC) later in life.

HISTORY

Rising skin cancer incidence

The overall annual incidence rate of cutaneous melanoma (CM) in the US rose from 6.4 per 100,000 to 14 per 100,000 between 1973 and 1994. The 120.5% increase in incidence rate and the 38.9% increase in mortality rate from CM during those 21 years made the early detection of CM an important public health issue.[3] For US men, the probability of developing invasive CM from birth to death is estimated to be one in 56 and for women it is estimated to be one in 80. In the late 1970s, the age-adjusted incidence of CM in whites was 11 per 100,000 for men and 10 per 100,000 for women; however, the incidence rose to 22 per 100,000 for men and 16 per 100,000 for women in the late 1990s.[4] While CM incidence rates in white men in the late 1990s were previously reported as being flat, reporting age-adjusted analysis showed a statistically significant increase since 1996. Reporting CMs may be delayed by up to 17 years. The delay for CM is greater than the time lag in reporting any other cancer. The delay accounts for the recently recognized 14% change between reporting age-adjusted and unadjusted cancer incidence for CM in whites regardless of sex.[3] CM age-adjusted incidence rates have increased by 4.1% per year since 1981. Mortality rates for white males begin to rise after age 50 and for those age 60 and above, the mortality rate has continued to increase from 1985 to 1994.

In the US, skin cancers, including CM and NMSC, BCC and squamous cell carcinoma (SCC), are the most common malignant neoplasms in the Caucasian population. The American Cancer Society estimates that the number of new cases of NMSC in 2004 will exceed 1.3 million, which is almost twice the number estimated in 1995. Since NMSCs are usually treated in outpatient settings and are not reported to cancer registries, exact incidence rates are not available for the US. An estimated 2300 people in the US will die from NMSC each year, primarily due to metastatic cutaneous SCC. While NMSC is likely to claim fewer lives than the 7810 deaths estimated for CM in 2004, considerable morbidity results from treatment. Since many NMSC arise on the frequently sun-exposed areas of the head and neck, surgical resection may result in significant disfigurement with impaired quality of life and social interaction. For all of the above reasons, the need for both primary and secondary prevention methods cannot be understated.

DESCRIPTION

Primary prevention of skin cancer: protection from ultraviolet radiation

Indoor tanning

The increasing skin cancer incidence is attributed to ultraviolet radiation exposure during the youth of people who are now adults. Behaviors such as intentional sunbathing, inadequate sun protection (e.g. lack or misuse of sunscreen/block and protective clothing), and the use of tanning lamps/salons by young individuals contribute to unprotected exposure. From 1986 to 1998, sunscreen use was increasing among adults and the use of indoor tanning among young people was also increasing. A series of studies examining indoor tanning usage in college students found usage rates for women consistently greater than 80% with approximately one-third of the women surveyed reporting frequent use, e.g. weekly.[5,6] Studies in high school populations report varying rates for males at 6–44% and for females at 20–70%. These studies also report that these students begin indoor tanning as early as 9 years old, with the majority reporting their first exposure by high school.[7] In 2001, the indoor tanning industry generated more than US$4 billion in revenues. The number of indoor tanning salon users grew 8% to over 27 million between 1998–1999, doubling in just the past decade. The North American Alliance of Tanning Salon Owners (NAATSO) reports in their mission statement the goal of doubling indoor tanning use in the next 5 years.

Widespread indoor tanning usage rates among young people is clearly a potential health risk because there is an 8:1 odds ratio for developing malignant CM for individuals younger than 36 years old who regularly indoor tan versus those who never do. At least seven case-control studies have reported significant positive associations between indoor tanning and increased risk of CM. The majority of these studies have documented some form of dose response relationship. Three of these studies have noted a greater CM risk for exposures several years before diagnosis than for more recent exposures. There is also consistent but not strong evidence suggesting that the younger the age of exposure the greater the risk for CM. More recently, these findings have been extended, and an association between indoor tanning and basal cell and squamous cell carcinoma has been reported.

Perceived benefit of tanning

Tanners are primarily attempting to achieve an improved appearance rather than perceiving indoor tanning as having health benefits. The next most common reason cited for tanning is that it gives the person a sense of relaxation and overall physical and psychological well-being. In general, knowledge of the health risks associated with tanning is *not* related to indoor tanning usage.[8,9]

Tanning behavior almost always begins in childhood as an unintentional byproduct of outdoor activity. Although there is evidence that some children begin to tan intentionally at relatively young ages, it is more typically initiated during the early teens. By adolescence, the majority of young people report finding tans attractive both in themselves and others. They also report the desire to be attractive as a critical variable in their decisions to tan. In theory, the perception that tanning is attractive occurs due to social learning and prior experience. In childhood, the child is socialized to view tanned skin as healthy-looking and untanned skin as unhealthy. By adolescence, this initial socialization is reinforced by the reactions of others. Their experience, in terms of others' comments and physical response to them, is that a tan is perceived as more desirable. This experience is further reinforced through modeling by the reaction that others within their peer group receive, as well as by the tanned image often being portrayed by media role models, to which adolescents are very attuned.

Not all adolescents however view a tan as more attractive. Some of this variability comes from differences in their actual versus ideal self-image and their social self-concept. Our skin is a critical element of our self-image.[10] Adolescents who define themselves as a 'tanned person', desire to be like a 'tanned person' or belong to social reference groups that define being tanned as part of group membership will be much more likely to tan. The perceived personal correlates of tanned vs pale skin by adolescents may form the basis for interventions that promote a natural appearance. Generally, tanned individuals are perceived as athletic, outdoor-loving, adventurous, popular, assertive, confident, and having more sexually appealing bodies, while pale individuals are rated as non-athletic, passive, uncertain, and having less sexually appealing bodies.

Adolescents perceive tanned skin as more attractive, perceive positive personal correlates of tanned skin, and frequently develop fantasies about what tanning will do for themselves socially, sexually, etc.[11] Therefore, it is not surprising that the initiation of tanning behavior typically begins during this time. The common historical reason cited is that tanning became attractive back in the 1920s when the economy changed such that laborers went from primarily working outdoors in the fields, etc. to working indoor in factories. Prior to this, tanned skin was associated with the working classes and pale skin was associated with the upper classes. After this time pale skin became associated with the working classes, while tan skin became associated with the leisure of the rich. While this hypothesis may be of historical interest, it is probably not a critical factor in tan perceptions among young people today. For adolescents today, tanning is associated with experiences at the beach and poolside. Both of these experiences are socially sanctioned environments where members of the opposite sex can mingle wearing minimal clothing. Sunbathing provides social benefits. Most adolescents engage in the behavior with their friends, at fun, socially arousing locations. Lying in the sun is also a relaxing, physically pleasurable activity for many people. In fact, for some light exposure from the sun has powerful mood enhancing effects.

Thus, while students cognitively recognize that tanning is not the 'best' overall choice, they base their decision to tan on more affective, non-cognitive factors.

Interventions to modify sun protection behaviors

Deterrence of deliberate tanning through education programs has been the major method of attempting to change risk behaviors of young individuals. The research has attempted to describe high-risk youth relative to others in terms of demographic variables, personality variables, general attitudinal variables, and topic knowledge. These studies support the notion that individual beliefs about sun-risk and sun-safe behaviors have a major influence on their intentional sunbathing and sunbathing consequences.[12]

School curriculum

Several interventions have in-depth educational curricula and thorough methodology examining short-term, long-term and process-based effects. With few minor exceptions, these studies report positive effects on attitudes and behavioral tendencies in their sample populations. Despite this, studies examining the quantity and frequency of youth sun-risk activities continue to report widespread rates of intentional sun exposure and low sun protection among young people. Although the demographic and personality variables that are important predictors of sun-risk behavior are known, such variables are not amenable to change in short-term intervention efforts. For example, attitudes toward sunbathing, sun protection, appearance, tanning, sunscreen, sun block and ultraviolet risk paired with normative beliefs and beliefs about risks have been found to be critical variables predicting numerous sun-risk and sun-safe behavioral outcome variables.

Parental role

According to the approach of our group formed by Drs Turrisi, Hillhouse and Robinson, to effectively reduce sunburns and sunburn severity one must decrease sunbathing behaviors while at the same time increasing the development of healthy attitudes concerning appearance, tanning, sunscreen, sun block, ultraviolet (UV) risk and perceptions about engaging in alternative activities. Parents in long-term relationships in the home may provide this dual approach. Specifically, parents who have good communication patterns with their children may guide their children through initiating conversations about skin cancer, high-risk behaviors and positive sun-safe behaviors. Parents serve as role models of sun protection for their children and identify sports figures, musicians, and other media figures with untanned skin as role models for the children.

Parents may reframe the sun protection health promotion message with their children. Young people often tend to discount health-related information, particularly when that information pertains to long-term consequences.

This effect is further bolstered by the adolescent's tendency to view people who worry about such things as future skin cancer as too passive, careful, non-adventurous, and not cool. Young people also have a well-documented sense of personal invulnerability, and a tendency to misperceive true risk when it goes against the desired behavior (tanning). The message from parents can emphasize what is gained now and what is lost in the future. The emphasis on the long-term benefits of sun protection decreasing the chance of getting skin cancer is shifted to talking about using daily sun protection now to have fewer or no painful burns.

'Tanning now means loss of the skin's health and beauty; you may get wrinkles in your 20s'. The role of adults in adolescent's health and disease prevention has been suggested as being even more influential than school curricula.

Adolescence is an important developmental period to introduce specific intervention programs aimed at reducing indoor tanning and sun exposure and to begin to learn how to recognize skin cancer. Young children from infancy until about age 8 to 9 are under the influence of their parents and have their sun protection provided by their parents. Enhanced sun protection in adolescence holds great potential to reduce the incidence of skin cancer. Improved SSE in adults has the potential to reduce mortality.

Host and environmental risk factors: the need for secondary prevention

Older age is associated with higher risk of developing both BCC and SCC. There is a rapid rise in incidence after age 40, with SCC increasing more rapidly than BCC. While the incidence for men and women are similar at early ages, after age 45 men develop NMSC two to three times more frequently than women. Even as the US CM incidence and mortality rates for younger age people and for women stabilized in recent years, the incidence and mortality rate for males age 60 and above continued to increase from 1985 to 1994. Some 75% of the thicker CMs with poor prognosis were in patients older than 50. It is expected that the US population of adults 65 and older will increase as much as 20% between 2010 and 2030; therefore, the number of people with skin cancer and the number of deaths it causes can be expected to continue to rise.

Skin cancer is more common in people with immunosuppressive diseases or with diseases that are controlled by chronic immunosuppressive therapy, e.g. survivors of non-Hodgkin's lymphoma, organ transplant patients, and those with rheumatoid arthritis. Among transplant recipients, the incidence of SCC is markedly increased in those with sun sensitive skin, a history of sun exposure, and clinical signs of photoaging. NMSCs usually appear three to seven years after the onset of chronic immunosuppressive therapy. Renal transplant patients with a functioning graft for more than 5 years have a relative risk of 6.5 of developing NMSC, which increases to 20 after more than 15 years. There is a 75% increased risk of CM among non-Hodgkin's lymphoma survivors and a

2- to 4-fold higher incidence in organ transplant patients undergoing immunosuppressive regimens.

The considerable variability in genetic susceptibility to developing skin cancer is attributed to the melanin content of skin and the skin's ability to tan in response to ultraviolet radiation exposure (UVR). Pale complexion, freckling, inability to tan, past severe sunburns and cumulative sun exposure, light eye color, northern European or Celtic heritage and red or blonde hair are strong predictors of NMSC, and all are related to the melanin content of the individual's epidermal cells. A family history or personal history of CM or NMSC is associated with an increased risk of developing other skin cancers. While families with multiple affected members account for about 10% of CM cases, the relative contributions of genetic and shared environmental risk factors are unknown. The familial tendency to develop NMSC may be related to the gene, MC1R, leading to red hair and sun sensitivity. The rates of NMSC for non-Hispanic whites were approximately 11 times greater than for Hispanics, who do not share the same phenotype. NMSC in Caucasians have a log-linear increasing incidence with age, which may be due to cumulative environmental ultraviolet radiation (UVR) exposure (Fig. 7.1).

Occupational and recreational patterns of sun exposure place those with genetic susceptibility at increased risk. NMSCs occur more frequently in residents of areas with high solar radiation, which is the reason for the clear latitudinal gradient in incidence rate. In 1996, the Arizona annual age-adjusted incidence rate of SCC for men was 270 per 100,000 and for women, 112 per 100,000; and of BCC for men, 935 per 100,000 and for women, 497 per 100,000.[4] In New Hampshire, the annual incidence rate of SCC for men was 97 per 100,000, for women, 32 per 100,000; and of BCC for men 310 per 100,000 and for women 166 per 100,000. SCCs occur on sun-exposed body locations with maximum exposure such as the head and neck, in people with a fair complexion, in

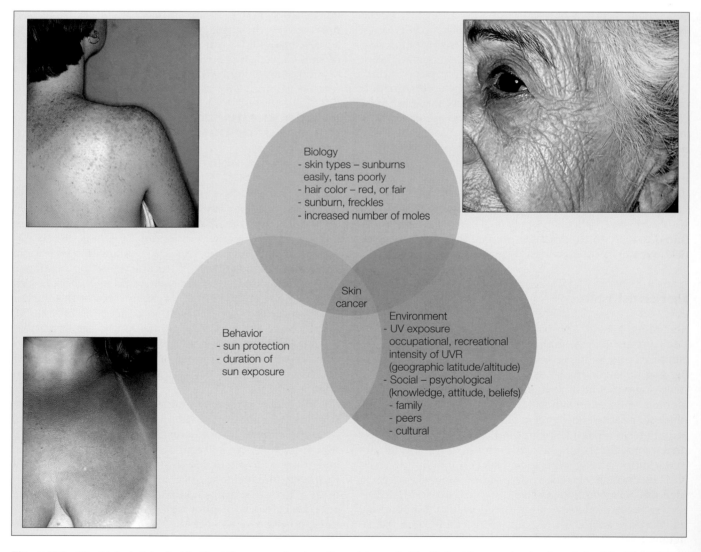

Figure 7.1 The biologic inherited traits of the person (such as the adolescent girl with freckles over her back and shoulders) form the base upon which the individual's occupation, intensity of ultraviolet radiation in their geographic location as well as their social and family normative beliefs regarding sun protection (such as the 90-year-old woman with a life-time of sun protection having no freckles) are laid establish their sun exposure behavioral patterns. After repetitive events of sunburns (young adult woman with sunburn of the chest) or chronic tanning over a period of years, skin cancer develops.

those with genetic disorders with increased sensitivity to UVR, in outdoor workers more commonly than in indoor workers, and more commonly in men than in women.

CM and BCC have a more complex relationship with sun exposure and appear to be associated with a history of sunburns, particularly in childhood. Migration studies show a higher rate of CM in those who migrate to a sunnier climate than those who remain in their own country, particularly if migration occurs in childhood. The risk of CM is higher in indoor workers than in outdoor workers. CM is more common in body areas with intermittent light exposure. BCC has a similar distribution pattern in the trunk and lower limbs, i.e. areas not so frequently exposed. Risk factors for the development of CM include having more than 50 moles (odds rate, OR 5.3–3.0), having one to four atypical nevi (OR 1.6–7.3), a family history of CM (OR 8), immunosuppression (OR 8) and personal history of CM, family history of CM and atypical moles (OR 35). Other risk factors for CM are red or light hair (OR 1.4–3.5), few (OR 1.9) or many solar lentigines (OR 3.5), very heavy sun exposure (OR 2.6), reported growth of a mole (OR 2.3), skin that does not tan easily (OR 1.98), and light skin color types (OR 1.4).

Both NMSC and CM occur in people with solar keratoses, sun-related precancerous lesions. Solar keratoses can be considered a marker of past excessive sun exposure. Case–control studies have shown solar keratoses to be a risk factor for both CM and NMSC. Thus the UVR exposure sustained by an adult in their youth places them at risk to develop skin cancer, both CM and NMSC, several decades later. For adults at risk of skin cancer who sustained unprotected sun exposure in childhood and adolescence, secondary prevention may prevent death and disfigurement.

Secondary prevention of skin cancer: early detection

Early detection is achieved by enhanced surveillance by the person who is at risk or their physicians. Many studies have documented that surveillance cases of CM detected in family settings are diagnosed at earlier stages than index cases.[14] Skin self-examination (SSE) is a form of secondary prevention, which includes early identification of risk factors or subclinical disease in people who have not yet developed symptoms. Those who perform SSE present for care at an earlier stage in the disease process, have 50% less advanced CM, and a significantly lower mortality from CM. It is estimated that SSE may reduce the death rate from CM by as much as 63%.[2] SSE could achieve some reduction in deaths from CM and reduce the physical and emotional burden of disease from both NMSC and CM.

Primary care physicians because of lack of confidence in their ability to detect skin cancers and inability to recognize risk factors may not routinely perform skin cancer screening. There are opportunities for case finding during the annual examination provided by primary care physicians; however, since the incidence of CM is lower than prostate and breast cancer, most physicians rarely have the opportunity to detect a CM. This hampers diagnostic accuracy and does not provide adequate reinforcement to physicians to perform skin cancer screening for their patients.

Therefore, the burden of early detection of CM falls to those who are at risk. Case finding by a physician might be expected to be more effective because it reaches patients, especially elderly men who have a higher mortality from CM than others, who are at risk and are least likely to practice SSE. However, people can perform self-examination more frequently (monthly on average) than screening by a physician and can note findings, particularly changes in size, border, or color of lesions, that may not be easily recognized by infrequent examinations.[15] Over 50% of CM patients detect their own CM and about 11% have the lesion found by a spouse. The caveat is that for people who escape early detection and/or progress to the advanced stage of the disease (Stage IV), there has been very little improvement in the survival rate over the last 20 years.

Factors that can influence the performance of SSE include: (1) individual host factors such as gender, age, sun sensitivity, impaired vision; (2) cognitive factors such as perception of risk, importance of skin cancer in light of comorbid disease, and knowledge of the warning signs of skin cancer; (3) social factors such as peer group norms, social norms, and social interactions; and (4) environmental factors such as skin cancer health promotion messages delivered by the media (Fig. 7.2). In those at risk of skin cancer because of having previous skin cancer or having more than 50 moles, the strongest predictors of SSE performance were attitude, having dermatology visits with skin biopsies and at least one skin cancer in the previous three years, and confidence in performance.[16] Other predictors of SSE performance were perceived risk, knowledge, younger age (40–59 years of age), being a woman, and asking a partner for help. Additional studies showed a greater likelihood of women performing SSE and the importance of physician recommendation to perform SSE.[17]

Theoretical models of social influence have stressed the role of peers in influencing a range of behaviors. For SSE, the relevant peer group is the partner who assists with performing the exam in locations that are difficult to see, e.g. back of scalp, back of legs or below the buttocks. The partner's and the person's perceptions of the benefit of SSE and risks of developing a skin cancer are probably both important to their acquiring the knowledge, skills, and abilities as well as providing post-performance reinforcement of the need to assist with performance. Once skin examination is initiated, the partner provides social reinforcement. Fulfillment of expectations by finding a worrisome lesion also reinforces SSE. Skin examination by a partner may be limited by privacy concerns, availability of a partner, or relationship with the partner (Fig. 7.3). Those who do not perform SSE may discount cognitively based information or place responsibility for early detection of skin cancer onto the physician.

Studies suggest that having a partner enhances the belief that they can perform the task for each other. Thus, the partner becomes a prominent influence for SSE performance by engaging in the process of assisting with the exam, helping to reach decisions about the lesion

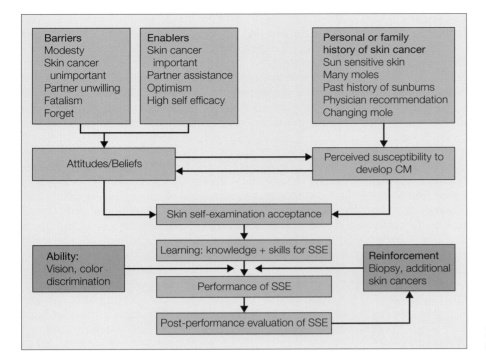

Figure 7.2 Behavioral model of skin self-examination (SSE) performance.

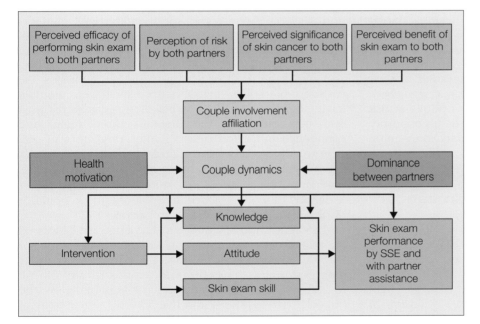

Figure 7.3 Model of reinforcement of skin self-examination by couples.

that is observed, and reinforcing the performance of SSE by the patient. The quality of the relationship between the patient and the partner may influence self-initiated and professionally assisted behavioral change (e.g. SSE). In prior research, relationship quality has correlated with a range of health behavior outcomes. In the context of partners with high affiliation, learning and behavioral change may be enhanced; conversely in dyads with low affiliation there may be no effect or a negative effect on learning and behavioral change.

FUTURE OUTLOOK

Primary and secondary prevention programs for skin cancer can make a significant difference in the mortality

and morbidity from skin cancer. Better strategies that enable change in the behaviors of those at risk to develop skin cancer are being developed. A promising approach is to improve the personal skin cancer risk perception of people. Recognition of solar keratoses as a warning signal of the individual's increased risk of developing skin cancer may lead to increased surveillance by SSE and physician examination.

Tanning attitudes are influencing the sun exposure and indoor tanning habits of our youth and young adults. Society wide attitudinal change in the perceived value of having a tan is an important enabler of attitudinal change for the individual. Since tanning is largely an affective driven decision in which the tanners often ignore or discount the cognitive-based information such as skin cancer risk and premature aging of the skin, societal attitude change promoting the appearance and healthy look of natural skin tones may set the stage for individual change. Societal attitudes are malleable as are the attitudes of individuals. Surveys in Australia showed that the appeal of tanned skin decreased following skin cancer education and prevention campaigns, which have been of greater magnitude and longer duration than those in the US.[18] In addition to educational campaigns, legislation and regulation may influence cultural attitudes toward risk taking behavior and effectively impact public health. An example of legislation changing behaviors in the US is the use of seat belts. Only 10–15% of US population used seat belts in the early 1980s. After seat belt legislation enactment and enforcement of mandatory seatbelt use and public education campaigns, the use in 1993 was 70%. Enacting youth access indoor tanning laws may spark societal changes that foster behavioral change.[19,20]

ACKNOWLEDGMENTS

Robert J Turrisi PhD, Professor and Director of Family Studies Research, Department of Psychology, Boise State University, Boise, Idaho, and Joel J Hillhouse PhD, Associate Professor, Department of Psychology, East Tennessee State University, Johnson City, Tennessee have worked with Dr Robinson in formulating the behavioral models of primary and secondary skin cancer prevention. The collaboration of all members of the group is represented in this work.

REFERENCES

1 Bandura A. Self-efficacy mechanism in physiological activation and health-promoting behavior. In: Madden J, Matthysse SP, Barchas J, eds. Adaptation, Learning and Affect. New York, NY: Raven Press; 1988.

2 Berwick M, Begg CM, Fine JA, Roush GC, Barnhill RL. Screening for cutaneous melanoma by skin self-examination. J Natl Cancer Inst 1996; 88:17–23.

3 Clegg LX, Feuer EJ, Midthune DN, Fay MP, Hankey BF. Impact of reporting delay and reporting error on cancer incidence rates and trends. J Natl Cancer Inst 2002; 94:1537–45.

4 DiFronzo LA, Wanek LA, Morton DL. Earlier diagnosis of second primary melanoma confirms the benefits of patient education and routine post-operative follow-up. Cancer 2001; 91:1520–4.

5 Hillhouse J, Turrisi R. Examination of the efficacy of an appearance focused intervention to reduce UV exposure. J Behav Med 2002; 25(4):395–409.

6 Hillhouse J, Turrisi R, Kastner M. Modeling tanning salon behavioral tendencies using appearance motivation and the theory of planned behavior. Health Educ Res 2000; 15:405–414.

7 Hillhouse J, Turrisi R, Holwiski F, McVeigh S. An examination of psychological variables relevant to artificial tanning tendencies. J Health Psychol 1999; 4(4):507–516.

8 Robinson JK, Rademaker AW, Sylvester J, Cook B. Summer sun exposure: Knowledge, attitudes, and behaviors of Midwest adolescents. Preventive Medicine 1997; 26:364–372.

9 Robinson JK, Fisher SG, Turrisi RJ. Predictors of skin self-examination performance. Cancer 2002; 95:135–46.

10 Robinson JK, Rigel DS, Amonette RA. What promotes skin self-examination? J Am Acad Derm 1998; 39:752–757.

11 Scotto J, Fears T, Kraemer K, Fraumeni J. Nonmelanoma skin cancer. In: Schottenfeld D, Fraumeni J, eds. Cancer Epidemiology and Prevention, 2nd edn. Oxford: Oxford University Press; 1996:1313–1330.

12 Turrisi R, Hillhouse J, Gebert C. Examination of cognitive variables relevant to sunbathing. J Behav Med 1998; 21(3):299–311.

13 Friedman RJ, Rigel DS, Kopf AW. Early detection of malignant melanoma. CA Cancer J Clin 1985; 35:130–151.

14 Greenlee RT, Hill-Harmon B, Murray T, Thun M. Cancer statistics. CA Cancer J Clin 2001; 51:15–36.

15 Hall HI, Miller DR, Rogers JD, Bewerse B. Update on incidence and mortality from melanoma in the United States. J Am Acad Derm 1999; 40:35–42.

16 Hillhouse JJ. A heuristic model of indoor tanning behavior in college students. Communication. 2002.

17 Hillhouse JJ, Stair A, Adler CM. Predictors of sunbathing and sunscreen use in college undergraduates. J Behav Med 1996; 19:543–561.

18 Buller DB, Borland R. Public education projects in skin cancer prevention: childcare, school and college-based. Clin Derm 1998; 16:447–459.

19 US Department of Transportation National Highway Traffic Safety Administration. Legislative Fact Sheet. US Department of Transportation National Highway Traffic Safety Administration, 2003; Available at http://www.nhtsa.dot.gov/people/injury/airbags/buckleplan/buckleup/legfac t.html (accessed May).

20 Nelson DE, Bolen J, Kresnow M. Trends in safety belt use by demographics and by type of state safety belt law, 1987 through 1993. Am J Public Health 1998; 88:245–249.

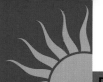

CHAPTER
8

Possible Precursors to Keratinocytic Epidermal Malignancies

Jeffrey P Callen

Key points

- Actinic keratoses are common and represent an early stage in the development of squamous cell carcinoma.
- Actinic keratoses serve as a marker of 'excess' sun exposure.
- Bowen's disease and its variants are intraepithelial malignancies and should be removed or destroyed once recognized.

INTRODUCTION

The recognition of lesions, conditions, or situations, which occur prior to the development of an epidermal malignancy may allow the prevention of the malignant process. Patients with these precursor lesions or conditions may be followed more carefully and even when malignancy does develop, it may be recognized and treated at an earlier stage and should be more easily cured. This chapter will deal with a variety of lesions, including actinic keratosis, radio-dermatitis, arsenic exposure, tar exposure, genetic pre-disposition, scarring processes and dermatoses, which may predispose to cancer formation.

ACTINIC KERATOSIS (SOLAR KERATOSIS)

Actinic keratoses are circumscribed, rough, epidermal lesions that develop on exposed skin surfaces that are primary due to chronic ultraviolet irradiation that may result from sun exposure or exposure to artificial light sources (e.g. tanning beds, ultraviolet light phototherapy or photochemotherapy).[1,2] Similar lesions may develop under the influence of radiation from radioactive sources such as X-ray therapy. (Radiodermatitis will be dealt with later in this chapter.)

The term actinic keratosis is relatively recent. It has been attributed to Hermann Pinkus and in 1959, Becker included it in his publication on Dermatological Nomenclature. Prior to that time the terms utilized included solar keratosis and senile keratosis.

The propensity to develop actinic keratoses is genetically influenced, with fair, blond-haired, blue-eyed individuals being more susceptible to solar damage. However, given (1) enough sun exposure (or UV exposure from an artificial source), and (2) enough time, most individuals would develop actinic keratoses. The widespread use of immunosuppressive therapies in the treatment of organ-donor recipients, cancer patients and inflammatory diseases has led to an increased number of patients and an increase in the number of lesions that occur on a given patient. With the advent of treatments for heart disease and cancer that improve our longevity, the prevalence of actinic keratoses continues to increase. Several other factors also influence to prevalence of actinic keratoses, including an increase in leisure time that is available for sun exposure, a shift of the population to the areas where sun exposure is more intense, and the use of artificial tanning beds.[3]

Historically, actinic keratoses have long been recognized as a side-effect of sun exposure in seamen or farmers. They have been referred to as solar keratosis previously, but since UV irradiation from artificial sources can cause them, it is best not to use this term. Also, a previous term used was senile keratosis. This term is no longer appropriate, because the lesions may occur at a relatively young age and because of the negative connotations implied to the patient. Traditionally, the lesions occur on sun-exposed surfaces, however, in today's society that can be almost any area of the body.

Actinic keratoses (AK) are epidermal neoplasms, consisting of altered epidermal keratinocytes. There is controversy regarding whether they should be classified as precursors to cancer or the earliest form of *in situ* cancer.[4] The risk that an individual lesion will become invasive has been estimated to be as high as 20%, or may be as low as 0.1%.[5] Despite the rate of this 'transformation' or 'progression', AKs possess changes that are identical to those found with invasive squamous cell carcinoma.[6] Therefore, all patients with AKs should be managed in some manner to prevent progression and observed for the frequently accompanying lesions such as basal cell carcinoma or *de novo* SCC. Biologically, the AK is considered to be a carcinoma *in situ*. The exact number of actinic keratoses that will invade through the basement membrane of the epidermis to become squamous cell carcinoma is dependent upon time; thus, if left untreated for enough time, it is possible that many actinic keratoses will progress to invasive squamous cell carcinomas.

The actinic keratosis is represented clinically by a scaly, rough lesion that is often better recognized by palpation than by inspection (Fig. 8.1). The lesion ranges from pinpoint size to large plaques (Fig. 8.2), but most lesions are between 3 and 6 mm in diameter. The AK may be flesh-colored, darkly pigmented, erythematous, tan or any hue in between these colors. AKs are often

93

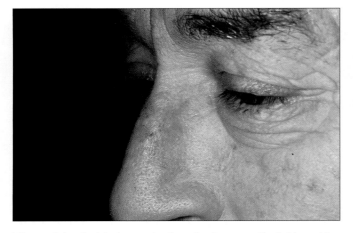

Figure 8.1 Actinic keratosis. A scaly plaque on the bridge of the nose.

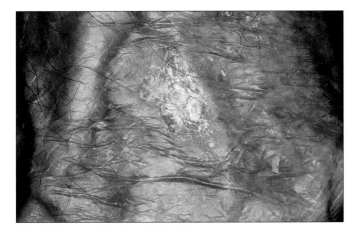

Figure 8.2 Actinic keratosis. A large, scaly plaque on the dorsum of the hand.

macular, particularly on the head and neck. On the arms and hands the lesions are thicker. Horn formation can occur on any area of the body (Fig. 8.3). The lesions may be sharply circumscribed, but more often they blend into the background skin gradually.

By definition, ultraviolet irradiation is the underlying etiologic factor for the actinic keratoses. However, the exact mechanism by which irradiation induces the lesion is not completely understood. Furthermore, it is not clear whether the damage involves only the epidermis or involves the dermis as well. Ultraviolet rays may affect the epidermal cells by causing DNA crosslinks known as thymidine dimers. In addition, it appears that mutation of a tumor suppressor gene, *p53* is very prevalent in both actinic keratoses and squamous cell carcinoma. Mutation of this gene allows cells damaged by sunlight to continue to grow and divide, while normal cells without a *p53* mutation when damaged by the same sunlight undergo apoptosis. This leaves space for the mutated cells to grow and thus cancer can begin to develop.[6] These cells then may not mature in a normal fashion and may eventually lead to a clone of cells that form the AK. Those factors that keep the dysplastic cells within the epidermis may well involve the immune surveillance system of the body. In addition, sunlight exposure is known to be immunosuppressive and this may play a role in the promotion of mutated cells as the normal mechanisms that would identify and destroy abnormal cells is lost or functions poorly. There is a delay of many years until development of the AK takes place; thus, it is unclear whether the keratinocytes or the surveillance system has the primary role.

There are several histopathologic pictures that may be found in actinic keratoses: a hypertrophic variant, an atrophic variant, a bowenoid variant, and a lichenoid variant.[4] The hypertrophic variant is the most common. Atrophic areas of epidermis are interspersed with areas of hyperkeratosis and papillomatosis. Cells throughout the suprabasal cell layer are irregularly arranged and have atypical, large, irregular, hyperchromatic nuclei. Individual cell keratinization may be present. Downward proliferation of the epidermis is present, but in all cases the basal lamina remain intact. The atrophic variant lacks the hyperkeratosis and papillomatosis. The bowenoid variant may truly not be different from that seen in Bowen's disease (see below); however, when the lesion is present on sun-exposed skin, some pathologists prefer to term the lesion a bowenoid actinic keratosis rather than call it Bowen's disease. Lastly, there is a variant in which there is a lymphohistiocytic infiltrate that hugs the epidermis with saw-toothing of the epidermis and some liquefactive degeneration of the basal cells is known as the lichenoid actinic keratosis. Whether this lichenoid AK is biologically or prognostically different is not known.

The main problem in differential diagnosis is the separation of an early squamous cell carcinoma from the actinic keratosis. This is usually not difficult. In addition, the hypertrophic lesions must be distinguished from warts and seborrheic keratoses. Usually this can be accomplished on the basis of the clinical correlation. Pigmented AKs must be differentiated from pigmented basal cell carcinomas and from malignant melanoma. When there is a question about the potential for melanoma, a full-thickness biopsy (punch or excision) should be performed.

Actinic keratoses, if left untreated, often persist. Regression may follow irritation of an individual lesion. In addition, the regular use of sunscreen has been demonstrated to allow regression of many lesions,[7] and a low-fat diet may also be associated with regression of existing lesions.[8] The major concern about prognosis is the potential of these lesions to become invasive squamous cell carcinomas, and for their presence to serve as a marker of photodamage that is associated with other cutaneous malignancies.

Treatment of the actinic keratosis is necessary, but the measures used should be conservative, cosmetically acceptable, and should not result in a great deal of morbidity. Discussions with the patient regarding the relationship of sun exposure should occur during most office visits, and a program of photoprotective measures including sun avoidance combined with an appropriate sunscreen regimen should be started. The patient should be told that the development of new lesions is common, but that the rate might be slowed with the use of sunscreens and use of other prudent measures.

Options for therapy of actinic keratoses include chemotherapeutic agents, surgical procedures, and irradiation.

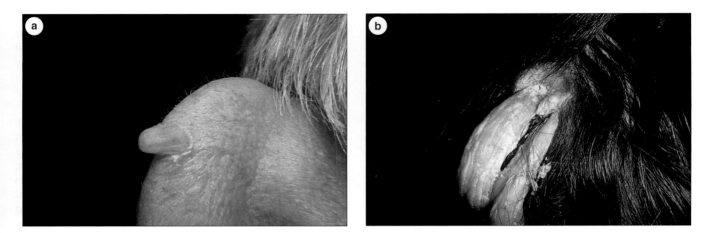

Figure 8.3 Cutaneous horns. Biopsy of these lesions revealed actinic keratosis.

Since the lesions are not yet invasive, irradiation is far too aggressive as an approach and should be avoided. Surgical or laser procedures, although effective, are not necessary and are expensive. Full-thickness excisions are only indicated if the dermatologic surgeon thinks that the cosmetic result warrants the procedure.

Actinic keratoses can be adequately treated with sharp curettage followed by electrodesiccation. This procedure allows the treating physician to obtain tissue for biopsy. Biopsy should be used whenever there is a question about the possibility of invasive carcinoma. Tissue removed by curettage (or any surgical method) should not be discarded. Although this form of treatment results in a cure in 99% of lesions, it frequently leaves residual hypopigmentation at the site of treatment. Furthermore, the procedure is much more costly to the patient, the insurance company and society. Therefore, use of other modalities should be considered.

Cryosurgery with liquid nitrogen, applied as a spray or using a cotton-tipped applicator, is effective therapy for most actinic keratoses. This procedure is the one that is performed most commonly as a treatment for an actinic keratosis by practicing dermatologists.[9] Depending on the depth of the freeze, dyspigmentation may result. The procedure is uncomfortable, but healing is prompt. Multiple lesions may be treated on an office visit. Follow-up in 4–6 weeks is indicated to be certain that the lesion has been eradicated. A variant that has been proposed is to utilize liquid nitrogen widely in an attempt to peel the skin and treat potential subclinical lesions. This 'cryo-peel' technique has not been tested and is not widely utilized in practice. Another similar method is the use of tri- or bichloracetic acid applied to the individual lesions. Although this method has lost favor, it can result in eradication of the lesions. This type of acid peel may also be used for widespread and possibly subclinical lesions.

Another destructive method that is available is the use of photodynamic therapy. This procedure involves the application of a photosensitizing compound followed by administration of the proper wavelength of irradiation. A system involving the application of aminolevulinic acid (ALA) followed about 12 hrs later with exposure to blue light was recently approved by the FDA, however this therapy involves two office visits and is associated with discomfort that is similar to cryosurgery. Although the resulting dyspigmentation may be less than with cryosurgery, this form of therapy has not been widely adopted due to socioeconomic factors.

Since many patients have multiple lesions present, and since the appearance of new lesions is common, methods that would eradicate lesions but also would prevent the development of new lesions would be ideal therapy. Topical chemotherapy was developed in the hope that this might be accomplished. Topical applications of 5-fluorouracil to the entire integument involved is useful in accomplishing this purpose. The medication is available in a cream or lotion form and in various concentrations from 1–5%. In addition, a newer formulation in a 'microsponge' system has also been approved by the FDA.[10] The medication is applied once daily and causes the lesion to become red and irritated. The irritation can be so intense that patients are uncomfortable; the lesions become exudative and patients are unable to maintain a normal social life because of their appearance (Fig. 8.4). 5-Fluorouracil treatment causes this reaction in areas of actinically damaged skin, which is clinically normal, and this reaction is believed to prevent the development of new lesions. The recommended length of treatment is between 3 and 8 weeks, but most patients are unable to tolerate more than 3 weeks of treatment because of the irritation. Topical corticosteroids may decrease the inflammatory reaction and are believed not to result in alteration of the efficacy.

Another potentially useful chemotherapy is topical tretinoin. In the early 1970s it was suggested that this agent might be of benefit for the treatment of actinic keratoses.[11] Subsequently, it has been advocated for the reversal of sun damage to the skin.[12] In a recent report from the University of Michigan, clinical AK lesions resolved with the use of topical tretinoin cream 0.1% applied daily for 4 months. Furthermore, the changes of epidermal dysplasia in 'normal' skin were reversed with therapy but not with the placebo cream. Thus, this topical therapy may have a role in treatment and also as a method of prevention. This aspect of topical tretinoin usage still needs to be further evaluated. Irritation,

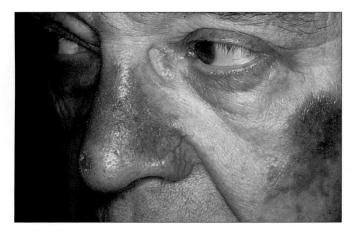

Figure 8.4 Irritant dermatitis following topical application of fluorouracil cream.

erythema, and dryness are side effects of the use of topical tretinoin. Another retinoid that might be useful in the future is adapalene. Currently this drug is available in a 0.1% concentration and is approved for therapy of acne vulgaris. However, preliminary reports of a 0.3% formulation suggest that it may be useful for the treatment of AK.[13]

Topical diclofenac, a nonsteroidal anti-inflammatory drug, has recently been approved for treatment of AK.[14] Daily application of this drug over a period of 3–6 months results in a statistically significant reduction in the number of AKs compared with placebo. The drug appears to be less irritating than 5-fluorouracil and imiquimod, but it must be used for a longer period of time.

Imiquimod is an immune response modifier that was developed initially for the treatment of genital warts and to date, this is its only FDA approved indication. However, there are multiple studies that have demonstrated its usefulness in the treatment of multiple AKs.[15–17] This drug may be applied as little as 2–3 times per week for up to 12 weeks. Salasche *et al.*[17] have recently demonstrated the effectiveness of imiquimod use in 4-week cycles with a 4-week rest period interspersed between each cycle. There is some possibility that this therapy might result in some immune enhancement and as well as the destruction of an individual lesion, the area treated may be altered in some manner that impedes the development of future AKs. In addition, like 5-fluorouracil, the application of imiquimod is associated with the appearance of inflamed skin that was presumed to contain a subclinical lesion. Therefore its use might result in a decrease in future development of AKs.

Lastly, in a recent publication, Grimaitre *et al.*[18] demonstrated that a topical preparation of colchicine was effective for a small group of patients with actinic keratoses. This agent needs to be tested in further studies before it is adopted.

The prognosis of the patient with actinic keratoses is generally good. The lesions may progress to carcinoma; the exact frequency of this transformation and the mechanisms of invasion are not clear. Furthermore, some AKs may spontaneously resolve. It is thought that SCCs that arise from an actinic keratosis rarely if ever

metastasize,[19] but these lesions (the AK) may occur in the presence of a spontaneously appearing SCC that can metastasize or in the presence of basal cell carcinomas that can be locally invasive. Thus, the recognition of a patient with actinic keratoses should alert the physician to treat these lesions, to advise the patient about limitation of further actinic damage, and to follow the patient for malignant lesions.

Actinic keratoses will continue to be a problem as the population ages and more immunosuppressive drugs are utilized for treatment of inflammatory diseases as well as for suppression for organ transplant recipients. We will need remittive therapies to complement our destructive methods. In addition, education about photoprotection beginning in grade school, must be part of the strategies for prevention that our national organizations advocate.

RADIATION-INDUCED KERATOSES

Premalignant keratoses can be induced by ionizing radiation used for either diagnostic or therapeutic purposes. In the early age of radiation therapy, improper shielding resulted in the delivery of large amounts of radiation to the skin.

Radiodermatitis, radiation-induced keratoses, and radiation-related carcinoma are currently induced by the use of radiation for (1) the treatment of internal malignancies, (2) the treatment of cutaneous malignancies, (3) the treatment of benign skin tumors, and (4) the treatment of benign inflammatory cutaneous conditions. Therapy of benign dermatoses with low doses of radiation (superficial X-ray or Grenz ray) is generally safe, but should be reserved for recalcitrant dermatoses only. Previously, in the 1950s the most common uses for X-ray therapy for cutaneous disease were for acne and hirsutism: today, recalcitrant hand dermatoses, chronic scalp psoriasis, and seborrhea are the most often treated dermatoses. The potential for malignant changes is related to the dose of X-ray given. The latent period between therapy and induction of the lesions can be as short as a few years or as long as 30 years.

Generally, the keratoses are preceded by a chronic radiodermatitis that has a cutaneous appearance similar to that seen from chronic sun exposure. The clinical lesion is identical to that seen with actinic keratoses and may take any of the forms described above. Histopathology of the epidermis in radiation-induced keratoses is similar, if not identical, to that observed with actinic keratosis. Possibly there are more elastotic changes in the dermis and a greater obliteration of vascular structures in radiation-induced keratoses. It appears that the prognosis of this lesion is more aggressive than that of the actinic keratosis, but quantification of this perception has not been proven.

Treatment options for radiodermatitis and radiation-induced keratoses are similar to those for actinic keratoses. Some physicians prefer to remove individual lesions with curettage and electrodesiccation or excision. The author does not use 5-fluorouracil in these patients; however, he believes that the use of topical tretinoin and possibly topical imiquimod may prove valuable in the future. Close follow-up of these patients is necessary.

ARSENICAL KERATOSES

Arsenical keratoses occur most often on the acral skin – in particular, on the volar surfaces. Arsenicals have several industrial and agricultural applications. Without proper precautions the worker may be exposed to large amounts of arsenic. The most common use is in insecticides, fungicides, herbicides, and defoliants. Arsenic trioxide was also used medicinally for the treatment of multiple conditions – in particular, psoriasis and asthmatic bronchitis. Lastly, arsenic is a contaminant in drinking water in some areas of the world. Arsenic has been linked through experimental studies to the development of cancer in animals. Epidemiological studies in humans also suggest that arsenic is related to the development of keratoses, squamous cell carcinoma, Bowen's disease, and superficial basal cell epithelioma.[20] The relationship between arsenic ingestion and internal malignancy is less clear; however, squamous cell carcinoma of the lung or bladder, or both, may be increased in persons exposed to arsenicals.

Clinically, arsenical keratoses are punctate palmar and/or plantar lesions. Usually there are hundreds of lesions present (Fig. 8.5). Similar lesions may occur on the dorsal surfaces as well. There is usually symmetrical involvement. The lesions grow but seem to reach some limiting size and then usually remain stable. Rapid change in growth may signify malignant degeneration and warrants close evaluation and removal of the lesion. The patients should be thoroughly examined, because multiple superficial basal cell carcinomas and multiple lesions of Bowen's disease may be found. The examiner should look through all hairy areas as well because these cancers do not have a solar relationship. The lesions of arsenical keratoses must be differentiated from warts and familial punctate palmar-plantar keratosis.

The histological features of the arsenical keratosis vary from the more benign to the frank *in situ* malignant changes seen in Bowen's disease. The lesions are multifocal, and thus changes of squamous intraepidermal neoplasia may co-exist with a basal cell carcinoma within the same specimen. The lesion has hyperkeratosis; it may be acanthotic and may lack the normal maturation seen in the normal epidermis. The cells may stain darkly, and dysplastic changes, division figures, and irregular arrangement are commonly observed. The differentiation of the arsenical keratosis from Bowen's disease often depends on clinical correlation.

Squamous cell carcinoma with the potential for metastasis can arise from arsenical keratoses, but the frequency of this occurrence is not clear. It has been estimated that this 'transformation' occurs in about 5% or less of the patients. The prognosis of patients with arsenical keratosis is determined by the rate of invasive squamous cell carcinoma and the potential for internal malignant disease.

Treatment of the patient with arsenical keratoses is difficult, primarily because of the large number of lesions present. In general, lesions that are symptomatic or that have undergone a rapid change should be treated. Cryotherapy, curettage, and electrodesiccation are preferred methods. Laser destruction and micrographically controlled surgery, although effective, are probably not indicated. The use of 5-fluorouracil has been reported, but adequate documentation that this therapy is effective in reversing the dysplastic nature of these deep lesions is not available. Ideally, a chemoprevention might be developed which might alter not only the risk of malignant degeneration but also alter the potential for internal malignant disease.

It is not clear what the future outlook is for arsenical keratoses, but it is likely that they have become much less common and will probably be seen less often.

BOWEN'S DISEASE AND ITS VARIANTS

Dr John Bowen is credited with the first description of this entity.[21] He believed it was a precancerous dermatosis because it was histopathologically characterized by atypical epithelial proliferation. Subsequently, this process has been recognized as an intraepidermal neoplasia of the skin which can occur on sun exposed or non-sun-exposed surfaces. It differs from a related process, the *in situ* squamous cell carcinoma, in its clinical and histopathologic characteristics. In addition, it differs from erythroplasia of Queyrat primarily in its clinical

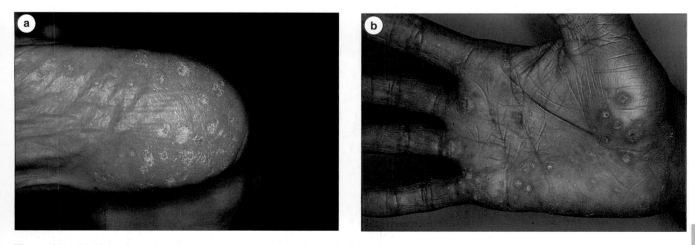

Figure 8.5 Multiple plantar keratoses are representative of arsenical keratoses.

characteristics. Controversies exist regarding the separation of Bowen's from non-Bowen's squamous intraepidermal neoplasia (SIN) and regarding the relationship of these processes to internal malignancy.

Bowen's disease is most often a slightly scaly, discrete, erythematous plaque with a sharp but often irregular or undulating border (Figs 8.6 and 8.7). The surface characteristics vary and include hyperkeratosis, fissures, dyspigmentation, erosions, and/or ulcerations. The distribution can vary from maximally or minimally exposed surfaces. The lesion usually grows in a slow but progressive manner. The lesions may be single or multiple. When the lesion occurs on an exposed surface, it is often accompanied by actinic damage of the surrounding skin, actinic keratoses, basal cell carcinomas, and/or squamous cell carcinomas. Patients with Bowen's disease may also have arsenical keratoses. This process usually occurs in people with fair skin.

Non-Bowen's squamous intraepidermal neoplasia may clinically represent the transitional stage between an actinic keratosis and a squamous cell carcinoma. Thus, the clinical characteristics are those of an actinic keratosis and include a scaly, poorly demarcated plaque. Erythema

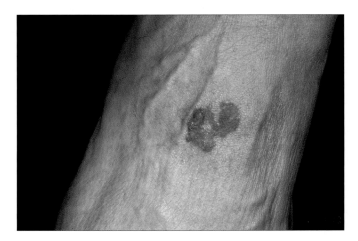

Figure 8.6 Bowen's disease. This plaque has a scaly surface with an undulating border.

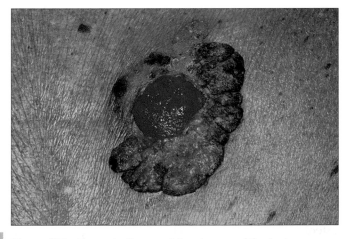

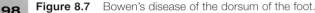

Figure 8.7 Bowen's disease of the dorsum of the foot.

or pigmentation may or may not be present. The lesions are often more easily palpated than visualized. These lesions usually occur on actinic damaged skin and often are accompanied by other premalignant and malignant skin lesions. This process is most often observed in people with fair skin.

Bowen's disease and non-Bowen's SIN have been linked in the literature to internal malignancy. The association has usually been characterized in groups of patients through retrospective analysis.[22–25] The frequency of internal malignancy in patients with these disorders has varied, but only one study from Scandinavia has failed to demonstrate an increase in the expected frequency of internal neoplasia. Despite this apparent relationship it appears that the concurrent recognition of the skin lesion and the internal neoplasm is extremely rare. In addition, the relationship of the skin lesion to the subsequent development of an internal malignancy has not been demonstrated. Furthermore, Arbesman and Ransohoff have recently analyzed the studies from a epidemiologist's view and have shown that the previous conclusions may not be valid.[24] Therefore, the patient with either Bowen's disease or non-Bowen's SIN does not warrant a malignancy evaluation.

Erythroplasia of Queyrat (EQ) generally occurs on the glans penis but may also occur on the shaft (Fig. 8.8), on the scrotum, or on the vulva. This disorder is almost always found in uncircumcised men. The lesion is usually solitary, and is characterized by a sharply defined, discrete, non-tender, erythematous plaque. The surface may be erosive or may have a slight scale. EQ usually occurs in people with fair skin, but may also occur in people with dark skin. EQ has not been associated with internal malignancy, nor has it been linked to arsenic ingestion. Thus, it appears that on clinical grounds this entity is best separated from Bowen's disease, even though it usually is histopathologically identical.

Bowen's disease has been linked to at least four potential etiologic agents: actinic damage, arsenic ingestion, radiation therapy and viral agents. Possibly a combination of these factors may be involved in some patients. The non-Bowen's SIN has been strongly linked to sun exposure, although an occasional patient will report the ingestion of arsenicals. Erythroplasia of Queyrat occurs most often in non-circumcised men and thus, it may be related to chronic irritation from retained secretions under the foreskin. In addition, it may be related to human papilloma virus infection.

Confirmation of the clinical diagnosis is made by histopathologic examination of a biopsy specimen. Bowen's disease should be suspected in any persistent, chronic plaque, particularly if therapy is not effective. Commonly, the clinical lesion was presumed to be psoriasis or a chronic eczema long before a biopsy was considered. In addition, the differential diagnosis includes superficial basal cell carcinoma, Paget's disease, and/or actinic keratosis. The histopathologic examination demonstrates a full thickness epidermal dysplasia with marked atypia in which individual cell dyskeratosis and increased mitoses are sharply defined from the contiguous normal epithelium. In contrast, non-Bowen's SIN has less nuclear pleomorphism, only slight to moderate

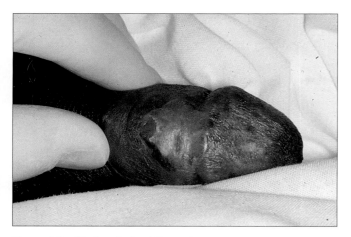

Figure 8.8 Erythroplasia of Queyrat.

dyskeratosis, limitation of the mitoses to the suprabasilar layer, and the dysplastic changes occur as a continuation from the surrounding epidermis. Clinically, this lesion may be difficult to differentiate from the related entities of actinic keratosis and invasive squamous cell carcinoma.

Erythroplasia of Queyrat must be differentiated from psoriasis, eczema, lichen planus, plasma cell balanitis (Zoon's), extramammary Paget's disease and fixed drug eruption. The histopathologic examination of a biopsy specimen will differentiate these processes and demonstrates changes identical to Bowen's disease.

The choices of therapy for these lesions include surgical excision, electrodesiccation and curettage, cryotherapy with liquid nitrogen, local irradiation, topical chemotherapy with 5-fluorouracil or imiquimod, laser surgery, and microscopically controlled surgery. The selection of one of these modalities for any given lesion is often arbitrary, with preference being given to those with which the physician is most familiar. For a small Bowen's disease lesion on the trunk or extremities, the author favors the use of electrodesiccation and curettage. For EQ, the author prefers either topical 5-fluorouracil, imiquimod or microscopically controlled surgery because they are least likely to result in functional impairment and/or mutilation of this vital structure. These lesions should be treated to resolution because if left untreated they can eventually become invasive and occasionally develop into metastatic squamous cell carcinoma.

TAR KERATOSIS

Keratosis and cancer of the skin that develop following chronic exposure to tar, pitch, coal, soot, and/or mineral oil products were among the first recognized occupational-related diseases; this discovery led to early understanding of chemical carcinogenesis. Tar keratoses are rare in the current climate of worker protection and workman's compensation. The lesions are keratotic or waxy and occur on skin that has other changes of tar exposure. Treatment of these lesions, which are often multiple, is similar to that for arsenical keratosis.

MISCELLANEOUS CONDITIONS THAT MAY BE PRECURSORS OF EPIDERMAL MALIGNANCIES

There are many cutaneous diseases or neoplasms, which may be associated with an eventual epithelial malignant neoplasm. In addition, several inherited conditions can predispose the patient to epithelial neoplasms. Xeroderma pigmentosa is a group of rare genetic syndromes in which there is a defect in DNA repair mechanisms. Thus, when solar irradiation injures the skin, the repair of DNA crosslinks cannot be accomplished and the patient develops malignancy at an early age. Another inherited condition is that of epidermodysplasia verruciformis. Patients with this rare condition develop multiple flat wart-like lesions. Recently, human papillomavirus (HPV) type V has been found in these lesions. About 20–25% of the patients develop a squamous cell carcinoma sometime in the course of the condition.

Infections due to human papillomavirus may play a role in the development of epidermal malignancy under a number of circumstances in addition to that involving epidermodysplasia verruciformis. The giant condyloma of Buschke–Lowenstein occurs on the genitalia and is thought to be caused by an HPV infection. Whether it is malignant at the onset or becomes malignant is the subject of some debate. Radiotherapy in this lesion should not be done because it may 'convert' into an aggressive invasive squamous cell carcinoma. Viruses have also been demonstrated in Bowenoid papulosis. Lastly, patients with renal or cardiac transplants are immunosuppressed and may develop multiple warts associated with their malignant skin tumours. In successful long-term transplants, an invasive squamous cell carcinoma can be responsible for the patient's death. Thus, close observation and therapy of all 'warty' lesions should be undertaken by the treating physician.

Porokeratosis is a group of disorders characterized by a distinct peripheral keratotic ridge, which corresponds to the coronoid lamella observed on histopathologic examination. There are at least five distinct variants of which two have been considered to have premalignant potential. Porokeratosis of Mibelli (classic porokeratosis) and its linear variant have been reported to have developed into squamous cell carcinomas in at least 20 patients. Disseminated superficial actinic porokeratosis (DSAP), which was first described by Chernosky, has also been reported to develop SCC within the lesions, but the frequency of malignant transformation seems to be much lower than with classical porokeratosis.[25] These lesions are viewed as potentially premalignant, and thus their destruction with either liquid nitrogen or topical 5-fluorouracil is desirable.

Scars that result from a number of injuries or from chronic irritation of the skin can predispose the patient to malignant epithelial neoplasms, in particular squamous cell carcinomas.[26] Classically the description of ulcerations within a burn scar is credited to Marjolin (Marjolin's ulcer). Similar lesions have complicated scars from frostbite, electrical injury, chronic sinuses or fistulas, chronic osteomyelitis, chronic stasis dermatitis, and scars following a variety of cutaneous infections.

The lesions that develop are almost always SCC, but the patient's prognosis depends on the risk of invasion and potential for metastases. In a large study of squamous cell carcinoma of the skin, Headington and Callen observed two histopathologic variants of SCC arising in scars: (1) an aggressive, invasive anaplastic lesion, and (2) a pattern similar to verrucous carcinoma. Patients with the former pattern frequently had metastases at the time of diagnosis, and the lesions were responsible for the patient's death. In contrast, those with a verrucous carcinoma pattern rarely had metastasis and were cured with local excisional surgery.

Erosive and/or scarring dermatoses have on rare occasions been associated with the development of cutaneous malignant disease. In general, as with scar cancer, the lesion is squamous cell carcinoma. The most often reported dermatoses complicated by cancer are discoid lupus erythematosus, scarring variants of epidermolysis bullosa (dystrophic bullous dermatosis), genital lichen sclerosus et atrophicus and its variant balanitis xerotica obliterans, and lichen planus. Observations regarding the histopathologic pattern as just described have not been made for these lesions due to the rarity of malignant changes within these already relatively rare disorders.

FUTURE OUTLOOK

The major issue relating to precursor lesions involves actinic keratoses. As the use of drugs and therapies that are immunomodulators, chemotherapeutic agents or immunosuppressive agents become more widespread for the management of patients with inflammatory diseases, cancer or organ transplantation, these lesions will more than likely become more prevalent and will be associated with a greater risk of progression to invasive squamous cell carcinoma. Early identification and treatment of these lesions will become increasingly more important. We will need remittive therapies to complement our destructive methods. In addition, education, beginning in grade school, must be part of the strategies that our national organizations advocate.

REFERENCES

1 Callen JP, Bickers DR, Moy RL. Actinic keratoses. J Am Acad Derm 1997; 36:650–653.

2 Leffell DJ. The scientific basis of skin cancer. J Am Acad Derm 2000; 42(1):18–22.

3 Cox NJ. Actinic keratosis induced by a sunbed. Brit Med J 1994; 308:977–978.

4 Cockerell CJ. Histopathology of incipient intraepidermal squamous cell carcinoma. J Am Acad Derm 2000; 42:11–17.

5 Glogau RG. The risk of progression to invasive disease. J Am Acad Derm 2000; 42(1):23–24.

6 Jonason AS, Kunala S, Price GJ, et al. Frequent clones of p53-mutated keratinocytes in normal human skin. Proc Natl Acad Sci USA 1996; 93:14025–14029.

7 Thompson SC, Jolley D, Marks R. Reduction of solar keratoses by regular sunscreen use. N Engl J Med 1993; 329:1147–1151.

8 Black HS, Herd JA, Goldberg LH, et al. Effect of a low-fat diet on the incidence of actinic keratosis. N Engl J Med 1994; 330:1272–1275.

9 Feldman SR, Fleischer AB Jr, Williford PM, Jorizzo JL. Destructive procedures are the standard of care for treatment of actinic keratoses. J Am Acad Derm 1999; 40:43–47.

10 Jorizzo J, Stewart D, Bucko A, Davis SA, Espy P, Hino P, et al. Randomized trial evaluating a new 0.5% fluorouracil formulation demonstrates efficacy after 1-, 2-, or 4-week treatment in patients with actinic keratosis. Cutis 2002; 70:335–339.

11 Baranco VP, Olson RL, Everett MA. Response of actinic keratosis to topical vitamin A acid. Cutis 1980; 6:681.

12 Weiss JS, Ellis CN, Headington JT, Tincoff T, Hamilton TA, Voorhees JJ. Topical tretinoin improves photoaged skin. A double-blind vehicle-controlled study. JAMA 1988; 259: 527–532.

13 Kang S, Goldfarb MT, Weiss JS, et al. Assessment of adapalene gel for the treatment of actinic keratoses and lentigines: a randomized trial. J Am Acad Dermatol 2003; 49:83–90.

14 Wolf JE Jr, Taylor JR, Tschen E, Kang S. Topical 3.0% diclofenac in 2.5% hyaluronan gel in the treatment of actinic keratoses. Int J Derm 2001; 40:709–713.

15 Walker JK, Koenig C. Is imiquimod effective and safe for actinic keratosis? J Fam Pr 2003; 52:184–185.

16 Stockfleth E, Meyer T, Benninghoff B, et al. A randomized, double-blind, vehicle-controlled study to assess 5% imiquimod cream for the treatment of multiple actinic keratoses. Arch Derm 2002; 138:1498–1502.

17 Salasche SJ, Levine N, Morrison L. Cycle therapy of actinic keratoses of the face and scalp with 5% topical imiquimod cream: An open-label trial. J Am Acad Derm 2002; 47:571–577.

18 Grimaitre M, Etienne A, Fathi M, Piletta PA, Saurat JH. Topical colchicine therapy for actinic keratoses. Dermatology 2000; 200:346–348.

19 Dinehart SM, Nelson-Adesokan P, Cockerell C, Russell S, Brown R. Metastatic cutaneous squamous cell carcinoma derived from actinic keratosis. Cancer 1997; 79:920–923.

20 Graham JH, Helwig EB. Cutaneous precancerous conditions in man. NCI Monogr 1963; 10:323.

21 Bowen JT. Precancerous dermatosis: A study of two cases of chronic atypical epithelial proliferation. J Cutan Dis Syph 1912; 30:241.

22 Callen JP, Headington J. Bowen's and non-Bowen's squamous intraepidermal neoplasia of the skin. Arch Derm 1980; 116:422–426.

23 Peterka ES, Lynch FW, Goltz RW. An association between Bowen's disease and internal cancer. Arch Derm 1961; 84:623–629.

24 Arbesman H, Ransohoff DF. Is Bowen's disease a predictor for the development of internal malignancy? JAMA 1987; 257:516–518.

25 Chernosky ME. Porokeratosis. Arch Derm 1986; 122:869–870.

26 Kaplan RP. Cancer complicating chronic ulcerative and scarring mucocutaneous disorders. Adv Derm 1987; 2:19.

CHAPTER

9

Basal Cell Carcinoma

Pearon G Lang and John C Maize Sr

Key points

- Basal cell carcinoma is the most common malignancy occurring in humans.
- Although most lesions are related to excess ultraviolet exposure, basal cell carcinoma is multifactorial in origin.
- Clinical–pathological correlation is critical when planning the treatment of a basal cell carcinoma.
- Basal cell carcinoma, if neglected or inappropriately managed, can cause significant morbidity and even death.
- Promising new treatment modalities include immune modulators, photodynamic therapy and drugs that address genetic defects.

INTRODUCTION

Currently, over 1,200,000 or more new cases of non-melanoma skin cancer (NMSC) are diagnosed in the US annually.[1] Of these, 75–80% are basal cell carcinomas (BCC). BCC is the most common cancer occurring in man.[2] Although BCCs rarely metastasize[3,4] and thus rarely cause death, they can result in significant morbidity. This is especially true if they are not correctly diagnosed and managed in a proper and timely manner.[5] BCCs are very common, and the incidence of skin cancer continues to rise and is no longer rare in young patients. Therefore, BCCs represent a significant health problem not only from the standpoint of patients' wellbeing but also from the perspective of healthcare dollars spent.[6]

HISTORY

Krompecher was the first to describe BCC and suggested that it arose from the basal cells of the epidermis.[7] Subsequently, a number of other theories were put forth as regards the site of origin of this tumor including the hair follicle and other appendageal structures. Others felt that the BCC was not a carcinoma but a nevoid tumor or hamartoma or that BCC derived from immature pluripotential cells which formed continuously during one's lifetime.[8]

EPIDEMIOLOGY

BCC is the most common cancer occurring in Caucasians. Some 75–80% of the new skin cancers diagnosed annually in the US are BCCs. Australia has the highest incidence of BCC with an annual incidence of 726 per 100,000.[9] In the past decade, significant increases in the incidence of BCC has been observed in Australia, Europe and the US.[1,9,10] Although BCC more commonly occurs in men, this sexual difference has become less pronounced in recent years. This finding may be a result of changes in the dress and lifestyle of women which has led to more gender balanced sun exposure. Increased sun exposure may also explain why BCC is no longer rare in young adults. With increasing emphasis on personal appearance, the desire for a 'beautiful year-round tan' and the availability of suntan parlors, the rapid rise in the incidence of BCC may continue. This trend may be augmented by depletion of the ozone layer, which filters out the carcinogenic rays of ultraviolet light (UVB).[11]

Metastasis of BCC is very rare. It has been estimated that from 0.0028%[3] to 0.1%[4] of BCCs will subsequently metastasize.

PATHOGENESIS

The most common factor involved in the pathogenesis of BCC is ultraviolet light (UVL). The closer one lives to the equator the greater the risk of developing BCC.[12–14] Fair-skinned individuals who burn easily and tan poorly are at greatest risk for developing BCC. Darkly pigmented persons and those who tan well are significantly less likely to develop such lesions.[13,15–19]

This protective role of skin pigmentation is well demonstrated in blacks with albinism. In contrast to normal blacks who rarely develop non-melanoma skin cancer,[20–22] those with albinism develop BCCs and other NMSC at an early age.[23–25] Although BCCs are unusual in blacks, these tumors have the same predilection for the head and neck as do BCCs in whites.[20–22]

Ultraviolet (UV) induced epidermal DNA damage is thought to be the primary carcinogenic event occurring in the development of BCC. Xeroderma pigmentosum (XP) is characterized by the development of NMSC at an early age. XP patients lack the ability to repair UVL induced DNA damage.[26-29] Using XP as a model, investigators have sought to determine if an inability to repair UVL induced DNA damage might also explain the genesis of skin cancer in non-XP patients. Although some studies have supported this theory,[29-33] there are enough inconsistencies from other studies[30,34] that, at this time, one cannot postulate that an inability to repair DNA, damaged by UV, could explain the development of *all* BCCs.

Cumulative lifetime UV exposure appears to increase the probability of developing BCC. However, recent studies also suggest that, like melanoma, intermittent intense sun exposure early in life leading to sunburn may be a risk factor.[35-39] The development and distribution of SCC may more accurately reflect cumulative sun damage than does that of BCC.[12,14,40] Approximately 20% of BCCs occur on non sun exposed skin[35-36] and up to one-third occur on areas of relatively less sun exposure.

UVL from sources besides sunlight including tanning beds[41-43] and UVL used for therapeutic purposes (PUVA)[44-46] may contribute to the development of BCC. There is an increase in the incidence of BCC in patients receiving PUVA therapy although a greater increase in the number of SCCs developing in these patients is also noted, as is the case in patients with lymphoma.[47]

UVL may mediate its carcinogenic effect not only by damaging epithelial DNA but also by creating an immune tolerant state in the skin.[48-58] In addition UVL may bring about the development of BCC through mutations in tumor suppressor gene p53 and other genes.[59-63] Mutations in p53 are thought to prevent the death of cells damaged by UVL, which would allow the propagation of these abnormal cell(s).[59,60]

Studies in patients with basal cell nevus syndrome (BCNS), (Fig. 9.1) suggest that another tumor suppressor gene, the patched gene, may play a role in the development of BCCs in these patients. The patched gene may also play a pathogenesis role in patients with sporadic BCCs.[64-66] This gene is located on the long arm of chromosome 9 (9q22). Its allelic loss or inactivation is associated with both sporadic occurring and BCNS associated BCCs. Several other syndromes are associated with the development of multiple BCCs including Bazex syndrome,[67] Rasmussen syndrome,[68] and the Rombo syndrome.[69]

Other environmental factors beyond UVL may lead to the development of BCC. Ionizing radiation given for benign conditions (e.g. tinea capitis, hirsutism, acne) in doses as low as 450 rads, has been associated with BCC formation.[70-72] The latency for tumor development is usually long and evidence of radiation damage need not be present.[70,71]

Arsenic exposure, especially to inorganic arsenic, has been associated with the development of multiple NMSC including BCC. Lesions most commonly occur on the trunk.[73-75] Sources of arsenic exposure include well water, pesticides (e.g. Paris green), medications (Fowler's solution, herbal remedies) and industry (mining, smelting, sheep dippings).[73]

Topical nitrogen mustard enhances photocarcinogenesis and is associated with a 14% incidence of cutaneous neoplasms including BCC involving both sun exposed and sun protected skin. The genital skin appears to be especially susceptible.

Scars may be the site of development of BCC.[76-81] The classical setting in which a BCC arises in a scar is an old vaccination scar.[79-81] BCC have also been reported to be associated with a thermal burn.[76] In contrast to SCCs, which arise in long standing burn scars (Marjolin's ulcer), the BCC lesion develops shortly after the injury ('acute burn carcinoma') suggesting that a clinically inapparent lesion may have already been present.[76-78]

BCC may arise in a nevus sebaceous.[82-83] Although occasionally observed in young persons,[82-83] these tumors usually arise in patients over 40 years of age.[82-83] Stromal induction may explain the development of basaloid proliferations and BCCs in this setting.[83]

HISTOGENESIS

Many theories have been proposed as to the site and cell of origin of the BCC.[84-90] These have included (1) basal cells of the epidermis, (2) basal cells of the epidermis and occasionally those of the infundibular and outer root sheath of the hair follicle, (3) dormant primordial epithelial germ cells, (4) pluripotential epithelial cells in the basal cell layer that persist throughout life, (5) cells of the pilosebaceous unit and (6) cells of other appendageal structures. This divergence of opinion may in part be explained by the histologic subtype of BCC studied and/or the area of tumor sampled. Histopathologically, most BCCs appear to arise from the epidermis and hair follicles.[87,88] Pinkus[89] suggested that BCCs and SCCs are derived from the same pluripotential epithelial cell and that other factors, such as stromal interaction, determine which type of tumor develops. This theory would explain the 'squamoid' changes seen in some BCCs and also why the metatypical BCC, histologically and biologically, demonstrates features of the SCC.[91-96]

Whether the BCC arises from the adult basal cell or a pluripotential cell may be entirely academic. Epidermal basal cells and germinative cells of appendageal structures share a common progenitor and since they contain the same genetic information (albeit partially repressed),

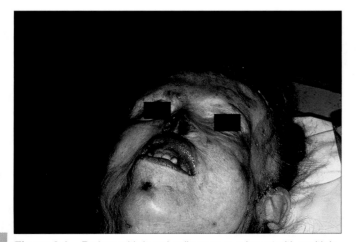

Figure 9.1 Patient with basal cell nevus syndrome with multiple BCCs present.

derepression by a transforming event could result in a pluripotential state. Thus, an epidermal basal cell could become more primitive or differentiate toward a malpighian cell or an appendageal-like structure.

A number of investigators have attempted to determine if the superficial multicentric BCC (SMBCC) is indeed multicentric. Zackheim[87] proposed a multicentric origin as did Sanderson,[97] who studied multiple sections from SBCCs. Madsen[98–100] however, on the basis of wax reconstructions of SBCCs, proposed a unicentric origin. A three-dimensional computer reconstruction of SBCCs has confirmed Madsen's theory[101] and Kimura[102] has also presented data that support a unicentric origin for the SBCC.

CLINICAL VARIANTS OF BASAL CELL CARCINOMA

Nodular BCC (noduloulcerative 'rodent ulcer')

This is the most common variant of BCC. Approximately 60% of all primary BCCs treated fall in this category. Typically, the lesion is a small pink or red, well-defined nodule with a translucent appearance and overlying telangiectasia (Figs 9.2, 9.3). As the lesion enlarges, ulceration may occur (noduloulcerative BCC). Melanin pigment may be present in variable amounts so that one may observe a few flecks of brown pigment or the lesion may be black or blue-black and may be confused with a melanocytic lesion (Fig. 9.4). Although slow growing, with the passage of time these tumors may reach a large size and extend deeply, destroying an eyelid, nose or ear. Thus the term 'rodent ulcer' originated because of the resemblance to tissue gnawed by a rat. In large lesions, tissue destruction and ulceration may dominate the picture so that the inexperienced clinician does not recognize the true nature of the ulcer. Careful examination, however, will often reveal at the edge of the ulcer an elevated translucent telangiectatic border.

Superficial (multicentric) BCC

Although this common variant of BCC is more commonly found on the trunk and extremities, the head and neck also may be affected. Typically the SBCC lesion is flat and pink or red (Fig. 9.5). A slight amount of scale may be present and there may be a thready translucent elevated border. Areas of spontaneous regression characterized by atrophy and hypopigmentation may be present. The diameter of the lesion varies from a few millimeters to several centimeters. Multiple lesions may be present. The lesion may be confused with a benign inflammatory condition such as nummular dermatitis and psoriasis. Variable amounts of pigment can be present leading to confusion with a melanocytic lesion. Initially, the growth pattern is primarily horizontal which accounts for the large size of these lesions. However, with the passage of time, these tumors can become deeply invasive with induration, ulceration and nodule formation. Extensive subclinical lateral spread accounts for the significant recurrence rate of these tumors after routine excision. Budding of tumor islands off the hair follicles can explain a recurrence after curettage and electro-desiccation or topical therapy.

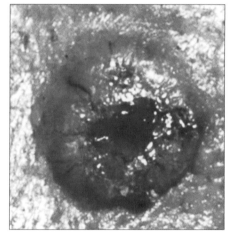

Figure 9.3 Nodulocystic basal cell carcinoma (closer view).

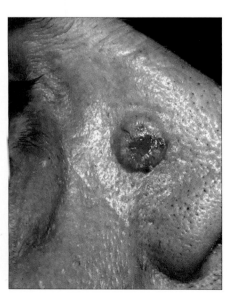

Figure 9.2 Nodulocystic basal cell carcinoma demonstrating classic rolled borders with telangiectasias.

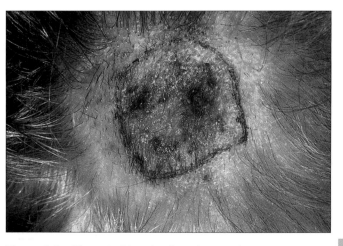

Figure 9.4 Pigmented basal cell carcinoma of the scalp.

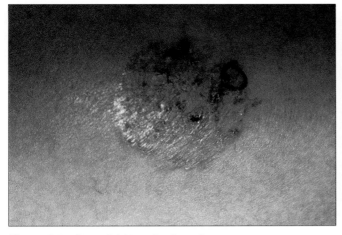

Figure 9.5 Superficial basal cell carcinoma.

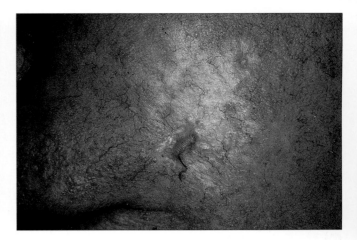

Figure 9.6 Morpheic basal cell carcinoma. Note the white plaque with telangiectasia. Lesion is extremely ill-defined.

Morpheaform BCC

The name for this variant of BCC is derived from its resemblance to a plaque of morphea (localized scleroderma). Typically, the lesion is indurated and ivory in color and there may be overlying telangiectasia (Figs 9.6, 9.7). Although the lesion has been likened to morphea, usually it is not difficult to distinguish between the two. Occasionally, however, metastatic carcinoma may be misdiagnosed clinically and histologically as a morpheaform BCC. The morpheaform BCC is noted for its subclinical spread and high recurrence rate after treatment.

Cystic BCC

Cystic degeneration in a BCC often is not clinically obvious and thus the lesion may appear to be a typical nodular BCC. However, in instances in which there are histologically marked cystic changes, the BCC clinically may have a clear or blue-gray cystic appearance and exude a clear fluid if punctured or cut.[103] If such a lesion is in the periorbital area, it may be confused with a hidrocystoma.

BCC with squamous metaplasia (basosquamous or metatypical carcinoma)

This is primarily a histologic variant of BCC and there are usually no clinical features that allow one to make the diagnosis preoperatively. Although controversial, this entity may biologically behave more like a SCC than a BCC.[91,92,95,96] and is much more aggressive and destructive in its behavior, more likely to metastasize and more likely to recur after treatment. Recurrent BCCs have been observed to acquire a more metatypical histologic appearance with each subsequent recurrence.[91,92,94,104] It has been estimated that the metatypical basal cell carcinoma constitutes 1 to 2.5% of all NMSC.[91,95,104,105]

When metastases occur with this variant of BCC, they may have the same microscopic appearance as the original tumor[92] or may resemble a poorly differentiated SCC.[91] The fact that some metastatic metatypical BCCs

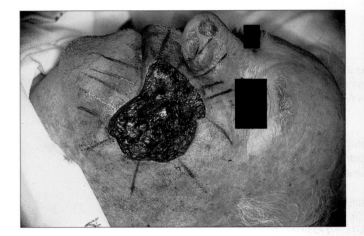

Figure 9.7 Surgical defect after Mohs surgery for lesion in Fig. 9.6. Note the extensive subclinical spread.

may have the histologic features of a SCC is in keeping with Fidler's concept that tumors with metastatic potential consist of a heterogenous population of cells, some with a greater potential for metastases than others.[93] Thus, the more squamoid cells in a metatypical BCC would have a greater potential for metastases and could give rise to a histologic picture of SCC in the seeded tissue. The incidence of metastases with this variant of BCC has been estimated to be as high as 9.7%.[91]

BCC with an aggressive (infiltrative or micronodular) growth pattern

These BCCs are notorious for their aggressive and destructive behavior, subclinical spread and high recurrence rate and it is therefore important to recognize these clinicopathologic variants. Up to 20% of all primary BCCs fall into this category. Clinically, these lesions are flat or only slightly elevated plaques (Figs 9.8–9.10) They are ill-defined in contrast to the purely nodular BCC. If there is a significant sclerosing stromal component (sclerosing BCC), they may present as a firm plaque and demonstrate some of the clinical features of a morphea-like BCC.

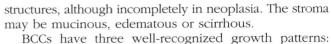

Premalignant fibroepithelioma of Pinkus

This is a rare variant of BCC, which has unique histologic features. In most instances, the lesion is situated on the lower back but it can occur elsewhere. The typical lesion is a smooth, slightly red, moderately firm nodule that may be pedunculated. Clinically the lesion resembles a fibroma.

HISTOLOGY OF BCC

BCCs are usually undifferentiated histologically, but some may show a degree of differentiation toward epithelial structures or adnexa. These neoplasms arise from the pluripotential germinative cells of the skin that reside in the basal layer of the epidermis or the epithelial structures of adnexa. BCCs have many different clinical and histologic appearances as may be expected in so common a neoplasm. The two major factors that influence the histologic appearance of basal cell carcinomas are the potential of its cells to differentiate and proliferate and the stromal response evoked by the epithelial component. Differentiation of neoplastic basal cells, just as of normal germinative basal cells in embryonic epidermis, may be toward follicular, sebaceous, eccrine or apocrine

structures, although incompletely in neoplasia. The stroma may be mucinous, edematous or scirrhous.

BCCs have three well-recognized growth patterns: (1) nodular, (2) superficial and (3) morpheic. The superficial and morpheic types each have a characteristic histopathologic picture that varies little from lesion to lesion. Nodular BCCs, however, may show many different histopathologic variants. The major ones have been classified as solid (primordial), keratotic (pilar), cystic and adenoid types. The adamantinoid and granular types are much rarer.[106]

Many nodular BCCs show secondary changes or unusual features. Some such changes are common and may have prognostic importance. A common finding is squamous differentiation. Some authors regard this as a metaplastic change that may correlate with a more aggressive biologic behavior.[92] Another common change is sclerosis of the stroma, which is usually found in recurrent lesions (especially in the deep portion) and renders them difficult to treat.[107]

Locally aggressive BCCs have been described that histologically show a diffuse, infiltrative pattern in the primary lesion that differs from the usually expansile nature of the nodular basal cell carcinoma.[108,109] This type of BCC is poorly circumscribed; the epithelial nests are widely separated from each other, show little palisading of the peripheral basal cells and often have a spiky shape. The well-developed stromal–parenchymal interaction that characterizes the usual nodular BCC is lacking. Some of these lesions have a central tumor nodule with infiltrative margins but others have no central nodular mass.

Classification

BCCs have also traditionally been histologically classified according to their degree and mode of differentiation, e.g. solid (primordial), adenoid, keratotic, pigmented and so forth. However, there is an accumulating body of evidence suggesting that the growth pattern of the neoplasm is more relevant than the degree of differentiation from the perspective of providing the clinician with information that may be helpful in planning the optimal

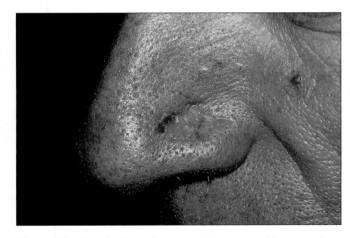

Figure 9.8 Basal cell carcinoma on alar crease with aggressive histologic growth pattern. Note flatness and ill-defined nature of the lesion.

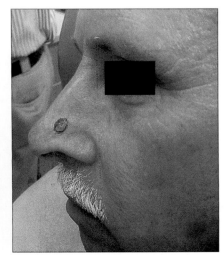

Figure 9.9 Patient with primary aggressive growth pattern basal cell carcinoma of the nose.

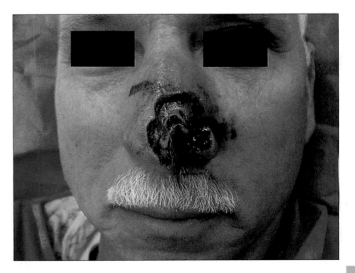

Figure 9.10 Patient in Fig. 9.9 at completion of Mohs surgery. Note extensive subclinical spread.

105

therapeutic procedure.[109–112] The classification in Table 9.1 is formulated primarily according to growth pattern and secondarily according to the type of differentiation.

Circumscribed basal cell carcinoma

The typical and most common BCC is the nodular or noduloulcerative type, which is a dome-shaped lesion. It is composed of irregularly sized and shaped islands of basaloid cells. Characteristically, the islands are relatively large and are aggregated in a cohesive cluster bound together by a fibrovascular stroma. The tumor margins are convex and the neoplasm grows in an expansile fashion. This tendency of the neoplasm to cohesiveness and expansile growth accounts for the circumscription of the tumor at the deep and lateral margins. The fact that the great majority of BCCs have a circumscribed growth pattern mainly accounts for their high cure rate. This type of BCC is usually symmetric and the margins can usually be easily determined clinically by inspection and palpation. Such lesions can be adequately treated by removal with a narrow margin of normal skin.[113]

Solid BCC

The solid BCC is composed primarily of large aggregates of basaloid cells with no evidence of differentiation toward any adnexal structure (Fig. 9.11). The cells are relatively uniform in size and have large nuclei with inapparent nucleoli and scant cytoplasm. The cell borders are not crisply defined as are those of squamous cell carcinoma (SCC) and it is often difficult to see intercellular bridges. Desmosomes are present, however, as has been readily demonstrated by electron microscopy and immunohistochemical studies and they can be visualized by light microscopy in about 60% of cases.[86,114,115] The cells at the periphery of the islands tend to align in a parallel array with the base of the cell contacting the basement membrane and the apex pointing inward toward the center of the island. This picket fence-like arrangement is referred to as palisading (Fig. 9.12). Mitotic figures are usually not found and, when present, usually appear normal. The large islands of basal cells often show central necrosis. This leads to the formation of lacunae, which contain amorphous debris and degenerated cells.

The islands of basaloid epithelial cells comprise the tumor parenchyma. They are embedded in a fibrovascular stroma that consists of plump fibroblasts in a meshwork of fine collagen fibers and abundant ground substance. The stroma serves a sustentacular role. The stroma often contains abundant mucin, especially adjacent to the islands of epithelial cells (Fig. 9.13). Because of the high content of glycosaminoglycans in the stroma which are removed during routine tissue processing, the stroma often pulls away from the palisaded row of basal cells at the edges of the islands thereby producing artefactual clefts. These clefts are found so regularly in paraffin-embedded specimens that they have taken on diagnostic importance.

Inflammation is not usually prominent in tumors that are not ulcerated. There often is a sparse to moderate infiltrate of mononuclear cells in the stroma with little or no exocytosis in the islands of basal cells. However, if

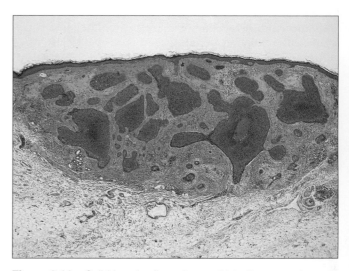

Figure 9.11 Solid basal cell carcinoma. Note the symmetry and circumscription of the tumor. It was composed predominantly of large islands of uniform cells. (H&E; original magnification × 25.)

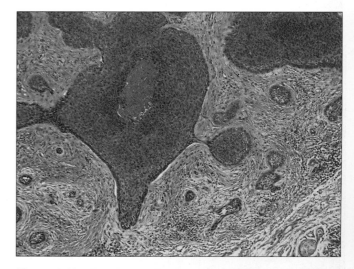

Figure 9.12 Prominent palisading of the outermost row of basal cells. Clear zone adjacent to the palisaded cells is due to loss of mucin from this area during tissue processing. (H&E; original magnification × 200.)

Table 9.1 Classification of basal cell carcinoma according to growth pattern	
Growth pattern	**Classification**
Circumscribed	• Cornifying (keratotic)
Solid	• Follicular
Undifferentiated	• Fibroepithelioma
With differentiation/metaplasia	• Diffuse
Basosquamous (metatypical)	• Superficial
Adamantinoid	• Morpheic
Granular	• Infiltrating
Sebaceous	• Micronodular
Adenoid	• Eccrine epithelioma
Cystic	• Apocrine epithelioma

the lesion becomes ulcerated, the inflammatory infiltrate becomes more pronounced and can be dense. Plasma cells are commonly found in the stroma of lesions from the face and scalp.

BCC with squamous metaplasia (basosquamous or metatypical carcinoma)

Some BCCs show regions with cellular features resembling SCC (Figs 9.14, 9.15). This type of BCC is composed of cells that are both basaloid and squamoid in appearance while retaining the typical organization of basal cell carcinoma. The presence of the stroma serves to distinguish BCC with squamous differentiation from SCC that does not evoke a stromal proliferation. There usually are some islands of basaloid tumor cells and others in which basal cells merge into a region composed of atypical squamoid cells. Some authors consider squamous metaplasia in BCC to be a sign of differentiation,[110,116] whereas others correlate this finding with the potential for more aggressive biologic behavior.[92]

Some solid BCCs demonstrate abortive differentiation. These neoplasms have abundant mucin in the inter-cellular spaces and the basal cells become stellate in shape. Cystic degeneration may occur in the center of some islands. There is a distinct palisade of the peripheral row of basal cells that maintain their normal morphology. This type of BCC may represent differentiation toward follicular sheath. Granular BCC is a rare variant of solid BCC in which several of the basal cell lobules are replaced by cells which have eccentric nuclei and cytoplasmic granules identical to the cells of granular cell tumor.[117] Some BCCs may show foci of differentiation toward sebaceous cells. If sebaceous differentiation is prominent, the neoplasm may be classified as a sebaceous epithelioma.[116] These lesions must be distinguished from clear cell BCC, in which the tumor cells have abundant cytoplasmic accumulations of glycogen.

Adenoid BCC

This type of BCC is characterized by interweaving cords and varying-sized islands of basal cells, which are sur-

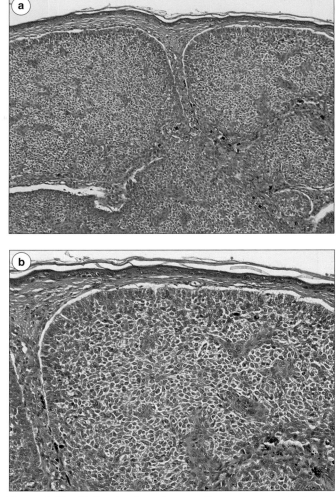

Figure 9.14 (a) Basal cell carcinoma with squamous metaplasia. This neoplasm has the usual organization of solid basal cell carcinoma. (H&E; original magnification × 40.) (b) At higher magnification it can be seen that many of the cells have abundant cytoplasm, are angulated rather than round and show intercellular bridges. (Hematoxylin-eosin; original magnification × 100.)

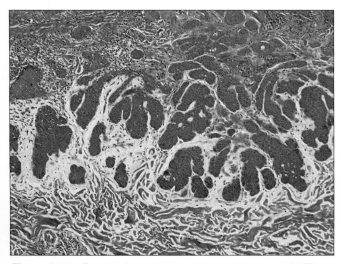

Figure 9.13 Basal cell carcinoma with myxoid stroma. (H&E; original magnification × 100.)

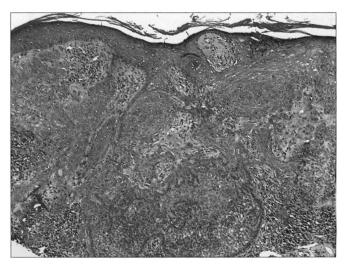

Figure 9.15 This basal cell carcinoma shows prominent squamous differentiation in the superficial portion of the tumor. The deeper portion shows more typically basaloid cells and prominent peripheral palisading. (Hematoxylin-eosin; original magnification × 100.)

rounded by a mucinous stroma (Fig. 9.16). The entrapment of the mucinous stroma between anastomosing strands of cells and within cell islands produces the appearance of gland-like or tubular structures. Sometimes the islands undergo cystic degeneration and are filled with mucin. Adenoid BCCs showing cystic change have been called adenocystic BCC. This term should probably be avoided because it may cause confusion with adenoid cystic carcinoma, which is a distinct entity unrelated to BCC.[118]

Cystic BCC

Microcysts are commonly found in islands of basal cells in solid BCCs. These are the result of necrosis of cells in the central portion of the islands.[86] Some BCCs show a unique histologic picture that merits the designation 'cystic'.[103] These uncommon tumors consist of one or a

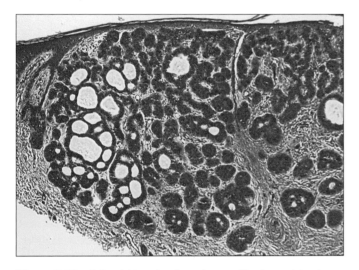

Figure 9.16 Adenoid basal cell carcinoma. The tumor islands are composed of basaloid epithelial cells surrounded by myxoid stroma. The arrangement of basaloid cells around the stroma focally resembles tubular structures. (H&E; original magnification × 40.)

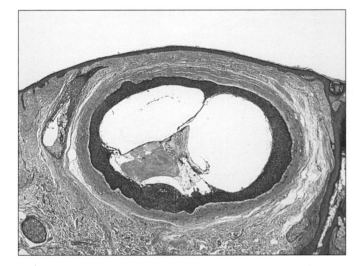

Figure 9.17 Cystic basal cell carcinoma. The bulk of this neoplasm is constituted of an exceptionally large island of basal cells which shows central cystic degeneration. (H&E; original magnification × 80.)

few exceptionally large islands of basal cells in which there is a large central lacuna containing amorphous debris and partially degenerated acantholytic epithelial cells (Fig. 9.17).

Cornifying (keratotic) BCC

Rarely, BCCs demonstrate the capacity to cornify. In such tumors the cornification takes place in the center of the islands of basaloid cells (Fig. 9.18). The keratin may be ortho- and/or parakeratotic. This change has been interpreted as evidence of follicular differentiation. Some examples of cornifying BCC show squamous metaplasia around the cornifying microcysts. These lesions can be distinguished from trichoepithelioma by the absence of abortive hair papilla formation in them, the unusual presence of stromal retraction around the islands of basaloid cells present and predominance of the epithelial component over the stromal component.

Follicular BCC (infundibulocystic BCC)

Follicular BCC is a peculiar variant that occurs on the face.[119,120] These lesions characteristically are small and are composed of aggregates of basaloid cells containing microcysts (Figs 9.19, 9.20). The microcysts have delicately laminated orthokeratotic material in them and often show squamoid metaplasia around the cysts. Some of the basaloid islands may rarely resemble hair follicles in telogen. They share features in common with trichoepithelioma, but they can be distinguished in several ways. In follicular BCC (in contrast to trichoepithelioma) the aggregates of cells frequently are in continuity with the epidermis, the stroma comprises the minority rather than the majority of the tumor, there are no foreign body reactions to keratin and structures reminiscent of hair papillae are lacking.

Fibroepithelioma

This type of BCC is composed of lace-like fronds of basaloid cells that anastomose in an edematous-appearing fibrous stroma (Fig. 9.21). The strands of basaloid cells emanate from the basal layer of the epidermis. The stroma

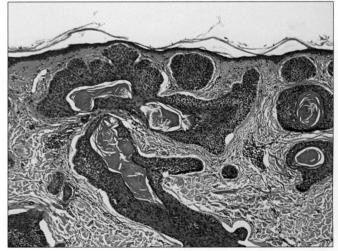

Figure 9.18 Cornifying basal cell carcinoma. There are central cystic structures containing masses of orthokeratin and a granular zone adjacent to the keratin. The structures resemble aberrant follicular units. (H&E; original magnification × 40.)

comprises the bulk of the lesion as opposed to adenoid BCCs, in which the stroma is much less prominent. Often there are more typical islands of basaloid cells with peripheral palisading. Microcysts are commonly present within the stroma.

Pigmented BCC

Melanin pigmentation may occur in all types of BCC with the possible exception of the morphea type. However, most pigmented BCCs are of the solid type (Fig. 9.22). In pigmented BCCs, melanocytes are interspersed among the basal cells and variable amounts of melanin are present within the cytoplasm of the neoplastic basal cells.[116] There are also numerous macrophages with melanin pigment in the stroma.[121]

BCC with a diffuse growth pattern

As opposed to the common nodular BCC which presents clinically as a dome-shaped lesion with fairly well-defined borders, lesions of the diffuse growth variant tend to be plaque-like or flat, spread horizontally in the skin and have poorly defined margins. These lesions tend to have a higher recurrence rate because they extend insidiously beyond the clinically visible or palpable border. Therefore, it is often difficult for the clinician to accurately gauge how much normal appearing tissue around the tumor must be sacrificed in order to achieve total removal.

Superficial BCC

Histologically, these tumors show horizontally arranged lobules of atypical basal cells in the papillary dermis that

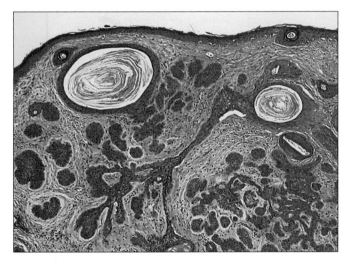

Figure 9.19 Basal cell carcinoma with follicular differentiation. This tumor is characteristically small, symmetric, well-circumscribed and superficial. Many of the aggregates of basaloid cells resemble telogen follicles. Microcysts are present (H&E; original magnification × 40.)

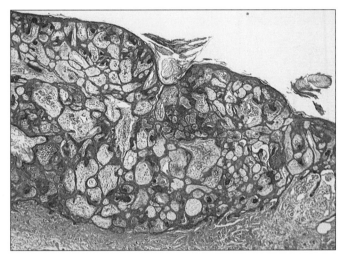

Figure 9.21 Fibroepithelioma. The bulk of this neoplasm is composed of the myxoid stroma. The epithelial component is made up mainly of anastomosing cords of basal cells. There is a fairly large aggregate of basal cells in the upper right corner beneath the epidermis. (H&E; original magnification × 40.)

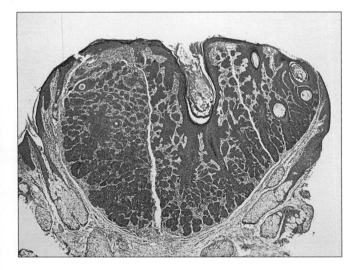

Figure 9.20 Basal cell carcinoma with follicular differentiation. This lesion shows occasional small horncysts and fissures in the stroma. (H&E; original magnification × 80.)

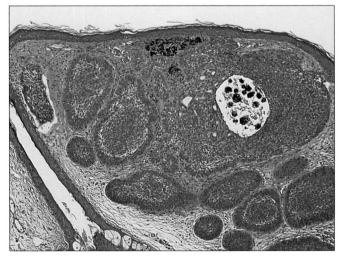

Figure 9.22 Pigmented basal cell carcinoma. This solid tumor shows many macrophages in the stroma and in the area of cystic necrosis that contain melanin pigment. (H&E; original magnification × 80).

have broad-based connections with the epidermis (Fig. 9.23). All islands of basal cells contact the epidermis. Therefore, there is no downward extension into the middle or deep dermis but rather only superficial centrifugal growth typically seen. The lobules of basal cells show palisading of the peripheral basal cells as do other types of BCC. A thin fibrovascular stroma, often with a host response of lymphocytes and histiocytes, underlies the tumor nests.

Morpheic BCC

Morpheic BCCs are notoriously difficult to treat because of their insidious centrifugal extensions, which make it difficult to determine margins by clinical inspection or palpation. Salasche and Ammonette found morphologic extensions averaging approximately 7 mm in these lesions.[122] The dense fibrous stroma, which comprises the majority of the tumor volume precludes treatment by curettage.

Morpheic BCCs often show no connection with the epidermis and the epithelial structures of adnexa are completely effaced. There are often cords, strands and small nests of basaloid cells enmeshed in a dense stroma of thickened collagen bundles (Figs 9.24, 9.25). Mucin is scant to absent, so there often is no evidence of retraction of the stroma from the epithelial cells. Because the nests and cords of cells are so thin, there is no palisading of the basal cells except in some of the small islands that may be present in some tumors. These strands and cords of cells most often are arranged parallel to the surface or at an acute angle to it.

Morpheic BCCs must be distinguished histologically from syringoma, desmoplastic trichoepithelioma and metastatic adenocarcinoma. Syringoma has as its hallmark small tubular epithelial structures embedded in a sclerotic stroma. However, in some sections (especially in those taken near the periphery of the lesion) the

lumina may not be evident and one sees only strands of epithelial cells in a dense collagenous stroma. Simply cutting and examining more sections will differentiate these lesions because the lumina will be found and morpheic BCCs never demonstrate lumina in the epithelial strands. Desmoplastic trichoepithelioma (Fig. 9.26) can also usually be distinguished from morpheic BCC[123] through the presence in these tumors of microcysts containing keratin, which are not found in morpheic BCCs.

Most problematic is distinguishing metastatic adenocarcinoma (especially breast carcinoma which may induce a scirrhous tissue reaction) from morpheic BCC. Careful examination of the tissue sections may reveal foci of glandular differentiation in metastatic adenocarcinoma or mucin droplets in the cytoplasm may be detectable

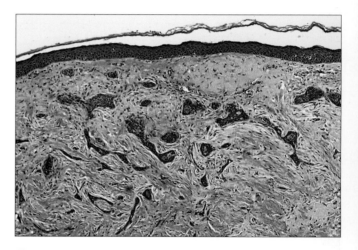

Figure 9.24 Morpheic basal cell carcinoma. The epithelial component is made up of small angulated nests, cords and strands of basal cells. These are surrounded by a dense collagenous stroma. Inflammation is characteristically sparse or absent and palisading is not present. There is usually no connection of the tumor islands with the epidermis. (H&E; original magnification × 80.)

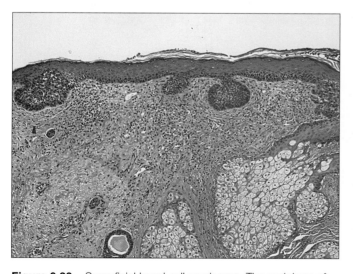

Figure 9.23 Superficial basal cell carcinoma. The periphery of the lesion is at the left. The 'shoulder' of the tumor is composed of horizontally oriented nests of basal cells that are connected to the epidermis. The stroma encases these islands. Evidence exists of regression in the central portion of the lesion, where there is fibrosis in the upper dermis and a dense host response of mononuclear cells. (H&E; original magnification × 40.)

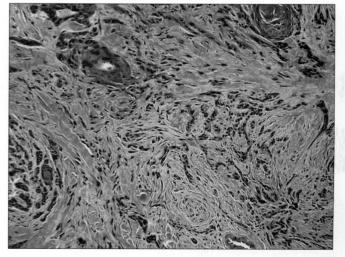

Figure 9.25 This morpheic basal cell carcinoma shows only strands of hyperchromatic basal cells in the abundant fibrotic stroma. It resembles metastatic scirrhous carcinoma of the breast. There is a focus of calcification at the far left. (H&E; original magnification × 80.)

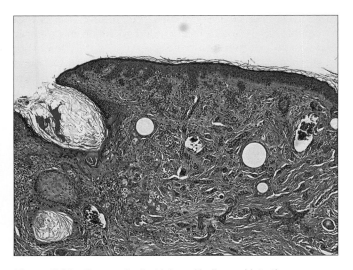

Figure 9.26 Desmoplastic trichoepithelioma. Note the horncysts and an abortive follicle. Horncysts and follicular differentiation are not found in morpheic basal cell carcinomas. (H&E; original magnification × 80).

with a mucicarmine stain. Furthermore, some metastatic adenocarcinomas will show the presence of carcino-embryonic antigen on staining by the immuno-peroxidase method whereas BCCs do not.

Infiltrating BCC

This term has been used to denote a peculiar type of BCC that, untreated, may pursue a particularly aggressive course of local tissue destruction.[108–110] In a series of unselected cases, this growth pattern was found to occur with approximately the same frequency as morpheic BCC.[124] These lesions lack a central cohesive mass of basal cell islands as seen in nodular BCC. Instead, they consist of elongated islands and cords of atypical basal cells that are widely separated spatially. The nests of tumor cells are often angulated and may be oriented almost perpendicular to the surface (Figs 9.27, 9.28). Palisading may be present but often is not well developed. The stroma may be mucinous, edematous or fibrotic. The dispersion of the tumor islands produces a poorly marginated flattish or plaque-like lesion. These

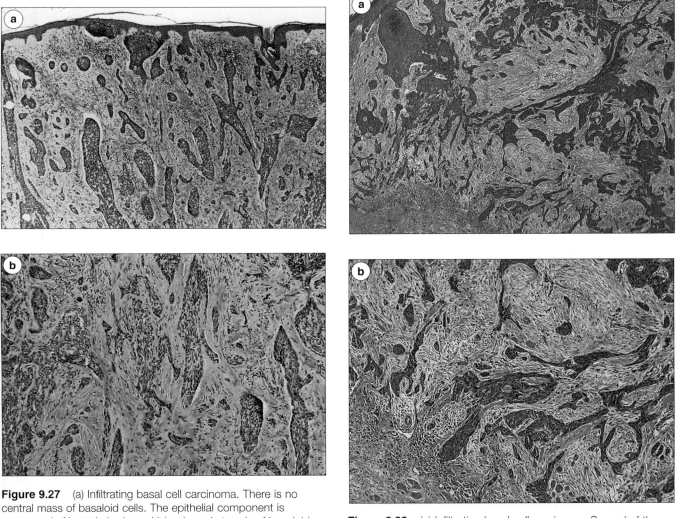

Figure 9.27 (a) Infiltrating basal cell carcinoma. There is no central mass of basaloid cells. The epithelial component is composed of irregularly shaped islands and strands of basaloid cells dispersed in the stroma. The tumor is a plaque with a flat surface. Note extensions into the subcutaneous fat. (H&E; original magnification × 40.) (b) The cellular aggregates have poorly developed palisading. (H&E; original magnification × 80.)

Figure 9.28 (a) Infiltrating basal cell carcinoma. Several of the aggregates of the tumor cells are oriented almost perpendicular to the flattish surface. (H&E; original magnification × 40.) (b) This lesion shows poorly developed palisading and squamous metaplasia. (H&E; original magnification × 80.)

tumors expand peripherally as do morpheic type BCCs but typically show simultaneous deep extension to underlying prominences of soft tissue whereas morpheic BCC usually remains confined to the reticular dermis.

Micronodular BCC

Micronodular BCC shares with infiltrating BCC the propensity for dispersion of the nests of epithelial cells. These neoplasms are made of small, round aggregates of basal cells rather than large aggregates as seen in solid BCCS.[110] Palisading is often well-developed. The islands approximate the size of hair bulbs. These lesions, too, usually are poorly defined and flat with indistinct borders and have the capacity to invade deeply. A unique aspect is the fact that the nests of cells at the deep aspect of the lesion often seem to be lying free in the tissue without surrounding stroma (Fig. 9.29). This may indicate that these clones have acquired an autonomous nature unlike ordinary solid BCCs, in which the epithelial component is intimately dependent upon the connective tissue stroma for its propagation.

It is not uncommon to see BCCs that have a mixture of growth patterns in varying combinations. For example, some lesions may have a micronodular component admixed with a solid component or a micronodular component with an infiltrative one. The presence of an infiltrative and/or micronodulary component along with a solid central or eccentric nodule indicates the potential for more aggressive local growth than in solid, purely nodular BCCs.[125]

Eccrine and apocrine epithelioma

Just as some BCCs may show follicular or sebaceous differentiation, others may show eccrine[126] or apocrine features,[127] although this presentation is much less common. Depending upon the individual lesion, eccrine epitheliomas may show a combination of fairly typical islands of BCCs, small cystic islands or syringoma-like areas in varying proportions within a scirrhous stroma

(Fig. 9.30). Eccrine epitheliomas, which have been found most commonly in the scalp, tend to recur as do other BCCs with a diffuse growth pattern.

Apocrine epithelioma is rare: only one case has been reported.[127] This case showed foci of glandular differentiation in the nests of basaloid cells, including some lumina with decapitation secretion. Enzyme histochemistry and electron microscopy confirmed the apocrine characteristics of this tumor, which pursued an aggressive clinical course requiring radical surgical extirpation.

Basaloid hyperplasia in dermatofibroma

There seems to be a stimulus for epidermal proliferation elaborated by the stromal cells in the dermis of dermatofibromas. Almost all dermatofibromas show epidermal hyperplasia with orthohyperkeratosis and peculiar elongation of the rete ridges, giving them a 'boot of Italy' appearance. Some dermatofibromas also show induction of hair germs from the base of the epidermis (Fig. 9.31). These buds of hyperplastic basal cells show peripheral palisading, are surrounded by a cellular myxoid stroma and resemble the basaloid lobules of superficial BCC. The small size and rounded contour of these buds are clues to their benign nature. Furthermore, usually only one or a few such buds are present in the lesion. The development of these hair germs bears no relationship to the type of dermatofibroma or the proximity of the fibroplasia to the epidermis.[128] In rare instances, however, true BCC evolves from the epidermis of dermatofibroma (Fig. 9.32). These neoplasms may be associated with epidermal ulceration. It is not known if such lesions develop from the hair germs or whether this is an independent phenomenon. Little is known about the biologic potential of these neoplasms.

Evolutionary histologic changes

Necrosis is common in islands of neoplastic basal cells. Sometimes entire islands of cells become necrotic. A

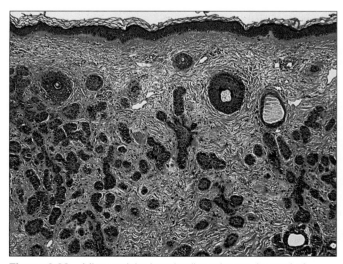

Figure 9.29 Micronodular basal cell carcinoma. Instead of large islands of basal cells, this variant is made up of small aggregates of cells. Palisading is often apparent around the periphery of the small nests, but stromal retraction is not usually present. (H&E; original magnification × 80.)

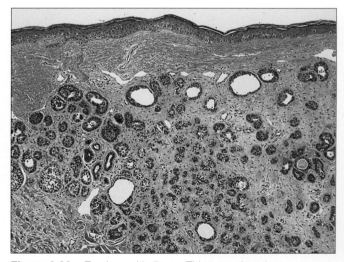

Figure 9.30 Eccrine epithelioma. This tumor has the organization and composition of a micronodular basal cell carcinoma, although several of the small aggregates of epithelial cells show central lumina. (H&E; original magnification × 40.)

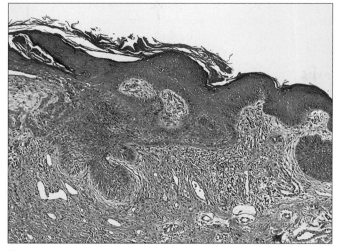

Figure 9.31 Dermatofibroma with induction of follicular germs. There are aggregates of basaloid cells emanating from the base of the epidermis; these show the organization of primitive follicles. (H&E; original magnification × 80.)

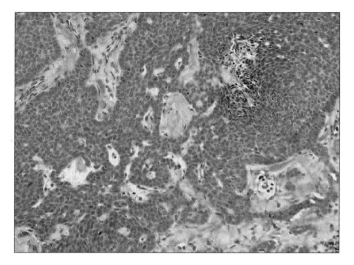

Figure 9.33 Small, pale-staining globules of amorphous material are present in the stroma adjacent to the basal cell aggregates. These globules are amyloid derived from necrotic tumor cells. (H&E; original magnification × 200.)

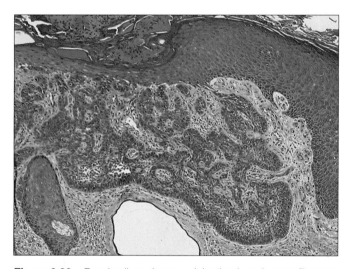

Figure 9.32 Basal cell carcinoma originating in a dermatofibroma. In this lesion the islands of basal cells are not showing any evidence of follicular differentiation, the islands are multifocal and the epidermis is ulcerated. (H&E; original magnification × 80.)

sequela of necrosis is dystrophic calcification. Calcium is commonly found in small aggregates in BCCs. On occasion, these calcium deposits serve as the nidus for metaplastic bone formation.

Partial regression may also occur in BCCs. Some investigators have noted regression in 20% of lesions.[129] Regression is characterized by a zone of fibrosis within the tumor. This is the result of the host immune response and of apoptosis. Areas of active regression show a dense mononuclear cell infiltrate around the lobules of basal cells. These contain many necrotic cells that can be identified by their pyknotic nuclei and eosinophilic cytoplasm.

Another finding associated with cell death in BCCs is the deposition of amyloid in the stroma (Fig. 9.33). It has been demonstrated that the amyloid in macular and lichen amyloidosis is the result of death of epidermal cells with the conversion of tonofilaments to amyloid

fibrils.[130] A similar phenomenon probably accounts for the common finding of amyloid globules in BCCs.[131]

Perineural and perifollicular extensions of BCC

Neoplasms often show a propensity to follow the paths of least resistance in their local growth. In the skin, nerves (Fig. 9.34) and hair follicles (Fig. 9.35) offer potential pathways along which BCC may extend beyond the main tumor body. Because these tumor extensions are not bulky, they are imperceptible to the physician during surgery and may be left behind to serve as a nidus for recurrence. Perifollicular extension is especially common on the scalp where there are terminal follicles that are deeply rooted in the subcutaneous tissue. An excision that does not extend deeply enough may result in tumor being buried in the base of the wound even though the main portion of the tumor has been adequately excised. It is important for the pathologist to scan the histologic sections for evidence of perineural and perifollicular extensions of BCC.

Ultrastructural features of BCC

By electron microscopy, undifferentiated basal cell carcinomas are composed of two cell types.[121] The major cell type has a large nucleus, sparse mitochondria and granular endoplasmic reticulum, abundant tonofilaments and prominent desmosomes. The second, less common cell type has dark granular cytoplasm and an irregular nucleus. The dark appearance of the cytoplasm results from a large number of free RNA particles. The morphologic features of undifferentiated BCC cells, therefore, are similar to normal epidermal basal and squamous cells. Pilar and eccrine differentiation may occur in some tumors. Some authors have found evidence of neuroendocrine differentiation in rare examples of BCC.[132–134]

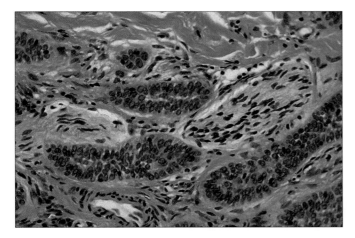

Figure 9.34 Neoplastic basal cells are present around nerve bundles in the dermis. Perineural extensions like these can go beyond the perceptible tumor margin. (H&E; original magnification × 200.)

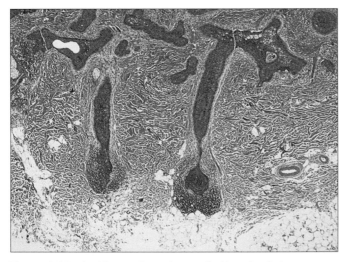

Figure 9.35 In this neoplasm the atypical basal cells have extended downward in the tracts of follicular units. (H&E; original magnification × 80.)

IMMUNOHISTOCHEMICAL FEATURES OF BCC

AE 1 is a monoclonal antikeratin antibody that has specificity for normal epidermal basal cells. BCCs show weak homogeneous staining with AE 1 by the peroxidase-antiperoxidase method.[135] Moss *et al.*[115] used monoclonal antibodies to desmoplakins to study various tumors for desmosome expression by immunofluorescence microscopy and demonstrated that desmosomes in BCC are detectable by this technique.

Stanley *et al.*[136] also used immunofluorescence to study the components of the basement membrane around the tumor aggregates in BCC. Laminin, type IV collagen and bullous pemphigoid antigen are definite protein components of normal epidermal basement membrane. Antibodies to laminin and to type IV collagen were found to react with the basement membrane around all tumor aggregates. Bullous pemphigoid antigen, which is produced by normal epidermal basal cells, was not detected strongly or continuously around the islands of neoplastic basal cells indicating that there is a selective defect of bullous pemphigoid antigen in the basement membrane of BCC. Alpha-smooth muscle actin has been documented in 66% of micronodular, 62% of morpheic and 0% of nodular BCC.[137] The presence of actin may be a marker for aggressive invasion in micronodular tumors. Expression of stromolysin 3, a member of the metalloproteinase family, is increased in deeply invasive BCC and morpheic BCC compared to the global rate of expression in BCC and may facilitate invasion.[138]

GROWTH, DEVELOPMENT, BIOLOGIC BEHAVIOR AND MODES OF SPREAD

The stroma appears to be important not only in the induction of BCC but also in its survival. In experimentally induced BCCs in animals, stromal changes precede the appearance of the tumor.[139] Transplantation of a BCC in the absence of its stroma often fails.[140–143]

This marked stromal dependence may explain why the BCC so rarely metastasizes. When cultured in vitro in the absence of their stroma, the tumor cells of the BCC differentiate toward keratinocytes and may form stratified squamous epithelium.[144,145] Experimentally induced BCCs, when transplanted into the uterus of a genetically compatible animal, may form normal epidermis.[146] These studies suggest that the stroma prevents the tumor cells of a BCC from differentiating toward keratinocytes and forming normal epidermis.[144–146] BCCs produce an angiogenic factor as an adequate blood supply is necessary for their survival.[147]

Statistical data predict a rapid doubling in the size of the BCC. However, clinical observation reveals a slow growth rate. This discrepancy may be partly due to the fact that most BCCs go through phases of growth and phases of regression. Which phase predominates determines the rapidity with which the tumor grows.[148] Regression may occur centrally or peripherally. During growth the stroma surrounding the tumor is thin and there is minimal inflammation while during regression the thickness of the stroma varies and there may be a marked inflammatory infiltrate present. In addition to regression, cell death, which approximates cell generation, probably also contributes to the slow growth of BCCs.[149–155]

Microfilaments are important for cell motility and are most commonly found in metastatic tumor cells and in tumor cells at the advancing edge of a carcinoma. Their frequency in BCC varies with the subtype of BCC, being most common in BCCs showing an infiltrative aggressive growth pattern.[156,157]

BCC has been found to contain increased amounts of type I collagenase,[158,159] with fibroblasts adjacent to the tumor acting as the source of this collagenase.[159] Nodular and SBCCs produce only type I collagenase whereas the more aggressive desmoplastic BCCs also produce type IV collagenase.[160] Type IV collagenase could be responsible for the gaps found in the basement membrane in this subtype of BCC and could explain more aggressive and invasive behavior.

Increased levels of prostaglandins PGE_2 and PGF_2 are much more marked in BCCs with an aggressive growth pattern.[161] Prostaglandins may influence the invasion and growth of the BCC by controlling collagenase production, suppressing the immune response or stimulating tumor growth.

As noted earlier, metastasis with BCC is very rare. This has been attributed to the stromal dependence of BCCs. Spread most commonly occurs via the lymphatics to regional nodes and via the bloodstream to the long bones and lungs. Other sites, including the skin, may be affected. Implantation in the lungs may also occur by aspiration of fragments of the tumor.

The primary tumor of metastatic BCCs is most commonly found on the head and neck, has usually been present many years and typically has a history of resistance to treatment. The primary tumor is often ulcerated and may be large, invasive and destructive and may show vascular invasion and perineural involvement. Any histologic subtype of BCC may give rise to metastases, but the adenoidal BCC and the metatypical BCC have been most commonly implicated. Interestingly, a review of the photomicrographs from these cases shows many of the BCCs demonstrating an infiltrative histologic growth pattern.

How certain BCCs acquire the ability to metastasize is not known. It has been suggested that a clone of cells may emerge which is capable of metastasis,[3,93] and/or that such patients may be immunologically impaired.[3,162,163]

Despite the rarity of metastases, BCCs can demonstrate aggressive local growth, spread and destruction. Conventional approaches teach that BCC is stromal-dependent. This suggests that BCCs always demonstrate islands of epithelial cells surrounded by a cellular myxoid stroma that resembles the stroma of the hair bulb. In many cases, BCCs demonstrating aggressive features can extend beyond the main body of the neoplasm as single epithelial cells. This extension is not dissimilar to the 'Indians in a file' array sometimes seen in metastatic carcinoma to skin. The atypical basaloid cells can be detected by immunocytochemistry utilizing antibodies to cytokeratins AE1 and AE3. In these cases, immunocyto-chemistry may be necessary to determine the adequacy of surgical margins.

Basal cell carcinoma growth almost always follows the "path of least resistance." It is for this reason that invasion of bone, cartilage and muscle is not common and is a late phenomenon. When BCC encounters these structures it will more often spread along the perichondrium,[105,164–166,168] periosteum,[105,164,166] fascia or tarsal plate.[105,166,167,169,170] This can partially explain the difficulty in the management of and higher than expected recurrence rate for BCCs of the eyelid,[166,167,169,170] ear,[164–166] nose,[166,171] and scalp.[172,173]

Embryonic fusion planes offer little resistance to the penetration of BCC. Such areas include the inner canthus, philtrum, mid-lower lip and chin, nasolabial sulcus (Figs 9.36, 9.37), preauricular area and retro-auricular sulcus[105,164–167,174,175] (Figs 9.38, 9.39). On the distal nose, the tumor may grow along the perichondrium until it comes to an area of articulating cartilages and then extend into the plane of soft tissue separating the cartilages (Figs 9.40, 9.41). Once in this plane, there can

be extensive spread of the tumor and destruction of normal tissue. On the superior nose, a BCC can infiltrate along the periosteum.[166] A BCC in the inner canthus can spread in the periosteum posteriorly along the medial wall of the orbit[166] (Figs 9.42–9.44). A BCC can also infiltrate along the periosteum down into the external auditory canal and can spread in this plane in the temple and malar areas sometimes resulting in extensive sub-clinical spread.[176]

The dermis serves as a barrier to the penetration of tumor. On the back the dermis is particularly thick and dense and it has been proposed that this is the reason why superficial BCCs are much more common on the trunk.[166] However, BCCs can spread laterally in the less dense upper dermis for some distance beyond what is thought to be the lateral margin of the tumor.[166] Basal cell carcinomas usually do not invade the subcutaneous

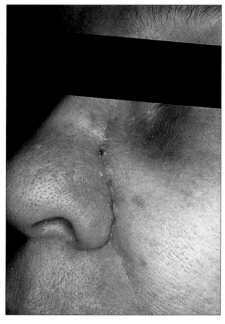

Figure 9.36
Patient with incompletely excised basal cell carcinoma of nasal-cheek sulcus. There had been three previous attempts at excision.

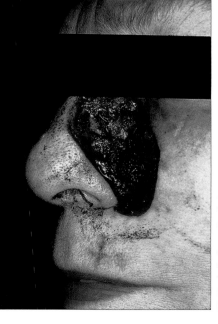

Figure 9.37
Surgical defect following Mohs surgery in patient in Fig. 9.36. Note extensive subclinical spread that is frequently seen with lesions in this location.

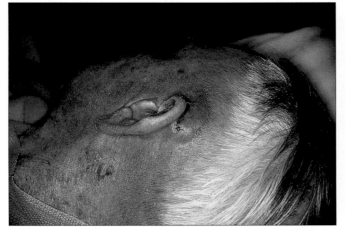

Figure 9.38 Recurrent basal cell carcinoma of postauricular sulcus. Tumor was buried by prior treatment.

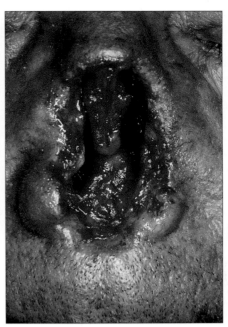

Figure 9.41 Patient shown in Fig. 9.40, following completion of Mohs surgery. Tumor had extended between the articulating cartilages.

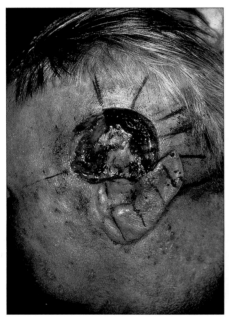

Figure 9.39 Surgical defect after Mohs surgery for lesion in Fig. 9.38. Note extensive subclinical spread.

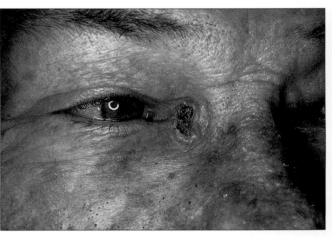

Figure 9.42 Primary basal cell carcinoma of inner canthus.

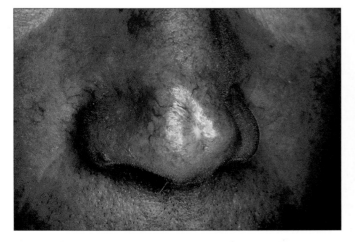

Figure 9.40 Patient with multiply recurrent basal cell carcinoma that had been managed by electrodesiccation and curettage.

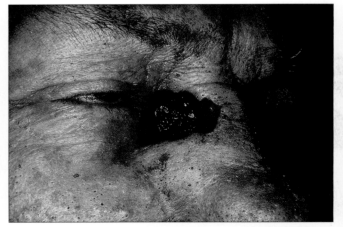

Figure 9.43 Lesion shown in Fig. 9.42 required three stages of Mohs surgery. Tumor extended posteriorly along medial wall of the orbit.

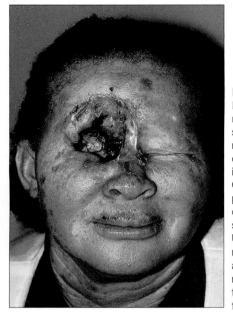

Figure 9.44
Patient who was referred for Mohs surgery for a recurrent basal cell carcinoma of the inner canthus. Clinically, the lesion preoperatively was comparable to that shown in Fig. 9.42. Ultimately, a multidisciplinary approach was required to render this patient tumor free.

fat because of its poor blood supply. If a BCC does invade fat, it travels down the fibrous septae that contain the blood vessels of this layer of the skin.[166] Basal cell carcinomas may invade the lymphatics and blood vessels of the skin, although this is uncommon. However, this does not appear to portend metastases.[166] Basal cell carcinomas occasionally spread along vessels.[166] Perineural spread is uncommon and usually is seen only with highly invasive BCCs of the infiltrative type.[166,177] The distance of spread may be limited or the tumor may travel a considerable distance and actually enter foramina.[177] The patient may complain of numbness, pain and paresthesias. Motor deficits also may be present.[177]

TREATMENT

Table 9.2 shows subtypes of BCC and their recommended treatment.

Overriding concepts

In managing the patient with a BCC, four goals should be kept in mind: (1) total removal or destruction of the BCC, (2) preservation of normal tissue, (3) preservation of function and (4) optimal cosmetic result. Although the clinician should try to achieve all these goals, the one goal of utmost importance is to rid the patient of the tumor. If this goal is not achieved, ultimately the other goals will not be met. Although a good cosmetic result is important, it should not become the major objective of therapy at the risk of not curing the patient. If it does, the consequences could be increased morbidity for the patient and a much greater cosmetic defect than would have resulted had adequate treatment been administered initially. This risk is well illustrated by Robins and Albom, who noted a high recurrence rate for BCCs in young women because cosmetic concerns had taken precedence over definitive treatment.[178]

Because BCCs grow slowly and rarely metastasize, they often are not given 'respect'. For example, a physician may decide to repeatedly curette and electrodesiccate a recurrent BCC because it does not appear deeply invasive and definitive therapy might disfigure the patient. Or alternatively, the physician may wish to spare an elderly patient the possible morbidity of a definitive surgical procedure. This approach ultimately can lead to the loss of an eye or nose. If the physician managing a patient with a recurrent BCC decides to use palliative therapy, the patient and family must be made aware that the treatment is not curative and informed consent must be obtained.

On the basis of a literature review, it may be difficult to decide which treatment modality is best in a given clinical situation since each author may report a series of patients for whom the treatment modality gave excellent results. When analyzing such studies one should be sure that the patient populations in the different studies are comparable and that follow-up is adequate. (Results should be evaluated in terms of 5-year cure rates.) One should also realize that the author(s) of the report usually have vast experience with the treatment modality they are advocating and that this same modality when used by someone less skilled might yield disappointing results. The difference in results may reflect the bias, skill and expertise of the different authors or it could reflect the skill and expertise of individuals such as the pathologist who determined whether the margins of excision were adequate.

In managing BCCs clinicians should employ those modalities with which they are most familiar and which they have found to be effective. This approach will usually produce the most satisfactory results. However, the clinician should avoid treating every BCC the same regardless of the location or type (i.e. treatment should be individualized). If the clinician is not skilled in the modality that will yield the best results for a particular patient, the patient should be referred. Although a comprehensive review of each treatment approach is provided elsewhere in this text, a description of their application in BCC is provided below.

The biopsy

Ideally, all BCCs should be biopsied before definitive therapy is carried out allowing for the selection of the most appropriate treatment modality. When a pretreatment biopsy is not deemed feasible or necessary and clinical diagnosis is certain, the clinician is justified in carrying out appropriate therapy. However, it is suggested that a specimen be submitted for pathologic examination at the time of treatment. If after reviewing the biopsy the clinician believes that the treatment carried out was inadequate, the patient can be recalled for additional therapy.

When the clinical diagnosis of BCC is not certain, a biopsy is mandatory before treatment is carried out. Other indications for a biopsy are determination of the histologic features of the BCC and its extent. This information not only allows selection of the most appropriate treatment modality but also may aid in the planning of therapy. Post-treatment biopsies are also helpful to

Table 9.2 Subtypes of basal cell carcinoma (BCC) and their recommended treatment

Type of BCC	Treatment options
Nodular ≤1 cm (not in high-risk area)	Curettage and electrodesiccation (lesion should not be deeply invasive) Cryosurgery Excision Radiation[a]
Nodular >1 cm (not in high-risk area)	Cryosurgery (may need to combine with curettage; use only for lesions ≤2 cm) Excision Radiation[a] Mohs surgery (especially if >2 cm)
Nodular (any size; high-risk area)	Mohs surgery[b] Excision Radiation (may want pre-and post-treatment biopsies)[a] Cryosurgery (may want pre- and post-treatment biopsies). Should be used only by someone with vast experience and skill; only for lesions ≤2 cm. May need to combine with curettage
Superficial (multicentric)	Shave excision with curettage Curettage and electrodesiccation 5% Imiquimod 5-Fluorouracil (may need to use with curettage or occlusion) Cryosurgery Excision Radiation (extremely superficial X-ray required; not a usual and preferred method of treatment)[a] Mohs surgery (if recurrent or large, e.g. >2 cm) Photodynamic therapy
Morpheaform	Mohs surgery[b] Excision (if Mohs surgery not available)
Aggressive growth pattern	Mohs surgery[b] Excision (if Mohs surgery not available) Radiation (may require pre- and post-treatment biopsies)[a]
'Field Fire'	Mohs surgery (allow wound to heal on its own if possible)[b] Excision, cryosurgery and radiation therapy not ideal alternatives; especially if possibly dealing with a recurrent BCC
Metatypical	Mohs surgery[b] Excision (if Mohs surgery not available) Radiation (may need pre- and post-treatment biopsies)[a]
Recurrent	Mohs surgery[b] Excision (if Mohs surgery not available)
Neurotropic	Mohs surgery[b] Excision (if Mohs surgery not available) Some of these patients may require postoperative radiation
Incompletely excised	Re-excise in conventional manner or by Mohs surgery
Unresectable and advanced disease	Cisplatin + doxorubicin + radiation
Metastases to regional nodes	Surgical removal of the nodes; may need to combine with radiation
Systemic metastases	Cisplatin + doxorubicin; may use with radiation when necessary

[a]Should not be used in younger patients. [b]Preferred treatment.

determine the adequacy of treatment when a blind modality such as cryosurgery or radiation therapy is used or if the lesion is treated topically. Curettings that are submitted for pathologic examination may be of limited value. Although they will confirm the diagnosis of BCC, they will not allow study of the histologic pattern or estimation of depth of penetration and therefore a punch or shave biopsy may provide a better diagnostic specimen. Caution should be used when shave biopsy is performed for BCCs with an aggressive growth pattern or for deeply buried recurrent BCCs since the tumor may be missed because there may be no tumor in the epidermis or

papillary dermis. In situations where there is the possibility of a deeply buried recurrent BCC, which may present as a subcutaneous mass, a deep punch or incisional biopsy may be required to make the diagnosis.

Methods of treatment

Curettage and electrodesiccation

Curettage and electrodesiccation (CE) is still the most common modality employed by dermatologists in the management of BCCs. As any other surgical modality, it must be done appropriately if the high cure rates reported in the literature are to be achieved.[179,180] Although some authors have suggested that CE should be performed a fixed number of times,[179–181] others[182] feel the procedure should be repeated only until a healthy base has been encountered.

In an attempt to improve the cosmetic results obtained with this modality, several investigators have omitted electrodesiccation.[183–186] This modification appears to eliminate hypertrophic scarring but does not avoid the risk of hypopigmentation.[183,184] The cure rate appears to be only slightly less than with CE.[184]

In order to achieve the high cure rates reported in the literature, not only must the technique be skillfully employed, but one must also carefully select the lesion to be treated.[179–181,183,184,187–190] As noted previously, the curette cannot ferret out BCC which (1) is enmeshed in a sclerotic stroma (i.e. recurrent BCC, morpheaform BCC, sclerosing BCC), (2) has an aggressive histologic growth pattern, (3) buds off or is concealed between pilosebaceous units (e.g. nose, scalp), (4) is deeply invasive (e.g. perineural, deep dermis, subcutaneous fat, perichondrium, periosteum) or (5) is in an area that is not firm or cannot be immobilized (e.g. lips, eyelids).

Caution needs to be used if CE is used in those areas at high risk for recurrence, i.e. embryonic fusion planes, scalp, ear, lips, eyelids, nose and temples. If, when curettage is performed on a BCC and a firm base cannot be reached, the tumor may have extensive subclinical spread and may not be adequately treated by this method. In this circumstance, the patient should have treatment by conventional excision or Mohs surgery.

A punch biopsy should be avoided for BCCs that are being considered for CE treatment because the curette will fall into the hole created by the punch biopsy and make curettage difficult and unreliable.[107,191] Many studies on CE have suggested that lesions as large as 2 cm (not SBCC) in diameter can be successfully treated.[179,182,187] Salasche[190] proposed that the upper limit should be 1 cm (excluding SBCC) because tumors more than 1 cm in diameter may penetrate deeply and extend beyond the clinically apparent margins, especially if located in a high-risk area.[107]

There have been several studies which have questioned the effectiveness of CE in the treatment of BCC of the head and neck.[188,192] Persistent tumor was detected in 30% to 47% of the BCCs on the head and neck[188,192] but in only 8% of those on the trunk and extremities.[192] In a study where all tumors were less than 1 cm in diameter and of the nodular type, persistent tumor was found most commonly in areas known for their high risk of recurrence, especially the nose and perinasal area.[188] Further studies are needed to better define the optimal tumors for treatment with CE.

In summary, CE appears best suited for well-defined exophytic, nodular BCCs less than 1 cm in diameter which are confined to the upper dermis and which are not situated in a high-risk area. This size limitation does not apply to SBCCs. The advantages of this modality are that it is easy to learn and perform, it is quick and it is suitable for the patient with multiple lesions. The disadvantage is that it can cause hypopigmentation and hypertrophic scarring (especially in young adults and on the trunk and extremities) which may not always be acceptable. However, the cosmetic result continues to improve with time[180] and the hypertrophic scar can be treated by topical or intralesional corticosteroids. CE done near mucocutaneous junctions (e.g. eyelids, lip) can also cause cosmetic deformities such as notching and ectropion. Unsuspected deep foci of BCC may be buried by CE and subsequently form a subdermal mass.[193]

Excision

Surgical excision offers the advantages of histologic control, rapid healing and optimal cosmetic result. Potentially, it can be used for all types of BCCs in all locations. However, it is time consuming, sacrifices some normal tissue and requires much more skill and training than does CE. It is less suitable for numerous lesions and reconstruction may be required to prevent or correct resultant cosmetic and functional defects.[191,194] The histologic control it offers in treating recurrent BCC,[195] morpheaform BCC,[122,196] BCCs with an aggressive histology,[197,198] and SBCC[109] and BCC in high-risk areas[194,199] is inferior to that achieved by Mohs surgery. Thus, recurrence rates are higher when these subtypes of BCC are treated by conventional excisional surgery. One modification that has been suggested to decrease the likelihood of marginal involvement in excisions is to curette the lesion prior to excising it. The principle on which this is based is that the curette will reveal subtle subclinical extensions not obvious to the naked eye.[200] Despite these limitations, it is the treatment of choice for difficult lesions if Mohs surgery is not available.

Although SBCC can be treated by excision, if the lesion is large, grafting may be necessary. Even when a primary closure is possible, healthy tissue still has to be sacrificed to achieve a good closure.[191] Moreover, since many SBCCs are located on the trunk and extremities, the patient may have a spreading scar which is larger and more unsightly than the scar left by CE or cryosurgery.

Margins for excision of BCCs have been suggested to be 3–5 mm margins for small primary BCCs and larger margins for large primary BCCs. For recurrent BCCs margins of 1.5–3.0 cm margins have been proposed.[201] Sexton and Maloney found that marginal involvement was much more likely when excising an aggressive growth pattern BCC as opposed to a nodular BCC.[201] Wolf and Zitelli[113] found that for 'well-defined' non-morpheaform BCCs 2 cm or less in diameter, 4 mm margins were required to eradicate 98% of the lesions. They found that the subclinical spread of the tumors was not equal in all directions and that for BCCs greater than 2 cm in size subclinical spread was so variable that no rigid recommendation for width of margin could be made. Given this data, for morpheaform BCCs, BCCs greater than 2 cm in size, those with an aggressive histologic growth pattern and those that are recurrent, if Mohs surgery is not chosen margins of 1 cm or greater may be necessary.

It is unusual for small primary BCCs to penetrate into the fat. Thus, if the excision is carried into fat, the depth of excision is usually adequate. However, large, longstanding BCCs, recurrent BCCs and those in high-risk areas may penetrate into the subcutaneous tissue and even more deeply.

Complications of excisional surgery include scarring, hypopigmentation, infection and cosmetic deformity. Excisional cosmetic results improve with the passage of time and scar revision is possible.[202]

In summary, excisional surgery offers histologic control and optimal cosmesis and can be utilized for the smallest and simplest or largest and most difficult of BCCs regardless of location.

Mohs micrographic surgery

Mohs surgery allows for the ultimate in histologic control and preservation of tissue during the removal of BCC.[203–206] It is the treatment of choice for large invasive BCCs; those with morpheaform or aggressive histologic features; those in high-risk areas; those which are recurrent;[203–206] those which exhibit perineural spread;[106] those that are ill-defined; those located in areas where maximal preservation of tissue is mandatory; and those which have been incompletely excised.

In addition to the disadvantages and complications associated with routine excisional surgery, Mohs surgery has the added disadvantage in some instances of being prolonged, time consuming and tedious for both the patient and surgeon. It is also not always readily available since special training, equipment and personnel are required. Although Mohs surgery is designed to deal with the most difficult of BCCs, if the tumor is extremely large and invasive the Mohs surgeon may need to call upon the expertise of other surgical disciplines in order to either eradicate the tumor or reconstruct the resultant defect.[207–210] When appropriately utilized for BCC, Mohs surgery is also cost effective[211] since: (1) the procedure is usually performed in an office setting as opposed to an operating room; (2) the Mohs surgeon serves both as surgeon and pathologist; and (3) with the high cure rate, the need to treat recurrences with their associated costs is less likely.

In recent years, some Mohs surgeons have used monoclonal antibodies to antigens expressed on neoplastic basal cells to aid in distinguishing tumor cells from normal epithelial structures as well as detecting tumor cells, which may not be readily visible with routine stain.[212–217] Although there are no specific tumor markers for BCC, the staining pattern with certain immunostains may help distinguish a BCC from adnexal structures.[215] These stains seem to be most helpful, however, when tracing out aggressive growth pattern BCCs with perineural involvement or when there is dense inflammation which makes detection of tumor cells with routine staining difficult, e.g. in patients with chronic lymphocytic leukemia.[213,214,216,217]

When using Mohs surgery to manage BCCs in patients with basal cell nevus syndrome, especially if they have numerous lesions, it may be impossible to get clear lateral margins without creating an inordinately large defect. In such circumstances, depending on the location of the tumor(s), one may have to settle for achieving clear deep margins only and simply follow the patient or use less invasive modalities to manage the epidermal component, (e.g. Imiquimod).

Radiation therapy

Radiation therapy is less frequently used in the management of BCC than in the past. However, radiation therapy remains a useful modality for the management of certain BCCs. To be effective, radiation therapy requires that the physician not only be knowledgeable in radiation principles but also well acquainted with the clinical and histopathologic features of BCCs. Skill in delineating the clinical extent of the BCC is critical. The high cure rates reported in the literature come from institutes in which the physicians are skilled and experienced in using radiation therapy for the treatment of skin cancer.

The major advantage cited for radiation therapy in the treatment of BCC is that it spares normal tissue, so it may spare the patient from undergoing a deforming surgical procedure which might necessitate reconstructive surgery. Consequently, radiation therapy is often advocated as the treatment of choice for BCCs of the nose, ear and periocular area because there is no need for reconstructive surgery and it prevents damage to the lacrimal collecting system.[218–223] Another advantage is that elderly patients who may be frail or in poor health and who might decline surgery usually are willing to have radiation therapy.[219] Radiation therapy can also be used in the patient who has an inoperable BCC. Although radiation therapy may not be curative, it may have considerable palliative benefit and improve the quality of life.[224] Radiation therapy may also be used as an adjunct to surgery in patients considered to be at high risk for recurrence.

Radiation therapy should not be used in younger patients.[218–221,225,226] Because of poor cosmetic results, radiation therapy is generally not recommended for the treatment of morpheaform BCCs.[199,218–221,225] Radiation therapy is said to be ill advised in the treatment of patients with basal cell nevus syndrome because of a fear of stimulating the development of additional BCCs.[227]

When properly executed, radiation therapy has resulted in five-year cure rates of 90 to 95%.[218–221,225] Not surprisingly, there is a decrease in cure rate as the size of the lesion increases.[199,224] The nose is the site with the highest recurrence rate.[199]

Although BCCs 1 cm or less in diameter can be effectively managed by a single dose of radiation, it is generally recommended that the dosage be fractionated, especially for larger lesions. The normal tissue will tolerate the radiation therapy much better and it is possible to deliver a larger total dosage of radiation to the BCC, thereby increasing the probability of cure. Fractionation is especially important if the BCC overlies bone or cartilage and will prevent complications and may produce a better cosmetic result.[218–221,225] The appearance of an irradiated area deteriorates with time and varies with the anatomic area treated. Often the area of irradiation will be characterized by atrophy, telangiectasia and hypopigmentation.[219,225] Scalp lesions generally are not irradiated because of the resultant alopecia.[225]

Although high cure rates have been reported for primary BCCs, the success rate in management of recurrent BCCs is not nearly as good. A 27% failure rate was noted when irradiating recurrent BCCs.[219] Undoubtedly this is because these lesions are ill-defined and/or have substantial subclinical extension. These same characteristics may be found in primary BCCs with an aggressive histologic growth pattern. Basal cell carcinomas 2 cm or greater in size and those occurring in high-risk areas also may exhibit significant subclinical spread which may result in a lower cure rate. To compensate for subclinical spread, wider margins of clinically normal skin need to be included in the field of irradiation. In the management of recurrent BCCs and high-risk primary BCCs, pretreatment biopsies to determine the extent and depth of these tumors may be advisable.[219] Under certain circumstances, post-treatment biopsies may also be appropriate.

Radiation therapy, as other treatment modalities, can result in buried tumor, which may grow for some time before it is clinically detected. In critical areas, such as the periocular area, this can be disastrous. With irradiation, erythema and sometimes oozing and crusting, is to be expected. This may be accompanied by itching, burning and crawling sensations. Subsequently, the area ulcerates and healing may require weeks to months, especially on the trunk and extremities.[219] If massive necrosis occurs following radiation therapy, one should suspect that much more tumor was present than was clinically suspected and biopsies should be done. Other complications of radiation therapy include comedones and chronic radiation dermatitis.[218]

In summary, radiation therapy has the advantages of sparing normal tissue, eliminating the need for reconstructive surgery and providing effective therapy for those too frail or unwilling to have surgery. On the other hand, it is a blind treatment technique that depends on the skill and experience of the therapist. For recurrent BCCs, large tumors, BCCs in high-risk areas and BCCs with an aggressive histologic growth pattern, there is a significant failure rate. Thus, great care in patient selection is required. Moreover, there is the inconvenience and expense of multiple treatments for a BCC that might have been treated surgically in a single office visit. Lastly, the cosmetic result deteriorates in time, in contrast to other therapies in which the scar's appearance improves with the passage of time.

Cryosurgery

When using cryosurgery in the management of a BCC, one must have the proper equipment and skill to use this modality effectively. In order to treat a BCC with cryosurgery, a cryoprobe or a liquid nitrogen spray unit is used. Discs and cotton-tipped swabs dipped in liquid nitrogen are not suitable for treating even the most superficial of BCCs.

Tumors overlying cartilage or bone may be frozen down to perichondrium or periosteum. (Clinically, when the freeze has reached this level the tissue will become fixed.)[228] For monitoring the breadth and depth of a freeze, measuring electrical impedance appears to be more accurate than monitoring tissue temperature.[229] In order to produce an adequate tumor kill, a double freeze-thaw cycle with a tissue temperature of −50°C is necessary.[229] The exception to this is the SBCC in which a single freeze is adequate for cure. As with all treatment modalities, it is necessary to include within the total area treated a margin of 'clinically normal' skin to compensate for subclinical spread.[229,230]

Opinion varies regarding the use of cryosurgery to treat BCCs with aggressive histologic features, recurrent BCCs, morpheaform BCCs, metatypical BCCs and BCCs located in high-risk areas.[229–234] Gage has suggested that sclerosing BCCs may not respond to cryosurgery because of their ill-defined nature and because nests of tumor cells are enmeshed in fibrous tissue that may insulate them.[232] Preoperative biopsies may be indicated to determine the depth and extent of the lesion. Post-treatment biopsies might also be useful to determine if the treatment has been adequate.[232] Cryosurgery may result in buried foci of tumor and is generally not recommended for BCCs of the scalp. If cryosurgery is used on the lower legs, the healing rate is slow, the cosmetic results often poor and the risk of infection is increased. When large tumors are treated, these may be debulked first and the base treated with cryosurgery.[232]

Cryosurgery may also be combined with curettage.[232,235] In addition to aiding in the removal of tumor, curettage also helps delineate subclinical extensions of the tumor.[232,234] Topical 5-FU has also been used preoperatively to help demonstrate the extent of the BCC.[234]

Cure rates as high as 97% have been achieved for nodular BCCs less than 1 cm in size[231] but there is a precipitous drop in cure rate for BCCs greater than 1 cm in diameter and for recurrent BCCs.[231,233] Cryosurgery may also be used for palliation.[228] Care must be taken when treating BCCs overlying superficial nerves (e.g. ulnar area, fingers) to avoid neuralgia and neuropathy. Although the neuropathy may persist for one to two years, it usually resolves.[234] Cure rates for cryosurgery in the management of primary BCCs 2 cm or less in size have been reported to be as high as 97 to 98%. Tumors greater than 2 cm in size, morpheaform BCCs, SBCCs, BCCs with an aggressive histologic growth pattern, BCCs in high-risk areas and recurrent BCCs show a higher recurrence rate (88%).[228,235] A relative contraindication to cryosurgery is a BCC greater than 3 cm in diameter (not SBCC).[234]

Pain occurs initially with freezing and as the thaw occurs. A depression may occur following cryosurgery. The most common locations for this complication are the tip of the nose, forehead, back, chest and ear.[234] If the tumor impinges on the vermilion of the upper lip or if the cartilage of the ear is involved, notching may occur.[228,234] Hypertrophic scars may appear four to six weeks after treatment.

In summary, cryosurgery is a modality which is tissue sparing and which can be utilized in patients who are in poor health or are taking anticoagulants or have pacemakers. When properly utilized it can give high cure rates for small nodular BCCs of the skin and eyelids. However, because it is a blind treatment modality, great caution needs to be exercised in managing high-risk lesions. Cosmetically, the results with cryosurgery are comparable to those achieved with CE.

Lasers

The carbon dioxide (CO_2) laser has been utilized in treatment of BCC. It can be used in its focused or incisional mode to excise the tumor and to create flaps to repair the resultant defect. Unlike electrosurgery, the CO_2 laser does not damage the specimen. Thus histologic examination of the specimen to determine the adequacy of the excision is not impaired. Added advantages of using the CO_2 laser for excisional surgery include the sealing of small blood vessels (thus creating a relatively bloodless field); the sealing of lymphatics and the sealing of nerves, which may minimize post-operative pain.[236,237] The CO_2 laser may also be used to remove cartilage or bone involved with tumor.[238]

Because it seals vessels, the CO_2 laser is ideal in the patient on anticoagulants or who has a pacemaker.[236] The CO_2 laser also sterilizes as it cuts and theoretically could decrease the risks of wound infection.[236]

The CO_2 laser has been used in its defocused vaporizing mode in conjunction with curettage to manage large or multiple SBCCs. High cure rates with minimal postoperative discomfort, rapid healing and usually excellent cosmesis have been reported.[237] Some 5% of patients, however, develop hypertrophic scars and hypopigmentation is common. Thus, using the CO_2 laser in this setting appears to offer no advantage over CE.

Photodynamic therapy

Photodynamic therapy (PDT) is still evolving as a therapeutic modality for BCC.[239-247] A photosensitizing agent, usually hematoporphyrin or a derivative of hematoporphyrin, is given intravenously,[239,240] applied topically,[241-243,245-248] or injected intralesionally.[240] To activate the agent, a light source is shone on the tumor or conducted through probes placed in the skin. This activates the photosensitizer, which subsequently causes necrosis of the tumor.

This necrosis may be associated with considerable discomfort. The area heals with a scar, but most patients find it acceptable. This therapy is based on the principle that the BCCr concentrates these photosensitizing agents relative to the surrounding normal skin. With intravenous therapy a generalized photosensitivity develops that may persist for up to one month.[239,240] With topical application of the photosensitizer, penetration is a problem, so that only thin lesions can be treated.[241,242,244] Although often yielding good cosmesis, the recurrence rate is significant (11–44%)[242,246] and multiple treatments may be required.

Despite its limitations, encouraging results have been reported with PDT and it will be interesting to watch the continuing evolution of this modality. It may prove to be especially useful in managing patients with multiple BCCs, e.g. patients with BCNS.

Immune response modifiers

The newest and most exciting advancement in the treatment of skin cancer has been the use of immune modulators. To date, the agent most commonly employed has been imiquimod 5% cream. Acting though Toll-like receptor 7, imiquimod induces the production of interferon alpha, tumor necrosis factor-alpha and a variety of other cytokines. It primarily targets antigen presenting cells such as monocytes, dendritic cells and epidermal Langerhans cells.[249,250]

Using a number of different regimens, encouraging responses have been reported in the treatment of primary nodular and superficial basal cell carcinomas.[251-261] Although ongoing studies will ultimately determine the efficacy of this modality and the ideal dosing regimen, currently it appears that once a day dosing for 5 days each week for 6 weeks is effective in most patients, especially in those with superficial basal cell carcinomas. As anticipated, there is a higher response rate for superficial basal cell carcinomas than for nodular BCCs (90% vs 76%).[256] Imiquimod may also prove to be a significant adjunct in the management of large superficial BCCs[261] and superficial BCCs in patients with multiple lesions.[257,260]

Interferon

Greenway and others have successfully managed primary nodular and SBCCs with intralesional interferon.[262-268] The agent most frequently used has been human recombinant α_2-interferon. A variety of dosing regimens have been employed but all require multiple injections over a significant time period. A sustained release form has also been successfully employed and has the added advantage of less frequent injections.[268] Side-effects include fever, malaise, rheumatic complaints, altered psyche, chills, transient decrease in the white count and pain and itching at the site of the injection. The long-term cure rate for this modality appears to be approximately 80%.[247] Besides requiring multiple visits, this modality also has the added disadvantage of being relatively expensive.

Topical chemotherapy

Topical 5-fluorouracil (5-FU) has limited usefulness in the management of BCC. It should be used only for treating SBCC.[269,270] Of the commercially available products, only the 5% concentration is suitable for the management of the SBCC, because the percutaneous penetration of 5-FU is variable and limited.[271-273] For this reason, 5-FU cannot be expected to be effective in eradicating invasive BCCs or BCCs with follicular involvement.[270,272,274,275] If 5-FU is used to treat an invasive BCC, the superficial component may be eliminated but the deeper component may be buried beneath scar and continue to grow until it develops into a subdermal mass with extensive subclinical spread.[269,270,273,276]

Curettage followed by topical 5-FU with occlusion, when used for SBCCs or 'thin' BCCs, appears to be more effective than topical 5-FU used only with occlusion, if treatment is carried out for only three weeks. This modification in conjunction with a 25% concentration of 5-FU demonstrated a 94% 5-year cure rate[272] with 80% of patients obtaining a good to excellent cosmetic result with topical 5-FU for SBCC superior to that seen with CE.[272] Side-effects from the use of topical 5-FU for SBCC include severe inflammation,[271] hyperpigmentation,[271] hypopigmentation,[272] and scarring.[272,274] Some 3% of patients become allergic to 5-FU, especially those with multiple lesions.[272] When used to treat SBCCs, topical 5% 5-FU is applied twice daily for no less than six weeks if not occluded or combined with curettage. Three months of treatment is often necessary to eradicate the tumor and discomfort can be significant. Because topical 5-FU can conceal clinically unsuspected deep foci of BCC and requires prolonged treatment and because it can produce considerable discomfort, its use should be reserved for patients with SBCCs for which no other treatment is practical. In addition to the management of SBCCs, it has been suggested that topical 5-FU may be of some prophylactic value in patients prone to developing multiple BCCs, e.g. basal cell nevus syndrome.[269,270]

Retinoids

Experience with the systemic retinoids, etretinate, isotretinoin and acitretin in the management of BCCs is limited.[277–279] Much of the data has come from the use of these agents in treating patients with the BCNS.[277,278] Doses of 4.5 mg/kg per day of isotretinoin and 1 mg/kg per day of etretinate are necessary to bring about regression of BCCs and even then most BCCs regress only partially.[279] These agents appear to have primarily a preventive effect.[277–279] Even for this preventive effect, significantly high doses of these agents are required (1.5 mg/kg per day for isotretinoin).[278,279] Consequently, many patients cannot tolerate these agents for prolonged periods. Once these agents are discontinued, relapse occurs.[277–279]

Systemic chemotherapy

Chemotherapy has been used both for the management of metastatic BCC and for the management of uncontrolled local disease. Metastatic BCC has a very poor prognosis when there is disseminated disease. Although occasional patients survive for years,[92] the usual period of survival is 10 to 20 months.[3,92]

If metastases are confined to the nodes, these may be successfully managed by surgery or surgery plus radiation therapy.[280–282] For disseminated metastases, including skeletal metastases, systemic chemotherapy alone or in conjunction with radiation therapy is indicated. Cisplatin, bleomycin, cyclophosphamide, 5-FU and vinblastine have been used.[280–282] Of these, cisplatin appears to be the most effective[282] and has been associated with long-term survival.[280–282] For advanced and unresectable BCCs, cisplatin and doxorubicin alone or in combination with radiation therapy, have proved to be excellent for palliation. This regimen is reasonably well tolerated and has yielded high response rates with prolonged disease control.[283–285]

Variables to consider in BCC management

When selecting the most appropriate modality for managing a BCC, a number of factors must be considered.

Age and cosmetic results

In the past, it was often assumed that elderly patients were not candidates for surgery and should be treated with radiation therapy. This is no longer the case. People not only live longer now, but they also usually enjoy a better quality of life and health. Consequently, an older individual need not be denied definitive surgery. For example, most elderly individuals can tolerate the removal of large or difficult BCCs by Mohs surgery, under local anesthesia.

Age also impacts cosmesis. Elderly individuals in general are less concerned about their appearance and thus more readily accept a scar from CE or cryosurgery. Younger individuals prefer an imperceptible scar that only excision can give. In addition, because the skin of the elderly is more forgiving, excellent cosmetic results may be obtained from CE in an older patient but a hypertrophic scar may occur in a younger patient. Radiation therapy is usually reserved for older individuals, because the cosmetic result deteriorates with time. There is a potential carcinogenic effect (albeit small) and because with the passage of time the chances of late radiation necrosis increase.

Number of lesions

If given enough time a surgeon may excise innumerable BCCs in a patient. However, this may be neither the most practical nor the best treatment. For example, treating multiple SBCCs with excision will be very time consuming, extensive healthy tissue will have to be sacrificed to get a good closure. What initially seems like a fine cosmetic result may eventuate in an ugly spreading scar. In this circumstance, any of three modalities – topical chemotherapy, cryosurgery or ED&C might be more practical and yield satisfactory therapeutic and cosmetic results.

Size of the lesion

The size of the lesion may be important from several standpoints. For example, if a patient has a 5 cm SBCC on the back which is excised and grafted, the cosmetic result will not be optimal. In such instances it might be better to consider topical chemotherapy, CE or cryosurgery. With large, invasive BCCs surgical excision or Mohs' surgery is generally the treatment of choice, although radiation therapy at times may be preferable.

Distinctness of the tumor borders

Those BCCs that are well demarcated and exophytic usually have a circumscribed nodular histology and can be managed by CE, cryosurgery, radiation therapy or excision with an anticipated high cure rate. However, those tumors that are ill-defined and flat or plaque-like usually demonstrate an aggressive growth pattern microscopically and are often best managed by Mohs surgery.

Primary versus recurrent BCC

Although histologic and anatomic factors need to be taken into consideration when managing a primary BCC, there are more treatment options available for a primary BCC than for a recurrent one. Similarly, with these treatment options there is a greater probability of curing a primary as opposed to a recurrent BCC. Numerous studies have shown that with standard modalities of treatment, there is a dramatic decline in cure rate for the recurrent as opposed to the primary BCC.[179,194,202,235] Only Mohs surgery, with its exact histologic control, offers patients with recurrent lesions a high likelihood of cure.[195,203–206] This is because these tumors are ill-defined, embedded in a sclerotic matrix and often demonstrate extensive subclinical spread.[195,196]

Anatomic location

As a rule of thumb, BCCs (not SBCC) in high-risk sites should be managed by Mohs surgery or routine surgical excision with histologic determination of the adequacy of the margins.

Besides subclinical spread, there may be other characteristics of an anatomic area that make a particular treatment modality unsuitable. For example, to perform effective curettage it is important to be able to immobilize the tissue. This is difficult on areas such as the lips or eyelids.[188] A chalazion clamp may be employed to give a more stable base when CE are done on the lips or lids. On the scalp and distal nose, areas rich in pilosebaceous units, BCCs may bud off hair follicles or lie between them and escape the curette. On the distal nose the deep dermis becomes so dense that tumor islands in this plane will not be completely removed by the curette.[188] Because of its rich vascularity, which causes difficulty in obtaining an adequate freeze and because of a high recurrence rate cryosurgeons prefer not to treat invasive BCCs of the scalp.[228] If a BCC on the leg is treated by cryosurgery, the healing time is markedly prolonged, there is a significant risk of infection and the cosmetic result is usually poor.[228] Although BCCs can be easily excised (on the trunk) spreading of the scar may result in a less than optimal cosmetic result when compared to another method of treatment. The cosmetic result obtained with radiation therapy for BCCs not located on the head and neck is usually poor; therefore, this modality, in general, should not be selected for treating BCCs of the trunk and extremities.[218,219]

Implications of the histologic growth pattern in the treatment of BCC

For years, clinicians have pondered whether the recurrent BCC is aggressive and elusive in its behavior from its onset or becomes that way because of treatment. In an attempt to answer this question, we studied the histologic evolution of the recurrent BCC.[110] In 65% of the BCCs studied the histology of the original tumor showed an aggressive growth pattern. Of the original tumors, only 24% showed a change to a more aggressive histologic picture. Thus, the majority of recurrent BCCs are aggressive from their onset and this can be predicted by carefully studying the histology of the tumor. Multiple studies[108,109,197,198,286,287] have demonstrated that BCCs which exhibit poor palisading and consist of infiltrating strands and micronodules of tumor are more likely to recur, invade deeply and widely and show aggressive biologic behavior. The stroma of these BCCs may[109] or may not[110,287] be sclerotic. Because BCCs with an aggressive histologic growth pattern exhibit marked subclinical spread,[110,287] and because they are capable of aggressive behavior and destruction, these tumors should not be treated by blind techniques but should be managed by conventional surgical excision or Mohs' surgery. Since conventional histopathologic examination of the excised specimen(s) may not detect some of the microscopic extensions of these tumors, a significant number of these lesions will recur after conventional surgical excision. CE have been shown to be ineffective in eradicating these tumors.[189]

Because of its tendency to recur, behave aggressively and metastasize, the metatypical BCC should not be treated by blind techniques. It should be managed by conventional surgical excision or Mohs surgery. The metatypical BCC may possess microscopic strands of tumor that routine pathologic examination may not detect. Thus, Mohs surgery is the preferred treatment. The morpheaform BCC is noted for its sometimes extensive subclinical extension[122,196] and again is best managed by a technique that employs histologic control, i.e. conventional surgical excision or Mohs surgery. Because microscopic extensions of this tumor may not be detected by conventional pathologic examination, Mohs surgery is the preferred treatment. Curettage is ineffective in the management of the morpheaform BCC because of the sclerotic stroma.[187,288]

The depth of penetration is also important in selecting a treatment modality. If the tumor extends into the deep dermis or subcutaneous fat, the curette cannot be relied upon to extirpate the tumor. Such tumors are best managed by conventional surgical excision or Mohs surgery.

Special situations

The 'Field Fire' BCC

This variant of BCC may be the result of a carcinogenic field effect or may represent a multifocal recurrent BCC. Clinically, it is not always possible to determine the margins of this variant; therefore, Mohs surgery, with its exacting histologic control and tissue sparing properties, is the treatment of choice. Management of the surgical defect should be conservative, with either healing by second intention or grafting of the area. Closures with dog-ear excisions or a flap may conceal tumor or introduce tumor cells into a tumor-free wound. If there is a known carcinogenic field effect and the area is limited in size (e.g. chronic radiation damage as the result of radiation therapy with which the patient was treated as a child for a small hemangioma of the nose), it may be best to excise all of the involved skin to prevent further tumor development.

Incompletely excised BCC

Based on several studies[289,290] some clinicians have elected not to re-excise BCCs when pathologic examination shows the margins of resection to be involved but instead simply follow the patient for signs of recurrence. This approach has been advocated because in the cited studies only one third of the presumably incompletely excised BCCs recurred. In cases in which the area was immediately re-excised, residual tumor was found in only 50% of the specimens.[289,291]

The explanation for why many incompletely excised BCCs do not recur is not totally clear. However, several hypotheses have been put forth. The most likely explanation is that those tumors which did not recur were indeed entirely excised, albeit with close margins.[290,292] Other possibilities are that an immune or inflammatory response eliminated the residual tumor[293] or that the residual tumor is so devitalized it cannot survive.[290,292]

As regards why residual tumor is not always found when the lesion is re-excised, in addition to the above explanations, it is probably that very little residual BCC was present in the re-excised specimen and it was undetected because of 'incomplete' histopathologic examination of the specimen.[291] Thus the clinician should not be dismayed if the pathologic report on the re-excision specimen shows no evidence of BCC.

Studies have shown a recurrence rate for incompletely excised BCCs as high as 86%.[293,294] Dellon et al.[293] have shown that an incompletely excised BCC with an aggressive growth pattern is more likely to recur than is one with a nodular growth pattern and have suggested that perhaps only incompletely excised BCCs with aggressive histology require immediate re-excision. However, any recurrent BCC, regardless of its histologic features, can behave aggressively[107,289,295,296] so it is suggested that every incompletely excised BCC should be reexcised.[294,296,297] In addition, by the time a BCC becomes clinically apparent, one may be seeing only the "tip of the iceberg." For this reason, whenever a major reconstruction is planned in the management of a BCC, it is mandatory to know that the BCC has been completely excised before the defect is reconstructed.

Perineural BCC

Perineural BCC is best managed by Mohs surgery, which allows the precise tracing out of the tumor. At times, this may entail the use of a multidisciplinary team. Hanke[177] has suggested that because of skip areas an additional layer of uninvolved tissue should be taken after the entire detectable tumor has been removed, but others do not take an additional layer of tissue once a tumor free wound has been achieved. Once the tumor has spread into the cranium, surgery is usually no longer feasible.[177] If the tumor has spread intracranially or the adequacy of surgery is questionable, radiation therapy can be administered.

Follow-up

Close follow-up is important in the management of patients with BCC. How frequently patients need to be seen will depend upon the severity of the cancer(s) treated, how much sun damage is present and how frequently and in what quantity they develop additional skin cancers and actinic keratoses. Although the majority of BCCs will recur within 5 years of treatment, a number of BCCs will recur after this period of time.[298] An additional benefit of following patients to detect recurrences is that many of these patients will subsequently develop new BCCs.[299–301] Often the patient will be unaware of the new lesions(s).[300,301] Some 20–33% of patients will develop a new BCC within a year of having been treated for the initial BCC and by the fifth year, up to 45% will develop an additional BCC.[301,302] Over a 5-year period (after treatment of an initial BCC), 20% of patients with Fitzpatrick types I or II skin who incur frequent sun exposure, will develop subsequent BCCs.[301]

FUTURE OUTLOOK

The most promising areas of ongoing research in BCC therapy would appear to be: (1) gene therapy, (2) photodynamic therapy and (3) the use of immune response modifiers.[303] One example of a potentially new therapeutic approach is the use of cyclopamine which is a potent stimulator of the patched gene. These agents may one day be used to treat patients with the BCNS who have a mutation in this gene or patients without this syndrome who, through loss of the protective effect of this gene, develop a BCC.[304–306] The family of immune response modifier agents is just beginning to be investigated. New compounds are being developed that have the potential to have even greater therapeutic efficacy. Another new experimental therapy is the topical use of an endonuclease in patients with xeroderma pigmentosum which has been shown to decrease the development of BCCs and actinic keratoses.[307]

Given the magnitude of BCC in the population, the future development of new diagnostic and therapeutic modalities for managing this most common of tumors will continue to increase in importance.

REFERENCES

1 Miller DL, Weinstock MA. Non melanoma skin cancer in the United States: Incidence. J Am Acad Derm 1994; 30:774–780.

2 Carter DM. Basal cell carcinoma. In: Fitzpatrick TB, Freedberg IM, Eisen AZ, et al. eds. Dermatology in General Medicine, 3rd edn. New York, NY: McGraw-Hill; 1987:759.

3 Mikhail GR, Nims LP, Kelly AP Jr, et al. Metastatic basal cell carcinoma. Review, pathogenesis and report of two cases. Arch Derm 1977; 113:1261–1269.

4 Domarus H Von, Steven PJ. Metastatic basal cell carcinoma. Report of five cases and review of 170 cases in the literature. J Am Acad Derm 1984; 10:1043–1060.

5 Jackson R, Adams RH. Horrifying basal cell carcinoma: A study of 33 cases and comparison with 435 non-horror cases and a report on four metastatic cases. J Surg Oncol 1973; 5:431–436.

6 Czarnecki D. The changing face of skin cancer in Australia. Int J Derm 1991; 30:715–717.

7 Krompecker E. Der Basalzellenkrebs. Jena: Fischer; 1903.

8 Lever WF. Tumors of the epidermal appendages. Classification of the Tumors of the Epidermal Appendages in Histopathology of the Skin, 4th edn. Philadelphia, PA: Lippincott; 1967:590–592.

9 Marks R. Trends in non melanocytic skin cancer treated in Australia: The second national survey. Int J Cancer 1993; 53:585–590.

10 Ko CB. The emerging epidemic of skin cancer. Br J Derm 1994; 130:269–272.

11 Fitzpatrick TB, Parrish JA. Haynes HA, et al. Ozone depletion and skin cancer. Dermatol Capsule Comment 1982; 4:10.

12 Auerbach H. Geographic variation in incidence of skin cancer in the United States. Public Health Rep 1961; 76:345.

13 Fears TR, Scotto J, Schneiderman MA. Mathematical models of age and ultraviolet effects on the incidence of skin cancer among whites in the United States. Am J Epidemiol 1977; 105:420–427.

14 Scotto J, Kopf AW, Urbach F. Nonmelanoma skin cancer among Caucasians in four areas of the United States. Cancer 1974; 34:1333–1338.

15 Vitaliano PP, Urbach F. The relative importance of risk factors in nonmelanoma carcinoma. Arch Derm 1980; 16:454–456.

16 Marshall DR. The clinical and pathological effects of prolonged solar exposure. Part II. The association with basal cell carcinoma. Aust NZ J Surg 1968; 38:89–97.

years later... Arch D 1978; A.D.D12–873.

80 Marmelzat WL. Malignant tumors in smallpox vaccination scars. A report of 24 cases. Arch Derm 1968; 97:400–406.

81 Feed WB, Wilson-Jones E. Malignant tumors as a late complication of vaccination. Arch Derm 1968; 98:132–135.

82 Domingo J, Helwig EB. Malignant neoplasms associated with nevus sebaceous of Jadassohn. J Am Acad Derm 1979; 1:545–556.

104 Conley J. Cancer of the skin of the nose. Arch Otolaryngol 1966; 84:55–60.

105 Levine HL, Bailin PL. Basal cell carcinoma of the head and neck. Identification of the high-risk patient. Laryngoscope 1980; 90:955–961.

106 Lever WF, Schaumburg-Lever G. Histopathology of the Skin, 6th edn. Philadelphia: Lippincott; 1983:562–575.

17 Oettle AG. Skin cancer in Africa. Natl Cancer Inst Monogr 1963; 10:197.

18 Quisenberry WB. Ethnic differences in skin cancer in Hawaii. Natl Cancer Inst Monogr 1963; 10:181.

19 Ten Seldam REJ. Skin cancer in Australia. Natl Cancer Inst Mongr 1963; 10:153.

20 Fleming ID, Barnwell JR, Burleson PE, et al. Skin cancer in black

and squamous cell carcinomas of the skin. Br J Cancer 1996; 73:1447–1454.

40 Diffey BL, Tate TJ, Davis A. Solar dosimetry of the face: The relationship of natural ultraviolet radiation exposure to basal cell carcinoma localization. Phys Med Bio 1979; 24:931–939.

41 Chen Y-T, Dubrow R, Zheh T, et al. Sunlamp use and the risk of

Cancer of the Skin

201 Sexton M, Jones DB, Maloney ME. Histologic pattern analysis of basal cell carcinoma. J Am Acad Derm 1990; 23:1118.

202 MacFarlane AW, Curley RK, Graham RM. Recurrence rates of basal cell carcinomas according to site, methods of removal, histological type and adequacy of excision. Br J Derm 1986; 115(Suppl):23.

203 Mohs FE. Carcinoma of the skin. A summary of therapeutic results. Chemosurgery: Microscopically Controlled Surgery for Skin Cancer. Springfield, IL: Charles C Thomas; 1978:153.

204 Robins P. Chemosurgery: My 15 years of experience. J Derm Surg Oncol 1981; 7:779–789.

205 Tromovitch TA, Stegman SJ. Microscopic-controlled excision of cutaneous tumors. Chemosurgery fresh tissue technique. Cancer 1978; 41:653–658.

206 Drake LA. Guidelines of cure for Mohs micrographic surgery. J Am Acad Derm 1995; 33:271.

207 Baker SR, Swanson NA, Grekin RC. An interdisciplinary approach to the management of basal cell carcinoma of the head and neck. J Derm Surg Oncol 1987; 13:1095–1106.

208 Levine H. Cutaneous carcinoma of the head and neck: Management of massive and previously uncontrolled lesions. Laryngoscope 1983; 93:87–105.

209 Levine H, Bailin P, Wood B, et al. Tissue conservation in the treatment of cutaneous neoplasms of the head and neck. Combined use of Mohs chemosurgical and conventional surgical techniques. Arch Otolaryngol 1979; 105:140–144.

210 Riefkohl R, Pollack S, Gerogiade GS. A rationale for the treatment of difficult basal cell and squamous cell carcinoma of the skin. Ann Plast Surg 1985; 15:99–104.

211 Cook J, Zitelli J. Mohs micrographic surgery: A cost analysis. J Am Acad Derm 1995; 39:698–703.

212 Morhenn VB, Roth S, Roth R. Use of monoclonal antibody (VM-2) plus the immunogold-silver technique to stain basal cell carcinoma cells. J Am Acad Derm 1987; 17:765–769.

213 Smeets NW, Stavast-Kooy AJ, Krekels GA, et al. Adjuvant cytokeratin staining in Mohs micrographic surgery for basal cell carcinoma. Derm Surg 2003; 29:375–377.

214 Kist D, Perkins W, Christ S, et al. Antihuman epithelial antigen (Ber-EP4) helps define basal cell carcinoma masked by inflammation. Derm Surg 1997; 23:1067–1070.

215 Krunic AL, Garrod DR, Viehman GE, et al. The use of antidesmoglein stains in Mohs micrographic surgery. A potential aid for the differentiation of basal cell carcinoma from horizontal sections of the hair follicle and folliculocentric basaloid proliferation. Derm Surg 1997; 23:463–468.

216 Ramnavain ND, Walker NP, Markey AC. Basal cell carcinoma: rapid techniques using cytokeratin markers to assist treatment by micrographic (Mohs) surgery. Br J Biomed Sci 1995; 52:184–187.

217 Jimenez FJ, Grchnik JM, Buchanan MD, et al. Immunohistochemical techniques in Mohs micrographic surgery: their potential use in the detection of neoplastic cells masked by inflammation. J Am Acad Dermatol 1995; 32:89–94.

218 Braun-Falco O, Lukacs S, Goldschmidt H. Dermatologic Radiotherapy. New York, NY: Springer; 1976:69.

219 Gladstein AH, Kopf AW, Bart RS. Radiotherapy of cutaneous malignancies. In: Goldschmidt H, ed. Physical Modalities in Dermatologic Therapy. Radiotherapy, Electrosurgery, Phototherapy, Cryosurgery. New York, NY: Springer-Verlag; 1978:95.

220 Chahbazian CM, Brown GS. Radiation therapy for carcinoma of the skin of the face and neck. Special considerations. JAMA 1980; 244:1135–1137.

221 Chahbazian CM, Brown GS. Skin cancer. In: Gilbert HA, ed. Modern Radiation Oncology Classic Literature and Current Management. Philadelphia. PA: Harper & Row; 1984:158.

222 Morrison WH, Garden AS, Ang KK. Radiation therapy for nonmelanoma skin carcinomas. Clin Plast Surg 1997; 24:719–729.

223 Leshin B, Yeatts P, Anscher M, et al. Management of periocular basal cell carcinoma: Mohs micrographic surgery verses radiotherapy. Surv Ophthalmol 1993; 38:193–212.

224 Hunter RD. Skin. In: Easson EC, Pointon RCS, eds. The Radiotherapy of Malignant Disease. New York, NY: Springer-Verlag; 1985:135.

225 Brady LW, Binnick SA, Fitzpatrick PJ. Skin cancer. In: Perez CA, Brady LW, eds. Principles and Practice of Radiation Oncology. Philadelphia: Lippincott; 1987:377.

226 Thissen MR, Neumann MH, Schouten LJ. A systematic review of treatment modalities for primary basal cell carcinomas. Arch Derm 1999; 135:1177–1183.

227 Gorlin RJ. Nevoid basal cell carcinoma syndrome. Medicine 1987; 66:98–113.

228 Zacarian SA. Cryosurgery for cancer of the skin. In: Zacarian SA, ed. Cryosurgery for Skin Cancer and Cutaneous Disorders. St Louis: Mosby; 1985:96.

229 Zacarian SA. Cryogenics: The cryolesion and the pathogenesis of cryonecrosis. In: Zacarian SA, ed. Cryosurgery for Skin Cancer and Cutaneous Disorders. St Louis, MO: Mosby; 1985:1.

230 Kuflik EG. Cryosurgery for cutaneous malignancy; an update. Derm Surg 1997; 23:1081–1087.

231 Fraunfelder FT. Cryosurgery of eyelid, conjunctival and intraocular tumors. In: Zacarian SA, ed. Cryosurgery for Skin Cancer and Cutaneous Disorders. St Louis, MO: Mosby; 1985:259.

232 Gage AA. Cryosurgery of advanced tumors of the head and neck. In: Zacarian SA, ed. Cryosurgery for Skin Cancer and Cutaneous Disorders. St Louis, MO: Mosby; 1985:163.

233 Kuflik EG. Cryosurgery for carcinoma of the eyelids. A 12-year experience. J Derm Surg Oncol 1985; 11:243–246.

234 Zacarian SA. Complications, indications and contraindications in cryosurgery. In: Zacarian SA, ed. Cryosurgery for Skin Cancer and Cutaneous Disorders. St Louis, MO: Mosby; 1985:283.

235 Spiller WF, Spiller RF. Cryosurgery and adjuvant surgical techniques for cutaneous carcinomas. In: Zacarian SA, ed. Cryosurgery for Skin Cancer and Cutaneous Disorders. St Louis, MO: Mosby; 1985:187.

236 Sacchini V, Lovo GF, Avioli N, et al. Carbon dioxide laser in scalp tumor surgery. Laser Surg Med 1984; 4:261–269.

237 Wheeland RG, Bailin PL, Ratz JL, et al. Carbon dioxide laser vaporization and curettage in the treatment of large or multiple superficial basal cell carcinomas. J Derm Surg Oncol 1987; 13:119–125.

238 Bailin PL, Ratz JL, Lutz-Nagey L. CO_2 laser modification of Mohs surgery. J Derm Surg Oncol 1981; 7:621–623.

239 Tse DT, Kersten RC, Anderson RL. Hematoporphyrin-derivative photoradiation therapy in managing nevoid basal cell carcinoma syndrome. A preliminary report. Arch Ophthalmol 1984; 102:990–994.

240 Waldow SM, Lobraico RV, Kohler IK, et al. Photodynamic therapy for treatment of malignant cutaneous lesions. Laser Surg Med 1987; 7:451–456.

241 Sacchini V, Melloni E, Marchesini R, et al. Preliminary clinical studies with PDT by topical TPPS. Administration in neoplastic skin lesions. Laser Surg Med 1987; 7:6–11.

242 Basset-Sequin N, Ibbotson S, Emestam L, et al. Photodynamic therapy using methylaminolevalinate is as efficacious as cryotherapy in primary superficial basal cell carcinoma but with better cosmetic outcome. American Academy Dermatology Annual Meeting, San Francisco, 2003.

243 Lue H, Salasche S, Kollias N, et al. Photodynamic therapy of non melanoma skin cancer with topical aminolevulinic acid: A clinical histologic study. Arch Derm 1995; 131:737–738.

244 Morton CA. Photodynamic therapy for basal cell carcinoma – tumor thickness a predictor of response. Br J Derm 1996; 135(Suppl):66.

245 Wang I, Bendsoe N, Klinteberg CAF, et al. Photodynamic therapy vs cryosurgery of basal cell carcinomas: results of a phase III clinical trial. Br J Derm 2001; 144:832–840.

246 Fink-Puches R, Soyer HP, Hofer A, et al. Longterm follow-up and histological changes of superficial non melanoma skin cancers treated with topical aminolevulinic acid photodynamic therapy. Arch Derm 1998; 134:821–826.

247 Vine JE. Skin cancer update. Treatment alternatives for basal cell and squamous cell carcinoma. N J Med 2001; 98:35–37.

248 Stockfleth E, Sterry W. New treatment modalities for basal cell carcinoma. Recent results. Cancer Res 2002; 160:259–268.

249 Stanley MA. Mechanism of action of imiquimod. Pap Rep 1999; 10:23–29.

250 Hemmi H, Kaisho T, Takeuchi O, et al. Small antiviral compounds activate immune cells via the TUR 7 MYD88-dependent signaling pathway. Nat Immunol 2002; 3:196–200.

251 Beatner KR, Geisse JK, Helman D, et al. Therapeutic response of basal cell carcinoma to the immune response modifier imiquimod 5% cream. J Am Acad Derm 1999; 41:1002–1007.

252 Marks R, Gebauer K, Shumiack S, et al. Imiquimod 5% cream in the treatment of superficial basal cell carcinoma: Results of a multicenter 6-week dose response trial. J Am Acad Derm 2001; 44:807–813.

253 Kagy MK, Amonette R. The use of imiquimod 5% cream for the treatment of superficial basal cell carcinomas in a basal cell nevus syndrome patient. Derm Surg 2000; 26:577–579.

254 Cowen E, Mercurio MG, Gaspari AA. An open case series of patients with basal cell carcinoma treated with topical 5% imiquimod cream. J Am Acad Derm 2002; 47(Suppl)(4):S240–S248.

255 Geisse JK, Rich P, Pandya A, et al. Imiquimod 5% cream for the treatment of superficial basal cell carcinoma: A double-blind randomized vehicle-controlled study. J Am Acad Derm 2002; 47:390–398.

256 Shumach S, Robinson J, Kossard S, et al. Efficacy of topical 5% imiquimod cream for the treatment of nodular basal cell carcinoma. Arch Derm 2002; 138:1165–1171.

257 Micali G, Pasquale R De, Caltabiano R. Topical imiquimod treatment of superficial and nodular basal cell carcinomas in patients affected by basal cell nevus syndrome: A preliminary report. J Derm Treat 2002; 3:123–127.

258 Salasche S. Imiquimod 5% cream: A new option for basal cell carcinoma. Int J Derm 2002; 41(Suppl)(1):16–20.

259 Kerr C. 'Rub-on' treatment for basal cell carcinoma. Lancet Oncol 2002; 3:201.

260 Drehs MM, Cock-Bolden F, Tanzi EL. Successful treatment of multiple superficial basal cell carcinomas with topical imiquimod: Case report and review of the literature. Derm Surg 2002; 28:427–429.

261 Chen TM, Rosen T, Orengo I. Treatment of a large superficial basal cell carcinoma with 5% imiquimod: A case report and review of the literature. Derm Surg 2002; 28:344–346.

262 Greenway HT, Cornell RC, Tanner DJ, et al. Treatment of basal cell carcinoma with intralesional interferon. J Am Acad Derm 1986; 15:437–443.

263 Cornell RC, Greenway HT, Tucker SB, et al. Intralesional interferon therapy for basal cell carcinoma. J Am Acad Derm 1990; 23:694–700.

264 Grob JJ, Collet AM, Munoz MH, et al. Treatment of large basal cell carcinomas with intralesional interferon-alpha-2a. Lancet 1988; 1:878–879.

265 Ikic D, Padovan IN, Pipic N, et al. Interferon therapy for basal cell carcinoma and squamous cell carcinoma. Int J Clin Pharm 1991; 29:342–346.

266 Alpsoy E, Yilmaz A, Easavian E, et al. Comparison of the effects of intralesional interferon alpha 2a and 2b in the treatment of basal cell carcinoma. J Derm 1996; 23:394–396.

267 Doga NB, Harmanyer Y, Baloglu H, et al. Intralesional alfa-2a interferon therapy for basal cell carcinoma. Cancer Lett 1995; 91:215–219.

268 Edwards L, Tucker SB, Perednia D, et al. The effect of an intralesional sustained release formulation of interferon alfa-2b on basal cell carcinomas. Arch Derm 1990; 126:1029–1032.

269 Goette DK. Topical chemotherapy with 5-fluorouracil. A review. J Am Acad Derm 1981; 4:633–649.

270 Klein E, Stoll HL, Miller E, et al. The effects of 5-fluorouracil (5-FU) ointment in the treatment of neoplastic dermatoses. Dermatologica 1970; 140(Suppl):21–33.

271 Ebner H. Treatment of skin epitheliomas with 5-fluorouracil (5FU) ointment. Influence of therapeutic design on recurrence of tumor. Dermatologica 1970; 140(Suppl):42–46.

272 Epstein E. Fluorouracil paste treatment of the basal cell carcinoma. Arch Derm 1985; 121:207–213.

273 Klostermann GG. Effects of 5-fluorouracil (5FU) ointment on normal and diseased skin. Histological findings and deep action. Dermatologica 1970; 140(Suppl):47.

274 Klein E, Stoll HL Jr, Milgrom H, et al. Tumors of the skin. Topical 5-fluorouracil for epidermal neoplasms. J Surg Oncol 1971; 3:331–349.

275 Reymann F. A follow-up study of treatment of basal cell carcinoma with 5-fluorouracil ointment. Dermatologica 1972; 144:205–208.

276 Mohs FE, Jones DL, Bloom RF. Tendency of fluorouracil to conceal deep foci of invasive basal cell carcinoma. Arch Derm 1978; 114:1021–1022

277 Crestofolini M, Zumiani G, Scappini P, et al: Aromatic retinoid in the chemoprevention of nevoid basal cell carcinoma syndrome. J Derm Surg Oncol 1984; 10:778–781.

278 Hodak E, Ginzburg A, David M, et al. Etretinate treatment of nevoid basal cell carcinoma syndrome. Therapeutic and chemopreventive effect. Int J Derm 1987; 26:606–609.

279 Peck GL. Topical tretinoin in actinic keratoses and basal cell carcinoma. J Am Acad Derm 1986; 15:829–835.

280 Coker DD, Elias EG, Viravathana T, et al: Chemotherapy for metastatic basal cell carcinoma. Arch Derm 1983; 119:44–50.

281 Hartman R, Hartman S, Green N. Long-term survival following bony metastases from basal cell carcinoma. Report of a case. Arch Derm 1986; 122:912–914.

282 Wieman TJ, Shiveley EH, Woodcock TM. Responsiveness of metastatic basal cell carcinoma to chemotherapy. A case report. Cancer 1983; 52:1583–1585.

283 Guthrie TH, McEleveen LJ, Porubsky ES, et al. Cisplatin and doxorubicin: An effective chemotherapy combination in the treatment of advanced basal cell and squamous cell carcinoma of the skin. Cancer 1985; 55:1629.

284 Guthrie TH, Porubsky ES. Successful systemic chemotherapy of advanced squamous and basal cell carcinoma of the skin with cis-diamine-dichloroplatinum III and doxorubicin. Laryngoscope 1982; 92:1298.

285 Robinson JK. Use of a combination of chemotherapy and radiation therapy in the management of advanced basal cell carcinoma of the head and neck. J Am Acad Derm 1987; 17:770.

286 Mehregan AH. Aggressive basal cell epithelioma on sunlight protected skin: Report of eight cases, one with pulmonary and bone metastases. Am J Derm 1983; 5:221.

287 Siegle RJ, MacMillan J, Pollack SV. Infiltrative basal cell carcinoma: A nonsclerosing subtype. J Derm Surg Oncol 1986; 12:830–836.

288 Crissey JT. Curettage and electrodesiccation as a method of treatment for epitheliomas of the skin. J Surg Oncol 1971; 3:287–290.

289 Pascal RP, Hobby LW, Lattes R, et al. Prognosis of 'incompletely excised' versus 'completely excised' basal cell carcinoma. Plast Reconstr Surg 1968; 41:328–332.

290 Gooding CA, White G, Yatsuhashi M. Significance of marginal extension in excised basal cell carcinoma. N Engl J Med 1965; 273:923.

291 Sarma DP, Griffing CC, Weilbaecher TG. Observations on the inadequately excised basal cell carcinomas. J Surg Oncol 1984; 25:79–80.

292 Jackson R. Why do basal cell carcinomas recur (or not recur) following treatment? J Surg Oncol 1974; 6:245–251.

293 Dellon AL, DeSilva S. Connolly M, et al. Prediction of recurrence in incompletely excised basal cell carcinoma. Plast Reconstr Surg 1985; 75:860–871.

294 Shanoff LB, Spira M, Hardy SA. Basal cell carcinoma. A statistical approach to rational management. Plast Reconstr Surg 1967; 39:619–624.

295 Hauben DJ, Zirkin H, Mahler D, et al. The biologic behavior of basal cell carcinoma: Analysis of recurrence in excised basal cell carcinoma II. Plast Reconstr Surg 1982; 69:110–116.

296 Koplin L, Zarem HA. Recurrent basal cell carcinoma: Review concerning the incidence, behavior and management of recurrent basal cell carcinoma with emphasis on the incompletely excised lesion. Plast Reconstr Surg 1980; 65:656–664.

297 Robinson JK. What are adequate treatment and follow-up care for nonmelanoma cutaneous cancer. Arch Derm 1987; 123:331–333.

298 Grover RW. Basal cell carcinoma. Arch Derm 1973; 107:138.

299 Bergstresser PR, Halprin KM. Multiple sequential skin cancers. The risk of skin cancer in patients with previous skin cancer. Arch Derm 1975; 111:995–996.

300 Epstein E. Value of follow-up after treatment of basal cell carcinoma. Arch Derm 1973; 108:798–800.

301 Robinson JK. Risk of developing another basal cell carcinoma. A 5-year prospective study. Cancer 1987; 60:118–120.

302 Marghoob A, et al. Risk of another basal cell carcinoma developing after treatment of a basal cell carcinoma. J Am Acad Derm 1993; 28:22–28.

303 Urosevic M, Dumminer R. Immunotherapy for non melanoma skin cancer: does it have a future? Cancer 2002; 94:477–485.

304 Taipale JP, Chen JK, Cooper MK, et al. Effects of oncogenic mutation in smoothened and patched can be reversed by cyclopamine. Nature 2000; 406:1005–1009.

305 Austerbaum M, Beech J, Epstein EH. Ultraviolet radiation mutagenesis of hedgehog pathway genes in basal cell carcinoma. J Invest Derm Symp Proc 1999; 4:41–45.

306 Miller SJ, Yu TC. Cyclopamine as a potential therapeutic agent for treatment of tumors relating to hedgehog pathway mutations. Derm Surg 2002; 28:187.

307 Yarosh D, Klein J, O'Connor A, et al. Effect of topically applied T4 endonuclease V in liposomes in skin cancer in xeroderma pigmentosum: A randomized study. Lancet 2001; 357:926–929.

CHAPTER
10

Squamous Cell Carcinoma

Tri H Nguyen and Jaeyoung Yoon

Key points

- Although 95% of squamous cell carcinomas (SCC) may be cured if diagnosed and treated early, a subset of tumors behave aggressively with high rates of recurrence and metastasis.
- Chronically immunosuppressed patients (organ transplant patients, lymphoproliferative malignancies) are vulnerable to developing high-risk squamous cell carcinomas. These patients should be closely monitored and aggressively treated.
- Therapies are most effective when clinical and histologic features are closely correlated.
- The approach to the staging and management of patients with regional disease is still evolving.
- Chemoprevention, biologic response modifiers and novel modifications of established therapies offer promising options for patients with cutaneous SCC.

INTRODUCTION AND HISTORY

Cutaneous squamous cell carcinoma (SCC) accounts for 10–20% of all skin malignancies and is the second most common skin cancer after basal cell carcinoma (BCC). The cell of origin is the epidermal keratinocyte, which undergoes malignant transformation with repeated ultraviolet (UV) induced mutations. It is extremely common in fair skinned individuals and fortunately has a better than 95% cure rate if detected and treated early. A subset of SCCs may be extremely aggressive with extensive tissue destruction, local recurrences, metastasis, and death. SCC is most consistently related to ultraviolet radiation (UVR) in its pathogenesis but may be varied in its presentation, both clinically and histologically.

EPIDEMIOLOGY

In the general population, BCCs outnumber SCCs 4:1. However, with their greater tendency to recur and metastasize, SCCs cause the majority of deaths among non-melanoma skin cancers (NMSC). SCC predominantly affects elderly white men and incidence increases markedly after the age of 40 (Fig. 10.1). Men are consistently affected 2–3 times more frequently than women. Outdoors occupation, less protective clothing, and a greater lifetime cumulative UVR exposure contribute to this gender gap.

Estimating incidence is difficult as health registries often exclude NMSC in their databases. Various rates, however, have been published for countries that are most affected (Table 10.1).[1-5] By far the highest incidence is found in Australia, where the two prerequisites for SCC are present; an intense UVR exposure level and a predominantly fair Caucasian population. Not surprisingly, the highest incidence of two other UV-associated malignancies; BCC and melanoma are also found in Australia.

What is most alarming about the rate of SCC is its continued increase, with a doubling in incidence over the last 40 years. After having a prior SCC, the 3-year cumulative risk of developing another SCC is 18%.[6] Interestingly, having a prior BCC does not connote the same risk, as the three-year risk of a subsequent SCC in these patients is substantially lower at 6%.

The contributions to the worldwide increase in SCC incidence are many. An improved living standard in industrialized nations has permitted more outdoor recreation and greater UVR exposure. Increasing public awareness of skin cancer warning signs and more frequent skin examinations has also resulted in earlier and more frequent detection of SCCs. As a result of the continuing ozone layer depletion, UVR is becoming progressively intense. There is a long latency period, however, between UV exposure and the development of skin cancers. The true impact of ozone depletion on skin cancer incidence will be more felt in the years ahead. Finally, the rising numbers of immunosuppressed patients is also contributing to the increase in SCCs. Whether internal (disease related, i.e. chronic lymphocytic leukemia (CLL) or acquired immunodeficiency syndrome (AIDS)), or external (medication related, i.e. organ transplant patients), immunosuppression is a fertile ground for skin cancer development.

A population especially susceptible to extraordinarily high rates of SCC is solid organ transplant recipients (OTR), which includes heart, lung, kidney, and pancreas recipients. As transplantation medicine becomes more successful and patients live longer, cutaneous carcinoma rather than organ failure becomes the primary battle. Patients after renal transplantation have a significantly increased risk for tumor development from 7% after the first year, to 45% after the 11th year, and culminating at 70% after 20 years.[7] The mean time interval to develop SCC from initial transplantation is 8 years[8] but this may be shortened by additional risk factors (Table 10.2). These patients have a three-fold overall increase in tumor formation and non-melanoma skin cancers (especially SCC) outnumber all other malignancies. Whereas the ratio of BCC:SCC in the general population is 4:1, this is

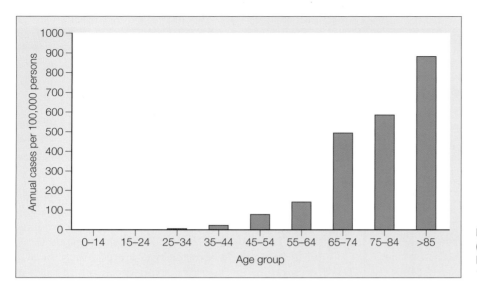

Figure 10.1 Squamous cell carcinoma (SCC) rates for first diagnosed tumors in Rochester, Minnesota between 1984 and 1992.[69]

reversed at 1:4 among transplant patients. Transplant patients have an increased risk of 65-fold for SCC, 84-fold for Kaposi's sarcoma, and a three-fold increase for melanoma.[9] Among solid organ recipients, heart transplant patients have a 2–3 times greater risk than renal transplants for developing SCCs while liver transplants have the lowest risk. In addition to having a greater risk of SCCs, almost half of transplant patients have multiple tumors on presentation. Their SCCs also behave more aggressively with higher rates of metastasis and death. Ong *et al.* showed that among Australian heart transplant patients surviving beyond the 4th year, skin cancers (particularly SCCs) were the cause of death in 27% of cases.[10] Clearly, more intense levels of immunosuppression result in a greater risk of tumor development. The medications in these patients may be directly carcinogenic, as in the case with azathioprine and cyclosporine. Indirectly, these agents also promote tumor growth by inhibiting cellular immunity and anti-tumor defenses. Not only are malignancies left unchecked, but viral infections that predispose to cancer are also uninhibited. A reduction of dose or an elimination of some immunosuppression (usually azathioprine) will greatly reduce the enormous tumor burden in some patients. The risk of organ rejection is real and should be balanced with the need for better tumor control. The duration and intensity of immunosuppression clearly raises the risk for SCC in these patients. Less clear is whether using newer immunosuppressive medications will reduce the skin cancer risk, as available studies show conflicting results. Patients with other causes of immunosuppression, such

as lymphoproliferative malignancies (lymphoma, CLL) and AIDS, are also at increased risk for aggressive SCCs.

PATHOGENESIS AND ETIOLOGY

The development of SCC is clearly multifactorial involving both genetic predisposition and environmental exposures. Multiple carcinogenic factors have been implicated, but the most convincing and important of these is ultraviolet radiation. Clinical and epidemiological evidence is compelling for the relationship between solar exposure and skin cancer development. Some 80% of SCCs occur

Table 10.2 Risk factors for SCC

General risk factors	Immunosuppression (in addition to general factors)
Fair skin (burns easily, never or rarely tan)	Duration of immunosuppression
Chronic cumulative UV exposure	Intensity of immunosuppression
Geography (closer to equator)	History of prior SCC
History of prior NMSC	Organ related (heart > kidney > liver): likely due to immunosuppression intensity
Age >50	>10 actinic keratoses
Male gender	
Genodermatoses (Table 10.3)	
Chronic scarring/inflammatory conditions (Table 10.3)	
Smoking (lip SCC)	
Chemical carcinogens	
Intense PUVA therapy (>300 treatments)	
Human papilloma virus infection (specific subtypes)	

Table 10.1   SCC incidence per 100,000 population by geography[1–5]

Geographic location	Men	Women
USA	81	26
South Wales	53	29.8
Netherlands	11	3
Australia	1332	755

on sun-exposed surfaces (head and neck, upper extremities). Patients at greatest risk are fair complexioned individuals who have relatively low constitutive melanin and who burn easily. Africans with oculocutaneous albinism have their protective melanin decreased to absent and suffer from significantly higher rates of SCC when compared with Africans without this disorder.[11] Among fair-skinned populations throughout the world, the highest incidence of SCC is in Australia, a country with intense perennial UVR exposure and where 92% of the population is of Caucasian descent.

Within the ultraviolet spectrum of solar energy, ultraviolet-B (UVB: 290–320 nm wavelength) is most closely implicated in the development of SCC. In laboratory animals, UVB is approximately 1000 times more potent than ultraviolet-A (UVA: 320–400 nm wavelength) in producing skin cancers. Although UVB is less abundant on the earth's surface and has less cutaneous penetration than UVA, it is more effective in producing genetic mutations. UVB is considered both an initiator and a promoter of cutaneous carcinogenesis. Absorption of UVB by deoxyribonucleic acid (DNA) within epidermal keratinocytes induces a unique DNA mutation at the site of pyrimidine dimers, which are adjacent pyrimidine nucleotides (C-C or T-C) on the same DNA strand.[12] This initiating event may result in errors during DNA replication and transcription, with the most deleterious damage occurring when tumor suppressor genes or oncogenes are affected. In xeroderma pigmentosum, a condition where the ability to repair these mutations is deficient, numerous skin cancers, including SCCs, develop.[13] Carcinogenesis is not a single event and usually requires multiple and cumulative transgressions. However, mutations in the single gene *p53* are present in 40–60% of all skin cancers. *p53* is a tumor suppressor gene involved in cell cycle regulation.[14] When *p53* encounters cells with DNA defects, it arrests cell growth at the G1 phase of the cell cycle to allow for DNA repair. With irreparable defects, *p53* induces cell death (apoptosis) and prevents replication and hence transmission of genetic mutations. Mutations in *p53*, therefore, may be the initiating event as they permit damaged cells to proliferate and possibly progress into cancer.[15] Indeed, UV-characteristic *p53* mutations have been found in both actinic keratoses (SCC precursors) and SCCs.

UVA, in addition to UVB, also appears to be important in the development of SCC. Although it is far less carcinogenic, tumors can be induced in laboratory animals when given large doses of UVA. Recent reports also show that patients who receive long term PUVA (Psoralen + UVA) therapy for conditions such as psoriasis have significantly increased rates of SCC.[16] This is particularly important as the vast majority, 90–99%, of the earth's ultraviolet radiation is in the form of UVA. Molecular studies show that UVA may not act as a tumor initiator, as UVB does, but rather as a tumor promoter to help expand initiated tumor cells through the modulation of protein kinase C, a signal transduction molecule.[17] More clear is UVA's role in cutaneous immunosuppression. UVA exposure suppresses both the induction and the elicitation of the immune response to a variety of antigens. Delayed hypersensitivity (DTH) responses such as contact dermatitis can be blocked by UVA, both prior to and after antigen sensitization. The mechanism of UVA immunosuppression is via cytokine (Interleukin-10) activation of suppressor T-cells that inhibit the induction of immunity.[18] It appears then that UVB and UVA work in concert for cutaneous carcinogenesis. UVB initiates keratinocyte DNA damage, which can lead to clonal proliferations of mutated cells, especially if *p53* protection is also dysfunctional from UVB injury. Immune rejection of these early malignancies is then impaired by chronic UVA induced immunosuppression, leading to progression of cancer.

Other causative factors for squamous cell carcinoma include chemical carcinogens. Well-documented agents include polycyclic aromatic hydrocarbons. These agents include soot, pitch and tar, shale oil and mineral oil. Occupational exposure to these agents has led to many well-recognized historical malignancies. Chimney sweep carcinoma of the scrotum and Mule Spinner's disease were both SCCs related to occupational exposure to soot and mineral oil respectively.

Arsenic is another important carcinogen in the development of cutaneous SCC. Arsenic is often ingested from two main sources, medicinal formulations and well water. Historically, oral Fowler's solution (potassium arsenite) was prescribed for the treatment of psoriasis and eczema. These patients developed both arsenical keratosis on the extremities and aggressive SCCs. Well water contaminated with high concentrations of trivalent inorganic arsenic is also associated with increased numbers of SCCs. These patients develop not only arsenical keratoses and SCC but also other cancers including BCCs and internal malignancies of the lung, urogenital region, and upper gastrointestinal tract.

Skin with previous injury or chronic dermatitis are also at increased risk for developing SCC. Breakdown of scars into ulcerated SCC was initially observed by Jean Nicholas Marjolin in the 1800s and was later described as 'Marjolin's ulcer'. Conditions predisposing to SCC include old scars caused by trauma (burns and frostbite) or chronic diseases, such as hidradenitis suppurativa and dystrophic epidermolysis bullosa (Table 10.3). Skin damaged by ionizing radiation, chronic thermal exposure, chronic inflammation, and lymphedema is also at risk. SCCs arising from such damaged skin are more aggressive with some studies citing a metastasis rate of 38% or higher. The cause for malignant degeneration at these sites and the increased aggression of these tumors is not clear at this time.

The oncogenic properties of human papilloma virus (HPV) have been well elucidated, especially in the development of cervical cancer. HPV proteins E6 and E7 may inhibit *p53* function directly and permit replication of malignant clones. Viral E6 protein may also act through *p53* independent mechanisms to prevent UV-induced apoptosis.[19] HPV is also associated with subtypes of cutaneous SCC. The most convincing relationship is HPV subtypes 6 and 11 and verrucous carcinoma of the perineum, also known as Buschke–Lowenstein tumor.[20] HPV 16 has been identified in many cases of nail bed SCC, but this relationship is less definitive. Viral particles have also been reported in keratoacanthomas. HPV in immunosuppressed patients may become uncontrollable infections leading to hundreds of verrucous

Table 10.3 Conditions predisposing to SCC

Chronic inflammatory conditions	Chronic infections	Chronic scarring conditions	Genetic syndromes
• Discoid lupus erythematosus • Erosive oral lichen planus • Lichen sclerosis et atrophicus • Lymphedema • Chronic leg ulcers	• Osteomyelitis • Follicular triad (acne conglobata, hidradenitis suppurativa, dissecting cellulitis of the scalp) • Chronic deep fungal infections • Lupus vulgaris • Lymphogranuloma venereum • Granuloma inguinale	• Burn scars • Thermal injury • Irradiated skin (ionizing radiation)	• Xeroderma pigmentosum • Oculocutaneous albinism • Epidermolysis bullosa dystrophica • Epidermodysplasia verruciformis • Fanconi's anemia • Dyskeratosis congenita • Rothmund–Thompson syndrome • Werner's syndrome • Chronic mucocutaneous candidiasis • KID syndrome (keratitis, ichthyosis, deafness)

nodules and an increase in SCCs. The widespread presence of HPV in both normal skin and malignant lesions makes causation difficult to prove for some associations.

CLINICAL FEATURES

The presentation of SCC will vary depending on the location, pigmentation background and clinical setting. The anatomic distribution of SCC is overwhelmingly on sun-exposed surfaces of fair skinned individuals. Approximately 70% are found on the head and neck and an additional 15% on the upper extremities. A smaller, yet significant portion, are found on sun-protected areas, such as the genitalia and buttock, suggesting that multiple factors in addition to solar irradiation are important for carcinogenesis. In organ transplant patients, 22% of invasive SCCs occur in normally covered locations (trunk and lower extremities).

For most fair-skinned patients, SCC will usually develop in a background of sun-damaged skin with surrounding actinic keratoses (AK). AK is the earliest precursor to SCC, showing similar keratinocyte atypia, UV-induced DNA damage (pyrimidine dimers), and UV-induced *p53* mutations. A suggested new name for AK is keratinocyte intraepidermal neoplasia (KIN), which reflects its malignant continuum with SCC.[21] AKs are rough, keratotic macules or papules found on sun-exposed skin. The borders are often ill-defined but may be well circumscribed in more hypertrophic lesions. Erythema may be present at the base and AKs are more easily felt than seen. Hypertrophic AK are thickened actinic keratoses that may be difficult to distinguish from early SCC. Other clinical variants of AK include the pigmented and lichenoid types. Disseminated superficial actinic porokeratosis (DSAP) and porokeratosis of Mibelli are two entities that may exhibit malignant potential for SCC. The risk of a single AK transforming into SCC ranges from a low of 0.24% to a high of 13%.[22,23] Although up to 25% of AK may spontaneously regress with sun protective measures,[23]

treatment is indicated for thicker or symptomatic lesions and for patients with prior SCCs or who are immunosuppressed. Rapid growth, induration, and erosions in an AK or porokeratosis, especially when associated with pain are often harbingers of SCC transformation. Most early SCCs will have a rough, adherent scale, characteristic of its keratin production. As the tumor progresses, it increases both in width and depth, resulting in a more palpable, firm, and adherent growth. Advanced SCCs can be nodular (Fig. 10.2) and/or ulcerated (Fig. 10.3). Larger tumors are more likely to be symptomatic with pain, ulceration, or weeping (Fig. 10.4). Paresthesias, dysesthesia, or motor nerve paresis may reflect underlying perineural spread but is a late manifestation. Only 40% of patients with perineural tumor have neurologic

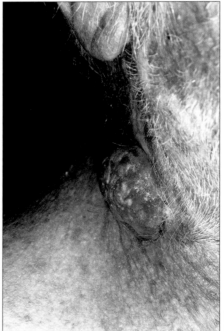

Figure 10.2 Large SCC nodule.

symptoms. Growth rate is variable with rapidly growing tumors having more aggressive features (deeper invasion, poor differentiation).

SCC in darker skin types is far less common, but is similarly a disease of elderly patients and is most often found on the face and legs. In this population, several differences are evident. SCC is 20% more common than BCC and SCC more frequently develops in sites of previous injury and scarring (Table 10.3). Native pigmentation may also confound diagnosis by masking inflammation and erythema. Tumors in covered locations are also eight times more common in darker skin types than in Caucasians, which often delays diagnosis until advanced stages. As a result, prognosis for SCC in black patients is worse, with one study citing a mortality rate of 18.4%.[24]

SCC of the lip is primarily limited to the lower lip and occurs predominantly in men. Lip SCCs are generally more aggressive with a higher metastasis rate than other facial locations.[25] The precursor setting for SCC of the lip is actinic cheilitis, where the vermillion border loses its definition and becomes dry, keratotic, atrophic, and irregularly hypopigmented (Fig. 10.5). Most lip SCCs occur on the vermillion border at midline or slightly lateral (Figs 10.6 and 10.7). Lesions at the oral commissure are especially aggressive and 20% of these lesions present with clinical lymphadenopathy. New erythema, induration, erosion, or elevation in previously stable actinic cheilitis

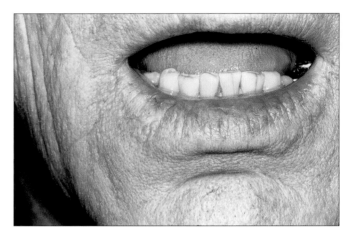

Figure 10.5   Actinic cheilitis.

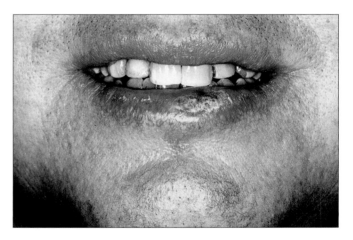

Figure 10.6   Lip SCC on the vermillion border at midline.

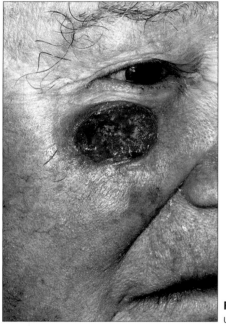

Figure 10.3   Large ulcerated SCC.

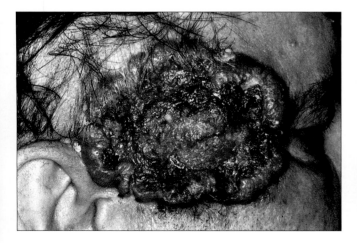

Figure 10.4   A larger SCC, more likely to be symptomatic with pain, ulceration, or weeping.

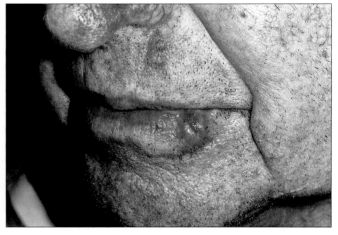

Figure 10.7   Lip SCC on the vermillion border, slightly lateral.

warrants a biopsy. Late changes include pain, ulceration, and nodular growth (Fig. 10.8). Lip SCC that is initially ulcerative often is poorly differentiated and invades early and deeply. Treatment of actinic cheilitis with CO_2 laser ablation can be preventive in deterring future SCCs. Cigarette smoking is an additional risk factor for lip SCC. A low threshold should be maintained in identifying and treating these tumors.

Intraoral SCCs are more difficult to diagnose. Common locations are the anterior floor of the mouth, anterior tongue (lateral and undersurface), and buccal vestibule (especially in tobacco chewers), (Figs 10.9 and 10.10). Intraorally, the counterpart to actinic cheilitis is leukoplakia, or white plaque. Not all leukoplakia lesions have similar malignant potential. Erythroplakia (reddish reticulation within a white plaque) has the highest risk for malignant degeneration. Signs and symptoms are similar for lip SCC except that intraoral lesions lack keratotic scale. Intraoral SCCs are even more aggressive than lip lesions and metastasis rates range from 20–70%. Behavioral risk factors include tobacco chewing and smoking, Betel nut chewing (Southeast Asian patients), reverse smoking (when the lighted end of a cigarette is placed intraorally), and alcohol.[26] Predisposing conditions such as human papilloma virus infections (especially HPV 16, 18),

erosive lichen planus, Plummer-Vinson syndrome (iron deficiency anemia, dysphagia, esophageal webs) and dyskeratosis congenita also increase the risk for oral SCC.

SCC found on the anogenital region is also more aggressive in nature (Figs 10.11 and 10.12). Associated symptoms and signs are irritation, pruritus, pain, and erythema, erosions, and intermittent bleeding. Maceration and lack of scale are typical of intertriginous areas. Penile tumors are usually on the glans (Fig. 10.13) and are associated with lack of circumcision, poor hygiene, and chronic inflammatory processes such as lichen sclerosis et atrophicus. Scrotal and vulvar SCCs have been closely associated with chronic occupational exposure to aromatic hydrocarbons such as mineral oil, pitch, and tar. Induration and ulceration rather than exophytic masses (late stage) are more characteristic of scrotal and vulvar SCC.

SCC of the digits predominantly affects elderly men. In the early days of X-rays, dentists often developed

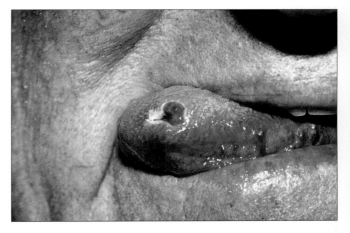

Figure 10.10 SCC of the tongue.

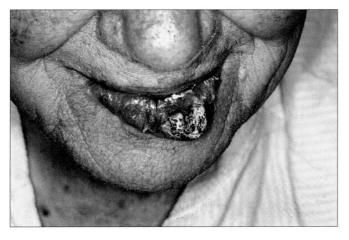

Figure 10.8 Lip SCC: Late changes include pain, ulceration and nodular growth.

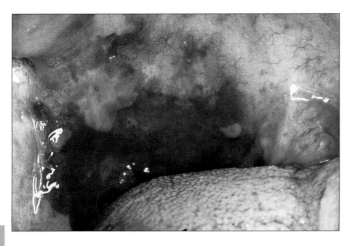

Figure 10.9 Oral SCC of soft palate.

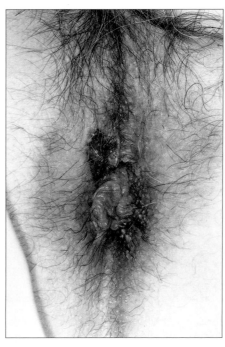

Figure 10.11
Perianal SCC.

digital SCCs from chronic exposure. Some subungual SCCs may be associated with HPV 16 but it is still unclear whether this is the causative agent. Tumors on the digits present similarly to those found on other cutaneous surfaces (Fig. 10.14). Proximal nail fold or subungual tumors, however, may mimic paronychia with swelling, erythema, and pain (Figs 10.15 and 10.16) and cause onychodystrophy. Chronic paronychia that is not responsive to antibiotics or antifungals should be evaluated for malignancy. Mohs micrographic surgery is particularly useful in preserving healthy tissue, and radical surgical amputation, as traditionally performed, should be avoided unless bone involvement is noted on X-ray.

Verrucous carcinoma is a low-grade subtype of SCC that rarely metastasizes. Clinically, it presents as a verrucous plaque or nodule and is often described as a 'cauliflower-like' growth (Fig. 10.12). If left untreated, these will develop into large verrucous tumors and may simulate deep fungal infections. Verrucous carcinoma is further distinguished by location: Buschke–Lowenstein tumor is found on the anogenital area (Fig. 10.12), Ackerman tumor on the oral mucosa, and epithelioma cuniculatum on the feet. Although metastasis is infrequent, the tumor can invade deeply and can cause significant local destruction. It has been associated with HPV 6 and 11, chronic inflammatory processes, persistent trauma, and chemical carcinogens such as chewing tobacco and Betel nuts. Anaplastic transformation into more aggressive behavior has been reported in verrucous carcinomas treated with radiation.[27]

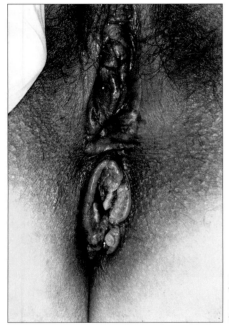

Figure 10.12
Verrucous carcinoma: Buschke–Lowenstein tumor.

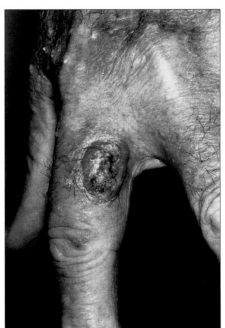

Figure 10.14
Digital SCC.

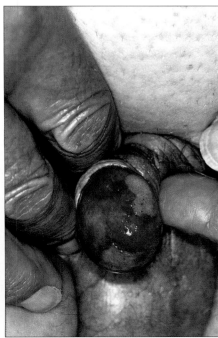

Figure 10.13
SCC on glans penis.

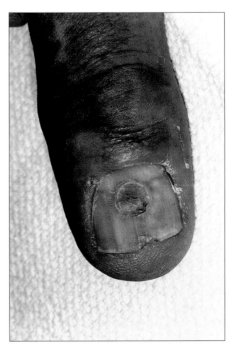

Figure 10.15   Nail bed SCC.

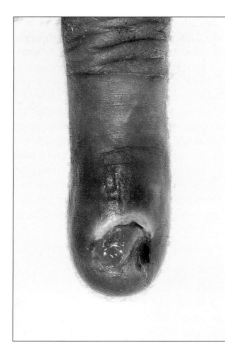

Figure 10.16
Periungual SCC.

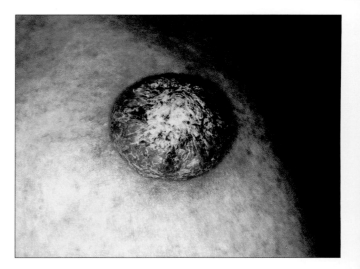

Figure 10.17   Keratoacanthoma.

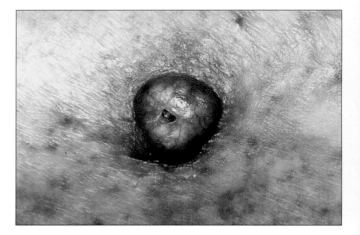

Figure 10.18   Another example of keratoacanthoma.

Keratoacanthoma (KA) is also known as a 'self healing squamous cell carcinoma'. It develops rapidly over several weeks, stabilizes in growth, and then spontaneously involutes over several months or even years with residual tissue destruction. Clinically, it is a dome shaped exophytic nodule with a central keratin crater that ranges from 1 to 3 cm in diameter (Figs 10.17 and 10.18). It is most often found on sun-exposed areas of elderly white men and may develop in areas of trauma or inflammation. Controversy exists on whether this is a spontaneously regressing benign tumor or a true malignancy. However, most practitioners consider and treat KA as a subtype of SCC and will recommend surgical excision over observation. A few of these tumors persist for many years and may cause disfiguring local destruction, especially on the face. Metastasizing KA has also been reported but may represent initial SCC from the onset. Multiple KAs are found in three clinical settings. In the familial Ferguson–Smith syndrome, multiple self-healing KAs develop in the second and third decade. With the Gryzbowski variant, hundreds of small miniature KAs erupt. Finally, in the Muir Torre syndrome, keratoacanthomas are found with cutaneous sebaceous tumors and visceral cancers, most commonly adenocarcinomas of the colon.[28]

Bowen's disease describes intraepidermal carcinoma or SCC in situ (Fig. 10.19). It presents clinically as a well-defined, thin, erythematous, scaly plaque and may be misdiagnosed as tinea, psoriasis, or nummular eczema. SCC *in situ* is known as erythroplasia of Queyrat when it is located on the penis (Fig. 10.20). Bowen's disease on sun-exposed areas is more common and is less aggressive compared to those in sun-protected areas. Intertriginous Bowen's may lack scale and instead may be moist and macerated. If left untreated, Bowen's disease may progress and become invasive, especially on the genitalia. When associated with arsenic exposure, Bowen's disease may occur with internal malignancies. Without

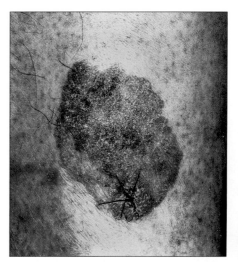

Figure 10.19
Bowen's disease.

arsenic ingestion, however, there is little evidence to link Bowen's disease with internal cancers.

Marjolin's ulcer is an eponym for SCC that arises from chronically scarred or inflamed skin (Fig. 10.21). Early diagnosis of these lesions is critical as they are particularly aggressive even early on. A new induration, elevation, or erosion in a stable scar is suspect. Tenderness, pruritus, and irritation may be associated symptoms. For pre-existing chronic ulcers or sinus tracts, diagnosis is more difficult. SCC may develop deep in the sinus tracts or be camouflaged in the existing ulcer. Biopsy is indicated for any chronic ulcer that has acutely changed in size (enlarged in width or elevation) or symptoms (pain or new malodorous discharge in the absence of infection). There is a long latency period of 20–30 years before SCC develops in these settings. Skin damaged by radiation has the shortest latency period to malignancy.

The metastasis of squamous cell carcinoma poses a significant problem as it portends a grim prognosis. Overall 5-year survival after regional metastasis is only 25%. SCC metastasizes primarily through the lymphatics and patients present with regional lymphadenopathy. In a subset of patients (CLL, OTR), multiple dermal in-transit metastases may occur before nodal spread (Fig. 10.22). Recurrent disease is often present at the time of lymph node involvement and distant visceral spread is rare without local or regional disease (Fig. 10.23). Most metastases (> 90%) will be evident within 3 years of initial diagnosis[25] with the parotid and cervical nodes most commonly involved. The overall risk of metastasis for SCC is in the range of 2–6%. This risk may rise to 47.3% depending on certain clinical and histologic factors (Table 10.4).[29] The true risk of recurrence and metastasis for each variable is unknown as studies have been retrospective and tumors often have multiple risk factors. However, certain trends can be established. Clinical variables include location, previous treatment, size, and immune status. In general, primary tumors located on sun-exposed areas have the lowest risk for distant spread. Exceptions include primary SCC of the ear (8.8% risk of metastasis) and lip (13.7% risk). Recurrence and size are major negative prognostic indicators. While primary SCC has an overall metastasis risk of 5.2%, this rises to 30.3% for recurrent tumors. SCC <2 cm in diameter have a metastasis rate of 9.1% compared with 30.3% for lesions ≥2 cm. Chronically immunosuppressed patients are also at a higher risk of developing metastasis. Histologic variables include degree of differentiation, depth of invasion, and perineural involvement.[29] Patients with poorly differentiated SCC have a higher risk of recurrence and metastasis. Lesions that invade deeper than 4 mm (Clark's level IV or greater) have a recurrence and metastasis rate of 17.2% and 45.7%. The worst histologic indicator may be perineural invasion, which has been shown to metastasize in 47.3% of cases.

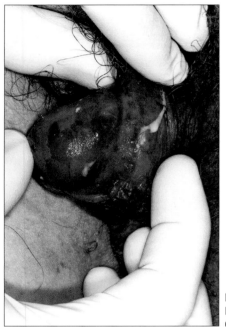

Figure 10.20
Erythroplasia of Queyrat.

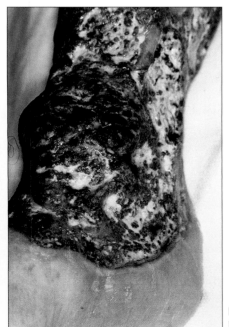

Figure 10.21
Marjolin's ulcer.

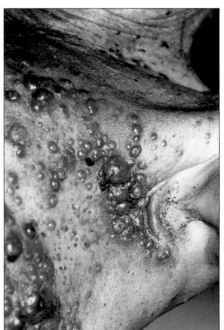

Figure 10.22
Multiple dermal in-transit metastases.

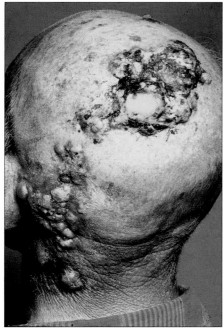

Figure 10.23
Metastatic SCC.

Table 10.4 Risk of recurrence and metastasis from clinical and histologic features[29]	Recurrence (%)	Metastasis (%)
Clinical features		
Anatomic location		
Sun-exposed skin	7.9	5.2
Scarred areas in sun-protected skin	n.a.	37.9
Lip	10.5	13.7
Ear	18.7	11.0
Size (diameter)		
<2 cm	7.4	9.1
>2 cm	15.2	30.3
Treatment history		
Primary	7.9	5.2
Recurrent	23.3	30.3
Immune status		
Immunosuppressed	13.4	8
Histologic features		
Differentiation		
Well-differentiated	13.6	9.2
Poorly-differentiated	28.6	32.8
Depth of invasion		
<4 mm (Clark level <IV)	5.3	6.7
>4 mm (Clark level ≥IV)	17.2	45.7
Nerve involvement		
Perineural invasion	47.2	47.3
n.a., not available.		

PATIENT EVALUATION, DIAGNOSIS AND DIFFERENTIAL DIAGNOSIS

The diagnosis of squamous cell carcinoma is most often straightforward and is based both on clinical presentation and histologic evaluation. Many biopsy techniques are available (shave, punch, incision, excision) and all should include deep dermis to evaluate the level of invasion. Therapy greatly depends on correlating clinical features with histologic findings.

The common differential diagnoses for SCC include hypertrophic actinic keratosis, verruca vulgaris, and inflamed or manipulated seborrheic keratosis. Consideration should be taken to biopsy chronic ulcers or suspected deep fungal infections as these may be indolent tumors. SCC on the penis may mimic candidal balanitis or psoriasis. Poor response to treatment should initiate a biopsy for a definitive diagnosis. SCC and verrucous carcinoma in the oral cavity may present variably and is especially difficult to distinguish from other mucosal lesions. A high level of suspicion should be maintained, as tumors on mucosal surfaces can often be more aggressive.

Patient history and physical should focus on identifying high risk factors. Prior radiation, pre-existing scars, prior treatment, immunosuppression, rapid growth and pain or paresthesia all warrant more detailed examination and staging. Patients should be staged according to American Joint Committee on Cancer (AJCC) criteria (Table 10.5). Relevant factors not listed in the AJCC system are histologic variables, such as differentiation, perineural spread and depth of invasion.

A complete skin examination is essential as not only are SCCs in covered areas more aggressive but also are more often missed. Skin should be examined with patients lying flat for maximal exposure and visibility. Examination of the oral cavity should not be overlooked, especially the anterior floor of the mouth and tongue.

Palpation or touch is key. Actinic keratoses are often palpable but not readily seen. Feeling the skin for keratotic papules is important in locating AK and noting their thickness. Palpating the perilesional skin for adherence, subcutaneous infiltration, and pain is necessary. The regional soft tissue should be palpated for in-transit metastases.

A lymphatic examination is mandatory for any invasive lesion and for patients with prior invasive or high risk SCC. Nose and cheek lesions usually drain to submandibular (submaxillary) nodes. Tumors on the lip and anterior mouth travel to submental nodes. Auricular lesions drain to postauricular nodes and those on the posterior scalp spread to occipital nodes. Anterior scalp, forehead, and temple SCC often travel to parotid nodes. Rarely, SCC may bypass primary nodes for secondary basins in the post cervical and jugular chains (behind and along the sternocleidomastoid muscle respectively). Occult metastasis is not infrequent. There is a 24–35% risk of occult cervical metastases when parotid nodes are positive (Fig. 10.24).[30] Conversely, in patients with cervical metastasis, there is an 18% risk of occult disease in the parotid nodes.[31] Even for a unilateral tumor, bilateral palpation is recommended as contralateral spread has been reported. Imaging studies are indicated either for clinically palpable nodes or for high-risk tumors (Table 10.4) without clinical nodes. Among imaging studies, CT scan is best for nodal evaluation and bony invasion.

Table 10.5 American Joint Committee on Cancer (AJCC) staging for squamous cell carcinoma

Primary tumor (T)	
TX	Primary tumor cannot be assessed
T0	No evidence of primary tumor
Tis	Carcinoma *in situ*
T1	Tumor 2 cm or less in the greatest diameter
T2	Tumor between 2 cm and 5 cm in the greatest diameter
T3	Tumor greater than 5 cm in the greatest diameter
T4	Tumor with deep invasion into cartilage, muscle or bone
Regional lymph node status (N)	
NX	Lymph nodes cannot be assessed
N0	No lymph node metastasis
N1	Lymph node metastasis
Distant metastasis (M)	
MX	Distant metastasis unable to be assessed
M0	No distant metastasis
M1	Distant metastasis
Stage groupings	
Stage 0	Tis, N0, M0
Stage 1	T1, N0, M0
Stage 2	T2–T3, N0, M0
Stage 3	T4, N0, M0 or Any T, N1, M0
Stage 4	Any T, Any N, M1

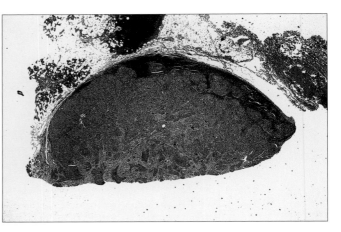

Figure 10.24 SCC lymph note occult metastasis.

PATHOLOGY

Pathology of SCC shows proliferation of eosinophilic squamous epithelial cells with anaplastic changes. Hypercellularity, increased nuclear-cytoplasmic ratios, hyperchromatism, prominent and increased nucleoli, disorganized architecture, and atypical mitoses are common to most malignancies as well as SCC. Keratinization may occur extracellularly as horn pearls or be seen within individual cells (Fig. 10.25). Superficially, there is epidermal hyperplasia and occasionally ulceration. Deeper, invasive SCC may be seen as bulging islands and nests or spiky strands and even single cells (Fig. 10.26). The latter pattern is characteristic of spindle cell SCC. Surrounding stroma of SCC may be desmoplastic. In all but the most poorly differentiated SCCs, desmosomal attachments and keratin production help identify its keratinocyte origin. *In-situ* SCC is entirely intra-epidermal (Fig. 10.27) while invasive lesions transgress the basement membrane. The boundary between hypertrophic actinic keratosis and squamous cell carcinoma in situ can be subtle and thought by many to be a progressive transition. AK and SCC *in situ* may have follicular extensions that should be noted as recurrences may occur with too superficial ablation.

Pseudoepitheliomatous hyperplasia (PEH) is well-differentiated epithelium that is proliferative epidermis, often seen during wound healing. Present at the periphery of wounds and ulcers, PEH may clinically and histologically simulate SCC. Features favoring PEH include its well differentiated, jagged vertically oriented epidermal extensions deep into the dermis, presence of lumen, and epidermal and dermal edema. Deeper sections or repeat biopsies are often needed to distinguish PEH from SCC.

SCC may be categorized as well, moderate, or poorly differentiated. In the Broder classification,[35] tumors are divided into four grades of differentiation, depending on the degree of keratinization (Table 10.6). Most clinically relevant are the two extremes of well versus poorly differentiated, as prognosis is markedly worse for the latter. Most metastatic SCCs are well-differentiated due to the greater overall numbers of well-differentiated tumors. However, a greater percentage of poorly-differentiated SCCs metastasize (17%) compared with their well-

Ultrasound is also useful for lymph nodes, especially if fine needle aspiration (FNA) is contemplated. MRI can delineate soft tissue spread and perineural disease. Plain radiographs or CT scan is necessary for digital tumors to assess bony involvement. A positron emission tomography (PET) scan is less useful for primary staging but has a role in the evaluation for an unknown primary, for assessing treatment response, and for determining persistent or recurrent disease.[32] Tumors must be ≥5 mm in diameter for detection by PET scans. A multidisciplinary approach is essential for patients with regional or distant disease.

A new tool in the staging of head and neck SCC (HNSCC) is sentinel lymph node mapping (SLNM). Motivated by the accuracy (99% identification), sensitivity (>95%), and false negative rate (2%) of SLNM for melanomas, SLNM is being applied to HNSCC. Despite the complexities of lymphatic drainage in the head and neck, 95% identification and 90% sensitivity may be achieved with HNSCC.[33] In a small study of high-risk cutaneous SCCs, Reschly *et al.* detected microscopic metastasis in four of nine (44%) clinically N0 patients. Prognostically, two of four sentinel node positive patients died of their disease while node negative patients were still alive at a short term follow up of 8 months.[34] Management for clinically N0 patients is controversial. What to do for these microscopically positive nodes (clinically N0 status) is also unclear. Although technically accurate, the use of SLNM in HNSCC is not the standard of care and should be part of well-designed clinical trials.

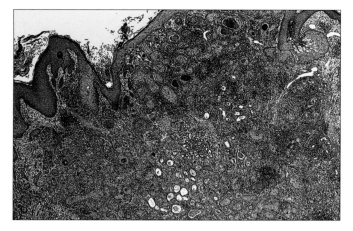

Figure 10.25 Acantholytic SCC with horn pearls.

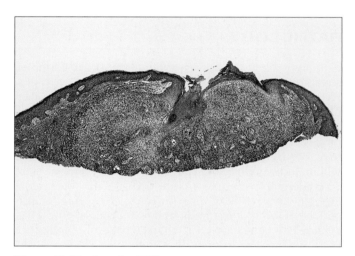

Figure 10.26 Invasive SCC.

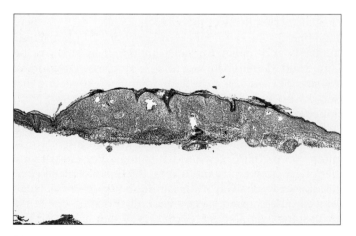

Figure 10.27 SCC *in situ*.

differentiated counterpart (0.6%).[36] Inflammation may be seen but is not a prognostic indicator. In patients with CLL, lymphocytic infiltrates can be pronounced. However, this inflammation is 75% B-cell predominant, leukemic in nature, and may greatly obscure histologic detection of SCC, especially under Mohs frozen sections.[37] The host immune response in CLL is dysfunctional.

Table 10.6 Broder's classification of squamous cell carcinoma differentiation

	Keratinization (%)
Grade 1	>75
Grade 2	50–75
Grade 3	25–50
Grade 4	<25

Several histological variants of squamous cell carcinoma have been characterized. These include acantholytic (adenoid, pseuodoglandular), spindle cell, and adenosquamous SCC. Acantholytic SCC is clinically indistinguishable from other SCCs. Histologically, it displays acantholysis centrally, which simulates a glandular appearance (Fig. 10.28). There is minimal evidence that acantholytic SCCs behave any more aggressively than other variants.

Spindle cell SCC is uncommon and presents most often on sun-exposed areas of elderly patients. Histologically, there is a dense proliferation of spindle cells with scant eosinophilic cytoplasm and large nuclei (Fig. 10.29). Tumor infiltration may be in strands or even single cells and cell borders are often ill defined. Histological identification may be difficult, and the spindle cell subtype may be impossible to distinguish from other spindle cell proliferations such as atypical fibroxanthoma, malignant melanoma or leiomyosarcoma. Immunohistochemical staining may be helpful in such cases. Spindle cell SCC usually expresses cytokeratin (Fig. 10.30). Atypical fibroxanthoma expresses vimentin, leiomyoscarcoma expresses desmin, and malignant melanoma typically expresses S-100 and Melan A. Due to the poor differentiation, this variant carries a worse prognosis.

Adenosquamous SCC is a rare variant that is often found on the genitalia and has also been known as mucoepidermoid carcinoma. It consists of a relatively well-differentiated SCC, which also has glandular cystic spaces that secrete mucin. Unlike the acantholytic subtype that only mimics glandular structures, adenosquamous SCC is actually glandular and contains mucin-secreting epithelium.

Verrucous carcinoma is considered a low-grade subtype of SCC and is found both in the oral cavity and the skin. Clinically, it is a slow growing, large warty appearing tumor. Histologically, the superficial portion also appears similar to a large verruca vulgaris with hyperkeratosis, papillomatosis, acanthosis and parakeratosis (Fig. 10.31). Proliferating well-differentiated keratinocytes have a deceptively benign appearance. Although an invasive component may not be seen, the rete ridges extend deep into the dermis in a pushing pattern. Identification of proliferating cell nuclear antigen (PCNA) at the borders may be helpful in distinguishing this growth from other SCC, which stains PCNA diffusely.[38]

Keratoacanthoma is clinically considered by most physicians to be a form of SCC. Histologic distinction between a KA and an SCC is often difficult. KA is a well-delineated, well-differentiated, symmetric proliferation of

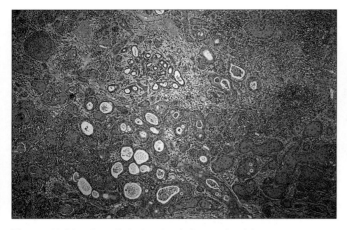

Figure 10.28 Acantholysis, simulating a glandular appearance.

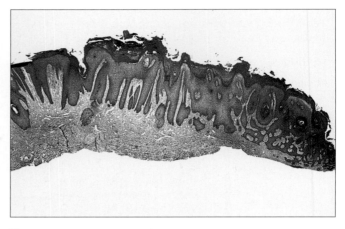

Figure 10.31 Verrucal carcinoma.

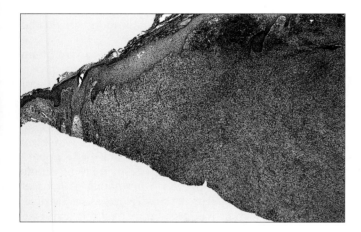

Figure 10.29 Spindle cell SCC.

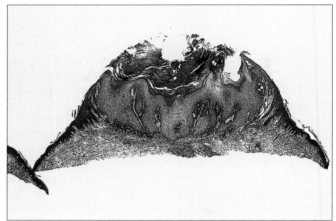

Figure 10.32 Keratoacanthoma.

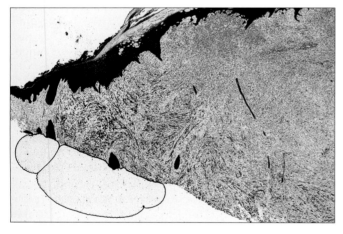

Figure 10.30 Spindle cell SCC (cytokeratin stain).

TREATMENT

Individual therapies for skin cancer are discussed in depth elsewhere in this book but their application in the treatment of SCC is reviewed here.

The vast majority of patients will present with localized disease (Stage I: N0, M0) and may be treated with a wide armamentarium of surgical and non-surgical modalities (Table 10.7). Treatment selection depends on multiple variables but an overriding priority is oncologic cure. Recurrent lesions become more difficult to cure and have more risk for metastasis. 42% of metastases occur along with persistence or recurrence of the primary tumor. The first chance at therapy is therefore also the best chance for cure. Therapeutic morbidity, cost, convenience, and patient preferences are other factors influencing treatment selection. Clinical (immune status, recurrence, location, size, symptoms) and histologic (invasiveness, differentiation) variables must be correlated to identify high-risk tumors. The management of invasive SCC in node negative patients is usually surgery. Elective node dissection with or without radiation should be considered for tumors that have a greater than 20% risk of metastasis based on clinical and histologic variables.[40] Depending on which nodes

squamous epithelium (Fig. 10.32). Superficially, there is often a cup shaped, keratin filled crater. There is minimal cellular atypia or mitosis. Sometimes a moderate neutrophilic and eosinophilic infiltrate is present in the adjacent dermis. Presence of peripherally located PCNA may also help to differentiate this tumor from squamous cell carcinoma.[39]

Table 10.7 Treatment options for localized squamous cell carcinoma	
Method	**Procedure/Agent**
Topical chemotherapy	Imiquimod 5-fluorouracil
Destruction (no margin control)	Cryotherapy Curettage and cryotherapy Electrodessication and curettage CO_2 laser ablation Photodynamic therapy Intralesional interferon Intralesional bleomycin Radiation therapy
Margin controlled resection	Excision Mohs micrographic surgery

are involved, parotidectomy (superficial or complete) and/or neck dissection with or without adjuvant radiation therapy is recommended although studies are mixed on which combinations are most effective. Treatment options may be divided into those that preclude versus those that permit histologic margin control. Cryotherapy, electrodessication and curettage (EDC), CO_2 laser ablation, chemotherapy, and radiotherapy all effect tumor destruction but preclude histologic evaluation. Excision and Mohs micrographic surgery (MMS), on the other hand, yield tissue for different methods of margin control. Guidelines of care for SCC are available from the American Academy of Dermatology (www.aad.org), National Comprehensive Cancer Network (www.nccn.org) and the International Transplant–Skin Cancer Collaborative.[41]

Cryotherapy is a time-proven and effective treatment for both benign and malignant cutaneous lesions. Liquid nitrogen, $-195.8°C$, is the most popular cryogen. For SCC, a cryogun spray is most effective at achieving the desired rapid tissue freeze to $-50°C$ and slow thaw that is most effective for tumor destruction. The 5-year cure rate for squamous cell carcinoma can be 94% or higher with proper tumor selection and technique.[42] Small (<1 cm), well-defined, well-differentiated, and superficially invasive SCCs are appropriate for cryotherapy. Debulking the tumor with curettage or tangential shave prior to cryotherapy will increase cryogen penetration and effectiveness.[43] Although tumors at any location may technically be treated, patients best tolerate cryotherapy to trunk and extremity lesions while those over joints or cartilage may cause considerable pain and chondronecrosis. Hair bearing skin should be avoided due to the risk of permanent alopecia. Transient burning, edema, and blistering are expected while hypopigmentation may be pronounced and permanent.

Electrodessication and curettage (EDC) is an experience dependent technique that is effective for superficial SCC. Tumor indications are similar to cryotherapy. EDC permits delineation of deep and superficial margins, as tumor tissue is friable and easily yields to the curette. Free margins (eyelids) or soft flexible contours (genitalia, lips, helical rim) are suboptimal locations, as they do not provide a firm surface for curettage. Lesions following punch biopsies may also be difficult to curette. Patients with implantable pacemakers and defibrillators require special precautions and monitoring for electrosurgery. Recurrent SCC or those with sclerotic stroma may be scar-like and not curette easily. Conversely, patients with atrophic skin (chronic prednisone, immunosuppression, severe actinic damage) may have excessive curettage destruction that is not tumor related. EDC may not reach SCC with follicular extensions. Cure rates as high as 98% have been reported in a treated series if proper tumor indications are followed.[44] EDC is highly technique dependent and cure rates improve with a practitioner's experience. If EDC extends down to subcutaneous fat, a deeply invasive tumor may be involved and these lesions should either be excised or treated with Mohs micrographic surgery for margin control. A hypopigmented, stellate scar of varying thickness is typical after EDC. This may be undesirable in locations above the neck.

CO_2 laser ablation is not usually used alone but along with curettage to destroy superficial SCC (in situ and up to papillary dermis). Continuous wave CO_2 is more destructive but provides less control of ablative depth than pulsed mode CO_2. Both are effective, however, in tumor control with sufficient passes. At least two CO_2 passes with curettage after each pass is most effective. Follicular tumor extensions are not effectively treated with CO_2. The best role for CO_2 is in treating actinic keratosis or in situ SCC noted on peripheral margins of excisions or Mohs frozen sections. Treated sites heal in several weeks with a hypopigmented, smooth scar. Like EDC, hypertrophic scarring may occur along the jaw line, mid-chest, and shoulders. CO_2 laser for SCC requires a high learning curve, expensive equipment and offers few advantages over other methods of nonspecific tissue destruction.

Radiation therapy (RT) is a non-surgical modality that can be effective as a primary or as an adjuvant treatment for SCC. Patients who are poor surgical candidates, who refuse surgery, and who have inoperable lesions may all benefit from primary treatment with RT. The five-year cure rate for primary SCC is approximately 90%.[29] RT should be avoided in younger patients (<55 years old) due to the long-term cosmetic morbidities and potential risk of SCC developing within the treated site. Radiation therapy has been associated with anaplastic transformation of oral verrucous carcinoma in some but not all studies.[27] Nevertheless, verrucous carcinoma is a radiosensitive tumor and partial to complete responses may be achieved with radiation alone.[45] For node negative but high-risk tumors, RT may be prophylactic while for node positive patients, RT may be an adjuvant to surgery for better tumor control. In patients with parotid node metastasis, superficial parotidectomy alone has a 25–63% tumor control rate compared to superficial parotidectomy combined with postoperative radiation therapy (80–89%).[46] Other studies, however, have not shown significant benefits for adjuvant RT in cervical and parotid disease.[47,48] Despite these inconsistencies, surgery with radiation is currently the standard of care for patients with regional nodal metastasis. Unfortunately, even with aggressive treatment with surgery and radiation, overall survival for patients with metastatic SCC remains poor. Pretreatment dynamic lymphoscintigraphy may define more accurately regions requiring treatment. Fractionated RT requires 3–5 treatments per week over 4–8 weeks. Intense inflammation, epidermal necrosis with desquamation, alopecia, pruritus, and pain occur acutely while sclerosis, atrophy, and poikiloderma develop after years. Bone and cartilage necrosis are serious complications but occur rarely. A lag time of 20 years is typical for SCC that arises within irradiated skin.

Surgical excision for SCC requires more skill and time, but it has several advantages. It is a versatile procedure that can treat small to larger tumors and from superficial to more invasive lesions. More importantly, histologic margin control is possible after tissue removal. Excision is best applied to tumors that have invaded beyond the papillary dermis.

Recommendations for SCC margins varied greatly until 1992, when Brodland and Zitelli published their pivotal study on appropriate margins for SCC based on tumor risk factors (diameter, location, depth of invasion, Broder's grade of differentiation). Using progressive 1 mm margins with Mohs micrographic surgery (MMS), the authors arrived at margins to achieve 95% tumor clearance.[49] For lower risk SCC (<2 cm, Grade I (well-differentiated), without subcutaneous fat invasion, located on trunk and extremities), margins of 4 mm achieved 95% clearance. However, for tumors that are greater than 2 cm in diameter, ≥Grade 2, invasive to fat, and high risk locations (central face, ears and pre and postauricular, temples, scalp, genitalia, hands and feet), a minimum of 6 mm margin was needed. Margins should be outlined beyond any visible perilesional erythema. Initial curettage prior to outlining safety margins may also enhance cure rates.

Advantages of excision include some degree of margin control and defect closure with a potentially better cosmetic outcome. Five-year cure rate with excision for primary SCC is 92%.[29] For recurrent SCC, 5-year cure rate is only 77%. Unfortunately, excisional margins for tumor clearance come at the expense of tissue sparing. Wider resection is acceptable on the trunk and extremities but can cause significant morbidity in critical locations (face, digits, shins, genitalia). Further, false negative histologic margins may occur with the traditional breadloaf method of evaluation.

Mohs micrographic surgery (MMS) has now become the standard of care for high-risk SCC without nodal disease. This technique, detailed elsewhere in this volume, has three key advantages. When compared with other treatments, MMS achieves the highest 5-year cure rate, maximally conserves healthy tissue, and is ambulatory, which permits faster patient recovery. The indications for MMS in SCC include large size (>2 cm), ill-defined borders, areas of high recurrence (lips, ears, nose, embryonal fusion planes of the central face), poor differentiation and recurrent or incompletely treated tumors. Mohs surgery is also the treatment of choice where tissue sparing is critical, such as the penis or digits where amputation was previously recommended. As with all techniques, the cure rate of MMS decreases as tumors become more aggressive or discontiguous.

A review of published studies since 1940 shows that Mohs micrographic surgery has the lowest 5-year recurrence rate for primary cutaneous SCC, 3.1% *vs* 7.9% for other treatment methods including electrodessication and curettage, radiation therapy, and excision.[29] In addition, it also has the lowest 5-year recurrence rate for high risk tumors when compared with other modalities for tumors on the lip, 2.3% (Mohs) *vs* 10.5% (non-Mohs), on the ear 5.3% (Mohs) *vs* 18.7% (non-Mohs) and recurrent tumors 10.0% (Mohs) *vs* 23.3% (non-Mohs).

Non-surgical therapies for SCC include topical chemotherapy, topical immune response modifiers (IRM) and photodynamic therapy (PDT). These are reserved for superficial SCC or precancerous AK. 5' fluorouracil (5FU) cream is a proven method for controlling AK. It can also be effective for SCC *in situ*. A newer option is imiquimod, which modulates immune cytokines to activate cytotoxic T-cells, which then has anti-viral and anti-tumor activities. Interferon-alpha, interleukins-1, 6, 8, 12 and tumor necrosis factor-alpha are all up regulated by imiquimod. Ongoing studies are investigating the safety of imiquimod in organ transplant patients. Both imiquimod and 5FU cream, alone or in combination, have been shown to eradicate Bowen's disease after prolonged application and can be as effective as traditional surgery.[50] These topical medications are especially helpful for SCC *in situ* of the perianal and genital area that are often difficult to treat surgically. Early case reports show efficacy using 5% imiquimod cream and 5% 5-fluorouracil up to 16 weeks as tolerated.[51,52] Currently, these topical regimens are recommended only for *in situ* lesions. Advantages include a non-invasive approach, patient convenience, minimal scarring or textural change, and the ability to treat adjacent precancers. Side effects include exuberant inflammation, pruritus, irritation, pain, and even erosions. These may be alleviated with occlusive moist wound care, temporary cessation of therapy, and low potency topical steroids.

Photodynamic therapy (PDT) is an effective approach to treat large numbers of AK.[53] A photosensitizer is applied either topically or systemically (intravenous) and patients are then exposed to light in the visible spectrum. Precancerous and malignant cells and follicular structures have a relatively selective uptake of photosensitizer compared with normal skin. The resulting photochemical reaction causes inflammation, ulceration and destruction of these lesions. Most commonly used photosensitizers are porphyrin metabolites, such as 5-aminolevulinic acid. Moderate to severe pain can be anticipated and patients need photoprotection for several days after therapy. Experience with PDT in SCC is minimal. Discrete SCC *in situ* responds well, but invasive SCC should not be treated with PDT.[53] Multiple superficial lesions are conveniently treated with PDT. For example, with numerous non-hypertrophic AK, PDT is advantageous in its ability to treat all lesions at once in one session. Isolated lesions, however, are more conveniently treated by other methods (EDC, cryotherapy).

Chemotherapy has traditionally been used as a primary treatment for inoperable SCC or as a salvage option for SCC failing surgery and radiation. A current trend is a neoadjuvant approach, in which systemic chemotherapy is given prior to surgery and/or radiation to reduce tumor volume and optimize chances for cure with the latter methods. Commonly used agents include cisplatin,

5-fluorouracil, bleomycin, and doxorubicin. Responses have ranged from partial (40–54%) to complete (28–31%) depending on the regimens.[54,55] Long-term remissions are possible especially when neoadjuvant chemotherapy is combined with surgery and radiation.

PREVENTION

The continued rise in SCC and the subsequent risk of further NMSC in patients with SCC warrant an effective prevention strategy. Recommendations include UVA and UVB photoprotection, regular self and physician skin examinations for early detection, patient education of skin cancer warning signs and aggressive treatment of actinic keratoses. Improper use of sunscreen is often responsible for continued UV exposure and sunburns. For patients with prior SCC, daily photoprotection must continue indefinitely.

Treatment of precancerous AK may prevent additional SCC. In one study where the histology of 459 squamous cell carcinomas were reviewed, 97% were found to have adjacent actinic keratoses.[56] Isolated actinic keratoses are effectively and simply treated with cryotherapy. For numerous or confluent AK, topical chemotherapy or PDT are excellent alternatives. These regimens have the benefit of treating both visible and subclinical lesions. Similar benefits are seen with regional chemical peels using various peeling agents (trichloroacetic acid, Jessner's solution). CO_2 laser ablation is an effective option for actinic cheilitis of the lower lip with low morbidity and excellent cosmesis.[57] Invasive SCC should first be treated prior to topical chemotherapy to prevent delays in diagnosis.

Systemic chemoprevention with oral retinoids may be an option for high-risk patients. Through nuclear retinoic acid receptors, retinoids regulate gene expression and affect cell growth and differentiation. Isotretinoin at 2 mg/kg was initially shown to reduce the 2-year risk of skin cancers by 63% in xeroderma pigmentosum patients.[58] Risk reduction is durable only with active therapy and discontinuation results in a return to pretreatment status. Renal transplant patients with SCC may also benefit from systemic retinoids. In a controlled study, only 11% (2 of 19) patients taking acitretin 30 mg/day developed SCC compared with 47% (9 of 19) of controls.[59] Side-effects of systemic retinoids include xerosis, eczema, hair loss, myalgia and lipid abnormalities. Long-term use of retinoids has been associated with skeletal toxicity and osteoporosis. Due to potential serious toxicities, chemoprevention with oral retinoids is currently recommended for patients in whom tumor control is difficult with conventional means. Retinoids have been combined with interferon in the treatment of both locally advanced and metastatic SCC. This combination has additive if not synergistic inhibition of cellular proliferation and angiogenesis.[60] Studies of retinoid-interferon treatment demonstrate both partial and complete responses in approximately 50% of patients with regional or metastatic disease.[47,61] Dose limiting side effects are mostly due to the interferon component. Unfortunately, responses are short in duration.

FUTURE OUTLOOK

Despite recent advances, cutaneous SCC remains an elusive malignancy. Current staging (AJCC system) for SCC is inadequate, as critical histologic variables such as perineural invasion, depth, differentiation, and histologic subtype are not considered. Unfortunately, the reporting of these features is inconsistent, and even among expert dermatopathologists there is debate to their individual prognostic significance. A useful staging system should aid in both prognosis and treatment. Microstaging of SCC needs to evolve towards the approach with malignant melanoma, where depth, ulceration, and sentinel node status critically influence prognosis and/or intervention. Microstaging may also benefit from new knowledge in tumor biology where cellular markers or genotype analysis may yield clues to aggressive tumor behavior. Rational staging requires a multi-institutional effort to prospectively identify these high-risk factors.

Mohs micrographic surgery continues to be the surgical gold standard for margin control and tissue sparing with localized disease. With proper tumor selection, non-invasive modalities are also effective. The management of locally advanced and regional disease, however, is more problematic. For those with macroscopic regional spread, the 'standard of care' is currently surgery with adjuvant radiation. This standard, however, is based on conflicting data and the benefit of radiation in certain settings is not proven. Even with surgery, approaches diverge. The extent of parotidectomy (superficial versus subtotal versus complete) is an issue of contention. Whether to treat the clinically negative neck if there is parotid disease or the parotid for cervical disease is also controversial given the real risk of occult spread. Accurate sentinel node mapping in the context of clinical trials may help to identify patients at risk for recurrence and metastasis.

Modifications of old techniques and medications are broadening the therapeutic arsenal for SCC. Capecitabine (Xeloda) is oral fluoropyrimidine 5-fluorouracil carbamate and is preferentially converted into 5-fluorouracil by tumor tissue. It is effective alone but is synergistic with other agents in the treatment of metastatic breast and colorectal cancer.[62–64] The potential for an oral form of 5-FU to treat cutaneous SCC is promising either as chemoprevention or as active therapy. Intralesional immunotherapy (interferon) and chemotherapy (bleomycin) is not new and can be curative for smaller tumors or palliative for inoperable lesions.[65] Electro-chemotherapy or electroporation therapy, however, is novel and applies electrical pulses to tumor sites following either intralesional or intravenous bleomycin. The electrical field increases local tissue permeability and enhances tumor penetration of bleomycin. Partial and complete responses have been achieved with primary basal cell and squamous cell carcinomas and metastatic melanomas.[66] Other new methods of drug delivery may increase the effectiveness of old therapies for SCC. For organ transplant recipients, the future is promising with rapamycin, a new immunosuppressive agent. At immunosuppressive doses, rapamycin has potent antitumor effects by inhibiting cellular proliferation and angiogenesis.[67] While preventing organ rejection,

OTR may simultaneously have tumor suppression benefits. Predicting which OTR will succumb to overwhelming cutaneous SCCs is an important and challenging task.

The greatest hope lies in effective chemoprevention. The use of imiquimod, tarazotene and anti-oxidants such as green tea extracts, vitamins C and E and cyclooxygenase (COX) inhibitors may one day greatly reduce the tumor burden in high-risk patients or even have a role in primary prevention.[68]

REFERENCES

1 Miller DL, Weinstock MA. Nonmelanoma skin cancer in the United States: Incidence. J Am Acad Dermatol 1994; 30:774–778.

2 Holme SA, Malinovszky K, Roberts DL. Changing trends in non-melanoma skin cancer in South Wales, 1988–98. Br J Dermatol 2000; 143:1224–1229.

3 Coebergh JW, Neumann HA, Vrints LW, van der Heijden L, Meijer WJ, Verhagen-Teulings MT. Trends in the incidence of non-melanoma skin cancer in the SE Netherlands 1975–1988: a registry-based study. Br J Dermatol 1991; 125:353–359.

4 Hannuksela-Svahn A, Pukkala E, Karvonen J. Basal cell skin carcinoma and other nonmelanoma skin cancers in Finland from 1956 through 1995. Arch Dermatol 1999; 135:781–786.

5 Buettner PG, Raasch BA. Incidence rates of skin cancer in Townsville, Australia. Int J Cancer 1998; 78:587–593.

6 Marcil I, Stern RS. Risk of developing a subsequent nonmelanoma skin cancer in patients with a history of nonmelanoma skin cancer: a critical review of the literature and meta-analysis. Arch Dermatol 2000; 136:1524–1530.

7 Bouwes Bavinck JN, Hardie DR, Green A, et al. The risk of skin cancer in renal transplant recipients in Queensland, Australia. A follow up study. Transplantation 1996; 61:715–721.

8 Ramsay HM, Fryer AA, Reece S, Smith AG, Harden PN. Clinical risk factors associated with nonmelanoma skin cancer in renal transplant recipients. Am J Kidney Dis 2000; 36:167–176.

9 Jensen P, Hansen S, Moller B, et al. Skin cancer in kidney and heart transplant recipients and different long-term immunosuppressive therapy regimens. J Am Acad Dermatol 1999; 40:177–186.

10 Ong CS, Keogh AM, Kossard S, Macdonald PS, Spratt PM. Skin cancer in Australia heart transplant recipients. J Am Acad Dermatol 1999; 40:27–34.

11 Kromberg JG, Castle D, Zwane EM, Jenkins T. Albinism and skin cancer in Southern Africa. Clin Genet 1989; 36:43–52.

12 Setlow RB, Carrier WL. Pyrimidine dimers in ultraviolet-irradiated DNAs. J Mol Biol 1966; 17:237–254.

13 Cleaver JE. Defective repair replication of DNA in xeroderma pigmentosum. Nature 1968; 218:652–656.

14 Sarasin A, Giglia-Maria G. p53 gene mutations in human skin cancers. Exp Dermatol 2002; 11:44–47.

15 Jiang W, Ananthaswamy HN, Muller HK, Kripke ML. p53 protects against skin cancer induction by UV-B radiation. Oncogene 1999; 18:4247–4253.

16 Studniberg HM, Weller P. PUVA, UVB, psoriasis, and nonmelanoma skin cancer. J Am Acad Dermatol 1993; 29:1013–1022.

17 Matsui MS, Leo VA De. Longwave ultraviolet radiation and promotion of skin cancer. Cancer Cell 1991; 3:8–12.

18 Nghiem DX, Kazimi N, Mitchell DL, et al. Mechanisms underlying the suppression of established immune responses by ultraviolet radiation. J Invest Dermatol 2002; 119:600–608.

19 Jackson R, Storey A. E6 protein from diverse cutaneous HPV types inhibit apoptosis in response to UV damage. Oncogene 2000; 19:592–598.

20 Schwartz RA, Nychay SG, Lyons M, Sciales CW, Lambert WC. Buschke–Lowenstein tumor: Verrucous carcinoma of the anogenitalia. Cutis 1991; 47:263–266.

21 Fu W, Cockerell CJ. The actinic (solar) keratosis: A 21st-century perspective. Arch Dermatol 2003; 139:66–70.

22 Graham JH. Selected precancerous skin and mucocutaneous lesions, in Neoplasms of skin and malignant melanoma. Chicago: Yearbooks; 1976:69.

23 Marks R, Foley P, Goodman G, Hage BH, Selwood TS. Spontaneous remission of solar keratoses: the case for conservative management. Br J Dermatol 1986; 115:649–655.

24 Mora RG, Perniciaro C. Cancer of the skin in blacks I. A review of 163 black patients with cutaneous squamous cell carcinoma. J Am Acad Dermatol 1981; 5:535–543.

25 Dinehart SM, Pollack SV. Metastases from squamous cell carcinoma of the skin and lip. J Am Acad Dermatol 1989; 21:241–248.

26 Neville BW, Day TA. Oral cancer and precancerous lesions. CA Cancer J Clin 2002; 52:195–215.

27 Perez CA, Kraus FT, Evans JC, Powers WE. Anaplastic transformation in verrucous carcinoma of the oral cavity after radiation therapy. Radiology 1966; 86:108.

28 Torre D. Multiple sebaceous tumors. Arch Dermatol 1968; 98:549–551.

29 Rowe DE, Carroll RJ, Day CL. Prognostic factors for local recurrence, metastasis, and survival rates in squamous cell carcinoma of the skin, ear, and lip. J Am Acad Dermatol 1992; 26:976–990.

30 Jackson GL, Ballantyne AJ. Role of parotidectomy for skin cancer of the head and neck. Am J Surg 1981; 142:464–469.

31 Lee K, McKean ME, McGregor IA. Metastatic patterns of squamous carcinoma in the parotid lymph nodes. Br J Plast Surg 1985; 38:6–10.

32 Hyde NC, Prvulovich E, Newman L, Waddington WA, Visvikis D, Ell P. A new approach to pre-treatment assessment of N0 neck in oral squamous cell carcinoma: the role of sentinel node biopsy and positron emission tomography. Oral Oncol 2003; 39:350–360.

33 Ross GL, Shoaib T, Soutar DS, et al. The first international conference on sentinel node biopsy in mucosal head and neck cancer and adoption of a multicenter trial protocol. Ann Surg Oncol 2002; 9:406–410.

34 Reschly MJ, Messina JL, Zaulyanov LL, Cruse W, Fenske NA. Utility of sentinel lymphadenectomy in management of patients with high risk cutaneous squamous cell carcinoma. Dermatol Surg 2003; 29:135–140.

35 Broder AC. Squamous-cell epithelioma of the skin. Ann Surg 1921; 73:141–160.

36 Breuninger H, Black B, Rassner G. Microstaging of squamous cell carcinomas. Am J Clin Pathol 1990; 94:624–627.

37 Mehrany K, Byrd DR, Roenigk RK, et al. Lymphocytic infiltrates and subepithelial tumor extension in patients with chronic leukemia and solid organ transplantation. Dermatol Surg 2003; 29:129–134.

38 Noel JC, Heenen M, Peny MO, et al. Proliferating cell nuclear antigen distribution in verrucous carcinoma of the skin. Br J Dermatol 1995; 133:868–873.

39 Phillips P, Helm KF. Proliferating cell nuclear antigen distribution in keratoacanthoma and squamous cell carcinoma. J Cutaneous Pathol 1993; 20:424–428.

40 Weiss MH, Harrison LB, Isaacs RS. Use of decision analysis in planning a management strategy for the stage N0 neck. Arch Otolaryngol Head Neck Surg 1994; 120:699–702.

41 Miller SJ. The national comprehensive cancer network (NCCN) guidelines of care for nonmelanoma skin cancers. Dermatol Surg 2000; 26:289–292.

42 Kuflik EG, Gage AA. The five year cure rate achieved by cryosurgery for skin cancer. J Am Acad Dermatol 1991; 24:1002–1004.

43 Nordin P. Curettage-cryosurgery for nonmelanoma skin cancer of the external ear: excellent 5-year results. Br J Dermatol 1999; 140:291–248.

44 Williamson GS, Jackson R. Treatment of squamous cell carcinoma of the skin by electrodessication and curettage. Can Med Assoc J 1964; 90:408–413.

45 Jyothirmayi R, Sankaranarayanan R, Varghese C, Jacob R, Nair MK. Radiotherapy in the treatment of verrucous carcinoma of the oral cavity. Oncology 1997; 33:124–128.

46 Taylor BW Jr, Brant TA, Mendenhall NP, et al. Carcinoma of the skin metastatic to parotid area lymph nodes. Head Neck 1991; 13:427–433.

47 Tacguchi T. Clinical studies of recombinant interferon-alpha (Roferon-A) in cancer patients. Cancer 1986; 57:175–178.

48 Khurana VG, Mentis DH, O'Brien CJ, Hurst TL, Stevens GN, Packham NA. Parotid and neck metastases from cutaneous squamous cell carcinoma of the head and neck. Am J Surg 1995; 170:446–450.

49 Brodland DG, Zitelli JA. Surgical margins for excision of primary cutaneous squamous cell carcinoma. J Am Acad Dermatol 1992; 27:241–248.

50 Mackenzie-Wood A, Kossard S, de Launey J, Wilkinson B, Owens ML. Imiquimod 5% cream in the treatment of Bowen's disease. J Am Acad Dermatol 2001; 44:462–470.

51 Pehouschek J, Smith KJ. Imiquimod and 5% fluorouracil therapy for anal and perianal squamous cell carcinoma in situ. Arch Dermatol 2001; 137:14–16.

52 Orengo I, Rosen T, Guill CK. Treatment of squamous cell carcinoma in situ of the penis with 5% imiquimod cream. A case report. J Am Acad Dermatol 2002; 47:S225–228.

53 Morton CA, Brown SB, Collins S, et al. Guidelines for topical photodynamic therapy: Report of a workshop of the British Photodermatology Group. Br J Dermatol 2002; 146:552–567.

54 Guthrie TH Jr, McElveen LJ, Porubsky ES, Harmon JD. Cisplatin and doxorubicin. An effective chemotherapy combination in treatment of advanced basal cell carcinoma and squamous cell carcinoma. Cancer 1985; 55:1629–1632.

55 Khansur T, Kennedy A. Cisplastin and 5-fluorouracil for advanced locoregional and metastatic squamous cell carcinoma of the skin. Cancer 1991; 67:2030–2032.

56 Hurwitz RM, Monger LE. Solar keratosis: an evolving squamous cell carcinoma. Benign malignant? Dermatologic Surgery 1995; 21:184.

57 Stanley RJ, Roenigk RK. Actinic cheilitis: Treatment with the carbon dioxide laser. Mayo Clin Proc 1988; 63:230–235.

58 Kraemer KH, DiGiovanna JJ, Moshell AN, Tarone RE, Peck GL. Prevention of skin cancer in xeroderma pigmentosum with the use of oral isotretinoin. N Engl J Med 1988; 318:1633–1637.

59 Bavinck JN, Tieben LM, Van der Woude FJ, et al. Prevention of skin cancer and reduction of keratotic skin lesions during acitretin therapy in renal transplant recipients: A double-blind, placebo-controlled study. J Clin Oncol 1995; 13:1933–1938.

60 Majewski S, Szmurlo A, Marczak M, Jablonska S, Bollag W. Synergistic effect of retinoids and interferon-alpha on tumor induced angiogenesis: anti-angiogenic effect on HPV-harboring tumor cell lines. Int J Cancer 1994; 57:81–85.

61 Toma S, Palumbo R, Vincenti M. Efficacy of recombinant alpha-interferon 2a and 13-cis-retinoic acid in the treatment of squamous cell carcinoma. Ann Oncol 1994; 5:463–465.

62 Tewes M, Schleucher N, Achterrath W. Capecitabine and irinotecan as first line chemotherapy in patients with metastatic colorectal cancer: results of an extended phase I study. Ann Oncol 2003; 14:1442–1448.

63 Kaklamani VG, Gradishar WJ. Role of capecitabine (Xeloda) in breast cancer. Expert Rev Anticancer Ther 2003; 3:137–144.

64 Yamaue H, Tanimura H, Kono N. Clinical efficacy of doxifluridine and correlation to in vitro sensitivity of anticancer drugs in patients with colorectal cancer. Anticancer Res 2003; 23:2559–2564.

65 Gomez De La Fuente E, Castano Suarez E, Vanaclocha Sebastian F, Rodriguez-Peralto JL, Iglesias Diez L. Verrucous carcinoma of the penis completely cured with shaving and intralesional interferon. Dermatology 2000; 200:152.

66 Burian M, Formanek M, Regele H. Electroporation therapy in head and neck cancer. Acta Otolaryngol 2003; 123:264–268.

67 Eisen HJ, Tuzcu EM, Dorent R, et al. RAD B253 Study Group. Everolimus for the prevention of allograft rejection and vasculopathy in cardiac-transplant recipients. N Engl J Med 2003; 349:847–858.

68 Bickers DR, Athar M. Novel approaches to chemoprevention of skin cancer. J Dermatol 2000; 27:691–695.

69 Gray DJ, Suman VJ, Su WP, Clay RP, Harmsen WS, Roenigk RK. Trends in the population-based incidence of squamous cell carcinoma of the skin first diagnosed between 1984 and 1992. Arch Dermatol 1997; 133:735–740.

CHAPTER

11

Bowenoid Papulosis

Marti Jill Rothe and Jane M Grant-Kels

Key points

- The term bowenoid papulosis was first presented in the literature by Kopf and Bart in 1977.
- Bowenoid papulosis most commonly presents as several to numerous wart-like papules affecting the genitals of young sexually active adults.
- Biopsy of bowenoid papulosis shows the histologic features of squamous cell carcinoma in situ.
- HPV genotype is detected in most lesions of bowenoid papulosis. HPV 16 is most commonly identified.
- Progression of bowenoid papulosis to invasive squamous cell carcinoma is unlikely.
- Bowenoid papulosis may be treated by a variety of surgical and medical modalities, alone or in combination. The topical immunomodulator imiquimod has recently been shown to be efficacious in the treatment of bowenoid papulosis.

INTRODUCTION

There is no other condition that better exemplifies the need for clinical-pathological correlation than bowenoid papulosis. Bowenoid papulosis lesions are banal in clinical appearance, while the biopsy of these lesions appears malignant. The true biologic potential of bowenoid papulosis lesions lies somewhere in the middle. Only when the clinical lesion and pathologic findings are closely correlated is one able to make the most appropriate diagnosis and institute the proper therapy.

In addition, bowenoid papulosis may help in the understanding of the potential etiologic role of viruses in oncology. The role of human papillomavirus (HPV) in cutaneous neoplasia has been well established. For example, condyloma acuminatum has been shown on occasion to evolve into or induce squamous cell carcinoma *in situ* or invasive squamous cell carcinoma. The relationship between bowenoid papulosis and HPV is another example of viral induced neoplasia and demonstrates that this oncogenic potential applies to the entire spectrum of squamous neoplasia.

HISTORY

The term bowenoid papulosis was first presented in the literature by Kopf and Bart in 1977.[1] Wade, Kopf and Ackerman further delineated the entity in additional publications in 1978[2] and 1979.[3] Other authors reported similar descriptions of wart-like papules with the histology of squamous cell carcinoma *in situ* during the 1970s.[4–8]

Epidemiology

Bowenoid papulosis most commonly affects young sexually active adults. There are rare pediatric reports including a 3-year-old, who was the victim of sexual abuse,[9] a 2-year-old with severe atopic dermatitis whose mother had a history of genital warts at the time of delivery,[10] and a 34-month-old with no obvious risk factor(s).[11] No racial predilection has been observed, although Wade *et al.* noted that the 11 patients in their initial series were Caucasian.[2] Twenty-seven of 28 affected men in Wade *et al.*'s subsequent report had been circumcised in infancy.[3] In contrast, 17 of 20 affected men in Porter *et al.*'s recently published series were uncircumcised.[12]

Often patients with bowenoid papulosis have a history of prior infectious or inflammatory genital dermatoses including condylomata acuminata, herpes simplex virus, psoriasis, lichen planus, and lichen sclerosus. HPV genotypes are usually identified in lesions of bowenoid papulosis. Obalek and colleagues detected cervical intraepithelial neoplasia (CIN) in three of five females with bowenoid papulosis; in two of the three with CIN, there was evidence of cervical HPV infection.[13] Penile papillomas (HPV negative) were diagnosed in the male sexual partner of a female with bowenoid papulosis and CIN with koilocytosis. In the same study, the sexual partner of five of six males with bowenoid papulosis had cervical HPV infection (cervical condylomata in two and CIN with HPV in three). In Rudlinger's series of eight women with bowenoid papulosis, four also had CIN.[14]

Immunosuppression related to pregnancy,[13] human immunodeficiency virus (HIV),[12] systemic medications (including for organ transplantation[15]), chronic renal insufficiency requiring hemodialysis[16] and atopic dermatitis[10] have been observed in some patients with bowenoid papulosis. Immunosuppression and advancing age are thought to be risk factors for progression of bowenoid papulosis to invasive squamous cell carcinoma.[5,13]

Pathogenesis and etiology

The link between HPV and bowenoid papulosis has been established via electron microscopy evidence of viral particles within lesions, immunoperoxidase and immunofluorescent techniques, and DNA hybridization. HPV genotype is detected in most lesions of bowenoid papulosis. HPV 16 is most commonly identified, but HPV types 6b, 18, 31–35, 39, 42, 48, 51–55 and 67 have also been detected.[17,18] Types 16, 18 and 33 are the most highly oncogenic, with HPV-16 and HPV-18 closely linked to cervical carcinoma.

Administration of HPV-16 vaccine to women negative for HPV-16 DNA and HPV-16 antibodies has been shown to reduce the incidence of HPV-16 infection and HPV-16 related CIN.[19] If a vaccination program were implemented for the general population, it is likely that the incidence of bowenoid papulosis would significantly decline.

Clinical features

Bowenoid papulosis is characterized by flat papules, which vary in color from pink to violaceous to reddish brown to deeply pigmented. The surface of the papules may be papillomatous, velvety, scaling, or smooth and glistening. Papules may be several or numerous and may coalesce to form plaques. Bowenoid papulosis may affect the shaft, glans, foreskin, inguinal fold, or perianal region in males and the vulva, perineum, and perianal region in females (Figs 11.1–11.4). Extragenital bowenoid papulosis has been described at various sites including the face,[20,21] neck,[22,23] trunk,[24] upper extremity,[24] and oral mucosa.[25]

Patients often present with bowenoid papulosis of many months to many years duration. Even in patients with longstanding lesions, progression to invasive squamous cell carcinoma is unlikely. Bowenoid papulosis

and invasive squamous cell carcinoma have rarely been reported to occur concomitantly.[26] When immunosuppression is reversed, bowenoid papulosis may spontaneously remit as has been observed after delivery in women affected during pregnancy[13] and after initiation of highly active anti-retroviral therapy (HAART).[12]

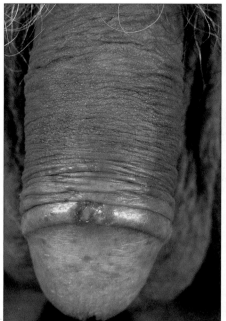

Figure 11.2
Bowenoid papulosis on the corona adjacent to a biopsy site (Image courtesy of New York University Department of Dermatology).

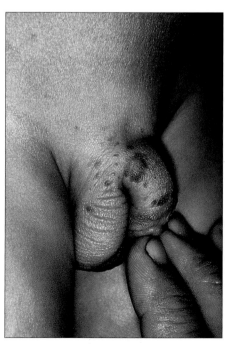

Figure 11.1
Multiple papules of bowenoid papulosis of the penile shaft and scrotum (Image courtesy of Yale Dermatology Residency Collection).

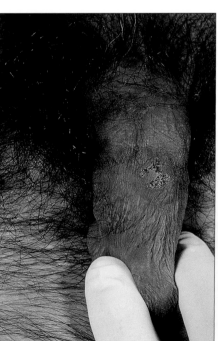

Figure 11.3
Multiple pigmented papules of bowenoid papulosis on the penile shaft (Image courtesy of New York University Department of Dermatology).

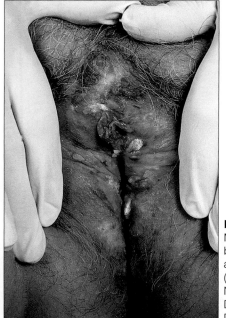

Figure 11.4
Multiple papules of bowenoid papulosis affecting the vulva (Image courtesy of New York University Department of Dermatology).

Patient evaluation, diagnosis and differential diagnosis

The diagnosis of bowenoid papulosis is established when characteristic clinical lesions show the histology of squamous cell carcinoma *in situ* on biopsy. Patients should be followed for any suggestion of invasive carcinoma such as crusting, ulceration, bleeding, or development of plaques. Patients with perianal involvement should be evaluated for anal intraepithelial neoplasia (AIN). Females affected with bowenoid papulosis should be evaluated for cervical HPV infection and CIN. Sexual

partners of patients with bowenoid papulosis should also be evaluated for evidence of HPV infection, CIN, and AIN. Affected patients and their partners require periodic reevaluation. HPV typing is an optional study which can be performed on lesional tissue and cervical and anal scrapings. The presence of more highly oncogenic genotypes may identify individuals who should have more frequent monitoring.

The clinical differential diagnosis of bowenoid papulosis includes condylomata acuminata, flat warts, seborrheic keratosis, epidermal nevus, granuloma annulare, melanocytic nevus, lichen planus, and psoriasis. Biopsy can readily differentiate bowenoid papulosis from these other diagnostic entities (Table 11.1).

Pathology

From scanning magnification the lesions of bowenoid papulosis have the architectural pattern of a condyloma acuminatum (Figs 11.5a, 11.5b, 11.6a). The epidermis is papillated and hyperplastic with focal hypergranulosis, arborization of the peripheral rete ridges, and dilated tortuous papillary blood vessels (Figs 11.5b, 11.6a). On occasion one can even discern focal vacuolization of the granular cell zone. Clinically pigmented lesions histologically also demonstrate dermal melanophages with or without epidermal hyperpigmentation (Fig. 11.7). However, on closer inspection of all lesions of bowenoid papulosis the cytologic changes within the epidermis resemble those of a squamous cell carcinoma *in situ* (Figs 11.5c, 11.6b). At all levels of the epidermis there are atypical keratinocytes in disarray demonstrating large, hyperchromatic and pleomorphic nuclei with eosinophilic cytoplasm as well as crowding of the epithelial nuclei (Figs 11.5c, 11.6b). Dyskeratotic keratinocytes, typical and atypical mitotic figures, multinucleated keratinocytes,

Table 11.1 Clinical differential diagnosis: diagnosis made by biopsy

	Clinical criteria	Histologic criteria
Condylomata acuminatum	Verrucous papules.	Papillated epidermal hyperplasia, parakeratosis, mitotic figures, vacuolated epithelial cells, arborization, no atypia, dilated tortuous capillaries.
Flat warts	Flat smooth papules.	Acanthosis, hyperkeratosis, vacuolization of epithelial cells, no atypia.
Seborrheic keratosis	Stuck on, brownish keratotic papules and plaques with plugging	Papillated acanthosis with hyperkeratosis and horn (pseudo)cysts
Epidermal nevus	Linearly arranged keratotic papules	Papillated acanthosis with hyperkeratosis
Granuloma annulare	Pale pink papules annularly arranged.	Palisaded granulomas with mucin.
Melanocytic nevus	Tan to brown papule.	Nests of melanocytic nevus cells.
Lichen planus	Flat topped violaceous papules with Wickham's striae.	Hyperkeratosis, acanthosis, wedge-shaped hypergranulosis, vacuolar alteration, band-like infiltrate.
Psoriasis	Red papules and plaques with silvery scale.	Psoriasiform epidermal hyperplasia, hyperkeratosis layered with neutrophils and mounds of parakeratosis, dilated tortuous capillaries.
Pearly penile papule	Small skin-colored papule.	Fibrosis, stellate fibroblasts, and increased number of dilated vascular spaces.

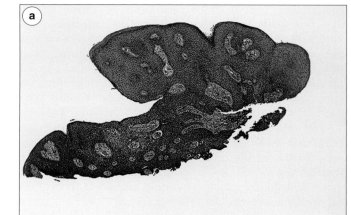

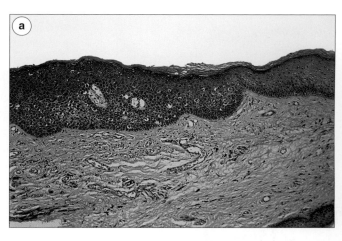

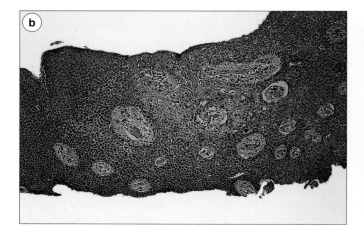

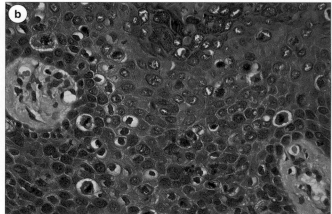

Figure 11.6 (a) Papillated epithelial hyperplasia with a suggestion of arborization of peripheral rete (×25; H&E). (b) High power view of epithelium demonstrating disarray, dyskeratosis, and mitotic figures (×100).

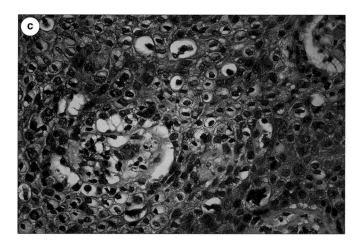

Figure 11.5 (a) Papillated and polypoid lesion of the penis (×10; H&E). (b) Higher magnification demonstrates hypergranulosis, arborization of the peripheral rete ridges, dilated and tortuous papillary blood vessels, and full thickness squamous atypia (×25). (c) High power view of cytologic atypia and mitotic figures at all levels of the epithelium (×100).

and hyperkeratosis with focal or confluent parakeratosis are prominent features. A superficial perivascular and often band-like lymphohistiocytic infiltrate is usually identified in the underlying dermis. The degree of cytologic atypia varies from lesion to lesion.

The histopathologic differential diagnosis includes Bowen's disease (Table 11.2). Lesions of Bowen's disease are usually broader, demonstrate confluent rather than focal parakeratosis, and generally show more prominent cytologic atypia with numerous atypical mitotic figures and multinucleated keratinocytes. Bowen's disease does not usually demonstrate hypergranulosis, dilated and tortuous papillary blood vessels, or papillated epidermal hyperplasia.

Another diagnostic entity that should be considered is that of a condyloma acuminatum that has been treated chemically with podophyllin resin. Podophyllin resin application results in necrotic keratinocytes and bizarre mitotic figures especially within the first 72 hrs after application. It has been reported that after 2 weeks, these changes are no longer present.[27]

In distinguishing among bowenoid papulosis, Bowen's disease and a podophyllum resin treated condyloma acuminata, clinical information should be obtained and clinical-pathological correlation must be applied before a definitive diagnosis can be established. On occasion a patient with multiple lesions consistent clinically with bowenoid papulosis or condyloma acuminatum may histologically show an admixture of lesions; i.e. some lesions histologically resemble Bowen's disease and represent bowenoid papulosis while others histologically demonstrate the changes only of a condyloma acuminatum.

Table 11.2 Pathologic differential diagnosis: diagnosis made by clinical pathologic correlation

	Clinical criteria	Histologic criteria
Bowen's disease	Red, scaling and/or crusting patch.	Confluent parakeratosis, acanthosis, full thickness epidermal atypia with mitoses.
Recently treated condyloma	History of condyloma recently treated with podophyllin resin.	Condyloma with necrotic keratinocytes and bizarre mitotic figures.
Bowenoid papulosis	Small red-brown papules, usually multiple in number, occasionally verrucoid.	Focal parakeratosis, acanthosis, and papillomatosis, full thickness epidermal atypia with mitoses.

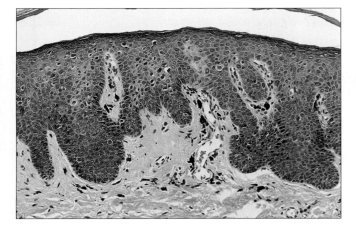

Figure 11.7 Histology of pigmented bowenoid papulosis demonstrating papillated epithelial hyperplasia with epidermal hyperpigmentation, full thickness squamous atypia and numerous underlying dermal melanophages (50×; H&E).

Treatment

The biologic potential of bowenoid papulosis directly impacts on treating these lesions. Although there have been reports of spontaneous regression of lesions, the regression is most commonly noted when an immunosuppressive state is reversed (like the end of pregnancy). On the opposite end of the spectrum are the reports of bowenoid papulosis progressing to invasive squamous cell carcinoma. Most bowenoid papulosis lesions usually follow a more benign course. However, since the majority of bowenoid papulosis lesions have historically been ablated by various techniques, the true biologic potential of bowenoid papulosis may not be completely appreciated. Ablation rather than conservative observation is usually chosen not only to remove any malignant potential that these lesions might possess but also to reduce the threat of both autoinoculation and inoculation to others with a viral-induced lesion.

Bowenoid papulosis may be treated by a variety of surgical and medical modalities, alone or in combination. Porter et al. recommend circumcision to eliminate a major risk factor for invasive carcinoma and HPV infection.[12] These authors also contend that circumcision facilitates follow-up and treatment of bowenoid papulosis. Partial or total vulvectomy may be performed as treatment in women but is rarely necessary. Local ablative options include shave removal, curettage, electrosurgery, cryo-

therapy, and laser (Nd:Yag or CO_2). Topical therapy alternatives include trichloroacetic acid, 5-fluorouracil, cidofovir,[28,29] and imiquimod.[30] One effective regimen has been the application of cidofovir 0.4% cream twice daily for 5 days, repeated every 15 days for 3 cycles. Imiquimod may be administered, as for genital warts, every other day and may show efficacy within 2–3 months. In HIV positive patients, surgical and topical therapy is generally ineffective until HAART is initiated.[12]

FUTURE OUTLOOK

The development of HPV vaccine, its successful trial in the prevention of HPV-16 infection and HPV-16 related CIN, and its possible future administration to the general population may ultimately reduce the incidence of bowenoid papulosis. Topical immunomodulatory therapy with imiquimod is a promising medical treatment for bowenoid papulosis.

REFERENCES

1 Kopf AW, Bart RS. Multiple bowenoid papules of the penis: A new entity? Tumor Conference No. 11. J Derm Surg Oncol 1977; 3:265–269.

2 Wade TR, Kopf AW, Ackerman AB. Bowenoid papulosis of the penis. Cancer 1978; 42:1890–1903.

3 Wade TR, Kopf AW, Ackerman AB. Bowenoid papulosis of the genitalia. Arch Derm 1979; 115:306–308.

4 Taylor DR, South DA. Bowenoid papulosis: A review. Cutis 1981; 27:92–98.

5 Schwartz RA, Janniger CK. Bowenoid papulosis. J Am Acad Derm 1991; 24:261–264.

6 Lloyd KM. Multicentric pigmented Bowen's disease of the groin. Arch Derm 1970; 101:48–51.

7 Lupulescu A, Mehregan AH, Rahbari H, et al. Venereal warts vs Bowen disease: a histologic and ultrastructural study of five cases. JAMA 1977; 237:2520–2522.

8 Katz HI, Posalaky Z, McGinley D. Pigmented penile papules with carcinoma in situ changes. Br J Derm 1978; 99:155–162.

9 Halasz C, Silvers D, Crum CP. Bowenoid papulosis in three-year-old girl. J Am Acad Derm 1986; 14:326–330.

10 Breneman DL, Lucky AW, Ostrow RS, et al. Bowenoid papulosis of the genitalia associated with human papillomavirus DNA type 16 in an infant with atopic dermatitis. Pediatr Derm 1985; 2:297–301.

11 Weitzner JM, Fields KW, Robinson MJ. Pediatric bowenoid papulosis: Risks and management. Pediatr Derm 1989; 6:303–305.

12 Porter WM, Francis N, Hawkins D, et al. Penile intraepithelial neoplasia: clinical spectrum and treatment of 35 cases. Br J Derm 2002; 147:1159–1165.

13 Obalek S, Jablonska S, Beaudenon S, et al. Bowenoid papulosis of the male and female genitalia: Risk of cervical neoplasia. J Am Acad Derm 1986; 14:433–444.

14 Rudlinger R. Bowenoid papulosis of the male and female genital tracts: Risk of cervical neoplasia. J Am Acad Derm 1987; 16:625–627.

15 Euvrard S, Kanitakis J, Chardonnet Y, et al. External anogenital lesions in organ transplant recipients. A clinicopathologic and virologic assessment. Arch Derm 1997; 133:175–178.

16 Gross G, Hagedorn M, Ikenberg H, et al. Bowenoid papulosis: Presence of human papillomavirus (HPV) structural antigens and of HPV 16-related DNA sequences. Arch Derm 1985; 121:858–863.

17 Park K-C, Kim K-H, Youn S-W, et al. Heterogeneity of human papillomavirus DNA in a patient with Bowenoid papulosis that progressed to squamous cell carcinoma. Br J Derm 1998; 139:1087–1091.

18 Yoneta A, Yamashita T, Jin H-Y, et al. Development of squamous cell carcinoma by two high-risk human papillomaviruses (HPVs), a novel HPV-67 and HPV-31 from bowenoid papulosis. Br J Derm 2000; 143:604–608.

19 Koutsky LA, Ault KA, Wheeler CM, et al. A controlled trial of a human papillomavirus type 16 vaccine. N Engl J Med 2002; 347:1645–1651.

20 Bart RS. Bowenoid papulosis of the chin. J Derm Surg Oncol 1984; 10:821–823.

21 Olhoffer IH, Davidson D, Longley J, et al. Facial bowenoid papulosis secondary to human papillomavirus type 16. Br J Derm 1999; 140:761–762.

22 Baron JM, Rubben A, Grussendorf-Conen E-I. HPV 18-induced pigmented bowenoid papulosis of the neck. J Am Acad Derm 1999; 40:633–634.

23 Johnson TM, Saluja A, Fader D, et al. Isolated extragenital bowenoid papulosis of the neck. J Am Acad Derm 1999; 41:867–870.

24 Papadopoulos AJ, Schwartz RA, Lefkowitz A, et al. Extragenital bowenoid papulosis associated with atypical human papillomavirus genotypes. J Cutan Med Surg 2002; 6:117–121.

25 Daley T, Birek C, Wysocki GP. Oral bowenoid lesions: Differential diagnosis and pathogenic insights. Oral Surg, Oral Med, Oral Pathol, Oral Radiol Endod 2000; 90:466–473.

26 Bergeron C, Naghashfar Z, Canaan C, et al. Human papillomavirus type 16 in intraepithelial neoplasia (bowenoid papulosis) and coexistent invasive carcinoma of the vulva. Int J Gynecol Pathol 1987; 6:1–11.

27 Wade TR, Ackerman AB. The effects of resin of podophyllin on condyloma acuminatum. Am J Derm 1984; 6:109–122.

28 Descamps V, Duval X, Grossin M, et al. Topical cidofovir for bowenoid papulosis in an HIV-infected patient. Br J Derm 2001; 144:642–643.

29 Snoeck R, Laethem Y Van, Clercq E De, et al. Treatment of bowenoid papulosis of the penis with local applications of cidofovir in a patient with acquired immunodeficiency syndrome. Arch Intern Med 2001; 161:2382–2384.

30 Petrow W, Gerdsen R, Uerlich M, et al. Successful topical immunotherapy of bowenoid papulosis with imiquimod. Br J Derm 2001; 145:1022–1023.

CHAPTER

12

Epidermodysplasia Verruciformis

Stefania Jablonska and Slavomir Majewski

Key points

- Epidermodysplasia verruciformis (EV) is a genetic lifelong disease associated with specific human papillomaviruses (HPV) and multiple skin cancers.
- Characteristic feature is immunotolerance towards own EVHPVs, which, due to genetic restriction, are not contagious for the general population.
- EV papillomavirus DNA is present in cutaneous cancers and benign epidermal proliferations also in the general population.
- EVHPVs enhancing keratinocyte proliferation were found also involved in the immunopathogenesis of psoriasis.

INTRODUCTION

This rare life-long, genetically determined disease, associated with specific human papillomavirus types (HPVs), is a model of cutaneous genetic carcinogenesis since over 50% of patients develop non-melanoma skin cancers. Although EVHPVs are not contagious for normal individuals due to genetic restriction, with the use of highly sensitive techniques the EV specific HPV DNA was found in skin cancers of the general population. This finding raised enormous interest in the disorder. Detection of EVHPV DNA in the bulge of the outer sheath of hair follicles[1] and in about 30% of the normal skin[2] indicates that EVHPVs are ubiquitous viruses which can produce cutaneous lesions only in genetically susceptible people. Moreover, recently DNA of potentially oncogenic EVHPVs was found in a high prevalence in psoriatic skin and in regenerating epidermal wounds.[3] Thus EVHPVs proved to be not only a cause of genetically determined cancers in EV patients, but are also involved in skin cancers and benign epidermal proliferations in the general population.

The term EV specific HPVs has been challenged since DNA of these ubiquitous HPVs was found in other malignant and benign proliferations. However cutaneous changes characteristic of EV are present exclusively in patients with EV, due to mutations of specific EV genes.[4]

HISTORY

EV was first described as genodermatosis by Lewandowsky and Lutz,[5] and as a model of viral cutaneous onco-

genesis in 1972.[6] The oncogenic EVHPV types were discovered in 1978.[7]

Epidemiology

The disease is rare due to the genetic restriction of EVHPVs in the general population. EVHPV DNA present in small amounts in the skin of immunosuppressed and immunocompetent populations, on activation, becomes expressed in proliferating keratinocytes and may be detected in malignant and premalignant lesions. Numerous warts, precancerous skin lesions and cutaneous cancers harboring EVHPV DNA are found in immunosuppressed individuals and the prevalence of these changes parallels the duration of immunosuppression.

Single cases of EV have been reported in all races from various countries, in Europe, Africa, Asia and both Americas. The disease is relatively more frequent in Africa. However, no exact statistical data are available. In black Africans the presentation has been described as multiple verruca seborrheica-like lesions.[8]

Etiopathogenesis

Etiology

EV is induced by specific benign and malignant EVHPVs, classified into a special branch of the phylogenetic tree of HPVs constructed on the basis of nucleotide homology.[9] Of about 20 characterized EVHPVs, high-risk HPV5 and HPV8 are predominantly associated with malignant tumors. Other EVHPVs (19, 17, 20 and 47) were detected in single tumors.

Benign lesions are associated with diverse EVHPVs.[10] A characteristic feature is a constant expression in tumors of E6 and E7 oncoproteins of oncogenic EVHPVs and a lack of integration of viral DNA into the host DNA.[10] Integration was reported exclusively in metastases[11] (which are extremely rare) occurring sometimes after application of co-cancerogens (e.g. X-ray therapy).

The role of EVHPVs in the pathogenesis of EV is substantiated by the presence in 25% of patients of specific antibodies to capsid (L1), and E6/E7 EVHPV5 proteins in over 70% of patients.[12] The antibodies are generated in response to activation of the life cycle of HPVs which become expressed in the proliferating keratinocytes of benign and malignant EV lesions.

157

Malignant transformation

The mechanism of cell transformation by oncogenic EVHPVs differs from that of high risk genital HPV16 and 18 because E6 of oncogenic EVHPV does not degrade *p53* protein,[13] and E7 oncoprotein has a very low transforming activity. A recent study found dysfunction of the *p53* gene in over 70% of invasive skin cancers and in over 50% of cancers *in situ*.[14] In EV patients, some *p53* mutations were characteristic for UVB- induced sun mutations as in the general population. However, some of them were found to be due to other mutagens, possibly EVHPVs. It is conceivable that the genetic defect determining high expression of E6/E7 proteins of oncogenic EVHPVs and leading to dysfunction of *p53*-dependent apoptosis could contribute to the tumor development. Thus malignant transformation depends both on host, i.e. genetics and immunity and on the environmental factors.

Genetics

Immunogenetic control of HPV infection is supported by an established association of cervical cancer with HLA-DRB1 haplotype. However, in our preliminary study on a large series of 57 EV patients, no positive association with DR-DQ haplotypes could be found. A high frequency of siblings and consanguineous marriages favors autosomal recessive mode of inheritance.[10] The susceptibility loci for EV were found localized to two chromosomes: EV1 on chromosome arm 17qter and EV2 on chromosome 2.[15] It should be stressed that both susceptibility loci for EV were found in regions containing psoriasis susceptibility loci. It is possible that other susceptibility loci for EV will be mapped also to other chromosomes since EV is polygenic and heterogenous disease. The recent most important finding is identification of two novel genes, named EVER 1 and EVER 2, whose mutations are responsible for the disease.[4] Polish patients with EV were found to have EVER 2 mutation. Characterization of these specific genes has made it possible to predict the susceptibility to the disease in the families of EV patients.

Immune abnormalities

The most important defect is immunosurveillance, leading to inability to eliminate own EVHPVs and HPV-transformed cells (i.e. to immunotolerance). Cell mediated immune responses, which are of special significance for natural defense against various pathogens, are in EV patients selectively defective towards infectious agents. However, this is usually preserved against other viruses and microbes since the patients are not prone to infections with no EVHPVs (e.g. genital warts). Characteristic for the disease is absence of cutaneous responses to locally applied sensitizers which is suggestive of a defect of local cellular immunity. However, the number and function of Langerhans cells in EV patients were found preserved.[16] Therefore, 'non specialist' cells (EVHPV infected keratinocytes) may act as their own antigen presenting cells. This, in absence of co-stimulatory signals, could lead to induction of immunotolerance with pronounced inhibition of cytotoxic T-cells[16] and natural killer cell activity[17] against the specific target. The specific cell mediated defect has recently been confirmed in *in vitro* study of T lymphocyte proliferative responses with the use of HPV5 virus like particles generated in baculovirus system. It was also found that peripheral blood mononuclear cells from EV patients did not respond to EVHPV5 VLP as measured by proliferative assay and INF-γ production. The levels of IL-18, a potent inducer of INF-γ production, were low whereas levels of immunosuppressive IL-10 were increased.

The local immunosurveillance appears to be of crucial importance as control mechanism of the infection with oncogenic HPVs, tumor development and formation of metastasis. High expression of mRNA for TNFα and TGFβ-1 have been found in the epidermis of EV lesions[18] and may have inhibitory effect on the infected keratinocytes leading also to depression of local immunosurveillance. TGFβ induces several protease inhibitors and decreases synthesis of enzymes degrading the extracellular matrix. This may contribute to limitation of progression of EV tumors and to absence of metastases if cancerogens are not applied.

The adverse effect on local immunosurveillance is mainly sun exposure. UVB induces formation of cis-isomer of urocanic acid (a UV absorbing component of the stratum corneum) which has a strong immunosuppressive activity.[19] UV-induced cytokines TGFβ-1, anti IL-1 are immunosuppressive, and TNFα in case of chronic sun exposure mediates specific immunotolerance through the soluble receptors. Characteristic *p53* 'sun' mutations and derangement of apoptosis may eventually lead to malignant transformation of cells harboring oncogenic EVHPVs. Therefore a characteristic feature of EV is malignant transformation, especially in sun-exposed areas.

Clinical features

Cutaneous manifestations

The first cutaneous manifestations of EV appear at the ages of 5–8 years, usually as very flat plane warts, localized mainly on the face and hands, spreading progressively all over the body (Fig. 12.1). Somewhat later, red plaques located mostly on the neck and trunk appear (Fig. 12.2). Skin changes are polymorphous. The plane wart-like lesions are often somewhat flatter, more abundant than plane warts in the general population, of various sizes and shapes, and sometimes confluent. There can also be brownish (Fig. 12.3), red and achromic plaques, and pityriasis versicolor-like lesions (Fig. 12.4). On the face and hands, wart-like lesions prevail. On the trunk, red plaques and pityriasis versicolor-like changes are seen. These benign manifestations are usually very widespread involving the face, trunk and extremities and may be generalized. The plane wart-like lesions not infrequently have a linear arrangement like warts in the general population (Koebner phenomenon). Some warts are more elevated and hyperkeratotic, similar to verrucae vulgaris. However, these display the cytopathic effect characteristic for plane warts induced by HPV3 in the general population and are found to harbor closely related HPV10/28. These lesions are referred to as intermediate warts,[20] which are more frequent in heavily immuno-suppressed patients.

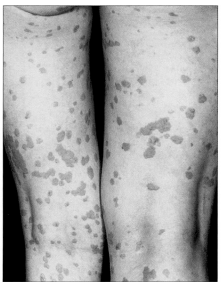

Figure 12.1 Plane wart-like lesions, more irregular, and more abundant than warts in the general population, mainly induced by EVHPV3. Some warts are confluent.

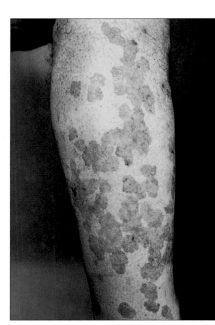

Figure 12.3 Large pigmented plaques with irregular outlines on the legs in a patient infected with EVHPV5 and HPV3.

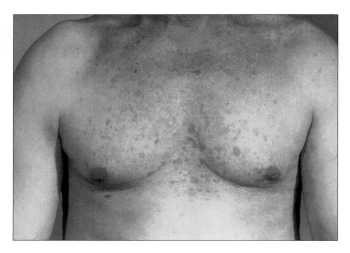

Figure 12.2 Widespread red plaques on the trunk induced by several EVHPVs, mainly EVHPV5.

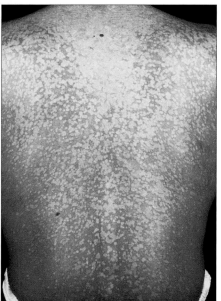

Figure 12.4 Pityriasis versicolor-like lesions, widespread on the trunk, found to be induced by several EVHPVs.

Unusual manifestations include:

- Very small, flat, disseminated, sometimes achromic papules without wart-like appearance.

- Papillomas and seborrhoic keratosis-like lesions, infrequently highly proliferative and pigmented, most often localized on the neck and in the inguinal region (Fig. 12.5). Lesions of this type were reported more often in black Africans,[8] however they can occur with lesser frequency in Caucasians.

- A combination of features of EV-specific lesions and plane or intermediate warts seen in the general population. The warts induced by HPV3/10/28 in EV patients are often more irregular, larger plaques. Some of these changes are polymorphous, typical of EV lesions induced by EV specific HPVs, characteristic pityriasis versicolor-like and red plaques. The mixed infection is sometimes seen in families of EV patients, in some members having prevailing lesions of EVHPV and in others having lesions seen of HPV3/10/28 type.

The patients having a mixed infection are most heavily immunosuppressed.[19] It could be presumed that due to the viral load by widespread infection with EVHPVs, the patients are more prone also to infection with HPV3 and related types, which are often associated with immunosuppression in non-EV patients.

Course of the disease

Although the disease starts usually in early childhood, the manifestations might be subtle. The flat wart-like lesions may be regarded just as warts in the general population and red plaques are not infrequently overlooked. Thus, some patients may not notice the benign lesions and claim that the disease started with the appearance of first premalignancies or malignancies in

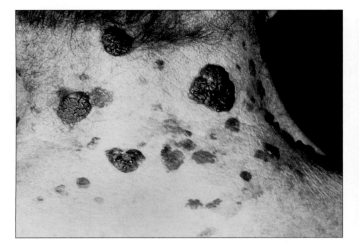

Figure 12.5 Pigmented papillomas and verruca seborrheica-like changes on the neck associated with EVHPV5.

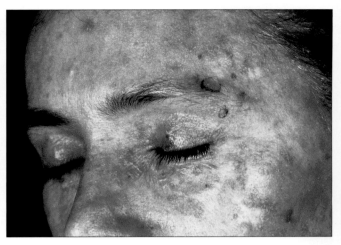

Figure 12.6 Wart-like lesions on the face, some larger, deeper, covered with crusts (early carcinoma *in situ*).

the third or fourth decade of life. The course of EV is diverse. Some cases are stabile, while others are progressive with steadily appearing new lesions.

Malignant transformation occurs in about half of the cases. In patients followed for up to 20 or more years, premalignant and malignant changes are detected at a more advanced age. Thus, the true incidence of cancer development in EV patients may be even higher than 50%.

Malignant neoplasms

Malignant conversion starts usually in the third decade. The preferential localization of tumors is the forehead and temporal areas, sites where actinic keratoses usually occur in the general population (Fig. 12.6). In patients with EV the first premalignancies have all the features of normal actinic keratoses but are often much more abundant, showing a higher degree of atypical features and dyskeratosis. Malignant transformation in EV patients occurs at much higher rate and at much younger age than in immunocompetent individuals. Premalignant lesions are hyperkeratotic, progressively deeper and larger, scaly and erosive (Fig. 12.7). The progression to malignancy is usually very slow but within a few years numerous tumors may develop. In some patients, the premalignant and early malignant changes are very abundant covering the whole forehead.

The rate of development of malignant tumors depends on the extent of infection with oncogenic EVHPVs and on the co-factors of oncogenesis including chronic sun exposure. Red plaques on the covered areas, as well as proliferative and seborrhoic wart-like papillomas localized on the neck and palpebra more rarely undergo malignant transformation.

EV tumors occur primarily on sun-exposed and/or traumatized areas: on the face, dorsal hands, in the inguinal and retroauricular folds (Fig. 12.8). Tumor growth is very slow. Cancers – although persistent – are usually only locally destructive with low metastatic potential. Mucous membranes are not involved and peri-

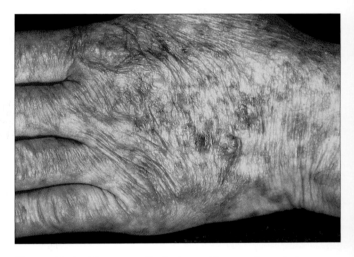

Figure 12.7 Plane wart-like lesions with premalignant changes and early carcinomas *in situ* developing from some warts.

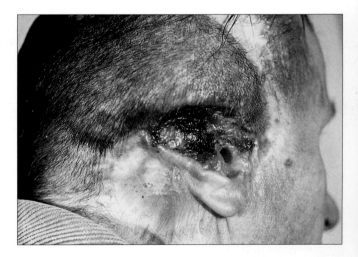

Figure 12.8 Invasive carcinoma in periauricular localization developed in primarily superficial tumors associated with several EVHPVs treated with X-rays.

orbital cancers do not destroy the globe of the eye (Fig. 12.9). Cancers localized on the lips do not spread into oral mucosa and generally do not metastasize if not treated with cancerogenic compounds. Metastatic cancers have been reported from Africa and Asia, usually in patients after radiotherapy for first malignancies. We have seen a sudden development of lip cancer in a patient with widespread HPV5-induced lesions after infection with herpes simplex, a co-factor of HPV oncogenesis. The healing was very fast and was complete in about 10 days after surgery, due probably to a very high prevalence of TGFβ in EV lesions.

Diagnosis

Diagnosis of epidermodysplasia verruciformis is based on clinical, histologic and virologic findings:

- The onset in childhood at the ages of 5–8 years.

- A lifelong persistence of cutaneous disease with no involvement of internal organs, mucous membranes and lymph nodes and a satisfactory general condition of the patient.

- Familial occurrence and consanguinity of the parents are often noted.

- Characteristic polymorphous cutaneous lesions: plane wart-like, red or brownish plaques, and pityriasis versicolor-like changes mainly on the trunk and neck.

- Appearance of premalignancies and malignancies characteristically on the sun exposed areas starting from the third decade.

- Slow tumor progression with a very low metastatic potential.

The diagnosis must be confirmed by biopsy, which demonstrates highly characteristic cytopathic effects in benign lesions (Fig. 12.10). Dyskeratotic, pleomorphic, Bowenoid-type changes in premalignant and malignant lesions involving the entire epidermis including hair follicles can also be noted. At the onset of malignant transformation the cytopathic effect starts to disappear.

Virological confirmation

Detection of EVHPV in the tissues is necessary since the cytopathic effect is similar in lesions induced by oncogenic and non oncogenic HPVs. A highly specific technique for this is the Southern blot test with the use of restriction enzymes and molecular hybridization *in situ* (Fig. 12.11). The most sensitive test is the polymerase chain reaction with the use of the specific or degenerate primers and sequencing of the reaction products. EV patients are usually infected with multiple oncogenic and non-oncogenic EVHPVs in different lesions (or even in the same lesion), and changes of various morphology may harbor the same types of EVHPVs (Fig. 12.12).

Genetic studies

Recent characterization of mutations of specific genes EVER1 and EVER2 provides confirmation for diagnosis.[4] Detection of these mutations allows the establishment

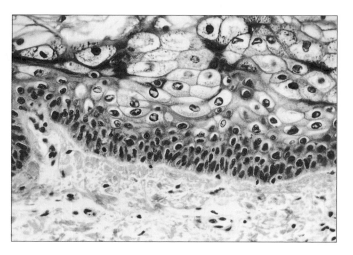

Figure 12.10 Characteristic cytopathic effect of EVHPV-induced lesion. Clarified dysplastic cells, starting suprabasally, with small pyknotic nuclei, replacing almost the entire epidermis.

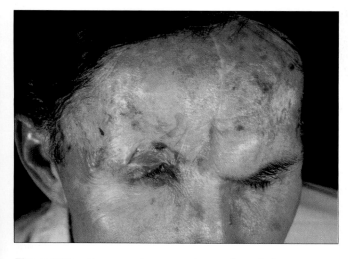

Figure 12.9 Numerous tumors and premalignant changes induced by EVHPV5 involving the entire forehead, with invasive carcinoma destroying the orbital area but sparing the eyeball.

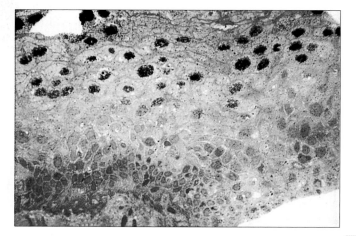

Figure 12.11 Molecular hybridization *in situ* showing abundant EVHPV5 DNA in the clarified cells.

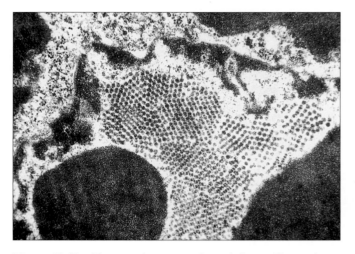

Figure 12.12 Electronmicroscopy of a red plaque. The nucleus and nucleolus are filled with viral particles; cytoplasm is almost devoid of organelles with prominent keratohyaline granules (×15.000).

of the diagnosis of EV in atypical, unclear, or very early familial or undeveloped cases.

Differential diagnosis

Clinical manifestations of EV induced by specific EVHPVs are highly characteristic. The differentiation is needed only in atypical cases, such as an exclusive presence of small whitish plaques, pigmented papillomas and 'verruca seborrheica' type of lesions.

Pityriasis versicolor-like changes are differentiated from pityriasis versicolor by the presence of a polymorphous eruption, mainly plane wart-like lesions and red or brownish plaques.

Clinical manifestations of the mixed variety of EV are diagnosed by a higher prevalence of HPV3-induced plane wart-like changes which might be difficult to recognize from widely disseminated long-lasting plane warts in immunosuppressed populations. This is particularly true when the characteristic EVHPV changes are slight and flat warts are prevailing. Only virologic study in these cases is helpful in disclosing EVHPVs since the histologic pattern without specific cytopathic effect is not contributory.

A lifelong infection of this type will be, in future, properly classified by the detection of specific genes EVER 1 and EVER 2 whose mutations occur only in EV patients. The genetic study has made it possible to diagnose EV in one of our familial cases, found to be infected – in contrast to the other family members – only with HPV3. In this patient lesions started to regress spontaneously after the delivery of her first child, and regressed completely within 8 months after the second delivery. No simultaneous inflammation was noted on all lesions, characteristic for regression of plane warts in the general population. The detection of specific gene EVER 2 also allowed for the recognition of EV in one girl with exclusively plane wart type lesions and EVHPV5 present only in a single wart, whose grand-

mother and two other members of the family had a severe form of EV induced by EVHPV5.

Pathology

A characteristic feature is the presence in the granular and upper spinous layers of large dysplastic cells with clarified cytoplasms and nucleoplasms (pyknotic nuclei) with prominent keratohyaline granules of various shapes and sizes (see Fig. 12.10). Dysplastic cells, often arranged in nests, start suprabasally replacing almost the entire epidermis. The horny layer is completely destroyed. This cytopathic effect, highly characteristic of EVHPVs, is present in all types of benign, even clinically atypical changes and does not occur in other diseases. The only exception to this finding is white sponge nevus which shows similar clarification of keratinocytes. However, the localization on mucosa excludes EV.

Premalignant lesions

Early malignant transformation starts as a downward proliferation of the epidermis containing pleomorphic, dyskeratotic cells, with hyperchromic large nuclei (sometimes multinucleated) showing Bowenoid dyskeratosis and variably numerous mitotic figures (Fig. 12.13). The cytopathic effect in very early premalignant lesions might be focally still preserved. However, this disappears with tumor progression. Some premalignant lesions have all the histologic features of actinic keratosis with atypical keratinocytes present throughout the entire epidermis and in the hair follicles, and with increased numbers of mitotic figures and atypical mitoses.

Neoplasms

Tumors developing from red plaques or premalignant lesions are squamous cell carcinomas (SCC) with preserved features of Bowenoid atypia and, more rarely, metatypic basal cell carcinomas (BCC). However, a basaloid histologic pattern can be found similar to BCC with the presence of Bowenoid dyskeratotic and pleomorphic cells. In some areas (not infrequently in hair follicles), these changes usually originate from actinic keratoses with pronounced Bowenoid-type dyskeratosis.

Malignant conversion starts within and around hair follicles (Fig. 12.14), which harbor EVHPV DNA.[1] This could provide an explanation for why actinic keratoses and EV tumors are mainly located on the forehead and in temporal areas which are sun exposed and abounding with hair follicles.

Treatment

There is no effective treatment since no known compound has been found to act directly on EVHPVs.

Experimental therapies

Systemic retinoids, having antiproliferative and antioncogenic activity, especially in combination with vitamin D3, may produce some transient improvement in early cancers and precancers but no clearing of EV lesions.

Thus the results are not satisfactory. However, in cases with prevailing HPV3 type lesions, this treatment may produce regression of plane-wart eruption. Systemic IFN-α was found to have a transient beneficial effect in some cases of mixed infection (EVHPVs and HPV3/10). However, the improvement only lasted up to 3 months after cessation of the therapy, when all lesions reappeared. IFNα and IFNγ have been tried systemically (and also locally) with unsatisfactory results although some lesions cleared or improved and the activity of the disease transiently decreased.

Local therapies

No local therapies are entirely effective, although pre-malignant lesions of actinic keratosis type can be cleared by application of 5-fluorouracil or 1% retinoic acid ointments. Since the lesions are usually very numerous, this therapy has limited practical application. However, the single early malignancies *in situ* of Bowen's type may be successfully treated with intralesional IFNα or β

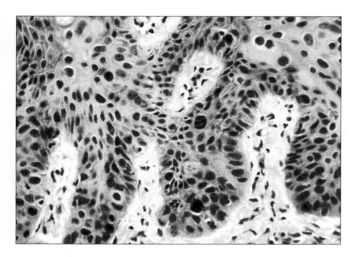

Figure 12.13 Early malignancy of actinic keratosis type with numerous dyskeratotic cells and abnormal mitoses at all levels of the epidermis (carcinoma *in situ* Bowen's type).

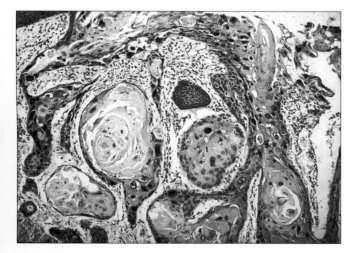

Figure 12.14 Carcinoma Bowen's type with numerous dyskeratotic and pleomorphic cells in and around hair follicles, which are partly filled with keratotic masses.

(10^6 MU, 3 times per week, for several weeks) or topical 5% imiquimod cream (3 times per week, for 16 weeks), in a regimen similar to that for BCC and Bowen's carcinoma *in situ* in immunocompetent individuals.

Malignant tumors should be treated by excision or laser surgery. Radiotherapy is strongly contraindicated.

Skin grafts

If almost the entire forehead is covered by early malignant lesions, Bowen's carcinoma *in situ* and actinic keratoses, which progressively become locally destructive and microinvasive. The only effective method is removal of the whole frontal skin followed by replacement with cutaneous graft taken from the inner, non-sun exposed sites of the arm (Fig. 12.15). We followed the graft life in six patients for over 20 years and we found that no malignancies developed in the grafted skin, while single benign EV lesions (red plaques) were noticed about 5–7 years after the skin transplantation.[21] This surgical procedure was life-saving for several patients. In addition, it provided an important insight into the EV oncogenesis: why the first benign lesions appear only at the ages of 5–8 years and the onset of cancers occurs so late (usually after over 20 years of disease duration) (Fig. 12.16) similar to genital cancers induced by high risk mucotropic HPVs.[22] The study provided also further confirmation of the harmful effect of chronic sun exposure.

Prophylaxis

Since there is no effective therapy for this genetic disease, it is highly important to avoid the genotoxic effects of sun and gamma radiation and to use the most potent sunscreens.

FUTURE OUTLOOK

Recent studies have disclosed multiple EVHPVs in 65 up to 90% of cancers of the transplant recipients, but also in 30–54% tumors of the general population.[23] In actinic keratoses, we found an even higher prevalence of EVHPVs (67%). Although various EVHPVs and some novel HPV DNA sequences were characterized in cutaneous malignancies, no one specific EVHPV type and no oncogenic HPV5 and HPV8 were found associated with skin cancers. Most importantly, no mRNA and no transforming oncoproteins E6 and E7, invariably present in tumors developing in EV patients, are detected in cancers of the general population and the associated EVHPVs are not oncogenic. Thus the causative role of EVHPVs in cutaneous oncogenesis in non-EV patients is still not fully documented.

However, the appearance of numerous warts, malignant and premalignant changes harboring EVHPV DNA in immunosuppressed populations is highly suggestive of some role of these viruses in cutaneous oncogenesis. The higher prevalence of EVHPVs in actinic keratoses than in cutaneous cancers would suggest that EVHPVs which have a weak transforming activity mainly enhance keratinocyte proliferation. In the

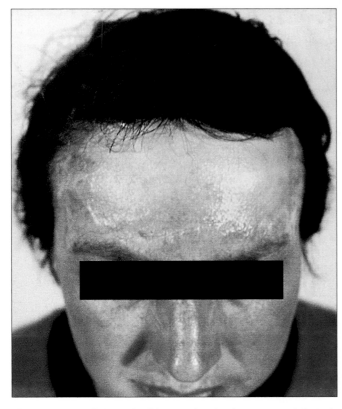

Figure 12.15 Skin graft of 2-year duration in a woman infected with multiple EVHPVs. The skin of the entire forehead covered with numerous premalignant and malignant changes was removed and replaced with grafted skin taken from the inner aspect of the arm. There are no red plaques within the graft.

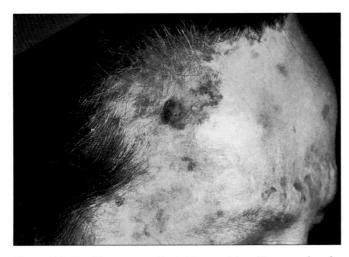

Figure 12.16 The same patient 15 years later, 17 years of graft life. Numerous premalignant lesions and a cancer around the graft. In grafted skin, single red plaques, which started to appear several years after the graft, did not convert into cancers.

later stages of oncogenesis, the chronic exposure to UV might be responsible for genetic instability, including $p53$ mutations.[22]

The most interesting new finding is detection of EVHPV DNA in benign keratinocyte proliferations, which is highly suggestive of the role of EV specific HPVs in other than EV skin disorders.[12] EVHPV DNA

was disclosed in over 90% of psoriatic plaques[3] and, in addition, specific antibodies to EV HPV5 L1 capsid protein and to oncoproteins E6/E7,[12] were found in patients with psoriasis. This finding favors the expression of EVHPV DNA and active lifecycle of EVHPVs. Activation of viral lifecycle might be responsible for sustained keratinocyte proliferations in psoriasis. Thus EVHPVs proved to be involved not only in the rare genetic disease epidermodysplasia verruciformis, but also in malignant and benign epidermal proliferations.[12,23] Future studies will better elucidate the relationship of EV and EVHPV to these disorders and may help us develop a better understanding of this disease.

REFERENCES

1 Boxman ILA, Berkhout RJM, Mulder LHC, et al. Detection of human papillomavirus DNA in plucked hairs from renal transplant recipients and healthy volunteers. J Invest Dermatol 1997; 108:712–715.

2 Astori G, Lavergne D, Benton C, et al. Human papillomaviruses are commonly found in normal skin of immunocompetent hosts. J Invest Derm 1998; 100:752–755.

3 Favre M, Orth G, Majewski S, et al. Psoriasis: a possible reservoir for human papillomavirus type 5, the virus associated with skin carcinomas of epidermodysplasia verruciformis. J Invest Derm 1998; 110:311–317.

4 Ramoz N, Rueda LA, Rueda B, et al. Mutations in two adjacent novel genes are associated with epidermodysplasia verruciformis. Nat Genet 2002; 32:579–581.

5 Lewandowsky F, Lutz W. Ein Fall einer bisher nicht beschriebenen Hauterkrankung (Epidermodysplasia verruciformis). Arch Derm Syph (Berlin) 1922; 141:193–203.

6 Jablonska S, Dabrowski J, Jakubowicz K. Epidermodysplasia verruciformis as a model in studies on the role of papovavirus in oncogenesis. Cancer Res 1972; 32:585–589.

7 Orth G, Jablonska S, Favre M, et al. Characterization of two types of human papillomaviruses in lesions of epidermodysplasia verruciformis. Proc Natl Acad Sci USA 1978; 75:1537–1541.

8 Jacyk WK, de Villiers EM. Epidermodysplasia verruciformis in Africans. Int J Derm 1993; 32:806–810.

9 Chan KW, Lam KY, Chan ACL, et al. Prevalence of human papillomavirus types 16 and 18 in penile carcinoma: a study of 41 cases using PCR. J Clin Pathol 1994; 47:823–826.

10 Orth G. Epidermodysplasia verruciformis. In: Salzman NP, Howley PM, eds. The Papovaviridae, Vol 2: The papillomaviruses. New York: Plenum Press; 1987:199–243.

11 Yabe Y, Sakai A, Hitsumoto T, et al. Human papillomavirus-5b DNA integrated in a metastatic tumor: cloning, nucleotide sequence and genomic organization. Int J Cancer 1999; 80:334–335.

12 Majewski S, Jablonska S. Possible involvement of epidemodysplasia veruciformis human papillomaviruses in the immunopathogenesis of psoriasis: a proposed hypothesis. Exp Dermatol 2003; 12:721–728.

13 Steger G, Pfister H. In vitro expressed HPV8 E6 protein does not bind $p53$. Arch Virol 1992; 125:355–360.

14 Padlewska K, Ramoz N, Cassonnet P, et al. Mutation and abnormal expression of the $p53$ gene in the viral skin carcinogenesis of epidermodysplasia verruciformis. J Invest Derm 2001; 117:935–942.

15 Ramoz N, Taieb A, Rueda LA, et al. Evidence for a nonallelic heterogeneity of epidermodysplasia verruciformis with two susceptibility loc mapped to chromosome regions 2p21-p24 and 17q25. J Invest Derm 2000; 114:1148–1153.

16 Cooper KD, Androphy EJ, Lowy D, et al. Antigen presentation and T-cell activation in epidermodysplasia verruciformis. J Invest Derm 1990; 94:769–776.

17 Majewski S, Malejczyk J, Jablonska S, et al. Natural cell-mediated cytctoxicity against various target cells in patients with epidermodysplasia verruciformis. J Am Acad Dermatol 1990; 22:423–427.

18 Majewski S, Hunzelmann N, Nischt R, et al. TGFB-1 and TNF expression in the epidermis of patients with epidermodysplasia verruciformis. J Invest Derm 1991; 97:862–867.

19 Majewski S, Jablonska S, Orth G. Epidermodysplasia verruciformis. Immunological and nonimmunological surveillance mechanisms: role in tumor progression. Clin Dermatol 1997; 15:321–334.

20 Obalek S, Favre M, Szymanczyk J, et al. Human papillomavirus (HPV) types specific of epidermodysplasia verruciformis detected in warts induced by HPV 3 or HPV 3-related types in immunosuppressed patients. J Invest Dermatol 1992; 98:936–941.

21 Majewski S, Jablonska S. Skin autografts in epidermodysplasia verruciformis: human papillomavirus-associated cutaneous changes need over 20 years for malignant conversion. Cancer Res 1997; 57:4214–4216.

22 Zur Hausen H. Papillomavirus infections – a major cause of human cancers. Biochim Biophys Acta Rev Cancer 1996; 1288:F55–78.

23 Majewski S, Jablonska S. Do epidermodysplasia verruciformis human papillomaviruses contribute to malignant and benign epidermal proliferations? Arch Derm 2002; 138:649–654.

CHAPTER
13

The Many Faces of Melanoma

Darrell S Rigel

The incidence of malignant melanoma continues to increase at an alarming rate. In the US, melanoma is the only major cancer where incidence is still rising and the reported incidence of melanoma may be lower than the actual rates.[1,2] In 2004 the lifetime risk for an American developing invasive malignant melanoma was 1 in 65 and, should the current rate of increase continue, will be 1 in 50 by the year 2010 (Fig. 13.1).

Melanoma is the most clear-cut form of cancer where early detection is a critical factor influencing survival. Patients diagnosed with melanoma in its earliest phase have an almost 100% chance of surviving their disease, while those with advanced disease at the time of diagnosis have an extremely poor prognosis. With incidence rates for this cancer continuing to rise, the importance of the clinician being able to recognize melanoma as early as possible has become even more essential.

However, melanoma can present clinically with many faces from the early lesions often described using the *ABCD* system (*A*symmetry, *B*order Irregularity, *C*olor variegation and *D*iameter >6 mm) to more advanced lesions demonstrating elevation, ulceration and bleeding. The purpose of the atlas is to depict many of the typical (and not so typical) presentations of melanoma to help augment the reader's diagnostic skills for earlier detection of this cancer.

REFERENCES

1 Merlino LA, Sullivan KJ, Whitaker DC, Lynch CF. The independent pathology laboratory as a reporting source for cutaneous melanoma incidence in Iowa, 1977–1994. J Am Acad Derm 1997; 37(4):578–585.

2 Wingo PA, Jamison PM, Hiatt RA, et al. Building the infrastructure for nationwide cancer surveillance and control – a comparison between the National Program of Cancer Registries (NPCR) and the Surveillance, Epidemiology and End Results (SEER) Program (United States). Cancer Causes Control 2003; 14(2):175–193.

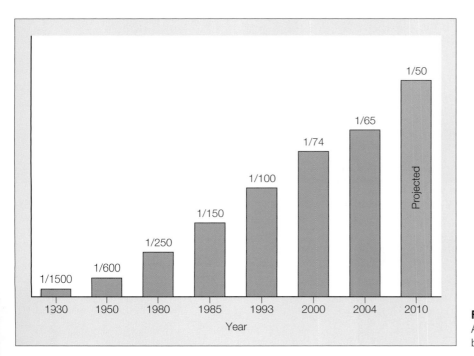

Figure 13.1 The lifetime risk of an American developing invasive melanoma by year.

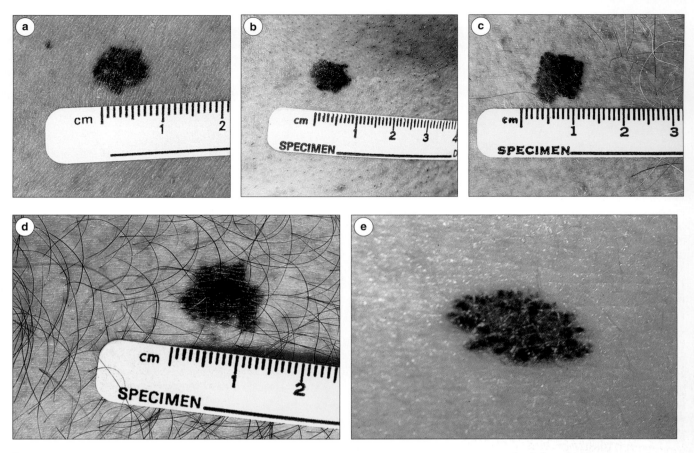

Figure 13.2 Early melanomas displaying the ABCD signs. (Images courtesy of New York University Department of Dermatology.)

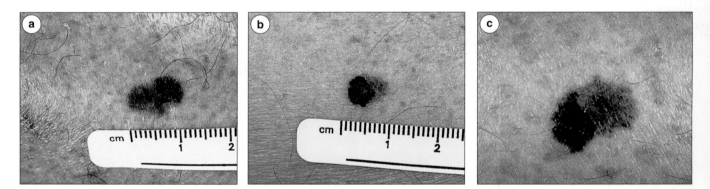

Figure 13.3 Melanoma arising in a pre-existing nevus. (Images (a) and (b) courtesy of New York University Department of Dermatology.)

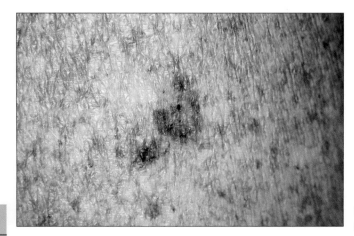

Figure 13.4 Desmoplastic melanoma with typical subtle presentation.

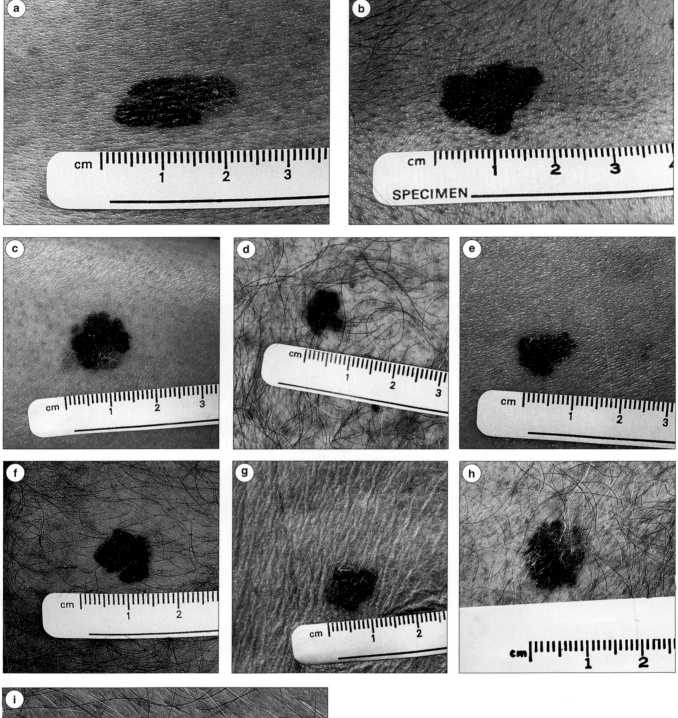

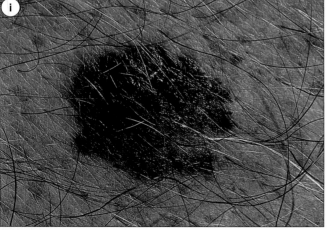

Figure 13.5 Advancing melanoma. (Images courtesy of New York University Department of Dermatology.)

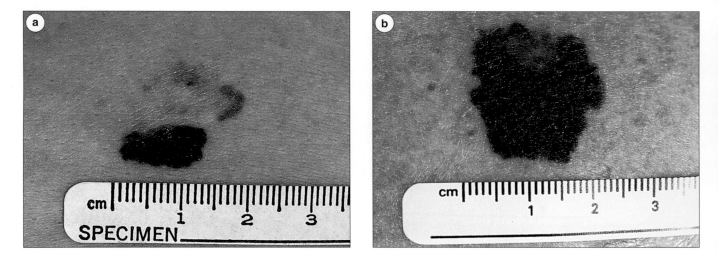

Figure 13.6   Melanoma with regression. Up to 20% of melanomas exhibit partial regression. (Images courtesy of New York University Department of Dermatology.)

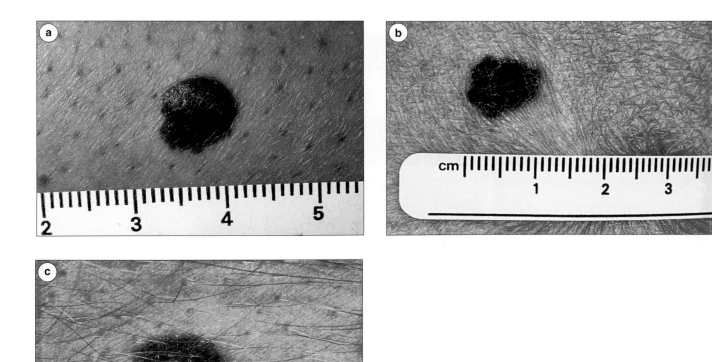

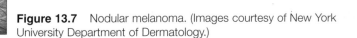

Figure 13.7   Nodular melanoma. (Images courtesy of New York University Department of Dermatology.)

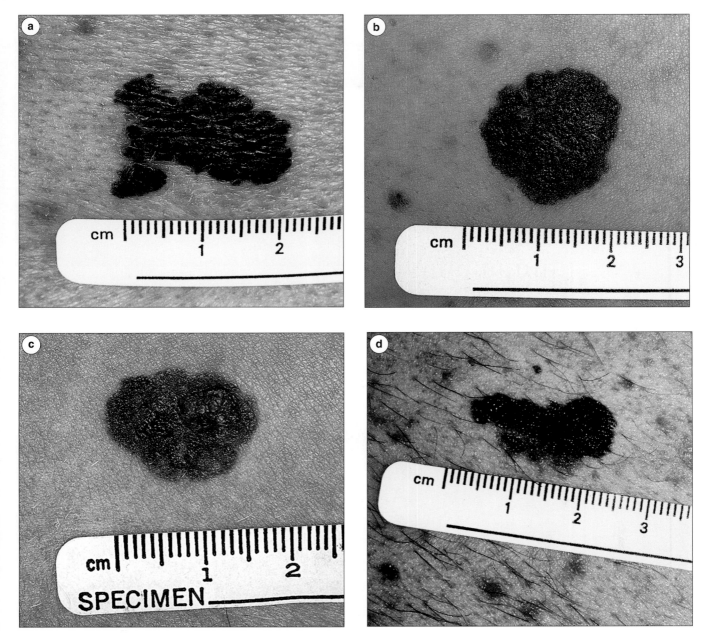

Figure 13.8   Later presentations of melanoma. (Images courtesy of New York University Department of Dermatology.)

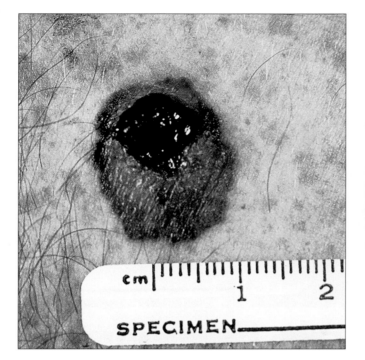

Figure 13.9 Melanoma with clinical ulceration (presence of this factor significantly worsens prognosis). (Image courtesy of New York University Department of Dermatology.)

Figure 13.10 Amelanotic melanoma. (Image courtesy of Jack Lesher MD.)

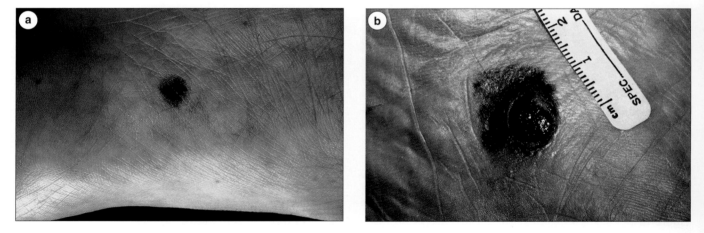

Figure 13.11 (a) Early melanoma on plantar surface – biopsy refused by patient. (b) 14 months later melanoma has progressed to vertical growth phase and nodule. Patient expired 4 months later. (Images courtesy of New York University Department of Dermatology.)

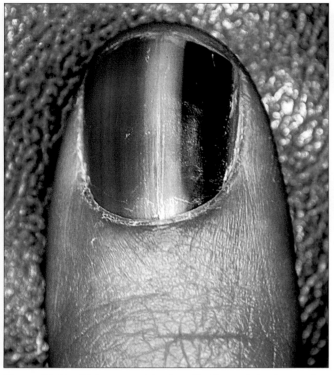

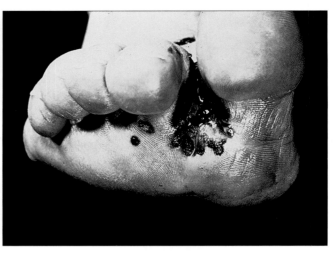

Figure 13.14   Melanoma of the foot with local metastatic lesions arising in the interdigital web. (Image courtesy of New York University Department of Dermatology.)

Figure 13.12   Melanoma arising in nail. Note subtle pigment in right side of proximal nail fold (Hutchinson's sign).

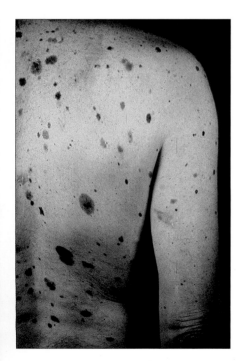

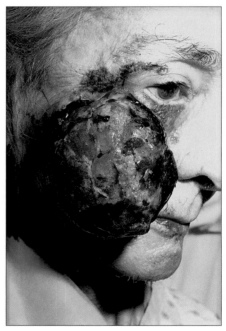

Figure 13.13
Patient with history of multiple primary melanomas who has "classic" dysplastic nevus syndrome. (Image courtesy of New York University Department of Dermatology.)

Figure 13.15
Advanced melanoma (52 mm thickness) of the cheek. (Image courtesy of New York University Department of Dermatology.)

CHAPTER
14

The Importance of Early Detection of Melanoma, Physician and Self-examination

Robert J Friedman

Key points

- Melanoma is the leading cause of death from diseases of the skin.
- The incidence of melanoma has tripled since 1980.
- Melanoma is completely curable if detected and resected early in its evolution.
- Education, coupled with regular physician examination of the entire integument and self-examination of the skin is a vitally important method of reducing deaths from melanoma.
- Most melanomas can be recognized using the *ABCD* method. A few smaller melanomas (6 mm or less in diameter) can be detected if one remembers that change in the diameter of a pigmented lesion over time in the presence of other clinical features of melanoma is an important clue to clinical diagnosis.
- "Melanoma writes its message in the skin with its own ink and it is there for all of us to see. Some see but do not comprehend".

INTRODUCTION

The leading cause of death from diseases of the skin is malignant melanoma. It is estimated that in 2004 in the US, at least 95,880 *new* cases of melanoma will be diagnosed.[1] About 7910 will die from melanoma in this country, one person for every hour of the year![1] The number of new cases of melanoma in 2004 will increase about 5% over that of 2003! At the current rate, about 1 in 65 Americans born this year will develop an *invasive* melanoma during their lifetime. This contrasts with about one in 1500 Americans born in 1935.[2] Melanoma is currently the 5th most prevalent cancer in men and the 7th most prevalent cancer in women in the US.[1]

These startling statistics coupled with the realization that survival of patients with melanoma is directly related to early detection points out the critical importance of detection of melanoma early in its biologic evolution and its prompt surgical removal in saving lives.[3–13] There are two ways to lower the morbidity and mortality from melanoma. First, and most directly, would be to identify and then eliminate the many, mostly unknown, factors which promote melanoma development (e.g. genetics, environmental (UVL, etc.), immunologic, viral, other carcinogens, etc.).[14] Aside from serious efforts related to reducing UVL exposure and, despite intensive efforts in

the world of basic and clinical research, little practical progress has been made. Thus, at this point in time, our efforts in terms of reducing melanoma-related morbidity and mortality lies in the realm of early detection of melanoma at a time in its evolution where its prognosis for cure is excellent.[1–14] Through education of both healthcare professionals and the lay public as to methods of identifying melanoma, routine physician-driven total cutaneous examinations and the teaching of patient self-examination, we can play a significant role in reducing deaths from melanoma.

HISTORY

The goal for every healthcare professional is to strive to increase our ability to detect melanoma at an early stage in its development and to promptly remove it. Historically, there is much data to support the fact that melanomas early in their development (*in situ* or very thin lesions) have an excellent prognosis.[8–12,15–17] The late Alexander Breslow in 1970 was the first to show that metastases generally did not occur in lesions <0.76 mm in thickness.[16] The fact that early melanomas have excellent prognoses has been repeatedly confirmed by many scientific investigators.[18–24] Our data from the NYU Melanoma Cooperative Group shows >99% 10-year survival for all patients with melanomas <0.76 mm in thickness contrasted to 48% for those melanomas measuring ≥3 mm in thickness.[14,25] Though rare exceptions do exist, it is clear that the thinner the melanoma and the earlier the surgical intervention, the better is the survival rate.[14] Thus, while it is clear that we as yet do not have the ability to prevent the development of melanoma, we surely have the ability to reduce to near zero, the death rate from melanoma.

In 1985, our group at the NYU School of Medicine first described a simple method of identifying most melanomas (the "ABCDs") along with a method of patient self-examination.[13] These tools, coupled with additional education from, and examination by other healthcare professionals can help in the identification of the vast majority of melanomas at a curable stage in their development.

Further, it is now known that patients having histories of a previous primary melanoma are at higher risk for developing a *second* primary melanoma (10–25 × greater than patients having no prior history of melanoma).[26] DiFronzo *et al.* at the John Wayne Cancer Institute[26] recently studied 51 patients who had an initial primary melanoma and who subsequently developed a second primary melanoma. The patients were followed regularly and all had well-conducted patient education sessions, including instruction in self-examination. The results of this study confirmed the importance of careful physician follow-up coupled with patient education and the practice of self-examination in that the mean thickness of the *second* primary melanomas in these patients was significantly *less* (0.63 mm) than that seen in the *initial* melanomas (1.32 mm).

In sum, there can clearly be a significant impact on melanoma mortality rates if healthcare providers practice regular total cutaneous examination thereby enhancing early detection. Further, historical data strongly supports the conclusion that healthcare providers also should instruct and counsel all patients, but particularly those patients at higher risk for melanoma (e.g. prior history of melanoma, family history of melanoma, presence of atypical (*dysplastic*) nevi, presence of large numbers (>100) of nevi) in careful self-examination of the skin.[14,26]

Epidemiology

Melanoma represents a significant and growing public health problem throughout the world.[1,27–30] While accounting for only about 4% of all skin cancers, melanoma accounts for nearly 80% of all deaths from skin cancer.[1] If one includes *in situ* lesions, about 1 in 37 Americans born this year will develop a melanoma during their lifetime. While the death rate has essentially flattened, most likely secondary to both physician and patient education and earlier detection and intervention, the incidence of melanoma within this country has more than tripled among Caucasians between 1980 and 2003.

The ever-increasing incidence of melanoma clearly is a product of our failure, as yet, to understand the patho-etiology of this malignancy. Hopefully, we will continue to develop a better understanding of the biology of melanoma and thus be better able to develop the preventive and other interventional strategies needed to impact on the increasing numbers of new melanomas each year. However, through worldwide educational programs, we have begun to impact of the morbidity and mortality from melanoma through detection of melanomas earlier in their evolution coupled with their relatively simple surgical removal. It is critical to continue along the pathway of early detection and appropriate intervention in our goal to reduce the number of deaths from melanoma to as close to zero as is possible.

Clinical features

Important factors in early diagnosis of melanoma

In order for the healthcare professional to make a clinical diagnosis of a possible melanoma as early in its course as possible, he/she must have a high index of suspicion for melanoma and a thorough knowledge of:

- The clinical features of early melanomas

- The clinical features of common pigmented lesions which must be differentiated from melanoma

- The characteristics and clinical features of variants of clinically atypical melanocytic nevi (*dysplastic nevi*) which may be more commonly seen in association with a higher risk for and/or association with melanoma

- Other factors that increase the risk for a patient developing melanoma (personal and/or family history of melanoma, presence of *dysplastic* nevi, presence of many (>100) melanocytic nevi, history of excessive sunburns, especially in childhood/adolescence, red/blonde hair, light eyes, fair complexion, freckling, etc.).

It is important that the healthcare professional alert such patients to a potential increased risk for melanoma and appropriately educate these patients in the early detection of melanoma, including self-examination.

Clinical characteristics of early melanoma

The clinically diagnostic features of early malignant melanoma are similar regardless of anatomic site.[15,31] The healthcare professional must keep in mind that while the clinical features of early melanoma to be described are generally present in most lesions, there are exceptions which need to be recognized. The vast majority of melanomas follow the *ABCD* rule originally described by our group at NYU in 1985.[13] In a currently ongoing clinical study[32] of some 200 patients having histologically proven melanoma, 91% of the clinical lesions had all of the ABCD clinical features. A smaller number of patients had lesions smaller than 6 mm in diameter, the smallest being 3.2 mm. Most lesions <6 mm in diameter were *in situ*, but several were minimally invasive to a maximum thickness of 0.58 mm. A few patients had amelanotic lesions and one patient had a small lesion lacking any of the ABCDs. Similar studies by others[33–38] have illustrated some of the other *exceptions* to the ABCD rule. However, the vast majority of early melanomas can be identified using the ABCD rule with the understanding that an important clue to diagnosis, regardless of actual diameter of the lesion, is a change (increase) in the diameter of any given lesion over time.

Thus, most early melanomas are (have):

- *Asymmetric* – they generally cannot be easily divided in half and have one half look like the other (Fig. 14.1).

- *Border irregularity* – the borders of most early melanomas are irregularly shaped (Fig. 14.2).

- *Color variability* – (Fig. 14.3) most early melanomas have a play in color ranging from subtle nuances of tans and browns, to areas of black and more rarely red, white (regression) and blue (deeper pigment). Keep in mind, most amelanotic melanomas will lack the play in color usually seen in pigmented melanomas. Sometimes, however, there may be some subtle pigmentation within the lesion, which helps the observer in making a diagnosis.

- *Diameter* – most early melanomas when they are clinically readily identified are ≥6 mm in diameter

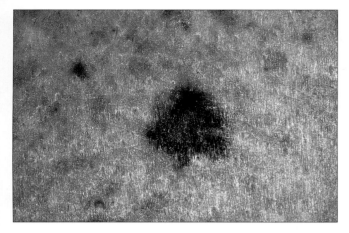

Figure 14.1 Malignant melanoma, *in situ,* chest illustrating significant clinical *asymmetry,* along with border irregularity and subtle variability in color. The lesion measures 7.2 mm in diameter.

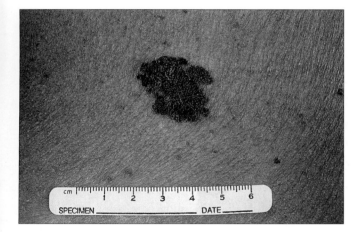

Figure 14.2 Malignant melanoma, predominantly *in situ,* but focally measuring approximately 0.22 mm in greatest thickness, trunk, illustrating classic *border irregularity*, coupled with lesion asymmetry and very subtle play in color from dark brown/black to medium brown. The lesion measures about 13 mm in greatest diameter. (Image courtesy of New York University Department of Dermatology.)

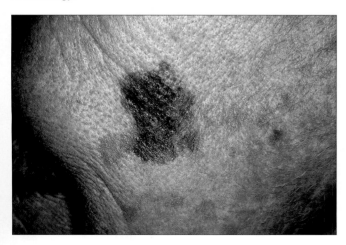

Figure 14.3 Malignant melanoma, predominantly *in situ* of face illustrating a play in color from tan to brown with a focal amelanotic (pink/red) component. There was a focal dermal component to this lesion measuring about 0.18 mm in thickness. The lesion is quite large measuring over 20 mm in diameter. It also exhibits lesion asymmetry and border irregularity. (Image courtesy of New York University Department of Dermatology.)

(Fig. 14.4). It is important to remember that all melanomas have a microscopic origin of one or more neoplastic melanocytes. Thus, there is a stage in the early evolution of melanoma where one or more of the ABCD criteria may be lacking. The most common missing criterion will be the *D,* in that a few melanomas will have diameters ≤6 mm. Thus, a good clue to an otherwise atypical pigmented lesion is remembering that malignant neoplasms *change over time.* Even in a smaller lesion, *a change in diameter over time in the presence of other clinically atypical features should arouse the observer's index of suspicion* (Fig 14.5).

A few clinical examples of the progression of melanoma from its early evolution to a more advanced lesion are illustrated (Figs 14.6 and 14.7) for comparison. While most of the more advanced lesions can be diagnosed using the ABCD rule, rare exceptions again exist for so-called *nodular* melanomas, for amelanotic melanomas, and a few other smaller melanomas. Keep in mind that healthcare professionals need to remind their patients that the more advanced lesions, while usually recognizable clinically, are associated with much poorer prognoses. In the educational process, we have found that illustrating the more advanced lesions is a helpful tool in that it emphasizes the importance of early detection (excellent prognosis with simple surgical intervention) of melanoma *vs* the detection of more advanced lesions (poor prognosis with complex surgical and oncologic intervention).

The early clinical diagnosis of melanoma has its basis not only in the clinical appearance of the lesion (physical examination), but also on the history and symptomatology. Change in a pre-existing melanocytic lesion or the development of a new pigmented lesion later in life (after the age of 40) are important features which should alert the patient to seek medical care, and the physician to use his/her skills and ancillary

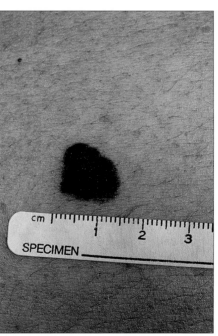

Figure 14.4
Malignant melanoma, trunk, measuring nearly 14 mm in diameter. The lesion was present for at least 2 years and was slowly growing. It measures about 0.4 mm in greatest thickness, with a sizeable component of the lesion still *in situ*. It too exhibits subtle asymmetry and border irregularity. There are subtle variations in pigmentation from brown to dark brown. (Image courtesy of New York University Department of Dermatology.)

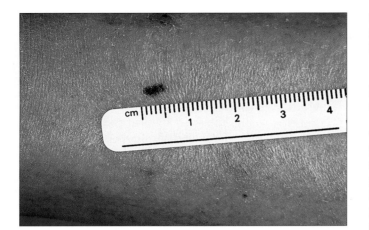

Figure 14.5 A small, approximately 4.5 mm in diameter pigmented macule of the leg which appeared within 6 months of biopsy as a small dark brown spot and grew to its current size over 3–4 months. The change in diameter prompted the patient to see a physician. Biopsy revealed a very early evolving melanoma, *in situ* in a lesion exhibiting subtle asymmetry of growth, irregularity of its border and color variability. This lesion is associated with 100% survival. (Image courtesy of New York University Department of Dermatology.)

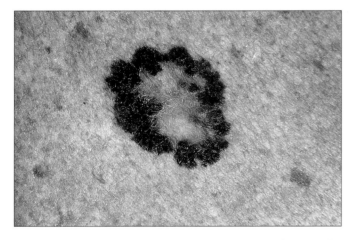

Figure 14.6 A large melanoma of the trunk present for several years exhibiting the ABCDs despite its plaque-like elevation peripherally and its rather dramatic zone of regression (pink-red) centrally. This lesion is associated with a poor prognosis. (Image courtesy of New York University Department of Dermatology.)

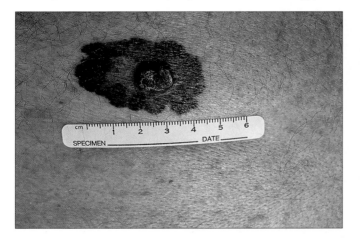

Figure 14.7 This large 4.5 cm plaque-like melanoma with nodule formation of the trunk again exhibits the ABCDs although more advanced. It is associated with a very poor prognosis. (Image courtesy of New York University Department of Dermatology.)

technologies to rule out the possibility of a melanoma. Other clinical *danger signs* seen in some melanomas are illustrated in Table 14.1.

Patient evaluation, diagnosis and differential diagnosis

The detection of early melanoma requires a partnership between the healthcare professional and the patient. Clearly, the patient has the opportunity on a daily basis to examine his/her skin, while the healthcare professional is limited to the one or two times per year that the patient may come into the office for a total cutaneous examination.

Thus, the successful partnership requires an initial extended visit whereby the healthcare professional and patient can discuss in depth the important issues of: (1) early detection of melanoma in terms of saving lives; (2) the salient clinical features that help distinguish benign melanocytic lesions and other non-melanocytic simulants from melanoma; (3) the art and skill of performing self-examination (discussed later in this chapter).

The healthcare professional must practice state-of-the-art medicine as relates to the clinical diagnosis of melanoma. This includes understanding the clinical features of melanoma, including the exceptional cases that do not fit into the norm, as well as the differential diagnosis of pigmented lesions of the skin. While in many cases, the differential diagnosis of melanoma can be done on the basis of clinical features alone, the use of both clinical total body imaging/photography and dermoscopy can be very useful adjuncts to accurate diagnosis.

Table 14.1 Clinical signs suggestive of malignant melanoma
Change in color Especially multiple shades of dark brown or black; red, white and blue; spread of color from the edge of the lesion into surrounding skin.
Change in size Especially sudden or continuous enlargement.
Change in shape Especially development of irregular margins.
Change in elevation Especially sudden elevation of a previously macular pigmented lesion.
Change in surface Especially scaliness, erosion, oozing, crusting, ulceration, bleeding.
Change in surrounding skin Especially redness, swelling, satellite pigmentations.
Change in sensation Especially itching, tenderness, pain.
Change in consistency Especially softening or friability.

The differential diagnosis of early melanoma

Common benign pigmented lesions

- *Simple lentigo* – a small (1–5 mm) pigmented macule. It is the initial stage of development of a common nevus (mole). The simple lentigo is a sharply defined, brown to black pigmented macule with regular or jagged edges that may appear anywhere on the surface of the skin. The pigmentation oftentimes has a reticulated (net-like) pattern. Such a lesion generally arises in childhood, but may appear later in life. Some simple lentigines are clinically indistinguishable from junctional nevi.

- *Junctional nevus* – a small (<6 mm) well circumscribed, pigmented macule, generally with a smooth surface, uniform pigmentation ranging from tan-light to brown to darker brown or even black. It may appear on any skin surface, but usually is seen on areas exposed to UV light. A junctional nevus usually appears during childhood, however may also be seen to occur in adolescence and young adulthood (<40). It may remain flat (junctional) throughout adult life or may undergo evolution into a compound or intradermal nevus as its cells proliferate and extend into the subjacent dermis. It is rare for a junctional nevus to develop in adults over the age of 40. Thus, both patients and their physicians should be alert for any new macular lesions appearing and growing in patients after the age of 40. Such lesions may actually represent early evolving melanomas.

- *Compound nevus* – generally a well circumscribed, small (<6 mm) slightly to substantially raised papule which is mostly uniformly pigmented with a range of color from skin colored, to tan to brown with either a rough or smooth surface. It may have hairs associated with it (which sometimes indicates a congenital origin). It usually develops in late childhood, adolescence, or early adulthood (<40).

- *Intradermal nevus* – generally a small (<6 mm), well circumscribed papule with generally uniform pigmentation from skin colored to tan to brown. They too, may be hypertrichotic and have either smooth or rough surfaces.

- *Solar lentigo* – generally a uniform tan to brown macule, but may have some play in color and thus may simulate melanoma, known to the lay public as a *liver spot*. It is found on sun-exposed skin in people with excessive sun exposure history.

- There may also be a genetic susceptibility in some patients. Common sites include the face, chest, dorsa of the hands and legs.

- *Seborrheic keratosis* – generally a verrucous round to ovoid, variably raised, light to darker brown to sometimes black, sharply demarcated papule, plaque or rarely nodule that varies in diameter from a few millimeters to several centimeters. It usually has a *dull* or *warty* surface and, oftentimes, has a *stuck-on* appearance. Seborrheic keratoses are found at the same sites as solar lentigines and are the end-stage in the development of such lesions. They oftentimes have a genetic component to their etiology. They are composed predominantly of proliferating keratinocytes and are *not* primarily melanocytic in origin.[14]

The differential diagnosis of pigmented lesions related to patient age

It is important to consider the age of the patient when making a differential diagnosis of a clinically pigmented lesion. It is rare for a child to develop a melanoma,[14,39–41] although such may be the case more frequently in familial melanoma. Other circumstances where melanomas are seen in childhood are those in which the melanoma arises in association with a congenital nevus (usually of the giant type).[42–46]

Ephelides (freckles), simple lentigines and junctional nevi are the most commonly identified pigmented lesions in children, a rarer variant of melanocytic nevus. The Spitz nevus can also be found in children. This lesion, if removed, shares some features in common with melanoma and should be diagnosed only by pathologists having extensive experience with this type of nevus.

Compound nevi generally develop in later childhood and adolescence, while intradermal nevi more commonly develop in young adulthood. The non-melanocytic pigmented lesions of the skin which can sometimes simulate melanoma, namely the solar lentigo and seborrheic keratosis, usually develop later in life (>35).

Melanoma is rare in childhood and increases with advancing age.[46–48] While the mean age for presentation of melanoma is about 50, any new pigmented lesion not fulfilling the criteria for diagnosis of the previously noted benign pigmented lesions in patients >40 should be a suspect for melanoma[47] or a *dysplastic* nevus (see below).

Atypical (dysplastic) nevi in the differential diagnosis of melanoma

There is increasing evidence[49–51] in the scientific literature that the presence in patients of certain clinically atypical melanocytic nevi (*dysplastic* nevi), may portend a higher risk for developing melanoma in such patients.[52–60] Furthermore, some of the *dysplastic* nevi themselves may develop melanoma within them (Fig. 14.8). Certainly, in many instances, these clinically atypical nevi may be difficult, if not impossible to distinguish from melanoma. In such cases, the health-care professional must call upon a number of useful adjuncts to diagnosis in making a decision as to whether any given lesion should be biopsied to rule out melanoma. These adjuncts include: (1) clinical experience, (2) comparison to prior photographs/digital images, (3) dermoscopy.[61,62] Issues related to dysplastic nevi are reviewed in depth in Chapter 16. We do not currently have all of the answers to the many questions which may arise in the determination of the differential diagnosis between melanoma and some *dysplastic* nevi. In such cases, where any question about diagnosis exists, an appropriate biopsy is mandatory.

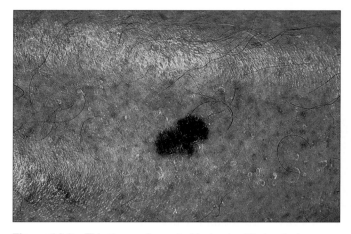

Figure 14.8   This 7 mm pigmented lesion had its beginnings with the uniformly brown pigmented lesion at the left lower portion of this clinical photograph. The darker brown, slightly asymmetric lesion with irregular borders at the upper right edge of the photograph developed over the past 5 or 6 months. Biopsy revealed a very early melanoma in situ arising in association with a compound melanocytic nevus having features of so-called *dysplastic* nevus.

Pathology of early melanoma

The vast majority of melanomas in the skin begin with a proliferation of single melanocytes along the dermo–epidermal junction.[15,31,63] However, the malignant changes of very early melanoma *in situ* may neither be apparent to the clinician ('too small') nor to the pathologist ('insufficient reproducible histologic criteria').

A melanoma of 1–2 mm in diameter may consist only of a small focus of an increased number of relatively normal appearing single melanocytes mostly along the dermo–epidermal junction. Clinically, such lesions may appear as a subtle tan-brown small macule with not much else to distinguish it as a tiny evolving melanoma. In time, a few cytologically atypical melanocytes may appear within the epidermis, again, mostly confined to the lower epidermis. These atypical melanocytes do not have a clinical counterpart. Thus, the small (<3 mm) melanoma *in situ* may clinically look like a slowly growing tan-brown macule with very subtle asymmetry of growth and border (the *A and B of the ABCDs*). As the evolution of the melanoma continues, a few melanocytes may be seen at higher levels of the epidermis and small nests may be present at and slightly above the dermo–epidermal junction. Single melanocytes usually predominate over nests.

The clinical counterpart of a 3–4 mm melanoma may vary from a lesion with subtle asymmetry (*A*) and a subtly irregular border (*B*), now with a bit more play in color (*C*) (usually subtle nuances of tan and brown) secondary to pigment within melanocytes at somewhat higher levels of the epidermis. These lesions may also demonstrate increased pigment within the nests of melanocytes both along the dermo–epidermal junction and somewhat above it. In some lesions, pigment-laden melanocytes may be present at higher levels of the epidermis, even into the cornified layer, giving a dark brown or even black appearance to parts of the lesion.

Keep in mind that while the clinical features of an evolving melanoma are much more apparent once the lesion measures ≥6 mm in diameter (*D*), in fact the lesion is subtly increasing in diameter from the point in time that it becomes clinically visible until such time that it develops enough of the clinical features which lead the observer to make a clinical diagnosis of melanoma. Thus the *change in diameter* (*D*) of any given pigmented lesion may be as important as the diameter itself.

After some variable amount of time (dependent on a number of factors including intrinsic tumor biology, host-immunologic response, etc.) and usually after the make-up of the neoplastic melanocytes is such that nests of melanocytes now predominate over single cells, atypical melanocytes may extend into the papillary dermis. Once the cells of the melanoma are in the dermis, the neoplasm generally continues to grow in a three-dimensional fashion, increasing in size both circumferentially, as well as in depth. At some point in this evolution, the neoplasm develops the competence for metastasis and may thus spread to other areas of the body eventually leading to the death of the patient.

While invasion (descent of the melanocytes of a melanoma from the epidermis into the subjacent dermis) may occur relatively early in the evolution of a melanoma (4 or 5 mm in diameter), many melanomas most certainly remain confined to the epidermis (*in situ*) for many months, years, or in some cases, for decades. Thus, one may see an *in situ* melanoma measuring 6 mm, 10 mm, 16 mm or, in some cases for melanomas of sun damaged skin of the head and neck ≥30 mm in diameter. The histology of these larger diameter melanomas oftentimes are seen with atypical melanocytes, arranged both singly and in nests throughout the epidermis, including extension far down epithelial adnexal structures. Regardless of their size, however, these wholly intra-epidermal melanomas are 100% curable as long as they are completely removed.

Maize and Ackerman[31] outlined the following histologic features (which correlate to the clinical ABCDs) of evolving melanoma (Fig. 14.9):

- Breadth usually greater than 6 mm by the time that the biopsy specimen had been taken.

- Asymmetry of growth of the neoplastic melanocytes (contributes to clinical asymmetry and enlarging diameter of the lesion).

- Poor circumscription – atypical melanocytes arranged as solitary units above the dermo–epidermal junction extend beyond the most peripheral discrete nest of melanocytes within the epidermis (contributes to both clinical asymmetry, border irregularity and enlarging diameter of the lesion).

- Increased number of single atypical melanocytes within the epidermis and epidermal adnexal structures, with single cells oftentimes predominating over nests (contributes to subtle play in clinical color of the lesion).

- Buck-shot scatter of melanocytes within the upper levels of the epidermis (contribute to the variation in browns and even black within the lesion).

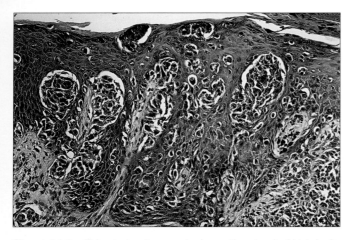

Figure 14.9 This photomicrograph shows the classical histologic changes of melanoma within the epidermis, namely: an increased number of single and nested melanocytes, some with cytologically atypical nuclei, arranged both along the dermo–epidermal junction and throughout all levels of the epidermis. The nests of melanocytes tend to vary in their sizes and shapes and focally tend toward confluence. Melanocytes are seen high up in the epidermis, even into the cornified layer. Single and nested atypical melanocytes can also be seen in the subjacent dermis. (× 250)

- Nests of melanocytes within the epidermis not equidistant (contributes to variation in clinical color).

- Variation in sizes and shapes of melanocytes (contributes to variation in clinical color of lesion).

- Irregularity in the shape of nests of melanocytes.

- Tendency of nests of melanocytes to confluence (contributes to concentration of pigmentation and thus, color changes).

For early *invasive* melanomas:

- Failure of maturation of atypical melanocytes with progressive descent into the dermis (contributes to clinical elevation of lesion, but not a sign of early, curable melanoma).

- Asymmetrical, patchy distribution of melanin pigment within the neoplasm (contributes to clinical play in color, including 'blue' in deeper lesions).

- Extension of atypical melanocytes far down epithelial structures of adnexa (in some cases).

- Asymmetrical distribution of inflammatory cell infiltrates (including melanophages) of variable densities with the neoplasm and at its base (contributes to clinical color variability, including browns, red, white and blue).

In sum, melanoma has its beginnings within the epidermis and may be difficult to diagnose both clinically and histologically until it reaches a certain size (≥6 mm). The clinical ABCD criteria have their basis in the histologic features seen in most evolving melanomas. Thus, in some circumstances, it is possible to clinically identify a lesion as probable melanoma substituting 'diameter enlarging' for the *D* of the ABCDs. It is important to realize that there will be exceptions to some of the rules (both clinical and histologic) some of the time. Clinical judgment and the use of newer technologies (imaging, dermoscopy, computerized image analysis)[64–66] may be helpful in such circumstances.

Treatment

The first step in diagnosis – the clinical examination

Dr Neville Davis eloquently stated, 'unlike other cancers, which are generally hidden from view, malignant melanoma writes its message in the skin with its own ink and it is there for all of us to see. Some see, but do not comprehend'.[67] It should be the goal of all those interested in skin cancer to help *everyone* from the highly trained surgical, medical and dermatologic oncologist, to the general dermatologist, plastic surgeon, general surgeon, obstetrician, ophthalmologist, internist, family practitioner, to the physician's assistant, nurse practitioner, registered nurse, to the podiatrist, the chiropractor, the beautician, barber, the lay public and anyone else who has the opportunity to look at the skin *to see, to comprehend and to act!*

Early detection of female breast cancer is made easier by examinations by their physicians and frequent self-examination by the patients themselves. Similarly, if melanoma is to be identified early in its evolution when it is small and curable, a partnership between the healthcare professional and the patient must occur. Complete and thorough total cutaneous examination should be done on all patients annually and in higher risk patients more frequently. Patients should be educated as to the clinical features of melanoma and on how to do self-examination of the skin.

Examination of the skin by the healthcare professional

The first step in the evaluation and examination of the skin centers on a thorough history which includes the following:

- General medical history

- Personal or family history of skin cancer, including melanoma

- Personal or family history of increased number of nevi (>100)

- Personal or family history of atypical (*dysplastic*) nevi

- Pharmaceutical history/drug allergies

- Social history, including sun exposure/sunburns during childhood and young adult life *vs* sun exposure currently.

Physical examination of the skin

The equipment required for physical examination of the skin consists of: (1) examination table (preferably one that allows the patient to lie flat), (2) source of bright light, (3) magnifying lens (2–4×), and (4) dermatoscope (for those physicians adept at dermoscopy).[3,13,14] The patient should be placed on the examination table with proper draping in place. When appropriate, it is advis-

able to have a nurse present during the examination of sensitive areas of the body. The patient should lie on the examination table and the entire anterior surface of the body, including the intertriginous areas, should be closely examined for the presence of any skin cancers/pigmented lesions. If the female patient wishes, examination of the genital areas can be done by their gynecologist with the understanding that the gynecologist will report any findings to the physician responsible for the skin examination.

Next, examine the entire posterior aspect of the body (including the intertriginous areas). The feet and hands should also be thoroughly examined, including areas between the toes and fingers. Be sure to examine the nailbeds for any evidence of skin cancer, including any abnormal pigmentation such as melanonychia striata (Fig. 14.10), which may indicate a nail matrix-based melanoma.

The scalp should also be thoroughly examined. There are two methods for thoroughly examining the scalp. One uses an ordinary blow dryer on a cool setting to better visualize the scalp. The other method is what we call the 'digital-visual' exam, uses the fingers to separate the hair and to palpate the scalp for any palpable lesions, coupled with a thorough visual exam of the surface of the scalp.

Any suspicious lesions should be carefully evaluated. Our group at NYU School of Medicine utilizes baseline total body digital photography for patients having many atypical nevi and/or a family history of melanoma. Such a system is helpful both for the patient and for the examining physician in terms of identifying new or changing pigmented lesions. In such cases, we utilize dermoscopy to help in the clinical classification of any pigmented lesion in question. Any lesion suggestive of melanoma is subject to biopsy *in toto*.

We recommend a complete annual examination of the skin by a physician for everyone, supplemented by additional physician-based examinations for those patients at higher risk for melanoma (personal history of melanoma, personal/family history of *dysplastic nevi* and family history of melanoma). Further, in such patients, it is recommended that a comprehensive program of patient education including a monthly self-examination be employed.

Self-examination of the skin

Routine self-examination of the skin is inexpensive (free), non-invasive, and lacks any danger. In our experience, it is important for the high risk patient to play a role and take some responsibility for his/her care as relates to the early detection of melanoma.[3,13,14] Performed correctly, the self-examination process reinforces the educational experience which occurs in the physicians' office at the time of the semi-annual or annual total cutaneous exam (Figs 14.11–14.18). In addition to the use of visual aids and information on self-examination, because we use digital photography, a copy of the digital photographs is given to the patient for use during the self-examination process. We find the use of a visual benchmark to be a great importance in terms of patient compliance. All patients are encouraged to call the office should they detect any new or changing lesions, which

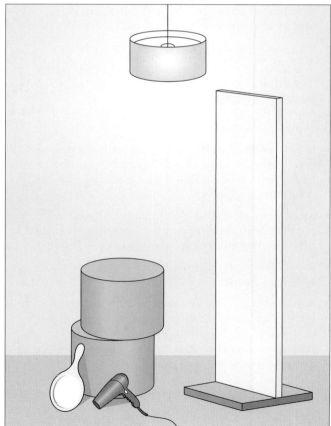

Figure 14.11 Make sure the room is well-lit and that you have nearby a full-length mirror, a hand-held mirror, a hand-held blow dryer and two chairs or stools. Undress completely. (Adapted from Friedman RJ, *et al.* Early detection of malignant melanoma: The role of physician-examination and self-examination of the skin. CA Cancer J Clin 1985; 35:130–151.)

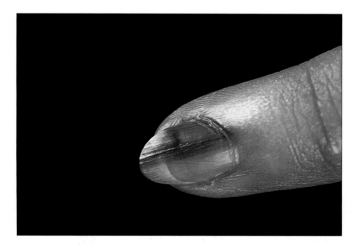

Figure 14.10 Melanonychia striata with subtle Hutchinson's sign at proximal nail fold. This melanoma *in situ* (on biopsy) is a clear exception to the ABCD rule. The clue to the diagnosis is a longitudinal band of pigmentation (of varying color in this patient) which has increased (historically) in width over time. The presence of a Hutchinson sign is key to making the diagnosis of melanoma (*vs* nevus) in this patient. The biopsy should be taken from the nail matrix.

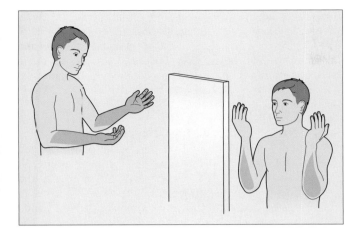

Figure 14.12   *Left*: Hold your hands with the palms face up, as shown in the drawing. Look at your palms, fingers, spaces between the fingers and forearms. Then turn your hands over and examine the backs of your hands, fingers, spaces between the fingers, fingernails, and forearms. *Right*: Now position yourself in front of the full-length mirror. Hold up your arms, bent at the elbows, with your palms facing you. In the mirror, look at the backs of your forearms and elbow. (Adapted from Friedman RJ, *et al*. Early detection of malignant melanoma: The role of physician-examination and self-examination of the skin. CA Cancer J Clin 1985; 35:130–151.)

they suspect might be melanoma. Earlier intervention, including biopsy, can then take place if indicated.

A thorough self-examination of the skin requires the patient to undress completely and, in the absence of a *partner* who can assist in the examination, a full-length mirror, a hand-held mirror, a hand-held blow dryer, two chairs and a well-lit room. Immediately after bathing is a good time for the examination. In women, we recommend that the self-examination occur at the same time that they are practicing self-examination of the breast.

The first few times, the patient should spend some time inspecting the entire surface of the skin. With experience, however, the self-examination should take but a few minutes. To visualize parts of the skin surface that may otherwise be difficult to see (e.g. some areas of the back, scalp and buttocks), the patient may find it helpful to elicit the help of a partner.

The self-examination process should be done in a stepwise fashion, as illustrated in Figures 14.11–14.18.[3,13,14] The patient should be advised to see his/her healthcare professional if there are any newly discovered or significantly changing lesions.

It is important to note that most melanomas are macular and grow in diameter for some time before they

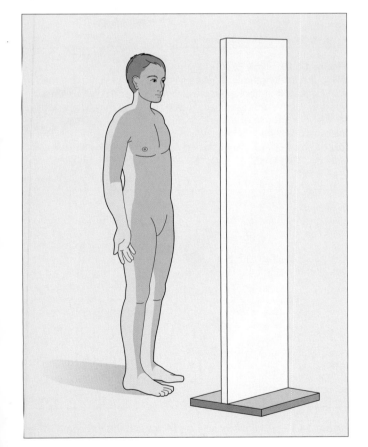

Figure 14.13   Again using the full-length mirror, observe the entire front of your body. In turn, look at your face, neck, and arms. Turn your palms to face the mirror and look at your upper arms. Then look at your chest and abdomen, pubic area, thighs and lower legs. (Adapted from Friedman RJ, *et al*. Early detection of malignant melanoma: The role of physician-examination and self-examination of the skin. CA Cancer J Clin 1985; 35:130–151.)

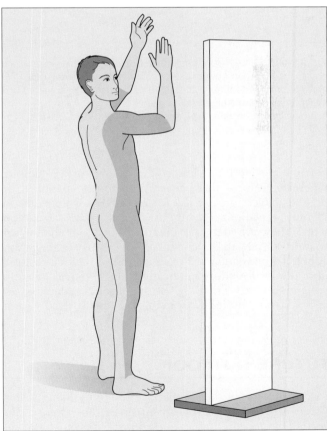

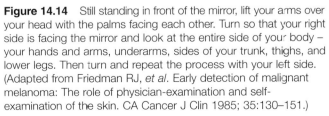

Figure 14.14   Still standing in front of the mirror, lift your arms over your head with the palms facing each other. Turn so that your right side is facing the mirror and look at the entire side of your body – your hands and arms, underarms, sides of your trunk, thighs, and lower legs. Then turn and repeat the process with your left side. (Adapted from Friedman RJ, *et al*. Early detection of malignant melanoma: The role of physician-examination and self-examination of the skin. CA Cancer J Clin 1985; 35:130–151.)

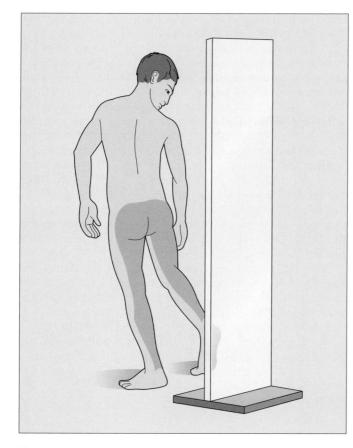

Figure 14.15 With your back toward the full-length mirror, look at your buttocks and the backs of your thighs and lower legs. (Adapted from Friedman RJ, *et al*. Early detection of malignant melanoma: The role of physician-examination and self-examination of the skin. CA Cancer J Clin 1985; 35:130–151.)

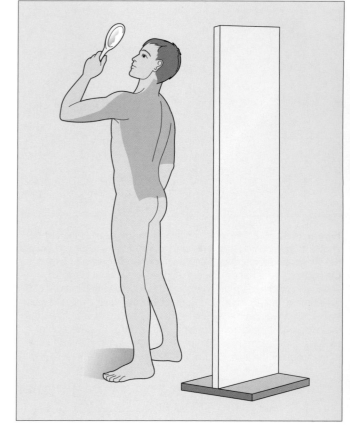

Figure 14.16 Now pick up the hand-held mirror. With your back still to the full-length mirror, examine the back of your neck, and your back and buttocks. Also examine the backs of your arms in this way. Some areas are hard to see, and you may find it helpful to ask your spouse or a friend to assist you. (Adapted from Friedman RJ, *et al*. Early detection of malignant melanoma: The role of physician-examination and self-examination of the skin. CA Cancer J Clin 1985; 35:130–151.)

become elevated. Flat lesions are nearly always curable, whereas lesions that develop plaques, papules or nodules have a greater risk for metastases. The goal is to identify melanomas early in their biologic evolution when they are flat and curable. The combination of routine physician-driven total cutaneous examination coupled with regular self-examination provides a realistic opportunity for the identification and removal of early melanomas, resulting in a significant reduction in morbidity and mortality from this potentially deadly form of skin cancer.

FUTURE OUTLOOK

Early detection of melanoma is a key to the cure of this potentially deadly neoplasm. At times, however, it can be difficult to differentiate melanoma from other clinical simulants, including so-called *dysplastic* nevi. Diagnostic accuracy can sometimes be improved through the use of dermoscopy,[62,64,68] but this technique may be difficult to learn and should only be used in those well skilled in this diagnostic tool. An important adjunctive medical device, which may prove to be vital in the clinical diagnosis of melanoma, is the use of computerized

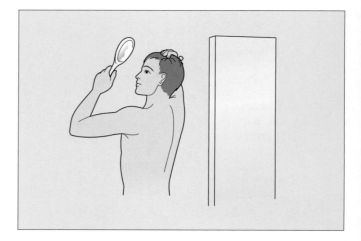

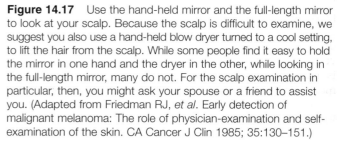

Figure 14.17 Use the hand-held mirror and the full-length mirror to look at your scalp. Because the scalp is difficult to examine, we suggest you also use a hand-held blow dryer turned to a cool setting, to lift the hair from the scalp. While some people find it easy to hold the mirror in one hand and the dryer in the other, while looking in the full-length mirror, many do not. For the scalp examination in particular, then, you might ask your spouse or a friend to assist you. (Adapted from Friedman RJ, *et al*. Early detection of malignant melanoma: The role of physician-examination and self-examination of the skin. CA Cancer J Clin 1985; 35:130–151.)

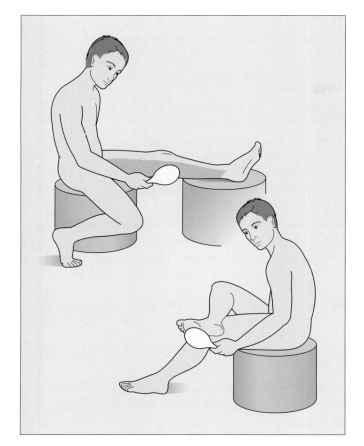

Figure 14.18 *Top:* Sit down and prop up one leg on a chair or stool in front of you as shown. Using the hand-held mirror, examine the inside of the propped-up leg, beginning at the groin area and moving the mirror down the leg to your foot. Repeat the procedure for your other leg. *Bottom*: Still sitting, cross one leg over the other. Use the hand-held mirror to examine the top of your foot, the toes, toenails, and spaces between the toes. Then look at the sole or bottom of your foot. Repeat the procedure for the other foot. (Adapted from Friedman RJ, *et al*. Early detection of malignant melanoma: The role of physician-examination and self-examination of the skin. CA Cancer J Clin 1985; 35:130–151.)

image analysis. Several such instruments are currently in clinical trials and recent evidence[64–66] suggests that computerized image analysis can improve the evaluation of pigmented skin lesions by identifying those lesions which might ordinarily have been missed using standard clinical tools, but are, in fact, early melanomas. This approach is discussed in further depth in Chapter 36.

The twenty-first century will most certainly be the time when we develop a thorough understanding of the pathobiology of melanoma. In the very near future, however, through the use of simple educational tools, including physician and patient education, routine physician-driven and patient-driven total cutaneous examinations, and through more complex tools such as dermoscopy, computerized image analysis, and real-time computerized image analysis of dermoscopic images, it is likely that we can succeed in our goal to reduce mortality from melanoma significantly.

Let us all heed the advice of Dr Neville Davis[67] and look for the signature of melanoma written in its own ink. It is there for all of us to see and to understand and it should be the goal of every healthcare professional to learn and teach to our patients the early clues to diagnosis. If we are successful, we can reduce the death rate from melanoma to near zero.

REFERENCES

1 Jemal A, Tiwari RC, Murray T, et al. Cancer Statistics 2004; CA Cancer J Clin 2004; 54:8–29.

2 Kopf AW, Rigel DS, Friedman RJ. The rising incidence and mortality rate of malignant melanoma. J Derm Surg Oncol 1982; 8:760–761.

3 Friedman RJ, Rigel DS, Silverman MK, et al. Malignant melanoma in the 1990s: The continued importance of early detection and the role of physician examination and self-examination of the skin. CA Cancer J Clin 1991; 41:201–226.

4 Ries LA, Hankey BS, Edwards BK. Cancer Statistics Review 1973–1978. NIH Publication No 90-2789. Division of Cancer Prevention and Control, National Cancer Institute, 1990.

5 Rigel DS, Kopf AW, Fredman RJ. The rate of malignant melanoma in the United States: Are we making an impact? J Am Acad Derm 1987; 17:1050–1053.

6 American Cancer Society. 1989 survey of physician's attitudes and practices in early cancer detection. CA Cancer J Clin 1990; 40:77–101.

7 Kopf AW. Prevention and early detection of skin cancer/melanoma. Cancer 1988; 62(8):1791–1795.

8 Mihm MC Jr, Fitzpatrick TB, Brown MM, et al. Early detection of primary cutaneous malignant melanoma: a color atlas. N Eng J Med 1973; 289:989–996.

9 Ackerman AB. Clinical diagnosis of malignant melanoma in situ. In: Ackerman AB, ed. Pathology of Malignant Melanoma. New York: Masson 1981:57–58.

10 Sober AJ, Fitzpatrick TB, Mihm MC Jr, et al. Early recognition of cutaneous melanoma. JAMA 1979; 242:2795–2799.

11 Breslow A. Prognostic factors in the treatment of cutaneous melanoma. J Cutan Pathol 1979; 6:208–212.

12 Clark WH Jr, From L, Bernardino E, et al. The histogenesis and biologic behavior of primary human malignant melanomas of the skin. Cancer Res 1969; 29:705–727.

13 Friedman RJ, Rigel DS, Kopf AW. Early detection of malignant melanoma: The role of physician examination and self-examination of the skin. CA Cancer J Clin 1985; 35:130–151.

14 Friedman RJ, Rigel DS, Kopf AW. Early detection of malignant melanoma: The role of physician examination and self-examination of the skin. In: Friedman RJ, Rigel DS, Kopf AW et al. Cancer of the Skin. Philadelphia, PA: WB Saunders; 1991:117–124.

15 Ackerman AB. Malignant melanoma: A unifying concept. Hum Pathol 1980; 11:591.

16 Breslow A. Thickness, cross sectional area and dept of invasion in the prognosis of cutaneous melanoma. Ann Surg 1970; 172:902–908.

17 Clark WH, Jr. Clinical diagnosis of cutaneous melanoma (editorial). JAMA 1976; 236:484.

18 Balch CM, Murad TM, Soong SJ, et al. A multifactorial analysis of melanoma: Prognostic histopathologic features comparing Clark's and Breslow's staging methods. Ann Surg 1978; 188:732–742.

19 Balch CM, Milton GW, Shaw HM, et al. Cutaneous Melanoma. Clinical Management and Treatment Results Worldwide. Philadelphia: JB Lippincott; 1985:63–70.

20 Breslow A, Cascinelli N, van der Esch EP, et al. Stage I melanoma of the limbs: assessment of prognosis by levels of invasion and maximal thickness. Tumori 1978; 64:273–281.

21 Day CL Jr, Sober AJ, Kopf AW, et al. A prognostic model for clinical Stage I melanoma of the trunk. Am J Surg 1981; 142:247–254.

22 Funk W, Schmoeckel C, Holzel D, et al. Prognostic classification of malignant melanoma by clinical criteria. Br J Derm 1984; 111:1129–1135.

23 McGovern VJ, Shaw HM, Milton GW, et al. Prognostic significance of the histologic features of malignant melanoma. Histopathology 1979; 3:385–393.

24 Wick MM, Sober AJ, Fitzpatrick TJ, et al. Clinical characteristics of early cutaneous melanoma. Cancer 1980; 45:2684–2691.

25 Rigel DS, Friedman RJ, Kopf AW, et al. Factors influencing survival in melanoma. Derm Clinics 1991:631–642.

26 DiFronzo LA, Wanek LA, Morton DL. Earlier diagnosis of second primary melanoma confirms the benefits of patient education and routine postoperative follow-up. Cancer 2001; 91:1520–1524.

27 Rigel DS, Carucci JA. Malignant melanoma: prevention, early detection, and treatment in the 21st century. CA Cancer J Clin 2000; 50:215–236.

28 National Center for Health Statistics. Division of Vital Statistics, Centers for Disease Control. National Center for Health Statistics, 2003. http://www.cdc,gov/nchs/nvss.htm.

29 Manual of the International Statistical Classification of Diseases. Injuries and Causes of Death, Vol. 1, 10th revision. Geneva, Switzerland: World Health Organization; 1992:1.

30 Perry C, Holten V Van, Muir C (eds). International Classification of Diseases for Oncology, 2nd edn. Geneva, Switzerland: World Health Organization; 1990.

31 Maize JC, Ackerman AB. Malignant Melanoma, in Pigmented Lesions of the Skin. Philadelphia: Lea & Febiger 1986:165–223.

32 Friedman RJ, Unpublished observations, 2003.

33 Shaw HM, McCarthy WH. Small-diameter malignant melanoma: A common diagnosis in New South Wales, Australia. J Am Acad Derm 1992; 27:679–682.

34 Schmoeckel C. Small malignant melanomas: clinicopathologic correlation and DNA ploidy analysis. J Am Acad Derm 1991; 24:1037.

35 Bergman R, Katz I, Lichtig C, et al. Malignant melanomas with histologic diameters less than 6 mm. J Am Acad Derm 1992; 26:462–466.

36 Kamino H, Kiryu H, Ratech H. Small malignant melanomas: clinicopathologic correlation and DNA ploidy analysis. J Am Acad Derm 1990; 22:1032–1038.

37 Howell JB. Spotting sinister spots. J Am Acad Derm 1986; 15:722–726.

38 Gonzalez A, West AJ, Pitha JV et al. Small diameter invasive melanomas: Clinical and pathologic characteristics. J Cutan Pathol 1996; 23:126–132.

39 Kopf AW, Mart RS, Rodriguez-Saints et al. (eds) In: Malignant Melanoma New York: Masson; 1979:152–153.

40 Loyal D. Malignant melanoma in infancy. JAMA 1967; 202:1153.

41 Trozac DJ, Rowland WD, Hu F. Metastatic malignant melanoma in prepubertal children. Pediatrics 1975; 55:191–196.

42 Kaplan EN. The risk of malignancy in large congenital nevi. Plast Reconstr Surg 1974; 53:421–426.

43 Kopf AW, Bart RS, Hennessey P. Congenital nevocytic nevi and malignant melanomas. J Am Acad Derm 1979; 1:123–127.

44 Mark GJ, Mihm MC Jr, Liteplo MG et al. Congenital melanocytic nevi of the small and garment type. Clinical, histologic, and ultrastructural studies. Hum Pathol 1973; 4:395–402.

45 Walton RG, Jacobs AH, Cox AJ. Pigmented lesions in newborn infants. Br J Derm 1976; 95:389–395.

46 Kopf AW, Bart RS, Rodriguez-Sains et al., eds. Malignant Melanoma. New York: Masson; 1979:1–3.

47 Jones RE Jr, Cash ME, Ackerman AB. Malignant melanomas mistaken histologically for junctional nevi. In: Ackerman AB, ed. Pathology of Malignant Melanoma, 1981:93–106.

48 Cutler SJ, Young JL, Jr, eds. Third National Cancer Survey: Incidence data. DHEW Publication No (NIH) 75–787. Monograph 41. Bethesda, Md: National Cancer Institute, 1975.

49 Ackerman AB. 'Dysplastic nevus' syndrome: Does a survey make it real? J Am Acad Derm 2003; 48:461–463.

50 Clark WH Jr, Ackerman AB. An exchange of views regarding the dysplastic nevus controversy. Semin Derm 1989; 8:229–250.

51 Piepkorn M, Meyer LJ, Goldgar D, et al. The dysplastic melanocytic nevus: a prevalent lesion that correlates poorly with clinical phenotype. J Am Acad Derm 1989; 20:407–415.

52 Clark WH Jr, Reimer RR, Greene M, et al. Origin of familial malignant melanoma from heritable melanocytic lesions. Arch Derm 1978; 114:732–738.

53 Crutcher WA, Sagebiel RW. Prevalence of dysplastic nevi in a community practice. Lancet 1984; 1:729.

54 Elder DE, Clark WH Jr, Elenitsas R, et al. The early and intermediate precursor lesions of tumor progression in the melanocytic system: common acquired nevi and atypical (dysplastic) nevi. Semin Diagn Pathol 1993; 10:18–35.

55 Greene MH, Tucker MA, Clark WH Jr, et al. Hereditary melanoma and the dysplastic nevus syndrome: the risk of cancers other than melanoma. J Am Acad Derm 1987; 16:792–797.

56 Lynch HT, Frichot BC III, Lynch JF. Familial atypical mole–melanoma syndrome. J Med Genet 1978; 15:352–356.

57 Mackie RM, McHenry P, Hole D. Accelerated detection with prospective surveillance for cutaneous melanoma in high risk groups. Lancet 1993; 341:1618–1620.

58 Marghoob AA, Kopf AW, Rigel DS, et al. Risk of cutaneous malignant melanoma in patients with 'classic' atypical-mole syndrome. A case control study. Arch Derm 1994; 130:993–998.

59 Metcalf JS, Maize JC. Clark's nevus. Semin Cutan Med Surg 1999; 18:43–46.

60 Rigel DS, Rivers JK, Friedman RJ, et al. Risk gradient for malignant melanoma in individuals with dysplastic naevi. Lancet 1988; 1:352–353.

61 Nachbar F, Stolz W, Merkle T, et al. The ABCD rule of dermoscopy. High prospective value in the diagnosis of doubtful melanocytic skin lesions. J Am Acad Derm 1994; 30:551–559.

62 Rao BK, Marghoob AA, Stolz W, et al. Can early melanoma be differentiated from atypical melanocytic nevi by in vivo techniques? Part I. Clinical and dermoscopic characteristics. Skin Res Tech 1997; 3:8–14.

63 Friedman RJ, Heilman ER, Gottlieb GJ, et al. Malignant melanoma: clinicopathologic correlations. In: Friedman RJ, Rigel DS, Kopf AW, et al., eds. Cancer of the Skin. Philadelphia: Saunders; 1991:148–175.

64 Kopf AW, Elbaum M, Provost N. The use of dermoscopy and digital imaging in the diagnosis of cutaneous melanoma. Skin Res Tech 1997; 3:1–7.

65 Gutkowicz-Krusin D, Elbaum M, Szwaykowski P, et al. Can early malignant melanoma be differentiated from atypical melanocytic nevus by in vivo techniques? II. Automatic machine vision classification. Skin Res Tech 1997; 3:15–22.

66 Jamora MJ, Wainwright BD, Meehan S, et al. Improved identification of potentially dangerous pigmented skin lesions by computerized image analysis. Arch Derm 2003; 139:195–198.

67 Davis N. Modern concepts of melanoma and its management. Ann Plast Surg 1978; 1:628–630.

68 Salopek TG, Kopf AW, Stefanato CM, et al. Differentiation of atypical moles (dysplastic nevi) from early melanomas by dermoscopy. Derm Clin 2001; 19:337–345.

Table 15.1 Factors associated with melanoma prognosis[97]

Clinical prognostic factors
  Age
  Gender
  Anatomic site
  Serum lactate dehydrogenase
  Distant metastasis

Histologic prognostic factors
  Tumor thickness
  Clark's level
  Ulceration
  Nodal status
  Sentinel lymph node status
  Tumor type
  Angiogenesis
  Vascular invasion
  Microsatellites
  Mitotic rate
  Regression
  Tumor infiltrating lymphocytes
  Growth patterns

Molecular and biochemical prognostic factors

Table 15.2 Melanoma survival vs Clark's level

Clark's level	Anatomic location of melanoma cells	10-year survival[7]
Level I	Confined to epidermis	99%
Level II	Penetrating the papillary dermis	96%
Level III	Filling the papillary dermis	90%
Level IV	Extending into the reticular dermis	67%
Level V	Invasion of the subcutis	26%

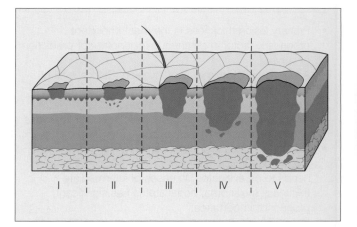

Figure 15.1 Clark's level measurement. Level I tumors are confined to the epidermis. Level II tumors penetrate into the papillary dermis. Level III tumors fill the papillary dermis. Level IV tumors extend into the reticular dermis. Level V tumors invade the subcutis.

Initially, it was observed by Clark *et al.* that the extent of anatomic tumor invasion by the primary tumor predicted the 10-year survival probability (Table 15.2).[7] The Clark classification involves staging the primary lesion based on anatomic level of invasion into the dermis or subcutaneous fat rather than based on its metric depth (Fig. 15.1). Ten-year survivals for patients with tumors extending to these levels were 99, 96, 90, 67 and 26% for levels I through V, respectively. Although Clark's levels introduced microanatomy as an important prognostic tool, tumor thickness has largely supplanted Clark's levels since it is a continuous variable and more accurate in its determinations. Tumor depth is reported as Breslow's thickness, a measure of the vertical depth of the tumor measured from the granular cell layer downward using an ocular micrometer (Figs 15.2, 15.3).[8] If the tumor is modeled as a sphere, the maximal thickness, as measured from the granular cell layer to the deepest component of the tumor, is mathematically related to the tumor volume. To date, tumor thickness remains the most powerful prognostic indicator that can be determined from evaluation of the primary melanoma itself.

More recent analyses have found that anatomic level of invasion does offer additional prognostic information in thin primary CMs; tumors of less than 1 mm depth but greater than Clark's level III have a worse prognosis than lesions of the same thickness with a Clark's level of III or less.[9] Furthermore, it has been shown that a Clark's level of III or higher is an independent predictor of positive sentinel lymph node biopsy.[10] Although current pathology reports for all CMs commonly include both Clark's level and Breslow thickness, in the future, perhaps, Clark's level will only need to be reported for tumors for which it is clinically significant (e.g. thinner tumors). Clark *et al.* extended the earlier observations and proposed that melanomas could be biologically

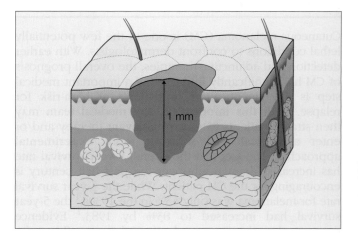

Figure 15.2 Breslow depth measurement. The tumor depth is measured from the granular layer to the deepest portion of the tumor.

distinguished based on their pattern of growth into those with radial growth phase (RGP; of lower metastatic potential) and those in vertical growth phase (VGP; of greater metastatic potential) (Fig. 15.4).[11] The biologic difference between these two phases of growth may account for some portion of the difference in survival rates between superficial and deep tumors.

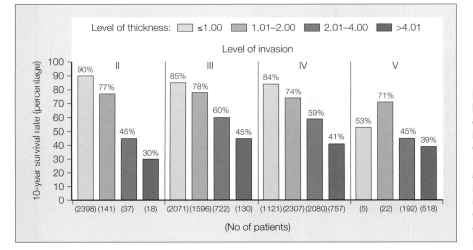

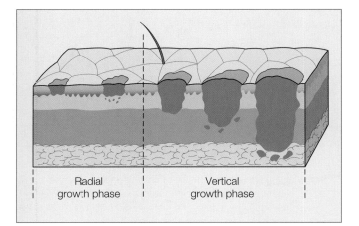

Figure 15.3 Breslow thickness, Clark's level and survival. Using the AJCC database, it is clear that Breslow thickness is more predictive of patient survival than Clark's level. However, lesions of less than 1 mm thickness and of Clark's level IV have a significantly worse prognosis than similar lesions with less anatomic invasion. (Reproduced with permission from Balch CM, et al. Cutaneous Melanoma, 4th edition. St Louis: Quality Medical Publishing; 2003.)

Figure 15.4 Melanoma growth phases. Tumors in vertical growth phase have a higher metastatic potential.

Tumor ulceration

Ulceration is the loss of continuity of the epithelium overlying the surface of the tumor and does not include traumatically induced ulceration (Fig. 15.5). Although the biology of ulceration remains speculative, it may be related to the inherent aggressiveness of the tumor itself or possibly other stromal factors, such as angiogenic support. For more than 20 years, it has been recognized that the presence microscopically of an ulcer in primary CM conveys a poorer prognosis.[12] Furthermore, greater width of ulceration carries with it an even poorer prognosis[13] and this seems particularly true for ulcers of greater than 3 mm width.[14] Because thicker lesions are more likely to be ulcerated, it might be logical to question whether ulceration is simply another marker for lesion thickness. However, multivariate analysis has shown the presence of an ulcer to be a significant prognostic factor even after accounting for lesion thickness.[15] Whereas Clark's level seems to be important in lesions less than 1 mm thick, it appears from the multivariate AJCC melanoma analysis that ulceration offers significant prognostic information for all invasive tumors regardless of thickness (Fig. 15.6). Ulceration is also the only feature of the primary tumor that has an

effect on outcome in stage III (node positive) disease.[15] This supports the notion that tumor ulceration may be an indicator of an aggressive biologic nature of individual melanoma cells originating from that tumor. Ulceration has been included in the 2002 AJCC staging system for melanoma.

Anatomic site

The anatomic location of a primary CM was shown to have a significant independent impact on survival in a multivariate analysis of the AJCC melanoma database of patients with stage I and II localized disease.[15] Lesions located on the head, neck and trunk had a risk ratio of 1.34 (95% CI 1.22–1.46) compared with those located on the extremities. Garbe et al have also found the importance of anatomic location in a multivariate analysis of 5093 patients.[16] The Pigmented Lesion Group at the University of Pennsylvania found anatomic site to be a useful variable in creating a CM prognostic model using multivariate analysis.[17] This model included tumor thickness, anatomic location (extremity excluding palmoplantar versus axial and palmoplantar) as well as patient characteristics such as age and sex (which will be addressed later in this chapter) (Table 15.3). This model was 50% more effective in predicting 10-year survival than was tumor thickness alone. These studies suggest that axial and acral lesions (i.e. hands/feet) carry a worse prognosis than non-acral extremity lesions.[18] The relatively rich lymphatic network of the axial anatomy may contribute to the apparent increased likelihood of metastases. Early detection failure may be partially responsible for the reduced prognosis at acral sites.

Mitotic rate

The mitotic rate in melanoma correlates directly with prognosis. In 1983, Schmoeckel *et al.* studied 585 cases of primary CM and found a correlation between mitotic rate and prognosis.[19] The mitotic index is defined as the number of mitoses per square millimeter multiplied by the lesion thickness.[20] Later, Kopf *et al.* showed that primary lesions with a thickness between 1.5 and 2.49 mm had an 84.1% 5-year survival overall, but that a subgroup with a mitotic index of 19 or greater had a 5-year survival of only 57.6%.[21] A recent study published

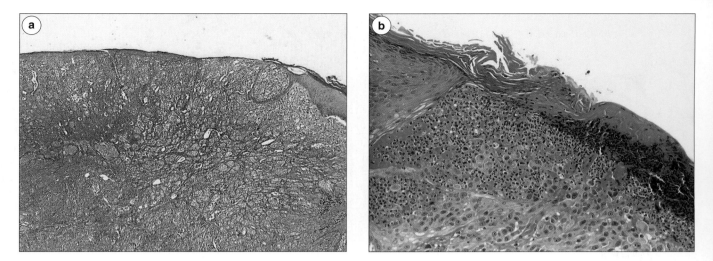

Figure 15.5 Ulceration. Photomicrographs illustrating (a) low and (b) high power views of ulceration. (Images courtesy of Dr Martin Mihm.)

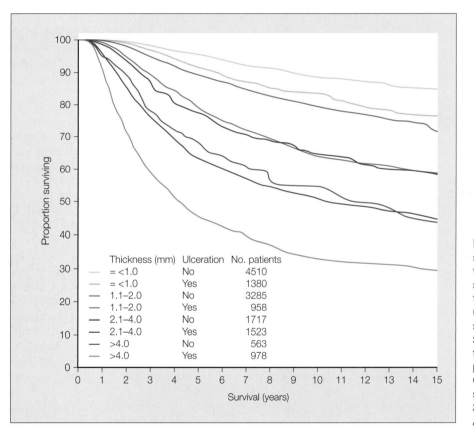

Thickness (mm)	Ulceration	No. patients
= <1.0	No	4510
= <1.0	Yes	1380
1.1–2.0	No	3285
1.1–2.0	Yes	958
2.1–4.0	No	1717
2.1–4.0	Yes	1523
>4.0	No	563
>4.0	Yes	978

Figure 15.6 Ulceration and patient survival. The survival curves show that tumor ulceration significantly affects patient survival even after controlling for tumor thickness. These data justify inclusion of ulceration into the new AJCC melanoma staging system. (From Balch CM, Soong SJ, Gershenwald JE, et al. Prognostic factors analysis of 17,600 melanoma patients: validation of the American Joint Committee on Cancer melanoma staging system. J Clin Oncol 2001; 19(16):3622–3634. Reprinted with permission from the American Society of Clinical Oncology.)

by Azzola *et al.* of 3661 CMs showed that tumor mitotic rate (TMR) was the second strongest independent prognostic factor after tumor thickness.[22] A higher number of mitoses predicted a poorer survival outcome. There was a profound and striking difference between the survival curves of patients with no mitoses compared with those with at least one mitosis. These authors suggest that future melanoma staging systems should include mitotic rate in the stratification. However, this would require the standardization of a method for mitotic rate calculation among pathologists.

Tumor infiltrating lymphocytes

Tumor infiltrating lymphocytes (TILs) were originally classified as brisk, non-brisk, or absent (Fig. 15.7).[23] TILs, when brisk, are thought to reflect a vigorous host response to the primary tumor and, thus, a better prognosis. Some have suggested that evaluation and categorization of TILs is subjective and that interobserver reliability is too low to demonstrate a correlation with survival; however, interobserver agreement seems to be quite high among pathologists who have been instructed in this simple classification.[24]

Table 15.3 Prognostic model

Variable	Probability of 10-year survival (95% CI)			
	Tumor with extremity location		Tumor with axis location*	
	Female patients	Male patients	Female patients	Male patients
Thickness <0.76 mm				
Age ≤60 years	0.99 (0.98 to 1.0)	0.98 (0.96 to 0.99)	0.97 (0.93 to 0.99)	0.94 (0.88 to 0.97)
Age >60 years	0.98 (0.95 to 0.99)	0.96 (0.89 to 0.98)	0.92 (0.82 to 0.96)	0.84 (0.70 to 0.93)
Thickness <0.76–1.69 mm				
Age ≤60 years	0.96 (0.92 to 0.98)	0.93 (0.85 to 0.97)	0.86 (0.76 to 0.92)	0.75 (0.62 to 0.84)
Age >60 years	0.90 (0.80 to 0.95)	0.81 (0.64 to 0.91)	0.67 (0.50 to 0.81)	0.50 (0.33 to 0.67)
Thickness 1.70–3.60 mm				
Age ≤60 years	0.89 (0.80 to 0.94)	0.80 (0.65 to 0.89)	0.65 (0.50 to 0.77)	0.48 (0.35 to 0.61)
Age >60 years	0.73 (0.57 to 0.85)	0.57 (0.38 to 0.75)	0.38 (0.24 to 0.55)	0.24 (0.14 to 0.37)
Thickness >3.60 mm				
Age ≤60 years	0.74 (0.53 to 0.87)	0.58 (0.36 to 0.77)	0.39 (0.21 to 0.60)	0.24 (0.13 to 0.40)
Age >60 years	0.48 (0.28 to 0.69)	0.32 (0.16 to 0.53)	0.18 (0.08 to 0.35)	0.10 (0.04 to 0.20)

*Axis location includes trunk, head and neck, and volar and subungual sites.
The factors used to predict survival in this model are tumor thickness, tumor location, patient age and patient sex. Use of this model was 50% more accurate in predicting 10-year survival than tumor thickness alone.17 (From Schuchter L, Schultz DJ, Synnestvedt M, et al. A prognostic model for predicting 10-year survival in patients with primary melanoma. The Pigmented Lesion Group. Ann Intern Med 1996; 125(5):369–375. Reprinted by permission of the American College of Physicians.)

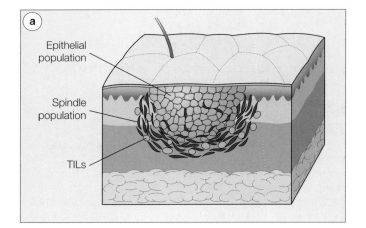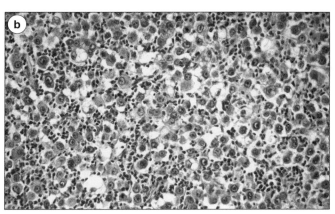

Figure 15.7 Tumor infiltrating lymphocytes. An illustrated example (a) of lymphocytic infiltration which is peripheral but non-brisk and a photomicrograph (b) showing a brisk lymphocytic infiltrate. (Image courtesy of Dr Martin Mihm.)

Recently, it has been shown that the absence of TILs is one of several tumor features that increase the risk of a positive sentinel lymph node biopsy.[25] Clemente *et al.* showed a very clear correlation between TILs status and survival in vertical growth phase melanoma. The 10-year survival rates were 55%, 45% and 27% for brisk, non-brisk and absent TILs, respectively, in the study. The hypothetical importance of immune surveillance in CM is one of the rationales for developing immunotherapeutic strategies to treat the disease.

Regression

Although regression is a relatively common feature observed in CM both clinically and histopathologically, its exact relationship to prognosis has not yet been clarified. Furthermore, there is no universal histopathologic definition of regression in primary CM. Although regression may, in theory, result from the host's immune response against the tumor, this has not been substantiated. There are data to suggest that regression confers an improved 10-year survival (87% vs 77%). However, regression is more common in thinner tumors and the statistical significance of this prognostic finding is lost when the tumors are controlled for lesion thickness.[26] Careful examination of 844 primary CMs stratifying for tumor thickness confirmed the lack of prognostic significance of regression.[27] In some studies, regression in the vertical growth phase has also been identified as a negative prognostic indicator.[23] One possible explanation is that regression causes a loss of visible tumor and consequent understaging. In these cases, correct staging would be based on the original tumor depth and would correlate with the worse prognosis seen in these tumors. This may explain the finding that regression is a significant risk factor for metastasis of thin (less than 1.0 mm deep) primary melanomas.[28] At the current time, more studies are needed to understand the affect of regression.

Angioinvasion and perineural invasion

The correlation between vascular invasion and poor prognosis in CM has been recognized for some time.[29] Kashani-Sabet et al. in a study of 526 patients with primary cutaneous melanoma showed that vascular invasion (defined as tumor cells within blood or lymphatic vessels) and uncertain vascular invasion (defined as melanoma cells immediately adjacent to the endothelium) correlate with recurrence and death as strongly as ulceration.[30] Niezabitowski et al., in a study of 93 consecutive melanoma patients, showed a significant link between vascular invasion and both overall and disease-free survival.[31] Furthermore, a disproportionate number of long-term survivors with very deep (>5 mm) melanomas have lesions that lack vascular invasion.[32] However, Massi et al. showed that for thick primary tumors (>3 mm Breslow thickness) vascular invasion predicted a higher risk of metastasis but did not affect survival.[33]

Transit of melanoma cells into either lymphatic channels or blood vessels is a prerequisite for metastases and angioinvasion may be histological documentation of this biological process. However, contrary to the expected finding, noting melanoma cells in the circulation using polymerase chain reaction (PCR) in patients of all stages of CM did not have any prognostic significance.[34]

Histologic type

Clark originally described three histologic subtypes of CM[7] to which a fourth subtype, the acral lentiginous subtype, is often added. While lentigo maligna melanoma, superficial spreading melanoma and acral lentiginous melanoma have an extended early horizontal growth phase, the fourth subtype, nodular melanoma, appears to exist only in the vertical growth phase. Although earlier studies suggested possible prognostic differences between CM subtypes, multivariate analyses have not shown histologic subtype to be of significant prognostic value after taking into account other prognostic clinical features.[35–38] Differences in 10-year survival amongst histologic types in univariate analysis appear to be accounted for by lesion thickness at diagnosis and anatomic location and are therefore lost in multivariate analysis.

A possible exception to the assertion that histologic subtype is not an independent prognostic variable is the desmoplastic neurotropic CM (DNCM), a subtype which accounts for less than 1% of all CMs.[39] This subtype appears to have a higher incidence of local recurrence than other subtypes. DNCM may arise beneath an overlying epidermal atypical melanocytic proliferation (usually lentigo maligna) or as a dermal nodule and shows both neuroid differentiation and a neurotropic and sometimes angiotropic growth pattern. These tumors are found most commonly on the head and neck and occur in males more often than females. DNCM appears to exhibit a higher rate of local recurrence although it is associated with a better prognosis compared to other subtypes if the tumor exceeds a depth of 5 mm.[32] However, as with all CMs, tumors that recur locally are at a greater risk for metastasis.[40] Thus, the tendency of these lesions to locally recur is worrisome. Overall, histologic type or 'growth pattern' is not considered to be an important independent predictor of metastasis or survival and is not used in the current AJCC staging system.

Histologic association with nevus

There is some evidence to suggest that CMs arising from a precursor nevus may have a better prognosis (95% compared with 85% of melanomas arising de novo).[41] It is not known why melanomas that appear histologically to be arising from a nevus have a better prognosis. One hypothesis is that a greater proportion of nodular CMs arise de novo from melanocytes not associated with a nevus and more superficial spreading CMs arise in nevi. Another possibility is that thicker lesions obliterate the nevic precursor skewing the data to make it appear that a nevus was never present in these more advanced lesions. Of course, it is possible that tumors that arise from nevi are biologically different and less aggressive, but this is yet to be established.

Patient characteristics affecting prognosis

Patient age

Advancing age has been shown in multiple studies to be a poor prognostic factor in patients with CM; however, some evidence suggests that correlation of age with decreased survival may be confounded by another direct relationship between age and tumor thickness.[42–45] Older patients, especially older men, tend to have thicker CMs at the time of diagnosis. Levine et al. hypothesized multiple possible reasons for the observed association of age with thickness including delayed diagnosis due to the presence of more pigmented lesions with age and a relative lack of concern about appearance amongst the elderly.[46] The Pigmented Lesion Group at the University of Pennsylvania showed that age greater than sixty years conferred an odds ratio for 10-year mortality of 3.0.[17] However, a follow-up study showed that prognosis based on tumor thickness alone was not significantly enhanced when a model incorporating thickness, age, sex and tumor location was applied.[47] Cohen et al. demonstrated that age remains an independent prognostic factor for melanoma-caused mortality even after accounting for differences in lesion thickness,[48] and Ferrone et al. showed that age was a significant independent risk factor for recurrence in high risk lesions (greater than 4.0 mm deep).[49] Age seems to be a significant prognostic factor for survival in melanoma in some studies. However, the relationship between age and melanoma prognosis is still tentative and further studies are warranted.

Patient gender

Gender appears to have little effect on the 2-year survival prognosis in patients with CM.[44] However, earlier studies suggested that women have a significantly better long-term prognosis.[43,50] Although women are more likely to have thinner lesions and lesions on the extremities rather than axial ones, female gender retains its favorable prognostic significance even after controlling for site and thickness.[51] The Pigmented Lesion Group at the University of Pennsylvania showed that female gender conferred an odds ratio for ten-year survival of 2.0.[17] In contrast, the Southwest Oncology Group (SWOG) found that, after controlling for all variables, the prognosis for both men and women were similar.[52]

Pregnancy

Although the mean thickness of pregnancy-associated melanomas may be significantly greater than that of non-pregnancy-associated tumors, melanomas that arise during pregnancy are not necessarily associated with a worse prognosis.[53,54] Because changes in nevus color occur in pregnancy especially in dysplastic nevi[55] and because melanomas are diagnosed with an increased thickness during this time, careful surveillance and early detection is critical.[56] To date, however, there are no conclusive studies to prove interactions between either pregnancy or hormonal therapy and melanoma prognosis. Psychosocial issues regarding childbearing in high-risk melanoma patients need to be carefully discussed with these patients so that a realistic understanding of their risks can be conveyed as a poor prognosis in patients with metastatic disease may affect a decision to undertake child-rearing.[57] Issues of melanoma and pregnancy are reviewed in Chapter 20.

Performance status

Performance status is a measure of a patient's ability to undertake physical activity and ranges from the ability to perform all strenuous activity to the ability to perform only activities of daily living to complete disability. Poor performance status has been consistently found to be a negative prognostic factor for survival in patients with stage IV disease. Recently, in an analysis of factors predicting survival in patients with stage IV disease treated with cytokine therapy, performance status was found to be a significant prognostic factor. In fact, all but one of the patients still alive at 2 years had the highest rating for performance status.[58] Manola et al. found in their meta-analysis of ECOG trials that performance status of 1 or more was associated with a relative risk of 1.49 for lengthened survival,[59] and Unger et al. found in their meta-analysis of SWOG trials that poor performance status was a predictor of worse survival with $P<0.001$.[52] Performance status should be considered in discussing treatment options with the stage IV melanoma patient.

Patient immune status

Immune surveillance is thought to be an important factor for controlling melanoma progression and this forms the basis for treatment approaches involving immuno-activation such as interferon and tumor vaccines. Patients with low white blood cell (WBC) counts have a decreased benefit from interferon therapy.[60] Rodrigues et al. demonstrated that HIV positive patients have a statistically significant poorer prognosis and showed a trend of an inverse relationship between time to first melanoma recurrence and CD4+ cell counts.[61] Despite the small numbers of patients, there is some evidence that metastatic skin cancer, including melanoma, may be associated with a poorer prognosis in organ transplant recipients.[62]

METASTASIS AND PROGNOSIS

Microscopic satellitosis and in transit metastases

Microscopic satellites are defined as discrete tumor nests measuring at least 0.05 mm in diameter that are separated from the main body of the tumor by normal reticular dermal collagen or subcutaneous fat (Fig. 15.8). This histologic finding could be considered to be either a feature of the primary tumor or a type of metastasis. We have chosen to discuss satellitosis in the context of metastatic tumor status because its prognostic import is similar to that of clinical satellitosis (clinically perceivable satellite tumor nodules) and of in transit metastases[63] and because microsatellites may represent 'within specimen' metastases as a result of intralymphatic invasion. Harrist et al. originally described the phenomenon of microscopic satellites and its independent correlation with an increased likelihood of nodal metastases.[64] This group found a decreased 5-year disease-free survival in melanomas with microscopic satellites (36% vs 89%).[65] Further study found the presence or absence of microscopic satellites to be one of the most important prognostic features for intermediate thickness melanoma[14] and retrospectively linked this feature to diminished survival.[66–68] The current AJCC

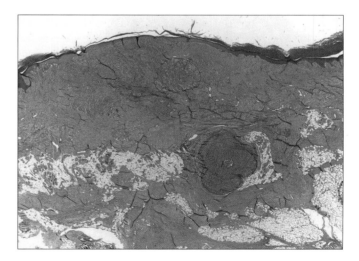

Figure 15.8 Microscopic satellites. This photomicrograph illustrates a microscopic satellite, defined as discrete tumor nests measuring at least 0.05 mm in diameter that are separated from the main body of the tumor by normal reticular dermal collagen or subcutaneous fat. This likely represents intralymphatic trapping of an *in transit* metastasis. (Image courtesy of Dr Martin Mihm.)

melanoma staging system groups clinical and microscopic satellitosis together with in-transit metastases (i.e. stage IIIB). Buzaid et al. found that the Kaplan–Meier survival curves of patients with either satellitosis, in transit metastases, or both were very similar.[69]

Local recurrence

True local recurrence should be distinguished from clinical satellitosis and/or in transit metastases in that it implies the recurrence of the primary tumor mass as a result of incomplete excision rather than the growth of an unresected distinct metastasis. However, it may be difficult to fully assess whether a recurrence in a scar is a result of an undetected satellite or represents a true local recurrence. When a tumor presents in the excision scar, it is likely the tumor would be classified as a local recurrence. Local recurrences occurring in patients who have had wide local excision of the primary tumor (with clear margins) most likely represent intra-lymphatic metastasis such as unresected satellitosis.[69] Local recurrences are probably associated with a poorer prognosis because many of these 'local' recurrences represent unresected satellites. In a sample of primary intermediate thickness (1–4 mm) CMs on the trunk, head, neck and distal extremities, those that recurred locally had a 9% 5-year survival compared to an 86% survival for those which did not recur locally.[70] Because the prognosis for patients with local recurrence after wide excision is similar to those with in transit metastases or satellitosis, the distinction between the three is arbitrary.[71]

Nodal metastatic disease

Regional lymph nodes represent the most common metastatic site in patients with CM. Nodal disease is currently categorized as either macroscopic (clinically apparent and pathologically confirmed) or microscopic (found only pathologically). Many patients with tumors that are at elevated risk for nodal metastases (i.e. >1.0 mm depth or Clark's level IV) now undergo sentinel lymph node biopsy to establish microscopic nodal status.[72] In this procedure, a vital dye and a radioactive dye are injected at the tumor site at the time of excision and traced to the node(s) where they are taken up; these node(s) are then excised and evaluated for metastatic disease. The information gained by doing this procedure can be used to (1) stage disease and refine prognosis and (2) guide the use of adjuvant interferon and (3) dictate stratification into clinical trials.[73,74] The sentinel node procedure also allows for the discovery of interval sentinel nodes, which are sentinel nodes that lie between the tumor and a traditional nodal basin (e.g. the axilla), that may be missed in a traditional elective lymphadenectomy.[75]

The sentinel lymph node status is one of the most powerful predictors of outcome.[76–81] In other words, patients with nodal involvement on sentinel lymph node biopsy exhibit a significantly worse prognosis compared to patients without nodal involvement. There is also some evidence that the tumor burden, measured as the largest diameter tumor nodule in a positive node, has further prognostic significance for the patient.[82] However, the number of nodal metastases was the most significant predictor of outcome in the AJCC analysis of patients with stage III disease.[15] White et al. found that patients with one positive node have a 53% overall 5-year survival and those with four or more had a 25% survival.[83]

Ulceration may be the only feature of primary CM tumor that affects the prognosis in stage III, node positive disease.[15] However, White et al. found that tumor thickness as well as ulceration were statistically significant predictors of survival in node positive disease.[83] Nodal disease with an unknown primary tumor appears to have a similar survival prognosis to nodal disease in cases with identified primary tumors.[84]

Distant metastases

The presence of distant metastases is the most ominous clinical finding for patients with CM and qualifies as stage IV disease. Patients with non-visceral distant metastases (i.e. to skin, subcutis, or non-regional lymph nodes) have a slightly better prognosis than those with visceral metastases.[69] It appears that patients with lung metastases have a better prognosis than those with metastases to other visceral sites and that having greater than one metastatic site carries a worse prognosis.[59] Balch et al. showed that the prognostic advantage of lung metastasis over other sites is transient and found similar survival rates for all visceral sites after one year.[15,85] This group found that the number of metastatic sites was the single most significant prognostic factor in patients with distant metastatic disease; for a single metastatic site, the 1-year survival rate was 36%, 13% for two sites and 0% for three or more sites.[85]

Serum lactate dehydrogenase level

An elevated serum lactate dehydrogenase (LDH) level was originally recognized as a marker for liver metastasis. LDH has since been found to be an independent prognostic factor in metastatic melanoma with elevated LDH conferring a relative risk for death of 1.89.[59] Eton et al. also found a normal LDH to be a favorable predictor of survival in patients with distant metastatic disease.[86] While LDH levels have definite prognostic significance in known metastatic disease, the benefit of screening LDH levels for patients with localized disease is not established. Other serum markers such as S100 protein[87] and alkaline phosphatase[59] show some limited promise for their potential in assessing prognosis.

AMERICAN JOINT COMMITTEE ON CANCER STAGING SYSTEM

Factors included in the new staging system

There are too many factors that have been linked to melanoma prognosis to include them all in a logical and practical staging system. Therefore, the AJCC Melanoma Staging Committee set forth certain goals in creating a unifying staging system:[88]

- the system must be useful for the diverse needs of all medical disciplines

- the criteria must incorporate results that were applicable worldwide

- the criteria must reflect the dominant prognostic factors consistently identified in Cox multivariate regression analyses

- the criteria must be relevant for use in standard clinical practice as well as in clinical trials

- the criteria must be simple and easy to identify so that patients can be correctly staged and chart reviews can be easily performed.

With these goals in mind, the new AJCC staging system was created.

Using this criteria, an evidence based approach to the classification of tumors, nodal status and metastatic disease (a TNM system) was created (Table 15.4). In this system, tumors are classified by thickness (slightly modified from the 1997 AJCC classification) and sub-classified by the presence of ulceration because of its relationship to prognosis.[15] The incorporation of ulceration represents a significant change from the 1997

Table 15.4   AJCC 2002 Revised Melanoma Staging

Stage	Histological features/TNM classification	1-year	Overall survival 5-year	10-year
0	Intraepithelial/in situ melanoma (TisN0M0)		100%	100%
A	≤1 mm without ulceration and Clark Level II/III (T1aN0M0)		95%	88%
IB	≤1 mm with ulceration or level IV/V (T1bN0M0)		91%	83%
	1.01–2 mm without ulceration (T2aN0M0)		89%	79%
IIA	1.01–2 mm with ulceration (T2bN0M0)		77%	64%
	2.01–4 mm without ulceration (T3aN0M0)		79%	64%
IIB	2.01–4 mm with ulceration (T3bN0M0)		63%	51%
	>4 mm without ulceration (T4aN0M0)		67%	54%
IIC	>4 mm with ulceration (T4bN0M0)		45%	32%
IIIA	Single regional nodal micrometastasis, nonulcerated primary (T1–4aN1aM0)		69%	63%
	2–3 microscopic regional nodes, nonulcerated primary (T1–4aN2aM0)		63%	57%
IIIB	Single regional nodal micrometastasis, ulcerated primary (T1–4bN1aM0)		53%	38%
	2–3 microscopic regional nodes, ulcerated primary (T1–4bN2aM0)		50%	36%
	Single regional nodal macrometastasis, nonulcerated primary (T1–4aN1bM0)		59%	48%
	2–3 macroscopic regional nodes, nonulcerated primary (T1–4aN2bM0)		46%	39%
	In-transit met(s)/satellite lesion(s) *without* metastatic lymph nodes (T1–4a/bN2cM0)		30–50%	
IIIC	Single microscopic regional node, ulcerated primary (T1–4bN1bM0)		29%	24%
	2–3 macroscopic regional nodes, ulcerated primary (T1–4bN2bM0)		24%	15%
	4 or more metastatic nodes, matted nodes/gross extracapsular extension, or in-transit met(s)/satellite(s) *and* metastatic nodes (anyTN3M0)		27%	18%
IV	Distant skin, subcutaneous, or nodal mets with normal LDH (any TanyNM1a)	59%	19%	16%
	Lung mets with normal LDH (anyTanyNM1B)	57%	7%	3%
	All other visceral mets with normal LDH or any distant mets with increased LDH (anyTanyNM1c)	41%	9%	6%

Below thickness is defined as the thickness of the lesion using an ocular micrometer to measure the total vertical height of the melanoma from the granular layer to the area of deepest penetration. The Clark's level refers to levels of invasion according to depth of penetration of the dermis. This categorization is based on survival data by Cox analysis.
Adapted with permission from Balch et al. Final Version of the American Joint Committee on Cancer Staging System for Cutaneous Melanoma. J Clin Oncol 2001; 19:3635–3548. Lippincott Williams & Wilkins.©

AJCC staging system. Nodal status is classified by the number of positive nodes (rather than nodal volume as previously) and whether they are microscopically identified (microscopic) or clinically palpable and pathologically confirmed (macroscopic). In-transit metastases and satellitosis are included in the nodal disease classification because they seem to biologically represent lymphatic spread and because they hold similar prognostic relevance.[69] Distant metastatic disease is separated into the following: (1) distant skin, soft tissue, or nodal metastases, (2) lung metastases with normal LDH, (3) other visceral metastases or either category 1 or 2 with elevated LDH. The importance of LDH in metastatic melanoma has been discussed.[59] The melanoma TNM categorization is based on survival data by Cox analysis;[15] finally, stage groupings were created using the TNM staging system based on prognoses using Cox analysis.[15]

Currrently, the AJCC melanoma staging system represents the most widely accepted algorithm for assessing melanoma prognosis.

FUTURE OUTLOOK

New classes of factors will play a significant role in assessing melanoma prognosis in the future.

DNA ploidy

Von Roenn *et al.* showed that DNA ploidy was strongly correlated with Breslow thickness and Clark's level.[89] This finding suggests that histologic and clinical features currently used in staging may be surrogate markers for tumor genotypes that directly determine biologic behavior. In a study of 177 CM patients with stage I melanoma, aneuploidy was linked to decreased disease-free survival, poorer survival prognosis and higher recurrence rates even after controlling for tumor thickness.[90] However, Zaloudik *et al.* were unable to find a link between DNA ploidy and outcome in a smaller study of 50 patients.[91] Polysomy for chromosome 7 was found in a higher percentage of metastatic CM than primary tumors or benign nevi.[92] This is possibly due to the overexpression of the epidermal growth factor receptor gene found on that chromosome.[92] DNA content analysis may be a clinically useful stratification method for melanoma in the future if the association with prognosis is more firmly established and tests become readily available.

Molecular prognostics

Numerous molecular markers have been proposed for the prognosis of CM and it is difficult to assess which of these will evolve and enter clinical practice in the future. It is exciting to imagine the use of genetic markers with known biologic relevance to tumor behavior on a cellular level. Carr *et al.* have used microarray expression analysis to identify genes for which the expression pattern is linked to melanoma progression.[93] One gene

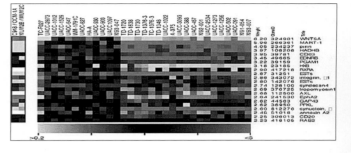

Figure 15.9 Differential gene expression in metastatic melanoma determined by microarray analysis. Microarray technology was used to identify the genes for which the expression correlates with metastasis. WNT5A, a gene tied to cell motility and invasiveness, was identified as a particularly suggestive marker for tumor progression. (Image courtesy of Dr Kristen Carr). (From Carr KM, Bittner M, Trent JM, eds. Gene-expression profiling in human cutaneous melanoma. Oncogene 2003; 22:3076–3080. Reprinted with permission from Nature Publishing Group.)

which was identified as being an important predictor of metastasis is WNT-5A (Fig. 15.9). Another marker that has recently received attention for its promise in the prediction of melanoma metastasis is *melastatin*.[94] Duncan *et al.* found that loss of melastatin expression was an independent negative prognostic factor for decreased eight-year disease-free survival in patients with stage I and II localized CM.[6] *Survivin*, an inhibitor of apoptosis, when expressed in sentinel lymph node metastases, was found to be a negative prognostic factor for patient outcome.[95] Another example of the use of advanced molecular techniques in the prognostication of CM is the use of reverse transcriptase polymerase chain reaction (RT-PCR) for tyrosinase mRNA to increase the sensitivity of sentinel node biopsies.[96] Although it is possible to detect a smaller number of metastatic melanoma cells in the sentinel node than could be recognized by standard histopathologic techniques, the use of this technique is not yet standard in centers performing sentinel node biopsies. The Sunbelt Melanoma Trial is directly addressing the role of RT-PCR in assessing nodal disease.

There are many candidate genes and new techniques that may be used to predict the biologic behavior of CM tumors and these are exciting and seemingly more direct and accurate ways to predict tumor behavior, detect metastatic disease and/or determine a tumor's likelihood of responding to specific targeted therapies. Establishment of the usefulness of these candidate genes in larger series of patients and verification by multivariate analyses remains to be done.

REFERENCES

1 Kopf AW, Rigel DS, Friedman RJ. The rising incidence and mortality rate of malignant melanoma. J Dermatol Surg Oncol 1982; 8(9):760–761.

2 Silverberg E. Cancer statistics. CA Cancer J Clin 1983; 33(1):9–25.

3 Berwick M, Dubin N, Luo ST, et al. No improvement in survival from melanoma diagnosed from 1973 to 1984. Int J Epidemiol 1994; 23(4):673–681.

4 Breslow A. Thickness, cross-sectional areas and depth of invasion in the prognosis of cutaneous melanoma. Ann Surg 1970; 172(5):902–908.

5 Kirkwood JM, Strawderman MH, Ernstoff MS, et al. Interferon alfa-2b adjuvant therapy of high-risk resected cutaneous melanoma: the Eastern Cooperative Oncology Group Trial EST 1684 [comment]. J Clin Oncol 1996; 14(1):7–17.

6 Duncan LM, Deeds J, Cronin FE, et al. Melastatin expression and prognosis in cutaneous malignant melanoma. J Clin Oncol 2001; 19(2):568–576.

7 Clark WH Jr, From L, Bernardino EA, et al. The histogenesis and biologic behavior of primary human malignant melanomas of the skin. Cancer Res 1969; 29(3):705–727.

8 Esch EP Van Der, Cascinelli N, Preda F, et al. Stage I melanoma of the skin: evaluation of prognosis according to histologic characteristics. Cancer 1981; 48(7):1668–1673.

9 Kelly JW, Sagebiel RW, Clyman S, et al. Thin level IV malignant melanoma. A subset in which level is the major prognostic indicator. Ann Surg 1985; 202(1):98–103.

10 McMasters KM, Wong SL, Edwards MJ, et al. Factors that predict the presence of sentinel lymph node metastasis in patients with melanoma. Surgery 2001; 130(2):151–156.

11 Clark WH Jr, Elder DE, Van Horn M. The biologic forms of malignant melanoma. Hum Pathol 1986; 17(5):443–450.

12 Balch CM, Wilkerson JA, Murad TM, et al. The prognostic significance of ulceration of cutaneous melanoma. Cancer 1980; 45(12):3012–3017.

13 Day CL Jr, Lew RA, Harrist TJ. Malignant melanoma prognostic factors 4: ulceration width. J Dermatol Surg Oncol 1984; 10(1):23–24.

14 Day CL Jr, Mihm MC Jr, Lew RA, et al. Prognostic factors for patients with clinical stage I melanoma of intermediate thickness (1.51 – 3.39 mm). A conceptual model for tumor growth and metastasis. Ann Surg 1982; 195(1):35–43.

15 Balch CM, Soong SJ, Gershenwald JE, et al. Prognostic factors analysis of 17,600 melanoma patients: validation of the American Joint Committee on Cancer melanoma staging system. J Clin Oncol 2001; 19(16):3622–3634.

16 Garbe C, Buttner P, Bertz J, et al. Primary cutaneous melanoma. Prognostic classification of anatomic location. Cancer 1995; 75(10):2492–2498.

17 Schuchter L, Schultz DJ, Synnestvedt M, et al. A prognostic model for predicting 10-year survival in patients with primary melanoma. The Pigmented Lesion Group [comment]. Ann Intern Med 1996; 125(5):369–375.

18 Bennett DR, Wasson D, MacArthur JD, et al. The effect of misdiagnosis and delay in diagnosis on clinical outcome in melanomas of the foot. J Am Coll Surg 1994; 179(3):279–284.

19 Schmoeckel C, Bockelbrink A, Bockelbrink H, et al. Low- and high-risk malignant melanoma – I. Evaluation of clinical and histological prognosticators in 585 cases. Eur J Cancer Clin Oncol 1983; 19(2):227–235.

20 Schmoeckel C, Braun-Falco O. Prognostic index in malignant melanoma. Arch Dermatol 1978; 114(6):871–873.

21 Kopf AW, Gross DF, Rogers GS, et al. Prognostic index for malignant melanoma. Cancer 1987; 59(6):1236–1241.

22 Azzola MF, Shaw HM, Thompson JF, et al. Tumor mitotic rate is a more powerful prognostic indicator than ulceration in patients with primary cutaneous melanoma: an analysis of 3661 patients from a single center. Cancer 2003; 97(6):1488–1498.

23 Clark WH Jr, Elder DE, Guerry D, et al. Model predicting survival in stage I melanoma based on tumor progression [comment]. J Natl Cancer Inst 1989; 81(24):1893–1904.

24 Busam KJ, Antonescu CR, Marghoob AA, et al. Histologic classification of tumor-infiltrating lymphocytes in primary cutaneous malignant melanoma. A study of interobserver agreement. Am J Clin Pathol 2001; 115(6):856–860.

25 Mraz-Gernhard S, Sagebiel RW, Kashani-Sabet M, et al. Prediction of sentinel lymph node micrometastasis by histological features in primary cutaneous malignant melanoma. Arch Dermatol 1998; 134(8):983–987.

26 Trau H, Kopf AW, Rigel DS, et al. Regression in malignant melanoma. J Am Acad Dermatol 1983; 8(3):363–368.

27 Kelly JW, Sagebiel RW, Blois MS. Regression in malignant melanoma. A histologic feature without independent prognostic significance. Cancer 1985; 56(9):2287–2291.

28 Guitart J, Lowe L, Piepkorn M, et al. Histological characteristics of metastasizing thin melanomas: a case–control study of 43 cases [comment]. Arch Dermatol 2002; 138(5):603–608.

29 Gilchrist KW, Gilbert E, Metter G, et al. Importance of microscopic vascular invasion in primary cutaneous malignant melanoma. Surgery. Gynecol Obstet 1977; 145(4):559–561.

30 Kashani-Sabet M, Sagebiel RW, Ferreira CM, et al. Vascular involvement in the prognosis of primary cutaneous melanoma [comment]. Arch Dermatol 2001; 137(9):1169–1173.

31 Niezabitowski A, Czajecki K, Ry SJ, et al. Prognostic evaluation of cutaneous malignant melanoma: a clinicopathologic and immunohistochemical study. J Surg Oncol 1999; 70(3):150–160.

32 Spatz A, Shaw HM, Crotty KA, et al. Analysis of histopathological factors associated with prolonged survival of 10 years or more for patients with thick melanomas (>5 mm). Histopathology 1998; 33(5):406–413.

33 Massi D, Borgognoni L, Franchi A, et al. Thick cutaneous malignant melanoma: a reappraisal of prognostic factors. Melanoma Res 2000; 10(2):153–164.

34 Palmieri G, Ascierto PA, Perrone F, et al. Prognostic value of circulating melanoma cells detected by reverse transcriptase-polymerase chain reaction [comment]. J Clin Oncol 2003; 21(5):767–773.

35 Day CL Jr, Sober AJ, Kopf AW, et al. A prognostic model for clinical stage I melanoma of the trunk. Location near the midline is not an independent risk factor for recurrent disease. Am J Surg 1981; 142(2):247–251.

36 Day CL Jr, Sober AJ, Kopf AW, et al. A prognostic model for clinical stage I melanoma of the upper extremity. The importance of anatomic subsites in predicting recurrent disease. Ann Surg 1981; 193(4):436–440.

37 Day CL Jr, Sober AJ, Kopf AW, et al. A prognostic model for clinical stage I melanoma of the lower extremity. Location on foot as independent risk factor for recurrent disease. Surgery 1981; 89(5):599–603.

38 Koh HK, Michalik E, Sober AJ, et al. Lentigo maligna melanoma has no better prognosis than other types of melanoma. J Clin Oncol 1984; 2(9):994–1001.

39 Carlson JA, Dickersin GR, Sober AJ, et al. Desmoplastic neurotropic melanoma. A clinicopathologic analysis of 28 cases. Cancer 1995; 75(2):478–494.

40 Jaroszewski DE, Pockaj BA, DiCaudo DJ, et al. The clinical behavior of desmoplastic melanoma. Am J Surg 2001; 182(6):590–595.

41 Friedman RJ, Rigel DS, Kopf AW, et al. Favorable prognosis for malignant melanomas associated with acquired melanocytic nevi. Arch Dermatol 1983; 119(6):455–462.

42 Cochran AJ. Method of assessing prognosis in patients with malignant melanoma. Lancet 1968; 2(7577):1062–1064.

43 Karjalainen S, Hakulinen T. Survival and prognostic factors of patients with skin melanoma. A regression-model analysis based on nationwide cancer registry data. Cancer 1988; 62(10):2274–2280.

44 Magnus K. Prognosis in malignant melanoma of the skin. Significance of stage of disease, anatomical site, sex, age and period of diagnosis. Cancer 1977; 40(1):389–397.

45 Osborne JE, Hutchinson PE. Clinical correlates of Breslow thickness of malignant melanoma. Br J Dermatol 2001; 144(3):476–483.

46 Levine J, Kopf AW, Rigel DS, et al. Correlation of thicknesses of superficial spreading malignant melanomas and ages of patients. J Dermatol Surg Oncol 1981; 7(4):311–316.

47 Margolis DJ, Halpern AC, Rebbeck T, et al. Validation of a melanoma prognostic model. Arch Dermatol 1998; 134(12):1597–1601.

48 Cohen HJ, Cox E, Manton K, et al. Malignant melanoma in the elderly. J Clin Oncol 1987; 5(1):100–106.

49 Ferrone CR, Panageas KS, Busam K, et al. Multivariate prognostic model for patients with thick cutaneous melanoma: importance of sentinel lymph node status. Ann Surg Oncol 2002; 9(7):637–645.

50 O'Doherty CJ, Prescott RJ, White H, et al. Sex differences in presentation of cutaneous malignant melanoma and in survival from stage I disease. Cancer 1986; 58(3):788–792.

51 Shaw HM, McGovern VJ, Milton GW, et al. Malignant melanoma: influence of site of lesion and age of patient in the female superiority in survival. Cancer 1980; 46(12):2731–2735.

52 Unger JM, Flaherty LE, Liu PY, et al. Gender and other survival predictors in patients with metastatic melanoma on Southwest Oncology Group trials. Cancer 2001; 91(6):1148–1155.

53 MacKie RM, Bufalino R, Morabito A, et al. Lack of effect of pregnancy on outcome of melanoma. For The World Health Organisation Melanoma Programme [comment]. Lancet 1991; 337(8742):653–655.

54 Travers RL, Sober AJ, Berwick M, et al. Increased thickness of pregnancy-associated melanoma. Br J Dermatol 1995; 132(6):876–883.

55 Ellis DL. Pregnancy and sex steroid hormone effects on nevi of patients with the dysplastic nevus syndrome. J Am Acad Dermatol 1991; 25(3):467–482.

56 Wrone DA, Duncan LM, Sober AJ. Melanoma and pregnancy: eight questions with discussion. J Gender Specific Med 1999; 2(4):52–54.

57 Borden EC. Melanoma and pregnancy. Semin Oncol 2000; 27(6):654–656.

58 Keilholz U, Martus P, Punt CJ, et al. Prognostic factors for survival and factors associated with long-term remission in patients with advanced melanoma receiving cytokine-based treatments: second analysis of a randomised EORTC Melanoma Group trial comparing interferon-alpha2a (IFNalpha) and interleukin 2 (IL-2) with or without cisplatin. Eur J Cancer 2002; 38(11):1501–1511.

59 Manola J, Atkins M, Ibrahim J, et al. Prognostic factors in metastatic melanoma: a pooled analysis of Eastern Cooperative Oncology Group trials. J Clin Oncol 2000; 18(22):3782–3793.

60 Salmoniere P de La, Grob JJ, Dreno B, et al. White blood cell count: a prognostic factor and possible subset indicator of optimal treatment with low-dose adjuvant interferon in primary melanoma. Clin Cancer Res 2000; 6(12):4713–4718.

61 Rodrigues LK, Klencke BJ, Vin-Christian K, et al. Altered clinical course of malignant melanoma in HIV-positive patients. Arch Dermatol 2002; 138(6):765–770.

62 Martinez JC, Otley CC, Stasko T, et al. Defining the clinical course of metastatic skin cancer in organ transplant recipients: a multicenter collaborative study. Arch Dermatol 2003; 139(3):301–306.

63 Haffner AC, Garbe C, Burg G, et al. The prognosis of primary and metastasising melanoma. An evaluation of the TNM classification in 2,495 patients. Br J Cancer 1992; 66(5):856–861.

64 Harrist TJ, Rigel DS, Day CL Jr, et al. Microscopic satellites are more highly associated with regional lymph node metastases than is primary melanoma thickness. Cancer 1984; 53(10):2183–2187.

65 Day CL Jr, Harrist TJ, Gorstein F, et al. Malignant melanoma. Prognostic significance of microscopic satellites in the reticular dermis and subcutaneous fat. Ann Surg 1981; 194(1):108–112.

66 Sober AJ, Day CL Jr, Fitzpatrick TB, et al. Early death from clinical stage I melanoma. J Invest Dermatol 1983; 80(Suppl):50–52.

67 Sober AJ, Day CL Jr, Fitzpatrick TB, et al. Factors associated with death from melanoma from 2 to 5 years following diagnosis in clinical stage I patients. J Invest Dermatol 1983; 80(Suppl):53–55.

68 Leon P, Daly JM, Synnestvedt M, et al. The prognostic implications of microscopic satellites in patients with clinical stage I melanoma. Arch Surg 1991; 126(12):1461–1468.

69 Buzaid AC, Ross MI, Balch CM, et al. Critical analysis of the current American Joint Committee on Cancer staging system for cutaneous melanoma and proposal of a new staging system [comment]. J Clin Oncol 1997; 15(3):1039–1051.

70 Balch CM, Soong SJ, Smith T, et al. Long-term results of a prospective surgical trial comparing 2 cm vs 4 cm excision margins for 740 patients with 1–4 mm melanomas [comment]. Ann Surg Oncol 2001; 8(2):101–108.

71 Gershenwald JE, Balch CM, Soong S, et al. Prognostic factors and natural history. In: Balch CM, ed. Cutaneous Melanoma, 2nd edn. Quality Medical Publishing, Inc. 2002:25–55.

72 Morton DL, Wen DR, Wong JH, et al. Technical details of intraoperative lymphatic mapping for early stage melanoma. Arch Surg 1992; 127(4):392–399.

73 McMasters KM, Reintgen DS, Ross MI, et al. Sentinel lymph node biopsy for melanoma: controversy despite widespread agreement. J Clin Oncol 2001; 19(11):2851–2855.

74 McMasters KM, Sober A, Kirkwood JM. Sentinel lymph node biopsy and adjuvant therapy for melanoma: evidence revisited [comment and author reply]. Arch Dermatol 2003; 139(1):99–100.

75 McMasters KM, Chao C, Wong SL, et al. Interval sentinel lymph nodes in melanoma. Arch Surg 2002; 547(9):543–549.

76 Essner R, Chung MH, Bleicher R, et al. Prognostic implications of thick (> or = 4 mm) melanoma in the era of intraoperative lymphatic mapping and sentinel lymphadenectomy [comment]. Ann Surg Oncol 2002; 9(8):754–761.

77 Gershenwald JE, Mansfield PF, Lee JE, et al. Role for lymphatic mapping and sentinel lymph node biopsy in patients with thick (> or = 4 mm) primary melanoma. Ann Surg Oncol 2000; 7(2):160–165.

78 Gershenwald JE, Thompson W, Mansfield PF, et al. Multi-institutional melanoma lymphatic mapping experience: the prognostic value of sentinel lymph node status in 612 stage I or II melanoma patients. J Clin Oncol 1999; 17(3):976–983.

79 Jansen L, Nieweg OE, Peterse JL, et al. Reliability of sentinel lymph node biopsy for staging melanoma [comment]. Br J Surg 2000; 87(4):484–489.

80 Shivers SC, Wang X, Li W, et al. Molecular staging of malignant melanoma: correlation with clinical outcome. JAMA 1998; 280(16):1410–1415.

81 Statius Muller MG, van Leeuwen PA, de Lange-De Klerk ES, et al. The sentinel lymph node status is an important factor for predicting clinical outcome in patients with Stage I or II cutaneous melanoma. Cancer 2001; 91(12):2401–2408.

82 Ranieri JM, Wagner JD, Azuaje R, et al. Prognostic importance of lymph node tumor burden in melanoma patients staged by sentinel node biopsy. Ann Surg Oncol 2002; 9(10):975–981.

83 White RR, Stanley WE, Johnson JL, et al. Long-term survival in 2,505 patients with melanoma with regional lymph node metastasis. Ann Surg 2002; 235(6):879–887.

84 Chang P, Knapper WH. Metastatic melanoma of unknown primary. Cancer 1982; 49(6):1106–1111.

85 Balch CM, Soong SJ, Murad TM, et al. A multifactorial analysis of melanoma. IV. Prognostic factors in 200 melanoma patients with distant metastases (stage III). J Clin Oncol 1983; 1(2):126–134.

86 Eton O, Legha SS, Moon TE, et al. Prognostic factors for survival of patients treated systemically for disseminated melanoma. J Clin Oncol 1998; 16(3):1103–1111.

87 Banfalvi T, Boldizsar M, Gergye M, et al. Comparison of prognostic significance of serum 5-S-Cysteinyldopa, LDH and S-100B protein in Stage III–IV malignant melanoma. Pathol Oncol Res 2002; 8(3):183–187.

88 Balch CM, Buzaid AC, Soong SJ, et al. Final version of the American Joint Committee on Cancer staging system for cutaneous melanoma. J Clin Oncol 2001; 19(16):3635–3648.

89 Von Roenn JH, Kheir SM, Wolter JM, et al. Significance of DNA abnormalities in primary malignant melanoma and nevi, a retrospective flow cytometric study. Cancer Res 1986; 46(6):3192–3195.

90 Kheir SM, Bines SD, Von Roenn JH, et al. Prognostic significance of DNA aneuploidy in stage I cutaneous melanoma. Ann Surg 1988; 207(4):455–461.

91 Zaloudik J, Moore M, Ghosh AK, et al. DNA content and MHC class II antigen expression in malignant melanoma: clinical course. J Clin Pathol 1988; 41(10):1078–1084.

92 Udart M, Utikal J, Krahn GM, et al. Chromosome 7 aneusomy. A marker for metastatic melanoma? Expression of the epidermal growth factor receptor gene and chromosome 7 aneusomy in nevi, primary malignant melanomas and metastases. Neoplasia (New York) 2001; 3(3):245–254.

93 Carr KM, Bittner M, Trent JM. Gene-expression profiling in human cutaneous melanoma. Oncogene 2003; 22(20):3076–3080.

94 Duncan LM, Deeds J, Hunter J, et al. Down-regulation of the novel gene melastatin correlates with potential for melanoma metastasis. Cancer Res 1998; 58(7):1515–1520.

95 Gradilone A, Gazzaniga P, Ribuffo D, et al. Survivin, bcl-2, bax and bcl-X gene expression in sentinel lymph nodes from melanoma patients. J Clin Oncol 2003; 21(2):306–312.

96 Sung J, Li W, Shivers S, et al. Molecular analysis in evaluating the sentinel node in malignant melanoma. Ann Surg Oncol 2001; 8(9):29S–30S.

97 Zettersten E, Shaikh L, Ramirez R, Kashani-Sabet M. Prognostic factors in primary cutaneous melanoma. Surg Clin N Am 2003; 83:61–75.

CHAPTER

16

Dysplastic Nevi

Thomas G Salopek and Robert J Friedman

Key points

- A dysplastic nevus is a distinct clinico-pathological entity that portends an increased risk for developing melanoma.
- The lesion falls on the tumor pathway that spans banal nevus at one end of the spectrum and melanoma at the other end. Despite this, dysplastic nevi rarely eventuate into melanoma.
- There appears to be a genetic basis for the condition, particularly in the context of familial melanoma.
- The condition can be readily diagnosed on clinical grounds alone, as such there is no need for histological confirmation.
- Removal of dysplastic nevi is only necessary when one can not reliably exclude melanoma.

INTRODUCTION

The single most important determinant of whether an individual is prone to develop melanoma (MM) or not, is the presence or absence of dysplastic nevi (DN). There are numerous epidemiological studies that confirm the significance of DN as markers for increased risk for developing MM. There is also irrefutable evidence both at the genomic and post-translational levels that supports the legitimacy of this lesion as a distinct entity separate from banal melanocytic nevi and MM. Biologically, DN represents a point on a continuum that spans benign nevus at one end of the spectrum, and MM at the other. Although they exist on the 'tumor progression pathway' to MM and have been well documented to occasionally progress to cancer, in most instances DN are benign lesions that infrequently eventuate to MM. The DN should be viewed not as an obligate precursor to MM, but rather as a phenotypic discriminator that identifies persons at increased risk for MM. Despite the overwhelming evidence at the clinical, epidemiologic, histologic and biologic levels, there are some researchers/experts who prefer to simply ignore the existence of DN.[1,2] As such, the importance and relevance of DN remains a highly contentious issue and one of the more controversial subjects in dermatology.[3] This chapter reviews the history behind DN, its epidemiology, biology and genetics, clinical features, pathology and provides guidelines on how to best manage individuals with these lesions.

HISTORY

In 1978, Clark and colleagues at the University of Pennsylvania described for the first time a previously unrecognized clinicopathological entity which identified persons at risk for MM.[4] They called their newly discovered disorder the 'B-K mole syndrome' in recognition of the two families that were studied, whose surnames began with the letters B and K. Since then various names have been used for this lesion and its corresponding syndrome. Unfortunately, the constant changing terminology and variable definitions of each have contributed to much of the confusion around this lesion. Terms that have been used or suggested include the DN (and syndrome), atypical mole (and syndrome), familial atypical multiple mole MM (FAMMM) syndrome, and Clark's nevus (and syndrome).[5–8] Similarly, multiple pathologic names have been assigned to the lesion. Many were simply histologic descriptors that failed to clarify matters and often perpetuated misunderstandings. These included 'pagetoid melanocytic proliferation', 'nevus with architectural disorder', 'atypical melanocytic proliferation' and 'intraepithelial melanocytic neoplasia'.[9–12]

Fourteen years after its initial description, the National Institute of Health in the US held a consensus development conference to resolve some of the controversy concerning DN. Experts from many disciplines of medicine convened in Bethesda, Maryland (27–29 January, 1992), to reach a consensus regarding the validity of this lesion and to make recommendations regarding the diagnosis and treatment of it and early MM.[10] The expert panel concluded that DN is a legitimate lesion representing an acquired pigmented tumor whose clinical and histologic appearance is different from common moles. Due to a lack of unanimity on the definition of dysplasia, the panel recommended the following: the term DN be replaced with atypical moles, that histologically they be diagnosed as nevi with architectural disorder, and that the syndrome for MM-prone families be called familial atypical mole and melanoma (FAM-M) syndrome. Their recommendations regarding terminology were never fully accepted by the medical community. Over the past 25 years, the term that is most frequently used by clinicians, pathologists and researchers is dysplastic nevus (and syndrome (DNS)), hence the reason for using this term throughout this chapter.

EPIDEMIOLOGY

The actual prevalence of DN is not known. Depending on whether clinical or histologic definitions were used to identify this lesion, the reported incidence rate has varied from as low as 2% to as high as 53%.[13,14] A more realistic number would suggest an incidence in the order of 2–8% for Caucasian populations.[15–17] Due to the interaction of genetic and environmental factors in the pathogenesis of DN it would be impossible to assign a more accurate figure. Bataille et al. have shown that even with a populations of a common genetic pool, sun-exposure can dramatically influence the incidence of DN.[15] They reported a prevalence of the 'atypical mole syndrome' phenotype in 6% of their studied population chronically exposed to sunlight vs 2% in the non-chronically sun-exposed cohort.

Multiple retrospective case–control studies have demonstrated a significant risk for MM in patients with DN (Table 16.1). The risk for MM is dependent on the number of DN present and other variables, but generally ranges between two- to 12-fold increase (if outliners listed in Table 16.1 are excluded).[15,18–27] Although DN are often a surrogate for the presence of numerous moles which portends its own inherent risk for MM, studies have shown that when corrected for numbers of nevi the risk for MM persists.[18,27]

Four prospective studies have confirmed an increased probability of developing MM in patients with DN.[28–31] The likelihood of MM was strongly influenced by whether there was a personal or family history of this cancer (Table 16.2). The relative risk for MM in patients with DN as compared with controls varied from 47–493. Furthermore, there have been two cohort, retrospective studies that examined the incidence of MM in patients with DNS.[32,33] Marghoob et al. compared the incidence of newly diagnosed MM in 287 patients with DNS versus 831 controls for a mean follow-up of 58 and 89 months, respectively. Based on their chart review of the two groups they estimated the 10-year cumulative risk for developing MM in the study population to be 10.7% vs 0.62% in the controls.[32] In a similar study, Halpern et al. reported a 71-fold increased incidence of MM in a cohort of 153 patients with DN followed for a minimum of 5 years compared with age-adjusted historical controls.[33]

PATHOGENESIS AND ETIOLOGY: GENETICS AND BIOLOGY

The strongest argument for the existence of DN as a distinct clinicopathological entity lies with its linkage with familial MM. In addition to being prone to develop MM, affected individuals often have multiple moles many of which are dysplastic clinically and histologically.[4,7] Pedigree mapping suggested that clustering of MM within these families was due to an autosomal dominantly inherited gene.[34] Several MM susceptibility genes have now been identified.[35] The first characterized gene located on the short arm of chromosome one (1p36)[36] has yet to be convincingly linked with MM.[37–39] Almost 15 years since its isolation, no gene product has been assigned to this segment of the chromosome, suggesting that it is of little importance in FAMMM syndrome. In fact, the original investigators have turned their attention to one of the other postulated genes.[40,41]

Researchers are currently focusing their attention on three other more likely candidate genes: the tumor suppressor gene p16/cyclin dependent kinase 2A (on chromosome 9p21 which is the most probable gene identified to date), an oncogene CDK4 (chromosome 12q14), and a second tumor suppressor gene p19 (also on chromosome 9p21).[35] Investigators from multiple centers around the world have demonstrated a strong linkage with the tumor suppressor gene p16.[41–48] The gene encodes for a cyclin dependent kinase that arrests cell proliferation at the G1 phase by binding to CDK 4 and 6, which in turn prevents the phosphorylation of the retinoblastoma protein.[49] A mutation of p16 results in phosphorylation of the retinoblastoma protein activating cell growth. In addition to being the gene most frequently associated with MM (approximately 40% of families with hereditary MM),[50] this gene has been linked with DN leading some to propose that CDKN2A is nevogenic.[48]

Using different techniques and approaches some researchers have demonstrated a linkage with p16,[51,52] while others have found no association.[50,53–55] This does not exclude the possibility of a genetic basis for DN. It simply highlights the heterogeneity of this condition and that its appearance is likely the consequence of a complex interaction between environmental and genetic factors, the latter possibly being polygenic.[15,56] One hypothesis suggests that DN are the result of inactivation of a single gene through the loss of both alleles, with loss of the first resulting in dysplasia, and the other in MM.[56] Conversely it is possible that the dysplastic-MM phenotype is dependent on two separate genes.[56,57] Inactivation of the first leads to dysplasia, and loss of the second to MM. Other genes including modifying genes that co-segregate with CDKN2A and increase the penetrance of the latter may also have a role in the expression of this phenotype.[48]

Several theories have been postulated to explain the increased frequency of mutations in p16 and other putative MM-DN genes. One theory contends that mutation is due to ultraviolet light-induced hyper-mutability of cells in patients with the DNS.[58] The other theory proposes an inherent instability of chromosomes as a consequence of a process known as 'microsatellite instability'.[59] The theories are not mutually exclusive, and it is possible that one alteration may influence the other.

From its earliest descriptions researchers have been aware of the presence of cytogenetic abnormalities in fibroblast and lymphocyte cell cultures obtained from patients with the DNS.[60,61] Many of the karyotypic changes seen were similar to those found in patients with Bloom's syndrome. For this reason it was suggested that DNS might represent a chromosomal instability disorder.[60] Subsequent work by Lynch et al. documented

Table 16.1 Relative risk for melanoma in patients with dysplastic nevi based on retrospective case–control studies

Country	Cases (n)	Controls (n)	Nevi (n)	RR	DN (n)	RR
Australia[18]	246	134	<16	1.0	Not adjusted for number of nevi	7.6
			16–30	1.3		
			31–45	1.7	Adjusted for number of nevi	7.7
			>45	0.8		
Australia[15]	183	162	<4	1.0	0	1.0
			5–9	0.9	1	1.3
			10–24	1.5	2	3.9
			25–49	4.2	>3	4.6
			50–99	4.5		
			>100	12.7		
France[19]	207	295	<10	1.0	>1	2.8
			11–20	1.2		
			21–40	3.8		
			41–80	3.5		
			81–120	4.1		
			>120	16.1		
Germany[20]	200	200	<10	1.0	0	1.0
			11–20	3.1	1–2	11.4
			21–40	2.3	>2	6.1
			41–60	7.3		
			>60	14.7		
Germany[21]	513	498	11–50	1.7	<4	1.6
			51–100	3.7	>4	6.1
			>100	7.6		
Scotland[22]	180	197	0	1.0	0	1.0
			1–9	0.8	1–4	5.2
			10–24	6.7	>5	5.7
			25–49	10.7		
			>50	53.9		
Scotland[23]	280	280	<20	1.0	<2	2.1
			>20 male	13.9	>3 male	4.5
			>20 female	6.7	>3 female	4.4
Sweden[24]	121	378	1–74	1.0	0	1.0
			75–149	1.2	1–2	2.5
			>150	2.6	>3	5.6
UK[15]	117	163	<4	1.0	0	1.0
			5–9	1.1	1	3.0
			10–24	1.5	2	1.4
			25–49	2.9	>3	51.7
			50–99	10.1		
			>100	16.5		
USA (CA)[25]	121	139	<10	1.0	0	1.0
			11–25	1.6	1–5	3.8
			26–50	4.4	>5	6.3
			51–100	5.4		
			>100	9.8		
USA (PA)[26]	105	181	<25	1.0	present vs	8.8
			>25	6.5	absent	
USA (PA and CA)[27]	716	1014	0	1.0	0	1.0
			1	1.3	1	3.8
			2–4	2.0	2–4	11
			5–9	3.7	5–9	8.6
			>10	7.2	>10	32

an increased frequency of chromosomal translocations, deletions, and inversions in cell cultures of DN and normal skin fibroblasts taken from two extended FAMMM kindreds.[62] The fact that chromosomal abnormalities were seen in fibroblasts, lymphocytes and melanocytes brings up the question of why individuals from MM-prone families with DN are only susceptible to MM and not other cancers?[63,64] It is possible that

Table 16.2   Prospective studies examining the incidence of melanoma in patients with dysplastic nevi

Country	History of melanoma	Patients (mean follow-up in patient months) (n)	Melanomas (n)	Relative risk
Without controls				
Scotland[29]	No	85 (6996)	5	92
	Personal	24 (2136)	4	91
	Family	7 (672)	6	444
USA (NY)[30]	No	281 (6876)	4	57
	Personal	66 (2242)	3	127
	Family	69 (1750)	4	214
	Personal & family	36 (911)	5	493
USA (NY)[31]	No	157 (8173)	4	53
	Personal	95 (4415)	4	74
	Family	89 (4132)	1	33
	Personal & family	16 (602)	1	137
With controls				
USA (CA)[28]	DN (no melanoma)	267 (16,020)	5	47
	Controls	2486 (149,160)	1	1

environmental factors, primarily exposure to ultraviolet light is responsible for this incongruity. When populations of a common genetic pool but different lifetime sun-exposure were compared for the frequency of the DNS phenotype, a three-fold increase in prevalence was noted in the habitually sun-exposed group supporting the role of sun exposure in nevogenesis.[15]

If ultraviolet radiation (UVR) is the initiating event in the expression of DN and MM, should there not be an increased incidence of non-melanocytic precancerous and cancerous skin lesions in these families? Although it would be expected that keratinocytes would have the same level of chromosomal instability as melanocytes, it has been shown that the former are more susceptible to UVR-induced apoptosis than melanocytes.[65] As the number of mutations increases, a threshold is reached that activates apoptosis within keratinocytes but not melanocytes, leading to their removal from the pool that could progress to skin cancer. In melanocytes, the relative resistance to apoptosis allows mutations to accumulate until one cell ultimately transforms into MM.

Since the early 1980s, researchers have been aware that cultured cells from FAMMM syndrome members exhibit an increased sensitivity to UVR.[66,67] These preliminary studies simply reported an increased cell death rate after exposure to ultraviolet light. However, due to the infancy of molecular biology at the time the investigators were unable to provide any explanations for this phenomenon. Subsequent studies demonstrated ultraviolet radiation associated hypermutability of chromosomes in these patients.[68,69] More recently it has been found that patients with DNS may have defective DNA repair systems for ultraviolet light-induced DNA damage.[70–72] To what extent these DNA repair systems participate in nevogenesis is not known. Other researchers using different methods for assessing DNA repair mechanisms were unable to confirm in these findings.[73–75]

A second possible explanation for the increased frequency of mutations in DN patients is the phenomenon known as microsatellite instability.[59] Microsatellites are simple sequence tandem repeats, usually 2–5 nucleotides in length. The repeat motifs are of variable number, from 8 to 50 and occur primarily in non-coding regions of the chromosome. They are stable and highly conserved from one generation to the next and in different cells from the same individual. Although their exact function remains a mystery, it has been proposed that they regulate gene expression and protein function. Mutations within these repetitive nucleotide sequences are known as microsatellite instability (MSI). These changes presumably develop secondary to decreased DNA repair capacity of the cell. Multiple studies have demonstrated variable amounts of MSI in melanocytic lesions. Benign nevi in general have little to no variability whereas DN and MM have increased amounts of MSI.[59,76,77] Though primarily found in non-coding regions, approximately 10% are found in coding sequences which results in cell dysfunction and possibly progression to cancer.

Almost every molecular, genetic (e.g. oncogenes and tumor suppressor genes), functional/biological, immunologic (e.g. surface antigens), biochemical (e.g. cytokines, growth factors and their receptors, adhesion molecules, cell growth regulators, apoptotic mechanisms, pigment synthesis, etc.) and structural abnormality that has been identified in MM has also been noted in dysplastic nevocytes.[78–88] Interestingly, the changes seen in DN place it somewhere between a benign nevus and MM supporting the theory of tumor progression along a pathway as has been proposed.[82,89,90] In the past it was common to assume that these changes were of causal importance in the pathogenesis of DN and its progression to MM. It is more likely that they are an epiphenomenon and are an expression of the genetic mutations outlined above.

CLINICAL FEATURES

DN is an acquired melanocytic nevus that clinically exhibits features also seen with MM. This definition, although imprecise and the source of much of the controversy around this lesion expresses those characteristics that set it apart from a common mole. To convey to colleagues and lay people features that specifically identify DN, some researchers have suggested the use of the ABCD rule of melanoma. It is the degree of each criterion that separates these two conditions.[91] It is obvious that there will be considerable overlap between DN and MM when this definition is used and that any distinction is quite subjective. Just as the ABCD rule of melanoma is inadequate in identifying all MM, so too is this description in encapsulating the essence of DN that permits its identification. It simply reflects biology of the lesion and that DN exists on a continuum which includes banal moles on one end of the spectrum and MM at the other extreme.[89,90]

Detractors claim that this is nonsense; that there can only be benign lesions or malignant lesions and 'nothing in between'.[92,93] This view of the world in simple black and white terms with absolute disregard for the gray areas (never mind the myriad of colors possible) goes against all the knowledge that has been acquired over the past 25 years concerning the genetics, molecular biology and tumor biology of this lesion.

Historically a DN was defined as a mole larger than 5 mm in diameter, variegated in pigmentation, and irregular in outline.[4] Since its original description more accurate features have been assigned that ensure its reproducibility. Researchers from Australia have emphasized the need for a macular component to the nevus and the presence of at least three of five criteria: an ill-defined or irregular border, irregularly distributed pigmentation, background of erythema and size >5 mm.[94] Tucker *et al.* have used similar clinical features to describe DN.[27] They stress that the mole should be greater than 5 mm in size and minimally elevated and

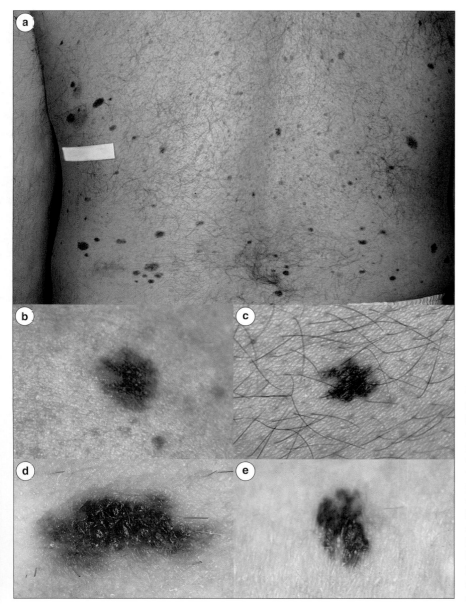

Figure 16.1 (a) A dysplastic nevus syndrome patient who had two previous invasive melanomas removed by local wide excision. The striking feature is the heterogeneity of his moles in terms of size, color and shape. (b–e) Close-up views of typical dysplastic nevi. They often mimic melanoma in that they can be variable in color (b) or exhibit prominent border irregularity and asymmetry (of color and outline), (c). Dysplastic nevi occasionally have a mammillated darker center with lighter colored macular component at the periphery (i.e. the 'shoulder') (d). Severe asymmetry and border irregularity with dark center (e).

should exhibit two of three other features: variable pigmentation, irregular or asymmetric outline, and indistinct borders. A striking feature of dysplastic moles is their heterogeneity in appearance. Moles of all shapes, colors and size may be seen (Fig. 16.1). Patients frequently have numerous moles, the majority of which are not dysplastic. DN are most commonly found on the trunk, however, it is not unusual to see them on the scalp or buttocks, typically sun-protected areas. Separating DN from MM clinically occasionally can be impossible as illustrated by the closely matched lesions in Figure 16.2. Even dermoscopy may at times be unable to make this distinction (Fig. 16.3). Histopathology evaluation is often required to make this distinction.

Using the aforementioned criteria one can often diagnose DN on clinical grounds alone. However, difficulties arise when one has to decide whether the patient has DNS versus an isolated DN. Although the latter is associated with a slightly increased risk for MM (~ two-fold), it is not as significant as being labeled with the full-blown syndrome which portends a markedly increased risk for MM. The NIH has suggested the following criteria for a diagnosis of familial atypical mole melanoma (FAM-M) syndrome: MM in one or more first or second degree relatives, the presence of a large number of moles (often >50) several of which are atypical, and moles that demonstrate distinct histologic features.[10] The Dutch Working Group requires the presence of three of the following five criteria to make a clinical diagnosis of DN (atypical mole): a mole >5 mm in diameter with a vague border, asymmetric shape, irregular pigmentation and red hue.[95] A patient is said to have DNS if there is a personal history of MM and one or more clinically dysplastic nevi.

British investigations have proposed the following scoring system to identify the 'atypical mole syndrome' (DN syndrome) phenotype: 100 or more nevi >2 mm (or 50 or more moles if <20 years of age, or >50 years of age); two or more atypical nevi (defined as a mole >5 mm, with an irregular or blurred edge, and irregular pigmentation); one or more nevi on the buttocks; and two or more on the dorsal feet (Table 16.3).[48] Each feature is worth one point. Patients with a score of two or higher have DNS. This scoring system is a revision of their earlier grading method which required the above feature plus the presence of one or more nevi on the anterior scalp and one or more iris nevi.[96] The earlier scoring system had been validated and shown to be easily learned by non-specialist health care professionals who would be involved in MM screening.[97] Although the revised scoring system is simpler than the original it has yet to be validated in a repeat study.

HISTOLOGY

The importance of pathology for the diagnosis of DN has diminished in recent years. As was previously mentioned, this diagnosis (as it relates to identifying individuals at risk for MM) can be readily made on clinical grounds. Therefore, there is no reason to perform a biopsy on a mole other than to rule out MM. This is not to say that the histology of this lesion is irrelevant. In fact the converse is true. It is essential that one be cognizant of its histologic appearance due to potential overlap and confusion with MM.

Critics of DN argue that the pathology of this lesion has never been adequately described nor have the terms used to delineate the histologic features of this lesion (e.g. dysplasia, cytological and architectural atypia, etc.) been precisely defined despite evidence to the contrary (Table 16.4).[1,98] Since the mid-1990s, there have been several well-designed studies that confirm the validity and reproducibility of the pathologic features of DN.

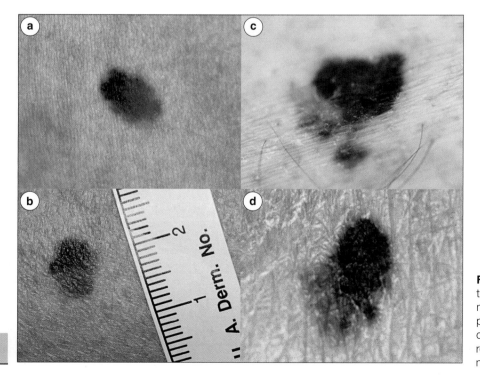

Figure 16.2 It can be extremely difficult to clinically differentiate dysplastic nevi from melanoma as the two closely matched pairs of lesions demonstrate. (a, b) dysplastic nevus and melanoma in situ, respectively; (c, d) dysplastic nevus and melanoma in situ, respectively.

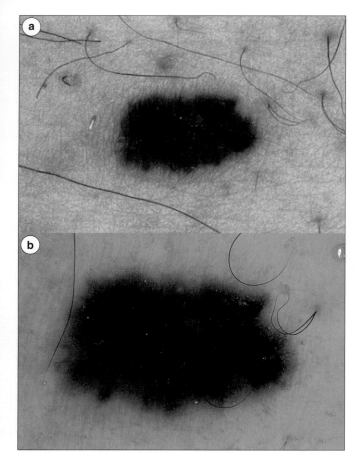

Figure 16.3 A severe dysplastic nevus that exhibited many of the features of (a) melanoma clinically and (b) dermoscopy; the distinction between the two only being possible on histology.

Table 16.4	Criteria for the histologic diagnosis of dysplastic nevus

Architecture
  Superficial plaque only (junctional), or plaque surrounding papule (compound)
  Nests bridge rete
  Nests at sides of rete
  Single cells between nests, nests predominate
  'Lentiginous' elongation of rete
  Anastomosis of rete
  Little or no pagetoid spread

Host responses
  Patchy lymphocytic infiltrate (bandlike lymphocytic response suggests melanoma)
  Eosinophilic fibroplasia
  Lamellar fibroplasia (rare)
  Prominent vessels (sometimes)

Cytology
  'Random' slight to moderate atypia
  Few, if any, mitoses
  Occasional macronucleoli
  Scattered epithelioid nevus cells
  Scattered cells with 'dusty' melanin pigment

Modified from Elder DE, Murphy GF. Melanocytic tumors of the skin. In: Rosai J, Sobin LH, eds. Atlas of Tumor Pathology; 3rd series, part 2. Washington, DC: Armed Forces Institute of Pathology; 1991.

Table 16.3	Revised dysplastic nevus syndrome score

Features	Score
100 or more nevi >2 mm (50 or more if under 20 or over 50 years of age)	1
2 or more atypical nevi	1
1 or more nevi on the buttocks	1
2 or more nevi on dorsal feet	1
Total score ≥2 = dysplastic nevus syndrome	

Reproduced from Bishop JA, et al. Genotype/phenotype and penetrance studies in melanoma families with germline CDKN2A mutations. J Invest Dermatol 2000; 114(1):28–33. Blackwell Publishing Ltd.

In 1993, the pathology subgroup of the EORTC Malignant Melanoma Cooperative Group reported a study that validated the histopathologic criteria used to diagnose DN.[100] In this study, ten dermatopathologists reviewed 50 cutaneous melanocytic lesions (including common nevi, DN and invasive and *in-situ* MM), and then scored each lesion semi-quantitatively using a standardized form of 20 defined histologic criteria. They found a high degree of concordance of diagnosis, with the most reproducible criteria for diagnosing DN being the presence of marked junctional proliferation, large melanocytic nuclei, irregular nests, and lympho-histiocytic infiltrate. If three or more of these features were present, they noted a sensitivity of 86% and specificity of 91% for making a diagnosis of DN. Based on their findings the authors devised a simplified approach to the diagnosis of melanocytic tumors which is outlined in Table 16.5.

A study by the Dysplastic Nevus Panel confirmed the reliability of the histopathologic diagnosis of melanocytic dysplasia.[101] A random sample of 112 melanocytic tumors (including common nevi, DN and MM) were graded on a five-point scale for the degree of atypia of the following histologic parameters: size of nucleus, variability in shape and size of the nucleus, chromatin staining, and features of the nucleolus and cytoplasm. Interrater reliability of the panelists (five dermatopathologists and two MM specialists) was measured by intraclass and Pearson correlation coef-ficients. They reported an acceptable level of concordance with intraclass and Pearson correlation coefficients of 0.67 and 0.67–0.84, respectively. Individual panel members were within one grade (on the five-point scale) of the mean of the study panel 88% of the time and, rarely, by two or more grades (3%). The authors concluded that it is possible to diagnose melanocytic dysplasia by well defined and agreed upon criteria, and that its severity graded with 'reasonable although imperfect reliability'.

Ideally, both cytological and architectural atypia should be present to make a diagnosis of DN histologically. Although these two features tend to be positively cor-related and somewhat interdependent, not infrequently one will see a lesion that exhibits a high score for one

Table 16.5 EORTC Malignant Melanoma Cooperative Group: diagnostic approach based on histological features of melanocytic tumors[100]

Morphological features	Diagnosis
None, or two or less of the features mentioned below for DN	Common nevus
≥3 of the following features: 　Marked junctional proliferation 　Irregular nests 　Large nuclei 　Lymphohistiocytic infiltrate	Dysplastic nevus
Pagetoid growth Continuous junctional proliferation	Melanoma *in situ*
Pagetoid growth Continuous junctional proliferation Invasion of markedly atypical melanocytes into the dermis	Superficial spreading melanoma

Table 16.6 Duke University grading system for dysplastic nevi[102]

Feature	Score 0	Score 1
Architectural disorder:		
Junctional component nested at both edges	Yes	No
Good overall symmetry	Yes	No
More than 5% of nests cohesive	Yes	No
Suprabasal spread prominent, or present at edge	No	Yes
Confluence of >50% of proliferation	No	Yes
Single-cell proliferation absent or focal	Yes	No
Sum total:	___	___
Cytologic atypia:		
Nuclei round or oval, and euchromatic	Yes	No
Nuclei > basal-layer keratinocyte nuclei	No	Yes
Nucleoli prominent	No	Yes
Cell diameter >2 × basal-layer keratinocyte nuclei	No	Yes
Sum total:	___	___

Key for architectural disorder: (0–1) = Mild; (2–3) = Moderate; (4–6) = Severe
Key for cytologic atypia: (0–1) = Mild; (2) = Moderate; (3–4) = Severe
Separate scores are obtained for architecture and cytology by assigning a value of 0 or 1 for each criterion and summing.

parameter and a low score for the other and vice versa.[102] Using a scoring system as proposed by Shea *et al.* it is possible to classify these lesions into mild, moderate or severe dysplasia (Table 16.6).[102] English researchers using slightly different histologic criteria came to the same conclusion that DN can be reliably segregated into high-grade (severe dysplasia) and low-grade (mild–moderate dysplasia) with a diagnostic accuracy of 99.5%.[103] By multivariate analyses they identified three nuclear variables (pleomorphism, heterogeneous chromatin and nucleolus prominence) and two architectural features (junctional symmetry, and presence and location of suprabasilar melanocytes) that were useful in categorizing DN along these lines.[103] It is important to remember that such classification has not been proven to be an indicator of degree of risk of evolution into MM and thus remains quite controversial.

MANAGEMENT

Patients with DNS can be challenging to manage. Despite this, the majority can be successfully treated by any dermatologist, and do not necessarily warrant referral to a pigmented lesion clinic. The latter should be considered if there is a strong family history of MM or if the patient has innumerable nevi that precludes satisfactory follow-up in the absence of total body photography and/or dermoscopy.

The management of DN centers around the following: (1) obtaining a detailed personal and family history for DN and MM, and performing a thorough examination of the skin; (2) regular follow-up; (3) the use of diagnostic aids for the early detection of MM including total body photography, dermoscopy, and/or digital imaging devices; (4) biopsy of any lesion suspected of being MM; (5) MM prophylaxis through sun-protection and sun-avoidance; and (6) nevi reduction for cosmetic reasons and possibly to prevent MM.

Personal and family history

Individuals diagnosed with DN should be questioned regarding any family history of DN and MM. Inquiries should take into consideration first-degree and second-degree relatives (i.e. parents, siblings, and offspring; grandparents, aunts, uncles and cousins, respectively). Reasons for pedigree mapping are two-fold: (1) the more family members affected with either entity the greater the risk for MM and therefore heightened need for more frequent follow-ups and (2) to make MM screening available to individuals who may be at similar increased risk for MM.

Unfortunately, relying on patient recall regarding their family history of MM or DN can be misleading. Weinstock *et al.* found that only about one in five supposed MMs in family members and first-degree relatives could be confirmed on medical records.[104] Furthermore, the adequacy of genetic surveys in identifying all individuals of a given family at increased risk for developing MM has recently been challenged.[105] Researchers from England attempted to correlate DNS phenotype with gene carrier status in five families with germline CDKN2A mutations, and found that there was a poor correlation between having an abnormal phenotype and carrying the mutant gene.[48] Although family members of the syndrome were three times more likely to be mutant gene carriers than their

relatives without the syndrome, there was considerable overlap between the gene carriers and non-carriers such that the DN phenotype did not sufficiently differentiate mutant carriers from those with a normal gene. The authors concluded that until there is a routine test for CDKN2A mutations, it would be prudent to screen all members of MM-prone families for this cancer. The feasibility of this recommendation has yet to be explored (see below).

Affected individuals should be screened regularly for MM, the frequency of which is dependent upon the risk for developing MM. Several different risk-stratifying systems have been proposed as a means to predict the probability of MM occurring. However, neither are routinely used or have gained universal acceptance (Tables 16.7 and 16.8).[30,106] A feature common to both grading systems is the stronger the family history of DN and MM, the greater the likelihood of developing this cancer. Instantly recognizable phenotypic traits are also useful in identifying individuals at risk for MM. These include the presence of numerous banal nevi, skin color, hair and eye color, sun sensitivity (specifically, propensity to develop sunburns and inability to tan), the history of other skin cancers and immunosuppression.[107,108]

The ideal frequency of follow-ups has yet to be established. Individuals with few moles and perhaps one or two DN can be reviewed every 6–12 months (or sooner if there is any reported change in their nevi). Individuals from MM-prone families should initially be screened every 3–6 months until the patient and physician are certain that the patient's nevi are stable in appearance.

Surveillance with total body photography has been shown to reduce the number of nevi that need to be removed for histologic assessment, and to result in the early detection of thin, potentially curable MM.[94,109] If the moles appear stable the interval between follow-up can ultimately be increased to once a year. It is important to appreciate that DN are dynamic throughout life. Although the majority of atypical moles remain stable in appearance,[41] they may exhibit increased atypia, decreased atypia or occasionally disappear altogether. Therefore, a change should not necessarily be construed as progression to MM.[110] Similarly it has been shown that dysplastic moles exhibit seasonal variations.[111] Each follow-up visit affords the physician the opportunity to educate the patient about the warning signs of MM, and to emphasize the need for routine self-skin examination (every 1–3 months) and the importance of preventing MM through sun-avoidance and sun-protection.

Not only are histologically proven DN uncommon in children,[112] MM appears to be a rare neoplasm in this population.[113] As such there is no need to see pre-pubescent children on a routine basis unless clinically warranted. Screening for MM should start during the teenage years or early twenties, and continue indefinitely, largely dependent on the probability of developing this cancer. Education of the younger patient population concerning the use of sun protection and early detection

Table 16.7 Rigel classification of melanoma risk for dysplastic nevus patients[30]	
Group	Score[a]
0	0
I	1
II	2
III	3+

[a]Scores are based on a point system as follows: personal history of MM = 1 point; family history of MM = 2 points per family member with MM.
(Reprinted with permission from Elsevier.)

Table 16.8 Kraemer classification of melanoma risk for dysplastic nevus syndrome[106]				
Type	Personal history		Family history	
	DN	MM	DN	MM
A	+	−	−	−
B	+	−	+	−
C	+	+	−	−
D1	+	+	+	−
	+	−	−	+
	+	−	+	+
D2	+	±	±	+ (>1)

Types A and C represent sporadic DNs. In type D1 only one blood relative in the entire family has MM (may be patient). In type D2 at least two blood relatives have MM (may include patient).
Modified nuclear pedigree consists of grandparents, parents, aunts, uncles, siblings and offspring. The same person may have both MM and AM.

may prove to be quite useful in both prevention of, and early intervention for, developing MM.

Physical examination

Physical examination should consist of a survey of the entire skin surface including intertriginous areas and scalp. Some physicians have suggested routine ophthalmologic examination to screen for ocular MM. It has been suggested that individuals with DNS are at increased risk for ocular MM.[114] While there has only been one case-controlled retrospective study that examined the possible association of ocular MM and DN, anecdotal reports in the literature suggest a positive correlation between the presence of DN and the development of ocular MM. Patients with uveal MM were only slightly more likely to have one or more atypical moles than not have one (RR=2.9; 95% confidence interval (CI) 1.2–6.3).[115] Interestingly, having blue or grey eye color (as opposed to brown colored eyes) results in a similar relative risk for ocular MM (RR=1.7 and 2.9, respectively).[116]

Diagnostic aids for melanoma

Patients with DNS frequently have hundreds of nevi. Although the majority may not be atypical in appearance, it can still be difficult to identify an individual suspicious nevus or new pigmented lesion among the plethora of moles. Total body photography has been well documented to be useful in this regard.[94,109] In this setting the only indicator of a potential problem may be photographic evidence that a pre-existing nevus has changed, or proof that a lesion was not there before.[117] Serial photography may be done with standard photographs, color slides, or digital imaging. The general trend in recent years has been to acquire and store total body photographs in digital format. Several computerized imaging systems are now commercially available (MoleMax; Molemap; Dermagraphix etc.) which minimize concerns about storage, archiving, and the retrieval of images.[118] With an almost unlimited storage capacity, computerized imaging permits the capture of as many pictures as desired for comparison purposes. In addition some of these systems are capable of analyzing a lesion dermoscopically (see below) and can provide an automated diagnosis in terms of the likelihood of a given lesion being MM or not. These systems are discussed in further depth in Chapter 36.

The primary advantage is the ability to detect change in a lesion, thereby reassuring the patient and physician that the lesion is likely benign. In this regard, use of these computer-based systems results in a substantial reduction of the number of moles that require biopsy. Although several studies have demonstrated the usefulness of photography in recognizing early MM,[119] health insurance companies have been reluctant to reimburse physicians/patients for the expense of this aid to follow-up. As a consequence total body photography often has been limited to specialized pigmented lesion clinics, academic institutions, or oncology-based dermatologists that have medical photographers readily available.

One of the more important advances in the early recognition of MM is dermoscopy. Numerous studies have shown that the clinical accuracy for MM can be markedly enhanced through dermoscopy.[120–123] Although there are no pathognomonic dermoscopic features to differentiate DN from MM unequivocally (similar to the clinical situation in which there can be considerable overlap in appearance between these two lesions) (Fig. 16.3), there are well described dermoscopic characteristics that should alert one to the possibility of MM, prompting a biopsy.[124] A dermoscopic classification of DN based on structural features and pigment distribution has been proposed by researchers from Europe which should help in recognition (Table 16.9).[125] In addition, there are several well established grading or scoring systems that have been devised to aid in differentiating MM from other pigmented lesions (these are summarized in Tables 16.10–16.12[126–128] and reviewed by the Consensus Net Meeting on Dermoscopy).[129]

Regrettably, dermatologists in North America have been somewhat slow to embrace this technology. Those who do not use dermoscopy argue that for typical MM, dermoscopy adds little to the clinical diagnosis.[130] It is

Table 16.9 Dermoscopic features of dysplastic nevi[125]

Structural	
Reticular	Prominent pigment network consisting of a regular mesh pattern, made up of thin lines
Globular	Presence of numerous globules or dots of variable size but evenly distributed
Homogeneous (structureless) pattern	Typical melanocytic features are missing, instead diffuse hypo- or hyper-pigmentation is seen
Combinations of the above	Reticular-globular; globular-homogeneous; reticular-homogeneous
Pigment distribution	
Central hypopigmentation	'Annular type' in which there is a structureless hypopigmented center ringed by a normal pigment network at the periphery
Central hyperpigmentation	As above but with a homogeneous dark brown center
Eccentric hypopigmentation	Peripherally located, hypopigmented structureless area
Eccentric hyperpigmentation	'Melanoma simulating type' in which there is a peripherally located hyperpigmented structureless area
Multifocal hypo- or hyper-pigmentation	Patchy and irregularly distributed homogenous areas, either hypopigmented or hyperpigmented

not 100% accurate, rather in the order of 80–90%. Furthermore, approximately 10% of MM are 'featureless' dermoscopically and therefore dermoscopy may not help in the early recognition of MM.[127] There is also a tendency for inexperienced users to over diagnose MM, resulting in an increased number of biopsies being performed.[131,132] Lastly, it has been suggested that if a lesion is atypical enough to warrant scrutiny by dermoscopy, it is likely equally suspicious to warrant histologic evaluation through biopsy.

Genetic counseling

With the completion of the human genome project in 2003 and the availability of DNA microarray technology, genetic testing has the potential to revolutionize the diagnosis of MM and conceivably prevent its development. In the future, it is envisioned that it will be possible to identify individuals at risk for MM not based on crude predictors such as phenotypic characteristics or the presence of DN, but by genetic testing.

It is estimated that approximately 10% of patients with MM will have one or more family members affected with this cancer.[64] While some familial cases result from similar environmental (sun exposure) risk factors, genetics likely play an important role. Those individuals who develop MM as a consequence of an MM susceptibility gene are reported to have 82–100%

Table 16.10 ABCD rule of dermatoscopy[126]

	Feature	Score	Weight
Asymmetry	In zero, one or two axes (color, structural components and shape are considered)	0–2	1.3
Border	Abrupt cut-off of pigment pattern in 0–8 segments	0–8	0.1
Color	Number of colors present which white, red, light- and dark-brown, slate-blue and black	1–6	0.5
Differential structures	Number of structural components present Possible: network, dots, globules, streaks and structureless areas	1–5	0.5

The weight score (Asymmetry x 1.3 + Border x 0.1 + Color x 0.5 + Differential structures x 0.5) is summed for the Total Dermoscopy Score (TDS). TDS = < 4.75 benign melanocytic nevus; TDS = 4.8–5.45 suspicious lesion for which excision or followup recommended; TDS >5.45 highly suspicious for melanoma.

Table 16.11 Menzies surface microscopy scoring system[127]

Negative features (should not be seen) = indicative of a benign lesion

Point and axial symmetry of pigmentation
Presence of only a single color

Positive features = indicative of melanoma

Asymmetry of pattern
Presence of >1 color
Any one of the following nine features: Blue-white veil; Multiple brown dots; Pseudopods; Radial streaming; Scar-like depigmentation; Peripheral black dots/globules; Multiple (5 or 6) colors; Multiple blue/gray dots; Broadened network

Table 16.12 ELM 7-point checklist[128]

Criteria	Points
Major criteria	
Atypical pigment network	2
Gray-blue areas	2
Atypical vascular pattern	2
Minor criteria	
Streaks	1
Blotches	1
Irregular dots and globules	1
Regression pattern	1

Seven point total score: <3 non-melanoma; ≥3 melanoma

'time-bomb' with its obvious deleterious effects on their quality of life. Furthermore, testing positive may raise legal issues as it relates to employability or insurability.

The American Society of Clinical Oncology (ASCO) does not currently recommend genetic testing for DN patients. Reasons for this include: (1) the role of MM susceptibility genes has not been adequately investigated and (2) it is unlikely that testing positively would alter or add to current management strategy. The Melanoma Genetic Consortium has taken a similar position, and presently only suggests genetic counseling as part of a research protocol.[133]

Removal of dysplastic nevi

It is indisputable that some DN progress to MM. There are several studies documenting this occurrence clinically based on sequential follow-up photography.[94,109,117] Similarly, histologically one may see evidence of DN in association with MM depending on how thoroughly one examines for its presence (20–25% of cases).[134,135] However, the overwhelming majority of DN *do not* eventuate into MM. A recent prospective study conducted over a 25-year period has reaffirmed the notion that these lesions are biologically benign, as the majority of DN either remain stable in appearance or regress. Few had changed in a manner that would cause concern for MM.[41] As a consequence, the idea of DN being a precursor lesion to MM has diminished over the past 10 years. DN should be primarily viewed as markers of an increased risk for developing MM. As DN can be consistently diagnosed on clinical grounds, there is no reason to remove them simply to confirm a diagnosis. A recent survey of American Academy of Dermatology members indicates that most dermatologists in the US follow this recommendation.[136] Although the original papers emphasized the need for confirmation by pathology, it has since been shown that there is little to be gained by doing such. Performing pathology does not help identify patients with DNS, nor does it segregate them into MM-risk groups.[103,137] The primary reason for doing a biopsy should be not to confirm a diagnosis of DN, but to exclude MM.

lifetime-risk for developing MM.[63,64] Therefore, it would be advisable to identify carriers of the gene to either prevent its development or at least allow for its early detection. Routine genetic testing, when it becomes available and is accurate, has been proposed as one method to identify individuals at risk for MM (see Chapter 21).

There are psychological implications of genetic testing for cancer-risk genes in individuals with DN. Patients who are found to be positive for a cancer predisposing gene may see themselves as a walking

Several studies have shown that prophylactically removing DN is largely an exercise in futility.[94,138] In a prospective study of 278 patients, with five or more atypical nevi, followed for a mean of 42 months, researchers from Australia attempted to address the cost-effectiveness of surveillance compared to prophylactic excision.[94] Over the study period, they identified 20 new MMs in 16 patients. Eleven were identified as a consequence of change in a pigmented lesion as compared with baseline photography. Nine of the lesions were detected by the patients or their partners. A total of 13 of the 20 MMs appeared to arise from new lesions, whereas only three developed from a pre-existing DN.

On further analysis of their findings, the authors surmised that they would have had to remove 5838 DN from their cohort population to have prevented three MMs. Besides being impractical, this management strategy would have been a prohibitively expensive form of preventive medicine. These researchers concluded that prophylactic excision of DN is an unsatisfactory alternative to follow-up as it does not provide sufficient risk-reduction to justify the cost and morbidity associated with this procedure.

Similarly, Cohen *et al.* have shown that wholesale removal is a poor substitute to regular follow-up.[138] Over a 4-year study interval, 190 patients segregated into two groups underwent prophylactic excision of multiple melanocytic nevi. One group consisted of 78 patients with a past history of primary cutaneous MM (Stages I and II), from whom 1630 moles were removed. The control group consisted of 112 patients without a prior history of MM, who had 1731 moles excised. In the MM cohort they detected 12 unsuspected MMs (nine *in situ* and three invasive), whereas in the control group, three unrecognized MMs *in situ* were detected as a result of their indiscriminate removal of moles. For the 15 MMs they had detected, they had to remove 3361 moles (i.e. one MM for every 224 moles). Even in their high-risk group (those with a past history of MM), they had to remove an unrealistic number of moles (136) for every MM identified by preventive excision. Lastly, a population-based estimate of the transformation rate of common melanocytic nevi into MM suggests that this is an exceedingly uncommon event (lifetime risk of 0.03% in men and 0.009% in women).[134]

The optimal method for removing DN has yet to be resolved. Traditionally, it was recommended that all suspicious pigmented lesions including DN be removed by excisional biopsy using 2 mm margins, as this provided the pathologist with optimal tissue for histologic assessment and ensured complete removal of the lesion if it was found to be a benign nevus.[139,140] A recent review of biopsy techniques for MM has shown that saucerization and deep shave biopsy in the majority of cases will provide adequate tissue for making a histologic diagnosis.[141] Although excisional biopsy was the most accurate method of biopsy, shave biopsy techniques were 88% accurate in determining maximal tumor thickness when compared with the microstaging parameters ascertained on local, wide excision specimens. Other researchers have reported a similar accuracy by deep shave excision by razor blade technique.[142]

Potential problems arise when the DN is reported as being incompletely excised. Total removal of suspicious lesions using the excisional or deep saucerization technique is typically recommended. Although these lesions are biologically benign, the tendency of pathologists has been to recommend re-excision particularly if there is significant cytological and architectural atypia in the biopsy specimen.[102,143] There may be some justification for this position. Despite rigid, reliable and reproducible histologic criteria for MM and DN, some pigmented lesions will have features that simply preclude definitive diagnosis. The dilemma pathologists face is distinguishing with certainty between a so-called severely dysplastic nevus and MM. Thus, complete removal of a clinically suspicious lesion in the first place may be a solution to this problem.

There has only been one study to examine the usefulness of re-excision of DN, in terms of frequency of residual nevus cells after re-excision, and for the possibility of a missed MM on the first biopsy.[144] Of 189 DN that were re-excised, 25% had evidence of residual nevus cells, and in one case the diagnosis was changed to MM, for a frequency of missed diagnosis of 0.5%. Although one of the authors feels obliged to re-excise incompletely removed severely dysplastic nevi, until a prospective randomized control study examining the natural evolution of such lesions is conducted the optimal method for managing this predicament will remain controversial. Reasons for advocating re-excision include medicolegal concerns (of a missed MM, particularly if the pathologist has recommended re-excision) and, to a lesser extent, because of anecdotal cases of malignant transformation arising from an incompletely excised DN (Fig. 16.4).

Cosmetic considerations

The current recommendation is to remove DN with surgical margins that ensure an optimal specimen for pathology. Regardless of the method used, all have the potential for leaving unsightly scars. This is particularly true since DN occur most commonly on the back where hyperplastic or keloidal scar formation is frequent. In an attempt to minimize this problem, other methods of ablation have been tried. These include systemic isotretinoin, topical tretinoin with or without topical hydrocortisone, topical 5-fluorouracil, and laser ablation.[145–151] Regrettably, none of these treatments results in the complete destruction of the nevus histologically or clinically.

The ability of lasers to target melanocytes by selective photothermolysis and thereby potentially avoid scar formation makes this a potentially attractive method of treating DN. To date, no laser consistently results in the complete destruction of melanocytic nevi. Most only ablate melanocytes within the epidermis and papillary dermis, leaving the deeper dermal melanocytes intact. There are theoretical risks that these nevocytes are at increased risk for malignant progression due to: (1) loss of the protective pigment layer above rending them more susceptible to the harmful effects of ultraviolet radiation, or (2) from the potential DNA damaging

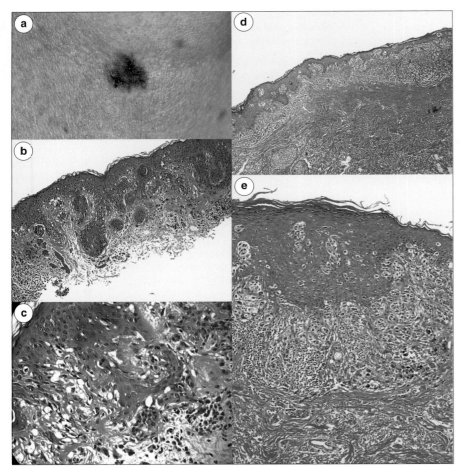

Figure 16.4 (a) A 52-year-old woman with a recurrent pigment lesion of the anterior neck at the site of a previous dysplastic nevus incompletely removed by shave biopsy 5 years earlier. (b) Low power view of the original biopsy in keeping with a dysplastic nevus. (c) High power view of the same lesion. (d) Low power view of the excisional biopsy specimen of the recurrent lesion illustrated in (a). (e) High power view of the same biopsy consistent with melanoma, Clark's level II, 0.3 mm.

effects of the laser light itself. Until there are long-term studies demonstrating the safety of lasers in the treatment of melanocytic nevi their use in this regard will remain controversial.[152]

Preventing dysplastic nevi

The appearance of DN requires the interaction of genetic and environmental factors.[15,153] Although it is impossible at present to alter our genetic make-up, in the not too distant future this may be possible through gene therapy. As a consequence, preventing the formation of DN currently rests with sun avoidance and protection (with clothing and sunblocks). Gallagher *et al.* have shown that regular sunscreen use in children can preclude the development of moles.[154] The development of DN and reduction of subsequent MM risk is unknown and remains a controversial area.[155]

CONCLUSIONS AND FUTURE OUTLOOK

Patients with DN can be challenging to manage. Not only is the clinician forced to contend with having to identify the proverbial needle in the haystack when it comes to detecting MM within a deluge of moles (many of which may be clinically atypical), the pathologist is similarly confronted with the dilemma of having to decide if a lesion is MM or simply DN.

In the future, it may be possible to distinguish MM from DN by automated digital imaging systems or through the use of dermoscopic or confocal surface microscopic appearance of a given lesion, thereby foregoing the need for a biopsy. Microarray DNA technology and genetic testing may allow for the absolute diagnosis of MM and the rapid identification of persons at risk for this cancer. Similarly, advances in gene therapy and proteomics as it pertains to the suppression of oncogenes, restoration of lost or inactive tumor suppressor genes, or the insertion of chemoprevention genes may make it possible one day to actually prevent MM. The rapidity at which advances are being made in these areas suggests that the management of DN may be radically different than outlined here in as short a period as the next 10–20 years.

REFERENCES

1 Ackerman AB, Mihara I. Dysplasia, dysplastic melanocytes, dysplastic nevi, the dysplastic nevus syndrome, and the relation between dysplastic nevi and malignant melanomas. Hum Pathol 1985; 16:87–91.

2 Annessi G, Cattaruzza MS, Abeni D, et al. Correlation between clinical atypia and histologic dysplasia in acquired melanocytic nevi. J Am Acad Derm 2001; 45:77–85.

3 Clark WH Jr, Ackerman AB. An exchange of views regarding the dysplastic nevus controversy. Semin Derm 1989; 8:229–250.

4 Clark WH Jr, Reimer RR, Greene M, et al. Origin of familial malignant melanomas from heritable melanocytic lesions. 'The B-K mole syndrome'. Arch Derm 1978; 114:732–738.

5 Elder DE, Goldman LI, Goldman SC, et al. Dysplastic nevus syndrome: a phenotypic association of sporadic cutaneous melanoma. Cancer 1980; 46:1787–1794.

6 Dowd P, Everall J. Atypical multiple mole melanoma syndrome. Br J Derm 1979; 101(17):32–33.

7 Lynch HT, Frichot BC 3rd, Lynch JF. Familial atypical multiple mole-melanoma syndrome. J Med Genet 1978; 15:352–356.

8 Ackerman AB, Milde P. Naming acquired melanocytic nevi. Common and dysplastic, normal and atypical, or Unna, Miescher, Spitz, and Clark? Am J Derm 1992; 14:447–453.

9 Sina B, Wood C. Atypical melanocytic proliferations. Am J Derm 1991; 13:317–319.

10 Consensus Statement. Diagnosis and treatment of early melanoma. NIH Consensus Development Conference, 27–29 January 1992.

11 Urso C, Giannini A, Bartolini M, et al. Histological analysis of intraepidermal proliferations of atypical melanocytes. Am J Derm 1990; 12:150–155.

12 Frankel KA. Intraepithelial melanocytic neoplasia: a classification by pattern analysis of proliferations of atypical melanocytes. Am J Derm 1987; 9:80–81.

13 Sander C, Tschochohei H, Hagedorn M. Epidemiology of dysplastic nevus. Hautarzt 1989; 40(12):758–760.

14 Piepkorn M, Meyer LJ, Goldgar D, et al. The dysplastic melanocytic nevus: a prevalent lesion that correlates poorly with clinical phenotype. J Am Acad Derm 1989; 20:407–415.

15 Bataille V, Grulich A, Sasieni P, et al. The association between naevi and melanoma in populations with different levels of sun exposure: a joint case–control study of melanoma in the UK and Australia. Br J Cancer 1998; 77:505–510.

16 Crutcher WA, Sagebiel RW. Prevalence of dysplastic naevi in a community practice. Lancet 1984; 1(8379):729.

17 Nordlund JJ, Kirkwood J, Forget BM, et al. Demographic study of clinically atypical (dysplastic) nevi in patients with melanoma and comparison subjects. Cancer Res 1985; 45(4):1855–1861.

18 Roush GC, Nordlund JJ, Forget B, et al. Independence of dysplastic nevi from total nevi in determining risk for nonfamilial melanoma. Prev Med 1988; 17(3):273–279.

19 Grob JJ, Gouvernet J, Aymar D, et al. Count of benign melanocytic nevi as a major indicator of risk for nonfamilial nodular and superficial spreading melanoma. Cancer 1990; 66(2):387–395.

20 Garbe C, Kruger S, Stadler R, et al. Markers and relative risk in a German population for developing malignant melanoma. Int J Derm 1989; 28(8):517–523.

21 Garbe C, Buttner P, Weiss J, et al. Associated factors in the prevalence of more than 50 common melanocytic nevi, atypical melanocytic nevi, and actinic lentigines: multicenter case–control study of the Central Malignant Melanoma Registry of the German Dermatological Society. J Invest Derm 1994; 102(5):700–705.

22 Swerdlow AJ, English J, MacKie RM, et al. Benign melanocytic naevi as a risk factor for malignant melanoma. Br Med J (Clin Res Ed) 1986; 292(6535):1555–1559.

23 MacKie RM, Aitchison TC, Freudenberger T. Risk factors for melanoma. Lancet 1989; 2(8668):928.

24 Augustsson A, Stierner U, Rosdahl I, Suurkula M. Common and dysplastic naevi as risk factors for cutaneous malignant melanoma in a Swedish population. Acta Derm Venereol 1991; 71(6):518–524.

25 Holly EA, Kelly JW, Shpall SN, Chiu SH. Number of melanocytic nevi as a major risk factor for malignant melanoma. J Am Acad Derm 1987; 17(3):459–468.

26 Halpern AC, Guerry D 4th, Elder DE, et al. Dysplastic nevi as risk markers of sporadic (nonfamilial) melanoma. A case–control study. Arch Derm 1991; 127(7):995–999.

27 Tucker MA, Halpern A, Holly EA, et al. Clinically recognized dysplastic nevi. A central risk factor for cutaneous melanoma. JAMA 1997; 277:1439–1444.

28 Schneider JS, Moore DH 2nd, Sagebiel RW. Risk factors for melanoma incidence in prospective follow-up. The importance of atypical (dysplastic) nevi. Arch Derm 1994; 130(8):1002–1007.

29 MacKie RM, McHenry P, Hole D. Accelerated detection with prospective surveillance for cutaneous malignant melanoma in high-risk groups. Lancet 1993; 341(8861):1618–1620.

30 Rigel DS, Rivers JK, Friedman RJ, et al. Risk gradient for malignant melanoma in individuals with dysplastic naevi. Lancet 1988; 1:352–353.

31 Tiersten AD, Grin CM, Kopf AW, et al. Prospective follow-up for malignant melanoma in patients with atypical-mole (dysplastic-nevus) syndrome. J Derm Surg Oncol 1991; 17(1):44–48.

32 Marghoob AA, Kopf AW, Rigel DS, et al. Risk of cutaneous malignant melanoma in patients with 'classic' atypical-mole syndrome. A case–control study. Arch Derm 1994; 130(8):993–998.

33 Halpern AC. Guerry D 4th, Elder DE, et al. A cohort study of melanoma in patients with dysplastic nevi. J Invest Derm 1993; 100(3):346S–349S.

34 Bale SJ, Chakravarti A, Greene MH. Cutaneous malignant melanoma and familial dysplastic nevi: evidence for autosomal dominance and pleiotropy. Am J Hum Genet 1986; 38(2):188–196.

35 Greene MH. The genetics of hereditary melanoma and nevi. 1998 update. Cancer 1999; 86(11):2464–2477.

36 Bale SJ, Dracopoli NC, Tucker MA, et al. Mapping the gene for hereditary cutaneous malignant melanoma-dysplastic nevus to chromosome 1p. N Engl J Med 1989; 320(21):1367–1372.

37 Haeringen A van, Bergman W, Nelen MR, et al. Exclusion of the dysplastic nevus syndrome (dysplastic neviS) locus from the short arm of chromosome 1 by linkage studies in Dutch families. Genomics 1989; 5(1):61–64.

38 Cannon-Albright LA, Goldgar DE, Wright EC, et al. Evidence against the reported linkage of the cutaneous melanoma-dysplastic nevus syndrome locus to chromosome 1p36. Am J Hum Genet 1990; 46(5):912–918.

39 Kefford RF, Salmon J, Shaw HM, et al. Hereditary melanoma in Australia. Variable association with dysplastic nevi and absence of genetic linkage to chromosome 1p. Cancer Genet Cytogenet 1991; 51(1):45–55.

40 Goldstein AM, Struewing JP, Chidambaram A, et al. Genotype–phenotype relationships in U.S. melanoma-prone families with CDKN2A and CDK4 mutations. J Natl Cancer Inst 2000; 92(12):1006–1010.

41 Tucker MA, Fraser MC, Goldstein AM, et al. A natural history of melanomas and dysplastic nevi: an atlas of lesions in melanoma-prone families. Cancer 2002; 94(12):3192–3209.

42 Gruis NA, Sandkuijl LA, Weber JL, et al. Linkage analysis in Dutch familial atypical multiple mole-melanoma (FAmelanomaM) syndrome families. Effect of naevus count. Melanoma Res 1993; 3:271–277.

43 Holland EA, Schmid H, Kefford RF, et al. CDKN2A (P16(INK4a)) and CDK4 mutation analysis in 131 Australian melanoma probands: effect of

family history and multiple primary melanomas. Genes Chromosomes Cancer 1999; 25:339–348.

44 MacKie RM, Andrew N, Lanyon WG, et al. CDKN2A germline mutations in U.K. patients with familial melanoma and multiple primary melanomas. J Invest Derm 1998; 111:269–272.

45 Newton Bishop JA, Bataille V, Pinney E, et al. Family studies in melanoma: identification of the atypical mole syndrome (AMS) phenotype. Melanoma Res 1994; 4:199–206.

46 Soufir N, Avril MF, Chompret A, et al. Prevalence of p16 and CDK4 germline mutations in 48 melanoma-prone families in France. Fr Familial Melanoma Study Group Hum Mol Genet 1998; 7:209–216.

47 Hussussian CJ, Struewing JP, Goldstein AM, et al. Germline p16 mutations in familial melanoma. Nat Genet 1994; 8:15–21.

48 Bishop JA, Wachsmuth RC, Harland M, et al. Genotype/phenotype and penetrance studies in melanoma families with germline CDKN2A mutations. J Invest Derm 2000; 114:28–33.

49 Serrano M, Hannon GJ, Beach D. A new regulatory motif in cell-cycle control causing specific inhibition of cyclin D/CDK4. Nature 1993; 366:704–707.

50 Ruiz A, Puig S, Malvehy J, et al. CDKN2A mutations in Spanish cutaneous malignant melanoma families and patients with multiple melanomas and other neoplasia. J Med Genet 1999; 36:490–493.

51 Hashemi J, Linder S, Platz A, et al. Melanoma development in relation to non-functional p16/INK4A protein and dysplastic naevus syndrome in Swedish melanoma kindreds. Melanoma Res 1999; 9:21–30.

52 Park WS, Vortmeyer AO, Pack S, et al. Allelic deletion at chromosome 9p21(p16) and 17p13(p53) in microdissected sporadic dysplastic nevus. Hum Pathol 1998; 29:127–130.

53 Goldstein AM, Martinez M, Tucker MA, Demenais F. Gene-covariate interaction between dysplastic nevi and the CDKN2A gene in American melanoma-prone families. Cancer Epidemiol Biomarkers Prev 2000; 9(9):889–894.

54 Gruis NA, Velden PA Van der, Bergman W, et al. Genetics of familial atypical multiple mole-melanoma (FAmelanomaM) syndrome in The Netherlands: how far have we come? Bull Cancer 1998; 85:627–630.

55 Puig S, Ruiz A, Castel T, et al. Inherited susceptibility to several cancers but absence of linkage between dysplastic nevus syndrome and CDKN2A in a melanoma family with a mutation in the CDKN2A (P16INK4A) gene. Hum Genet 1997; 101:359–364.

56 Hussein MR, Wood GS. Molecular aspects of melanocytic dysplastic nevi. J Mol Diagn 2002; 4(2):71–80.

57 Traupe H, Macher E, Hamm H, Happle R. Mutation rate estimates are not compatible with autosomal dominant inheritance of the dysplastic nevus 'syndrome'. Am J Med Genet 1989; 32(2):155–157.

58 Perera MI, Um KI, Greene MH, et al. Hereditary dysplastic nevus syndrome: lymphoid cell ultraviolet hypermutability in association with increased melanoma susceptibility. Cancer Res 1986; 46(2):1005–1009.

59 Hussein MR, Sun M, Tuthill RJ, et al. Comprehensive analysis of 112 melanocytic skin lesions demonstrates microsatellite instability in melanomas and dysplastic nevi, but not in benign nevi. J Cutan Pathol 2001; 28:343–350.

60 Caporaso N, Greene MH, Tsai S, et al. Cytogenetics in hereditary malignant melanoma and dysplastic nevus syndrome: is dysplastic nevus syndrome a chromosome instability disorder? Cancer Genet Cytogenet 1987; 24:299–314.

61 Jaspers NG, Roza-de Jongh EJ, Donselaar IG, et al: Sister chromatid exchanges, hyperdiploidy and chromosomal rearrangements studied in cells from melanoma-prone individuals belonging to families with the dysplastic nevus syndrome. Cancer Genet Cytogenet 1987; 24:33–43.

62 Lynch HT, Fusaro RM, Sandberg AA, et al. Chromosome instability and the FAmelanomaM syndrome. Cancer Genet Cytogenet 1993; 71:27–39.

63 Greene MH, Tucker MA, Clark WH Jr, et al. Hereditary melanoma and the dysplastic nevus syndrome: the risk of cancers other than melanoma. J Am Acad Derm 1987; 16:792–797.

64 Tucker MA, Fraser MC, Goldstein AM, et al. Risk of melanoma and other cancers in melanoma-prone families. J Invest Derm 1993; 100:350S–355S.

65 Gilchrest BA, Eller MS, Geller AC, et al. The pathogenesis of melanoma induced by ultraviolet radiation. N Engl J Med 1999; 340:1341–1348.

66 Ramsay RG, Chen P, Imray FP, et al. Familial melanoma associated with dominant ultraviolet radiation sensitivity. Cancer Res 1982; 42:2909–2912.

67 Smith PJ, Greene MH, Devlin DA, et al. Abnormal sensitivity to UV-radiation in cultured skin fibroblasts from patients with hereditary cutaneous malignant melanoma and dysplastic nevus syndrome. Int J Cancer 1982; 30:39–45.

68 Jung EG, Bohnert E, Boonen H. Dysplastic nevus syndrome: ultraviolet hypermutability confirmed in vitro by elevated sister chromatid exchanges. Dermatologica 1986; 173(6):297–300.

69 Seetharam S, Waters HL, Seidman melanoma, Kraemer KH. Ultraviolet mutagenesis in a plasmid vector replicated in lymphoid cells from patient with the melanoma-prone disorder dysplastic nevus syndrome. Cancer Res 1989; 49(21):5918–5921.

70 Moriwaki SI, Tarone RE, Tucker MA, et al. Hypermutability of UV-treated plasmids in dysplastic nevus/familial melanoma cell lines. Cancer Res 1997; 57:4637–4641.

71 Abrahams PJ, Houweling A, Cornelissen-Steijger PD, et al. Impaired dysplastic neviA repair capacity in skin fibroblasts from various hereditary cancer-prone syndromes. Mutat Res 1998; 407:189–201.

72 Noz KC, Bauwens M, Buul PP van, et al. Comet assay demonstrates a higher ultraviolet B sensitivity to dysplastic neviA damage in dysplastic nevi cells than in common melanocytic nevus cells and foreskin melanocytes. J Invest Derm 1996; 106:1198–1202.

73 Runger TM, Epe B, Moller K, et al. Repair of directly and indirectly UV-induced dysplastic neviA lesions and of dysplastic neviA double-strand breaks in cells from skin cancer-prone patients with the disorders dysplastic nevi syndrome or basal cell nevus syndrome. Recent Results Cancer Res 1997; 143:337–351.

74 Thielmann HW, Popanda O, Edler L, et al. dysplastic neviA repair synthesis following irradiation with 254-nm and 312-nm ultraviolet light is not diminished in fibroblasts from patients with dysplastic nevus syndrome. J Cancer Res Clin Oncol 1995; 121:327–337.

75 Hansson J, Loow H. Normal reactivation of plasmid DNA inactivated by UV irradiation by lymphocytes from individuals with hereditary dysplastic naevus syndrome. Melanoma Res 1994; 4(3):163–167.

76 Rubben A, Bogdan I, Grussendorf-Conen EI, et al. Loss of heterozygosity and microsatellite instability in acquired melanocytic nevi: towards a molecular definition of the dysplastic nevus. Recent Results Cancer Res 2002; 160:100–110.

77 Birindelli S, Tragni G, Bartoli C, et al. Detection of microsatellite alterations in the spectrum of melanocytic nevi in patients with or without individual or family history of melanoma. Int J Cancer 2000; 15(86):255–261.

78 Wang Y, Rao U, Mascari R, et al. Molecular analysis of melanoma precursor lesions. Cell Growth Differ 1996; 7:1733–1740.

79 Platz A, Ringborg U, Grafstrom E, et al. Immunohistochemical analysis of the N-ras p21 and the p53 proteins in naevi, primary tumours and metastases of human cutaneous malignant melanoma: increased immunopositivity in hereditary melanoma. Melanoma Res 1995; 5:101–106.

80 Nanney LB, Coffey RJ Jr, Ellis DL. Expression and distribution of transforming growth factor-alpha within melanocytic lesions. J Invest Derm 1994; 103:707–714.

81 Moretti S, Martini L, Berti E, et al. Adhesion molecule profile and malignancy of melanocytic lesions. Melanoma Res 1993; 3:235–239.

82 Meier F, Satyamoorthy K, Nesbit M, et al. Molecular events in melanoma development and progression. Front Biosci 1998; 3:D1005–D1010.

83 Lazzaro B, Strassburg A. Tumor antigen expression in compound dysplastic nevi and superficial spreading melanoma defined by a panel of nevomelanoma monoclonal antibodies. Hybridoma 1996; 15:141–146.

84 Fleming MG, Howe SF, Candel AG. Immunohistochemical localization of cytokines in nevi. Am J Derm 1992; 14:496–503.

85 Ewanowich C, Brynes RK, Medeiros L, et al. Cyclin D1 expression in dysplastic nevi: an immunohistochemical study. Arch Pathol Lab Med 2001; 125:208–210.

86 Elder DE, Herlyn M. Antigens associated with tumor progression in melanocytic neoplasia. Pigm Cell Res Suppl 1992; 2:136–143.

87 Ahmed AA, Nordlind K, Hedblad M, et al. Interleukin (IL)-1 alpha- and -1 beta-, IL-6-, and tumor necrosis factor-alpha-like immunoreactivities in human common and dysplastic nevocellular nevi and malignant melanoma. Am J Derm 1995; 17:222–229.

88 Salopek TG, Yamada K, Ito S, Jimbow K. Dysplastic melanocytic nevi contain high levels of pheomelanin: quantitative comparison of pheomelanin/eumelanin levels between normal skin, common nevi, and dysplastic nevi. Pigm Cell Res 1991; 4(4):172–179.

89 Elder DE, Clark WH Jr, Elenitsas R, et al. The early and intermediate precursor lesions of tumor progression in the melanocytic system: common acquired nevi and atypical (dysplastic) nevi. Semin Diagn Pathol 1993; 10(1):18–35.

90 Clark WH. Tumour progression and the nature of cancer. Br J Cancer 1991; 64(4):631–644.

91 McBride A, Rivers JK, Kopf AW, et al. Clinical features of dysplastic nevi. Derm Clin 1991; 9(4):717–722.

92 Nieland ML. 'Dysplastic nevus' syndrome: does a survey make it real? J Am Acad Derm 2003; 48(3):463–464.

93 Ackerman AB. 'Dysplastic nevus' syndrome: does a survey make it real? J Am Acad Derm 2003; 48(3):461–463.

94 Kelly JW, Yeatman JM, Regalia C, et al. A high incidence of melanoma found in patients with multiple dysplastic naevi by photographic surveillance. Med J Aust 1997; 167:191–194.

95 Bergman W, Voorst Vader PC van, Ruiter DJ. Dysplastic nevi and the risk of melanoma: a guideline for patient care. Nederlandse Melanoom Werkgroep van de Vereniging voor Integrale Kankercentra. Ned Tijdschr Geneeskd 1997; 141:2010–2014.

96 Newton JA. Familial melanoma. Clin Exp Derm 1993; 18:5–11.

97 Bishop JA, Bradburn M, Bergman W, et al. Teaching non-specialist health care professionals how to identify the atypical mole syndrome phenotype: a multinational study. Br J Derm 2000; 142:331–337.

98 Ackerman AB. Dysplastic nevus. Am J Surg Pathol 2000; 24:757–758.

99 Elder DE, Murphy GF. Melanocytic tumors of the skin. In: Rosai J, Sobin LH, eds. Atlas of Tumor Pathology; 3rd series, part 2. Washington, DC: Armed Forces Institute of Pathology; 1991.

100 de Wit PE. van't Hof-Grootenboer B, Ruiter DJ, et al. Validity of the histopathological criteria used for diagnosing dysplastic naevi. An interobserver study by the pathology subgroup of the EORTC Malignant Melanoma Cooperative Group. Eur J Cancer 1993; 29A(6):831–839.

101 Weinstock MA, Barnhill RL, Rhodes AR, et al. Reliability of the histopathologic diagnosis of melanocytic dysplasia. Dysplastic Nevus Panel Arch Derm 1997; 133:953–958.

102 Shea CR, Vollmer RT, Prieto VG. Correlating architectural disorder and cytologic atypia in Clark (dysplastic) melanocytic nevi. Hum Pathol 1999; 30:500–505.

103 Pozo L, Naase M, Cerio R, et al. Critical analysis of histologic criteria for grading atypical (dysplastic) melanocytic nevi. Am J Clin Pathol 2001; 115:194–204.

104 Weinstock MA, Brodsky GL. Bias in the assessment of family history of melanoma and its association with dysplastic nevi in a case–control study. J Clin Epidemiol 1998; 51(12):1299–1303.

105 Wachsmuth RC, Harland M, Bishop JA. The atypical-mole syndrome and predisposition to melanoma. N Engl J Med 1998; 339:348–349.

106 Kraemer KH, Greene MH. Dysplastic nevus syndrome. Familial and sporadic precursors of cutaneous melanoma. Derm Clin 1985; 3(2):225–237.

107 Koh HK. Cutaneous melanoma. N Engl J Med 1991; 325:171–182.

108 Marghoob AA, Slade J, Salopek TG, et al. Basal cell and squamous cell carcinomas are important risk factors for cutaneous malignant melanoma. Screening implications. Cancer 1995; 75(2):707–714.

109 Slue W, Kopf AW, Rivers JK. Total-body photographs of dysplastic nevi. Arch Derm 1988; 124:1239–1243.

110 Halpern AC. Guerry D 4th, Elder DE, et al. Natural history of dysplastic nevi. J Am Acad Derm 1993b; 29:51–57.

111 Stanganelli I, Rafanelli S, Bucchi L. Seasonal prevalence of digital epiluminescence microscopy patterns in acquired melanocytic nevi. J Am Acad Derm 1996; 34(3):460–464.

112 Haley JC, Hood AF, Chuang TY, Rasmussen J. The frequency of histologically dysplastic nevi in 199 pediatric patients. Pediatr Derm 2000; 17(4):266–269.

113 Schmid-Wendtner MH, Berking C, et al. Cutaneous melanoma in childhood and adolescence: an analysis of 36 patients. J Am Acad Derm 2002; 46(6):874–879.

114 Rodriguez-Sains RS. Ocular findings in patients with dysplastic nevus syndrome. Ophthalmology 1986; 93(5):661–665.

115 Hees CL van, Boer A de, Jager MJ, et al. Are atypical nevi a risk factor for uveal melanoma? A case–control study. J Invest Derm 1994; 103(2):202–205.

116 Vajdic CM, Kricker A, Giblin M, et al. Eye color and cutaneous nevi predict risk of ocular melanoma in Australia. Int J Cancer 2001; 92(6):906–912.

117 Lucas CR, Sanders LL, Murray JC, et al. Early melanoma detection: Nonuniform dermoscopic features and growth. J Am Acad Derm 2003; 48(5):663–671.

118 Marghoob AA, Swindle LD, Moricz CZ, et al. Instruments and new technologies for the in vivo diagnosis of melanoma. J Am Acad Dermatol 2003; 49:777–797.

119 Rhodes AR. Intervention strategy to prevent lethal cutaneous melanoma: use of dermatologic photography to aid surveillance of high-risk persons. J Am Acad Derm 1998; 39:262–267.

120 Binder M, Puespoeck-Schwarz M, Steiner A, et al. Epiluminescence microscopy of small pigmented skin lesions: short-term formal training

improves the diagnostic performance of dermatologists. J Am Acad Derm 1997; 36:197–202.

121 Nachbar F, Stolz W, Merkle T, et al. The ABCD rule of dermatoscopy. High prospective value in the diagnosis of doubtful melanocytic skin lesions. J Am Acad Derm 1994; 30:551–559.

122 Nilles M, Boedeker RH, Schill WB. Surface microscopy of naevi and melanoma – clues to melanoma. Br J Derm 1994; 130:349–355.

123 Steiner A, Binder M, Schemper M, et al. Statistical evaluation of epiluminescence microscopy criteria for melanocytic pigmented skin lesions. J Am Acad Derm 1993; 29:581–588.

124 Salopek TG, Kopf AW, Stefanato CM, et al. Differentiation of atypical moles (dysplastic nevi) from early melanomas by dermoscopy. Derm Clin 2001; 19:337–345.

125 Hofmann-Wellenhof R, Blum A, Wolf IH, et al. Dermoscopic classification of Clark's nevi (atypical melanocytic nevi). Clin Derm 2002; 20(3):255–258.

126 Stolz W, Braun-Falco O, Bilek P, et al. Color Atlas of Dermatoscopy. Oxford: Blackwell Science; 1994.

127 Menzies SW, Ingvar C, Crotty KA, McCarthy WH. Frequency and morphologic characteristics of invasive melanomas lacking specific surface microscopic features. Arch Derm 1996; 132(10):1178–1182.

128 Argenziano G, Fabbrocini G, Carli P, et al. Epiluminescence microscopy for the diagnosis of doubtful melanocytic skin lesions. Comparison of the ABCD rule of dermatoscopy and a new 7-point checklist based on pattern analysis. Arch Derm 1998; 134(12):1563–1570.

129 Argenziano G, Soyer HP, Chimenti S, et al. Dermoscopy of pigmented skin lesions: results of a consensus meeting via the Internet. J Am Acad Derm 2003; 48(5):679–693.

130 Mayer J. Systematic review of the diagnostic accuracy of dermatoscopy in detecting malignant melanoma. Med J Aust 1997; 167:206–210.

131 Binder M, Schwarz M, Winkler A, et al. Epiluminescence microscopy: A useful tool for the diagnosis of pigmented skin lesions for formally trained dermatologists. Arch Derm 1995; 131:286–291.

132 Rao BK, Marghoob AA, Stolz W, et al. Can early malignant melanoma be differentiated from atypical melanocytic nevi by in vivo techniques? Part I. Clinical and dermoscopic characteristics. Skin Res Technol 1997; 3:8–14.

133 Kefford RF, Newton Bishop JA, Bergman W, et al. Counseling and dysplastic nevi testing for individuals perceived to be genetically predisposed to melanoma: A consensus statement of the Melanoma Genetics Consortium. J Clin Oncol 1999; 17:3245–3251.

134 Sagebiel RW. Melanocytic nevi in histologic association with primary cutaneous melanoma of superficial spreading and nodular types: effect of tumor thickness. J Invest Derm 1993; 100(3):322S–325S.

135 Tsao H, Bevona C, Goggins W, Quinn T. The transformation rate of moles (melanocytic nevi) into cutaneous melanoma: a population-based estimate. Arch Derm 2003; 139(3):282–288.

136 Tripp JM, Kopf AW, Marghoob AA, Bart RS. Management of dysplastic nevi: a survey of fellows of the American Academy of Dermatology. J Am Acad Derm 2002; 46(5):674–682.

137 Mooi WJ. The dysplastic naevus. J Clin Pathol 1997; 50:711–715.

138 Cohen MH, Cohen BJ, Shotkin JD, et al. Surgical prophylaxis of malignant melanoma. Ann Surg 1991; 213:308–314.

139 Ho VC, Sober AJ, Balch CM. Biopsy techniques. In: Balch CM, Houghton AN, Sober AJ, Soong S, eds. Cutaneous Melanoma, 3rd edition, St Louis, MO: Quality Medical Publishing, Inc.; 1998:135–140.

140 Swanson NA, Lee KK, Gorman A, Lee HN. Biopsy techniques. Diagnosis of melanoma. Derm Clin 2002; 20(4):677–680.

141 Ng PC, Barzilai DA, Ismail SA, et al. Evaluating invasive cutaneous melanoma: is the initial biopsy representative of the final depth? J Am Acad Derm 2003; 48(3):420–424.

142 Gambichler T, Senger E, Rapp S, et al. Deep shave excision of macular melanocytic nevi with the razor blade biopsy technique. Derm Surg 2000; 26:662–666.

143 Metcalf JS, Maize JC. Clark's nevus. Semin Cutan Med Surg 1999; 18:43–46.

144 Cohen LM, Hodge SJ, Owen LG, et al. Atypical melanocytic nevi. Clinical and histopathologic predictors of residual tumor at reexcision. J Am Acad Derm 1992; 27:701–706.

145 Bondi EE, Clark WH Jr, Elder D, et al. Topical chemotherapy of dysplastic melanocytic nevi with 5% fluorouracil. Arch Derm 1981; 117:89–92.

146 Edwards L, Jaffe P. The effect of topical tretinoin on dysplastic nevi. A preliminary trial. Arch Derm 1990; 126:494–499.

147 Halpern AC, Schuchter LM, Elder DE, et al. Effects of topical tretinoin on dysplastic nevi. J Clin Oncol 1994; 12:1028–1035.

148 Meyskens FL Jr, Edwards L, Levine NS. Role of topical tretinoin in melanoma and dysplastic nevi. J Am Acad Derm 1986; 15:822–825.

149 Stam-Posthuma JJ. Vink J, le Cessie S, et al: Effect of topical tretinoin under occlusion on atypical naevi. Melanoma Res 1998; 8:539–548.

150 Edwards L, Meyskens F, Levine N. Effect of oral isotretinoin on dysplastic nevi. J Am Acad Derm 1989; 20:257–260.

151 Duke D, Byers HR, Sober AJ, et al. Treatment of benign and atypical nevi with the normal-mode ruby laser and the Q-switched ruby laser: clinical improvement but failure to completely eliminate nevomelanocytes. Arch Derm 1999; 135:290–296.

152 Stratigos AJ, Dover JS, Arndt KA. Laser treatment of pigmented lesions – 2000: how far have we gone? Arch Derm 2000; 136:915–921.

153 Kelly JW, Rivers JK, MacLennan R, Harrison S, Lewis AE, Tate BJ. Sunlight: a major factor associated with the development of melanocytic nevi in Australian schoolchildren. J Am Acad Derm 1994; 30:40–48.

154 Gallagher RP, Rivers JK, Lee TK, et al. Broad-spectrum sunscreen use and the development of new nevi in white children: A randomized controlled trial. JAMA 2000; 283:2955–2960.

155 Bigby M. The sunscreen and melanoma controversy. Arch Derm 1999; 135:1526–1527.

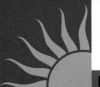

CHAPTER

17

Congenital Melanocytic Nevi

Ashfaq A Marghoob

Key points

- Congenital melanocytic nevi can have medical, cosmetic and psychological sequelae.
- Melanoma can develop in association with any congenital melanocytic nevus.
- Risk for developing melanoma is greatest for individuals with large congenital melanocytic nevi.
- Melanoma can develop in cutaneous or extra-cutaneous sites.
- Individuals with large congenital melanocytic nevi, multiple smaller congenital melanocytic nevi or many satellite nevi are at risk for neurocutaneous melanocytosis.
- Management of congenital melanocytic nevi requires balancing issues surrounding cosmesis and prevention of melanoma.

INTRODUCTION

Congenital melanocytic nevi (CMN) are nevomelanocytic nevi whose presence is determined *in utero*. They are usually evident at birth, but some CMN may not be apparent at birth due to a lack of visible pigment. These 'tardive' CMN may slowly develop pigment over time, often within the first 2 years of life. Those nevi with congenital features in which the history of their 'presence since birth' cannot be verified are termed congenital-nevus-like nevi (CNLN).

CMN may be cosmetically disfiguring, can occasionally give rise to melanoma, can suggest the presence of neurocutaneous melanocytosis (NCM) and may rarely be associated with other medical problems such as the tethered cord syndrome. Physicians are frequently asked to render advice on the management of these nevi. This advice must be tailored for each patient and each CMN, taking into consideration the risk for developing malignancy, risk for developing symptomatic NCM, cosmetic implications of having the CMN, cosmetic implications of any resultant surgical scars from the removal of the CMN, adverse effects that the CMN may have on psychosocial development and the adverse effects and long-term sequelae of any surgical intervention.

EPIDEMIOLOGY

It is estimated that between 1 and 6% of infants are born with a CMN and between 2 and 6% of the population have a CNLN. Crude incidence estimates suggest that approximately 1 in 100 infants are born with a small CMN; 1 in 1000 are born with a medium-sized CMN; 1 in 20,000 are born with a large CMN and 1 in 500,000 are born with a very large (giant) CMN.

PATHOGENESIS AND ETIOLOGY

CMN form during early embryogenesis, between the fifth and twenty-fourth week of gestation. Though there are reported cases of familial clustering of CMN, most

Figure 17.1 Melanocytic differentiation pathway. The melanocytic stem cell migrates from the neural crest to the leptomeninges and embryonic dermis. Subsequently, melanocytes migrate from the dermis to the epidermis. Dysregulation in the timing of the migration process may determine the depth to which nevomelanocytes can be found. The timing of melanogenesis may determine when the CMN will develop clinically visible pigment.

221

occur sporadically. Some have suggested that CMN may be inherited in a paradominant fashion. This would imply that heterozygous individuals would be phenotypically normal and the trait would manifest only if allelic loss (loss of heterozygosity) occurred during early embryogenesis, giving rise to a patchy area of homozygous or hemizygous cells. Research is beginning to shed some light on the etiology of CMN (Fig. 17.1). It is theorized that during embryogenesis, a morphogenic error in the neuroectoderm results in the dysregulated growth of melanoblasts/melanocytes.[1] In addition, the melanoblasts, which normally migrate from the neural

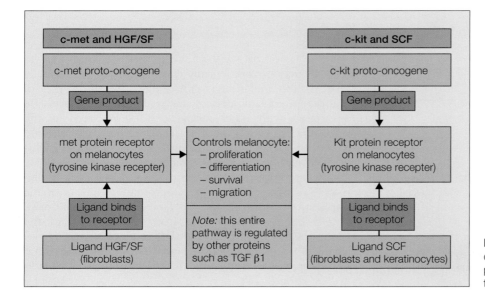

Figure 17.2 Melanocyte proliferation, differentiation, survival and migration are partly under the control of c-met, c-kit and their respective ligands.

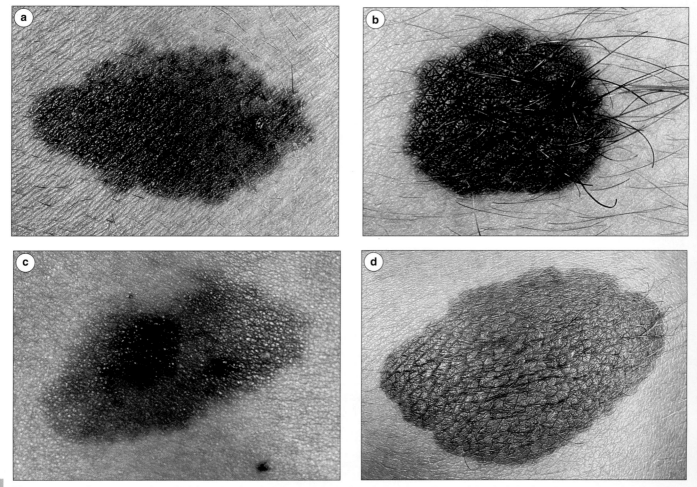

Figure 17.3 Small to medium CMN tend to be sharply demarcated and often have hypertrichosis (a,b,d) and a mamillated surface (d). Some CMN can have multiple shades of brown color (c).

crest to the leptomeninges and integument, do so in a dysregulated pattern.[2] The timing of melanocyte migration may determine the depth to which nevus cells are present within the integument). The timing of melanogenesis may determine when the nevus becomes visible, thereby explaining why some CMN are not apparent at birth (tardive).

Perturbations in migration, proliferation and/or differentiation of the neural crest derived melanoblasts may be linked to the c-met and/or c-kit proto-oncogene, which controls the expression of the tyrosine-kinase receptors met and kit on melanocytes, respectively (Fig. 17.2). The met receptor binds hepatocyte growth factor/scatter factor (HGF/SF) and the kit receptor binds stem cell factor (SCF). If the met or kit receptors or their respective ligands, HGF/SF and SCF, are over expressed, the result may be the formation of CMN and/or NCM.[1,3] It is believed that HGF/SF and SCF, both of which are found on fibroblasts and keratinocytes, serve partly as chemotactic agents, guiding the migration of those melanoblasts that express met and/or kit. Besides controlling melanocyte migration, these two ligands may also control melanocyte proliferation, differentiation and survival.[4] Receptor-ligand pathways are further regulated by other proteins such as transforming growth factor β1.[4] It is interesting to note that the c-met proto-oncogene may also play a role in the development of melanoma and rhabdomyosarcomas which occur at a higher than expected frequency in patients with large CMN.[1,5,6] In addition, kit can activate the N-ras oncogene which may be a risk factor for melanoma formation in large CMN.[7]

CLINICAL FEATURES/NATURAL HISTORY

CMN usually present as round to oval, fairly homogeneous, brown, multi-shaded pigmented lesions with sharply demarcated borders, often with a mammillated surface and hypertrichosis (Fig. 17.3). However, some CMN, especially the larger ones, can be heterogeneous displaying multiple colors, irregular topography and a nodular (neurotized – see section on histology) to rugous surface (Fig. 17.4). Although most CMN are symmetric with regular borders, some may be asymmetric with irregular borders and thereby resemble melanoma (Fig. 17.5).

Most CMN grow in proportion to the growth of the child, except during early infancy when some CMN can grow rapidly. With the passage of time, CMN may get darker, lighter, lose pigmentation, become more heterogeneous, become more homogeneous, develop a nodular surface or, rarely, regress (Fig. 17.6).[8] Most of these changes occur symmetrically and globally throughout the lesion. Although some alterations are normal, focal changes should be viewed with some caution.

CMN present in a continuum of sizes ranging from small to very large. There are several definitions of what constitutes a small, medium and large CMN (Table 17.1). Reasons for classifying CMN by size include the risk for developing melanoma, level of surgical complexity involved, as well as other complications which may be roughly proportional to their size. CMN are classified as 'large' if the greatest diameter of the lesion, in adulthood, is 20 cm or more; 'medium' if its greatest diameter measures between 1.5 and 19.9 cm; and 'small' if it measures less than 1.5 cm. Assuming proportionate expansion of body surface area, a 9 to 12 cm CMN on the head or a 6 to 7 cm CMN on the body of an infant will measure approximately 20 cm in adulthood.[9,10] The very large CMN, with diameters greater than 50 cm, are also known as 'giant' or 'garment nevi' (Fig. 17.7).

CMN are usually asymptomatic. However, the larger CMN on occasion can be associated with symptoms of pruritus, paraesthesias, temperature sensitivity and tenderness. The skin overlying a CMN can develop xerosis and it may sometimes lack the ability to produce sufficient sweat in response to heat.

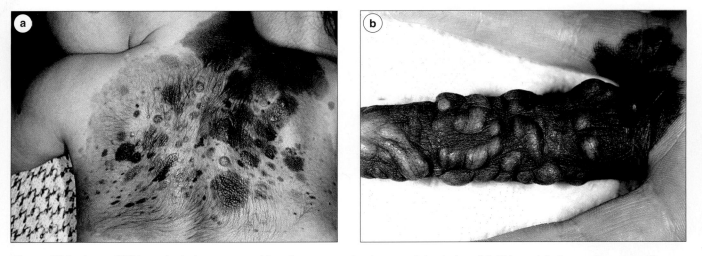

Figure 17.4 Large CMN can be heterogeneous (a) and some can develop a nodular surface (b). This nodularity usually represents neurotization.

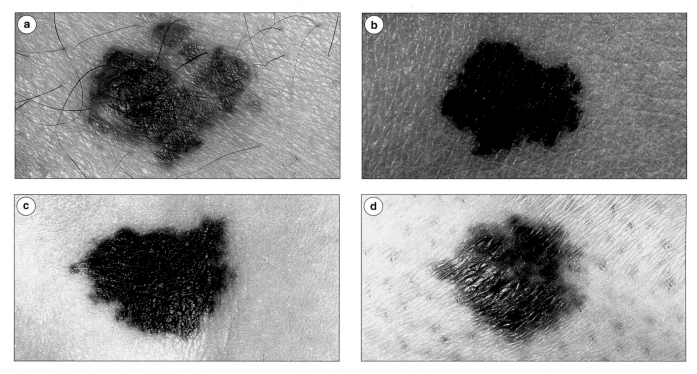

Figure 17.5 Examples of CMN, which possess some of the 'abcd' features of melanoma.

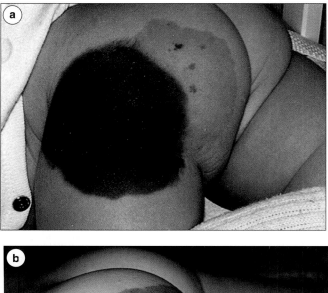

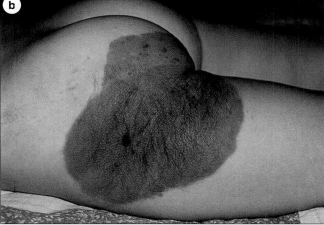

Figure 17.6 Over 60% of CMN will change over time. This is an example of a LCMN that has become lighter. (a) 4 months of age; (b) 4 years of age.

Table 17.1   Size definitions for congenital melanocytic nevi (CMN)

Size	Definition
Small	• A CMN less than 1.5 cm in greatest diameter • A CMN that can be completely excised and the defect closed primarily in a single operation
Medium	• A CMN 1.5 to 19.9 cm in greatest diameter • A CMN that can be completely excised, but the resulting surgical defect cannot be closed primarily; e.g. flaps, grafts, or tissue expanders are required
Large (Giant)	• A CMN 20 cm or more in greatest diameter • A CMN involving a major part of an anatomical area such as a face or hand • A CMN that covers greater than 1% of the cutaneous surface. (Greater than 0.5% if on the head and neck) • A CMN on the head and neck that is at least the size of a palm. CMN in most other anatomical sites need to be at least twice the size of a palm • A CMN that is 900 cm² or more in area • A CMN that covers at least 5% of the body surface area • A CMN that requires serial or staged excisions for its complete removal

Knowledge of the classic dermoscopy features of CMN can aid in the clinical evaluation of these lesions.[11] Most CMN can be classified into one of four dermoscopic patterns: (1) reticular (network) (Fig. 17.8); (2) globular (i.e. cobblestone) (Fig. 17.9); (3) reticularglobular (i.e. globules placed centrally and network placed peripherally) (Fig. 17.10) and (4) diffuse pigmentation with or without remnant network structures and/or globules (Fig. 17.11). The overall dermoscopic arrangement of the pigment and structures is symmetric and homogeneous.

Other dermoscopic features commonly seen in CMN include milia cysts, hypertrichosis and perifollicular hyperpigmentation or hypopigmentation. CMN that deviate from the commonly known dermoscopic patterns, develop focal dermoscopic changes during sequential follow-up, or reveal a multi-component dermoscopic pattern should be viewed with caution. A combined approach of clinical evaluation coupled with dermoscopic evaluation has been shown to be useful in the follow-up of CMN.

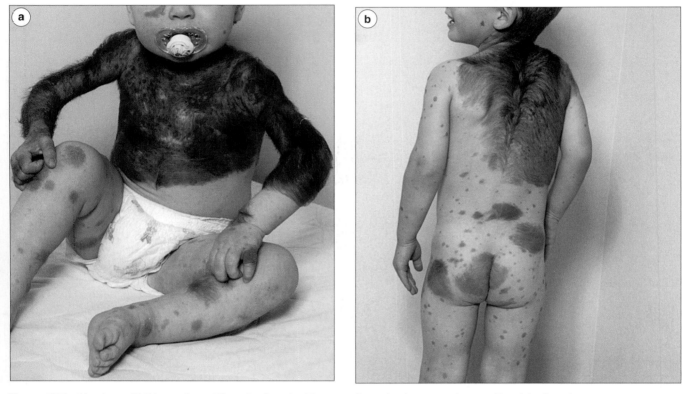

Figure 17.7   Very large CMN are often >50 cm in diameter. These nevi are also known as 'garment' or 'giant' nevi.

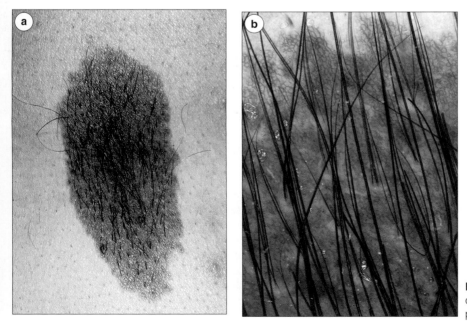

Figure 17.8   CMN with the clinical feature of hypertrichosis (a) and dermoscopic pattern of reticulated network (b).

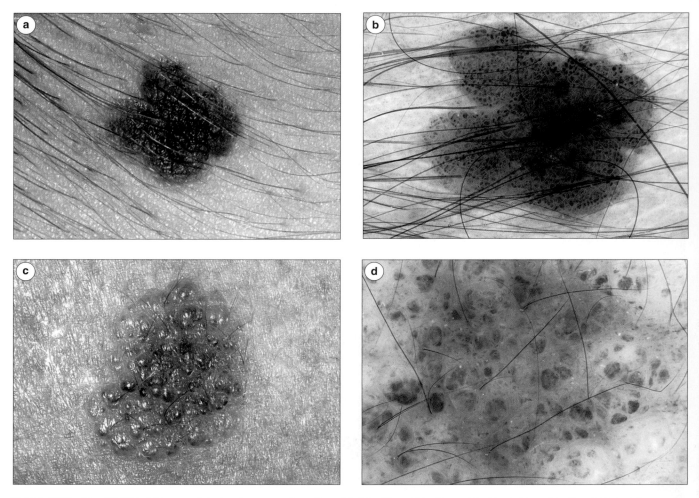

Figure 17.9 The CMN in (a) has a globular dermoscopic pattern (b). (c) with cobblestone globules seen under dermoscopy (d).

PATIENT EVALUATION, DIAGNOSIS AND DIFFERENTIAL DIAGNOSIS

Any melanocytic nevus documented to be present at birth is a CMN. CNLN can be characterized as congenital based on some or all of the following: the timing of its appearance (i.e. within 2 years of life), the clinical/dermoscopic appearance, the patient history and/or the histology of the nevus, if available.

The differential diagnosis for CMN may include café-au-lait macule, Becker's nevus, dysplastic nevus, melanoma, nevus of Ota/Ito, Mongolian spot and speckled lentiginous nevus.

CMN can have medical, cosmetic and psychological ramifications. Behavioral and emotional problems are reported to occur in as many as 30% of patients with large CMN.[12] The psychological burden on patients and parents may stem from the cosmetic appearance of the CMN, the anxiety associated with the knowledge that complications such as melanoma can develop, the discomfort associated with the often multiple staged surgical treatments rendered (Fig. 17.12a) and the cosmetic appearance of resulting scars (Fig. 17.12b).[12] In addition, some CMN and/or nevi excision scars may develop tenderness, pruritus and/or skin fragility thus adding to the patient's discomfort.

Melanoma can develop within any CMN.[13] However the risk for developing melanoma appears to correlate with the size of the nevus. In turn, the size of the nevus frequently correlates with the depth of penetration of the nevus cells and the total number of nevomelanocytes present within the nevus.[14] Individuals at greatest risk are those with large CMN. The nevus cells in large CMN are frequently found to penetrate deep into the dermis or beyond. The estimated lifetime risk for developing melanoma in patients with large CMN is between 4.5 and 10% and the relative risk is between 101 and 1046. Individuals with large CMN can develop melanoma at any age (Fig. 17.13). However, 70% of the melanomas are diagnosed in children under the age of 10. 45% of primary melanomas develop in association with the large nevus and 31% develop within the central nervous system. 24% of patients with large CMN who have melanoma present with metastatic disease in which the primary site of the melanoma cannot be found. In some of these patients, the focus of the primary melanoma is 'hidden' somewhere within their large CMN. In fact, two-thirds of melanomas forming within large CMN develop subepidermally (i.e. non-epidermal sites), making their clinical detection challenging (Table 17.2).[15] Biopsy of growths that develop within large CMN, particularly those found during early infancy (i.e. proliferative

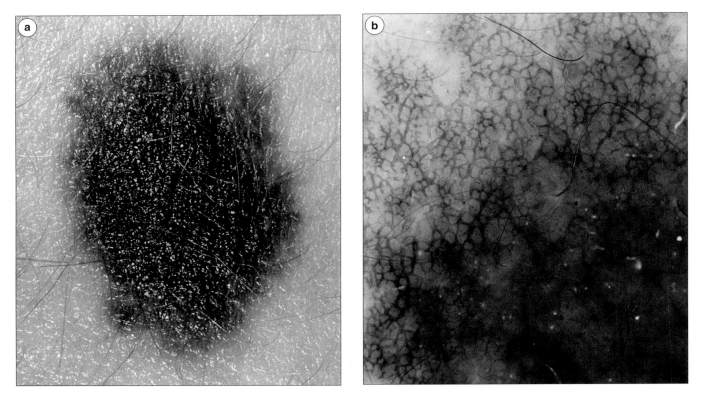

Figure 17.10 CMN (a) revealing a reticulo-globular pattern with reticulation at the periphery and globules placed centrally (b).

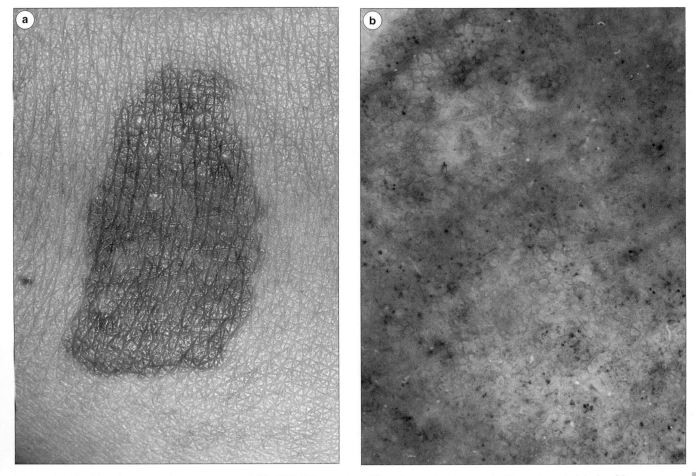

Figure 17.11 The dermoscopic appearance of this CMN (a) reveals a diffuse brown background with scattered globules (b).

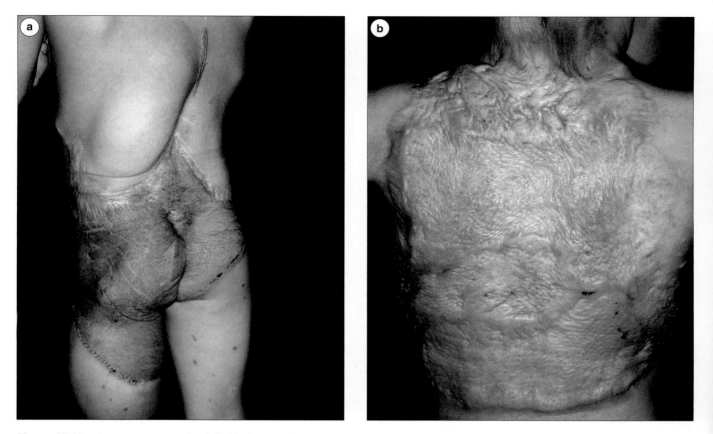

Figure 17.12   Attempts at removing LCMN often requires the placement of tissue expanders (a) and multi-staged surgical excisions. The poor cosmetic appearance of scars and discomfort from scarring is sometimes unavoidable (b).

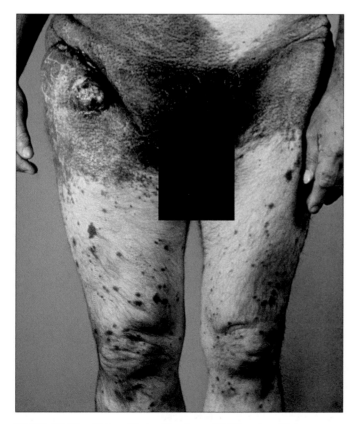

Figure 17.13   This patient with a large CMN and multiple satellite nevi developed a melanoma within the large nevus on the right thigh. Melanomas developing in large CMN can develop at any age, however most develop in early childhood. (Image courtesy of Dr Alfred Kopf.)

nodules), may yield some histological features in common with melanoma, yet behave in a clinically benign fashion.[16] The clinical and histological differentiation between true melanoma and its simulants can at times be difficult and together with patient selection/referral bias may partly explain the overestimated melanoma risks previously reported of 42%. Evaluating nevus biopsy specimens for DNA content, cell cycle aberrations, clonality, gene mutations and/or the over or under expression of specific proteins may someday aid in differentiating melanoma from its simulants.[17] Though it is clear that patients with large CMN are at increased risk for developing melanoma, this risk may not be equal for all patients (Fig. 17.14). There may be differences in risk between large and very large CMN (Fig. 17.14 a vs c), superficial and deep penetrating CMN (Fig. 17.14 a vs d), macular and rugose CMN (Fig. 17.14 a vs d) and homogeneous and heterogeneous CMN (Fig. 17.14 a vs b). Only continued prospective clinical follow-up will help better identify those at greatest risk.

Individuals with large CMN are also at risk for NCM, an entity in which the leptomeninges contain excessive amounts of melanocytes and melanin.[10,18] Malignant degeneration of these melanocytes results in development of primary central nervous system melanomas. However, benign proliferation of melanocytes within the leptomeninges can also result in serious complications such as mass effect or obstructive hydrocephalus secondary to cisternal blockage and destruction of arachnoid villi. This results in increased CSF pressure and neurological symptoms, eventuating in death if not

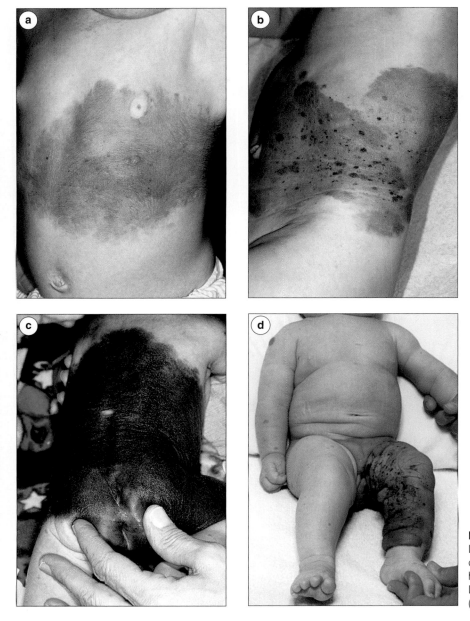

Figure 17.14 These four patients with LCMN may not all be at the same risk for developing melanoma. (a) light brown, thin, homogeneous LCMN; (b) heterogeneous LCMN. (c) very large CMN (giant nevus); (d) raised, rugose LCMN.

corrected. The 5-year cumulative risk for developing melanoma, NCM, or both melanoma and NCM in individuals with large CMN is 2.3%, 2.5% and 3.3%, respectively.[18] Patients with large CMN at greatest risk for developing melanoma and/or NCM are those in whom the large CMN is in para-vertebral or axial locations such as the back, head or neck.[6,10] However, recent data suggests that the most important factor correlated to NCM is the presence of many (i.e. greater than 20) satellite melanocytic nevi, irrespective of the anatomical location of the large CMN (Fig. 17.15). This may also explain why patients with multiple medium-sized CMN (Fig. 17.16), or with multiple satellite nevi only are also at increased risk for developing NCM.[19,20] Despite the fact that thousands of satellite nevi have been followed, no melanoma has ever been reported to have developed within one of these satellite nevi.[6]

CMN that are less than 20 cm in diameter have a reported lifetime risk for developing melanoma of between 0 and 4.9%. Recent studies evaluating medium-sized CMN did not reveal an increased risk for melanoma developing in nevi of this size. However, there are many case reports and series of cases that clearly show that melanomas can and do develop in CMN that are less than 20 cm in diameter and therefore these lesions require monitoring (Fig. 17.17).[21] Melanomas developing in smaller CMN tend to develop at or after puberty. These melanomas also tend to develop at the dermo-epidermal junction thus making their clinical detection easier than for those that develop in the dermis (Table 17.2). For CMN less than 1.5 cm in diameter the risk for developing melanoma is considered to be low enough that prophylactic removal of these lesions is not warranted. However, if a small CMN develops suspicious changes, becomes symptomatic, or is irregular, then an excisional biopsy may be justified.

Finally, CMN overlying the sacral area may rarely be associated with underlying spinal dysraphism and the

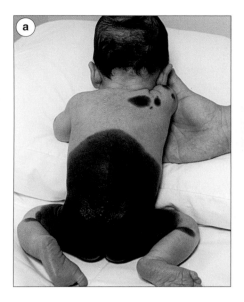
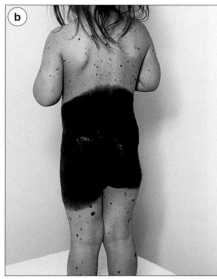

Figure 17.15 Patients with LCMN located on the posterior axis (para-spinal) are at increased risk, by univariate analysis, for developing NCM. However, when evaluated by multivariate analysis the only factor that is significantly correlated with NCM is the number of satellite CMN. Thus, although both patients (a and b) have LCMN located on the posterior axis, the patient in (b) is at higher risk for NCM based on presence of an increased number of satellite nevi.

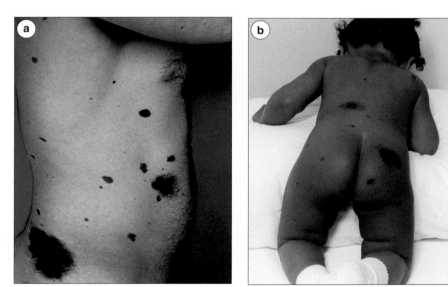

Figure 17.16 Patients with (a) multiple satellite nevi or with (b) three or more medium-sized CMN are at increased risk for NCM.

tethered cord syndrome (Fig. 17.14c). It is important to make this diagnosis early in life, surgically sever the connection of the spinal cord to the integument and thereby avert irreversible nerve injury.

PATHOLOGY AND HISTOLOGY

Nevo-melanocytes differ from normal melanocytes in that they lack the ability to transfer pigment. Histologic features thought to be characteristic of CMN are listed in Table 17.3. However, due to the presence of considerable histologic overlap between CMN and acquired nevi, the two are sometimes indistinguishable.[22,23] A diagnosis of CMN is favored when nevus cells are present among collagen bundles either singly or in single files, are present in the lower two-thirds of the reticular dermis, and when nevus cells involve appendages, nerves and vessels within the lower two-thirds of the reticular

dermis or subcutis. However, the absence of such involvement does not preclude a congenital origin since nevo-melanocytes in some CMN may be located only superficially. There does appear to be a distinct correlation between the size of a CMN and the depth of nevus cell infiltration.[14] In addition, nevus cells typically display a pattern of 'maturation' extending from superficial to deeper layers of the dermis. Maturation is the tendency for diminished nesting and dispersion of nevus cells among collagen bundles with increasing depth. There also tends to be a progressive, although slight, reduction in cell and nuclear sizes.

Subsets of large CMN are characterized by spindle cells with neuroidal differentiation resembling neural tubules or pseudomeissnerian structures. Commonly, the neuroidal pattern appears as highly cellular whorls of schwannian tissue deep within the dermis. In addition, some large CMN may exhibit a variety of other patterns suggesting that they are hamartomas of neural crest

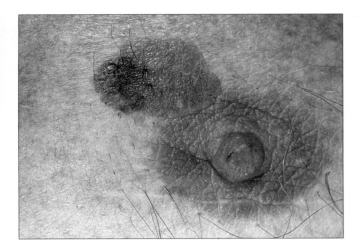

Figure 17.17 This 70-year-old male with a small CMN developed an *in situ*/microinvasive melanoma at the edge of the CMN. The melanoma developed at the dermo-epidermal junction. The nevus was confirmed to be present since birth by history and by the identification of the nevus on baby photographs.

Table 17.2   Frequently asked questions regarding CMN of varying sizes

CMN size	Small and medium	Large
What is the reported lifetime risk for developing melanoma?	• 0–4.9%	• 4.5–10%
Where do melanomas develop?	• within the CMN • CNS (if ≥3 CMN present)	• within the CMN • CNS • other (i.e. retroperitoneal)
If melanoma develops within the CMN, where does it start?	• dermo-epidermal junction • peripheral edge of the CMN	• anywhere within the CMN including below the dermo-epidermal junction (i.e. dermis)
What is the ease of diagnosing cutaneous melanoma?	• since melanomas tend to develop at the dermo-epidermal junction, they can be easily recognized clinically and diagnosed early	• since many melanomas develop deep within the CMN, the clinical recognition of • early melanoma is difficult
When do most melanomas develop?	• at or after puberty	• before puberty
Who is at increased risk for NCM?	• patients with ≥3 CMN	• CMN located in axial locations (i.e. head and neck, midline back) • patients with multiple satellite CMN
What are the management options?	• clinical follow-up • monthly self skin examination • cosmetic improvement (make-up, lasers, excision) • prophylactic removal	• clinical follow-up • monthly self skin examination • cosmetic improvement (make-up, lasers, excision, dermabrasion) • prophylactic removal
If prophylactic removal is decided upon, when should it be done and what methods are available?	• removal can be planned at anytime up to puberty • excision (simple or serial, with or without skin grafts or tissue expanders)	• treatment should be rendered early in life • excision (simple or serial, with or without skin grafts or tissue expanders) • curettage in neonatal period?
Aids to the detection of early melanoma? (If prophylactic excision is not an option or if portions of the nevus are not excised)	• clinical inspection • dermoscopy • baseline photographs used during follow-up examinations to help detect subtle changes • confocal laser microscopy	• clinical inspection • palpation • baseline photographs to help detect subtle changes • dermoscopy? • confocal laser microscopy?
What complications other than melanoma can develop?	• cosmetic issues due to CMN or surgical scars • psychosocial	• cosmetic issues due to CMN or surgical scars • psychosocial • other malignancies (i.e. rhabdomyosarcoma) • symptoms (i.e. pruritus, tenderness, skin fragility)
What laboratory tests or consultations should be considered?	• dermatologist • plastic surgeon • psychologist	• dermatologist • plastic surgeon • pediatric neurologist • psychologist • MRI of brain (radiologist)
All patients should be instructed on the importance of sun avoidance and sun protection.		

Table 17.3 Characteristic histologic features of nevus cells of congenital melanocytic nevi

In lower two-thirds of reticular dermis as single cells or in Indian files.
In subcutaneous septa as single cells or in Indian files.
In subcutaneous fat as single cells or in nests.
Within sebaceous glands and blood vessel walls, and as nests in nerves, at any level of dermis or subcutis.
Within arrectores pilorum, hair follicles, and eccrine ducts and intimately apposed to lymphatics, in lower two-thirds of reticular dermis.
Involving many units of one type of appendage, nerve, or vessel.
Involving more than one type of appendage, nerve, or vessel.
Arrayed in perivascular and perieccrine distribution, mimicking an inflammatory infiltrate.
Paradoxically sparing perifollicular adventitia.
In dense sheets obscuring reticular dermal collagen, appendages, nerves and vessels.
Eliciting little stromal response when arrayed as single cells or in single files.
Possessing oval vesicular nuclei at both superficial and deep levels.

differentiation. Heterologous elements such as cartilage, bone, adipose tissue, vascular malformation, hemangioma, lymphangioma, mastocytoma and schwannoma may be present.

MANAGEMENT

General

The management of CMN needs to be tailored for each patient. The nevus location, nevus size, cosmetic issues regarding the nevus or resultant surgical scars, risk of anesthesia, risk of surgery, psychological implications, risk of melanoma and risk of NCM all need to be taken into account in this decision making process. Surgical removal of CMN, especially large or clinically atypical CMN, may lower the risk for developing cutaneous melanoma, however, this has not been confirmed in any controlled study. Analysis of previous studies, arranged chronologically by year of publication, reveals a progressive decline in the reported risk of melanoma developing in large CMN. Study design, selection bias, awareness of the importance of ultraviolet protection and the introduction of sunscreens may, in part, explain some of this apparent decline in the melanoma risk associated with large CMN. In addition, over the last 30 years, great strides have been made in improving the safety of general anesthesia and surgical techniques. The routine use of tissue expanders and skin grafts has made removal of larger CMN more feasible and many patients (or their parents) elect to have their CMN excised in an attempt to improve the cosmetic appearance and/or reduce the risk of melanoma. The fact that many patients

undergo complete or partial removal of their large CMN may be another variable that can explain the decline in melanoma risk observed over time. However, most excisions cannot eliminate the risk of melanoma completely, since it is frequently impossible or impractical to remove every nevus cell and melanomas can develop from remnant nevus cells.[15] Furthermore, surgical excision does not eliminate the risk of developing extra-cutaneous melanomas as can occur in patients with NCM. If surgical excision is selected as the treatment of choice, it should ideally address the risk of malignant transformation, achieve satisfactory cosmetic results and maintain adequate function. Although other surgical interventions such as curettage, dermabrasion and lasers may improve the cosmetic appearance of CMN, they do not adequately address the risk of developing melanoma or pseudo-melanoma (recurrent nevus) from nevus remnants located in the dermis. Furthermore, it may be difficult to detect changes indicative of melanoma and problematic to differentiate between melanoma and pseudo-melanoma in CMN treated in this fashion. Finally, some patients and their families have unrealistic expectations regarding the cosmetic outcome after surgery. These individuals should be informed that although surgery may sometimes improve the cosmetic appearance, some patients may be left with scars that can also be unattractive and/or uncomfortable (Fig. 17.12).

An alternative to prophylactic excision, especially for those nevi that are uniform, light colored, even textured and without nodules, is periodic clinical surveillance. Patient and family involvement can aid in the early detection of melanoma via performance of monthly self-skin examinations. Any changes suspicious for melanoma should be biopsied and appropriately treated. To avoid the false positive diagnosis of melanoma, which can result in unnecessary surgery and other possible therapies, it is recommended that all biopsies be evaluated by pathologists experienced in the evaluation of pigmented lesions. It is important to remember that erosions (Fig. 17.18a) and proliferative nodules (Fig. 17.18b), which are often seen in large CMN within the first few weeks of the patient's life, are not necessarily signs of cancer and most will heal and/or disappear over time. Baseline clinical and sometimes dermoscopic photographs of the nevus can be utilized for comparison during subsequent skin examinations in an attempt to detect subtle changes within these nevi. Changing lesions can be further evaluated by *in vivo* techniques such as dermoscopy or confocal laser microscopy.[24] Dermoscopy may help detect small foci of melanoma within a CMN, thus directing clinicians and pathologists in evaluating the most appropriate area (Fig. 17.19a).[25] This may potentially avoid sampling error resulting in the false negative diagnosis of malignancy. Confocal laser microscopy, which utilizes a near infrared laser beam, is a new experimental *in vivo* imaging technique that provides near histological horizontal microscopic section images of the epidermis, dermoepidermal junction and papillary dermis. This technique may prove to be useful in evaluating CMN suspect for having developed melanoma (Fig. 17.19b,c). However, it is important to appreciate that both dermoscopy and confocal microscopy can evaluate skin to the depth of the

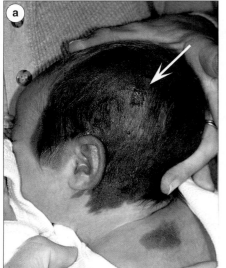

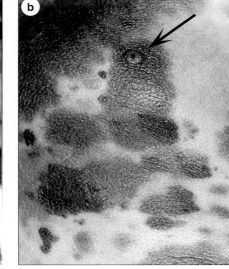

Figure 17.18 Erosions (a) and proliferative nodules (b) within LCMN can often be observed during early infancy.

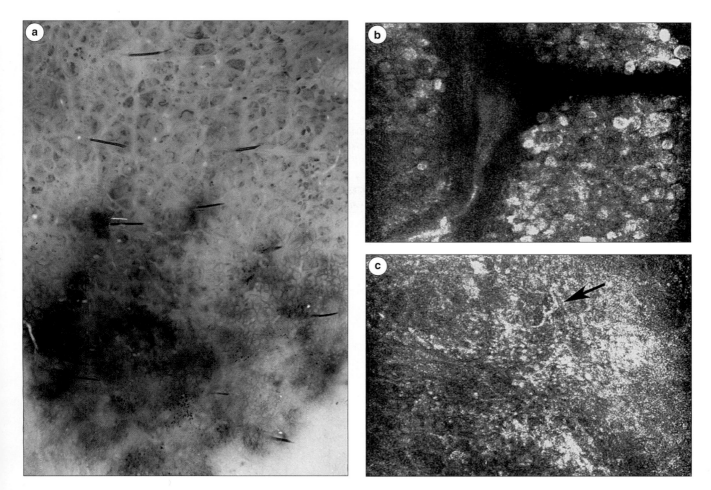

Figure 17.19 Dermoscopy (a) of the lesion in figure 17.17 showing the dermoscopic features of a CMN with homogeneous distribution of globules (cobblestone pattern) on the superior pole of the image. On the inferior pole one observes irregular black dots, blue-gray areas, and thickened reticulation all of which are commonly seen in melanoma (a). The confocal image of the CMN portion of the lesion reveals the normal rete ridge pattern at the dermo-epidermal junction and nests of round nevomelanocytes in the papillary dermis, a feature often seen in CMN (b). The confocal image of the melanoma portion of the lesion reveals the loss of the normal rete ridge pattern; single cells predominate over nests; and pagetoid spread of melanocytes (c). The arrow points to one of the irregular, pagetoid and dendritic melanocytes located in the epidermis (c). The combination of large dendritic melanocytes in the epidermis in conjunction with a loss of the normal architecture is frequently observed in melanoma viewed under confocal laser microscopy.

papillary dermis. Thus, these techniques can provide useful information when evaluating smaller and/or superficial CMN, since most melanomas that develop in these nevi occur at the dermo-epidermal junction. On the other hand, both dermoscopy and confocal laser microscopy have limited utility in the evaluation of changes occurring in the dermis of large or deeply penetrating CMN. Lesions suggestive of melanoma on clinical inspection, palpation, dermoscopy or confocal laser microscopy should be promptly biopsied.

It is important to inform patients and/or caregivers that sunburns increase the risk of developing melanoma within nevi. Thus all patients should be instructed on proper sun avoidance and sun protection techniques. CMN present on exposed skin can be concealed with cover-up foundation and cosmetics, many of which contain sunscreens. CMN on non-exposed skin can be protected from ultraviolet light by use of sun-protective clothing and sun-protective swimwear with ultraviolet protection factor (UPF) 50 or more. Future developments in chemoprevention with improved sunscreen formulations, development of compounds that help repair ultraviolet damaged DNA[26] and the development of compounds that can prevent ultraviolet damage may also help decrease the risk of developing melanoma.[27] Patients with large CMN should be informed that the skin overlying the nevus may be fragile and often lacks the normal skin barrier functions found in normal skin. Thus, the involved skin can easily become xerotic, which in turn can cause pruritus. Diligent use of moisturizers applied on a regular basis may help control these symptoms.

For those patients at increased risk for NCM, obtaining a screening MRI scan of the brain should be considered.[28,29] However, it is important to note that approximately 23% of neurologically asymptomatic patients with large CMN will have a positive MRI scan revealing changes suggestive of NCM, but a very small percentage of them will actually develop symptomatic NCM.[30] On the other hand, a normal MRI scan does not exclude the possibility of developing symptoms, though the chance of this is small. Some physicians recommend obtaining serial MRI scans in asymptomatic patients at risk for developing NCM. Thorough neurological examinations can also be used in the assessment of patients at risk for developing NCM. Serial neurological examinations may be a substitute for MRI scans in following these individuals. There are some physicians and patients who question the necessity of obtaining screening MRI scans since there are no treatments available for asymptomatic NCM. However, knowledge of a positive MRI scan may affect the management decisions regarding timing of surgery, and a negative MRI scan may help alleviate some anxieties. Patients with symptomatic NCM, on the other hand, should have MRI scans performed to determine whether they may be candidates for medical intervention (i.e. ventriculo-peritoneal shunt placement, surgical excision, radiation therapy, experimental therapy with interferon, chemotherapy and/or retinoids) to help alleviate their symptoms. In addition to brain MRI scan, patients with large or medium-sized nevi overlying the lumbosacral area may require an MRI scan of the spine to rule out spinal anomalies such as the tethered cord syndrome.[31]

Treatment modalities

Treatment interventions include full-thickness excisions, partial-thickness excisions, dermabrasions, curettage, laser treatment and chemical peels. Improving the cosmetic appearance frequently requires the use of a combination of different treatment interventions. In terms of preventing the development of melanoma (prophylactic removal), any of the above-mentioned procedures will reduce the overall number of melanocytes which theoretically should lower the risk of melanoma. However, with the exception of full-thickness surgical excision, these procedures do not adequately address the risk for developing melanoma within the deep dermis or subcutis. As with any treatment, the risk and benefits of each treatment modality should be discussed with the patient or guardian. Patients and their parents also need to be informed of the psychological and cosmetic burden frequently placed on patients with large or multiple smaller CMN. This burden may not be eliminated by surgery because the scars from surgery may also be cosmetically disfiguring, although it appears that most patients or their parents prefer the scars to the nevus (Fig. 17.20).[12] Furthermore, between 50% and 75% of patients with large CMN, if given the opportunity, would elect to have an operation to remove the CMN. Finally, cosmetic cover-up foundation make-up such as Dermablend can be used to help conceal exposed nevus and/or scars (Fig. 17.21). These products have an added benefit in that most also contain a sunscreen.

Surgical excision

Most small CMN can easily be excised and the resulting defect repaired in a relatively simple manner. Larger lesions require individualization, depending on their size, location and depth. Serial excisions, tissue expanders and skin grafts each have a place in the surgical management of LCMN. As with any treatment, the possible complications involved with surgery need to be considered, such as infection, bleeding and risk of general anesthesia. One study, evaluating the risk for developing melanoma, risk of general anesthesia and psychosocial factors, deemed that the best timing for surgical excision is between 6 and 9 months of age or between 8 and 12 years of age. Based on the age groups at highest risk for melanoma, prophylactic excision of LCMN should be performed early in life, whereas prophylactic excisions of small CMN can be delayed until later years. However, the best surgical results, from a cosmetic perspective, are obtained when excisions are performed prior to age 2. The improved cosmetic results obtained from early surgical excision needs to be weighed against the higher likelihood of nevus recurrence along the scar margins when excisions are performed early. It is presumed that this high rate of nevus recurrence is based on the theory that nevo-genesis is not complete until at least 2 years of age.

Prophylactic excision should be contemplated for LCMN that are atypical, nodular or thickened. These lesions are difficult to follow clinically even in the presence of baseline photographs. If prophylactic complete excision is not possible then attempts should be made to excise the most infiltrated, thickened or multinodular component

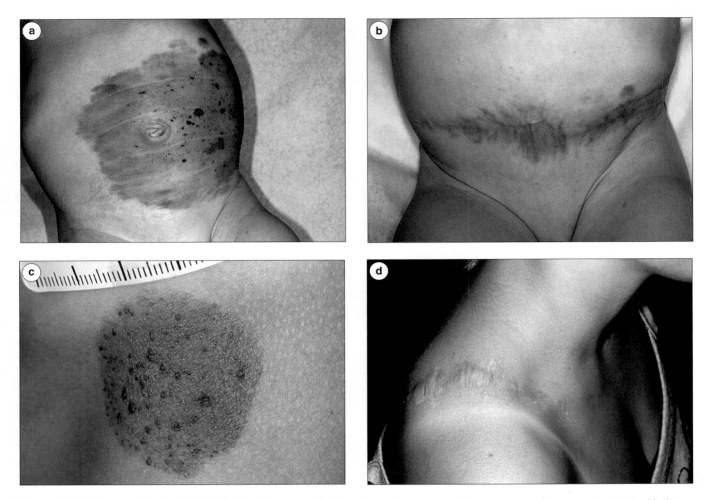

Figure 17.20   The parents of patient (a) decided to remove the LCMN for primarily cosmetic concerns and were very content with the results (b). Patient (c) decided to remove the CMN mainly for prophylactic reasons, despite knowing the low risk for developing melanoma and was unhappy with the surgical scar (d).

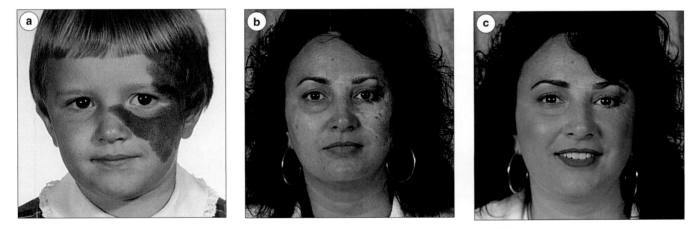

Figure 17.21   Cosmetic coverup can help conceal nevus, nevus remnants and scars. (a) Large CMN. (b) Surgical scar from removal of the CMN. (c) Cosmetic cover-up concealing the scar.

of the nevus. The reason for this is that melanoma can be difficult to detect in these thickened areas.

Dermabrasion

Dermabrasion, which removes the epidermis and part of the dermis, eliminates the superficial nevus cells. In

an attempt to remove as many nevus cells as possible, it has been suggested that dermabrasion be performed during infancy. This is based on the fact that dermabrasion becomes more difficult as the epidermal and dermal elements become more adherent with age and on the belief, held by some, that nevus cells migrate

235

down into the deeper layers of the skin over time. Dermabrasion may reduce the degree of pigmentation and improve the cosmetic appearance. The remaining deep dermal and subcutaneous nevus cells are eventually covered by scar tissue. The post dermabraded skin is usually thinner, more fragile, tender and has reduced hair density.[32] Some believe that the reduced pigmentation following dermabrasion may allow for easier detection of color changes indicative of melanoma in the deeper layers.

Curettage

Treatment of CMN with curettage consists of curetting through a natural cleavage plane that separates the highly nevus populated upper dermis from the relatively less nevus populated deeper dermis.[33] Unfortunately, this cleavage plane is present only during the first few weeks of life, thus limiting the time frame within which this procedure can be performed with reasonably good results and raises the issue of whether the potential cosmetic success of the operation outweighs the risk of anesthesia at this young age. On the other hand, since curettage of larger CMN can often be done as a single procedure, it may offer a reduction in operative risk compared to multiple serial excisions. When performed by experienced operators, curettage can result in acceptable cosmesis. One study demonstrated that for non-scalp CMN the functional and cosmetic results from curettage were superior or equivalent to surgical excision.[33] The post-curettaged dermis is replaced by sclerotic and dense connective tissue.

Chemical peel

Chemical peels with agents such as phenol have been utilized by some to treat CMN. Deep chemical peels can result in the reduction of the number of melanocytes and may be an option for those lesions that are surgically unresectable and cosmetically disfiguring.[34] CMN most suitable for treatment by chemical peel are those with lighter pigmentation and those with nevus cells confined to the epidermis and superficial dermis. Potential side-effects of phenol include cardiac and renal toxicity, which need to be considered before embarking on this treatment modality.

Laser

Lasers can be utilized in the treatment of some CMN with most patients requiring multiple laser treatments before achieving acceptable cosmetic results. Carbon dioxide (CO_2) lasers vaporize tissue resulting in scarring and thus should be considered surgical procedures akin to dermabrasion. Commonly used lasers that do not vaporize tissue include normal mode ruby, Q-switched ruby, Q-switched alexandrite (755 nm) and Q-switched neodymium:yttrium-aluminum-garnet (Nd:YAG) (532 and 1064 nm).[35] The Q-switched ruby laser is the most popular laser used to treat CMN. The specificity of the Q-switched ruby laser is due to its 694 nm wavelength, which is selectively absorbed by melanin.[36] In addition, the laser produces a 20-ns pulse duration that approximates the thermal relaxation time for melanosomes, thereby confining the energy to the targeted cells and resulting in the thermal destruction of melanocytes. Q-switched ruby lasers have recently been shown to lighten CMN that because of location, size, or depth of nevo-melanocytes were not amenable to surgical excision. This form of treatment is attractive because of its low potential for scarring and its ability to decrease the pigmentation thereby improving the cosmetic outcome. Preliminary histological data show that treatment with Q-switched lasers can achieve significant reduction of papillary dermal melanocytes resulting in reduction of visible pigment.[37] Partial repigmentation however, does occur in most patients resulting in a final pigment clearance of approximately 50%.[37] The degree of pigment clearance and melanocyte destruction can potentially be enhanced by utilizing a combination of different lasers.[38,39]

Lasers can also be utilized to help eliminate the hypertrichosis that so commonly occurs on CMN. However, whether lasers are used for hair removal or nevus 'removal', one must contemplate the possibility of adverse long-term sequelae. Lasers work by applying heat energy to melanocytes and it is currently unknown whether this heat energy can be potentially mutagenic.

MANAGEMENT OPTIONS

All patients with CMN and their parents should be instructed in the technique of self-skin examination, which should be performed on a monthly basis. They need to be educated on the warning signs of melanoma including change in color, size, shape and symptoms. If a change is noted it should be brought to the attention of their physician. All patients should be instructed to avoid excessive ultraviolet light exposure and to use sun-protective clothing and sunscreens. Patients with LCMN, whether excised or not, should be followed for life with complete skin examinations, review of systems, palpation of lymph nodes and neurological examinations to search for primary or metastatic melanoma. In addition, the nevus and scars, if any, should be palpated for the detection of subcutaneous lumps.

Large congenital melanocytic nevi

Key issues regarding the management of larger sized CMN are presented in Figures 17.22–17.26. Figure 17.22 provides an overview. Figure 17.23 provides information on individuals with large CMN lacking suspicious areas that have a normal neurological examination. Figure 17.24 provides information on individuals with a normal neurological examination but large CMN displaying 'atypical' areas. Figure 17.25 provides information on individuals whose examination is suggestive of NCM. Patients with symptomatic NCM should be evaluated to determine whether their symptoms can be alleviated by neurosurgical procedures such as placement of a ventriculo-peritoneal (VP) shunt. However, the VP shunt may also provide a conduit for leptomeningeal melanocyte migration from the leptomeninges to the peritoneal cavity.[40] Patients with symptomatic NCM whose symptoms are progressive tend to have a poor prognosis and should be spared aggressive prophylactic cutaneous surgery, at least until their status improves. Patients with symptomatic NCM whose symptoms are improving may ultimately have a relatively good prognosis and thus can be managed as outlined in Figures 17.23 and 17.24. Figure 17.26 provides information on screening magnetic resonance imaging (MRI). MRI scans can be utilized as a screening tool to detect asymptomatic NCM in high-risk individuals, such as those with LCMN and many satellite nevi. The timing of when a screening MRI is performed may be very important. It appears that myelin protein can obscure subtle deposits of melanocytes.[29] Thus, it may be best to obtain a screening MRI in early infancy (birth to 4 months of age) before the brain has myelinized. Individuals with a normal MRI scan can be managed as outlined in Figures 17.23 and 17.24. Asymptomatic individuals with an MRI scan suggestive of NCM should be followed closely and elective surgeries delayed until the status of the patient is known. Preliminary data suggests that only a small proportion of these individuals will actually develop symptomatic disease. Those with a good prognosis (i.e. stable or improving MRI findings) can be managed as outlined in Figures 17.23 and 17.24. Those with a poor prognosis (i.e. progressive changes on MRI scans or development of symptomatic NCM) should be managed as described in Figure 17.25.

Small and medium congenital melanocytic nevi

An algorithm delineating an approach to the management of patients with small to medium-sized CMN is presented in Figure 17.27. The management of small and medium-sized CMN remains controversial. Since it is rare for smaller CMN to undergo malignant transformation during childhood, many physicians agree that these lesions generally need not be considered for excision until later in life. However, CMN under 20 cm in diameter that may warrant excision at an earlier age include relatively large medium-sized lesions and those with unusual morphologic features, such as thickened lobular or cerebriform appearance, that would otherwise compromise the ability to clinically follow the lesion.

Homogeneous and symmetric smaller CMN can be followed during childhood with routine physician follow-up, self-skin examinations, baseline photographs and dermoscopy. If a change is noted on any of the aforementioned examinations, the lesion should be evaluated for biopsy. The decision to proceed with elective 'prophylactic' excision can be delayed until the child can actively participate in the decision making process and is old enough to tolerate the procedure under local anesthesia. Prophylactic excision should be considered if examination of the lesion and the follow-up is burdensome to the patient or family. Prophylactic removal should also be considered if the patient or the parents' anxiety level is very high regarding the follow-up of these nevi or their potential risk for developing melanoma. If the nevus is not excised then photographs and periodic follow-up, especially after the age of 12 years, is recommended.

CONCLUSION AND FUTURE OUTLOOK

In conclusion, the care of patients with CMN often requires a multidisciplinary approach involving pediatricians, family physicians, internists, dermatologists, psychologists, plastic surgeons, neurologists and radiologists. The cosmetic and psychosocial issues combined with the knowledge of the increased risk of developing melanoma and/or NCM is a burden that many of these patients and their families have to carry. It is important for physicians to help them come to terms with these issues. Although the precise risks for melanoma in patients with CMN are not known, including the added risk resulting from sun exposure, all patients and/or family members should be instructed on sun avoidance and sun protection. Routine examinations, aided by photographic documentation, may enable early diagnosis and treatment should melanoma develop. Furthermore, patients and families should be reminded that though melanoma, NCM or other complications can develop, the majority of affected individuals will not develop any complications. At times, psychological consultation is useful in gaining a better

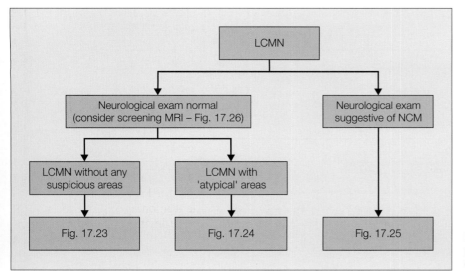

Figure 17.22 Overview of the key issues regarding the management of larger-sized CMN.

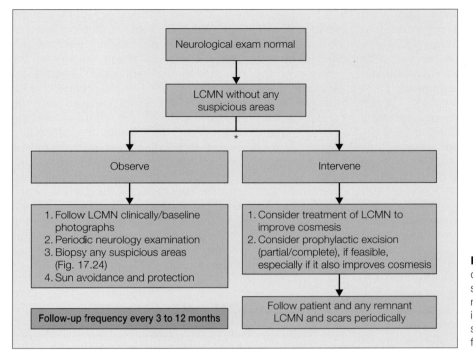

Figure 17.23 Management information on individuals with large CMN lacking suspicious areas that have a normal neurological examination. *Factors influencing therapeutic intervention include size, location, patient anxiety, aesthetic and functional tradeoffs, etc.

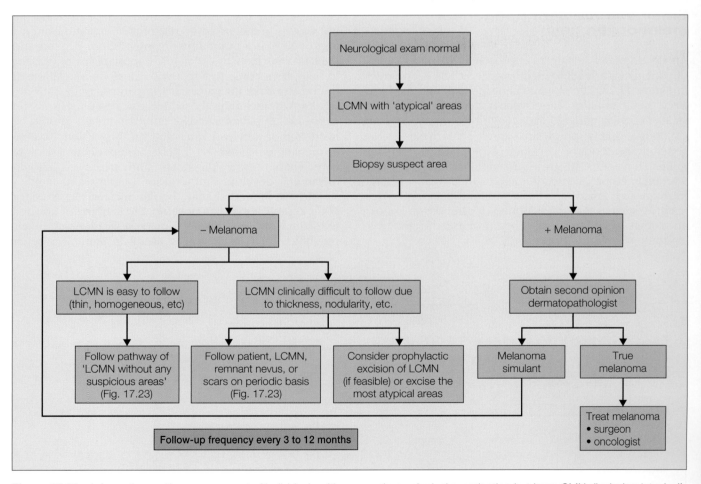

Figure 17.24 Information on the management of individuals with a normal neurological examination but large CMN displaying 'atypical' areas.

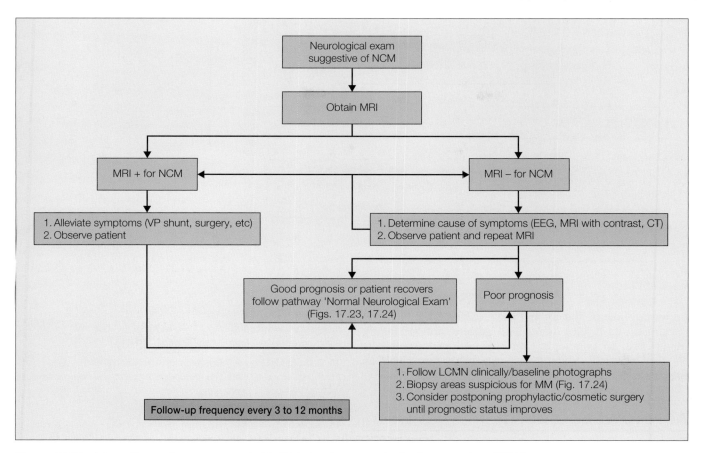

Figure 17.25 Information on the management of individuals whose examination is suggestive of NCM.

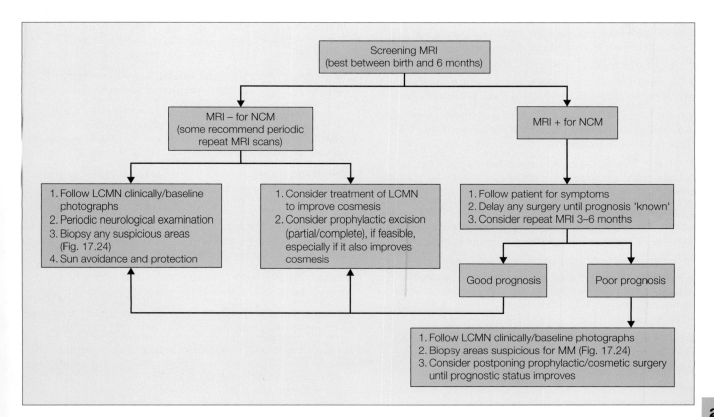

Figure 17.26 Information on screening MRI.

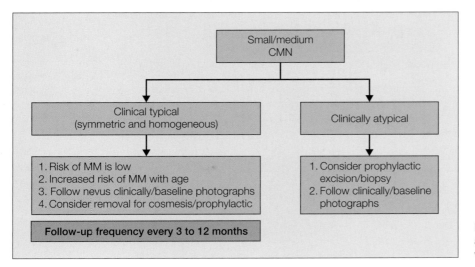

Figure 17.27   An algorithm delineating an approach to the management of patients with small to medium-sized CMN.

understanding of the impact that a CMN may have on psychosocial development. The patient and/or family might wish to contact a CMN support group such as Nevus Outreach (www.nevus.org) or Nevus Network (www.nevusnetwork.org).

ACKNOWLEDGMENT

I would like to thank Daphne Demas for preparing the images for this chapter.

REFERENCES

1 Takayama H, Nagashima Y, Hara M, et al. Immunohistochemical detection of the c-met proto-oncogene product in the congenital melanocytic nevus of an infant with neurocutaneous melanosis. J Am Acad Derm 2001; 44:538–540.

2 Cramer SF. The melanocytic differentiation pathway in congenital melanocytic nevi: theoretical considerations. Pediat Pathol 1988; 8:253–265.

3 Kos L, Aronzon A, Takayama H, et al. Hepatocyte growth factor/scatter factor-Met signaling in neural crest-derived melanocyte development. Pigment Cell Res 1999; 12:13–21.

4 Kawakami T, Soma Y, Kawa Y, et al. Transforming growth factor β1 regulates melanocyte proliferation and differentiation in mouse neural crest cells via stem cell factor/KIT signaling. J Invest Derm 2002; 118:471–478.

5 Natali PG, Nicotra MR, DiRenzo MF, et al. Expression of the c-Met/HGF receptor in human melanocytic neoplasms: demonstration of the relationship to malignant melanoma tumour progression. Br J Cancer 1993; 68:746–750.

6 DeDavid M, Orlow SJ, Provost N, et al. A study of large congenital melanocytic nevi and associated malignant melanomas: review of cases in the New York University Registry and the world literature. J Am Acad Derm 1997; 36:409–416.

7 Papp T, Pemsel H, Zimmermann R, et al. Mutational analysis of the N-ras, p53, p16INK4a, CDK4, and MC1R genes in human congenital melanocytic naevi. J Med Genet 1999; 36:610–614.

8 Egan CL, Oliveria SA, Elenitsas R, et al. Cutaneous melanoma risk and phenotypic changes in large congenital nevi: a follow-up study of 46 patients. J Am Acad Derm 1998; 39(6):923–932.

9 Marghoob AA, Schoenbach SP, Kopf AW, et al. Large congenital melanocytic nevi and the risk for the development of malignant melanoma: a prospective study. Arch Derm 1996; 132:170–175.

10 DeDavid M, Orlow SJ, Provost N, et al. Neurocutaneous melanosis: clinical features of large congenital melanocytic nevi in patients with manifest central nervous system melanosis. J Am Acad Derm 1996; 35:529–538.

11 Seidenari S, Pellacani G. Surface microscopy features of congenital nevi. Clin Derm 2002; 20:263–267.

12 Koot HM, DeWaard-van der Spek F, Peer CD, et al. Psychosocial sequelae in 29 children with giant congenital melanocytic naevi. Clin Exp Derm 2000; 25:589–593.

13 Ceballos P, Ruiz-Maldonado R, Mihm M. Melanoma in children. N Engl J Med 1995; 332:656–662.

14 Barnhill RL, Fleischli M. Histologic features of congenital melanocytic nevi in infants 1 year of age or younger. J Am Acad Derm 1995; 33:780–785.

15 Rhodes AR, Wood WC, Sober AJ, et al. Nonepidermal origin of malignant melanoma associated with giant congenital nevocellular nevus. Plast Reconstr Surg 1981; 67:782–790.

16 Mancianti M, Clark WH, Hayes FN, et al. Malignant melanoma simulants arising in congenital melanocytic nevi do not show experimental evidence for a malignant phenotype. Am J Pathol 1990; 136:817–829.

17 Bastian BC, Xiong J, Frieden IJ, et al. Genetic changes in neoplasms arising in congenital melanocytic nevi. Differences between nodular proliferations and melanomas. Am J Pathol 2002; 161:1163–1169.

18 Bittencourt FV, Marghoob AA, Kopf AW, et al. Large congenital melanocytic nevi and the risk for development of malignant melanoma and neurocutaneous melanocytosis. Pediatrics 2000; 106:736–741.

19 Kodonaga JN, Frieden IJ. Neurocutaneous melanosis: definition and review of the literature. J Am Acad Derm 1991; 24:747–755.

20 Reyes-Mugica M, Chou P, Byrd S, et al. Nevomelanocytic proliferations in the central nervous system of children. Cancer 1993; 73:227–285.

21 Illig C, Weidener F, Hundeiker H, et al. Congenital nevi less than or equal to 10 cm as precursors to melanoma: 52 cases, a review, and a new conception. Arch Derm 1985; 121:1274–1281.

22 Cribier BJ, Santinelli F, Grosshans E. Lack of clinical-pathological correlation in the diagnosis of congenital naevi. Br J Derm 1999; 141:1004–1009.

23 Mark GJ, Mihm MC, Litelpo MG, Reed RJ, Clark WH. Congenital melanocytic nevi of the small and garment type. Clinical, histologic, and ultrastructural studies. Hum Pathol 1973; 4:395–418.

24 Langley R, Rajadhyaksha M, Dwyer P, et al. Confocal scanning laser microscopy of benign and malignant melanocytic skin lesions in vivo. J Am Acad Derm 2001; 45:365–376.

25 Bauer J, Metzler G, Rassner G, et al. Dermatoscopy turns histopathologist's attention to the suspicious area in melanocytic lesions. Arch Derm 2001; 137:1338–1340.

26 Yarosh D, Klein J, O'Connor A, et al. Effect of topically applied T4 endonuclease V in liposomes on skin cancer in xeroderma pigmentosum: a randomized study. Lancet 2001; 357:926–929.

27 Salti GI, Kichina JV, DasGupta TK, et al. Betulinic acid reduces ultraviolet-C-induced DNA breakage in congenital melanocytic naeval cells: evidence for a potential role as a chemopreventive agent. Melanoma Res 2001; 11:99–104.

28 Frieden IJ, Williams ML, Barkovich AJ. Giant congenital melanocytic nevi: brain magnetic resonance findings in neurologically asymptomatic children. J Am Acad Derm 1994; 31:423–429.

29 Barkovich AJ, Frieden IJ, Williams ML. MR of neurocutaneous melanosis. AJNR Am J Neuroradiol 1994; 15:859–867.

30 Foster RD, Williams ML, Barkovich AJ, et al. Giant congenital melanocytic nevi: the significance of neurocutaneous melanosis in neurologically asymptomatic children. Plast Reconstr Surg 2001; 107:933–941.

31 Humphreys RP. Clinical evaluation of cutaneous lesions of the back: spinal signatures that do not go away. Clin Neurosurg 1996; 43:175–187.

32 Bohn J, Svensson H, Aberg M. Dermabrasion of large congenital melanocytic naevi in neonates. Scand J Plast Reconstr Surg Hand Surg 2000; 34(4):321–326.

33 DeRaeve LE, Roseeuw DI. Curettage of giant congenital melanocytic nevi in neonates. A decade later. Arch Derm 2002; 138:943–947.

34 Hopkins JD, Smith AW, Jackson IT. Adjunctive treatment of congenital pigmented nevi with phenol chemical peel. Plast Reconstr Surg 2000; 105(1):1–11.

35 Imayama S, Ueda S. Long- and short-term histological observations of congenital nevi treated with the normal-mode ruby laser. Arch Derm 1999; 135(10):1211–1218.

36 Grevelink JM, Leeuwen RL van, Anderson RR, Byers HR. Clinical and histological responses of congenital melanocytic nevi after single treatment with Q-switched lasers. Arch Derm 1997; 133(3):349–353.

37 Waldorf HA, Kauvar ANB, Geronemus RG. Treatment of small and medium congenital nevi with the Q-Switched Ruby Laser. Arch Derm 1996; 132:301–304.

38 Duke D, Byers HR, Sober AJ, Anderson RR, Grevelink JM. Treatment of benign and atypical nevi with the normal-mode ruby laser and the Q-switched ruby laser: clinical improvement but failure to completely eliminate nevomelanocytes. Arch Derm 1999; 135(3):290–296.

39 Kono T, Nozaki M, Chan HH, Sasaki K, Kwon SG. Combined use of normal mode and Q-switched ruby lasers in the treatment of congenital melanocytic naevi. Br J Plast Surg 2001; 54(7):640–643.

40 Faillace WJ, Okawara SH, Mcdonald JV. Neurocutaneous melanosis with extensive intracerebral and spinal cord involvement. Report of two cases. J Neurosurg 1984; 61(4):782–785.

CHAPTER
18

Pathology of Melanoma: New Concepts

Jennifer Cather, J Christian Cather and Clay J Cockerell

Key points

- It is essential that clinicians understand the appropriate methods for biopsy of lesions that are highly suspect for melanoma as well as those that are less likely to but could represent melanoma.
- Histopathologists who diagnose cutaneous melanoma must have appropriate training and must be aware of the many different histologic variants and the simulators of melanoma.
- Special stains and other techniques are valuable adjuncts to routine histology but no stain or special technique alone can distinguish between a benign nevus and melanoma.
- The ability to assess melanoma prognosis based on histologic features alone is somewhat limited. Breslow's thickness remains the most reliable individual prognostic factor.

INTRODUCTION

The American Cancer Society estimates that over 55,100 new cases of invasive melanoma will be diagnosed in the US in 2004.[1] One in 65 individuals born in the US in 2004 will develop invasive melanoma over the course of their lifetime. Given the large number of melanomas, more unusual clinical and histologic variants are being observed. Thus, it is important for both clinicians and histopathologists to be well versed in the pathologic features of cutaneous melanoma.

CLINICAL FEATURES

Cutaneous melanoma may have many clinical appearances with corresponding histopathological correlates. While most early lesions demonstrate the 'ABCDs' that have been described, others may be unusual and manifest either some or none of these features. While most are either patches, plaques, nodules or tumors, some may be polypoid with a stalk.[2] Most lesions are greater than 6 mm in diameter when diagnosed but lesions much smaller than this are well-recognized.

Desmoplastic melanoma is a rare variant that is notoriously difficult to diagnose clinically and histologically. It usually presents subtly as a pigmented or skin-colored indurated patch, papule or plaque on sun-exposed skin. Lesions are usually described clinically as 'fibroma' or 'scar'.

Fortunately, less than 2% of melanomas are amelanotic as these pose the most difficulty in clinical diagnosis.[3] They are pink or skin-colored patches, plaques or nodules that may be ulcerated. They are often mistaken for pyogenic granuloma, basal cell carcinoma, nevi or fibromas. A clue to the diagnosis may be a hint of pigmentation at the periphery which may be easier to appreciate with dermoscopy.[4] Dermoscopy also commonly shows small red dots evenly distributed or grouped on a whitish or pink-red background.[4]

Verrucous melanoma is a variant that was first described in 1967[5] as hyperkeratotic pigmented lesions that are usually on the extremities (71%).[6] Clinically, they are usually misdiagnosed as benign lesions such as seborrheic keratosis, verruca, nevus and Spitz nevus.[7–9]

Rarely, melanoma may arise in association with blue nevi or arise *de novo* but clinically resemble blue nevi.[10] Most of these lesions are present for many years before diagnosis and may elude suspicion because they tend to grow slowly and involve the deep dermis rather than the epidermis. The clinicopathologic correlations of melanoma variants are critical in the effective management of melanoma.

HISTOLOGIC DIAGNOSIS OF MELANOMA

Natural history of melanoma: clinical and histologic aspects

Although some controversy exists about how melanoma develops and evolves, a pathway that has been proposed by Ackerman is considered by many to be the most valid.[11,12] According to this hypothesis, an oncogenic stimulus, usually chronic ultraviolet irradiation, occurs within one or more melanocytes in the epidermis at the dermoepidermal junction. Melanocytes then begin to proliferate initially as solitary units at the junction and are manifest as scattered, single hyperchromatic cells with a cleft or halo surrounding them. Clinically, there may be only a very light tan macule or the process may be invisible (Fig. 18.1).

Over time, these melanocytes become more numerous and begin to coalesce and form small nests although they are still confined to the dermoepidermal junction. There may also be involvement of adnexal structures such as acrotrichia and acrosyringia. At this

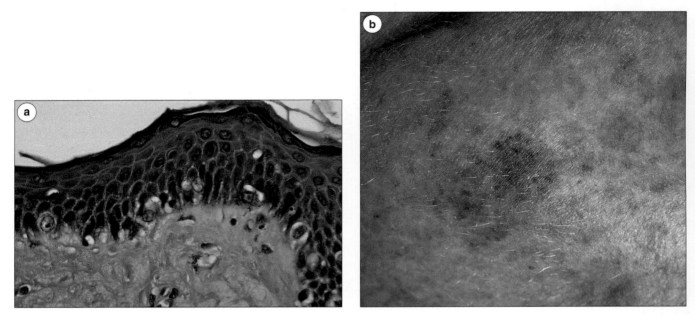

Figure 18.1 Natural history of melanoma. Melanoma begins with a proliferation of slightly atypical melanocytes arranged as solitary units at the dermo-epidermal junction, usually on sun damaged skin as depicted here. The distance between melanocytes varies. Atypical melanocytes are manifest as small, hyperchromatic cells with clear haloes surrounding them (Hematoxylin and eosin, original magnification ×100.) Clinically, there may be no lesion visible or only a very faint tan macule, as in this photograph.

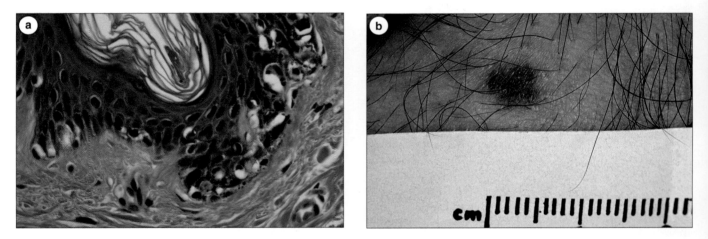

Figure 18.2 Natural history of melanoma. As melanoma evolves, the number of atypical melanocytes increases, their nuclei become more atypical and melanocytes are present above the dermo-epidermal junction and within the epithelium of adnexal structures. Clinically, these are usually tan macules usually up to 4 mm in diameter. They may be quite nondescript and as such, biopsies may not be performed at this stage. (H&E, original magnification ×100.)

point, there is often a tan to brown macule that ranges from 3 to 4 mm in diameter but again, it usually is not significantly atypical (Fig. 18.2). As the tumor progresses, more nests of atypical melanocytes develop at the dermoepidermal junction and solitary atypical melanocytes are distributed over these nests throughout the epidermis.[13] Nests also begin to be present above the junction. Clinically, such lesions may appear darker brown and shades of black may be seen which correlates with the presence of melanin in upper levels of the epidermis and in the cornified layer. They may still be quite small, approximately 3–4 mm in diameter at this stage, although they may be somewhat larger (Fig. 18.3). Some of the architectural features of melanoma may begin to be visible at this time, namely slight

asymmetry and irregular borders and as such, a biopsy may be performed.

As the lesion progresses, there is even more involvement of the epidermis with nests and single atypical melanocytes throughout and involving adnexal structures. Neoplastic melanocytes also involve the papillary dermis initially in small foci but over time, there is more extensive involvement and it becomes filled and expanded (Figs 18.4, 18.5). At this stage, lesions are usually greater than 6 mm in diameter and now demonstrate the 'ABCDs' of melanoma in most cases. Most lesions at this stage are still macular or only slightly elevated although skin markings are often obliterated.

If not recognized and treated at this stage, lesions may progress to involve deeper structures such as the

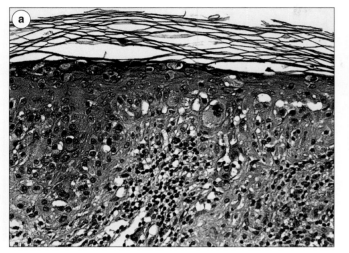
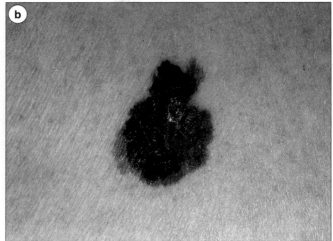

Figure 18.3 Natural history of melanoma. In time, nests of atypical melanocytes form at the dermo-epidermal junction that are distributed non-uniformly and begin to coalesce. More atypical melanocytes, both singly and in nests, are present throughout the epicermis giving rise to the 'buckshot scatter' pattern. Clinically, these lesions are usually tan with foci of black, have irregular borders and are usually greater than 6 mm in diameter. This represents melanoma in situ. (H&E, original magnification ×100.)

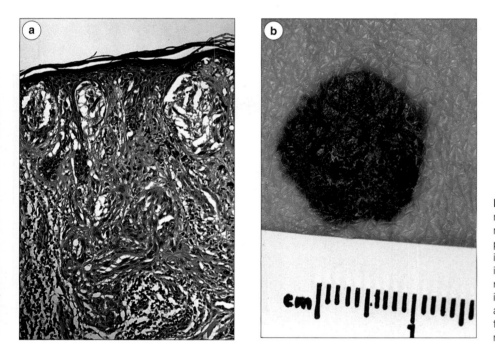

Figure 18.4 Natural history of melanoma. In this melanoma, although most of the atypical melanocytes are present throughout the epidermis, there is a small nest of atypical melanocytes in the papillary dermis. Clinically, this represents melanoma with early dermal involvement and would usually have an appearance that has been described by the mnemonic, 'ABCD'. (H&E, original magnification ×100.)

reticular dermis and subcutaneous fat. This may be accompanied by additional clinical features including nodule formation, ulceration and colors such as red, blue and white, the latter associated with the presence of regression (Fig. 18.6). All of these features signify more advanced lesions and are associated with poor prognosis.[14] Finally, metastasis may develop and many different organs can be involved. Usually, regional lymph nodes are involved first although local 'satellite' cutaneous metastasis may occur as an initial manifestation of metastatic disease.

Different clinical and histologic manifestations are seen depending on which sites are involved. In cutaneous metastases of melanoma, histologically there are aggregates of atypical neoplastic melanocytes in the dermis usually without contiguity with the epidermis (Fig. 18.7). These may be nodular aggregates or cords and strands of cells between and among dermal collagen bundles. There may also be involvement of the superficial papillary dermis in so-called 'epidermotropic' metastases. Blood vessels and lymphatics also often contain neoplastic cells and there may be involvement of nerves. Clinically, these may appear as intracutaneous or subcutaneous nodules that range in color from that of normal skin to jet black. When lymph nodes are involved clinically, there is usually one or more firm nodules that develop in a lymph node chain or group that may be fixed to underlying structures. Histologically, there is usually replacement of the lymph node architecture by atypical neoplastic melanocytes.

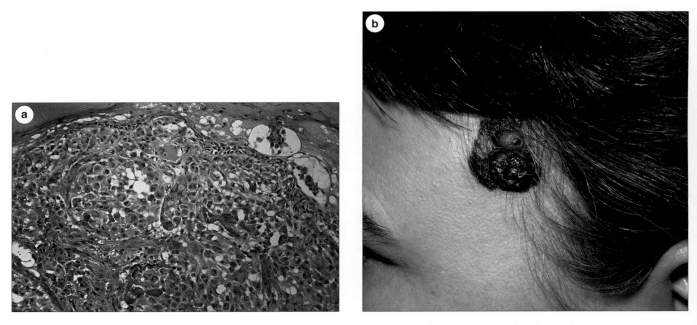

Figure 18.5 Natural history of melanoma. In this lesion, there are extensive nests of melanocytes in the dermis that vary in size and shape and are confluent. Melanocytes are more atypical. Neoplastic melanocytes in the epidermis are confluent. Clinically such lesions are readily recognizable as melanoma in the vast majority of cases. When the dermis is involved extensively, the prognosis is poorer. (H&E, original magnification ×100.)

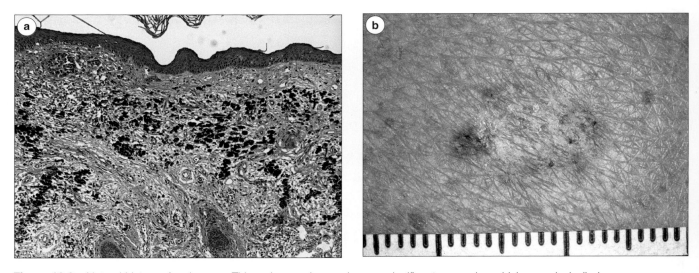

Figure 18.6 Natural history of melanoma. This melanoma has undergone significant regression which, paradoxically, is a poor prognostic sign. The papillary dermis is thickened and demonstrates fibroplasia, telangiectases, scattered lymphocytes and melanophages. The epidermis is thinned and the retia are effaced and lacking the normal undulating pattern. There is one residual nest of melanocytes in the upper left portion of the lesion. Clinically such lesions have the appearance of a gray or white area either within a recognizable melanoma or without visible residual neoplasm. (H&E, original magnification ×100.)

Although this pathway describes melanoma that develops *de novo*, approximately 25% of melanomas develop in association with nevi. This has led some workers to propose a pathway that describes 'precursor' lesions.[15] However, melanoma may arise in virtually any melanocytic nevus, especially giant congenital nevi so it remains important for clinicians to evaluate all nevi carefully for changes that may signal the development of melanoma within them and perform directed biopsies when appropriate.

Clark and colleagues described a model of progression of melanoma where a 'radial' growth phase is followed by a 'vertical' growth phase.[16] The radial growth phase is characterized by malignant melanocytes proliferating in the epidermis and papillary dermis at which time the cells do not have the ability to metastasize. These same cells have limited capacity for growth in cell culture.[17,18] Melanomas in this phase are considered to be biologically less aggressive than those of the vertical growth phase in which there is more extensive involvement of the dermis. Melanocytes from lesions in this phase have the capacity for immortality in cell culture.[18] However, there are significant exceptions to this model including nodular melanomas which have a very short or no radial growth

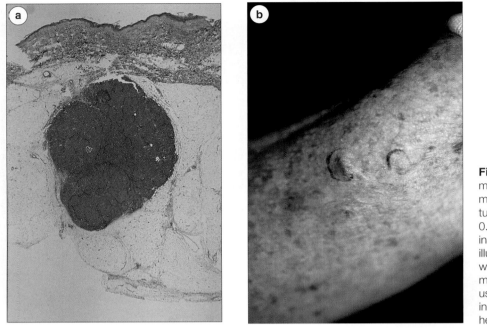

Figure 18.7 Natural history of melanoma. This represents a cutaneous metastasis of melanoma. When the tumor reaches a thickness greater than 0.76 mm, the potential for metastasis increases significantly. In the lesion illustrated, there is a dermal nodule that was comprised of sheets of atypical melanocytes. Clinically, such lesions are usually dermal nodules that may range in color to blue or black as depicted here. (H&E, original magnification ×100.)

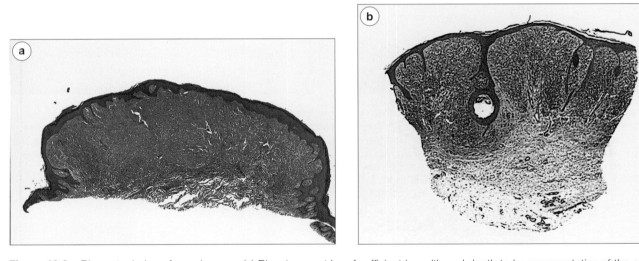

Figure 18.8 Biopsy technique for melanoma. (a) Biopsies must be of sufficient breadth and depth to be representative of the entire process to allow for assessment of histologic features. While excision technique is preferable, saucerization such as depicted here may be adequate if it extends into the deep reticular dermis over the bulk of the sample. (H&E, original magnification ×20.) (b) Small punch biopsies do not always obtain representative specimens and pose a significant risk for misdiagnosis as in the case of this nevoid melanoma. (H&E, original magnification ×20.)

phase[15,19] and metastasizing thin melanomas without a vertical growth phase. Furthermore, recent studies have demonstrated that cells of acrolentiginous melanoma demonstrates genotypic features of metastatic melanoma while confined to the epidermis.[20] As such, the assignment of radial and vertical growth phases for melanoma has fallen into disfavor by some.

Recent molecular studies suggest that some 'dysplastic' nevi may represent intermediate lesions in a multi-step melanoma tumorigenesis pathway.[21] Alterations of some tumor suppressor genes, oncogenes, mismatch repair proteins, extracellular matrix proteins, and growth factors are common to both lesions. However, such work remains quite controversial and speculative.

Biopsy technique

The accurate histologic diagnosis of melanoma requires an appropriate biopsy that is representative of the lesion in question and allows for the microscopic evaluation of as many diagnostic criteria as possible. Many of these are architectural such as breadth of the lesion, symmetry and circumscription. Accordingly, biopsies should be of sufficient breadth and depth to be representative of the entire process and allow for assessment of these features (Fig. 18.8a, b). Furthermore, specimens must be intact and must be processed well. Fragmented specimens or those that are deteriorated or damaged in processing are often not interpretable. Specimens that do not meet

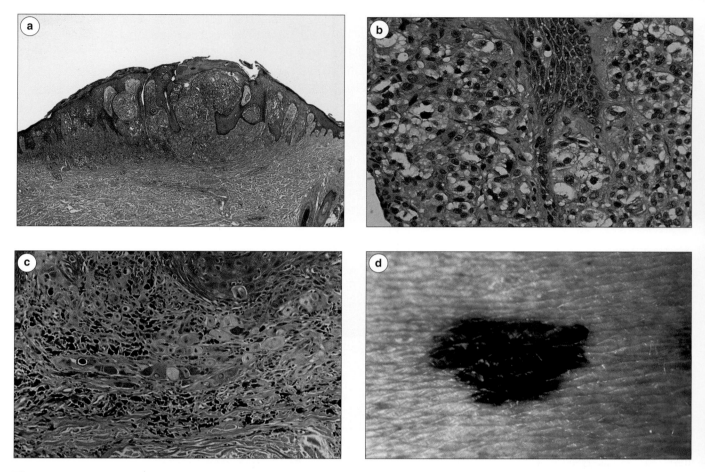

Figure 18.9 Classic melanoma. (a) At low magnification, there is a broad (>1 cm), poorly circumscribed, asymmetrical neoplasm. Note the asymmetric distribution of melanin and the variability in the size and shape of the nests of melanocytes. (H&E, original magnification ×20.) (b) At higher magnification, single melanocytes present within adnexal epithelium and throughout the epidermis is readily visible. The poor circumscription is readily appreciated. (H&E, original magnification ×100.) (c) Centrally, atypical melanocytes in the dermis are seen. Note the absence of maturation and the scattered mitotic figures. (H&E, original magnification ×100.) (d) The clinical picture of the melanoma from which these photomicrographs were produced. Note the asymmetry, indistinct borders and color irregularity. The lesion measured more than 1 cm in diameter. While some sub-classify these into clinical subtypes, the most important factor with regard to prognosis remains tumor thickness.

these criteria may fail to reveal diagnostic areas resulting in misdiagnoses. Furthermore, a number of entities may simulate melanoma both clinically as well as histologically so that if representative biopsies are not submitted, erroneous diagnoses may well be rendered.

Since the most important prognostic factor for melanoma is the thickness of the lesion, a non-representative biopsy could potentially yield false information on which treatment planning is based. A retrospective review of 145 cutaneous melanomas demonstrated that initial diagnostic biopsies performed using non-excisional shave or punch biopsies technique were 88% accurate with Breslow depth greater than or equal to subsequent excision Breslow depth. Saucerization biopsies were more accurate than punch biopsies less than 5 mm in diameter for melanomas less than 1 mm thick. Excisional biopsy was found to be the most accurate method of biopsy. However, in lesions that do not demonstrate classic features of melanoma or are located in areas where complete excision is difficult to perform, this technique is not practical. Therefore, saucerization biopsy is preferable to superficial shave or punch biopsy

for primary cutaneous melanoma when an initial sample is taken for diagnosis.[22]

Additionally, Hsu and Cockerell reviewed 1123 histologically-proven cutaneous melanomas and found significant diagnostic discrepancy between initial punch biopsies and re-excision specimens. While excisional biopsy and saucerization shave biopsy demonstrated near 100% accuracy, punch technique was only 86.5% accurate. Due to the inherent intra-lesional heterogeneity of cutaneous melanoma, the authors conclude small punch biopsies do not always obtain representative specimens and subject the patient to a significant risk of misdiagnosis.[23]

Histopathologic criteria for melanoma

A 'unifying concept' regarding the histologic classification of melanomas based on both architectural and cytologic features has been proposed by Ackerman. *Architectural* characteristics include an asymmetric, poorly circumscribed lesion composed of melanocytes that are irregularly distributed, singly or in nests, in the epidermis (Pagetoid spread), adnexa, and dermis. Melanocytes are present above the dermo-epidermal junction and may form irregular nests which may become confluent (Fig. 18.9). The nests and individual melanocytes lack maturation with progressive descent into the dermis. Additionally, the distribution of melanin is irregularly distributed in the lesion within the epidermis, dermis and adnexa. *Cytologic* characteristics include the presence of atypical melanocytes, necrotic melanocytes and melanocytes in mitosis.[24]

Pathologic features of different clinical forms of cutaneous melanoma

Superficial spreading melanoma
This variant usually displays the characteristic features mentioned above although it commonly demonstrates prominent spread of large atypical melanocytes with abundant pale cytoplasm throughout the epidermis.

Melanoma *in situ* (lentigo maligna)
It is now recognized that virtually all forms of melanoma have a stage in which the neoplasm is confined to the epidermis. Lentigo maligna refers to a subtype in which lesions are virtually always present on sun-damaged skin of older individuals. They are characterized histologically by an increased number of atypical melanocytes arranged singly and in nests distributed irregularly at the dermoepidermal junction and above it. Atypical melanocytes are often present within hair follicles and appendageal structures. The epidermis is often thin and atrophic with loss of retia. There is usually abundant solar elastosis. There may be an infiltrate of lymphocytes in the superficial dermis that may be lichenoid and may cause it to appear similar to a benign lichenoid keratosis on low magnification evaluation.

The histologic evaluation of margin involvement of these lesions may be difficult because of diffuse melanocytic proliferation that is present as a consequence of longstanding sun-damage.[25] In contrast to true persistent melanoma, the number of melanocytes per unit area is less and nests of melanocytes are not generally seen. In some cases, however, the distinction may be impossible without clinical correlation.

Nodular melanoma
As virtually all melanomas progress through an *in situ* stage, if left untreated, they may all eventually progress to involve the dermis and may form papules or nodules clinically. One form tends to involve the dermis at a relatively early point in time in contrast to others that tend to remain confined to the epidermis. However, some contend that since thickness is the most important prognostic variable, a nodule appearing in a melanoma is a sign of metastatic potential rather than a distinct subtype of melanoma.[24,26,27]

Acrolentiginous melanoma
In contrast to the other forms of melanoma mentioned above, these lesions tend to have a greater number of dendritic melanocytes with dendrites extending into the upper layers of the epidermis on volar skin. Initially, the degree of cytologic atypia may be minimal. Later, melanocytes may become more spindle or pagetoid in appearance with prominent pleomorphism (Fig. 18.10). In time, involvement of the dermis and deeper structures is seen.

Desmoplastic melanoma
Since the diagnosis of desmoplastic melanoma (DM) is rarely made clinically, the dermatopathologist must have a high index of suspicion of this lesion. Virtually all lesions are advanced by the time of biopsy. There are several histologic variants of this lesion. In one form, melanocytes are delicate and spindle in shape and are arranged in fascicles in the upper dermis. The cells may demonstrate minimal atypia and may simulate a neural neoplasm such as neurofibroma. There is also often a myxoid stroma. Another variant demonstrates prominent thickness of collagen in the dermis with admixed spindle and sometimes epithelioid cells displaying features quite similar to a scar or fibroma. This is important as many of these lesions have been previously biopsied and there may indeed be scar tissue admixed with the neoplasm. A third variant is comprised of abundant strikingly atypical spindle and/or epithelioid cells arranged in sheets or fascicles. This variant contains abundant pleomorphic cells with hyperchromatic and bizarre nuclei.[28] Most lesions have a component of melanoma *in situ* in the overlying epidermis but this may be absent in over 20% of cases. They can arise in association with a preexisting melanoma of another type or may arise *de novo*. They also usually have nodular aggregates of lymphocytes scattered throughout the dermis.

Perineural invasion is more common in DM and is responsible for recurrence and spread along nerves (Fig. 18.11). Immunohistochemistry (see Table 18.1) is often necessary to distinguish desmoplastic melanoma from other entities included in the histologic differential diagnosis as the spindle cells may be poorly differentiated. S-100 protein is the most useful stain as it is almost uniformly positive although occasionally only weakly. Stains for Mart-1 and HMB-45 antigen are often negative.

Verrucous melanoma
This lesion is often considered a variant of superficial spreading melanoma and is characterized by having an exophytic papilliferous growth pattern (Fig. 18.12).[9] Pseudo-epitheliomatous hyperplasia and overlying hyperkeratosis are prominent features which may obscure the underlying melanoma cells that exhibit varying degrees of cellular pleomorphism at the dermoepidermal junction and beneath it.[7] Blessing *et al.* reviewed 20 cases and found 10% had been given benign diagnosis; however, eight patients had metastases, and seven died of their disease. The Breslow depth and Clark level may be difficult to determine given the papilliferous architecture.[7] Kuehnl-Petzoldt *et al.* reported that reliable Clark's levels could be assigned in only two-thirds of these neoplasms as well.[6] It is important to recognize this variant as it may easily be confused with squamous cell carcinoma or other benign epithelial proliferations.

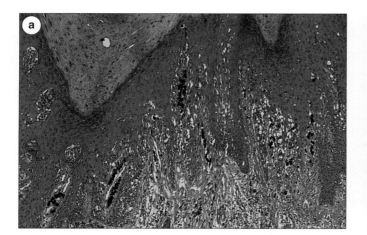

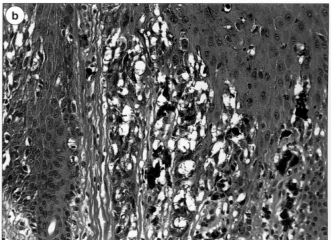

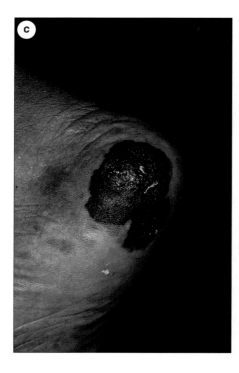

Figure 18.10 Acrolentiginous melanoma. (a) There is a proliferation of atypical, somewhat spindle and dendritic melanocytes at the dermo-epidermal junction and above it with irregular acanthosis. Scattered atypical melanocytes are in the upper dermis as well. (H&E, original magnification ×40.) (b) Higher magnification demonstrates the atypical cytologic features of the melanocytes. (H&E, original magnification ×100.) (c) Clinically, these lesions often appear as black patches or plaques that may develop nodules.

Animal melanoma

Crowson *et al.* encountered six patients with this rare dermal-based melanocytic neoplasm. The lesions are comprised of sheets of heavily pigmented epithelioid or spindle cells with numerous melanophages in the dermis. Mitoses are infrequent.[35] The amount of pigment present makes the cytology difficult to evaluate. They may be confused with heavily pigmented blue nevi although the diffuse architecture and deep extension are features that allow the diagnosis to be rendered.

Nevoid melanoma

At scanning magnification these lesions resemble ordinary compound or dermal nevi, however, pleomorphism and impaired maturation, asymmetry as well as mitoses are clues that aid in the diagnosis (Fig. 18.13).[36] Such lesions in the past have been referred to as 'minimal deviation melanoma', although this term is being used far less frequently today.

Malignant blue 'nevus'

Malignant blue nevus is a misnomer that refers to either *de novo* melanoma that simulates a cellular blue nevus or melanoma that arises in association with a blue nevus. These lesions are similar to animal melanoma in that they are characterized by large, deep proliferations of melanocytes with 'sheet-like' growth patterns. Individual cells are epithelioid or spindle in shape and demonstrate mitoses, necrosis, nuclear atypia, pleomorphism, hyperchromasia, and prominent nucleoli. Pigmented dendritic cells are seen in virtually all lesions.[10]

Clear-cell soft part sarcoma

Clear-cell sarcoma (CCS), also known as melanoma of soft parts (MSP) is a very rare variant of melanoma that has features of a soft tissue sarcoma. These lesions are deep at presentation and have a soft tissue location primarily. Genetically, they have a characteristic translocation of t(12;22)(q13;q12) involving EWS and ATF1 genes. Histologically, they are characterized by a

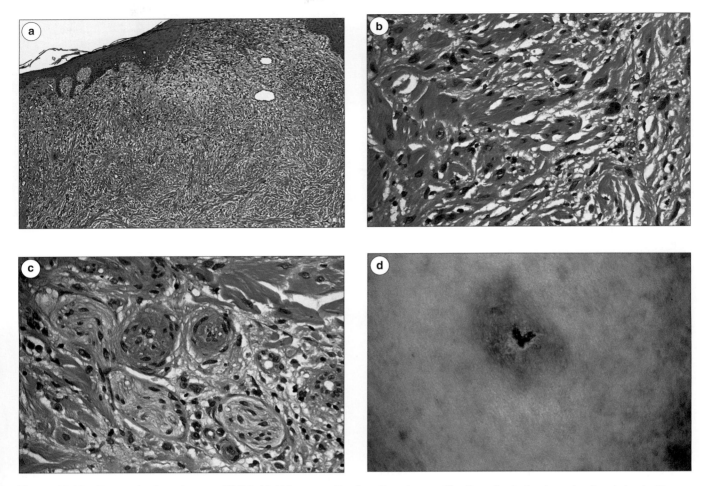

Figure 18.11 Desmoplastic melanoma (DMM). (a) At low magnification, there is a proliferation of spindle-shaped cells admixed with collagen and blood vessels in the dermis. (H&E, original magnification ×40.) (b) At higher magnification, the spindle cells can be seen to be pleomorphic and atypical. They are arranged in loose fascicles admixed with collagen bundles. (H&E, original magnification ×200.) (c) Neoplastic cells are arranged in a concentric fashion around cutaneous nerves, a feature commonly seen in this variant. (H&E, original magnification ×200.) (d) Clinical photograph of DMM. Note the nondescript nature of the lesion and its appearance more similar to that of a scarring process.

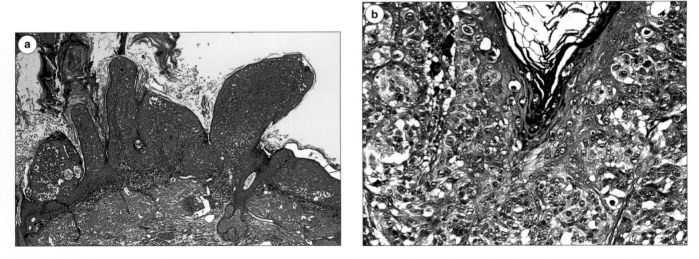

Figure 18.12 Verrucous melanoma. (a) At low magnification, marked verrucous hyperplasia of the epidermis is seen, simulating a verruca or epithelial neoplasm. Nests of melanocytes fill the dermis. (H&E, original magnification ×20.) (b) At higher magnification, the atypia of the melanocytes is readily appreciated. (H&E, original magnification ×100.)

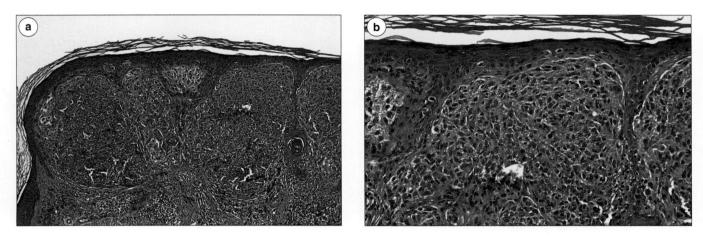

Figure 18.13 Nevoid melanoma. (a) At low magnification, there is a largely symmetrical lesion with relatively minimal pigment. Note the similarity to a benign nevus. (H&E, original magnification ×40.) (b) At higher magnification, there are pleomorphism, scattered mitotic figures and impaired maturation of melanocytes. (H&E, ×100.)

diffuse neoplasm of atypical, pleomorphic clear staining cells arranged in sheets and focally in nests. Usually minimal epidermal involvement is seen. The presence of melanin is variable. Neoplastic cells demonstrate immunoreactivity for S100 protein and HMB45 antigen. Because of their deep extension, they have a propensity for regional lymph node and widespread metastases.

'Spitzoid' melanoma

Spitz's nevus and melanoma are known histologic simulators of one another. Features that favor the diagnosis of melanoma over Spitz's nevus include asymmetry, failure of maturation, deep mitoses, lack of Kamino bodies and necrosis *en masse*. Furthermore, 'spitzoid' lesions in adults should be considered melanoma if there are virtually any features more consistent with the diagnosis of melanoma while the reverse is true of similar lesions in children (especially prepubertal children).

Sarcomatoid melanoma

Occasionally, melanoma may have features that simulate a spindle cell or epithelioid cell sarcoma (Fig. 18.14). Such lesions are extremely poorly differentiated and are characterized by diffuse sheets of anaplastic cells with ulceration and necrosis *en masse*. Immunoperoxidase stains are necessary to render an accurate diagnosis.

Spindle cell melanoma

Some melanomas may be characterized by a proliferation of spindle shaped melanocytes arranged in fascicles and sheets yet they do not demonstrate the diffuse and deep nature of the so-called sarcomatoid melanoma or of desmoplastic melanoma. Many of these lesions still demonstrate features that suggest melanoma such as involvement of the epidermis, pagetoid spread of melanocytes, nesting and melanin. However, because they are poorly differentiated, they must be distinguished from other malignant neoplasms of the skin that may demonstrate a spindle cell morphology including spindle cell squamous cell carcinoma and atypical fibroxanthoma. As with the other poorly differentiated variants of melanoma, immunoperoxidase stains are required to render a precise diagnosis.

Melanoma in children

Melanoma is quite rare in childhood and the diagnosis should only be made when virtually every feature of melanoma is present both clinically and histologically. The head-and-neck region is most commonly involved, and there is a male predominance (74% of cases). Most melanomas in children arise from large or giant congenital nevi although transplacental origin may be seen on occasion. They have histologic features that are identical with melanomas in adults, namely, asymmetry, atypical melanocytes, mitoses, pagetoid spread and failure of maturation with progressive depth. The diagnosis is more difficult when the lesions demonstrate a 'spitzoid' morphology as most such lesions represent Spitz's nevus. When spitzoid lesions in children have poor maturation, mitoses near their bases and have wide, deep areas, usually wider than superficially, the diagnosis of melanoma should be strongly considered. In questionable cases, excision with appropriate margins and possibly performance of sentinel lymphadenectomy is generally recommended. The prognosis for childhood melanoma is usually poor – 40% mortality rate by 18 months.[37]

Special problems in the histologic diagnosis of cutaneous melanoma

There are a number of problems that may cause difficulty in the diagnosis of melanoma other than those described above. Some of these represent 'simulators' of melanoma while others are problems associated with certain settings in which melanoma may develop or may be altered by other factors.

Nevi on 'special' sites

Melanocytic nevi located on certain body sites may closely simulate melanoma and it is important not to overdiagnose melanoma in these circumstances. Some of these sites include the breast, the scalp (especially in children), the ear, the umbilicus, the perineal and genital area and flexural sites such as the axilla, neck, popliteal and antecubital fossa (Fig. 18.15a, b). Features that may cause difficulty in diagnosis include large size of

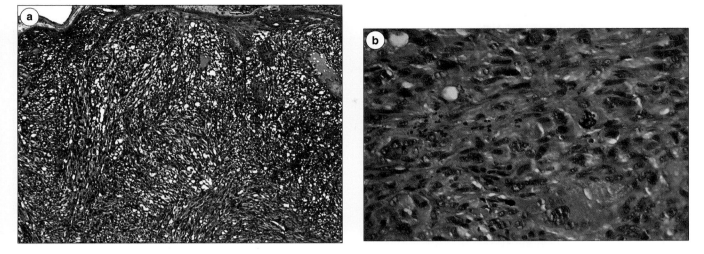

Figure 18.14 Sarcomatoid melanoma. (a) There is a diffuse neoplasm comprised of poorly differentiated spindle and epithelioid neoplastic cells. (H&E, original magnification ×40.) (b) Higher magnification demonstrates the atypical features and the undifferentiated nature of the cells. Immunohistochemical stains are required in cases such as these to characterize the nature of the process. (H&E, original magnification ×200.)

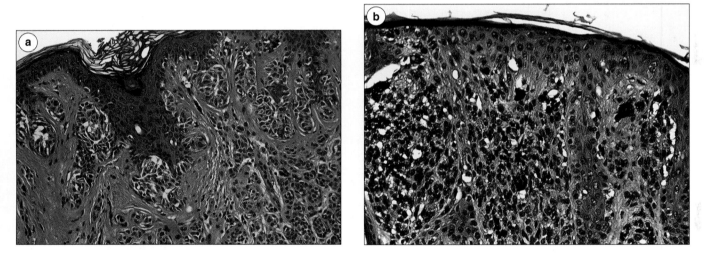

Figure 18.15 Compound 'dysplastic' nevus of the pubic area. (a) There is a symmetrical proliferation of nests and individual melanocytes at the dermoepidermal junction and in the upper dermis. Individual melanocytes are larger than usual and have abundant cytoplasm. (H&E, original magnification ×20.) (b) With higher magnification, slight pagetoid spread of melanocytes in the epidermis can be appreciated although no mitoses are present. This is a lesion that may simulate melanoma histologically. (H&E, original magnification ×100.)

individual melanocytes, large nests of melanocytes and slight pagetoid spread of melanocytes in the epidermis. Nevi that develop on genital areas affected by lichen sclerosus et atrophicus may demonstrate even more pagetoid spread and atypia.

Congenital nevi biopsied in neonates

Congenital nevi are biopsied shortly after birth and rarely up to 2 to 3 years of age may simulate melanoma due to pagetoid spread of melanocytes throughout the epidermis and large size of melanocytes with abundant cytoplasm. This is thought to be a consequence of migration of evolving nevus cells (melanoblasts) through the epidermis. As congenital nevi mature, the single cells in the epidermis become arranged as nests and then become situated at the dermoepidermal junction and in the dermis. Although there is a prominent intraepidermal melanocytic pro-

liferation, there are also nests of typical appearing melanocytes arranged in nests in the dermis between and among collagen bundles and around adnexal structures characteristic of a congenital nevus. Clinical correlation is also valuable in making an accurate diagnosis.

Congenital melanoblastic proliferation

Occasionally in congenital nevi, there may be nodular aggregations of small melanocytes that are hyperchromatic that may be relatively large. Such proliferations may simulate melanoma because of some pleomorphism and the presence of mitoses. The key to the diagnosis is that the process is virtually always symmetrical and well circumscribed and demonstrates evidence of maturation. Furthermore, this lesion is usually always present at birth and matures with age. Some may undergo complete regression.

253

Persistent (recurrent) nevi

Previously biopsied nevi or those that may have been damaged by trauma such as shaving may develop histologic features that simulate melanoma. Melanocytes in the epidermis may be large, may coalesce and may be present at all levels of the epidermis including the granular and cornified layer. Scattered mitotic figures may also be seen. There is also scar tissue in the dermis and the atypical changes are confined to the epidermis directly over the scar (Fig. 18.16). If the melanocytic proliferation extends beyond the margin of the scar, the diagnosis of melanoma should be considered. There may also be nests of nevus cells in the dermis beneath or within the scar, which is a clue to the diagnosis. Clinical correlation is important as the changes may simulate melanoma quite closely and it is often valuable to review histologic sections from the prior biopsy if possible. If not, it might be reasonable to recommend conservative re-excision.

Single cell melanocytic proliferations

Proliferation of single melanocytes in the epidermis may simulate melanoma in situ as it begins in this fashion. Single melanocytic proliferation may be observed in a number of different settings including overlying congenital nevi (Fig. 18.17), on sun damaged skin, on the eyelid, in the epidermis overlying fibrous papules, within solar lentigines and on mucocutaneous sites such as in the nail unit. Most of these examples do not demonstrate the density and number of melanocytes per unit area that is seen in melanoma in situ. Furthermore, in coincidental melanocytic proliferation, there are usually no nests. The presence of an obvious congenital nevus in the dermis beneath the epidermal proliferation allows the diagnosis to be rendered with certainty. Clinical correlation is also valuable as most of these lesions demonstrate no visible pigmented lesion. This is especially important when dealing with excision margins of melanoma.

Artifact from Monsel's solution

Monsel's solution (ferrous subsulfate) is a styptic used to control bleeding in outpatient settings and is commonly used by dermatologists when performing a biopsy. Because of the iron, it has a brown color and when applied to the skin, the iron-containing crystals are engulfed by histiocytes. These may simulate atypical melanocytes and as such, melanoma.[38] Careful inspection reveals that the pigment is refractile like hemosiderin and that the cells themselves are not significantly pleomorphic or atypical.

Regressed melanoma

When melanoma undergoes regression, there is a characteristic pattern of dermal fibrosis in the upper dermis with telangiectases, lymphocytes and abundant

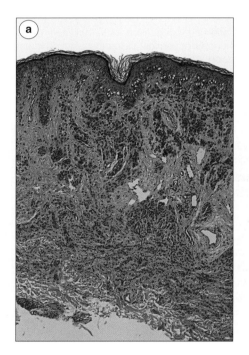

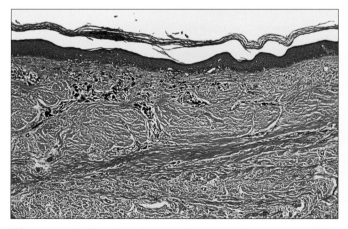

Figure 18.16 Persistent (recurrent) nevus. Melanocytes overlying the scar of a previously biopsied nevus are often large, somewhat atypical and may demonstrate pagetoid spread thereby simulating melanoma. There is often evidence of residual nevus in the specimen and the unusual features are confined to the epidermis directly over the scar and not to the side of it. The presence of a scar in the dermis should prompt the review of prior records and biopsy specimens when possible. In this case, there was a history of a previously biopsied 'dysplastic' nevus at this site. (H&E, ×40.)

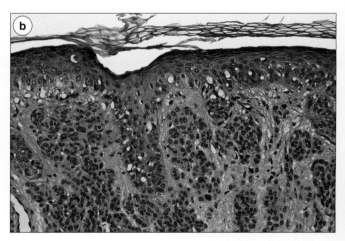

Figure 18.17 Congenital nevus with intraepidermal melanocytic proliferation. (a) Proliferations of single melanocytes are often seen in the epidermis overlying the dermal component of congenital nevi which may simulate melanoma in situ. (H&E, ×20.) (b) The density of epidermal melanocytes is less than that seen in melanoma and they are virtually always seen overlying the dermal nevus component. (H&E, ×100.)

melanophages. The stroma is fibromucinous and differs from fibroplasia seen in scars. The fibrosis is broad and mirrors the original melanoma that was present previously. There may be scattered single melanocytes remaining in the epidermis or a few nests of atypical melanocytes in the fibrotic dermis (Fig. 18.7a).

Metastatic melanoma

Most metastases of melanoma are characterized by atypical melanocytes in the deep dermis or subcutis either in nodules or diffusely in cords and strands. Occasionally, melanoma may involve the superficial dermis as well as the epidermis. These lesions may be quite small which may cause confusion with nevi or primary melanoma. They are often as deep as they are broad and melanocytes are atypical with mitoses seen throughout.

Another form of metastatic melanoma is characterized by atypical but delicate pigmented spindle or dendritic melanocytes in the dermis. These may simulate blue nevi. The fact that they usually develop relatively rapidly and demonstrate some atypia with occasional mitoses allows the diagnosis to be made.

TECHNIQUES TO IMPROVE ACCURACY OF HISTOPATHOLOGIC DIAGNOSIS OF MELANOMA

Special stains and immunohistochemical stains

For poorly differentiated tumors or amelanotic melanomas, a silver stain such as the Fontana–Masson stain for melanin in conjunction with specialized immunohistochemical stains may be useful (Table 18.1 and Fig. 18.18). Stains directed against S-100 protein are the most sensitive marker for melanocytic lesions and are useful in determining melanocytic differentiation (Table 18.2[39] and Fig. 18.19). While commonly referred to as 'S-100 protein', this actually refers to a family of proteins that are soluble in 100% ammonium sulfate, hence 'S-100'. Commercially available antibodies to S-100 protein are typically specific to S-100B polypeptide chains.[40] Recently, efforts have been made to use differential staining patterns to different S-100 polypeptide chains in melanocytic neoplasms in attempts to differentiate between Spitz nevi and melanoma. Ribe et al. examined S-100 protein expression in 42 Spitz nevi and 105 melanomas. All of the Spitz nevi stained with monoclonal antibodies to S-100A6 whereas only 35 of the 105 melanomas were stained.[40] While somewhat promising, these results are not specific enough for this marker to be used to reliably differentiate between these two lesions. A pan-melanoma cocktail containing HMB 45, MART-1 and tyrosinase has a high sensitivity for all forms of melanoma and is a complementary marker to polyclonal S-100 protein.[39]

Stains directed to S-100 protein highlight Langerhans cells, some neural neoplasms, lipocytes, chondrocytes as well as some others so it is important to be aware that positive staining is not necessarily diagnostic of melanocytic differentiation. This is especially true when attempting to differentiate desmoplastic melanoma from scar tissue. Chorny found positive S-100 staining in 9 of 10 scars from previously biopsied non-melanocytic neoplasms in the spindle cell component. Re-excision scars from previously biopsied nevomelanocytic lesions also stain for S-100 protein.[41] Thus, evaluation of the histologic pattern as well as clinical features in addition to immunohistochemical staining are essential.

Cytogenetics

Cytogenetics may prove useful in the future to achieve a higher level of specificity in the diagnosis of melanoma. Comparative genomic hybridization has been used to detect chromosomal abnormalities that helped differentiate two atypical spitzoid lesions, one of which was

Table 18.1	Immunohistochemical stains
S-100	Polyclonal protein found in melanocytes, Langerhans cells and neural tumors. Sensitivity is better than any of the monoclonal antibodies; however not specific. Melanomas very rarely can be S-100 negative and require cocktails of multiple antibodies
HMB-45	Monoclonal antibody that stains stimulated melanocytes. Highly sensitive for cutaneous melanoma; however it does not stain desmoplastic melanoma.[29]
MART-1	Melanoma antigen recognized by T cells (Mart-1) monoclonal antibody. Staining for Mart-1 antigen cannot be used to differentiate benign melanocytic nevi from malignant melanoma.[30]
Tyrosinase	Tyrosinase functions in melanin synthesis (catalyzes the conversion of tyrosine to dihydroxyphenylalanine).[31] Monoclonal antibody to tyrosinase is less sensitive for amelanotic melanomas compared with HMB-45.[32]
NKIC3	Monoclonal antibody with less general sensitivity than S-100 and less sensitivity with spindle cell melanomas.[33]
Pan melanoma cocktail	HMB 45, MART-1 and tyrosinase
CD10 antigen	A neutral endopeptidase expressed by a variety of mesenchymal tumors including a subset of malignant melanomas. CD10 antigen is upregulated during the process of metastasis in melanomas. In 72 melanomas, only 6 of 28 (21.4%) primary skin melanomas expressed CD10 compared with metastatic melanomas to skin (18/26; 69%) and lymph nodes (11/18; 61%) (28 primary skin, 26 metastatic to the skin and 18 lymph node metastases). The CD10 antigen was expressed by 18 of the 26 (69%) and 11 of the 18 (61%) melanomas metastatic to the skin or lymph nodes, respectively; in contrast, only 6 of the 28 primary melanomas (21.4%).[34]

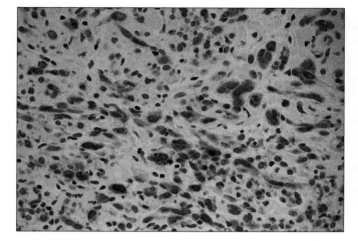

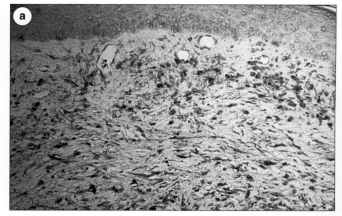

Figure 18.18 Immunohistochemical staining of melanoma. Mart-1 stain highlights melanoma cells in the dermis of this melanoma. Mart-1 is expressed in both benign and malignant melanocytic neoplasms but not in the majority of desmoplastic melanomas. (Mart-1, alkaline phosphatase method, original magnification ×200.)

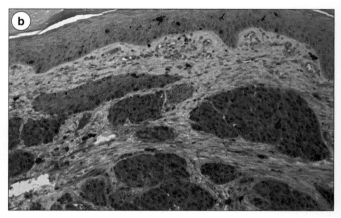

Table 18.2 Staining characteristics of cutaneous lesions[39]

	S-100	HMB-45	MART-1	Cocktail	Tyro
SCCa n=10	–	–	–	–	–
BCCa n=10	–	–	–	–	–
Benign nevi	+	a	+	+	+
Primary melanoma n=50	+	46/50	47/50	49/50	49/50
Metastatic melanoma n=20	+	17/20	19/20	+	+
Desmoplastic melanoma n=5	+	3/5 positive			

aHMB-45 labelled all junctional and compound nevi, 5/8 intradermal nevi and 5/7 blue nevi.

Figure 18.19 Immunohistochemical staining of melanoma. In these 2 slides, immunoreactivity for S-100 is demonstrated by two methods. (a) Both dermal nests and epidermal Langerhans cells are highlighted. (S-100 immunostain, streptavidin alkaline phosphatase, original magnification ×100.) (b) S-100 labeling of neoplastic cells in a case of desmoplastic melanoma using immunoperoxidase with 3-amino-9-ethylcarbazole (AEC) counterstained with hematoxylin. (S-100 immunostain, original magnification ×100.)

found to represent a Spitz nevus and the other was found to be melanoma.[42] Polymerase chain reaction has been used to detect the mRNA transcripts of tyrosinase and MelanA/MART-1.[43] Microarray assays are research tools that have been used to compare gene expression in melanoma and nevi. Microarray gene chip technology allows simultaneous evaluation of thousands of genes and thereby detects which genes are being expressed in different specimens. Seykora *et al.* discovered several genes involved with cellular proliferation that were upregulated in melanoma specimens relative to nevi using this new technology.[44] Its practical clinical relevance has yet to be determined.

Proliferation markers

Various malignancies have been found to have identifiable proliferation markers that can aid in diagnosis and prognosis. Several studies have investigated the role of melanocytic cellular antigens as markers of proliferation. Ki-67 is a nuclear antigen expressed during periods of cellular growth. However, it is not expressed during non-proliferating stages (G0 and early G1). Antibodies to Ki-67 have been used to label melanocytes in an effort to correlate the rate of proliferation with histologic malignancy.

Smolle and colleagues examined 25 melanocytic skin tumors using antibodies to Ki-67 on fresh frozen tissue. Using the parameter of 'growth fraction' (percentage of positively stained nuclei to total nuclei), statistically significant differences were found between nevi, primary melanomas and malignant melanomas.[45] Similarly, Li *et al.* used MIB1, another antibody to Ki-67, which is able to stain nuclear antigen on formalin-fixed, paraffin-embedded specimens and is therefore useful in archival tissues.[46] 72 lesions were retrospectively evaluated using MIB1 staining. These lesions included compound nevi, dysplastic nevi, Spitz nevi and malignant melanomas. Using the percentage of positively stained cells, the researchers were able to discriminate between benign lesions and melanomas with statistical significance.[47]

Others have described MIB1 staining as a useful adjunct to HMB-45 in the differentiation of nevoid malignant melanoma from benign melanocytic lesions.[48] Lastly, Boni *et al.* found that MIB1 expression was significantly higher in primary melanomas (Breslow depth >1.5 mm) that metastasized.[46] Nevertheless, there is significant overlap between lesions with greater and lesser numbers of cells that stain positively so that this technique cannot be used to reliably differentiate between benign and malignant lesions alone. More studies will be required before this technique can be recommended for widespread use.

DIFFERENTIAL DIAGNOSIS

For differential diagnosis, see Table 18.3.[49–51] Lesions that may pose difficulty in diagnosis clinically or histologically are:

- Dysplastic nevi
- Amelanotic melanoma (Fig. 18.20a, b)
- Deeply pigmented melanocytic lesions
- Lesions in scars (Fig. 18.21a, b)
- Lesions arising in blue nevi
- Lesions arising in congenital nevi
- Lesions arising on scalp or genitalia
- 'Collision' tumors

Staging and prognosis

Histologic features related to prognosis

Breslow's depth
In 1970, Alexander Breslow evaluated the histologic depth of melanoma as it relates to prognosis. Melanoma excision specimens were obtained from 98 patients. After 5 years, 71 of the patients remained disease free while 27 developed metastatic or recurrent disease. An ocular micrometer was used to measure from the skin surface to the deepest level of extension of the tumor. There was no recurrence or metastasis in those patients whose maximum tumor thickness was less than 0.76 mm (n=38).[52] Breslow thickness, defined as the depth from the granular layer to the deepest level of neoplasm, has subsequently been determined by multiple studies to be the most important prognostic indicator of survival in primary cutaneous melanomas.[14,53]

As with any technique, there are a number of limitations. In some areas such as near volar skin, the epidermis may be quite thick and contribute significantly to this measurement imparting an artificially higher number than if the lesion were present at another site. Conversely, at sites where the skin is very thin such as the eyelid, thin lesions may extend into the deep dermis or subcutis and may have a worse prognosis than might be expected. Furthermore, thickness measurements are subjective and can vary from one histopathologist to another. This can be a consequence of the section that

Table 18.3 Differential diagnosis	
Clinical	**Histologic**
• Blue nevus (cellular or common)	• Dermatofibroma with atypical cells
• Carbon tattoo	• Dysplastic nevus
• Congenital nevus	• Leiomyosarcomas[51]
• Dermatofibroma	• Neurofibroma
• Dysplastic nevus	• Pagetoid neoplasms
• Intracorneal hemorrhage	• Pigmented atypical fibroxanthoma[49]
• Kaposi's sarcoma	• Scar
• Lentigo	• Spindle cell neoplasms[51]
• Pigmented atypical fibroxanthoma[49]	• Spitz nevus
• Pigmented basal cell carcinoma	
• Pigmented Bowen's disease	
• Pyogenic granuloma	
• Scar	
• Seborrheic keratosis[50]	
• Solar lentigo	
• Spindle cell nevus of Reed	
• Spitz nevus	
• Tag	
• Tinea nigra	
• Wart	

was cut or even in variation between microscopes. It should also be remembered that re-excision specimens may reveal areas that are thicker than in the original biopsy specimen. Thus, thickness measurements, while providing important information, their absolute value should not be overemphasized. For example, there is little significance between a lesion of 1.0 mm in thickness and one that is 1.2 mm in thickness.

Because of wide variation in prognosis and many exceptions to prognostic variables based on histologic evaluation alone, they must be taken as only general guidelines. Because none of them are as reliable as thickness, many dermatopathologists do not routinely include them in pathology reports.

Clark's levels
In 1969, Clark *et al.* proposed a schema where a melanoma is described by its anatomical depth of involvement.[54] Clark's levels are as follows:

I – Confined to the epidermis (*in situ*)

II – Neoplasm to the papillary dermis, but not filling the papillary dermis

III – Neoplasm present to level of the junction between the papillary and reticular dermis (filling the papillary dermis)

IV – Neoplasm extending into the reticular dermis

V – Neoplasm extending into the subcutaneous fat

Clark's level derives most of its prognostic value from a secondary correlation with tumor thickness.[55] Balch and co-workers reported the 5-year survival for 17,600 patients

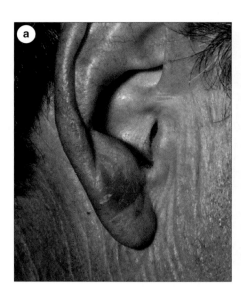

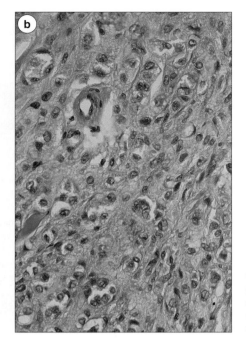

Figure 18.20 Amelanotic melanoma. (a) This hypopigmented, erythematous papule on the external ear of a middle-aged man proved to represent melanoma (b) when biopsied. (H&E, original magnification ×200.)

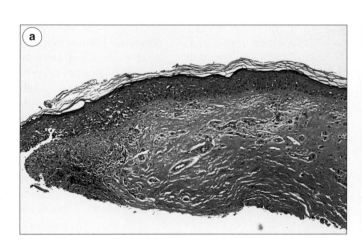

Figure 18.21 Melanoma *in situ* overlying a scar. (a) In contrast to persistent nevi, persistent melanoma usually demonstrate cardinal architectural features of melanoma and the changes in the epidermis are not confined to the area above the scar. (H&E, original magnification ×40.) (b) This pigmented lesion overlying the scarred area proved to be a melanoma.

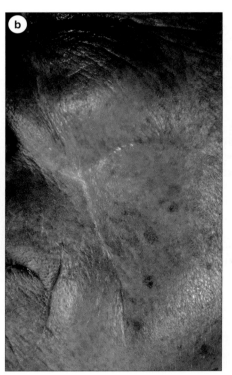

with melanoma was dictated by tumor thickness. However, Clark's level was significant within the subgroup of patients with melanomas <1 mm. In these thin tumors, Clark's level IV or V invasion was significantly predictive of survival.[14,56] The 2002 American Joint Committee on Cancer staging system for cutaneous melanoma includes Clark's level for thin melanomas only.[14]

Clark's levels should not be confused with melanoma stage. Historically, Stage I includes those where involvement is limited to within a 5 cm zone around the primary site. Stage II indicates involvement of the regional lymph node basin. Stage III includes those with two or more

lymph node basins involved or disseminated metastases to the skin or visceral sites. Revisions to the staging of melanoma were made in 2002 by the American Joint Committee on Cancer.

Ulceration

Ulceration is defined histologically as loss of epidermis and some of the dermis. In 1980, Balch and coworkers evaluated the prognostic significance of melanoma ulceration on 5-year survival. They found a decrease in survival associated with ulcerated (55%) compared with non-ulcerated melanomas (80%) in Stage I melanoma patients. In Stage II the decrease in survival fell from 53 to 12% 5-year survival. These trends remained even when corrected for thickness as ulceration is virtually always confined to thicker melanomas.[57,58] Balch later evaluated 5-year survival data from 17,600 melanoma patients. Cox regression analysis found ulceration and thickness to be the most powerful predictors of survival.[14] Because of these findings, ulceration was added to the revised 2002 American Joint Committee on Cancer melanoma staging system.[59] In this system, the presence of ulceration 'upstages' the melanoma to the next worst prognostic level.[60]

There are a number of problems with ulceration as a prognostic variable, however. The definition of ulceration as applied to melanoma is highly subjective. True ulceration in a neoplasm is a manifestation of the lesion outgrowing its blood supply and is almost always associated with zones of necrosis (Fig. 18.22). Such neoplasms are usually quite thick and are highly proliferative and as such, have higher metastatic potential. The current use of ulceration as a prognostic variable is problematic in that it does not define the extent of ulceration of a lesion and does not discriminate between lesions that may have been previously traumatized or biopsied. Furthermore, no recommendations are made with respect to how much of a lesion needs to be evaluated to search for ulceration. In our opinion, ulceration occurs in a subset of thick, nodular lesions and when it is extensive, it is a marker of a more aggressive lesion. It is not present in thin or *in situ* lesions and caution is advised in reporting tiny, microscopic foci of ulceration or erosion that may have been induced by trauma or a prior procedure as that may impart a worse prognosis to the patient when it is not truly indicated.

Tumor infiltrating lymphocytes

In 1989, Clark, Elder and coworkers demonstrated that tumor infiltrating lymphocytes were independent predictors of 8-year survival. Infiltrating lymphocytes patterns are described as 'brisk, non-brisk and absent'. A 'brisk' infiltrating lymphocyte pattern was associated with improved prognosis. A 'brisk' pattern was defined as a dense infiltrate of lymphocytes that was present both within the substance of the neoplasm as well as its periphery.[61] Tuthill *et al.* supported tumor infiltrating lymphocytes' independent role in survival prediction in their study of 259 patients.[62] Although there has been criticism regarding lack of histologic criteria and standardization, one study demonstrated good agreement between inexperienced observers after a brief tutorial with written guidelines.[63] Nevertheless, this remains controversial and is not generally reported by most dermatopathologists today.

Regression

There are conflicting reports on the prognostic significance of regression. Regression is defined as destruction of melanoma cells with replacement by fibrous tissue, blood vessels and melanophages. Regression may be detected clinically as gray or whitish areas either within a melanoma or without obvious residual melanoma. Guitart and co-workers performed a case–control study of 43 cases investigating the histological characteristics found in metastasizing thin melanomas. Extensive regression was found in 42% of the patients with thin melanomas compared with 5% in controls.[64] Another study examined 103 patients with thin melanomas less than 0.76 mm thick. Of the 103 patients, 30 had histologic evidence of regression. Six of the patients with regression died of metastatic disease. All of these six patients had greater than 77% regression. The remaining 24 patients in the partial regression group remained living at the end of the three year study and most had regression less than 50% (mean 29.9%). No metastasis occurred in the 73 patients who had thin melanomas without regression.[65] There is speculation that these lesions are thin because they have undergone regression and may have once represented deeper and therefore more aggressive melanomas.

Complete regression of melanoma has also been shown to be associated with metastatic disease and worsened prognosis. Patients may present with metastatic

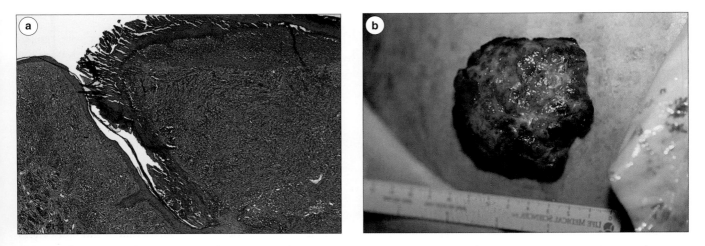

Figure 18.22 Ulceration in melanoma. (a) This thick melanoma demonstrates ulceration with marked necrosis. It is important to distinguish ulceration from excoriation or biopsy-related erosion as this does not represent true ulceration, which is a manifestation of the neoplasm outgrowing its blood supply. (b) Such lesions as the one illustrated here, tend to have worse prognoses. (H&E, original magnification ×40.)

disease and when they are evaluated, are found to have a gray or white area that when biopsied reveals features of complete regression of melanoma.

Histologic satellite metastases

In 1981, Day and co-workers defined microscopic satellites as 'discrete tumor nests greater than 0.05 mm in diameter that were separated from the main body of the melanoma by normal reticular dermal collagen or subcutaneous fat'. They reviewed histologic sections of 596 patients with stage I melanoma. The 5-year disease free survival for patients with 'microscopic satellites' was 36%. Patients without satellites had a survival rate of 89%.[66]

The prognostic power of microscopic satellites spurred their inclusion in the revised 2002 American Joint Committee on Cancer melanoma staging system.[59]

Mitotic rate

A study evaluating 3661 patients from the Sydney Melanoma Unit database investigated the prognostic value of tumor mitotic rate (mitosis/mm^2). Patients with tumor mitotic rate of zero mitoses/mm^2 had a significantly improved survival when compared with those with one or more mitoses. Regression analysis demonstrated that tumor mitotic rate was less predictive of survival than tumor thickness but had improved predictive ability relative to ulceration.[67]

Sentinel lymph node biopsy

During the 1970s, several large prospective studies were undertaken to evaluate the role of elective lymph node dissection at the time of wide resection of malignant melanoma. The rationale for lymph node dissection was based on the clinical observation that lymph node involvement usually preceded more widespread metastatic disease. Therefore, many believed that removal of regional lymph nodes might prevent metastasis. Cascinelli recently reviewed the long-term results of several World Health Organization (WHO) trials conducted between 1967–1989. Overall, there was no survival benefit to elective lymphadenectomy.[68]

However, a 5-year WHO study that evaluated 240 patients with melanomas on the trunk greater than 1.5 mm did reveal useful prognosis data. Although multivariate analysis demonstrated no impact on survival, it demonstrated that prognosis was improved in patients with clinically unsuspected lymph nodes that were histologically positive. Therefore, although no benefit could be found for elective lymph node dissection, the histologic status of the lymph nodes could yield significant survival prognostic data.[69]

In 1992, Morton et al. advocated 'sentinel lymph node (SLN) biopsy' as a less invasive means for determining occult metastasis to anatomically related skin draining lymph nodes.[70] Initially, intra-operative lymphatic mapping with sentinel node biopsy was performed using isosulfan blue dye.[71] Modern sentinel node biopsy uses lymphatic mapping to identify the specific draining node or nodes that are at greatest risk for micrometastasis. Intra-operative histopathologic evaluation of the involved node provides prognostic information that can guide therapy.[72] If no evidence of metastasis is found, wide excision of the melanoma is performed; however, if nodal metastasis is discovered, wide excision is combined with lymphadenectomy.[73] The lymphadenectomy is performed for local regional control as noted above, it does not confer an improved prognosis.

Muller et al. investigated the prognostic significance of the sentinel lymph node biopsy. They evaluated 263 patients with stage I or II melanoma who had undergone sentinel lymph node biopsy. Tumor-positive nodes were found in 20% of the patients, and this was associated with a 49% 5-year survival rate. In contrast, the tumor-free sentinel node group had a 91% disease-free survival rate. Sentinel lymph node status was found to be the most powerful predictor of survival for melanoma patients.[74] Thus, the presence of sentinel lymph node positive for melanoma correlates with a worsened prognosis and is an indication that metastasis has occurred from the primary neoplasm. Other studies have also corroborated the prognostic significance of the sentinel node biopsy.[75,76]

A small study (n=46) involving patients who had SLN biopsies for melanomas less than or equal to 1 mm in depth found three patients (7%) had positive sentinel lymph nodes or micrometastatic disease. Positive sentinel lymph node was associated with a Clark level of III or more ($P \leq 0.07$). Therefore, these authors advocate sentinel lymph node biopsy for melanomas <1 mm if Clark level is III or more.[77]

Molecular staging has also been performed on sentinel lymph node tissue. Of 114 patients with stage I or II melanoma who underwent SLN biopsy and were followed an average of 28 months, 23 (20%) had pathologically positive SLNs which were also RT-PCR positive for tyrosine messenger RNA, evidence of melanoma involvement. Forty-seven of the 91 histologically negative lymph nodes were also RT-PCR positive. There was a recurrence rate among 14 (61%) of the 23 patients who were both pathologically and RT-PCR positive and a recurrence rate in 1 (2%) of 44 patients who were both pathologically and RT-PCR negative. For patients who were upstaged by the molecular assay (pathologically negative, RT-PCR positive), there was a recurrence rate among 6 (13%) of 47 patients. In both univariate and multivariate regression analyses, the histological and RT-PCR status of the SLNs were the best predictors of disease-free survival.[78,79]

The 2002 revised American Joint Committee on Cancer staging system for cutaneous melanoma incorporates the powerful prognostic significance of the sentinel lymph node. Additionally, the sentinel node biopsy can be useful to determine the metastatic potential of diagnostically difficult melanocytic tumors. Many primary cutaneous melanocytic neoplasms are difficult to diagnose with certainty by routine light microscopy. In some cases, completely excising such lesions could be mutilating and therefore an increase in the diagnosis sensitivity is needed.

Kelley and Cockerell proposed that sentinel lymphadenectomy be considered in patients with melanocytic neoplasms of uncertain behavior that are 1.0 mm or more in thickness. If positive, the suspicion of malignancy is greater and a complete excision is justifiable.[80] Su et al. reviewed 18 cases of borderline spitzoid lesions in which the patient had undergone sentinel node biopsy. Eight of the patients had positive nodes and were offered adjuvant therapy that they may not have received had sentinel node biopsy not been performed.[81]

When examining SLN, benign intraparenchymal nevus cells in clusters or few cells up to 2.1 mm aggregates may occasionally be noted. These benign melanocytes lack mitotic figures and lymphatic or vascular involvement. Additionally, the nevus cell aggregates express S-100 protein and/or MART-1 but not gp100 protein (HMB-45) or Ki-67 (<1%).[82] Another entity which may cause confusion when examining SLN is the presence of tattoo pigment.[83]

FUTURE OUTLOOK

One of the main challenges regarding the diagnosis and treatment of melanoma lies at the histologic level. As noted throughout this manuscript, there may be significant difficulty in rendering an accurate diagnosis of melanoma histologically. Furthermore, the ability to prognosticate based on histologic findings is limited. In the future, techniques will be available that allow for more accurate diagnoses to be rendered quickly using biometric assays and techniques that can be used in conjunction with routine histology. Furthermore, techniques will likely be developed that allow for more accurate prediction of prognosis and likelihood of metastasis based on features such as the genotype of the melanoma coupled with immunologic profiles of the patient. Finally, with intense educational efforts that are ongoing, it is hoped that the ultimate goals of earlier diagnosis and ultimately prevention will be achieved.

ACKNOWLEDGMENT

We are grateful to Dr Lydia Essary for compiling the photographs for this chapter.

REFERENCES

1 Jemal A, Murray T, Samuels A, Ghafoor A, Ward E, Thun MJ. Cancer statistics, 2004. CA Cancer J Clin 2004; 54(1):5–26.

2 Plotnick H, Rachmaninoff N, VandenBerg HJ, Jr. Polypoid melanoma: a virulent variant of nodular melanoma. Report of three cases and literature review. J Am Acad Derm 1990; 23(5):880–884.

3 Giuliano AE, Cochran AJ, Morton DL. Melanoma from unknown primary site and amelanotic melanoma. Semin Oncol 1982; 9(4):442–447.

4 Bono A, Maurichi A, Moglia D, et al. Clinical and dermatoscopic diagnosis of early amelanotic melanoma. Melanoma Res 2001; 11(5):491–494.

5 Montgomery RM. Differential diagnosis and treatment of warts. West Med Med J West 1967; 1:34–36.

6 Kuehnl-Petzoldt C, Berger H, Wiebelt H. Verrucous-keratotic variations of malignant melanoma: a clinicopathological study. Am J Derm 1982; 4(5):403–410.

7 Blessing K, Evans AT, al-Nafussi A. Verrucous naevoid and keratotic malignant melanoma: a clinico-pathological study of 20 cases. Histopathology 1993; 23(5):453–458.

8 Suster S, Ronnen M, Bubis JJ. Verrucous pseudonevoid melanoma. J Surg Oncol 1987; 36(2):134–137.

9 Steiner A, Konrad K, Pehamberger H, Wolff K. Verrucous malignant melanoma. Arch Derm 1988; 124(10):1534–1537.

10 Granter SR, McKee PH, Calonje E, Mihm MC Jr, Busam K. Melanoma associated with blue nevus and melanoma mimicking cellular blue nevus: a clinicopathologic study of 10 cases on the spectrum of so-called 'malignant blue nevus'. Am J Surg Pathol 2001; 25(3):316–323.

11 Ackerman AB. Malignant melanoma: a unifying concept. Hum Pathol 1980; 11(6):591–595.

12 Ackerman AB, David KM. A unifying concept of malignant melanoma: biologic aspects. Hum Pathol 1986; 17(5):438–440.

13 Bono A, Bartoli C, Moglia D, et al. Small melanomas: a clinical study on 270 consecutive cases of cutaneous melanoma. Melanoma Res 1999; 9(6):583–586.

14 Balch CM, Soong SJ, Gershenwald JE, et al. Prognostic factors analysis of 17,600 melanoma patients: validation of the American Joint Committee on Cancer melanoma staging system. J Clin Oncol 2001; 19(16):3622–3634.

15 Clark WH Jr, Elder DE, Guerry D 4th, et al. A study of tumor progression: the precursor lesions of superficial spreading and nodular melanoma. Hum Pathol 1984; 15(12):1147–1165.

16 Clark WH Jr, Elder DE, and Van Horn M. The biologic forms of malignant melanoma. Hum Pathol 1986; 17(5):443–450.

17 Elder DE, Guerry D 4th, Epstein MN, et al. Invasive malignant melanomas lacking competence for metastasis. Am J Derm 1984; 6(Suppl):55–61.

18 Herlyn M, Clark WH, Rodeck U, Mancianti ML, Jambrosic J, Koprowski H. Biology of tumor progression in human melanocytes. Lab Invest 1987; 56(5):461–474.

19 Barnhill RL, Mihm MC Jr. The histopathology of cutaneous malignant melanoma. Semin Diagn Pathol 1993; 10(1):47–75.

20 Su WP. Malignant melanoma: basic approach to clinicopathologic correlation. Mayo Clin Proc 1997; 72(3):267–272.

21 Hussein MR, Wood GS. Molecular aspects of melanocytic dysplastic nevi. J Mol Diagn 2002; 4(2):71–80.

22 Ng PC, Barzilai DA, Ismail SA, Averitte RL Jr, Gilliam AC. Evaluating invasive cutaneous melanoma: is the initial biopsy representative of the final depth? J Am Acad Derm 2003; 48(3):420–424.

23 Hsu M, Wisiniewski K, Tsai S, Cockerell CJ. Punch biopsy of melanocytic neoplasms: A poorly recognized pitfall in the diagnosis of cutaneous malignant melanoma. Am J Dermatopathol 2003; in press.

24 Ackerman AB. Malignant melanoma. A unifying concept. Am J Derm 1980; 2(4):309–313.

25 Florell SR, Boucher KM, Leachman SA, et al. Histopathologic recognition of involved margins of lentigo maligna excised by staged excision: an interobserver comparison study. Arch Derm 2003; 139(5):595–604.

26 Heenan PJ. Nodular melanoma is not a distinct entity. Arch Derm 2003; 139(3):387–388.

27 Chamberlain AJ, Fritschi L, Giles GG, Dowling JP, Kelly JW. Nodular type and older age as the most significant associations of thick melanoma in Victoria, Australia. Arch Derm 2002; 138(5):609–614.

28 From L, Hanna W, Kahn HJ, Gruss J, Marks A, Baumal R. Origin of the desmoplasia in desmoplastic malignant melanoma. Hum Pathol 1983; 14(12):1072–1080.

29 Orchard GE. Comparison of immunohistochemical labelling of melanocyte differentiation antibodies melan-A, tyrosinase and HMB 45 with NKIC3 and S100 protein in the evaluation of benign naevi and malignant melanoma. Histochem J 2000; 32(8):475–481.

30 Mehregan DR, Hamzavi I. Staining of melanocytic neoplasms by melanoma antigen recognized by T cells. Am J Derm 2000; 22(3):247–250.

31 Liu V, Mihm MC. Pathology of malignant melanoma. Surg Clin North Am 2003; 83(1):31–60.

32 Boyle JL, Haupt HM, Stern JB, Multhaupt HA. Tyrosinase expression in malignant melanoma, desmoplastic melanoma, and peripheral nerve tumors. Arch Pathol Lab Med 2002; 126(7):816–822.

33 Fernando SS, Johnson S, Bate J. Immunohistochemical analysis of cutaneous malignant melanoma: comparison of S-100 protein, HMB-45 monoclonal antibody and NKI/C3 monoclonal antibody. Pathology 1994; 26(1):16–19.

34 Kanitakis J, Narvaez D, Claudy A. Differential expression of the CD10 antigen (neutral endopeptidase) in primary versus metastatic malignant melanomas of the skin. Melanoma Res 2002; 12(3):241–244.

35 Crowson AN, Magro CM, Mihm MC Jr. Malignant melanoma with prominent pigment synthesis: 'animal type' melanoma – a clinical and histological study of six cases with a consideration of other melanocytic neoplasms with prominent pigment synthesis. Hum Pathol 1999; 30(5):543–550.

36 Zembowicz A, McCusker M, Chiarelli C, et al. Morphological analysis of nevoid melanoma: a study of 20 cases with a review of the literature. Am J Derm 2001; 23(3):167–175.

37 Richardson SK, Tannous ZS, Mihm MC, Jr. Congenital and infantile melanoma: review of the literature and report of an uncommon variant, pigment-synthesizing melanoma. J Am Acad Derm 2002; 47(1):77–90.

38 Duray PH, Livolsi VA. Recurrent dysplastic nevus following shave excision. J Derm Surg Oncol 1984; 10(10):811–815.

39 Orchard G. Evaluation of melanocytic neoplasms: application of a pan-melanoma antibody cocktail. Br J Biomed Sci 2002; 59(4):196–202.

40 Ribe A, McNutt NS. S100A6 protein expression is different in Spitz nevi and melanomas. Mod Pathol 2003; 16(5):505–511.

41 Chorny JA, Barr RJ. S100-positive spindle cells in scars: a diagnostic pitfall in the re-excision of desmoplastic melanoma. Am J Derm 2002; 24(4):309–312.

42 Takata M, Maruo K, Kageshita T, et al. Two cases of unusual acral melanocytic tumors: illustration of molecular cytogenetics as a diagnostic tool. Hum Pathol 2003; 34(1):89–92.

43 Schittek B, Bodingbauer Y, Ellwanger U, Blaheta HJ, Garbe C. Amplification of MelanA messenger RNA in addition to tyrosinase increases sensitivity of melanoma cell detection in peripheral blood and is associated with the clinical stage and prognosis of malignant melanoma. Br J Derm 1999; 141(1):30–36.

44 Seykora JT, Jih D, Elenitsas R, Horng WH, Elder DE. Gene expression profiling of melanocytic lesions. Am J Derm 2003; 25(1):6–11.

45 Smole J, Soyer HP, Kerl H. Proliferation activity of cutaneous melanocytic tumors defined by ki-67 monoclonal antibody. Am J Derm 1989; 11(4):301–307.

46 Bon R, Doguoglu A, Burg G, Muller B, Dummer R. MIB-1 immunoreactivity correlates with metastatic dissemination in primary thick cutaneous melanoma. J Am Acad Derm 1996; 35:416–418.

47 Li LX, Crotty KA, McCarthy SW, Palmer AA, Kril JJ. A zonal comparison of MIB1-Ki67 immunoreactivity in benign and malignant melanocytic lesions. Am J Derm 2000; 22(6):489–495.

48 McNutt NS, Urmacher C, Hakimian J, Hoss DM, Lugo J. Nevoid malignant melanoma: morphologic patterns and immunohistochemical reactivity. J Cutan Pathol 1995; 22(6):502–517.

49 Diaz-Cascajo C, Weyers W, Borghi S. Pigmented atypical fibroxanthoma: a tumor that may be easily mistaken for malignant melanoma. Am J Derm 2003; 25(1):1–5.

50 Izikson L, Sober AJ, Mihm MC Jr, Zembowicz A. Prevalence of melanoma clinically resembling seborrheic keratosis: analysis of 9204 cases. Arch Derm 2002; 138(12):1562–1566.

51 King R, Googe PB, Weilbaecher KN, Mihm MC Jr, Fisher DE. Microphthalmia transcription factor expression in cutaneous benign, malignant melanocytic, and nonmelanocytic tumors. Am J Surg Pathol 2001; 25(1):51–57.

52 Breslow A. Thickness, cross-sectional areas and depth of invasion in the prognosis of cutaneous melanoma. Ann Surg 1970; 172(5):902–908.

53 Barnhill RL, Fine JA, Roush GC, Berwick M. Predicting five-year outcome for patients with cutaneous melanoma in a population-based study. Cancer 1996; 78(3):427–432.

54 Clark WH Jr, From L, Bernardino EA, Mihm MC. The histogenesis and biologic behavior of primary human malignant melanomas of the skin. Cancer Res 1969; 29(3):705–727.

55 Maize JC. Primary cutaneous malignant melanoma. J Am Acad Derm 1983; 8(6):857–863.

56 Zetterstein E, Shaikh L, Ramirez R, Kashani-Sabet M. Prognostic factors in primary cutaneous melanoma. Surg Clin North Am 2003; 83(1):61–75.

57 Balch CM, Wilkerson JA, Murad TM, Soong SJ, Ingalls AL, Maddox WA. The prognostic significance of ulceration of cutaneous melanoma. Cancer 1980; 45(12):3012–3017.

58 Rigel DS, Friedman RJ, Kopf AW, Silverman MK. Factors influencing survival in melanoma. Derm Clin 1991; 9(4):631–642.

59 Balch CM, Buzaid AC, Soong SJ, et al. Final version of the American Joint Committee on Cancer staging system for cutaneous melanoma. J Clin Oncol 2001; 19(16):3635–3648.

60 Kanzler MH, Swetter SM. Malignant melanoma. J Am Acad Derm 2003; 48(5):780–783.

61 Clark WH Jr, Elder DE, Guerry D 4th, et al. Model predicting survival in stage I melanoma based on tumor progression. J Natl Cancer Inst 1989; 81(24):1893–1904.

62 Tuthill RJ, Unger JM, Liu PY, et al. Risk assessment in localized primary cutaneous melanoma: a Southwest Oncology Group study evaluating nine factors and a test of the Clark logistic regression prediction model. Am J Clin Pathol 2002; 118(4):504–511.

63 Busam KJ, Antonescu CR, Marghoob AA, et al. Histologic classification of tumor-infiltrating lymphocytes in primary cutaneous malignant melanoma. A study of interobserver agreement. Am J Clin Pathol 2001; 115(6):856–860.

64 Guitart J, Lowe L, Piepkorn M, et al. Histological characteristics of metastasizing thin melanomas: a case–control study of 43 cases. Arch Derm 2002; 138(5):603–608.

65 Ronan SG, Eng AM, Briele HA, Shioura NN, Das Gupta TK. Thin malignant melanomas with regression and metastases. Arch Derm 1987; 123(10):1326–1330.

66 Day CL Jr, Harrist TJ, Gorstein F, et al. Malignant melanoma. Prognostic significance of 'microscopic satellites' in the reticular dermis and subcutaneous fat. Ann Surg 1981; 194(1):108–112.

67 Azzola MF, Shaw HM, Thompson JF, et al. Tumor mitotic rate is a more powerful prognostic indicator than ulceration in patients with primary cutaneous melanoma: an analysis of 3661 patients from a single center.

Cancer 2003; 97(6):1488–1498.

68 Cascinelli N, Santinami M, Maurichi A, Patuzzo R, Pennacchioli E. World Health Organization experience in the treatment of melanoma. Surg Clin North Am 2003; 83(2):405–416.

69 Cascinelli N, Morabito A, Santinami M, MacKie RM, Belli F. Immediate or delayed dissection of regional nodes in patients with melanoma of the trunk: a randomised trial. WHO Melanoma Programme. Lancet 1998; 351(9105):793–796.

70 Cochran AJ, Wen DR, Morton DL. Management of the regional lymph nodes in patients with cutaneous malignant melanoma. World J Surg 1992; 16(2):214–221.

71 Rousseau DL Jr, Ross MI, Johnson MM, et al. Revised American joint committee on cancer staging criteria accurately predict sentinel lymph node positivity in clinically node-negative melanoma patients. Ann Surg Oncol 2003; 10(5):569–574.

72 Uren RF, Howman-Giles R, Thompson JF. Patterns of lymphatic drainage from the skin in patients with melanoma. J Nucl Med 2003; 44(4):570–582.

73 Shapiro RL. Surgical approaches to malignant melanoma. Practical guidelines. Derm Clin 2002; 20(4):681–699.

74 Statius Muller MG, van Leeuwen PA, de Lange-De Klerk ES, et al. The sentinel lymph node status is an important factor for predicting clinical outcome in patients with Stage I or II cutaneous melanoma. Cancer 2001; 91(12):2401–2408.

75 Gershenwald JE, Thompson W, Mansfield PF, et al. Multi-institutional melanoma lymphatic mapping experience: the prognostic value of sentinel lymph node status in 612 stage I or II melanoma patients. J Clin Oncol 1999; 17(3):976–983.

76 Vuylsteke RJ, van Leeuwen PA, Statius Muller MG, Gietema HA, Kragt DR, Meijer S. Clinical outcome of stage I/II melanoma patients after selective sentinel lymph node dissection: long-term follow-up results. J Clin Oncol 2003; 21(6):1057–1065.

77 Lowe JB, Hurst E, Moley JF, Cornelius LA. Sentinel lymph node biopsy in patients with thin melanoma. Arch Derm 2003; 139(5):617–621.

78 Shivers SC, Wang X, Li W, et al. Molecular staging of malignant melanoma: correlation with clinical outcome. JAMA 1998; 280(16):1410–1415.

79 Goydos JS, Patel KN, Shih WJ, et al. Patterns of recurrence in patients with melanoma and histologically negative but RT-PCR-positive sentinel lymph nodes. J Am Coll Surg 2003; 196(2):196–205.

80 Kelley SW, Cockerell CJ. Sentinel lymph node biopsy as an adjunct to management of histologically difficult to diagnose melanocytic lesions: a proposal. J Am Acad Derm 2000; 42(3):527–530.

81 Su LD, Fullen DR, Sondak VK, Johnson TM, Lowe L. Sentinel lymph node biopsy for patients with problematic spitzoid melanocytic lesions: a report on 18 patients. Cancer 2003; 97(2):499–507.

82 Biddle DA, Evans HL, Kemp BL, et al. Intraparenchymal nevus cell aggregates in lymph nodes: a possible diagnostic pitfall with malignant melanoma and carcinoma. Am J Surg Pathol 2003; 27(5):673–681.

83 Friedman T, Westreich M, Mozes SN, Dorenbaum A, Herman O. Tattoo pigment in lymph nodes mimicking metastatic malignant melanoma. Plast Reconstr Surg 2003; 111(6):2120–2122.

CHAPTER
19

Management of the Patient with Melanoma

Carol L Huang and Allan C Halpern

Key points

- Melanoma is the deadliest form of skin cancer.
- Prevention and early detection are the keys to reducing morbidity and mortality.
- Treatment should be tailored to the needs of each individual patient.
- Surgical excision is the cornerstone of melanoma management.
- Sentinel lymph node biopsy is currently a staging and prognostic tool in the management of melanoma.
- Adjuvant therapy should be considered in patients at high risk of recurrence.
- Single drug chemotherapy remains the standard treatment for advanced metastatic disease. Clinical trials should be strongly considered for patients with metastatic melanoma.
- Regular follow-up and skin self-examinations and sun protection are important in patients with history of melanoma.

INTRODUCTION

Importance of early effective treatment

The incidence and mortality of melanoma has continued to rise steadily over the past few decades. Currently, the lifetime risk of developing melanoma is 1 in 65 and the projected risk by 2010 is that 1 in 50 Americans will develop melanoma in their lifetime.[1] Emphasis on prevention and early detection are the keys to reducing melanoma morbidity and mortality.[2] Optimal management of a patient diagnosed with melanoma requires consideration of multiple factors and decisions regarding management of the primary site, staging procedures, adjuvant therapy, and follow-up. There are several varying guidelines for melanoma management that have been set forth by different organizations, including the National Comprehensive Cancer Network (NCCN), American Academy of Dermatology, Society of Surgical Oncology and the British Association of Dermatologists.[3–6] The significant variations among these different published guidelines highlight the absence of a single 'evidence based' approach for managing melanoma patients (Table 19.1). Treatment should be tailored to the needs of each individual patient. This chapter presents a generalized approach to the surgical

management (excision margins) for melanoma, the diagnostic and staging work-up, follow-up recommendations and adjuvant treatment options.

Diagnosis

The diagnosis of melanoma begins with a biopsy of the suspected primary lesion. Ideally, an excisional biopsy should be performed to avoid sampling error and to obtain precise prognostic information. However, for most thin melanomas, the depth of the lesion as measured from a shave biopsy does not differ from that measured from definitive excision.[7] There is no data to suggest that incising a melanoma results in a worsening prognosis due to trauma related tumor cell metastasis. Once the diagnosis has been established with histopathologic confirmation, staging work-up and treatment options are considered, taking into account the prognostic attributes such as thickness of the lesion, location, and overall medical condition of the patient (Table 19.2). The new American Joint Committee on Cancer (AJCC) staging classification is listed in Table 19.3.[8] Work-up, treatment and follow-up guidelines take into consideration the stage of the patient's disease.

Staging

Staging of a melanoma patient requires a thorough history and physical examination. A problem oriented physical examination should include a complete skin and lymph node examination and assessment of any abnormalities detected on a thorough review of systems. Suspicious signs, symptoms and physical findings (e.g. in-transit metastases, satellite lesions, and palpable lymph nodes) warrant additional laboratory studies, imaging studies, and possible histological confirmation. The AJCC staging classification takes into account the status of lymph node involvement for those who undergo lymphatic mapping. Accurate staging provides important prognostic and survival information as listed in Table 19.4.[8] Patients with melanomas <1.0 mm do not need specific blood work or imaging studies to search for occult metastases. For patients with melanomas >1.0 mm, baseline laboratory values including complete blood count (CBC), lactic dehydrogenase (LDH), other liver function tests and chest X-ray (CXR) have been suggested by some guidelines as part of the initial work-up, but are very low yield. Routine imaging studies are not indicated in patients with stage I or II disease. In

265

Table 19.1   Published guidelines for managing patients with melanoma

		Margins	Work-up	Follow-up
AAD	*In situ*	0.5 cm	H&P*; CXR, LDH (optional)	General recommendations not stage specific, should be based on individual risk. H&P 1–4×/year for 2 years then 1–2×/year. Directed laboratory and imaging studies.
	<2 mm	1.0 cm		
	>2 mm	2.0 cm		
	Stage III	Not discussed	Not discussed	Not discussed
	Stage IV	Not discussed	Not discussed	Not discussed
NCCN	*In situ*	0.5 cm	None	Not discussed
	<1 mm	1.0 cm	None	H&P every 6 months for 2 years, then yearly
	1–4 mm	1–2.0 cm	Consider sentinel lymph node biopsy (SLNB); CXR, liver function tests (LFT) (optional)	H&P 3–6 months for 3 years, then 6–12 months for 2 years. CXR, LFT every 6–12 months (optional)
	>4 mm	≥2.0 cm		
	Stage III	Excision and lymph node dissection	LFT, CXR; pelvic and otherCT if indicated	H&P 3–6 months for 3 years then 4–12 months for 2 years, then yearly CXR, CBC, LFT every 3–12 months (optional), CT scans as indicated
	Stage IV	Excision and focal resection	LFT, CXR; CT scans if indicated	Not discussed
BAD	*In situ*	0.2–0.5 cm	None	Self-examination, no follow-up required
	<1 mm	1 cm	None	H&P every 3 months for 3 years
	1–2 mm	1–2 cm	Stage II; Consider SLNB	H&P every 3 months for 3 years, then every 6 months for 2 years
	2.1–4 mm	2–3 cm	Stage IIB and up; LFT, LDH, CBC, CXR, liver ultrasound, CT chest, abdomen, pelvis	
	>4 mm	2–3 cm		
	Stage III	Excision and lymph node dissection		Not discussed
	Stage IV	Excision and resection when possible		Not discussed

*H&P includes review of systems, symptoms directed exam, full skin examination and lymph node examination
AAD, American Academy of Dermatology; NCCN, National Comprehensive Cancer Network; BAD, British Association of Dermatologists.

Table 19.2   Suggested recommendations for managing patients with melanoma

Stage*	Work up	Surgical treatment	Systemic therapy	Follow-up
Stage 0	H&P	Excision	None	Lifelong follow-up at least yearly
Stage IA	H&P; CXR and LDH (optional)	Excision	None	H&P every 6 months for 2 years, then yearly
Stage IB–II	H&P; CXR and LDH (optional)	Excision — No SLNB; SNLB — (+) LN (complete dissection) / (–) LN	Consider adjuvant treatment in clinical trial or adjuvant α IFN	H&P every 3–6 months for 3 years, then 6–12 months for 2 years, then yearly CXR, LDH (optional). Directed laboratory and imaging studies as indicated
Stage III	CXR, LDH; CT/MRI/PET if indicated	Excision and complete LN dissection**	Consider adjuvant treatment in clinical trial or adjuvant α IFN	H&P every 3–6 months for 3 years then 4–12 months for 2 years then yearly. Laboratory and imaging studies as indicated
Stage IV	CXR, LDH; CT/MRI/PET if indicated	Consider resection of solitary or limited disease	Clinical trial Chemotherapy Biochemotherapy Interferon	CXR, CBC, LDH every 3–12 months (optional), imaging studies as indicated

*Stage at presentation
** For special cases when excision is not feasible, treatment options include: hyperthermic limb perfusion, XRT and systemic chemotherapy.
H&P includes review of systems, complete skin and lymph node examination and a symptoms directed physical examination.

patients with more advanced stage disease, radiologic imaging and LDH levels may be used to monitor the progression or recurrence of metastatic disease. An elevated serum lactic dehydrogenase (LDH) level on two separate occasions, at least 24 hrs apart, is an indication of metastatic disease based on the new AJCC staging classification, if there are no other obvious causes. It can also be followed as a marker for disease activity. Although very sensitive, an elevated LDH can be quite non-specific. For this reason, there is little evidence to support the usefulness of this test. However, LDH testing is relatively inexpensive and provides a baseline for future reference.

Radiologic and nuclear imaging studies may be useful in the evaluation and guiding the management of stage III and IV patients who have nodal or metastatic disease. CT scans and more recently PET scans are commonly used to evaluate symptoms or abnormalities noted on follow-up examinations.

Surgical management

The cornerstone of treatment for primary melanoma is excisional surgery with margins based on Breslow thickness. Generally accepted surgical margins for excision are listed in Table 19.5. Margins may be modified to accommodate individual anatomic or cosmetic considerations (Fig. 19.1). The preferred treatment for lentigo maligna is complete surgical excision. However, the large size of many of these lesions coupled with their common occurrence on the face of elderly patients, warrants consideration of radiation therapy, cryotherapy, topical therapy, or observation in some cases of lentigo maligna (Fig. 19.2).

Table 19.3   AJCC staging for melanoma[8]

0		In-situ
IA		≤1.0 mm, no ulceration
IB		≤1.0 mm with ulceration 1.01–2.0 mm, no ulceration
IIA		1.01–2.0 mm with ulceration 2.01–4.0 mm, no ulceration
IIB		2.01–4.0 mm with ulceration >4.0 mm, no ulceration
IIC		>4.0 mm with ulceration
IIIA		Non-ulcerated primary tumor (T1–T4a) with ≤3 nodal *micromets*
IIIB		Non-ulcerated primary tumor (T1–T4a) with ≤3 *macromets* Any primary tumor (T1–T4b) with ≤3 nodal *micromets* Any T with in transit or satellite
IIIC		Any T with ≤3 *macromets* Any T with ≥4 nodes
IV	M1a	Distant skin, subcutaneous or nodal mets with normal LDH
	M1b	Lung metastasis with normal LDH
	M1c	All other visceral metastasis with normal LDH or Any distant metastasis with elevated LDH

Table 19.4   Survival data (%) for melanoma[8]

		1 Year	5 Year	10 Year
IA			95	88
IB			90	80
IIA			78	65
IIB			65	50
IIC			45	32
IIIA			65	60
IIIB			50	40
IIIC			25	20
IV	M1a	59	19	16
	M1b	57	7	3
	M1c	41	10	6

Stage I, II – worse prognosis with ulceration, increasing thickness, age, axial location, being male.
Stage III – worse with increasing number of nodes, macrometastasis, ulceration of primary tumor.
Stage IV – depends on site, but differences are minimal.
Mets to the lung only has 1-year survival advantage over other visceral mets.

Table 19.5   Current recommendations for surgical margins for melanoma[3]

In situ	0.5 cm
<1 mm	1.0 cm
1.01–4 mm	2.0 cm
>4 mm	≥2.0 cm

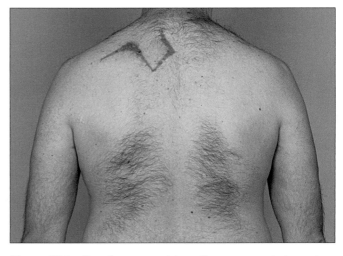

Figure 19.1   Scar from an excision with recommended margins.

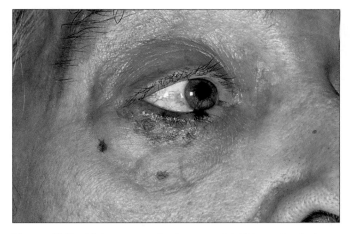

Figure 19.2 Melanoma on the lower eyelid. This anatomical location precludes excision with suggested margins.

Table 19.6   Risk factors for positive sentinel lymph node[9]
Thick primary tumor
Ulceration
Clark level IV+

For patients with Stage IA disease (i.e. thin melanomas <1.0 mm without negative prognostic attributes such as ulceration, Clark's level IV–V, or extensive regression), wide local excision is sufficient treatment. For patients with Stage IB–II disease (i.e. intermediate and thick lesions (>1.0 mm) without clinical evidence of nodal involvement), sentinel lymph node biopsy should be considered in conjunction with wide local excision.

Lymphatic mapping with sentinel lymph node biopsies (SLNB) have become a common procedure performed at the time of wide local excision to identify regional nodal metastases for melanomas greater than 1 mm in thickness. It is also considered for patients with thinner melanomas with high risk characteristics, (listed in Table 19.6) including Clark's level IV or greater, presence of ulceration, or evidence of regression. The procedure is useful in identifying patients with positive sentinel nodes for early therapeutic lymph node dissection as well as stratifying more precisely the candidates for clinical trials and those who are most likely to benefit from adjuvant therapy. It is known that lymph node status in general is an excellent prognostic indicator of recurrence and survival and number of positive regional nodes noted on dissection relate directly to prognosis (Fig. 19.3). The tumor status of the sentinel node(s) is a very significant prognostic factor (Fig. 19.4) and may be even a better predictor of survival than tumor thickness. Approximately 20% of sentinel lymph nodes are positive for melanoma, ranging from 12–36% in the literature.[9] With newer molecular staging using reverse transcriptase-PCR, sensitivity of detecting positive nodes is greater. The probability of recurrence as well as overall survival are influenced by the RT-PCR status of the sentinel lymph node. Patients with a sentinel lymph node negative for metastasis by H&E staining but positive with RT-PCR have an intermediate probability of recurrence and overall survival compared to patients with metastases found on both H&E staining and RT-PCR and patients negative for metastases on both H&E staining and RT-PCR.[10] This suggests that RT-PCR is more sensitive in detecting metastases. However, there is significant variability in the type and number of markers used. In addition, with more recent long term follow-up data, even the patients who had negative

sentinel lymph nodes by both H&E staining and RT-PCR have probability of survival <100%.[11] Predictive factors for a positive sentinel lymph node include primary melanomas with greater thickness, ulceration, and high mitotic index >5/hpf. Currently, SLNB is primarily a staging and prognostic tool with no proven therapeutic value or survival benefit.

Patients who do not have evidence of melanoma in the sentinel lymph nodes are spared additional surgery. Patients with melanoma micrometastases found on sentinel lymph node biopsy typically undergo complete, therapeutic lymphadenectomy of the affected lymph node basin, and then consideration for adjuvant therapy with interferon (IFN)-α or participation in clinical trials. Patients with clinical evidence of regional lymph node metastases are evaluated with fine needle aspiration or lymph node biopsy. Patients with histologically proven lymph node metastases are treated with therapeutic lymphadenectomy. For patients who have extracapsular nodal disease, regional local control of tumor growth can present a significant challenge. In this setting, lymphadenectomy should be performed with consideration of adjuvant radiation therapy to the nodal basin.

Adjuvant therapy

Adjuvant therapy should be considered for patients at high risk for recurrence, particularly those with thick primary tumors and/or positive lymph nodes. Multiple approaches to adjuvant therapy including chemotherapy, immunotherapy, or vaccine therapy have been studied in this setting. Randomized studies of adjuvant treatment using Bacillus Calmette-Guerin (BCG), *Corynebacterium parvum*, DTIC, Levamisole, Vitamin A, or Megestrol acetate alone or in combination have generally failed to show any benefit in disease free or overall survival. Small subsets of isolated positive results have not been corroborated.

A study of high dose interferon-α given for one full year in patients with Stage IIB and III disease found a median increase in overall survival from 2.8 years to 3.8 years in treated patients.[12] This initial study formed the basis for FDA approval of high dose IFN for the adjuvant treatment of melanoma. There was significant toxicity associated with high dose IFN therapy, however, a Q-TWiST analysis (quality of life adjusted survival time)[13] found that the treated group still had a gain of 8.9 months without relapse and 7 months of overall survival time compared to the observation group.[14] Two other trials using high dose IFN showed improvement only in disease free survival in patients with positive nodal disease.[15,16] In a large trial comparing high dose IFN, low dose IFN, and observation, there was no difference in

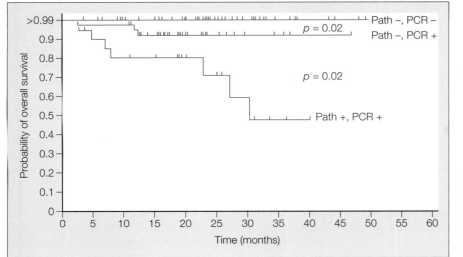

Figure 19.3 Survival vs sentinel lymph node status. (Reproduced from Shivers SC *et al.* Molecular staging of malignant melanoma: correlation with clinical outcome. JAMA 1998; 280:1410–1415. Copyright © 1998 American Medical Association. All rights reserved.)

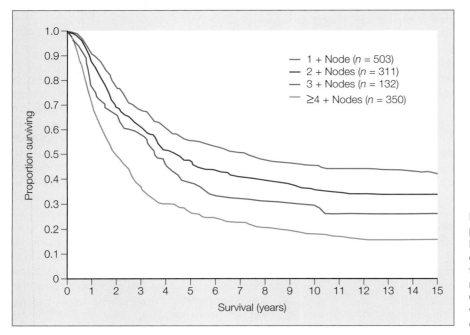

Figure 19.4 Survival vs number of positive lymph nodes. (Reproduced from Balch, CM *et al.* Prognostic factors analysis of 17,600 melanoma patients: validation of the American Joint Committee on Cancer melanoma staging system. J Clin Oncol 2001; 19:3622–3634. Reprinted with permission from the American Society of Clinical Oncology.)

overall survival between the treatment groups. There was only a marginally significant increase in relapse free survival in the high dose IFN group compared to the observation group.[17] A trial comparing high dose IFN and GM2-KLH/QS-21 vaccines revealed significant increases of disease free and overall survival with IFN.[17]

Low dose IFN, although better tolerated, was ineffective in increasing disease free or overall survival in patients with positive or negative lymph nodes.[18,19] Two other studies using low dose IFN in patients with primary melanomas >1.5 mm and negative lymph nodes showed prolonged disease free but not overall survival.[20,21] In summary, high dose IFN has prolonged relapse free and overall survival in some patients with significant associated toxicity, but low dose IFN has not been proven to be beneficial to overall survival.

Adjuvant vaccine therapy has been shown to be beneficial in a limited number of patients. However, to date, no vaccine has demonstrated significant survival benefit when prospectively compared with high dose IFN or observation. Randomized, prospective studies have yet to show any significant increase in overall survival.[22,23] This may be a function of the different types of vaccines available and small study population. A variety of antigens can be used to stimulate an immune response. Vaccines can be targeted to a single antigen or to multiple antigens; agents utilized for vaccination have included whole cells, cell lysates, shed antigens, gangliosides, or peptides. In patients who develop an anti-tumor (humoral and/or cellular) response to a particular vaccine, disease free and overall survival have been improved.[24] Patients not improving on one vaccine may have success with a different antigen. Additional on-going trials are in progress to further evaluate the value of various vaccines. Recent areas of research include the use of dendritic cells, RNA and DNA for vaccination. Please see chapter on Vaccine therapy in this text for detailed discussion of adjuvant vaccine treatment.

Management of the patient with metastatic disease

Limited in-transit metastatic disease can be managed with excision, carbon dioxide laser ablation, or intra-lesional immunotherapy with dinitrochlorobenzene (DNCB) or IFN. These have all been shown to be effective in local control of limited in-transit disease. Hyperthermic isolated limb perfusion (HILP) is a treatment option for patients with more extensive in-transit metastatic disease. This can be done using melphalan as a single agent or in combination with tumor necrosis factor (TNF); cisplatin or DTIC.[3] While HILP has not been associated with significant improvement in overall survival, it can have dramatic palliative effects and avoid the need for amputation in some patients with extensive limb involvement. Radiation therapy is another less effective alternative palliative therapy in this setting.

In patients with metastatic melanoma distant to the local/regional site, curative resection of relatively stable remote nodal and soft-tissue lesions, as well as isolated visceral lesions should be considered. In symptomatic patients, palliative resection may also be appropriate. The lung is the most common visceral site of metastasis that is potentially curable with the resection of isolated lesions. Prolonged survival among some patients treated with surgical resection of limited liver, pulmonary, or brain metastases has also been reported.[25–27] Palliative radiation therapy is an option in the setting of inoperable brain metastases, prolonging survival by 1–2 months.

Systemic chemotherapy with dacarbazine (DTIC) remains the mainstay of therapy for patients with extensive distant metastatic disease. Response rates are generally low (20%) and median duration of responses approaches 1 year. Complete responses are rare, usually less than 5%. While several combination chemotherapy regimens have been evaluated over the years, none have demonstrated consistent improvements in survival compared to single agent DTIC.[28,29] Temazolamide, an analog of DTIC in oral formulation, with improved CNS penetration has recently become available. Response rates to Temazolamide have been similar to DTIC. Combination treatments have been compared to single agent. In a large trial with 240 patients, DTIC was compared to the Dartmouth regimen (dacarbazine, cisplatin, carmustine, and tamoxifen) and no survival difference was found. There was a small, non-significant increase in tumor response in patient who received the Dartmouth regimen, however, it was accompanied by greater bone marrow suppression, nausea, vomiting, and fatigue.[30] Another approach to therapy of distant metastatic disease has been the use of immuno 'biotherapies' specifically IFN and IL-2 either alone or in combination with multidrug chemotherapy. IL-2, which is also FDA approved, has an overall response rate of 15–20% and can yield durable remissions in 6% of patients.[31] DTIC with IFN-alpha did not have better response or survival rates when compared to DTIC alone, but did have significant increase in toxicity.[29] DTIC with IL-2 had response rates of 13–33%, which is in the same range as DTIC alone. Histamine dihydrochloride is an agent that has been used for metastatic melanoma in combination with IL-2 for its inhibition of reactive oxygen species.[32,33] A study comparing treatment with histamine dihydrochloride plus IL-2 versus IL-2 alone showed that histamine is an effective adjunct with significant prolongation of survival in patients with liver metastases.[32] One study with IFN-alpha + IL-2 + cisplatin, vinblastine and DTIC yielded a 60% response rate with 21% complete response, however, there was significant toxicity.[34] Follow-up studies have failed to duplicate these dramatic results.

Vaccine therapy in advanced disease is well tolerated with low toxicity. Initial trials had promising results with some patients having increased disease free and overall survival when compared to historical controls. However, in a prospective trial comparing vaccine to chemotherapy there was no survival advantage but there was significantly less toxicity.[35] The biologic agents and vaccines seem to benefit fewer people when compared with chemotherapy, however, for patients who do have complete responses, they are durable. Vitiligo in the course of immunotherapy has been associated with improved outcome.

Follow-up

Regular skin examinations are very important in patients with melanoma because they are at increased risk for getting another primary melanoma. Approximately 1–8% of patients with melanoma will develop subsequent primary melanomas.[36] The proper use of sunscreens and sun-protective clothing including sunglasses and hats should be highly encouraged. All patients should be instructed in self-examination and return for routine physician surveillance for additional primary lesions. One retrospective study concluded that skin self-examination has the potential to reduce melanoma mortality by 63%.[37] Patient education on self skin-examination includes information on the ABCD changes of lesions and instruction on how to perform a thorough total body skin-examination. New lesions may arise *de novo* or transform from existing nevi (Figs 19.5 and 19.6).[38] Individuals with very prominent and/or atypical nevi may benefit from having their cutaneous surface photographed.[39] These photographs can serve as a baseline to which future skin examinations can be compared (Fig. 19.7). They can assist in the detection of sometimes subtle changes in size, shape and color of the numerous nevi (Figs 19.8 and 19.9). Any new, changing, or symptomatic pigmented lesions should be examined closely and possibly biopsied.

Patients with invasive primary malignant melanoma need regular follow-up for assessment of metastasis (Table 19.7).[40] A thorough review of systems and physical examination including lymph node exam should be performed on all follow-up visits. Initially, patients with melanoma should be followed closely every 2–3 months. Although recurrences can occur at anytime, even as far out as 10–20 years from the primary, the greatest risk is in the 2 years following diagnosis. Therefore, surveillance is most important in the period immediately following treatment. After those first two years, if the patient remains free of disease, the interval between follow-up visits can be spaced out to between 6 month and 1 year

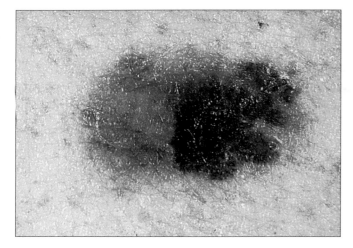

Figure 19.5 Clinical photo of a melanoma arising from a dysplastic nevus.

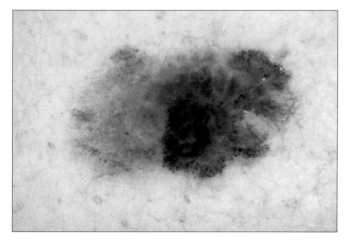

Figure 19.6 Dermoscopic photo of the same melanoma arising from a dysplastic nevus.

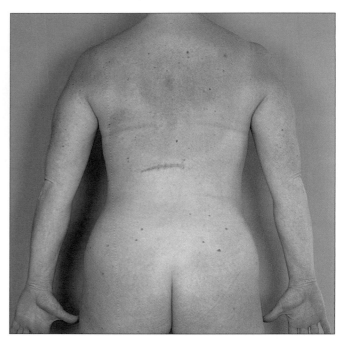

Figure 19.7 One image from total body photographs allowing multiple nevi to be followed for changes.

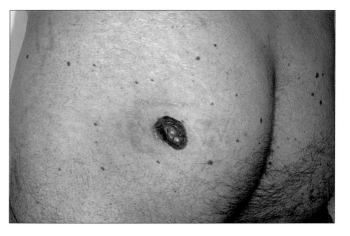

Figure 19.8 Nodular melanoma in a background of homogenous nevi.

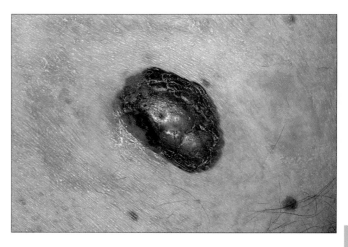

Figure 19.9 Close-up of the nodular melanoma.

depending on individual risk factors. Time to recurrence for patients with node-negative disease varies inversely with the thickness of the primary tumor.[41] Thus, patients with thin melanomas can potentially recur years after initial diagnosis. Every patient with history of melanoma should be examined at least yearly. In addition, because of the risk of a melanoma patient developing an additional unrelated primary melanoma (approximately 5%) these patients must be carefully examined for the development of new, suspicious lesions.

The prognosis of a pregnant patient with melanoma appears to be similar to that of a non-pregnant patient. Issues related to melanoma and pregnancy are covered in greater depth in Chapter 20. The 10-year disease-free and overall survival for Stage I and II patients is not statistically different between the two groups.[42] Some studies have shown that pregnant women present with thicker melanomas, however, the etiology is unclear. Hormonal factors influencing the growth of pigmented lesions have been suggested, but no particular link has been established. It is possible that changing lesions are observed during a pregnancy, but biopsy and diagnosis are delayed. It is best to examine pregnant patients more

Table 19.7 Risk factors for recurrence[40]
Number of positive lymph nodes
Older age
Thick primary tumor

Table 19.8 Common sites of recurrence and metastases[45,46]
Skin
Lymph nodes
Lung
Brain
Liver

frequently and biopsy any suspicious lesions without delay. Also, alternative techniques to oral contraceptive are often suggested to melanoma patients of child-bearing age. There are no studies that suggest the use of hormone replacement therapy worsens subsequent prognosis in these patients.

Follow-up laboratory and imaging studies are guided by history, review of systems and symptoms, as well as findings on a complete skin examination and lymph node evaluation.[43] Most recurrences are found on physical examination or may produce symptoms that are revealed on review of systems. A smaller percentage of metastases are found on CXR.[44] The first site of metastases is most commonly the skin and subcutaneous tissue, followed by lymph nodes, lung, liver, and brain (Table 19.8).[45,46] In general, men and older patients have a worse prognosis than women and younger patients.

It is also of great importance to provide psychosocial support for a patient diagnosed with melanoma. It is a serious, potentially fatal cancer that can be a source of great anxiety and fear for the patient and his/her family. Frequent follow-up visits in the period immediately after diagnosis can provide reassurance and comfort from careful surveillance.

FUTURE OUTLOOK

As more cellular and molecular prognostic factors are identified, better stratification of patients will be obtained leading to better customization of therapy such as surgical margins, node dissections and follow up regimens. However, until this occurs, early detection and treatment will remain the cornerstone of the effective management of the patient with melanoma.

Genetic testing for inherited predisposition to melanoma is currently available as a research tool, of limited clinical utility. Two major melanoma susceptibility genes, CDKN2A and CDK4, have been identified to date. The CDKN2A gene located on chromosome 9p21 encodes two cell-cycle regulatory proteins, p16INK4A and p14ARF. Carriers of inherited mutations in the genes confer an increased risk of melanoma. However, only a very small percentage (less than 1–2%) of all melanomas can be attributed to inherited mutations in these genes. Most patients will not have a CDKN2A mutation. It is most likely in individuals from high-risk families with strong family history (three or more affected members). Even among these families, less than half will have the mutation. There is also uncertainty on the penetrance of the mutation. Some non-carriers may still develop melanoma and have higher risk then the general population, while some gene carriers may not develop melanoma. Testing for DNA status does not change prevention, surveillance, or management of patients and their families at this point. Sun protection, self-examinations and regular physician follow-ups should still be advocated for all individuals. At this time, the Melanoma Genetics Consortium does not recommend routine genetic testing other than in defined research programs.[47]

REFERENCES

1 Jemal A, Murray T, Samuels A, et al. Cancer statistics. CA Cancer J Clin 2003; 53:5–26.

2 Rigel DS, Carucci JA. Malignant melanoma: prevention, early detection, and treatment in the 21st century. CA Cancer J Clin 2000; 50:215–236.

3 Houghton A, Coit D, Bloomer W, et al. NCCN melanoma practice guidelines. Natl Compr Cancer Network Oncol (Huntingt) 1998; 12:153–177.

4 Coit D, Wallack M, Balch C. Society of Surgical Oncology practice guidelines. Melanoma surgical practice guidelines. Oncology (Huntingt) 1997; 11:1317–1323.

5 Roberts DL, Anstey AV, Barlow RJ, et al. U.K. guidelines for the management of cutaneous melanoma. Br J Derm 2002; 146:7–17.

6 Sober AJ, Chuang TY, Duvic M, et al. Guidelines of care for primary cutaneous melanoma. J Am Acad Derm 2001; 45:579–586.

7 Ng PC, Barzilai DA, Ismail SA, et al. Evaluating invasive cutaneous melanoma: is the initial biopsy representative of the final depth? J Am Acad Derm 2003; 48:420–424.

8 Balch CM, Buzaid AC, Soong SJ, et al. Final version of the American Joint Committee on Cancer Staging System for cutaneous melanoma. J Clin Oncol 2001; 19:3635–3648.

9 Gershenwald JE, Thompson W, Mansfield PF, et al. Multi-institutional melanoma lymphatic mapping experience: the prognostic value of sentinel lymph node status in 612 stage I or II melanoma patients. J Clin Oncol 1999; 17:976–983.

10 Shivers S, Wang X, Li W, et al. Molecular staging of malignant melanoma. Correlation with clinical outcome. JAMA 1998; 16:1410–1415.

11 Kuo C, Hoon D, Tekeuchi H, et al. Prediction of disease outcome in melanoma patients by molecular analysis of paraffin-embedded sentinel lymph nodes. J Clin Oncol 2003; 19:1–7.

12 Kirkwood JM, Strawderman MH, Ernstoff MS, et al. Interferon alfa-2b adjuvant therapy of high-risk resected cutaneous melanoma: the Eastern Cooperative Oncology Group Trial EST 1684. J Clin Oncol 1996; 14:7–17.

13 Agarwala SS, Kirkwood JM. Adjuvant therapy of melanoma. Semin Surg Oncol 1998; 14:302–310.

14 Cole BF, Gelber RD, Kirkwood JM, et al. Quality-of-life-adjusted survival analysis of interferon alfa-2b adjuvant treatment of high-risk resected cutaneous melanoma: an Eastern Cooperative Oncology Group study. J Clin Oncol 1996; 14:2666–2673.

15 Creagan ET, Dalton RJ, Ahmann DL, et al. Randomized, surgical adjuvant clinical trial of recombinant interferon alfa-2a in selected patients with malignant melanoma. J Clin Oncol 1995; 13:2776–2783.

16 Kirkwood JM, Ibrahim JG, Sondak VK, et al. High- and low-dose interferon alfa-2b in high-risk melanoma: first analysis of intergroup trial E1690/S9111/C9190. J Clin Oncol 2000; 18:2444–2458.

17 Kirkwood JM, Ibrahim JG, Sosman JA, et al. High-dose interferon alfa-2b significantly prolongs relapse-free and overall survival compared with the GM2-KLH/QS-21 vaccine in patients with resected stage IIB-III melanoma: results of intergroup trial E1694/S9512/C509801. J Clin Oncol 2001; 19:2370–2380.

18 Inman JL, Russell GB, Savage P, et al. Low-dose adjuvant interferon for stage III malignant melanoma. Am Surg 2003; 69:127–130.

19 Cascinelli N, Belli F, MacKie RM, et al. Effect of long-term adjuvant therapy with interferon alpha-2a in patients with regional node metastases from cutaneous melanoma: a randomised trial. Lancet 2001; 358:866–869.

20 Grob JJDB, Salmoniere P de la, Delaunay M, et al. Randomised trial of interferon alpha-2a as adjuvant therapy in resected primary melanoma thicker than 1.5 mm without clinically detectable node metastases. French Cooperative Group on Melanoma. Lancet 1998; 351:1905–1910.

21 Pehamberger H, Soyer HP, Steiner A, et al. Adjuvant interferon alfa-2a treatment in resected primary stage II cutaneous melanoma. Austrian Malignant Melanoma Coop Group. J Clin Oncol 1998; 16:1425–1429.

22 Hersey P, Coates AS, McCarthy WH, et al. Adjuvant immunotherapy of patients with high-risk melanoma using vaccinia viral lysates of melanoma: results of a randomized trial. J Clin Oncol 2002; 20:4181–4190.

23 Wallack MK, Sivanandham M, Balch CM, et al. Surgical adjuvant active specific immunotherapy for patients with stage III melanoma: the final analysis of data from a phase III, randomized, double-blind, multicenter vaccinia melanoma oncolysate trial. J Am Coll Surg 1998; 187:69–77.

24 Bystryn JC, Zeleniuch-Jacquotte A, Oratz R, et al. Double-blind trial of a polyvalent, shed-antigen, melanoma vaccine. Clin Cancer Res 2001; 7:1882–1887.

25 Leo F, Cagini L, Rocmans P, et al. Lung metastases from melanoma: when is surgical treatment warranted? Br J Cancer 2000; 83:569–572.

26 Essner R. Surgical treatment of malignant melanoma. Surg Clin North Am 2003; 83:109–156.

27 Wronski M, Arbit E. Surgical treatment of brain metastases from melanoma: a retrospective study of 91 patients. J Neurosurg 2000; 93:9–18.

28 Falkson CI, Ibrahim J, Kirkwood JM, et al. Phase III trial of dacarbazine versus dacarbazine with interferon alpha-2b versus dacarbazine with tamoxifen versus dacarbazine with interferon alpha-2b and tamoxifen in patients with metastatic malignant melanoma: an Eastern Cooperative Oncology Group study. J Clin Oncol 1998; 16:1743–1751.

29 Young AM, Marsden J, Goodman A, et al. Prospective randomized comparison of dacarbazine (DTIC) versus DTIC plus interferon-alpha (IFN-alpha) in metastatic melanoma. Clin Oncol (R Coll Radiol) 2001; 13:458–465.

30 Chapman PB, Einhorn LH, Meyers ML, et al. Phase III multicenter randomized trial of the Dartmouth regimen versus dacarbazine in patients with metastatic melanoma. J Clin Oncol 1999; 17:2745–2751.

31 Agarwala S. Improving survival in patients with high-risk and metastatic melanoma: immunotherapy leads the way. Am J Clin Derm 2003; 4:333–346.

32 Agarwala SS, Glaspy J, O'Day SJ, et al. Results from a randomized phase III study comparing combined treatment with histamine dihydrochloride plus interleukin-2 versus interleukin-2 alone in patients with metastatic melanoma. J Clin Oncol 2002; 20:125–133.

33 Agarwala SS, Sabbagh MH. Histamine dihydrochloride: inhibiting oxidants and synergising IL-2-mediated immune activation in the tumour microenvironment. Expert Opin Biol Ther 2001; 1:869–879.

34 Legha SS, Ring S, Eton O, et al. Development of a biochemotherapy regimen with concurrent administration of cisplatin, vinblastine, dacarbazine, interferon alfa, and interleukin-2 for patients with metastatic melanoma. J Clin Oncol 1998; 16:1752–1759.

35 Mitchell MS. Perspective on allogeneic melanoma lysates in active specific immunotherapy. Semin Oncol 1998; 25:623–635.

36 Stam-Posthuma JJ, Duinen C van, Scheffer E, et al. Multiple primary melanomas. J Am Acad Derm 2001; 44:22–27.

37 Berwick M, Begg CB, Fine J, et al. Screening for cutaneous melanoma by skin self-examination. J Natl Cancer Inst 1996; 88:17–23.

38 Marks R, Dorevitch AP, Mason G. Do all melanomas come from 'moles'? A study of the histological association between melanocytic naevi and melanoma. Australas J Dermatol 1990; 31:77–80.

39 Halpern AC. The use of whole body photography in a pigmented lesion clinic. Derm Surg 2000; 26:1175–1180.

40 Clary BM, Brady MS, Lewis JJ, Coit DG. Sentinel lymph node biopsy in the management of patients with primary cutaneous melanoma: Review of a large single-institutional experience with an emphasis on recurrence. Ann Surg 2001; 233:250–258.

41 Romero JB, Stefanato CM, Kopf AW, et al. Follow-up recommendations for patients with stage I malignant melanoma. J Derm Surg Oncol 1994; 20:175–178.

42 Daryanani D, Plukker JT, Hullu JA De, et al. Pregnancy and early-stage melanoma. Cancer 2003; 97:2248–2253.

43 Huang CL, Provost N, Marghoob AA, et al. Laboratory tests and imaging studies in patients with cutaneous malignant melanoma. J Am Acad Derm 1998; 39:451–463.

44 Mooney MM, Kulas M, McKinley B, et al. Impact on survival by method of recurrence detection in stage I and II cutaneous melanoma. Ann Surg Oncol 1998; 5:54–63.

45 Balch CM, Soong SJ, Murad TM, et al. A multifactorial analysis of melanoma. IV. Prognostic factors in 200 melanoma patients with distant metastases (stage III). J Clin Oncol 1983; 1:126–134.

46 Hwu WJ, Balch CM, Houghton AN. Diagnosis of stage IV disease. In: Balch CM, Houghton AN, Sober AJ, Soong SJ, eds. Cutaneous Melanoma, 4th edn. St. Louis: Quality Medical Publishing; 2003:523–546.

47 Kefford RF, Newton-Bishop JA, Bergman W, Tucker MA. Counseling and DNA testing for individuals perceived to be genetically predisposed to melanoma: A Consensus Statement of the Melanoma Genetics Consortium. J Clin Oncol 1999; 17:3245–3251.

CHAPTER
20 Pregnancy and Melanoma

Caron M Grin, Marcia S Driscoll and David Polsky

Key points

- Pregnancy does not have an adverse effect on the prognosis of patients with Stage I/II melanoma.
- Recommendations for these patients regarding future pregnancies should be based on the prognostic factors for the given tumor.
- There is some evidence that pregnant patients are diagnosed with thicker melanomas compared with non-pregnant controls and this finding needs further study.

INTRODUCTION

There has been significant controversy regarding the relationship between pregnancy and malignant melanoma (MM). The origin of this concern arises from case reports published over the past 50 years, suggesting a poor prognosis for women developing MM during pregnancy and from observations that MM may be a hormonally-responsive tumor. This has become an increasingly important issue as more women delay childbearing until the fourth or even fifth decade of life. As the age-specific incidence of MM increases during these decades, a rising incidence of MM during pregnancy may be seen in the coming years.

HISTORY

The controversy concerning the influence of pregnancy on the prognosis of MM began with multiple case reports dating back to 1951. Pack and Scharnagel[1] reviewed 1050 cases of MM and reported that of 10 patients diagnosed with MM during pregnancy, five died within 30 months of diagnosis. Another 11 patients noted changes in nevi during pregnancy and were subsequently diagnosed with MM in the postpartum period. Two of these women died of widely metastatic disease within 3 years and one was noted to have probable brain metastases. These investigators concluded that "some benign nevi are incited to undergo malignant degeneration during pregnancy ... such melanomas grow with unusual rapidity and metastasize widely ... the prognosis of pregnant women with melanoma is bad and few cures are obtained". In 1954, Byrd and McGanity[2] stated that the risk of pregnancy, in women with a history of MM, was significant enough to 'justify surgical sterilization in

those women who were amenable to terminating their child bearing career'.

In addition to case reports, there were observations which supported a relationship between hormones and MM, including: the rare occurrence of MM before puberty, the increasing incidence of MM during the childbearing years, the darkening and enlargement of nevi during pregnancy, the presence of receptors for estrogen and progesterone in some MMs, the augmentation of MM cell growth in tissue culture on addition of steroid hormones and the enhancement of MM growth in mice after administration of estrogen. However, over the past several years, data from recent laboratory and clinical studies have been unable to substantiate the above hypotheses and observations.

EPIDEMIOLOGY

One-third of women with MM are of child-bearing age at the time of diagnosis. The incidence of MM during pregnancy is estimated as 2.6 cases per 1000 births.[3] MM is one of the most common cancers diagnosed during pregnancy, representing 8% of all malignancies occurring during pregnancy. MM is the most likely tumor to metastasize to the placenta although this is still a rare occurrence. If transplacental metastases occur, there is a 25% risk that the fetus will be affected.[4]

PATHOGENESIS AND ETIOLOGY

It has been hypothesized that there may be some factor associated with pregnancy that could affect MM. However, it is unknown if there is a specific pregnancy-related hormone that could affect MM cell proliferation and the induction of angiogenesis. Numerous investigators have studied the binding of estrogen, progesterone, androgens and glucocorticoids to MM in tissue culture utilizing various techniques. If binding did occur, it was at a low level and most of the binding seen in MM was not to true receptors. Recent laboratory studies utilizing monoclonal antibody techniques, which are likely to have greater specificity than the previous studies, did not detect estrogen receptors in benign nevi, primary MM, metastatic MM, or pregnancy-associated MM.[5–7] Two groups of investigators[8,9] have recently studied placenta growth factor (PlGF), a member of the platelet-derived growth factor family. While both groups found that human melanoma cell lines secrete PlGF, only one group[8] observed MM cell proliferation in response to PlGF.

In addition to laboratory investigations, endocrine manipulation with anti-estrogens such as tamoxifen, have been ineffective in the treatment of patients with MM. Likewise, several epidemiologic studies have not demonstrated an increased risk for MM in women who have taken oral contraceptive pills.[10]

CLINICAL FEATURES AND PROGNOSIS

Influence of pregnancy on the prognosis of MM

Several controlled studies have shown no significant difference in survival rates in women diagnosed with localized MM (American Joint Committee on Cancer Stage I or II) while pregnant compared with non-pregnant women with MM[11–17] and these studies have been reviewed in detail in a previous review[16] (Table 20.1). Duke University investigators, in both of their

studies,[11,14] however, observed that the disease-free interval (DFI) was significantly shortened in patients diagnosed during pregnancy, attributable to a shortened time to nodal metastases. These investigators postulated that the shortened DFI, without effect on overall survival, was due to either insufficient duration of patient follow-up, or that pregnancy increases risk for recurrence of MM without an effect on survival.

A recently published study followed 46 women, diagnosed with MM during pregnancy, for approximately 10 years after diagnosis. There was no significant difference in overall survival rates for patients with Stage I or Stage II MM compared with the control group of non-pregnant patients. The pregnant women did have thicker melanomas at the time of diagnosis. However, this difference was not statistically significant.[17]

Two controlled studies[15,18] addressed the effect of *prior* pregnancies on the prognosis of MM. There was no significant difference in prognosis for women who had prior pregnancies compared with those who had never been pregnant. Likewise, only two controlled studies[11,15]

Table 20.1 Malignant melanoma during pregnancy: Case–control studies[16]

Authors	Patients (n)	Control groups	AJCC stage of disease	Mean thickness of primary lesion (mm)	Duration of follow-up	Effect of pregnancy on survival	Effect of pregnancy on disease-free interval (DFI)
Reintgen et al.[11]	58	Not pregnant at time of dx or within 5 years of dx (n=585)	I or II	Study group: 1.90; Controls: 1.51 SD not stated	5 year (mean)	No	Yes (shorter DFI in study group, P=0.04)
McManamny et al.[12]	23	Not pregnant at time of dx or after dx (n=243)	I or II	Study group: 1.62 (survived); 2.62 (died). Controls: 1.72 (survived); 3.96 (died) NS	2 months–20 years	No	No
Wong et al.[13]	66	Controls: Not pregnant at time of dx (n=619). Matched controls: Not pregnant at time of dx and matched for age, tumor thickness, site of primary lesion and histopathologic type (n=66)	I or II	Study group: 1.24; Controls: 1.28 Matched controls: 1.06. SD not stated	Not stated	No	Actuarial DFI curves not generated. Study group: 37.7 months. Matched controls: 27.3 months. SD not stated
Slinguff et al.[14]	88	Not pregnant at time of dx (n=79)	I or II	Study group: 1.87; Controls: 1.75. SD not stated	6 years (mean)	No	Yes (shorter DFI in study group, P=0.039)
	100	Not pregnant at time of dx (n=86)	All stages	Study group: 2.17; Controls: 1.52 SD, P=0.052	6 years (mean)	No	Yes (shorter DFI in study group, P=0.028)
Mackie et al.[15]	92	Not pregnant at time of dx (n=143)	I or II	Study group: 2.38; Controls: 1.96. SD, P=0.002	Not stated	No	No
Daryanani et al.[17]	46	Not pregnant at time of dx (n = 368)	I or II	Study group: 2.0 Control: 1.7 NS	9 years	No	No

AJCC, American Joint Committee on Cancer; dx, diagnosis; SD, significant difference; NS, not significantly different.

addressed the effect of *subsequent* pregnancies on the prognosis of MM. Both studies found no significant difference in survival or DFI in women who became pregnant after being diagnosed with MM compared to women who did not have a subsequent pregnancy. Based on the above controlled studies, pregnancy before, after, or during the time of diagnosis of Stage I or II MM does not appear to influence overall survival.

Features of MM and nevi during pregnancy

Three studies[14,15,19] have observed a significantly increased tumor thickness in pregnancy-associated MM. There are several possible explanations for this observation. There may be a specific pregnancy-related hormone that accelerates MM growth, although this has not been clearly demonstrated as of yet. Second, there may be a delay in diagnosis of MM during pregnancy. Regarding this possibility, it has been often stated that nevi typically darken and enlarge during pregnancy. However, few studies have investigated changes in nevi during pregnancy. In two studies[20,21] that addressed this issue, the changes were reported by the patients themselves and on further examination most of these changes occurred in non-melanocytic lesions rather than in melanocytic nevi.[20] Of 129 nevi studied, only 8 (6.2%) changed from the first to third trimester: four nevi increased by 1 mm and four decreased by 1 mm (Table 20.2).[22] Larger prospective studies need to be performed, but one should not assume that all changes in nevi during pregnancy are physiologic. Biopsy of changing nevi during pregnancy should not be delayed.

Placental and fetal metastases

MM in the newborn can develop: (1) through transplacental spread (metastasis to the fetus), (2) within a large congenital nevus (3) as part of neurocutaneous melanosis, or (4) *de novo* in the skin. Only a small number of MM metastatic to the placenta and/or fetus have been reported.[23–25] All of the pregnant women had widely metastatic MM and died within 6 months of delivery. MM was present in 7 of 20 newborns or fetuses: five of the seven affected newborns or fetuses died within 11 months as a result of widely metastatic disease and the remaining affected infants had spontaneous resolution of disease. Metastasis to the placenta does not necessarily result in metastasis to the fetus. It is estimated that in those cases with placental metastases, 25% of newborns will be affected. Invasion of the chorionic villi does not predict fetal involvement; in the ten cases where intravillous invasion was observed, only two developed MM.

PATIENT EVALUATION AND DIAGNOSIS

In general, the evaluation of the pregnant patient with MM is similar to that for the non-pregnant patient. However, there are some special concerns that must be addressed to protect the wellbeing of the fetus.

Since the early diagnosis and treatment of MM is crucial to improved prognosis and survival, biopsy of suspicious pigmented lesions during pregnancy should not be delayed. In patients with multiple dysplastic nevi (atypical-mole syndrome), photographic documentation at the beginning of pregnancy can be helpful in establishing a baseline for subsequent comparison throughout the pregnancy. Follow-up visits each trimester are often recommended to detect any changes.

Once the diagnosis of MM is made, then a wide excision under local anesthesia is indicated. Avoidance of general anesthesia is the rule during pregnancy. If the tumor is associated with a high risk for recurrence, then sentinel lymph node mapping and biopsy (SLN) should be considered. There is controversy concerning the safety of SLN in pregnancy. Squatrito and Harlow[26] recommended the use of the blue dye technique alone, if the nodal drainage basin is predictable and avoidance of the radiolabeled technique during pregnancy. In contrast, Nicklas and Baker[27] felt that the amount of radiation associated with the technetium tracer is very small and that this technique could be used safely in pregnancy. At the University of Michigan, SLN biopsy is done with radiocolloid alone because of the concern of anaphylactic reactions to blue dye.[28] Shapiro[29] concluded that the accuracy and safety of intraoperative lymphatic mapping using vital blue dye and/or radiolabeled technetium sulfur colloid and selective lymphadenectomy is unclear and recommended that regional lymph node procedures be performed only if palpable nodal metastases arise, or after completion of pregnancy.

In pregnant patients where there is high risk for distant metastases, imaging studies may be considered. Radiographs of the chest may be performed safely in the pregnant patients with appropriate shielding. Ultrasonography may also be safely used. However, CT

Table 20.2 Changes in size of melanocytic nevi during pregnancy					
Authors	Patients (*n*)	No of nevi photographed (Back)	Mean no. of nevi per patient (Back)	No. of nevi changed from 1st to 3rd trimester	Nature of changes in nevi. Mean change in size = 0.
Pennoyer et al.[21]	22	129	5.86	8/129 (6.22)	4 nevi increased in size by 1 mm; 4 nevi decreased in size by 1 mm.

scanning with IV contrast is generally not recommended in early pregnancy because of the risk of brain injury to the fetus, which is highest between 8 and 15 weeks of age. While MRI has been considered relatively safe, avoidance in the first trimester is recommended because of its unknown risks.

PATHOLOGY

The pathology of MM in pregnant patients is the same as that for non-pregnant patients. The only exception is the finding of increased tumor thickness of MM in pregnant women compared with non-pregnant women as discussed earlier in this chapter.

It is important that the placenta of pregnant women with MM be examined microscopically as well as grossly for the presence of metastases. Multiple sections may be required to detect small foci of tumor.[24]

TREATMENT

Melanoma in the pregnant patient

In general, the recommendations for the pregnant patient should be based on the same prognostic factors established for the non-pregnant patient. Treatment of the pregnant patient with stages I or II MM should include wide excision and consideration of sentinel lymph node biopsy. In contrast, the treatment regimen for the pregnant patient with advanced disease (stages III, IV) needs to be individualized (Fig. 20.1) and take into

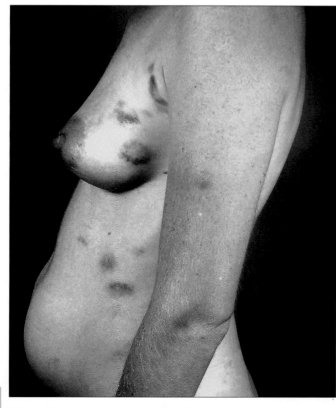

Figure 20.1 Pregnant patient with MM metastases.

consideration the safety of the fetus. While the benefits of interferon for MM are continually debated, this treatment has been safely used during pregnancy. In contrast, the use of chemotherapy has been associated with an increased incidence of spontaneous abortion in the first month of pregnancy and with an increased risk of mental retardation when used later in pregnancy.

Subsequent pregnancy, oral contraceptives and hormone replacement therapy

One of the most common questions regarding MM and pregnancy is whether to postpone or avoid a subsequent pregnancy after the diagnosis of MM. To date, there is no evidence that pregnancy has an adverse effect on MM outcome. When advising a MM patient whether to become pregnant, one must consider how the established prognosis for that given MM affects the life expectancy of the mother. If the patient has been diagnosed with a tumor with a high risk for recurrence, then perhaps a waiting period of 2–3 years is reasonable as the majority of recurrences will occur during this time. If however a patient is diagnosed with an early, thin MM, then there is no reason to delay a subsequent pregnancy.

How should these patients with MM be advised concerning the use of oral contraceptives (OCs) or hormone replacement therapy (HRT)? Most of the studies concerning exogenous hormones and MM focus on the relationship between exposure to OCs and the incidence of MM. Only one[30] of 17 studies showed a significantly increased risk for development of MM in patients who had ever taken OCs.[30–46] There were several studies[31–35] that found an increased risk for MM in specific subsets of patients. All of the studies suggesting an increased risk for MM in women taking OCs had inadequate controls for potential confounding variables, such as sun exposure and/or included a small number of cases. There was little evidence for increasing risk for MM with increasing duration of OC exposure which would be expected if there were a strong relationship between OC use and risk for MM.

There are few studies that address the incidence of MM in patients taking HRT. Seven[30,32,35,38,39,42,48] of eight studies have *not* found an enhanced risk for MM in patients taking HRT. The sole study[47] which reported an increased risk for MM in patients taking HRT had significant design limitations. It did not consider sun exposure in the analysis and did not show a trend of increasing risk of MM associated with increasing duration of HRT use.

The data that would be most beneficial to have to make a specific clinical recommendation for these patients (i.e. studies of the effect of OCs or HRT on the prognosis of patients who have MM) are limited in the medical literature. Shaw and colleagues[49–51] reported a slightly, but not significantly, better 5-year survival rate in 113 patients with MM who were taking OCs compared with 237 patients not taking OCs. However, these investigators did not address tumor thickness in their analysis and there were more patients with regional and distant metastases among nonusers of OCs.

Mackie and Bray recently published a study of 206 women with a history of MM. 83 of the patients received HRT and 123 never took HRT after diagnosis. There was no adverse effect of HRT on prognosis. Rather, there was a suggestion that those who took HRT may have had an improved outcome.[50]

In summary, based on existing evidence, *exogenous* hormones do not appear to influence the development of MM or to adversely affect prognosis. This evidence, combined with the lack of effect of *endogenous* hormones (in pregnancy) on the prognosis of MM, leads to the following recommendation: women with MM who have a strong medical indication for OCs or HRT and do not have reasonable alternatives, should not have OCs or HRT withheld.

FUTURE OUTLOOK

At current rates, about 25% of MMs occur in women of childbearing age and this fraction should increase as more women choose to defer pregnancy. The current management recommendations are based upon a small number of studies and conflicting data exists. Future studies in this important area are needed to better define the association between MM, pregnancy and hormones.

REFERENCES

1 Pack GT, Scharnagel IM. The prognosis for malignant melanoma in the pregnant women. Cancer 1951; 4:324–334.

2 Byrd BF, McGanity WJ. The effect of pregnancy on the clinical course of malignant melanoma. South Med J 1954; 47:196–200.

3 Pavlidis NA. Coexistence of pregnancy and malignancy. Oncologist 2002; 7:279–287.

4 Anderson JF, Kent S, Machin GA. Maternal malignant melanoma with placental metastases: a case report with literature review. Pediatr Pathol 1989; 9:35–42.

5 Flowers JL, Seigler HF, McCarty KS, et al. Absence of estrogen receptors in human melanoma as evaluated by a monoclonal antiestrogen receptor antibody. Arch Derm 1987; 123:764–765.

6 Lecavalier MA, From L, Gaid N. Absence of estrogen receptors in dysplastic nevi and malignant melanoma. J Am Acad Derm 1990; 23:242–246.

7 Duncan LM, Travers RL, Koerner FC, et al. Estrogen and progesterone receptor analysis in pregnancy-associated melanoma: absence of immunohistochemically detectable hormone receptors. Hum Pathol 1994; 25:36–41.

8 Lacal PM, Failla CM, Pagani E, et al. Human melanoma cells secrete and respond to placenta growth factor and vascular endothelial growth factor. J Invest Derm 2000; 115:1000–1007.

9 Graeven U, Rodeck U, Karpinski S, et al. Expression patterns of placenta growth factor in human melanocytic cell lines. J Invest Derm 2000; 115:118–123.

10 Holly EA, Cress RD, Ahn DK. Cutaneous melanoma in women: III. Reproductive factors and oral contraceptive use. Am J Epidemiol 1995; 141:943–950.

11 Reintgen DS, McCarty KS, Vollmer R, et al. Malignant melanoma and pregnancy. Cancer 1985; 55:1340–1344.

12 McManamny DS, Moss ALH, Pocock PV, et al. Melanoma and pregnancy: a long term follow-up. Br J Obstet Gynecol 1989; 96:1419–1423.

13 Wong JH, Stern EE, Kopald KH, et al. Prognostic significance of pregnancy in stage I melanoma. Arch Surg 1989; 124:1227–1231.

14 Slinguff CL Jr, Reintgen DS, Vollmer RT, et al. Malignant melanoma arising during pregnancy: a study of 100 patients. Ann Surg 1990; 211:552–559.

15 MacKie RM, Bufalino R, Morabito A, et al. Lack of effect of pregnancy on outcome of melanoma. Lancet 1991; 337:653–655.

16 Driscoll MS, Grin-Jorgensen CM, Grant-Kels JM. Does pregnancy influence the prognosis of malignant melanoma? J Am Acad Derm 1993; 29:619–630.

17 Daryanani D, Plukker JT, Hullu JA De, et al. Pregnancy and early-stage melanoma. Cancer 2003; 97:2248–2253.

18 Bork K, Brauninger W. Prior pregnancy and melanoma survival. Arch Derm 1986; 122:1097.

19 Travers RL, Sober AJ, Berwick M, et al. Increased thickness of pregnancy-associated melanoma. Br J Derm 1995; 132:876–883.

20 Foucar E, Bentley TJ, Laube DW, et al. A histopathologic examination of nevocellular nevi in pregnancy. Arch Derm 1985; 121:350–354.

21 Sanchez JL, Figueroa LD, Rodriguez E. Behavior of melanocytic nevi during pregnancy. Am J Derm 1984; 6(suppl)(1):89–91.

22 Pennoyer JW, Grin CM, Driscoll MS, et al. Changes in size of melanocytic nevi during pregnancy. J Am Acad Derm 1997; 36:378–382.

23 Ferreira CMM, Maceira JMP, Coelho JMCO. Melanoma and pregnancy with placental metastases: report of a case. Am J Derm 1998; 20:403–407.

24 Baergen RN, Johnson D, Moore T, et al. Maternal melanoma metastatic to the placenta: a case report and review of the literature. Arch Pathol Lab Med 1997; 121:508–511.

25 Alexander A, Harris RM, Grossman D, et al. Vulvar melanoma: diffuse melanosis and metastasis to the placenta. J Am Acad Dermatol 2004; 50:293–298.

26 Squatrito RC, Harlow SP. Melanoma complicating pregnancy. Obstet Gynecol Clin N Amer 1998; 25:407–416.

27 Nicklas AH, Baker ME. Imaging strategies in the pregnant cancer patient. Semin Oncol 2000; 27:623–632.

28 Schwartz JL, Mozurkewich EL, Johnson TM. Current management of patients with melanoma who are pregnant, want to get pregnant, or do not want to get pregnant. Cancer 2003; 97:2130–2133.

29 Shapiro RL. Surgical approaches to malignant melanoma: practical guidelines. Derm Clin 2002; 20:681–699.

30 Beral V, Ramcharan S, Faris R. Malignant melanoma and oral contraceptive use among women in California. Br J Cancer 1977; 36:804–809.

31 Adam SA, Sheaves SA, Wright NH, et al. A case–control study of the possible association between oral contraceptives and malignant melanoma. Br J Cancer 1981; 44:45–50.

32 Holly EA, Weiss NS, Liff JM. Cutaneous melanoma in relation to exogenous hormones and reproductive factors. J Natl Cancer Inst 1983; 70:827–831.

33 Lê MG, Cabanes PA, Desvignes V, et al. Oral contraceptive use and the risk of cutaneous malignant melanoma in a case–control study of French women. Cancer Causes Control 1992; 3:199–205.

34 Palmer JR, Rosenberg L, Strom BL, et al. Oral contraceptive use and risk of cutaneous malignant melanoma. Cancer Causes Contr 1992; 3:547–554.

35 Beral V, Evans S, Shaw H, et al. Oral contraceptive use and malignant melanoma in Australia. Br J Cancer 1984; 50:681–685.

36 Hannaford PC, Villard-Mackintosh L, Vessey MP, et al. Br J Cancer 1991; 63:430–433.

37 Zanetti R, Franceschi S, Rosso S, et al. Cutaneous malignant melanoma in females: the role of hormonal and reproductive factors. Int J Epidemiol 1990; 19:522–526.

38 Osterlind A, Tucker MA, Stone BJ, et al. The Danish case–control study of cutaneous malignant melanoma. III. Hormonal and reproductive factors in women. Int J Cancer 1988; 42:821–824.

39 Gallagher RP, Elwood JM, Hill GB, et al. Reproductive factors, oral contraceptives and risk of malignant melanoma: Western Canada melanoma study. Br J Cancer 1985; 52:901–907.

40 Green A, Bain C. Hormonal factors and melanoma in women. Med J Aust 1985; 142:446–448.

41 Helmrich SP, Rosenberg L, Kaufman DW, et al. Lack of an elevated risk of malignant melanoma in relation to oral contraceptive use. J Natl Cancer Inst 1984; 72:617–620.

42 Holman CDJ, Armstrong BK, Heenan PJ. Cutaneous malignant melanoma in females: exogenous sex hormones and reproductive factors. Br J Cancer 1984; 50:673–680.

43 Bain C, Hennekens CH, Speizer FE, et al. Oral contraceptive use and malignant melanoma. J Natl Cancer Inst 1982; 68:537–539.

44 Holly EA, Cress RD, Ahn DK. Cutaneous melanoma in women. II. Reproductive factors and oral contraceptive use. Am J Epidemiol 1995; 141:943–950.

45 Westerdahl J, Jonsson N, Ingvar C, et al. Risk of malignant melanoma in relation to drug intake, alcohol, smoking and hormonal factors. Br J Cancer 1996; 73:1126–1131.

46 Smith MA, Fine JA, Barnhill RL, et al. Hormonal and reproductive influences and risk of melanoma in women. Int J Epidemiol 1998; 27:751–757.

47 Holly EA, Cress RD, Ahn DK. Cutaneous melanoma in women: ovulatory life, menopause and use of exogenous estrogens. Cancer Epidemiol Biomarkers Prev 1994; 3:661–668.

48 Persson I, Yuen J, Berkvist L, et al. Cancer incidence and mortality in women receiving estrogen and estrogen-progestin replacement therapy: long-term follow-up of a Swedish cohort. Int J Cancer 1996; 67:327–332.

49 Shaw HM, Milton GW, Farago G, et al. Endocrine influences on survival from malignant melanoma. Cancer 1976; 42:669–677.

50 Mackie RM, Bray CA. Hormone replacement therapy after surgery for Stage 1 or 2 cutaneous melanoma. Br J Cancer 2004; 90:770–772.

51 Mackie RM. Pregnancy and exogenous hormones in patients with cutaneous malignant melanoma. Curr Opin Oncol 1999; 11:129–131.

CHAPTER

21 Genetic Testing for Melanoma

Sancy A Leachman, Katrina Lowstuter and Lisa M Wadge

Key points

- Genetic testing for hereditary melanoma should take place within research protocols to improve data collection and future health outcomes.
- Clinical genetic testing may be successfully performed outside of a research protocol as long as attention is paid to patient selection, education and counseling needs, valid test interpretation and alteration of medical management in the appropriate individuals.
- All patients receiving genetic testing should have pre- and post-test counseling
- Candidates for genetic testing include melanoma patients with a strong (about 10% or more) pre-test probability of having a *p16* mutation.
- Carriers of a pathogenic *p16* mutation should receive aggressive melanoma surveillance and be educated about the risk of pancreatic cancer, including the possibility of participating in pancreatic cancer surveillance programs.

INTRODUCTION

The majority of melanomas seen by practitioners are associated with a combination of environmental and sporadic mutational factors and are not part of a hereditary syndrome. (See Table 21.1 for hereditary and non-hereditary melanoma risk factors.[1–14]) However, about 10% of melanoma presents in familial clusters,[15,16] suggesting that an inherited mutation, a shared environmental exposure, or both, are contributing to pathogenesis (Fig. 21.1). Melanoma patients who fall into this 'familial' category are at 30–70-fold higher risk of developing melanoma than the general population and therefore represent a very high-risk group.[17] Improved methods to identify, screen and prevent melanoma in these high-risk individuals are needed. Genetic testing is one mechanism of identifying a subset of particularly high-risk patients so that additional clinical resources can be devoted to their care, even in fast-paced outpatient practices.

To date, there have been three high penetrance genes definitively associated with hereditary melanoma (for an excellent review, see Hayward 2003).[16] These genes encode cyclin-dependent kinase inhibitor 2A (*CDKN2A, INK4a, MTS1, p16*), cyclin-dependent kinase 4 (*CDK4*) and alternate reading frame protein (*ARF, p14*).[15–17] Of these three, *p16* is currently the major melanoma

susceptibility gene accounting for approximately 20–40% of hereditary melanoma, or approximately 0.2–2% of all melanomas[15–19] (Fig. 21.1). Pathogenic mutations in *p16* are associated with a dramatic increase in the risk for melanoma (up to 76% lifetime risk in the US) and also an increased risk for pancreatic cancer in some families[20–22] (Fig. 21.2). In contrast, mutations in *ARF* and *CDK4* are rare and have been associated with only a handful of hereditary melanoma families.[23–27] At the present time, *p16* remains the major melanoma predisposition gene and this chapter will primarily discuss the role of mutation testing for this gene.

Genetic testing for *p16* is available clinically through several laboratories (*www.genetests.org*).[28] However, availability is only one component in offering a genetic test. When introducing a genetic test into clinical medicine, the fundamental question is whether there is value added by using a genetic as well as a traditional approach to assessment. This question continues to be debated for melanoma genetic testing. There is no governing body that determines when a genetic test is ready for clinical application. Therefore, clinicians are currently responsible for assessing the value of *p16* genetic testing for their patients. The primary goal of this chapter is to identify the major issues associated with clinical *p16* genetic testing and to prepare clinicians to utilize *p16* genetic testing when indicated.

HISTORY

p16 was first identified as a melanoma predisposition gene in 1994[29,30] and has been studied extensively since that time.[31] *p16* is located on chromosome 9p21 and is a tumor suppressor gene that regulates cellular proliferation and growth by inhibiting retinoblastoma phosphorylation and entry into the cell cycle.[31–33] *p16*-associated melanoma is inherited in an autosomal dominant pattern and was identified at approximately the same time as the breast cancer susceptibly genes *BRCA1* and *BRCA2*. However, clinical genetic testing for melanoma has lagged behind that of clinical breast cancer genetic testing, which started in 1996.

There has been controversy about the clinical use of *p16* genetic testing.[17,34–36] The International Melanoma Genetics Consortium advocates that genetic testing for *p16* be conducted only as part of a research protocol. Hansen *et al.*[34] discuss the alternative viewpoint that clinical genetic testing may be successfully performed outside of a research protocol, as long as attention is paid to patient selection, patient education and counseling needs, valid

Table 21.1 Relative risk for developing melanoma*	
Risk factor	**Approximate/estimated relative risk**
Member of melanoma prone family, personal history of melanoma, dysplastic nevi	500[1]
Member of a melanoma prone family, no personal history of melanoma, dysplastic nevi	184[2]
Member of melanoma prone family[a]	Up to 35–70[3]
Previous primary cutaneous melanoma	8.5[4]
Family history of melanoma[b]	2–3[5]
Skin Type I	1.4[6]
Freckling	2–3[6–8]
Blue eyes	1.6[6,7]
Red hair	2.4–4[6,7]
History of blistering sunburn	2–3[6,7]
≥ 6 atypical nevi[c]	6.3[9]
≥10 dysplastic nevi[c,d]	12[10]
100 or more nevi[c]	3.1–16.5[9,11–13]
5 nevi > 5mm[c]	10[14]
≥ 5 nevi on buttocks	10.9[11,14]

*Relative risk indicates degree of increased risk compared to the general population.
[a]Multiple affected relatives on the same side of the family
[b]One or more affected first-degree relatives
[c]Personal history of nevi present without a family history of melanoma
[d]Relative risk in the UK population
(Reproduced with permission from Hansen CG, et al. Clinical genetic testing for melanoma. Lancet Oncol 2004; in press.)

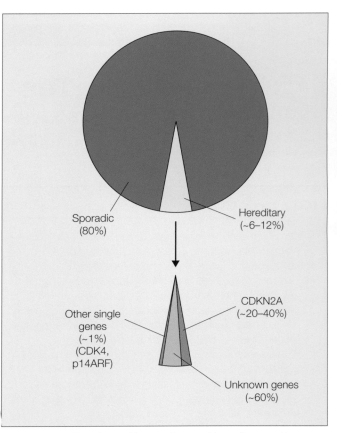

Figure 21.1 Pie chart with prevalence of hereditary melanoma and *p16* mutation in hereditary melanoma. (Adapted with permission from Hansen CG, et al. Clinical genetic testing for melanoma. Lancet Oncol 2004; in press.)

test interpretation and alteration of medical management in the appropriate individuals.

Historically, as genetic tests enter the clinical realm they are evaluated by a set of three specific criteria (established by The American Society of Clinical Oncology, ASCO) in order to determine if clinical use is appropriate.[37,38] These criteria include: (1) the individual has personal or family features suggestive of a genetic cancer susceptibility condition; (2) the test can be adequately interpreted; and (3) the results will aid in diagnosis or influence the medical or surgical management of the patient or family members at hereditary risk of cancer. Hansen *et al*.[34] have reviewed the current status of *p16* genetic testing with regard to ASCO recommendations and have concluded that careful transition of *p16* genetic testing into clinical practice is reasonable.

DESCRIPTION

This chapter focuses on three major issues associated with the transition of *p16* testing into the clinical realm: (1) *p16* genetic testing and ASCO recommendations;

(2) risks and benefits of clinical *p16* genetic testing; and (3) implementation of *p16* genetic testing into clinical practice.

p16 genetic testing and ASCO recommendations

The purpose of the first ASCO criterion is to determine whether individuals can be identified as appropriate candidates for testing based upon personal or family features suggestive of the genetic cancer susceptibility condition. In the case of hereditary melanoma, there are several such subpopulations of melanoma patients that can be identified (Table 21.2). The patient categories listed in Table 21.2 represent specific populations that have a greater than 10% pre-test probability of carrying a *p16* mutation,[17,39–41] a probability previously suggested by ASCO as reasonable for testing.[37] It is important to note that early age of onset and the presence of multiple or atypical nevi without a strong family history of melanoma have not been associated with a greater than 10% pre-test probability of *p16* mutation.[42] Therefore neither young individuals nor individuals with the atypical mole syndrome should be considered for clinical testing at this time unless they also have a personal or family history of melanoma. Accurate identification of patients that qualify as candidates for genetic testing is crucial for appropriate application of the *p16* genetic test.

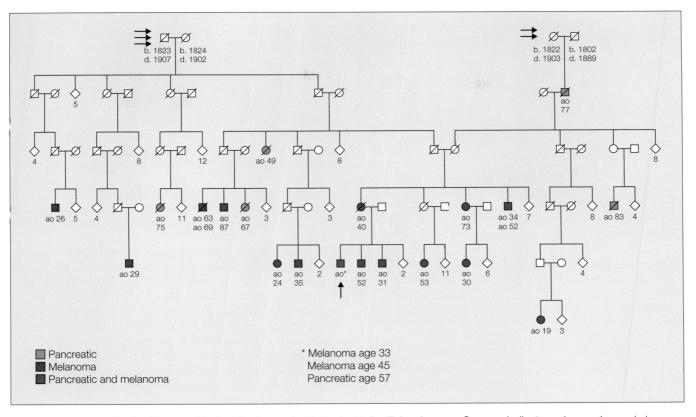

Figure 21.2 Large Utah Melanoma Kindred Pedigree of a kindred with familial melanoma. Squares indicate male members; circles, female members; diamonds a group of unaffected members, with the number of members in each group indicated below each symbol; and slashes, dead. (From Parker JF, Florell SR, Alexander A, et al. Pancreatic carcinoma surveillance in patients with familial melanoma. Arch Dermatol 2003; 139:1019–1025. Copyright © 2003 American Medical Association. All rights reserved.)

ASCO criterion 2 requires that the genetic test be interpretable. CLIA approved *p16* genetic tests are experimentally validated and sequence-based,[28] which is the current 'gold standard' for clinical genetic testing. Thus, *p16* genetic testing is interpretable from a technical perspective. One of three possible results can be expected from *p16* mutation testing. The patient can have no detectable mutation (negative), can have a mutation known to be associated with hereditary melanoma (positive, or pathogenic), or can have a mutation with an undetermined association to hereditary melanoma (uncertain significance). Although interpretation of these test results can be challenging, sufficient data is available to permit good risk estimation.[20,34] By most measures of interpretability and relative to other clinical genetic tests, *p16* can be adequately interpreted in a clinical setting as long as practitioners refer patients to a genetic counselor (or other healthcare provider) trained to explain the results in understandable terms.

The final criterion of ASCO is that the results of genetic testing should have an impact on medical management.[37,38] The lifetime risk to carriers of *p16* mutations appears to be about 53 times that of the general population and 33 times that of non-carriers in *p16* families. In contrast, the lifetime risk to non-carriers in mutation-carrying families appears to be about 1.7-fold higher than the general population.[34] In circumstances where the risk to carriers is dramatically higher than the risk to non-carriers and physician time and money for screening is limited, it is logical to direct increased efforts toward the population at the highest risk. Studies have demonstrated that increased skin cancer screening and surveillance through physician office visits and self-skin examination practices result in earlier detection of thinner melanomas.[43-45] In addition, Robinson et al. have shown that the performance of self-skin examinations is directly correlated with the patient's understanding of personal risk.[44,45] Although further investigation is needed, these data suggest that *p16* mutation carriers will benefit from increased physician screening and aggressive education on prevention and early detection strategies.

It is also becoming apparent that some *p16* mutation carriers may be at an increased risk for pancreatic cancer and they should be educated about this risk and potentially referred to pancreatic cancer surveillance programs.[21,22,46,47] Overall, knowledge of a patient's *p16* mutation status will encourage clinicians to offer improved care to these high-risk melanoma patients.

Risks and benefits to clinical *p16* genetic testing

Organizations such as ASCO recommend that the risks and benefits of genetic testing be thoroughly addressed as part of the pre-test informed consent counseling session. Potential risks involved with *p16* clinical genetic testing include: insurance and employment discrimination, disruption of family relationships, and survivor guilt and false sense of security in non-carriers.[35,36] These

Table 21.2 Features associated with at least a 10% probability of carrying a *p16* mutation

Features	Probability of carrying a *p16* mutation (%)
Melanoma patient with 2 or more family members with melanoma	20–40[3]
Melanoma patient with a family member who has multiple primary melanomas	45[26]
Melanoma patient with a family history of melanoma and pancreatic cancer	45[26]
An individual with multiple primary melanoma, regardless of family history	10–15[27,28]
First-degree relatives of a proven *p16* mutation carrier	≈50
(Reproduced with permission from Hansen CG, et al. Clinical genetic testing for melanoma. Lancet Oncol 2004; in press.)	

concerns are universal to genetic cancer testing and in general have been addressed by the genetic and oncology communities. Experience with other hereditary cancer syndromes suggests that the fear of insurance discrimination may be more perceived than real. Cases of insurance discrimination are largely anecdotal and attempts to quantify them are often limited to measuring behaviors such as eligible patients declining genetic testing based on discrimination fears.[48]

Data also exists regarding the development of a false sense of security in non-carrier individuals. Studies suggest that non-carrier women in hereditary breast cancer families do not appear to develop a false sense of security (as documented by the observation that they generally maintain appropriate screening activities).[49,50] Fortunately, the field of melanoma genetics can benefit from the extensive experience of the genetic and oncology communities to minimize the potential risks prior to testing.

There are also recognized benefits from genetic testing. The benefits to individuals who test positive may include: increased motivation to follow prevention and surveillance strategies, resolution of uncertainty about the etiology of their melanoma and for provision of information to family members. The primary benefit to individuals who test negative (in a family with an established *p16* mutation) is reduction in anxiety for self and children. The risk–benefit profile for *p16* genetic testing must be determined on a case-by-case basis.

Implementation of *p16* genetic testing into clinical practice

Figure 21.3 gives details of the implementation of *p16* genetic testing into clinical practice.

Step 1: Patient selection

Table 21.2 shows the patient populations that should be considered for *p16* genetic testing. It should be emphasized that the subpopulations of melanoma patients detailed in Table 21.2 represent a very small proportion (<2%) of melanoma patients. Furthermore, only an affected member of a family should initially be tested, except in very rare circumstances, because of the difficulty in interpreting a negative test result in an unaffected patient (i.e. such a patient could be a non-carrier in a *p16* mutation family, or either a carrier or non-carrier in a family with a mutation in another gene other than *p16*). If a pathogenic *p16* mutation is confirmed in an affected individual, first-degree relatives become candidates for *p16* testing regardless of their melanoma status.

Genetic testing of minors under the age of 18 has generally been discouraged for adult onset cancer conditions. However, because childhood sunburns play a particularly important role in the pathogenesis of melanoma and because exposure to UV light increases the penetrance of *p16* mutations; an argument can be made for testing children when they are capable of providing assent. Testing of children has the potential to increase compliance with photo-protection and screening strategies during the most vulnerable time of life. This issue needs to be addressed further in the setting of familial melanoma.

Step 2: Informed consent

It is critical that anyone considering *p16* genetic testing in the clinical setting has the ability to provide appropriate counseling and follow-up. In most cases this is accomplished by referral to a trained genetic counselor or an academic institution. Physicians can identify genetic counseling services in their area through *www.nsgc.org/resourcelink.asp* or the National Cancer Institute's website, *www.cancer.gov*. The genetic and oncology communities recommend that informed consent for cancer susceptibility testing be an ongoing process of education and counseling in which providers elicit individual, family and community values. During the consent process, decision making is shared, the style of information disclosure is individualized and specific content areas are discussed. Content areas should include a description of the limitations and burdens of genetic testing, the potential psychological and social implications of learning genetic information and all the risks and benefits discussed in the previous section.

After completion of informed consent each patient should understand the purpose of the test, the logistics of the test and interpretations of the possible results. Possible test results and their interpretation will often differ depending on whether or not a specific gene mutation has been previously identified in the patient's family. Finally, informed consent should also include options for medical follow-up, privacy and confidentiality of test results and alternatives to testing.[51] An example of an informed consent document, containing the recommended elements, is shown in Figure 21.4.

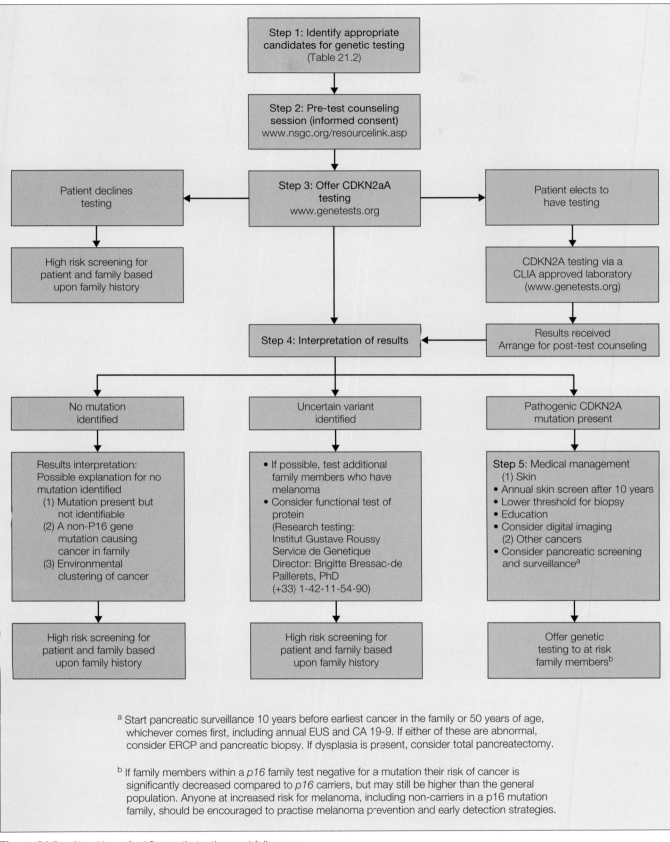

Figure 21.3 Algorithm of *p16* genetic testing and follow-up.

CONSENT TO TEST FOR P16 GENE FOR MELANOMA SUSCEPTIBILITY
UNKNOWN MUTATION

You have requested laboratory testing to look for a gene change that increases the risk for developing melanoma skin cancer, and possibly other types of cancer. The gene that will be analyzed is called p16 (also known as CDKN2A). The genetic test is called DNA sequencing and is done on a blood sample. If you are found to have inherited a mutation in this gene (a change in the gene that makes it work incorrectly), it may help explain why you have developed cancer or may mean that you will develop cancer in the future, although the test cannot usually predict if or when this will happen. You have been counseled regarding the risks, limitations and benefits of knowing your test results and have had your questions answered. Following are some of the key points that have been shared during that discussion:

ABOUT THE TEST
The test is done from a small sample of your blood. Blood is drawn by placing a small needle into a vein in the arm. The risks of blood drawing are minimal and include superficial bruising, bleeding from the site of the puncture, and uneasiness associated with needles. The laboratory used for this test is a clinical laboratory approved by the Clinical Laboratories Improvement Amendment. Every effort is made to assure quality control in the laboratory, but undetected laboratory errors can occur.

POSSIBLE RESULTS OF THE TEST
There are three possible results to this test:

1. A significant mutation is found in the p16 gene. This type of gene change is associated with an increased risk of developing melanoma and possibly pancreatic and nervous system cancers.
2. A change of unknown significance is found in the p16 gene. At this time we do not know whether these types of changes alter the risk of developing melanoma or other cancers.
3. No evidence of a mutation is found in the p16 gene. In this case, it is possible that a) the p16 gene is not functioning properly, but a mutation cannot be detected by the current test; b) there is a gene mutation in another, as yet unidentified, melanoma susceptibility gene; c) that no inherited risk for melanoma is present and the melanomas in you or your family were due to other causes.

RISKS OF THE TEST
In addition to the physical risk of drawing blood, which is described above, there may also be emotional or social risks associated with genetic testing.
☐ Emotional risks include the psychological stress that may come from knowing your DNA results. Finding that you do not carry the gene mutation can produce guilt as well as joy. Finding that you do carry the gene mutation can cause feelings of depression, futility, and distress. Finding that you carry the gene may also cause feelings of guilt about the possibility of passing the mutation on to your children.
☐ Social risks include the possibility of employment or insurance discrimination. Although it is unlikely that a person will be dropped from a current health insurance policy, insurance companies may increase costs of insurance policies for healthy individuals with an identified mutation in one of these genes. In applying for new insurance policies, some people may be asked about the results of any genetic testing. In addition, some policies require that insurance companies be able to access medical records in which test results may be found. However, federal laws such as the Health Insurance Portability and Accountability Act (HIPAA) and state laws such as the Utah genetic privacy law also offer protection from discrimination in health insurance based on genetic information.

LIMITATIONS OF THE TEST
The decision to test this particular gene has been made based on information that you have provided about your personal and family's medical history. If this information is incomplete or inaccurate, the wrong gene may be tested, and negative test results may be falsely reassuring. Also, other genes can cause inherited cancer. It is possible that the cancer in your family is caused by a mutation in a different gene, and in that case, this test will not detect it.

Sometimes testing may be unable to find a mutation in a gene, even when one is present. Therefore, negative test results do not mean that your risk of cancer, specifically melanoma, is zero. In fact, if a mutation is not found, your and your family's risk of cancer would continue to be assessed based on your family and personal history. In addition, test results of uncertain significance can occur, meaning that it is unknown whether or not the change is a true mutation causing an increased risk of cancer.

Our understanding about cancer syndromes and their management is changing rapidly. There is still uncertainty about the medical recommendations for people who have p16 mutations. The p16 gene is just one of many factors influencing melanoma risk, and we are still learning how p16 gene mutations interact with these other factors. The best treatment or prevention options for people who test positive may not yet be known, but when you learn your results, specific current information will also be provided to you.

BENEFITS OF THE TEST
The benefits of testing include better knowledge about your risk of melanoma and possibly pancreatic cancer, and the opportunity to use this information in your future health care planning as we learn more about how to best care for people who carry p16 mutations as well as those who do not (see above limitations to this test). Finding that you carry the gene mutation may help you take measures to prevent cancer or reduce the severity of cancer in the future, such as having more frequent skin examinations with your doctor, checking your own skin more regularly, or limiting your sun exposure.

Figure 21.4 Example of 'Informed Consent Document' for *p16* genetic testing.

(b)

If this test is able to identify an inherited p16 gene mutation in you, other family members would also be at risk for carrying this mutation and testing would be available to identify whether or not they have inherited the mutation or not.

LEARNING YOUR RESULTS
The information obtained from your genetic test will only be told to you by a physician or genetic counselor. Your genetic information will be kept confidential, and no information about your genetic test will be released to anyone without your written permission. We encourage you to share this genetic information with the doctor who will be providing your routine health care.

VOLUNTARY NATURE OF THE TEST
Participation in genetic testing is completely voluntary. Not having this test will involve no penalty or loss of benefits to which you are otherwise entitled. Even after the test is complete, you may choose to not learn your test results, and you will still receive the same standard of care that you otherwise would have received.

FINANCIAL RESPONSIBILITY:
Genetic testing for the p16 gene is $_____ for the first member of your family. If a genetic mutation is found, testing for each additional family member is $_____. _____(Laboratory Name) will bill you directly for the cost of the testing. Your health care plan may not fully cover payment for this testing. You will be personally responsible for paying for the test.

You will be given a copy of this signed and dated consent form.

With the above information, and after having the chance to have all of my questions answered to my satisfaction, I request that my blood be drawn for genetic testing of the p16 melanoma susceptibility gene.

Signature: _____ Witness: _____

Date: _____ Date: _____

Physician's/Counselor's Statement:

I have explained DNA testing to this person. I have addressed the items outlined above, and I have given them the opportunity to have their questions answered.

Signature: _____ Date: _____

Figure 21.4, cont'd.

Step 3: *p16* mutation testing

Once a patient has given informed consent, testing may proceed. Whenever possible, *p16* genetic testing should take place within research protocols to improve data collection and future health outcomes. It is appreciated that this may not always be possible for a variety of logistical reasons. When clinical testing outside a research setting is performed, only CLIA-certified laboratories should be utilized. Such laboratories can be identified at *www.genetests.org*.

Step 4: Result interpretation and post-test counseling

If a *pathogenic mutation* is detected, patients should be counseled using the latest available risk estimation data about their increased risk for melanoma and possibly pancreatic cancer. It should be noted that the confidence intervals for penetrance in *p16* mutation carriers is large, making risk estimation imprecise. Although even the lowest estimates of risk (31–96% by age 80, 95% confidence interval (CI)) are substantially higher than that of the general population,[29] the large range in risk should be addressed in pre- and post-test genetic counseling sessions. The fact that not all *p16* mutation carriers appear to be at risk for pancreatic cancer should

also be discussed.[21] The data demonstrates an increased penetrance seen in *p16* carriers living in UV-rich environments which should be utilized to emphasize the need for future photo protection strategies. Educational materials regarding prevention and early detection should be provided to the patient and follow-up plans should be arranged in conjunction with their physician.

If a *negative result* is obtained, there are three possibilities that should be explained to the patient: (1) a mutation may be present, but is not detectable by the current methodology, (2) a different, non-*p16* mutation is responsible for their hereditary predisposition, or (3) the familial clustering is environmentally induced rather than inherited. If the family history is compelling or the patient is interested in pursuing further testing, *ARF* and/or *CDK4* mutation testing can be considered on a research basis, but this should be done through an established research protocol. At present *CDK4* and *ARF* mutation testing is outside the realm of clinical practice.

If a mutation of *uncertain significance* is detected, additional family members can also be tested to determine if the mutation segregates with melanoma (which would suggest pathogenicity) or does not segregate with melanoma (which would suggest a polymorphism). If the mutation appears to be pathogenic, functional testing of *p16* can be performed on a research basis to evaluate CDK4 binding of *p16*.[52] Despite these options, it is still often impossible to determine whether a mutation of uncertain significance is pathogenic or benign and patients should be made aware of this fact prior to testing.

Step 5: Management of the *p16* mutation carrier

Identified carriers of a pathogenic *p16* mutation should be managed aggressively to prevent and detect melanoma at the earliest stage possible. Mutation carriers should receive total body skin examinations beginning at age 10. Follow-up examinations should be performed every six months until nevi are stable and annually thereafter. The level of surveillance for non-carriers within a *p16* mutation family should be similar to that of other high-risk groups such as patients with red hair or extensive sun exposure but do not require the examination intensity needed for *p16* mutation carriers. However, it should be noted that the International Melanoma Consortium recommends the aggressive surveillance strategy above for all family members regardless of genetic status.[17] In families that may have a mutation in a different (non-*p16*) gene, every member of the family should be treated as if they are a mutation carrier. Additional effort should be made to encourage self-skin examination and sun protection in the *p16* mutation carriers. A lower threshold for biopsy should be considered and the use of longitudinal photography or digital imaging should be used whenever possible in mutation carriers.

All *p16* mutation carriers should be warned of a possible increased risk of pancreatic cancer and should be educated about the early signs and symptoms of the disease. Increased surveillance for pancreatic cancer may be warranted in certain *p16* mutation carriers and includes an annual endoscopic ultrasound (EUS) or spiral CT confirmed by an ERCP when necessary.[21,22,46] Although endoscopic pancreatic cancer screening is aggressive and currently not appropriate or efficacious in the general population, it is reported to be cost-effective in high-risk pancreatic cancer families.[46] Pancreatic cancer screening should only be performed as part of a research protocol or by physicians with expertise in these procedures. Specific recommendations for the management of both mutation positive and negative individuals should continue to emerge from the results of future studies. Clearly, anyone at increased risk for melanoma, including non-carriers in a *p16* mutation family, should be encouraged to practice melanoma prevention and early detection strategies, but *p16* mutation carriers can be targeted to receive the most aggressive surveillance strategies possible.

FUTURE OUTLOOK

Clinical genetic testing for hereditary cancers, such as breast and colon cancer, is proving to be an excellent adjunct to clinical care for patients with a genetic predisposition to these diseases. This is likely to be true for melanoma in the future as well. Historic precedent from

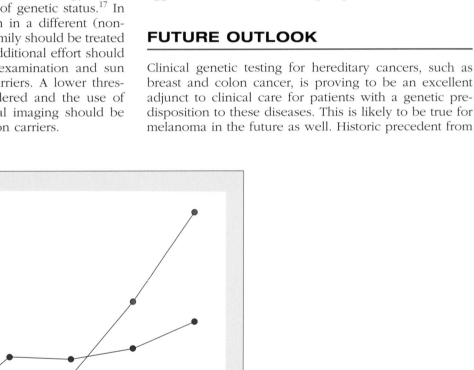

	1996 baseline	1997	1998	1999	2000	2001	2002
Total clinical	10	200	246	580	978	1900	2980
Total research	100	31	88	186	182	203	255

	1997 baseline	1998	1999	2000	2001	2002
Total clinical	10	12	29	49	95	149
Total research	10	28	60	59	66	82

Figure 21.5 Graph detailing relative levels of clinical and research testing at Myriad Genetics, Inc for BRCA 1 and 2 from 1997 to 2002. (Adapted from a presentation by Sancy Leachman MD PhD at the American Academy of Dermatology meeting in 2003.)

hereditary breast and colon cancer indicates that clinical genetic testing for melanoma will proceed despite concerns. Therefore, clinicians should be prepared to identify the appropriate patient populations for genetic testing, to refer those patients for genetic counseling and to consider changes in their management based on mutational status.

The initiation of clinical testing for *BRCA1* and *BRCA2* has led to a dramatic increase in the number of tests performed (Fig. 21.5) and has substantially enhanced the understanding of the gene defect. We predict that initiation of clinical genetic testing for melanoma will have similar beneficial effects, especially in enhancing our understanding of pathogenic mutations versus polymorphisms and in the relationship between *p16* mutations and other cancers. This increased knowledge base will permit improved risk stratification for patients. Furthermore, as test results become available to patients, it is likely to increase participation in ongoing research protocols and clinical trials for this subset of patients. For example, carefully designed clinical trials could be performed to determine the appropriate post-test management of patients. In addition, as increased numbers of patients begin to receive the results of *p16* testing, it will become clear whether this information is helpful in increasing compliance with prevention and early detection strategies in the carriers and in reducing the anxiety felt by non-carriers. Finally, as melanoma chemoprevention trials are initiated, *p16* mutation carriers might prove to be an extremely valuable cohort due to the high rate at which they develop melanoma.

While there is much to learn about the genetics of melanoma, there is currently enough knowledge available to allow clinicians and patients to determine if genetic testing would be beneficial in their unique situation. Furthermore, the potential benefit of clinical genetic testing for melanoma appears to be as great as genetic testing for other hereditary cancer syndromes. Clinical *p16* genetic testing represents a major step forward in the application of molecular medicine to the clinical care of high-risk melanoma patients. For families that carry a *p16* mutation, this test offers them valuable insight into the etiology and pathogenesis of their condition. In the face of imminent clinical availability of *p16* testing, the challenge remains to proceed with caution without losing site of the enormous potential this test may have for the prevention and early detection of a deadly disease.

ACKNOWLEDGMENT

We wish to thank the following for generous support of this work: Huntsman Cancer Foundation and The Tom C Mathews Jr Familial Melanoma Research Clinic. We would like to acknowledge thoughtful contributions from Ken Boucher PhD, University of Utah, Huntsman Cancer Institute and Christopher B Hansen MD, University of Utah Department of Dermatology.

REFERENCES

1 Kraemer KH, Tucker M, Tarone R, Elder DE, Clark WHJ. Risk of cutaneous melanoma in dysplastic nevus syndrome types A and B. N Engl J Med 1986; 315:1615–1616.

2 Greene MH, Clark WH Jr, Tucker MA, Kraemer KH, Elder DE, Fraser MC. The prospective diagnosis of malignant melanoma in a population at high risk: hereditary melanoma and the dysplastic nevus syndrome. Ann Intern Med. 1985; 102:458–465.

3 Goldstein AM, Tucker MA. Genetic epidemiology of familial melanoma. Dermatol Clin 1995; 13:605–612.

4 Tucker MA, Boice JD Jr, Hoffman DA. Second cancer following cutaneous melanoma and cancers of the brain, thyroid, connective tissue, bone, and eye in Connecticut, 1935-82. Natl Cancer Inst Monogr 1985; 68:161–189.

5 Ford D, Bliss JM, Swerdlow AJ, et al. Risk of cutaneous melanoma associated with a family history of the disease. The International Melanoma Analysis Group (IMAGE). Int J Cancer 1995; 62:377–381.

6 Marrett LD, King WD, Walter SD, et al. Use of host factors to identify people at high risk for cutaneous malignant melanoma. Can Med Assoc J 1992; 147: 445–453.

7 Bliss JM, Ford D, Swerdlow AJ, et al. Risk of cutaneous melanoma associated with pigmentation characteristics and freckling: systematic overview of 10 case-control studies. The International Melanoma Analysis Group (IMAGE). Int J Cancer 1995; 62:367–376.

8 Gallagher RP, Elwood JM, Hill GB. Risk factors for cutaneous malignant melanoma: the Western Canada Melanoma Study. Recent Results Cancer Res 1986; 102:38–55

9 Holly EA, Kelly JW, Shpall SN, Chiu SH. Number of melanocytic nevi as a major risk factor for malignant melanoma. J Am Acad Dermatol 1987; 17:459–468

10 Tucker MA, Halpern A, Holly EA, et al. Clinically recognized dysplastic nevi: a central risk factor for cutaneous melanoma. JAMA 1997; 277:1439–1444.

11 Bataille V, Bishop JA, Sasieni P, et al. Risk of cutaneous melanoma in relation to the numbers, types and sites of naevi: a case control study. Br J Cancer 1996; 73:1605–1611.

12 Kanzler MH, Mraz-Gernhard S. Primary cutaneous malignant melanoma and its precursor lesions: Diagnostic and therapeutic overview. J Am Acad Dermatol 2001; 45:260–276.

13 Bataille V, Grulich A, Sasieni P, et al. The association between naevi and melanoma in populations with different levels of sun exposure: a joint case–control study of melanoma in the UK and Australia. Br J Cancer 1998; 77:505–510.

14 Grob H, Gouvernet J, Aymar D, et al. Count of benign melanocytic nevi as a major indicator of risk for non-familial nodular and superficial spreading melanoma. Cancer 1990; 66:387–395.

15 Tucker MA, Goldstein AM. Melanoma etiology: where are we? Oncogene 2003; 22:3042–3052.

16 Hayward NK. Genetics of melanoma predisposition. Oncogene 2003; 22:3053–3062.

17 Kefford RF, Newton Bishop JA, Bergman W, Tucker MA. Counseling and DNA testing for individuals perceived to be genetically predisposed to melanoma: A consensus statement of the Melanoma Genetic Consortium. J Clin Oncol 1999; 17:3245–3251.

18 Piepkorn M. Melanoma genetics: An update with focus on the CDKN2A(p16)/ARF tumor suppressors. J Am Acad Derm 2000; 42:705–722.

19 Aitken J, Welch J, Duffy D, et al. CDKN2A variants in a population-based sample of Queensland families with melanoma. J Natl Cancer Inst 1999; 91(5):446–452.

20 Bishop DT, Demenais F, Goldstein AM, et al. Geographic variation in the penetrance of CDKN2A mutations for melanoma. J Natl Cancer Inst 2002; 94:894–903.

21 Rulyak SJ, Brentnall TA, Lynch HT, Austin MA. Characterization of the neoplastic phenotype in the familial atypical multiple-mole melanoma-pancreatic carcinoma syndrome. Cancer 2003; 98(4):798–804.

22 Parker JF, Florell SR, Alexander A, et al. Pancreatic carcinoma surveillance in patients with familial melanoma. Arch Derm 2003; 139:1019–1025.

23 Zuo L, Weger J, Yang Q, et al. Germline mutations in the p16INK4a binding domain of CDK4 in familial melanoma. Nat Genet 1996; 12:97–99.

24 Soufir N, Avril MF, Chompret A, et al. Prevalence of p16 and CDK4 germline mutations in 48 melanoma-prone families in France. Fr Familial Melanoma Study Group Hum Mol Genet 1998; 7:209–216.

25 Randerson-Moor JA, Harland M, Williams S, et al. A germline deletion of p14(ARF) but not CDKN2A in a melanoma-neural system tumour syndrome family. Hum Mol Genet 2001; 10:55–62.

26 Hewitt C, Lee Wu C, Evans G, et al. Germline mutation of ARF in a melanoma kindred. Hum Mol Genet 2002; 11:1273–1279.

27 Rizos H, Puig S, Badenas C, et al. A melanoma-associated germline mutation in exon 1beta inactivates p14ARF. Oncogene 2001; 20:5543–5547.

28 Genetests (funded by NIH, HRSA and DOE). Available at www.genetests.org. Accessed June 2003.

29 Kamb A, Shattuck-Eidens D, Eeles R, et al. Analysis of the p16 gene (CDKN2) as a candidate for the chromosome 9p melanoma susceptibility locus. Nat Genet 1994; 8:23–26.

30 Hussussian CJ, Struewing JP, Goldstein AM, et al. Germline p16 mutations in familial melanoma. Nat Genet 1994; 8:15–21.

31 Ruas M, Peters G. The p16INK4a/CDKN2A tumor suppressor and its relatives. Biochim Biophys Acta 1998; 1378:F115–F177.

32 Cannon-Albright LA, Goldgar DE, Neuhausen S, et al. Localization of the 9p melanoma susceptibility locus (MLM) to a 2-cM region between D9S736 and D9S171. Genomics 1994; 23(1):265–268.

33 Sviderskaya EV, Gray-Schopfer VC, Hill SP, et al. p16/cyclin-dependent kinase inhibitor 2A deficiency in human melanocyte senescence, apoptosis and immortalization: possible implications for melanoma progression. J Natl Cancer Inst 2003; 95:723–732.

34 Hansen CB, Wadge LM, Lowstuter K, Boucher K, Leachman SA. Clinical genetic testing for melanoma. Lancet Oncol 2004; submitted.

35 Kefford R, Bishop JN, Tucker M, et al. Genetic testing for melanoma. Lancet Oncol 2002; 3:653–654.

36 Kefford RF, Mann GJ. Is there a role for genetic testing in patients with melanoma. Curr Opin Oncol 2003; 15:157–161.

37 Statement of the American Society of Clinical Oncology. Genetic testing for cancer susceptibility. J Clin Oncol 1996; 14:1730–1736.

38 American Society of Clinical Oncology Policy Statement Update. Genetic testing for cancer susceptibility. J Clin Oncol 2003; 21:2003.

39 Mantelli M, Barile M, Ciotti P, et al. High prevalence of the G101W germline mutation in CDKN2A (P16ink4a) gene in 62 Italian malignant melanoma families. Am J Med Genet 2002; 107:214–221.

40 Hashemi J, Platz A, Ueno T, et al. CDKN2A germ-line mutations in individuals with multiple cutaneous melanomas. Cancer Res 2000; 60:6864–6867.

41 Monzon J, Liu L, Brill H, et al. CDKN2A mutations in multiple primary melanomas. N Engl J Med 1998; 338:879–887.

42 Tsao H, Zhang X, Kwitkiwiski K, et al. Low prevalence of germline CDKN2A and CDK4 mutations in patients with early-onset melanoma. Arch Derm 2000; 136:1118–1122.

43 Carli P, Giorgi V De, Palli D, et al. Dermatologist detection and skin self-examination are associated with thinner melanomas: results from a survey of the Italian Multidisciplinary Group on Melanoma. Arch Derm 2003; 139:607–612.

44 Robinson JK, Fisher SG, Turrisi RJ. Predictors of skin self-examination performance. Cancer 2002; 95:135–146.

45 Robinson JK, Rigel DS, Amonette RA. What promotes skin self-examination? J Am Acad Derm 1998; 38:752–757.

46 Rulyak SJ, Kimmey MB, Veenstra DL, Brentnall TA. Cost-effectiveness of pancreatic cancer screening in familial pancreatic cancer kindreds. Gastrointest Endosc 2003; 57:23–29.

47 Goldstein AM, Fraser MC, Struewing JP. Increased risk of pancreatic cancer in melanoma-prone kindreds with p16INK4 mutations. N Engl J Med 1995; 333:970–974.

48 Peterson E, Milliron KJ, Lewis KE, et al. Health insurance and discrimination concerns and BRCA 1/2 testing in a clinic population. Cancer Epidemiology. Biomarkers Prev 2002; 11:79–87.

49 Botkin JR, Smith KR, Croyle RT, et al. Genetic testing for a BRCA1 mutation: Prophylactic surgery and screening behavior in women 2 years post testing. Amer J Med Gen 2003; 118A:201–209.

50 Peshkin BN, Schwartz MD, Isaacs C, et al. Utilization of breast cancer screening in a clinically based sample of women after BRCA1/2 testing. Cancer Epidemiol Biomarkers Prev 2002; 11:1115–1118.

51 Geller G, Botkin JR, Green MJ, et al. Genetic testing for susceptibility to adult-onset cancer. The process and content of informed consent. JAMA 1997; 277:1467–1474.

52 Institut Gustave Roussy Service de Genetique. Contact Bridgitte Bressac-de Paillerets. Accessed. Institut Gustave Roussy Service de Genetique; 2003.

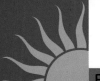

CHAPTER

22 Adnexal Cancers of the Skin

Babar Rao and Rebecca Lintner

Key points

- Rare tumors that arise in the four subtypes of skin appendages.
- Due to the rarity of these tumors, many are misdiagnosed as more common skin cancers.
- Treatment includes wide local excision or Mohs surgery.
- Follow up extremely important due to the tendency of the neoplasms to recur.

INTRODUCTION

Adnexal carcinomas are rare tumors that arise in the four subtypes of skin appendages, namely, the hair, eccrine glands, apocrine glands and sebaceous glands. The tumors may arise *de novo* or may occur secondary to malignant transformation within their benign counterpart. Due to the rarity of such tumors (many with less than 100 reported cases), it is possible that many are misdiagnosed as more common skin cancers such as basal cell carcinomas and squamous cell carcinomas. When viewing such questionable lesions it is important for the pathologist to consider an adnexal neoplasm due to the high rate of local recurrence, local invasion and capability of visceral metastases. Diagnosis is made in most cases by biopsy. The main differential diagnoses are that of basal cell carcinoma and of cutaneous metastases from another cancer. In order to rule out metastatic adnexal carcinoma, clinical correlation may be necessary. For some subtypes, special histopathologic staining may be helpful. Treatment for adnexal carcinoma includes wide local excision or Mohs surgery. Follow-up is extremely important due to the tendency of the neoplasms to recur. For the more aggressive tumors, lymph node dissection and screening for metastatic disease may be advisable. Due to the small number of reported metastatic cases, there exists few protocols for the treatment of metastatic disease.

TUMORS ARISING FROM HAIR APPENDAGEAL STRUCTURES

Carcinomas arising from the hair follicle are exceedingly rare. The tumors are related to benign counterparts and often arise via malignant transformation. A few carcinomas arising in hair follicles arise *de novo*. The majority of the neoplasms are aggressive and may metastasize both regionally and to distant organ sites.

Pilomatrix carcinoma

The pilomatrix carcinoma is a rare malignant counterpart of pilomatrixoma that may be locally aggressive or metastatic. There are about 63 well-documented cases of pilomatrix carcinoma.[1] The pilomatrix carcinoma may arise either from malignant transformation of its benign counterpart, the pilomatricoma, or may arise *de novo*.[2] Malignant transformation in pilomatricomas was not described until 1980, when Lopansri and Mihm reported what they claimed to be the first case of malignant pilomatrixoma.[3] These authors created the term *pilomatrix carcinoma* or *calcifying epitheliocarcinoma of Malherbe* to describe the lesions. Clinically, the pilomatrix carcinoma is locally aggressive and has a tendency to recur. Distant metastases often to the lungs have been reported.[4,5]

Clinically the tumor is a deep firm nodule that is covered with normal skin. Occasionally it can be superficial, either occurring as a blue-red/dark red nodule with or without ulceration (Fig. 22.1).

The differentiation of these tumors from benign pilomatricomas depends on the careful review of microscopic features, which may or may not be identifiable in individual biopsy specimens.[6] Since both pilomatricoma and pilomatrix carcinoma may exhibit increased mitotic activity, the architectural features on scanning magnification are often useful in diagnosis.[7] Histologically the tumor has numerous large anaplastic hyperchromatic basal cells with numerous mitoses which are most evident at the periphery.[3] The central portion of the tumor may resemble the benign counterpart with eosinophilic shadow cells.[8] The center may also contain areas of necrotic debris.[9] DNA content flow cytometry of an isolated pilomatrix carcinoma show neither aneuploid peaks nor high proliferative fractions (Figs 22.2, 22.3).[6]

The differential diagnosis of pilomatrix carcinoma includes basal cell carcinoma with matrical differentiation, which has several features in common with both pilomatrix carcinoma and its benign counterpart, the pilomatricoma. These tumors typically present in the sixth to seventh decade of life and are composed histologically of aggregates of 'shadow' cells intermingled with relative monomorphic basaloid cells with peripheral palisading of nuclei, cystic spaces filled with fibrinous material, retraction spaces between the neoplastic lobules and the stroma and a desmoplastic stroma surrounding the tumor nests.[10,11]

Treatment of the pilomatrix carcinoma involves wide excision of the tumor as well as close follow-up due to their tendency to recur. Currently, other treatment modalities such as radiation or chemotherapy have not been widely used.

Malignant proliferating trichilemmal tumor

Malignant transformation of a proliferating trichilemmal cyst is a rare occurrence. Although the proliferating trichilemmal cyst is a locally aggressive tumor and may be potentially malignant, malignant transformation and distant metastasis are unusual.[12] Malignant transformation is indicated by rapid enlargement of the tumor.[13] Metastasis tends to be to regional lymph nodes, but reports of generalized metastasis do exist, most of which have led to a fatal outcome.[14–16]

Clinically the tumors have a 3:1 female predominance and occur most commonly on the scalp, followed by the trunk (Figs 22.4, 22.5).[12] They can grow into a large lobulated mass that may ulcerate and thus can resemble a squamous cell carcinoma.

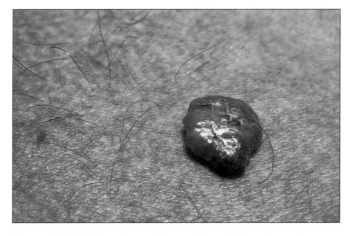

Figure 22.1 Pilomatrix carcinoma. Superficial erythematous nodule with smooth overlying skin. (Image courtesy of New York University Department of Dermatology.)

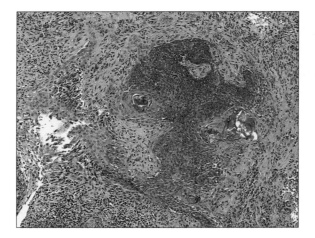

Figure 22.2 Pilomatrix carcinoma, low magnification. Large anaplastic tumor with basaloid cells in the middle, and eosinophilic (shadow) cells at the periphery. (Image courtesy of Dr Jag Bhawan, Boston University Dermatology Department.)

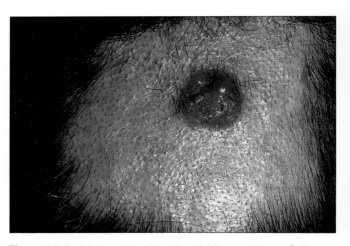

Figure 22.4 Malignant proliferating trichilemmal tumor. Solitary erythematous nodule on scalp. (Image courtesy of New York University Department of Dermatology.)

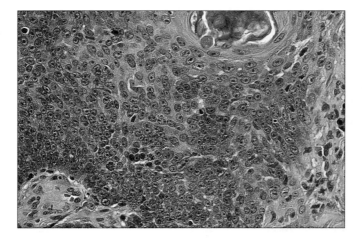

Figure 22.3 Pilomatrix carcinoma, high magnification. Numerous mitosis in hyperchromatic basaloid cells. (Image courtesy of Dr Jag Bhawan, Boston University Dermatology Department.)

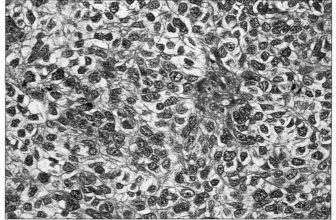

Figure 22.5 Malignant proliferating trichilemmal tumor, high magnification. Clear glycogenitated cells with atypical and mitotic areas. (Image courtesy of Dr Jag Bhawan, Boston University Dermatology Department.)

Histologically, the tumor shows severe atypia with invasion of surrounding tissue.[13] These tumors should be treated with wide local excision and close follow up (Fig. 22.6).

Trichilemmal carcinoma

Trichilemmal carcinoma originates from the external root sheath of the hair follicle and is the malignant form of the trichilemmoma. It often arises on the face of elderly individuals in areas of sun exposure. It is a solitary fixed nodule that may ulcerate.[17] Reports of trichilemmal carcinoma arising in preexisting lesions such as burn scars and solar keratoses have been reported.[18,19] Clinically, the lesion may resemble a squamous cell carcinoma, basal cell carcinoma, nodular amelanotic melanoma or keratoacanthoma (Fig. 22.7).[20]

Histologically, the tumor is usually invasive and contains atypical cells filled with a clear glycogenated cytoplasm demonstrating peripheral palisading and hyaline basement membranes. There are foci of trichilemmal keratinization and cytologic atypia is widespread (Fig. 22.8).[21] In a study of DNA flow cytometry aneuploidy was found in 9 out of 10 lesions.[22]

The tumor generally has an indolent course and wide excision is recommended and shown to be curative.[17]

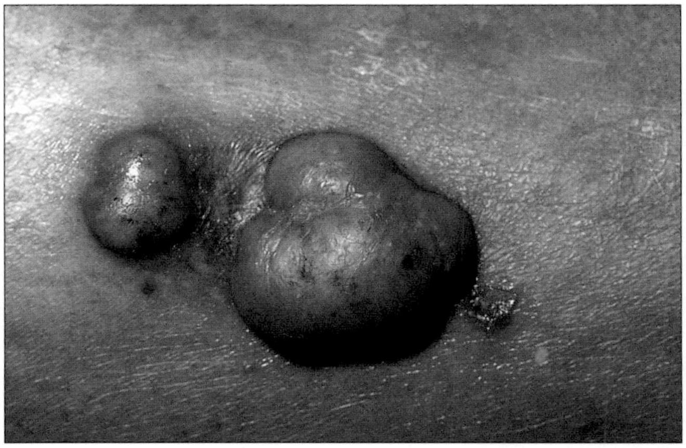

Trichoblastic carcinoma

The term 'trichoblastic' carcinoma was coined by Regauer et al. to describe an aggressively behaving malignant trichogenic tumor arising in a trichoblastoma.[23] The tumor is exceedingly rare and few cases are reported in the literature.[24–26] Clinically the tumor has been reported as a deep dermal nodule which may present with rapid enlargement and pain (Fig. 22.9).[27]

Histologically tumors contain solid and lobular proliferations of small basaloid cells with focal nuclear pleomorphism and large, round nuclei surrounding preexisting trichogenic structures and spindle cell proliferations in sweeping fascicles or tightly packed

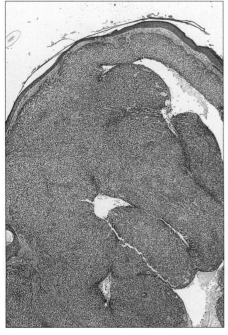

Figure 22.6 Trichilemmal carcinoma. Firm, skin-colored nodules. (Image courtesy of New York University Department of Dermatology.)

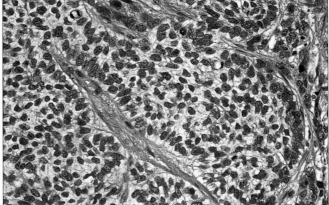

Figure 22.8 Trichilemmal carcinoma, high magnification. Small, clear cells with atypia and peripheral basaloid cells. (Image courtesy of Dr Jag Bhawan, Boston University Dermatology Department.)

Figure 22.7 Trichilemmal carcinoma, low magnification. Large endophytic proliferation of small clear cells. (Image courtesy of Dr Jag Bhawan, Boston University Dermatology Department.)

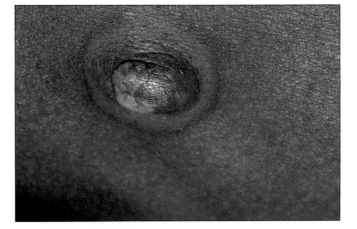

Figure 22.9 Trichoblastic carcinoma. A firm dermal nodule. (Image courtesy of New York University Department of Dermatology.)

nests. The neoplasm can be highly vascularized with extensive hemorrhagic cystic necrosis. Abundant regular and pathologic mitoses as well as apoptotic cells may be observed.[27] Histologic differential diagnosis includes basal cell carcinoma.

The tumor is highly aggressive and by all reports has infiltrated local structures at the time of diagnosis.[26,27]

TUMORS ARISING FROM ECCRINE ADNEXAL STRUCTURES

Many of the following neoplasms arise from their benign counterpart.

Malignant eccrine poroma/ porocarcinoma

This neoplasm was first described in 1963 by Pinkus and Mehregan as a glycogen rich malignant tumor.[28] The eccrine porocarcinoma is the most common eccrine carcinoma and constitutes approximately half of all eccrine adenocarcinomas.[29] Approximately 50% of eccrine porocarcinomas arise via malignant transformation in pre-existing poromas. Clinically they may resemble squamous cell carcinoma, basal cell carcinoma, malignant melanoma, granuloma pyogenicum or an unusual nevus (Fig. 22.10).[30] The tumor usually occurs on the legs or feet of older adults and may appear as a localized nodule, verrucous neoplasm, or ulceration, or may extend into the surrounding epidermis.[28,31] Occasionally, the tumor may be associated with visceral metastases most often to the lung and lymph nodes, but breast, ureter, uterus, bladder, long bones, visceral lymphatic metastases and peritoneal seedlings have been reported.[28,32]

Histologically, the tumor is composed of anaplastic cells with hyperchromatic nuclei and multiple mitoses. The tumor forms duct-like lumina with Alcian blue reactive acid mucopolysaccharide within the duct-like structures (Figs 22.11, 22.12). The cells do not demonstrate palisading,

which may help to differentiate from basal cell carcinoma.[33]

The eccrine porocarcinoma is an aggressive tumor. Treatment involves wide local excision and evaluation of metastasis to nodes and visceral organs. A new therapeutic protocol using isotretinoin and (alpha)-interferon has recently been introduced for the treatment of metastatic porocarcinoma and has proven to be promising.[34–36]

Malignant eccrine spiradenoma

Malignant eccrine spiradenoma usually arises in a preexisting benign eccrine spiradenoma that has been present for an average of at least twenty years. The tumor has been reported in head and neck region, the lower extremities, the torso, the upper extremities and the labia (in females). Most occur in the sixth and seventh decades of life. Clinically the tumor may present with

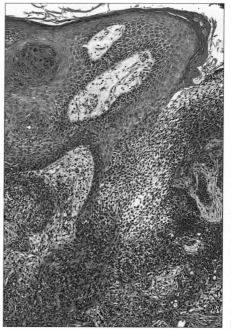

Figure 22.11 Malignant eccrine poroma, low magnification. Large trabeculated tumor composed of vacuolated and basaloid cells. (Image courtesy of Dr Jag Bhawan, Boston University Dermatology Department.)

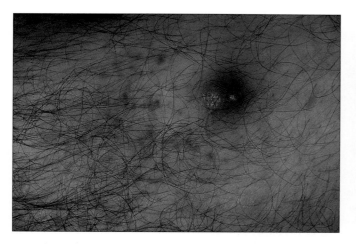

Figure 22.10 Malignant eccrine poroma. Slightly erythematous/ pigmented nodule. (Image courtesy of New York University Department of Dermatology.)

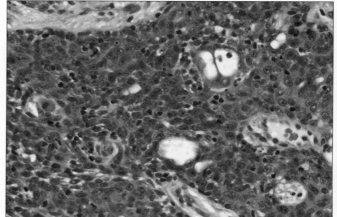

Figure 22.12 Malignant eccrine poroma, high magnification. Ductal differentiation and atypical cells with mitosis. (Image courtesy of Dr Jag Bhawan, Boston University Dermatology Department.)

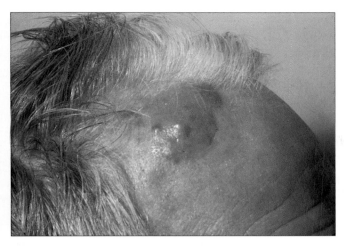

Figure 22.13 Malignant eccrine spiradenoma. Firm, solitary nodule on scalp. (Image courtesy of New York University Department of Dermatology.)

pain and enlargement of an existing lesion, often a solitary intradermal nodule (Fig. 22.13). A large percentage of tumors have local occurrences but lethal metastases have been reported.[37]

Histologically, the malignant elements of the tumor may merge with those of a benign eccrine spiradenoma. In some tumors, the malignant elements demonstrate a lobular, nested and trabecular growth pattern, ductal differentiation and associated ectatic vascular spaces mimicking some of the features seen in benign spiradenoma. The tumor shows two distinctive morphologic patterns. In the first, malignant features are easily detectable at low power and include a sheetlike growth pattern, loss of normal lobular architecture and variable necrosis. In the second, loss of the dual cell population, variable pleomorphism and frequent mitoses are seen at a high power, but at lower power the tumor resembles a benign spiradenoma. Additional histologic features may include squamous morulus, oncocyte-like features, sarcomatous changes and conspicuous myxoid stroma.[38–40]

Treatment currently involves wide local excision and close follow up, although tumor shrinkage with hormonal therapy in patients with estrogen receptor-positive tumors have been reported.[41]

Malignant nodular hidradenoma

Malignant nodular hidradenomas are rare and most often arise *de novo*, although transformation of nodular hidradenoma into its malignant counterpart has been reported.[42] The tumor is highly aggressive, tends to invade the surrounding tissue and has a high incidence of distant metastases.[43] Clinically the tumor present as an intradermal nodule on the head, trunk or extremities. The tumors often arise in middle-aged adults, but cases in adolescents have been reported.[44]

Histologically, the tumor is asymmetrical and invades into the surrounding tissue occasionally with invasion into surrounding vessels or lymphatics.[43] The ill-defined, epithelial neoformation, is formed by lobules of clear polygonal cells at the deep dermis and subcutaneous

tissue; groups of cells with a basaloid aspect may exist and may be mildly atypical.[44]

Since the tumor is highly aggressive and has the capability of fatal metastases, wide excision and lymph node dissection is recommended.

Malignant chondroid syringoma

Malignant chondroid syringoma most often arises *de novo*, but cases of malignant transformation of benign chondroid syringomas have been reported.[44] The tumor is most often located on the extremities and the torso of middle-aged adults with an approximate 2:1 female-to-male ratio. The tumor is often noticed after a period of rapid growth and is highly aggressive. Approximately half of the reported tumors have metastasized to regional lymph nodes and almost one-half have been reported to have distant metastases.[45]

Histologically, the tumor is composed of gland-like elements with two or more rows of cuboidal cells morphologically within a matrix of varying appearance showing basophilic chondroid substance, foamy material, or eosinophilic hyaline material.[46] Malignancy is indicated by cellular pleomorphism, mitoses, islands of tumor cells, necrosis and invasion into surrounding tissues.[46]

The treatment of choice is wide surgical excision, evaluation for metastases and postoperative external beam radiation therapy for metastatic lesions.[46]

The following eccrine-derived carcinomas arise *de novo* and have no benign counterpart. These tumors are locally aggressive and have a tendency to recur. In some subtypes, visceral metastases has been reported, but are rare. Regional node metastases are also reported for some subtypes, but they too are uncommon.

Syringoid eccrine carcinoma

Syringoid eccrine carcinoma was first described in 1969 as a basal-cell tumor with eccrine differentiation. The tumors usually present as an asymptomatic nodule or plaque either on the head or extremities in middle-aged adults.[47] The tumors are locally invasive and recurrence is common but metastases are rare.[48]

Histologically syringoid eccrine carcinoma is characterized by dermal invasion of a tubulocystic proliferation with a dense fibrovascular stroma. In some cases, the tumor extends into the subcutaneous tissues. Perineural infiltration, mitotic activity and nuclear pleomorphism indicate the neoplasm's malignancy. It contains ductal, cystic and comma-like epithelial elements like the benign syringoma. Eccrine enzymes such as phosphorylase and succinic dehydrogenase are found on histochemical staining.[49,50] The most difficult differential diagnosis is the differentiation of syringoid eccrine carcinoma from cutaneous metastases of some adenocarcinomas. Immunohistochemical features are not useful in making this differentiation. When differentiating the tumor from adenoid basal-cell carcinoma, the expression of CEA indicates that the tumor is a sweat gland neoplasm.[50]

Treatment includes wide local excision and close follow-up for recurrence.

Microcystic adnexal carcinoma

Microcystic adnexal carcinoma is a locally aggressive tumor that most commonly arises in middle-aged adults, but cases in ages from 20–76 years have been reported.[51] It usually presents as a pale yellow nodule or plaque with ill-defined borders. It grows slowly and may take as many as 30 years to evolve.[52] It is commonly found in the nasolabial and periorbital areas of the face. Other reported locations include the axilla, buttock and scalp (Figs 22.14–22.16).[52,53] The tumor is locally aggressive with dermal invasion as well as infiltration of subcutaneous tissue and skeletal muscle. Perineural invasion is common.[54] Local recurrence is also common and has been reported in up to 40% of patients. Metastatic disease has not been reported, however one case of regional lymph node involvement has been noted due to direct extension of the tumor.[52]

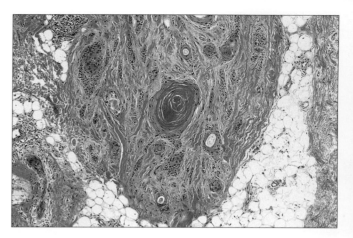

Figure 22.16 Microcystic adnexal carcinoma, high magnification. Nests and cords of small dark cells invading deep into subcutaneous tissue. (Image courtesy of Dr Jag Bhawan, Boston University Dermatology Department.)

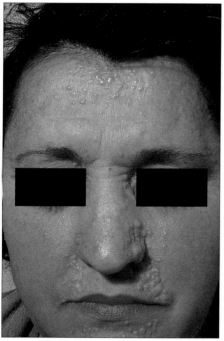

Figure 22.14 Microcystic adnexal carcinoma. A pale plaque with ill-defined borders. (Image courtesy of New York University Department of Dermatology.)

Histologically the tumor is composed of epithelial islands or nests in an eosinophilic, fibrotic stroma, which infiltrate the surrounding dermis and often the subcutaneous tissue. Perineural invasion is common. The upper dermis contains prominent keratinous cysts with ducts and gland-like structures in the middle and deep areas. Areas of ductal differentiation are also present.[55,56] The glandular structures of the tumor stain positive for carcinoembryonic antigen.[57] The tumor is likely to be confused with benign eccrine tumors such as desmoplastic trichoepithelioma, trichoadenoma, syringoma and morpheaform basal cell carcinoma.[56]

Currently, the recommended treatment is removal by Mohs microscopic surgery with close follow-up for recurrence.[58] Primary or postoperative radiotherapy has not been shown to reduce the recurrence rate.[56]

Mucinous adenocystic (eccrine) carcinoma

Mucinous adenocystic (eccrine) carcinoma was first described in 1971 as a primary mucinous carcinoma of the eccrine glands.[59] The tumor presents clinically as either a superficial raised nodule or a subcutaneous lesion. The tumor is most often located in the eyelid but may also be found on other areas of the face or scalp.[60] Lesions on the vulva have been reported.[61] The tumor most often arises in males aged 50–70. It has a tendency to locally recur, but metastases are very rare (Fig. 22.17).[62]

Histologically, the tumor is composed of cords, nests and ducts of light and dark staining epithelial cells separated by clear mucin containing areas.[63] Cells are strongly positive for periodic acid-Schiff stain and for Alcian blue at pH 2.5. The mucinous material is resistant to diastase and hyaluronidase but is sensitive to digestion with sialidase. These findings indicate that the mucinous material is most likely sialomucin.[64]

The major differential diagnosis that must be considered is that of metastatic carcinoma from the breast, gastrointestinal tract, ovary and lung. Both clinical and

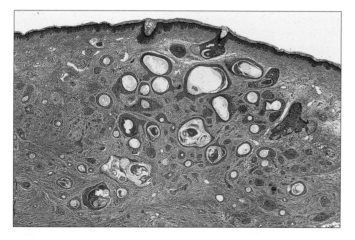

Figure 22.15 Microcystic adnexal carcinoma, low magnification. Large, deep tumor with nests and cysts containing light and dark cells. (Image courtesy of Dr Jag Bhawan, Boston University Dermatology Department.)

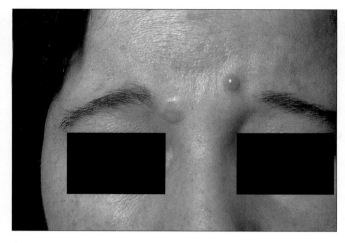

Figure 22.17 Mucinous adenocystic (eccrine) carcinoma. Superficial skin-colored nodule. (Image courtesy of New York University Department of Dermatology.)

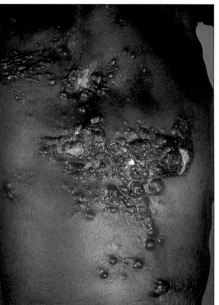

Figure 22.18 Adenoid cystic carcinoma. Multiple smooth papules and nodules on chest. (Image courtesy of New York University Department of Dermatology.)

histopathologic data are useful in this differentiation. Metastatic disease often has more atypical cells and is usually found between collagen bundles at the margin of the nodule.[65] It is also more common for metastases from carcinomas of the large intestine to involve the anterior abdominal wall and for metastases of the breast to involve the anterior chest wall.[66] Histochemically, metastatic gastrointestinal carcinomas are usually positive with Alcian blue stain at pH 1 and 0.4 whereas mucinous adenocystic (eccrine) carcinoma reacts positively with Alcian blue stain at pH 2.5 but not at pH 1 or 0.4.[63]

Treatment of mucinous adenocystic (eccrine) carcinoma involves wide local excision and close follow-up for recurrence. Both mammography and colonoscopy should be considered to rule out metastatic disease from the breast or colon.

Adenoid cystic carcinoma

Primary cutaneous adenoid cystic carcinomas were first described by Boggio in 1975.[67] The tumors are exceedingly rare with less than 50 reported in the literature.[68] The tumor appears most often on the scalp of middle-aged to elderly adults with an increased female incidence (Fig. 22.18).[69] The tumor has a high local recurrence rate.[70] Metastases are uncommon but have been reported both to local lymph nodes and to distant sites such as the lung.[71–73]

Histologically, primary cutaneous adenoid cystic carcinoma is composed of basaloid cells with round hyperchromatic nuclei and small amounts of cytoplasm. The tumor invades the dermis and subcutaneous tissue with variable cribriform, tubular, cystic and solid patterns of growth. Nuclear atypia is not prominent. Cylinders and eosinophilic globules are often observed and perineural invasion is common.[74] Histologically, the tumor must be differentiated from adenoid basal cell carcinoma which displays peripheral palisading as well as lack of epidermal continuity.[75]

Reports of immunohistochemical data for the tumor differ. In a recent review by Kato *et al.* neoplastic cells were positive for keratin and S-100 protein in 67 to 83% of reported cases and carcinoembryonic antigen stain has been reported to be positive in half of reported cases.[75]

Treatment involves wide local excision and close follow-up for recurrence. Microscopically controlled surgery has also been used as a treatment modality.[76] Radiotherapy is reported to aid in local control of the tumor in other organs.[77] Thus, this approach may be applicable to lesions of cutaneous origin. Combination chemotherapy with adriamycin and cisplatin has been effective in the treatment of metastatic disease.[78]

Aggressive digital papillary adenocarcinoma

Aggressive digital papillary adenocarcinoma is a rare tumor that is frequently misdiagnosed. They were first described by Helwig in 1984.[79] The tumor commonly affects middle-aged white males. Clinically they present as a solitary, slowly enlarging nodule usually on the volar surface of a digit, between the nailbed and the interphalangeal joint. Tumors on the palm, toe, sole, calf and webspace have been reported. Occasionally the lesions become tender, ulcerate and bleed. Local recurrence is common and metastatic disease can occur. Most metastases are to the lung and may result in death.[80]

Histologically the tumor has a mixed tubuloalveolar and papillary pattern with a fibrocollagenous stroma and focal squamous metaplasia (Fig. 22.19). Kao *et al.* indicate that increased cellular atypia, mitotic activity, bone invasion and tumor necrosis correspond with more aggressive behavior.[81] Duke *et al.*, in a review of 67 case reports of aggressive digital papillary adenocarcinoma and the low grade aggressive digital papillary adenoma, found that the criteria defined by Kao did not predict tumor behavior. They concluded that the distinction be-

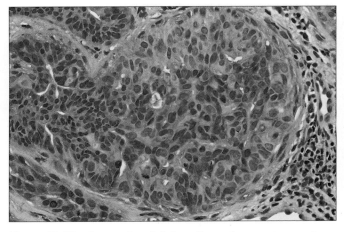

Figure 22.19 Aggressive digital papillary adenocarcinoma. An area with lobular and papillary pattern and focal squamous metaplasia. (Image courtesy of Dr Jag Bhawan, Boston University Dermatology Department.)

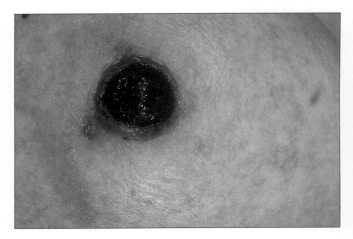

Figure 22.20 Mucoepidermoid (low grade adenosquamous carcinoma). An erythematous ulcerated mucous nodule. (Image courtesy of New York University Department of Dermatology.)

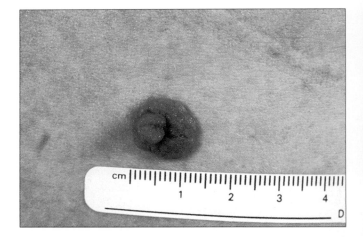

Figure 22.21 Apocrine carcinoma. A firm erythematous nodule. (Image courtesy of New York University Department of Dermatology.)

tween aggressive digital papillary adenoma and adenocarcinoma could not reliably be made on a histologic basis and therefore there was no low grade counterpart of the adenosarcoma.[81] Clinical correlation is necessary to rule out metastatic adenocarcinoma, particularly of the breast, colon, or thyroid but it should be noted that it is unusual for an invasive papillary breast carcinoma to metastasize.[82]

Treatment involves wide local excision as well as work up for possible metastatic disease. Aggressive surgical therapy for limited metastatic disease may be beneficial but no effective treatment for extensive metastatic disease exists at this time.

Mucoepidermoid (low-grade adenosquamous carcinoma)

Mucoepidermoid carcinomas occur most commonly in salivary glands, but rare reports of primary cutaneous lesions have been reported (Fig. 22.20).[83] The tumors are composed of various proportions of both mucus-secreting cells and epidermoid-type cells. Mohs micrographic surgery, or surgical excision are the treatments of choice.

TUMORS ARISING FROM APOCRINE ADNEXAL STRUCTURES

Apocrine carcinoma

Apocrine gland carcinoma originates from either normal or modified apocrine glands (ceruminous and Moll). Normal apocrine glands are located most commonly in the axilla, medial aspect of the upper arm and lateral breast.[84] The majority of reported cases of apocrine carcinoma are located in the axillae, followed by the anogenital region. Rare cases of apocrine gland carcinoma has been reported in the scalp, lip, ear, eyelid, trunk, foot, toe and finger (Fig. 22.21).[85–87] Clinically, the lesion is an asymptomatic indolent skin-colored firm or cystic nodule. The tumor has a high rate of local recurrence and reports of rare lymph node invasion and widespread metastases do exist.[88,89]

Histologically apocrine carcinoma may range from poorly differentiated to well differentiated.[90] Tumor cells are larger than normal apocrine cells and may contain iron-positive granules within the cytoplasm. Poorly differentiated tumors demonstrate poor glandular formation but varying degrees of differentiation may be seen within the same tumor. Glandular patterns include papillary, complex glandular, anastomosing tubular, solid cellular sheets and cord-like infiltration with desmoplasia (Figs 22.22, 22.23). Apocrine carcinoma must be differentiated from other more common benign and malignant forms of sweat gland neoplasms, such as metastatic breast carcinoma, metastatic disease from other sites, melanoma, lymphoma, benign apocrine disease/neoplasm, or ectopic benign breast tissue. The presence of mature apocrine glands high in the dermis, with a transitional zone between normal glands and the presence of intracytoplasmic iron granules may help to distinguish apocrine carcinoma.[91]

Additional histologic criteria that may differentiate apocrine carcinoma include decapitation secretion, periodic acid-Schiff-positive diastase-resistant material in the cells or lumenae and immunoreactivity with gross cystic disease fluid protein 15.[88]

Initial diagnosis may include a core biopsy or fine-needle aspiration of the tumor, followed by wide local excision. Mohs micrographic surgery may be effective in small lesions such as those on the finger or eyelid. The role of either lymphadenectomy or adjuvant therapy has not been adequately addressed in the literature. Chamberlin *et al.* suggest the consideration of adjuvant radiotherapy if the tumor is unusually large (>5 cm), the margins of resection are positive or close (<1 cm), or the tumor is moderately to poorly differentiated or exhibits other aggressive histologic characteristics such as vascular or lymphatic invasion. They also suggest adjuvant radiotherapy to the draining lymph node basin if there is evidence of extensive lymph node involvement (>4 lymph nodes).[92]

TUMORS ARISING FROM SEBACEOUS GLANDS

Sebaceous carcinoma

Sebaceous carcinoma is a rare, aggressive, malignant tumor derived from the adnexal epithelium of sebaceous glands.[92] Sebaceous carcinomas are divided into two main variants, ocular and extraocular. Clinically, ocular sebaceous carcinoma is a more aggressive tumor with a higher rate of metastases.[93] Extraocular sebaceous carcinomas are uncommon and comprise only about 25% of reported cases of sebaceous carcinomas.[94] They are found mostly on the head and neck, where the sebaceous glands are most numerable. Cases of tumors on the external genitalia, foot, trunk and hand have been reported.[95–98] Clinically the tumor occurs in older adults with a wide range in size. It usually presents as a pink to red nodule that may bleed (Figs 22.24, 22.25).[94,99] Tumors are aggressive and have a tendency to recur.

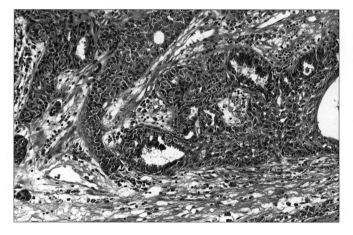

Figure 22.22 Apocrine carcinoma, low magnification. Anaplastic, lobulated and glandular tumor with apocrine differentiation and hyperchromatic/atypical cells. (Image courtesy of Dr Jag Bhawan, Boston University Dermatology Department.)

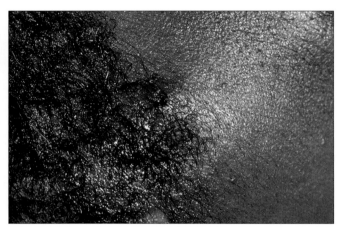

Figure 22.24 Sebaceous carcinoma. Erythematous indurated plaque. (Image courtesy of New York University Department of Dermatology.)

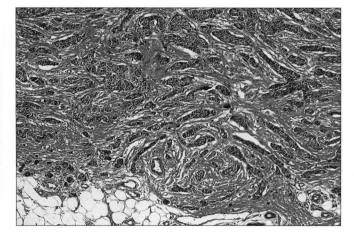

Figure 22.23 Apocrine carcinoma, high magnification. Deep invasion by glandular cords and sheets and desmoplasia. (Image courtesy of Dr Jag Bhawan, Boston University Dermatology Department.)

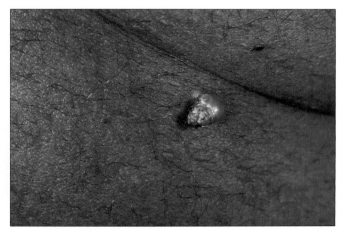

Figure 22.25 Sebaceous carcinoma. An ulcerated firm nodule. (Image courtesy of New York University Department of Dermatology.)

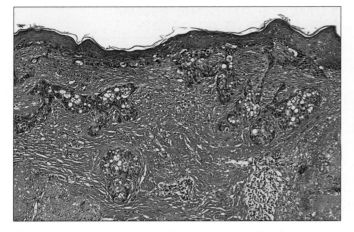

Figure 22.26 Sebaceous carcinoma, low magnification. Asymmetrical wide proliferation of sebaceous and basaloid cells. (Image courtesy of Dr Jag Bhawan, Boston University Dermatology Department.)

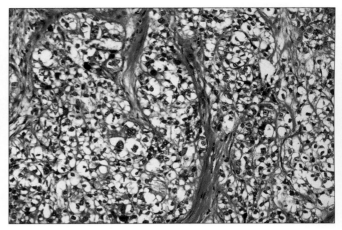

Figure 22.27 Sebaceous carcinoma, high magnification. Anaplastic tumor sebaceous cells with numerous mitosis. (Image courtesy of Dr Jag Bhawan, Boston University Dermatology Department.)

Moreno *et al.* in a review of literature found only 22 cases of metastasizing extraocular sebaceous carcinoma often to regional lymph nodes. Widespread metastatic disease is uncommon, but reports do exist, with nine reports of death due to visceral metastases.[100]

Histopathologically, the tumor is poorly circumscribed and asymmetric. It is composed of irregularly sized and shaped aggregations of atypical sebocytes. In the well-differentiated form sebaceous ductal structures with a crenulated eosinophilic cuticle, characteristic of ducts, are oftentimes seen.[101] The lesion is often epidermal, but dermal lesions, often exhibiting vascular and perineural involvement, have been reported (Figs 22.26, 22.27).[98,102] Oil-Red-O or Sudan IV lipid stains are positive as are immunohistochemical stains such as EMA or LeuM1.[102,103] Intracytoplasmic lipid droplets in neoplastic cells may be visible on electron microscopic examination, as evidence of sebaceous differentiation.[98,103]

Basal cell carcinoma with sebaceous differentiation is part of the histological differential diagnosis of sebaceous carcinoma. In sebaceous carcinoma the tumor cells are more eosinophilic and often show pagetoid spread.[94] The differential diagnosis also includes cutaneous metastases from internal malignancies such as renal, breast, bladder and prostatic carcinoma or melanoma. Periodic acid-Schiff (PAS) and mucicarmine histochemical staining and immunohistochemical antigens such as prostatic specific antigen for prostatic carcinoma or S-100 and HMB-45 for melanoma may be helpful in differentiating sebaceous carcinoma from other tumors.[103,104]

Wide surgical excision, with or without regional lymphadenectomy or evaluation of metastatic spread is the recommended treatment.[105] Excision and/or radiotherapy and/or chemotherapy are indicated in patients with metastatic disease.[105]

FUTURE OUTLOOK

The rarity of most adnexal tumors leads to problems in accurately assessing prognosis and the effectiveness of various therapeutic interventions. The evaluation of existing meta-analyses of adnexal tumor studies may help to enhance further understanding in this area.

REFERENCES

1 Hardisson D, Linares MD, Cuevas-Santos J, Contreras F. Pilomatrix carcinoma: a clinicopathologic study of six cases and review of the literature. Am J Derm 2001; 23(5):394–401.

2 Wood MG, Parhizzar B, Beerman H. Malignant pilomatricoma. Arch Derm 1984; 120:770.

3 Lopansri S, Mihm MC Jr. Pilomatrix carcinoma or calcifying epitheliocarcinoma of Malherbe. Cancer 1980; 45:2368–2373.

4 Gould E, Kurzon R, Kowalcyk AP, et al. Pilomatrix carcinoma with pulmonary metastases. Report of a case. Cancer 1984; 54:370–372.

5 Mir R, Cortes E, Papantoniou PA, et al. Metastatic trichomatrical carcinoma. Arch Pathol Lab Med 1986; 110:660–663.

6 Rabkin MS, Wittwer CT, Soong VY. Flow cytometric DNA content analysis of a case of pilomatrix carcinoma showing multiple recurrences and invasion of the cranial vault. J Am Acad Derm 1990; 23:104–108.

7 Ackerman AB, Viragh PA De, Chongchitnant N. Matrical carcinoma. In: Neoplasms with follicular differentiation. Philadelphia, PA: Lea & Febiger; 1993:661–675.

8 Weedon D, Bell J, Mayze J. Matrical carcinoma of the skin. J Cutan Pathol 1980; 7:39.

9 Green DE, Sanusi ID, Fowler MR. Pilomatrix carcinoma. J Am Acad Dermatol 1987; 17(2):264–270.

10 Aloi FG, Molinero A, Pippione M. Basal cell carcinoma with matrical differentiation. Matrical carcinoma. Am J Derm 1988; 10:509–513.

11 Ambrojo P, Aguilar A, Simón P, et al. Basal cell carcinoma with matrical differentiation. Am J Derm 1992; 14:293–297.

12 Sau P, Graham JH, Helwig EB. Proliferating epithelial cysts: clinicopathological analysis of 96 cases. J Cutan Pathol 1995; 22:394–406.

13 Mehregan AH, Lee KC. Malignant proliferating trichilemmal tumors: report of three cases. J Derm Surg Oncol 1987; 13:1339–1342.

14 Amaral AMP, Nascimento AG, Goellner JR. Proliferating pilar (trichilemmal) cyst: report of two cases, one with carcinomatous transformation and one with distant metastases. Arch Pathol Lab Med 1934; 108:808–810.

15 Mori O, Hachisuka H, Sasay Y. Proliferating trichilemmal cyst with a spindle cell carcinoma. Am J Derm 1990; 12:479–484.

16 Park BS, Yang SG, Cho KH. Malignant proliferating trichilemmal tumor showing distant metastases. Am J Derm 1997; 19:536–539.

17 Reis JP, Tellechea O, Cunha MF, Baptista AP. Trichilemmal carcinoma: review of 8 cases. J Cutan Pathol 1993; 20:44–49.

18 Misago N, Tanaka T, Kohda H. Trichilemmal carcinoma occurring in a lesion of solar keratosis. J Derm 1993; 20:358–364.

19 Ko T, Tada H, Hatoko M, Muramatsu T, et al. Trichilemmal carcinoma developing in a burn scar: a report of two cases. J Derm 1996; 23:463–468.

20 Chan KO, Lim IJ, Baladas HG, Tan WT. Multiple tumour presentation of trichilemmal carcinoma. Br J Plast Surg 1999; 52:665–667.

21 Schell H, Haneke E. Tricholemmales karzinom. Bericht uber 11 falle. Hautarzt 1985; 37:384.

22 Hashimoto Y, Matsuo S, Iizuka H. A DNA-flow cytometric analysis of trichilemmal carcinoma, proliferating trichilemmal cyst and trichilemmal cyst. Acta Derm Venereol 1994; 74:358–360.

23 Regauer S, Beham-Schmid C, Okcu M, Hartner E, Mannweiler S. Trichoblastic carcinoma ('malignant trichoblastoma') with lymphatic and hematogenous metastases. Mod Pathol 2000; 13:673–678.

24 Hunt SJ, Abell E. Malignant hair matrix tumor ('malignant trichoepithelioma') arising in the setting of multiple hereditary trichoepithelioma. Am J Derm 1991; 13:275–281.

25 Sau P, Lupton GP, Graham JH. Trichogerminoma: a report of 14 cases. J Cutan Pathol 1992; 19:357–365.

26 Rofagha R, Usmani AS, Vadmal M, Hessel AB, et al. Trichoblastic carcinoma: a report of two cases of a deeply infiltrative trichoblastic neoplasm. Derm Surg 2001; 27:663–666.

27 Regauer S, Beham-Schmid C, Okcu M, Hartner E, et al. Trichoblastic carcinoma ('malignant trichoblastoma') with lymphatic and hematogenous metastases. Mod Pathol 2000; 13:673–678.

28 Pinkus H, Mehregan AH. Epidermotropic eccrine carcinoma. Arch Derm 1963; 88:597–606.

29 Ryan JF, Darley CR, Pollock DJ. Malignant eccrine poroma: Report of three cases. J Clin Pathol 1986; 39:1099–1104.

30 Snow SN, Reizner GT. Eccrine porocarcinoma of the face. J Am Acad Derm 1992; 27:306–311.

31 Cooper PH. Carcinomas of sweat glands. Pathol Ann 1987; 22:83–124.

32 Kolde G, Macher E, Grundmann E. Metastasising eccrine porocarcinoma: Report of two cases with fatal outcome. Pathol Res Pr 1991; 187:477–481.

33 Mehregan AH, Hashinoto K, Hamayoon R. Eccrine adenocarcinoma: A clinicopathologic study of 35 cases. Arch Derm 1983; 119:104–113.

34 Barzi AS, Ruggeri S, Recchia F, Bertoldi I. Malignant metastatic eccrine poroma: Proposal for a new therapeutic protocol. Derm Surg 1997; 23:267–272.

35 Friedland M, Bajracharya A, Arlin Z. Malignant eccrine poroma and isotretinoin (letter). Ann Intern Med 1984; 100:614.

36 Roach MIII. A malignant eccrine poroma responds to isotretinoin (13-cis-retinoic acid). Ann Intern Med 1983; 99:486–488.

37 Tay JS, Tapen EM, Solari PG. Malignant eccrine spiradenoma. Case report and review of the literature. Am J Clin Oncol 1997; 20:552–557.

38 Rosborough D. Malignant mixed tumors of skin. Br J Surg 1963; 50:697–699.

39 McKee PH, Fletcher CDM, Stavrinos P, Pambakian H. Carcinosarcoma arising in eccrine spiradenoma. A clinicopathologic and immuno-histochemical study of two cases. Am J Derm 1990; 12:335–343.

40 Granter SR, Seeger K, Calonje E, Busam K, McKee PH. Malignant eccrine spiradenoma (spiradenocarcinoma): a clinicopathologic study of 12 cases. Am J Derm 2000; 22:97–103.

41 Sridhar KS, Benedetto P, Otrakji CL, Charyulu KK. Response of eccrine adenocarcinoma to tamoxifen. Cancer 1989; 64:366–370.

42 Mambo NC. The significance of atypical nuclear changes in benign eccrine acrospiomas: a clinical and pathological study of 18 cases. J Cutan Pathol 1984; 11:35.

43 Toma G De, Plocco M, Nicolanti V, et al. Malignant nodular hidradenoma. A clinical case [review, in Italian]. Minerva Chirurgica 2000; 55(3):185–187.

44 Metzler G, Schaumburg-Lever G, Hornstein O, Rassner G. Malignant chondroid syringoma: immunohistopathology. Am J Derm 1996; 18(1):83–89.

45 Barnett MD, Wallack MK, Zuretti A, et al. Recurrent malignant chondroid syringoma of the foot: a case report and review of the literature [review]. Am J Clin Oncol 2000; 23(3):227–232.

46 Hirsch P, Helwig EB. Chondroid syringoma: mixed tumor of the skin, salivary gland type. Arch Derm 1961; 84:835–847.

47 Freeman RG, Winkelmann RK. Basal cell tumor with eccrine differentiation (eccrine epithelioma). Arch Derm 1969; 100:234–242.

48 Mehregan AH, Hashimoto K, Rahbari H. Eccrine adenocarcinoma. A clinicopathologic study of 35 cases. Arch Derm 1983; 119(2):104–114.

49 Swanson PE, Cherwitz DL, Neumann MP, Wick MR. Eccrine sweat gland carcinoma: an histologic and immunohistochemical study of 32 cases. J Cutan Pathol 1987; 14:65–86.

50 Malmusi M, Collina G. Syringoid eccrine carcinoma: a case report. Am J Derm 1997; 19(5):533–535.

51 Cooper PH, Mills SE, Leonard DD, et al. Sclerosing sweat duct (syringomatous) carcinoma. Am J Surg Pathol 1985; 9:422–433.

52 Santa Cruz DJ. Sweat gland carcinoma: a comprehensive review. Semin Diagn Pathol 1987; 4:38–74.

53 Chow WC, Cockerell CJ, Geronemus RG. Microcystic adnexal carcinoma of the scalp. J Derm Surg Oncol 1989; 15:768–773.

54 Let Boit PE, Sexton M. Microcystic adnexal carcinoma of the skin. A reappraisal of the differentiation and differential diagnosis of an under recognized neoplasm. J Am Acad Derm 1993; 29:609–618.

55 Sabhikhi AK, Rao CR, Kumar RV, Hazarika D. Microcystic adnexal carcinoma. Int J Dermatol 1997; 36:134–136.

56 Pujol RM, LeBoit PE, Su WP. Microcystic adnexal carcinoma with extensive sebaceous differentiation. Am J Derm 1997; 19:358–362.

57 Nickoloff BJ, Fleischmann HE, Carmel J, Wood CC, Roth RJ. Microcystic adnexal carcinoma. Immunohistologic observations suggesting dual (pilar and eccrine) differentiation. Arch Derm 1986; 122:290–294.

58 Fleischmann HE, Roth FJ, Wood C, et al. Microcystic adnexal carcinoma treated with microscopically controlled excision. J Derm Surg Oncol 1984; 10:873–875.

59 Mendoza S. Helwig EB. Mucinous (adenocystic) carcinoma of the skin. Arch Derm 1971; 103:68–78.

60 Snow SN, Reizner GT. Mucinous eccrine carcinoma of the eyelid. Cancer 1992; 70:2099–2104.

61 Rahilly MA, Beattie GJ, Lessels AM. Mucinous eccrine carcinoma of the vulva with neuroendocrine differentiation. Histopathology 1995; 27:82–86.

62 Snow SN, Reizner GT. Mucinous eccrine carcinoma of the eyelid. Cancer 1992; 70:2099–2104.

63 Weber PJ, Hevia O, Gretzula JC, Rabinovitz HC. Primary mucinous carcinoma. J Derm Surg Oncol 1988; 14:170–172.

64 Abe S, Matsumoto Y, Fujita T. Primary mucinous carcinoma of the skin. Plast Reconstr Surg 1997; 99:1160–1164.

65 Bellezza G, Sidoni A, Bucciarelli E. Primary mucinous carcinoma of the skin. Am J Derm 2000; 22:166–170.

66 Brownstein MH, Helwig EB. Metastatic tumors of the skin. Cancer 1972; 29:1298–1307.

67 Boggio R. Adenoid cystic carcinoma of the scalp. Arch Derm 1975; 111:793–794.

68 Urso C. Primary cutaneous adenoid cystic carcinoma. Am J Derm 1999; 21:400.

69 Kato N, Yasukawa K, Onozuka T. Primary cutaneous adenoid cystic carcinoma with lymph node metastasis. Am J Derm 1998; 20:571–577.

70 Irvine AD, Kenny B, Walsh MY, Burrows D. Primary cutaneous adenoid cystic carcinoma. Clin Exper Derm 1996; 21:249–250.

71 Chu SS, Chang YL, Lou PJ. Primary cutaneous adenoid cystic carcinoma with regional lymph node metastasis. J Laryng Otol 2001; 115:673–675.

72 Sanderson KV, Batten JE. Adenoid cystic carcinoma of the scalp with pulmonary metastasis. Proc R Soc Med 1975; 68:649–650.

73 Chang SE, Ahn SJ, Choi JH, et al. Primary adenoid cystic carcinoma of skin with lung metastasis. J Am Acad Derm 1999; 40:640–642.

74 Kato N, Yasukawa K, Onozuka T. Primary cutaneous adenoid cystic carcinoma with lymph node metastasis. Am J Derm 20:571–577.

75 Headington JT, Teears R, Niederhuber JE, Slinger RP. Primary adenoid cystic carcinoma of skin. Arch Derm 1978; 114:421–424.

76 Lang PG Jr, Metcalf JS, Maize JC. Recurrent adenoid cystic carcinoma of the skin managed by microscopically controlled surgery (Mohs surgery). J Derm Surg Oncol 1986; 12:395–398.

77 Skibba JL, Hurley JD, Ravelo HV. Complete response of a metastatic adenoid cystic carcinoma of the parotid gland to chemotherapy. Cancer 1981; 47:2543–2548.

78 Petursson SR. Adenoid cystic carcinoma of the esophagus. Complete response to combination chemotherapy. Cancer 1986; 57:1464–1467.

79 Helwig EB. Eccrine acrospiroma. J Cutan Pathol 1984; 11:415–420.

80 Kao GF, Helwig EB, Graham JH. Aggressive digital papillary adenoma and adenocarcinoma. A clinicopathological study of 57 patients, with histochemical, immunopathological and ultrastructural observations. J Cutan Pathol 1987; 14:129–146.

81 Duke WH, Sherrod TT, Lupton GP. Aggressive digital papillary adenocarcinoma (aggressive digital papillary adenoma and adenocarcinoma revisited). Am J Surg Pathol 2000; 24:775–784.

82 Inaloz HS, Patel GK, Knight AG. An aggressive treatment for aggressive digital papillary adenocarcinoma. Cutis 2002; 69:179–182.

83 Yen A, Sanchez RL, Fearneyhough P, Tschen J, Wagner RF Jr. Mucoepidermoid carcinoma with cutaneous presentation. J Am Acad Derm 1997; 37:340–342.

84 Stout AP, Cooley SGE. Carcinoma of sweat glands. Cancer 1951; 4:521–535.

85 Jacyk WK, Requena L, Sanchez Yus E, Judd MJ. Tubular apocrine carcinoma arising in a nevus sebaceus of Jadassohn. Am J Derm 1998; 20:389–392.

86 Hayes MM, Matisic JP, Weir L. Apocrine carcinoma of the lip: a case report including immunohistochemical and ultrastructural study, discussion of differential diagnosis and review of the literature. Oral Surgery, Oral Medicine, Oral Pathology. Oral Radiol Endo 1996; 82:193–199.

87 Paties C, Taccagni GL, Papotti M, et al. Apocrine carcinoma of the skin. A clinicopathologic, immunocytochemical and ultrastructural study. Cancer 1993; 71:375–381.

88 Dhawan SS, Nanda VS, Grekin S, Rabinovitz HS. Apocrine adenocarcinoma: a case report and review of the literature. J Derm Surg Oncol 1990; 16:468–470.

89 Baes H, Suurmond D. Apocrine sweat gland carcinoma. Br J Derm 1970; 83:483.

90 Warkel RL, Helwig EB. Apocrine gland adenoma and adenocarcinoma of the axilla. Arch Dematol 1978; 114:198.

91 Chamberlain RS, Huber K, White JC, Travaglino-Parda R. Apocrine gland carcinoma of the axilla: review of the literature and recommendations for treatment. Am J Clin Oncol 1999; 22:131–135.

92 Nelson BR, Hamlet KR, Gillard M, et al. Sebaceous carcinoma. J Am Acad Derm 1995; 33:1–15.

93 Rao NA, Hidayat AA, McLean IW, et al. Sebaceous carcinoma of the ocular adnexa: a clinicopathologic study of 104 cases, with five-year follow-up data. Hum Pathol 1982; 13:113–122.

94 Wick MR, Goellner JR, Wolfe JT, et al. Adnexal carcinomas of the skin. II. Extraocular sebaceous carcinomas. Cancer 1985; 56:1163–1172.

95 Kane HD, Squire MA, Kallet HA. Sebaceous carcinoma of the foot. Case presentation and discussion. J Am Podiatry Assoc 1984; 74:120–124.

96 Escalonilla P, Grilli R, Canamero M, et al. Sebaceous carcinoma of the vulva. Am J Derm 1999; 21:468–472.

97 Oka K, Katsumata M. Intraepidermal sebaceous carcinoma: a case report. Dermatologica 1990; 180:181–185.

98 Rulon DB, Helwig EB. Cutaneous sebaceous neoplasms. Cancer 1974; 33:82–102.

99 Heenan PJ, Waring PM, Crocker AD. Massive cutaneous tumor of the scalp. Australas J Derm 1990; 31:115–116.

100 Moreno C, Jacyk WK, Judd MJ, Requena L. Highly aggressive extraocular sebaceous carcinoma. Am J Derm 2001; 23:450–455.

101 Steffen C, Ackerman AB. Sebaceous carcinoma. In: Neoplasms with Sebaceous Differentiation. Philadelphia, PA: Lea & Febiger; 1994:487–574.

102 Wolfe JT, Wick MR, Campbell RJ. Sebaceous carcinoma of the oculocutaneous adnexa and extraocular skin. In: Pathology of Unusual Malignant Cutaneous Tumors. New York, NY: Marcel Dekker; 1985:77–106.

103 Kawamoto M, Fukuda Y, Kamoi S, Sugisaki Y, Yamanaka N. Sebaceous carcinoma of the vulva. Pathol Intern 1995; 45:767–773.

104 Escalonilla P, Grilli R, Canamero M, et al. Sebaceous carcinoma of the vulva. Am J Derm 1999; 21:468–472.

105 Nelson BR, Hamlet KR, Gillard M, Railan D, Johnson TM. Sebaceous carcinoma. J Am Acad Derm 1995; 33:1–15.

CHAPTER
23 Paget's Disease

George Niedt

Key points

- Paget's disease is a form of intraepidermal adenccarcinoma.
- It may occur in the breast (mammary Paget's disease) or other sites such as vulva, scrotum and perianal regions (extra mammary Paget's disease).
- It usually presents as a persistent, eczematous dermatitis and does not resemble a neoplasm clinically.
- Histologically, the differential diagnosis includes malignant melanoma and squamous cell carcinoma among others. Distinguishing these entities is usually straightforward using routine immunohistochemical techniques.
- Mammary Paget's disease is nearly always associated with an underlying carcinoma.
- Extra mammary Paget's disease is sometimes associated with an underlying carcinoma.
- Treatment, in general is surgical and prognosis is largely dependent on the type and extent of underlying carcinoma.

INTRODUCTION

Paget's disease is an unusual form of intraepidermal adenocarcinoma.

It is a relatively rare condition, which is difficult to diagnose, as the clinical picture is usually that of an eczematous process and not a neoplasm. Paget's disease usually presents as a scaly, erythematous plaque sometimes with a discernible nodule. Paget's disease is traditionally divided into two types. Mammary Paget's disease, which represents a manifestation of an underlying carcinoma of the breast and extramammary Paget's disease, which may not be associated with underlying carcinoma.

MAMMARY PAGET'S DISEASE

HISTORY

Paget's disease was described by Sir James Paget in 1874.[1] Paget, a British surgeon, was one of the great Victorian physicians. Two major diseases have been associated with his name: Paget's disease of the bone and Paget's disease of the breast.

James Paget was born the eighth of 16 children in a well-to-do family in Great Yarmouth, England, in 1814. At the age of 20 Paget entered St Bartholomew's Hospital, in London, where he spent most of his life. As a first year student at St Bartholomew's he noted white specks in the muscle of the cadaver which he was dissecting and was the first to discover the causative organisms of trichinosis. He had a successful private practice, becoming surgeon to both Queen Victoria and the Prince of Wales. A terrific lecturer, he maintained friendships with such notables as Louis Pasteur, Florence Nightingale and Charles Darwin. Paget noted the association of an eczematous condition of the nipple with underlying breast carcinoma in 1874. The histology of this disease was described by Thin in 1881,[2] who believed it represented carcinoma and not eczema.

EPIDEMIOLOGY

Paget's disease is present in approximately 1–2% of patients with breast carcinoma. About half of the patients will have an underlying palpable breast tumor and of those who have a palpable underlying tumor, approximately half will have lymph node metastasis. In patients who present with Paget's disease without a clinically evident underlying tumor, less than 40% of cases will show invasive carcinoma and axillary lymph node metastasis will be seen in approximately 10%. In rare cases Paget's disease may be seen in men. There seem to be no predisposing clinical or epidemiologic factors for Paget's disease.

PATHOGENESIS AND ETIOLOGY

Over the years, the pathogenesis of Paget's disease has presented a source of controversy. In past years, Paget's disease was regarded as an inflammatory process, originating in the epidermis and inducing an underlying breast carcinoma. This may stem from Sir James Paget's original description of the lesion in which he compared it with carcinomas of other sites, like scrotum, which develop after chronic irritation.

It is clear now that from its inception, Paget's disease of the nipple represents intraepidermal adenocarcinoma of the breast. Immunohistochemical studies reveal positive staining for low molecular weight keratins, breast mucin, ck7, her-2/neu and ema in Paget's disease in a manner similar to that which would be expected in mammary carcinoma. Estrogen and progesterone receptors may

303

also be present in Paget's disease. In addition, conventional histochemical staining for mucins are positive in Paget's disease of the nipple and electron microscopic examination reveals evidence of glandular differentiation in these cells. When these findings are considered with the fact that the vast majority of cases of Paget's disease of the nipple is associated with an underlying intraductal or invasive breast carcinoma, there can be no other conclusion: Paget's disease of the nipple represents an extension of underlying adenocarcinoma of the breast.

CLINICAL FEATURES

Clinically, the diagnosis of mammary Paget's disease may be difficult. Mammary Paget's disease generally presents as an eczematous process.[3] In one study, approximately 39% of patient's presented with eczema, 37% with bleeding, 32% with ulcer and 22% with a breast mass.[4] Many of these patients had symptoms for more than 4 months. Patients may also complain of pain, burning or itching. Clinical examination will reveal an erythematous scaly patch or plaque, which may involve only the nipple or may extend to the areola or surrounding skin (Figs 23.1 and 23.2). Approximately half of the patients will have a palpable underlying breast mass. Patients may give a history of mammary carcinoma. The lesion may be excoriated and patients may rarely present with small vesicles. There may be evidence of ulceration or discharge and the lesion can range in size from less than 0.5 cm to many cm. There may be invagination of the nipple, but this is due to underlying carcinoma. The disease is generally unilateral.

PATIENT EVALUATION, DIAGNOSIS AND DIFFERENTIAL DIAGNOSIS

The initial examination of a patient with a clinical suspicion for Paget's disease should include careful examination of the skin of both breasts, a breast exam to search for any underlying mass and an examination of the axillary lymph nodes. Clinically, the differential diagnosis may include an eczematous process and a dermatophyte infection. However, KOH preparations will be negative and the patient will not respond to anti-fungal or topical steroid therapy. Erosive adenomatosis of the nipple may also present with an ulcerated lesion of the nipple. This usually does not have an associated plaque-like area but it may be associated with a small underlying mass. Other neoplasms, which may simulate Paget's disease, include Bowen's disease and malignant melanoma.

If the process is recalcitrant to topical steroid therapy, after a brief trial, then either a scraping or biopsy should be obtained. Of course, if there is a palpable underlying mass, a biopsy should be obtained immediately of the superficial skin. Another simple way to diagnose Paget's disease of the nipple is by use of a scraping of the nipple with subsequent cytological evaluation.[5] A scraping may be performed when material is smeared on a slide with a scalpel or spatula in a manner analogous to a pap or Tzanck smear. These smears may be preserved in

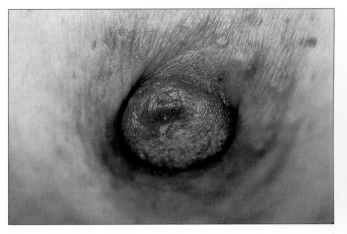

Figure 23.1 Paget's disease of the nipple: There is slight scaling and erosion of the nipple. (Image courtesy of Dr Marc Grossman.)

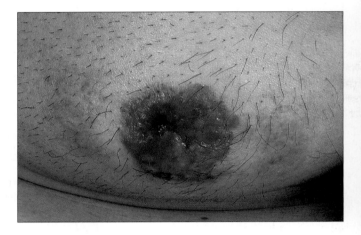

Figure 23.2 Paget's disease of the male breast.

alcohol or sprayed with fixative. As an alternative air dried smears may be examined by use of modified Giemsa stain. A fine needle aspiration of any underlying mass may also yield a diagnosis of adenocarcinoma of the breast. Conventional biopsy may be performed using a variety of techniques including the shave or punch technique. It is not necessary to obtain a significant amount of dermis to diagnose Paget's disease as the epidermal changes are diagnostic.

A detailed knowledge of the anatomy and drainage of the breast duct system is important before attempting an excision of these lesions. Dermatologists may not feel comfortable doing a biopsy of the underlying breast mass or a needle aspirate of the mass. Therefore, referral to a surgeon who is comfortable with such procedures should be arranged. Once the diagnosis of Paget's disease has been established, the work up of the disease will depend on the extent and type of underlying breast carcinoma. Mammography will be indicated to locate non-palpable breast masses. Surgical biopsy and/or excision will be necessary to diagnose the type of underlying carcinoma.

PATHOLOGY

The histology of Paget's disease is so characteristic, that the term 'Pagetoid' has been used to describe the histologic appearance of other neoplasms, which simulate Paget's disease. The hallmark of Paget's disease is the presence of so-called Pagetoid cells. These have abundant pale cytoplasm, which is paler than that of the surrounding keratinocytes. These cells may be arranged singly, or in nests, at all levels of the epidermis (pagetoid pattern) (Figs 23.3 and 23.4).[6] In some instances, the cells may be so densely packed, that the lesion may simulate a squamous cell carcinoma *in situ*. In other instances, the cells may actually form small glandular structures within the epidermis (Fig. 23.4). As the biopsies are usually from the nipple, there will be surrounding changes of normal nipple skin, such as of smooth muscle, normal breast ducts and sebaceous glands. The Paget cells may extend down ductal structures.

Histologically, there are a number of diseases which mimic Paget's disease, the most common of which are malignant melanoma *in situ* and squamous cell carcinoma *in situ*. Malignant melanoma may be differentiated from Paget's disease because the cells in Paget's disease are generally located above the basilar layer, while the cells of malignant melanoma *in situ* often originate from the basilar layer. In addition, melanoma *in situ* may exhibit nests of melanocytes at the dermal–epidermal junction. Squamous cell carcinoma *in situ* will usually exhibit full thickness atypia of the epidermis in some areas. Also, close histologic inspection of these cells will reveal that the cells of squamous cell carcinoma *in situ* will often contain keratohyaline granules as they progress through the granular layer of the epidermis. Occasionally, a seborrheic keratosis which has been irritated may show a nesting pattern, which mimics Paget's disease. The cells of an irritated seborrheic keratosis will not exhibit cytologic atypia and will usually be covered by an orthokeratotic horn. There may be typical changes of seborrheic keratosis adjacent to these areas of irritation. Toker cell (clear cell) hyperplasia may simulate Paget's disease.[7] In

this condition, vacuolated keratinocytes are present within the epidermis. These cells lack cytologic atypia and exhibit intercellular bridges. In erosive adenomatosis[3] of the nipple there are clusters of duct-like structures lined by apocrine type epithelium. Some of these may contain papillary structures. There is no proliferation of cells within the epidermis. Mucin stains such as Alcian blue, mucicarmine and PAS will demonstrate mucin in the Paget's cells.

Because of the difficulty in some cases of differentiating Paget's disease from malignant melanoma *in situ* and squamous cell carcinoma *in situ*, immunohistochemical studies may be performed. These studies usually confirm the diagnosis. A panel of antibodies, which includes s100 protein, melan A, low and high molecular weight cytokeratins and carcinoembryonic antigen, will usually suffice. Using this simple panel of antibodies, melanomas are usually positive for s100 protein and melan A and negative for the other antibodies. Squamous cell carcinoma *in situ* is generally positive for high molecular weight cytokeratins and sometimes for low molecular weight cytokeratins but negative for the other antibodies. Paget's disease is usually positive for carcinoembryonic antigen and low molecular weight keratin. Immunohistochemical markers for prognosis of breast carcinoma may be performed on lesions of Paget's disease including her-2/neu and estrogen and progesterone receptors. However, the literature indicates that the percentage of cases positive for the latter two receptors appear to be less in Paget's disease than in underlying breast carcinomas.

TREATMENT

As with other forms of breast cancer, debate persists as to the appropriate treatment of Paget's disease of the breast. Generally, treatment is based on whether or not there is an underlying mass. In patients who have an underlying breast mass, treatment is generally directed at treating the underlying carcinoma. The traditional treatment has been mastectomy with axillary lymph node dissection. In patients who have no evidence radiologically

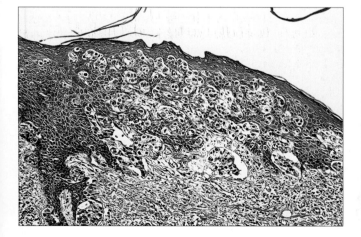

Figure 23.3 Paget's disease of the nipple: The sections show clusters of pale cells forming duct-like structures within the epidermis. (Image courtesy of Dr Hanina Hibshoosh.)

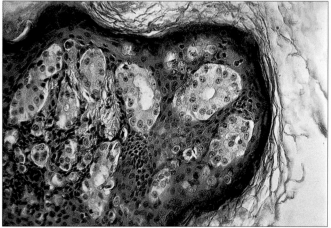

Figure 23.4 Paget's disease of the nipple: The sections show large cells with pale cytoplasm at all levels of the epidermis. (Image courtesy of Dr Marc Grossman.)

of multifocal disease, it has been proposed that breast conserving therapy can be considered with postoperative irradiation if margins are negative.[4] However, patients who have multifocal disease or with positive margins should be treated with mastectomy.

Treatment of patients with Paget's disease without an underlying mass is more problematic. A number of studies have supported a conservative approach to these patients.[8,9] The problem with this approach is that even in cases without a palpable mass, there is often underlying carcinoma and this carcinoma is frequently multifocal (73% in one study).[10] If there is an underlying breast mass, the prognosis is significantly worse. In one study, the 5-year survival for patients with an underlying nodule was only 38%, while that for patients without a palpable nodule was 92%.[11]

In summary, conservative management, including excision of the nipple areola complex, excision of the underlying breast mass and radiotherapy may be attempted, but the mainstay of therapy for Paget's disease remains mastectomy (either radical or modified) with removal of lymph nodes. Radiation therapy alone should probably be reserved only for patients who refuse mastectomy or who are unable to undergo a surgical procedure. From the dermatologist's point of view, the most important treatment is referral to a physician who can perform the appropriate surgical removal of the lesion.

EXTRA MAMMARY PAGET'S DISEASE

INTRODUCTION

Extra mammary Paget's disease is a relatively uncommon form of cancer, which masquerades as an eczematous dermatitis. This disease is a form of intraepidermal adenocarcinoma. Unlike Paget's disease of the nipple, extra mammary Paget's disease is usually not associated with an underlying carcinoma although, in a substantial minority of cases, there may be one.

This disease can be difficult to treat because usually it is fairly widespread, it may be multifocal and there may be an underlying carcinoma. It can also be difficult to diagnose because of its similarity to an inflammatory skin disease. Thus, it may be unsuspected until it is biopsied. Although it may occur nearly anywhere on the body, characteristic locations include the perianal region and vulva.

HISTORY

Sir James Paget was the first to notice a correlation between an eczematous dermatitis of the nipple and underlying breast carcinoma. Although he did not publish the first case of extra mammary Paget's disease, James Paget did examine the first patient and make the diagnosis. In 1888, Crocker[12] described this patient with Paget's disease affecting the scrotum and penis. This patient had an eczematous eruption, which was asso-ciated with an underlying carcinoma. In 1893, Darier also reported a case of the 'maladie de Paget' in the perianal and scrotal region.[13]

EPIDEMIOLOGY

Extramammary Paget's disease is primarily a disease of middle aged to elderly women. In Chanda's review of 196 cases,[14] 150 of the cases were reported in women. The age range was from 47 to 87. There appears to be no racial or ethnic predisposition to the disease. Approximately 26% of the patients die of the disease.

The disease is a relatively uncommon entity with only 196 cases reported in the English literature during the years 1962 to 1982. There appears to be no geographical disposition. However, one paper suggests the disease in China is more common in males.[15]

PATHOGENESIS AND ETIOLOGY

The pathogenesis of extra mammary Paget's disease is controversial. It has been proposed that this disease represents an intraepidermal adenocarcinoma, a primary adenocarcinoma of sweat ducts and an epidermal manifestation of a dermal sweat gland carcinoma. For most cases of extra mammary Paget's disease the pathogenesis is unknown.

There are at least three types of extra mammary Paget's disease. The least controversial type of extra mammary Paget's disease is that associated with visceral malignancy. The most common underlying visceral malignancy is an adenocarcinoma of the anal canal or rectum. However, extra mammary Paget's disease has been associated with carcinomas of the bladder, cervix, sebaceous glands and apocrine glands. In these instances, the Paget's disease represents either a direct extension of the carcinoma via either ductal structures, epithelium or metastases. The immunohistochemical profile of this type of Paget's disease is similar to that of the underlying carcinoma. This type is most commonly found in the perianal region.

In Chanda's review, 24% of patients with extra mammary Paget's disease had an associated underlying cutaneous adenocarcinoma.[14] However, other series would contradict this finding. In one series, only two examples of invasive sweat gland carcinoma were found in more than 100 cases of extra mammary Paget's disease.[16] Nonetheless, it is clear that a minority of cases of extra mammary Paget's disease is associated with underlying sweat gland carcinoma. It is debated whether the carcinoma originates from the epidermal ductal cells and subsequently spreads into the dermis or originates from an underlying sweat gland carcinoma and spreads to the epidermis.

The third type of extra mammary Paget's disease is that in which there is no associated invasive carcinoma. This represents the majority of cases of extra mammary Paget's disease. Some authors have used this observation to support the hypothesis that the Paget's disease arises within the epidermis, possibly from an intraepidermal portion of a ductal structure, probably an apocrine duct (as Paget's disease preferentially occurs in places where apocrine glands are known to exist). Other authors feel that even though it cannot be demonstrated histologically, Paget's disease more likely arises from a duct or gland and spreads upward through the epidermis. Because of the numerous ducts within the epidermis, they believe that it not always possible to find the individual duct which gives rise to the Paget's disease. As there is no reliable histochemical method for differentiating between eccrine, apocrine and ductal cells, the precise pathogenesis of most cases of extra mammary Paget's disease remains enigmatic.

Even in cases where there is no direct extension of an underlying carcinoma, Paget's disease of the skin appears to be associated with a high risk of coexistent malignancy. It may represent a cutaneous marker of malignancy similar to Bowen's disease of the skin. Some 20% of patients will have an underlying internal malignancy.[14]

CLINICAL FEATURES

Extra mammary Paget's disease has a similar clinical appearance to mammary Paget's disease. Patients usually complain of pruritis[14] and may also complain of burning, or pain. Physical exam reveals an erythematous, sometimes scaly patch or plaque. It usually occurs in the vulva, perianal (Figs 23.5–23.7) or scrotal regions. Unusual sites include periaural, axillary and periorbital regions. The patient may or may not have a history of underlying carcinoma. In contrast to mammary Paget's disease, there is usually no evidence of an underlying mass. In exceptional cases, the lesion may be ulcerated.

PATIENT EVALUATION, DIAGNOSIS AND DIFFERENTIAL DIAGNOSIS

Generally, initial consideration will be that of an inflammatory dermatosis. The initial clinical evaluation would generally be oriented toward treating and diagnosing an inflammatory dermatosis. The differential diagnosis includes an eczematous dermatitis such as a nummular

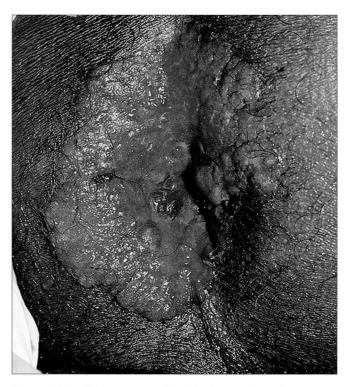

Figure 23.6 Extra mammary Paget's disease: A much more extensive lesion of extra mammary Paget's disease with erosion and surrounding lichen simplex chronicus. (Image courtesy of Dr Marc Grossman.)

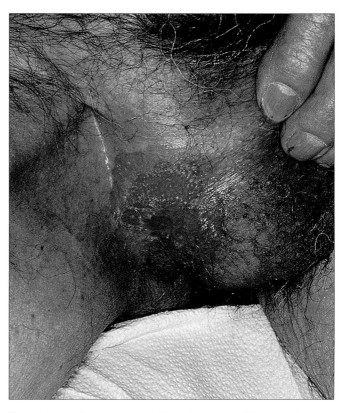

Figure 23.7 Extra mammary Paget's disease: There is an erythematous patch, which is partly eroded in the scrotal region. (Image courtesy of Dr Marc Grossman.)

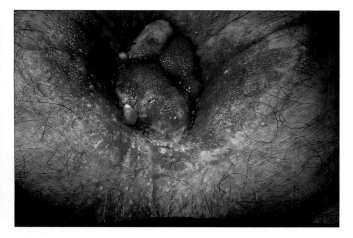

Figure 23.5 Extramammary Paget's disease: Perianal Paget's disease. The hemorrhoidal appearing lesion turned out to be adenocarcinoma. (Image courtesy of Dr Harvey Weinberg.)

dermatitis, or a contact dermatitis. However, in Paget's disease, there will be no response to topical steroid therapy or to removal of any possible irritant or contactant. Another clinical consideration might include a dermatophyte infection. However, KOH preparations will be negative and the lesion will be unresponsive to antifungal therapy. A drug eruption might also be included in the differential diagnosis but the lesion will persist despite any alteration in drug regimen.

The clinical differential diagnosis also includes squamous cell carcinoma *in situ* (Bowen's disease). Both Bowen's disease and extra mammary Paget's disease will persist after therapy for an inflammatory dermatosis. Persistent rash in a characteristic region (inguinal, scrotal, perianal and vulvar) should prompt a biopsy. Any sort of biopsy of the conventional type (punch, shave, or excisional) should confirm the diagnosis.

PATHOLOGY

Extra mammary Paget's disease usually has a characteristic histology, which is similar to that of Paget's disease of the breast.[6] Sections stained with hematoxylin and eosin stain will demonstrate the presence of single and clustered pale enlarged cells throughout the epidermis (Figs 23.8 and 23.9). In some cases, these cells may actually form glandular structures. In most cases, these cells will stain positively for mucin.

The histologic differential diagnosis includes malignant melanoma *in situ* and Pagetoid squamous cell carcinoma *in situ*. By light microscopy these diseases can usually be differentiated. In the case of malignant melanoma *in situ*, there are often nests of cells at the dermal-epidermal junction, spindle and epithelioid shaped cells may be present, there may be melanin pigment and there may be a pre-existing nevus or underlying invasive melanoma. Squamous cell carcinoma *in situ* generally reveals some areas in which there is full thickness atypia of squamous cells within the epidermis. A helpful clue to making this diagnosis of extra mammary Paget's disease by light microscopy is the presence of keratohyaline granules within the atypical cells as they extend through the granular layer. Another histologic simulant of extra mammary Paget's disease is an irritated seborrheic keratosis. Generally, these lack significant atypia and often show adjacent changes of classic seborrheic keratosis.

Nonetheless, immunohistochemical studies are often used to confirm the diagnosis. Malignant melanoma generally stains with s100 protein, HMB45 and melan A. Squamous cell carcinoma *in situ* is usually positive for high molecular weight cytokeratins. Extramammary Paget's disease on the other hand is usually positive for low molecular weight cytokeratins and carcinoembryonic antigen. A panel of s100 protein, high and low molecular weight cytokeratins and CEA is usually sufficient to establish the diagnosis.

Other immunohistochemical studies are often helpful in determining whether there is underlying carcinoma. Cases without underlying carcinoma generally stain positively for gross cystic disease fluid protein-15.[17] Cytokeratin 7 is positive in most types of extra mammary

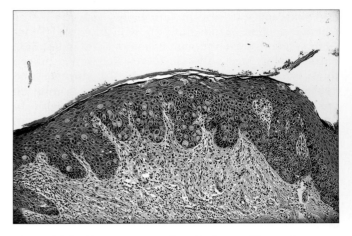

Figure 23.8 Extra mammary Paget's disease: The sections show pale cells at all levels of the epidermis (low magnification).

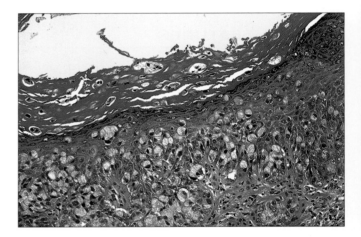

Figure 23.9 Extra mammary Paget's disease: The sections show pale cells at all levels of the epidermis. Some of the cells are clustered. Some cells exhibit a signet ring type of morphology (high magnification).

Paget's disease, however, in cases with underlying anal carcinoma, ck20 has also been reported to be positive.[18,19] Cases with underlying urethelial carcinoma have been reported to be positive for uroplakin.[20] It is incumbent upon the histopathologist to be aware that these antibodies may help in determining whether there is underlying carcinoma and if so, what the site of such carcinoma may be.

TREATMENT

The treatment for extra mammary Paget's disease must be directed at both the Paget's disease itself and the underlying carcinoma. Once the diagnosis has been established, Paget's disease is generally treated by surgical excision. It does not appear to respond to topical 5-fluorouracil (5-FU) therapy, however, topical 5-FU therapy may be used to map out and assist in obtaining a surgical margin.[21] After a diagnosis of extra mammary Paget's disease, the patient must be evaluated for the presence of underlying carcinoma. This evaluation will vary depending on the site of the disease. The evaluation of any patient with Paget's disease should include a thorough physical examination including examination of lymph nodes. For Paget's disease in the vulvar region, a pelvic exam with a search for any clue to underlying cervical carcinoma should be undertaken. The pelvic exam will also help to evaluate the extent of the Paget's disease. In this region, consideration of an underlying urethelial carcinoma must also be given. In the perianal region, a digital rectal exam followed by examination of the anus and sigmoid part of the colon is essential. Biopsy of any suspicious regions, including areas which may clinically resemble hemorrhoids, is recommended.

Once the patient has been evaluated for the presence of an underlying carcinoma, the therapy for Paget's disease will be determined by the presence or absence of such carcinoma. In patients with underlying carcinoma, therapy will be directed at removing that carcinoma whether it be an anal carcinoma, transitional cell carcinoma, or other carcinoma. The Paget's disease itself must also be removed.

Surgical therapy remains the mainstay of treatment for extra mammary Paget's disease. A number of studies support an approach of wide local excision to prevent recurrence.[22] Paget's disease of the vulva has generally been treated with radical vulvectomy, though good results have been obtained in treating patients with skinning vulvectomy or hemivulvectomy particularly when intra-operative frozen sections are examined to determine margins.[23] Patients with Paget's disease of the anus also appear to do best when treated with wide local excision. Nonetheless, cases have been treated with Moh's micrographic surgery.[24] This technique may help to decrease the high rate of recurrence of this disease.

In some cases surgical treatment may be refused or inappropriate. Radiation and chemotherapy have been tried as alternative modes of treatment.[25] Imiquod has also been reported to be successful in treatment of extra mammary Paget's disease.[26] The numbers of patients treated with these alternative modes of therapy are small and the results should be viewed with some skepticism. Nonetheless, these approaches may provide alternatives for patients who are not surgical candidates.

FUTURE OUTLOOK

The etiology and underlying cause of Paget's disease remains an enigma. Future studies will hopefully identify genetic and histologic markers to aid in the accurate diagnosis of this disease and better recognize those at risk.

REFERENCES

1 Paget J. On diseases of the mammary areola proceeding cancer of the mammary gland. St. Bartholomew Hospital Report. St Bartholomew Hospital Report 1874; 10:87–89.

2 Thin G. Malignant papillary dermatitis of the nipple and the breast tumor with which it is found associated. BMJ 1881:760–763.

3 Rosen PP. Paget's disease of the nipple. In: Rosen, ed. Rosen's Breast Pathology. London: Lippincott Raven; 1997:493–506.

4 Sakorafas GH, Blanchard DK, Sarr MG, Farley DR. Paget's disease of the breast: A clinical perspective. Langenbecks Arch Surg 2001; 386(6):444–450.

5 Samarasingle D, Frost R, Sterrett G, et al. Cytological diagnosis of Paget's disease of the nipple by scrape smears: A report of 5 cases. Diagn Cytopathol 1993; 9(3):291–295.

6 Jones RE, Austin C, Ackerman AB. Extra mammary Paget's disease: A critical examination. Am J Derm 1979; 1(2):101–132.

7 Toker C. Clear cells of the nipple epidermis. Cancer 1970; 25(3):601–610.

8 Kollmorgen DR, Varansi JS, Edge SB, Carson WE. Paget's disease of the breast, a 33 year experience. J Amer Col Surg 1998; 187(2):171–177.

9 Polgar C, Borzars S, Covacks T, Phodor J. Breast conserving therapy for Paget's disease of the nipple: A prospective European organization for research and treatment of cancer study of 61 patients. Cancer 2002; 94(6):1904–1905.

10 Yeni JH, Wick MR, Philpott GW, et al. Underlying pathology in mammary Paget's disease. Ann Surg Pathol 1997; 4(4):287–292.

11 Salvadori B, Saraselle G, Saccozzi R. Analysis of 100 cases of Paget's disease of the breast. Tumor 1976; 62(5):529–535.

12 Crocker HR. Paget's disease affecting the scrotum and penis. Trans Path Soc Lond 1988; 40:187–191.

13 Darier J, Couillaud P. Surum Cas De Maladie de Paget's de la region Helen Perineoanale et scrotale. Societe Francaise de Dermatologie et de Syphilligraphie 1893; 4:25–31.

14 Chanda JJ. Extramammary Paget's disease: prognosis in relationship to internal malignancy. J Amer Acad Derm 1985; 13(6):1009–1014.

15 Chang YT, Lieu HM, Wong CK. Extramammary Paget's disease: a report of 22 cases in Chinese males. J Derm 1996; 5:320–324.

16 Wick MR, Goellner JR, Wolfe JT 3rd, Su WP. Vulvar sweat gland carcinomas: Arch Path Lab Med 1985; 109(1):43–47.

17 Kohler S, Smoller BR. Gross cystic disease fluid protein-15 reactivity in extramammary Paget's disease with and without associated internal malignancy. Am J Dermatopathol 1996; 8:118–123.

18 Ohnishi T, Watanabbi S. The use of cytokeratin 7 and 20 in the diagnosis of primary and secondary extramammary Paget's disease: Br J Dermatol 142(2):243.

19 Goldblum J, Hart W. Perianal Paget's disease: A histologic and immunohistochemical study of 11 cases with and without associated rectal carcinoma. Amer J Surg Pathol 1998; 22: 170–179.

20 Brown HM, Wilkenson EJ. Uroplakin-III to distinguish primary vulva Paget's disease from Paget's disease secondary to urethelial carcinoma. Hum Pathol 2002; 33(5):545–548.

21 Eliezri YD, Silvers DN, Horan DB. Role of preoperative topical 5-fluorouracil in preparation for Mohs micrographic surgery of extramammary Paget's disease: J Am Acad Dermat 1987; 17(3):497–505.

22 Zolo JD. Zeitonic: The Roswell Park Cancer Institute experience with extramammary Paget's disease. Br J Derm 2000; 142(1):59–65.

23 Curtin JP, Rubin SC, Jones WB, et al. Paget's disease of the vulva. Gyn Oncol 39(3):374–377.

24 Coldiron BM, Goldsmith BA, Robinson JK. Surgical treatment of extramammary Paget's disease. A report of six cases and a re-examination of Moh's micrographic surgery compared with conventional surgical excision. Cancer 1991; 67(4):933–938.

25 Floun RF, Lancaster KJ, McCormick K, et al. Radiotherapy for perianal Paget's disease. Clin Oncol 2002; 14(4):272–284.

26 Zampogna JC, Flowers FP, Roth WI, Haffenein AM. Treatment of primary limited cutaneous extramammary Paget's disease with topical imiquimod monotherapy: Two case reports. J Amer Acad Derm 2002; 47(suppl)(4):229–235.

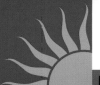

CHAPTER
24

Sarcomas of the Skin

David R Guillén and Clay J Cockerell

Key points

- Sarcoma of the skin comprises several rare entities that can afflict patients of any age, including infants and children.
- Cutaneous sarcomas most commonly present as nodules or plaques; however, variant presentations can simulate inflammatory conditions or developmental malformations, respectively.
- Epithelioid sarcoma is an aggressive neoplasm that can simulate an inflammatory process both clinically and histologically.
- Immunohistochemical, cytogenetic, molecular diagnostic, ultrastructural and radiological studies complement histopathologic or cytopathologic evaluation of these tumors.
- Cutaneous sarcomas are composed of neoplastic spindle, round or epithelioid cells; their histopathologic differential diagnosis includes benign neoplasms and reactive proliferations.
- Complete surgical excision is the mainstay of therapy, and Mohs micrographic surgical technique has proven superior to conventional surgical excision, particularly for cutaneous sarcomas that are likely to recur, such as dermatofibrosarcoma protuberans (DFSP).
- Radiotherapy is effective and appropriate adjuvant therapy in some settings.
- Patients with metastatic DFSP have had variable responses to imatinib mesylate (Gleevec™).

INTRODUCTION

The term *cutaneous sarcoma* refers to non-epithelial primary skin neoplasms that are locally aggressive or have the capacity to metastasize. This category comprises tumors showing evidence of mesenchymal differentiation, but by convention it also includes neural neoplasms. Thus, cutaneous sarcomas are composed of cells that resemble fibrocytes, smooth muscle cells, adipocytes, vascular endothelial cells, skeletal muscle cells, chondrocytes, osteocytes or Schwann cells, among other cell types. This complex category of skin cancer includes a large number of uncommon tumors. Because a detailed discussion of each entity is beyond the scope of this chapter, we have taken an integrative approach, emphasizing common themes in clinical presentation,

evaluation, diagnosis and treatment. The discussion here focuses on primary cutaneous tumors except in those instances where it is useful to contrast the cutaneous tumor with its deeper subcutaneous, subfascial or visceral counterpart. Abbreviations used in this chapter are listed in Table 24.1. Vascular neoplasms are considered separately elsewhere in this volume.

HISTORY

Modern concepts of cutaneous sarcomas emerged gradually from small case series in tandem with the development of special techniques such as electron microscopy, immunohistochemistry, cytogenetics and molecular biology. In 1924, Darier and Ferrand recognized the high local recurrence rate of the tumor now known as dermatofibrosarcoma protuberans (DFSP). The relatively good prognosis of atypical fibroxanthoma (AFX) did not appear commensurate with its striking nuclear pleomorphism such that terms coined in the 1960s erroneously suggested a *pseudosarcomatous* process. Only subsequently was its metastatic potential recognized. In their seminal 1964 article in *Cancer*, Stout and Hill described the natural history of superficial leiomyosarcoma (LMS). The higher metastatic rate of subcutaneous tumors relative to their dermal counterparts was noted, thereby anticipating the current practice of considering cutaneous tumors separately.[1]

EPIDEMIOLOGY

National cancer registries do not report cutaneous sarcomas as a separate category. These tumors are variously categorized as 'non-melanoma skin cancer', 'sarcoma', or 'miscellaneous tumors'; under the first two headings, the relatively uncommon primary cutaneous sarcomas would be overshadowed by cutaneous carcinomas and subfascial sarcomas, respectively. As one example, DFSP is included under the more general heading 'low grade fibrosarcoma' in the Swedish Cancer Registry of 1999, which lists the crude incidence rate for this category as 30 per 100,000 persons per year. It therefore appears that the impact of cutaneous sarcoma has not been rigorously defined. Nevertheless, physicians who treat skin cancer will certainly encounter the more common sarcomas during the course of their professional careers.

Table 24.1	Abbreviations
AFX	Atypical fibroxanthoma
BL	Benign lipoblastoma
CCS	Clear cell sarcoma
CK	Cytokeratin(s)
DF	Dermatofibroma
DFSP	Dermatofibrosarcoma protuberans
FS-DFSP	Fibrosarcomatous dermatofibrosarcoma protuberans
EMC	Extraskeletal myxoid chondrosarcoma
EpS	Epithelioid sarcoma
EwS	Ewing sarcoma
GCF	Giant cell fibroblastoma
IHC	Immunohistochemical
LMS	Leiomyosarcoma
LPS	Liposarcoma
MFH	Malignant fibrous histiocytoma
MMS	Mohs micrographic surgery
MPNST	Malignant peripheral nerve sheath tumor
NFas	Nodular fasciitis
OssFMT	Ossifying fibromyxoid tumor
PlexFHT	Plexiform fibrohistiocytic tumor
PNET	Peripheral primitive neuroectodermal tumor
RMS	Rhabdomyosarcoma

PATHOGENESIS AND ETIOLOGY

Sarcomatous elements rarely arise *secondarily* within epithelial skin cancers, most commonly squamous cell carcinoma. This phenomenon, termed *metaplastic carcinoma* or *carcinosarcoma*, suggests neoplastic transformation and divergent differentiation of pluripotential cells.

The frequent association of AFX with marked solar elastosis has long suggested a causative role for actinic irradiation. This hypothesis has been substantiated in part by the demonstration of CC→TT dimeric transitions in the mutated *p53* gene of some cases of AFX, a genetic alteration that points to ultraviolet-induced damage. Prior therapeutic irradiation for cancer also predisposes to the development of cutaneous sarcoma including pediatric patients treated with high-dose irradiation of central nervous system and visceral malignancies. Post-irradiation cutaneous sarcomas in adults include AFX and DFSP; the latter has been reported following cutaneous irradiation for basal cell carcinoma. DFSP has also been reported in the setting of post-transplant immunosuppression, suggesting that loss of immune surveillance is another important factor in tumorigenesis.

Recent investigation of the pathogenesis of cutaneous sarcomas has implicated a variety of oncogenic events. Cytogenetic studies of DFSP and giant cell fibroblastoma have reproducibly demonstrated a characteristic translocation between chromosomes 17 and 22, t(17;22). This results in fusion of a portion of the collagen gene *COL1A1* to the platelet-derived growth factor-beta gene,

PDGFB.[2] The fusion product, which retains growth factor activity, is overexpressed. DFSP tumor cells express the PDGFB-receptor, which sets the stage for an autocrine loop. Expression of the *bcl-2* oncoprotein has been found in benign and malignant spindle cell tumors, including fibrocytic, fibrohistiocytic and neural neoplasms such as malignant peripheral nerve sheath tumor (MPNST), malignant fibrous histiocytoma and low-grade fibromyxoid sarcoma. Mutations in the *N-ras* oncogene have been identified in an epithelioid sarcoma that widely metastasized to both cutaneous and visceral sites and resulted in death. Abnormalities of insulin receptors and post-receptor cellular metabolism have been identified in a variety of lipomatous tumors including liposarcoma.

CLINICAL FEATURES

Clinical presentation

Common presentations

AFX, DFSP and LMS constitute the vast majority of superficial sarcomas that present as true cutaneous tumors. AFX commonly occurs as a nodule, often ulcerated, on sun-exposed skin of elderly individuals (Fig. 24.1), but approximately one-quarter of cases occur on the trunk and extremities of younger adults. DFSP presents across the age spectrum (including infants and children) as a slowly growing, firm irregular plaque fixed to the skin but mobile over the deep fascia and containing protuberant nodules (Fig. 24.2). The trunk is the most common site in some series, but all locations of the head and neck and of the extremities have been reported. Unusual presentations include the depressed indurated plaque of non-protuberant ('atrophic') DFSP[3] and pedunculated lesions that closely simulate neurofibromas or fibroepithelial polyps.[4] LMS, which affects adults of all ages, including younger adults, develops as a papulonodule that is usually misdiagnosed clinically because of its nondescript appearance (Fig. 24.3); indeed, the clinical impression may be that of a banal lesion, such as an epidermoid cyst.

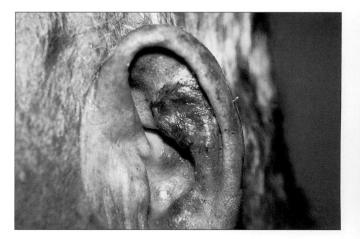

Figure 24.1 Atypical fibroxanthoma of the pinna in an elderly patient. (Image courtesy of Clinical Images Library of the Department of Dermatology at UT Southwestern Medical Center, Dallas, TX.)

Tumors on the extremities

Epithelioid sarcoma (EpS) and clear cell sarcoma (CCS) generally affect acral sites. A distal extremity tumor of the flexor surface of a digit or of the hand or foot of a young man suggests the possibility of EpS, but the tumor does not arise exclusively in the extremities, and EpS of genital sites in both sexes have been described. EpS can simulate Dupuytren's contracture. Not infrequently, EpS can present as a chronic ulcer for which the clinical differential diagnosis includes infectious processes.[5] A tumor of the foot and specifically of the ankle raises the possibility of CCS, which can also affect other periarticular locations of either the upper or lower extremities. Ossifying fibromyxoid tumor (OssFMT) tends to occur on the proximal extremities of adults and plexiform fibrohistiocytic tumor (PlexFHT) on the upper extremities of children and young adults. The superficial fibromatoses – palmar (Dupuytren's), plantar (Ledderhose's) and penile (Peyronie's) – present as firm plaques or contractures and have a tendency to recur locally but never metastasize; a full discussion of this group of disorders is beyond the scope of this chapter.

Lipomatous tumors

The rare primary cutaneous liposarcoma (LPS) has demonstrated some predilection for the scalp of elderly individuals in small series, although the possibility of metastatic LPS must be excluded clinically. Because of their macroscopic and histological similarities to mature adipose tissue, well-differentiated LPS can simulate common lipomas clinically. Recent rapid growth of a tumor that arises from a longstanding subcutaneous mass can herald dedifferentiation of an atypical lipomatous tumor (well-differentiated LPS). Multicentricity alone should not lead to presumption of malignancy, especially if symmetric and slowly progressive, as is often the case for benign lipomatous tumors such as angiolipomas and spindle cell/pleomorphic lipomas.

Pediatric patients

Sarcomatous skin tumors in pediatric patients raise additional considerations. Early DFSP can present as a red-blue plaque that resembles a vascular malformation. This is an especially important pitfall with DFSP arising in infants in whom a malformative process might be the favored clinical diagnosis. In this clinical setting, histopathologic evaluation is critical. Cutaneous metastasis may be the first manifestation of deep soft tissue or osseous sarcomas such as RMS, neuroblastoma, osteosarcoma, Ewing sarcoma (EwS) and peripheral primitive neuroectodermal tumor (PNET).[6] 'Blueberry muffin'-like eruptions in neonates or infants have been described in the setting of viral infection (TORCH syndrome) but can also be due to widespread cutaneous metastases of alveolar RMS from a soft tissue primary.[7] Rhabdomyosarcoma can rarely present as a cutaneous primary in patients of any age group but this is a diagnosis of exclusion; as with DFSP, congenital RMS has presented as a deforming mass that simulated a congenital malformation.[8]

Special situations

Cutaneous sarcomas rarely arise within congenital melanocytic nevi. Unlike deep MPNST, which most often arises from large nerve trunks in the setting of type I neurofibromatosis, cutaneous MPNST has been reported in the absence of either a large associated nerve trunk or the stigmata of neurofibromatosis.[9]

Natural history

In general, cutaneous sarcomas are associated with the capacity for local recurrence and low metastatic potential. When it occurs, metastasis is often preceded by local recurrence, and both local recurrence and metastasis can occur after many years. This generalization holds true for the most common cutaneous sarcomas – DFSP, AFX and LMS – each of which is associated with metastatic rates in the single digit percent range (approximately 4% for DFSP). Similar clinical behavior characterizes many, though not all, of the rarer cutaneous sarcomas. For instance, the few reported cases of cutaneous LPS,

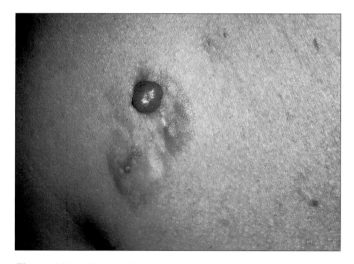

Figure 24.2 Dermatofibrosarcoma protuberans on the trunk of a young adult. Note the protuberant nodule within the otherwise flat irregular plaque. Tentacle-like processes of tumor can extend up to 10 cm beyond its clinically appreciable extent. (Image courtesy of Clinical Images Library of the Department of Dermatology at UT Southwestern Medical Center, Dallas, TX.)

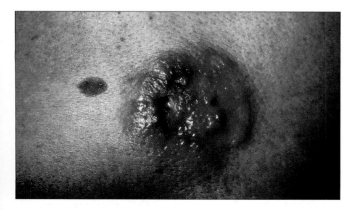

Figure 24.3 Leiomyosarcoma. Although the clinical finding of an ulcerated nodule suggests a malignant diagnosis, there are no specific clinical features pointing to the diagnosis LMS.

including high-grade tumors of the pleomorphic subtype, have recurred locally but have not metastasized. While less aggressive than its more deeply seated counterpart, primary cutaneous PNET has occasionally resulted in metastasis and death.[10] However, a small series of the related primary cutaneous EwS reported no local recurrence or metastasis.[11] OssFMT and parachordoma have been classified by some experts as benign but both have the capacity to recur locally and rarely to metastasize.

An important exception to the above generalizations is EpS, which is particularly aggressive even when superficial. Patients can rapidly develop regional lymph node involvement and distant bony or pulmonary metastases, often within 1 year of the initial diagnosis.

Tumor progression is exemplified by the development of fibrosarcomatous areas within DFSP (FS-DFSP). Earlier studies associated this phenomenon with higher rates of distant metastasis to lung, bone and soft tissue and death.[12] However, a recent study suggests that the outcome of completely resected FS-DFSP may in fact be similar to that of conventional DFSP.[13] Progression of OssFMT to well-differentiated osteosarcoma and of well-differentiated to dedifferentiated LPS have also been reported.

Patient evaluation

Biopsy technique

Histopathologic diagnosis is essential and requires a representative specimen. Evaluation of a small biopsy specimen may be non-diagnostic or indeterminate. Especially in the case of EpS, resemblance to palisaded granulomatous processes can lead to misdiagnosis; a high clinical index of suspicion for EpS should prompt re-biopsy in any persistent, growing or ulcerated nodule or plaque at an acral site. A similar principle applies for other cutaneous sarcomas and other anatomic sites. The diagnosis of well differentiated LPS may not be suspected because such tumors may closely resemble common lipomas; therefore, before embarking on an unsuitable treatment for LPS, such as liposuction, biopsy confirmation is important. The orientation of an incisional biopsy procedure should be carefully planned so as to be easily encompassed by the subsequent excision.

Radiological evaluation

DFSP demonstrates similar signal attenuation to that of skeletal muscle on computed tomography (CT) and non-specifically prolonged T1 and T2 relaxation times on magnetic resonance imaging (MRI). MRI is particularly helpful in detecting subclinical tumor extension, which can be considerable in DFSP, EpS and subcutaneous malignant fibrous histiocytoma (MFH). Although MRI can suggest the likely composition of a tumor, it cannot distinguish between tumors of similar composition, such as lipoma and atypical lipomatous tumor; similarly, those variants of lipoma (e.g. spindle cell lipoma) and LPS with minimal mature fat cannot be distinguished radiologically from other soft tissue tumors. Approximately 80% of OssFMTs show a characteristic peripheral rim of calcification.

DIAGNOSIS

Histopathology

Hypercellular spindle cell tumors

Classic AFX is composed of haphazardly arranged, pleomorphic spindle and giant cells, often with a high mitotic rate and many abnormal mitotic figures (Fig. 24.4). In rare cases, a marked lymphocytic inflammatory infiltrate can partly obscure the neoplastic cells. Pleomorphic tumors histologically identical to AFX but centered in the subcutis are best classified as subcutaneous MFH. Cutaneous sarcomas of almost any subtype can exhibit similarly pleomorphic or hypercellular proliferations of spindle cells: LMS (Fig. 24.5), high-grade fibrosarcoma (e.g. high-grade FS-DFSP), EpS with a predominantly spindle cell pattern, pleomorphic LPS, pleomorphic RMS, and high-grade osteosarcoma, among others. In distinguishing among these, a diligent search should be made for evidence of specific differentiation by careful routine microscopic examination and judicious use of immunohistochemical stains.

Monomorphic spindle cell tumors

Classic DFSP is composed of relatively small, uniform spindle cells arranged at least focally in a distinctly storiform pattern. Similar proliferations of uniform spindle cells, though without the characteristic storiform arrangement, characterize FS-DFSP, superficial fibromatoses, desmoid fibromatosis, small cell AFX, spindle cell LPS, MPNST and the exceedingly rare primary cutaneous synovial sarcoma. Compared with conventional DFSP, FS-DFSP shows greater hypercellularity, fascicular arrangement, necrosis and generally higher mitotic rates. Scattered pigmented spindle or stellate cells can be found in DFSP (referred to as Bednar tumor), FS-DFSP or giant

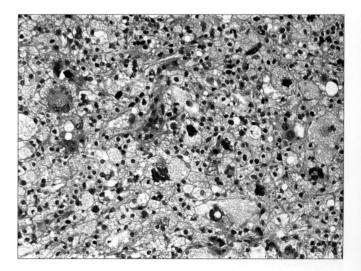

Figure 24.4 Atypical fibroxanthoma. In this portion of the tumor, pleomorphic tumor giant cells and round mononuclear cells with abundant, finely vacuolated cytoplasm predominate. Note the very coarse chromatin, lobulated and irregular nuclear contours, occasional intranuclear cytoplasmic pseudoinclusions and scattered mitotic figures. (Image courtesy of Robert Quirey MD, Dallas, TX.)

cell fibroblastoma (GCF). The histology of MPNST is that of a mitotically active spindle cell population with variable arrangement in fascicles, geographic necrosis and hypercellular areas predominantly around vessels (*peritheliomatous* pattern).

Hypocellularity

Low neoplastic cell density characterizes GCF and many myxoid neoplasms such as myxoid DFSP (Fig. 24.6), myxoid LPS (Fig. 24.7), low-grade fibromyxoid sarcoma and low- and intermediate-grade areas of myxofibro-sarcoma.[14]

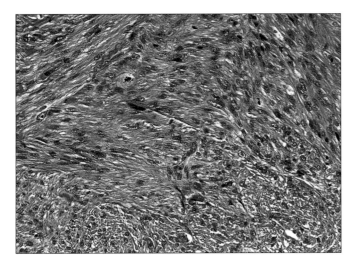

Figure 24.5 Leiomyosarcoma. Fascicles of neoplastic cells intersect perpendicularly, a common feature of LMS. Within fascicles, elongated atypical nuclei with coarse chromatin are aligned parallel to one another and are associated with characteristically eosinophilic cytoplasm, occasional paranuclear vacuoles and scattered mitotic figures. (Image courtesy of Robert Quirey MD, Dallas, TX.)

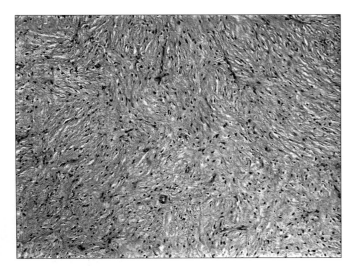

Figure 24.6 Myxoid DFSP. Small, slightly curved nuclei are scattered throughout a delicate, lightly basophilic myxoid matrix; the similarity to neurofibroma is striking. Other portions of the tumor showed infiltration of subcutaneous adipose tissue characteristic of DFSP. (Image courtesy of David Stewart MD, Dallas, TX.)

Round cell morphology

Round cell tumors that are composed of crowded primitive cells with scant cytoplasm include embryonal RMS, alveolar RMS, EwS, PNET, MPNST and round cell LPS. In ossifying fibromyxoid tumor (OssFMT), nests or cords of round to fusiform cells are surrounded by a myxoid to collagenous stroma. OssFMT with greater cellularity and/or mitotic activity has been referred to as 'atypical' or 'malignant' but, in fact, both the conventional and hypercellular types can recur and rarely metastasize. Similar round to spindle cell morphology is seen in parachordoma, which also contains vacuolated cells similar to the physaliferous cells of chordoma.

Epithelioid morphology

EpS and rarely other cutaneous sarcomas exhibit epithelioid cell morphology, that is, round or polygonal cells with prominent, often eosinophilic cytoplasm and distinct cell boundaries (Fig. 24.8). Epithelioid variants have been described for LMS, angiosarcoma and MPNST.

Granular cell morphology

Tumors characterized by granular cells have coarsely granular eosinophilic cytoplasm, which is a non-specific phenotype by light microscopy that correlates with the presence ultrastructurally of abundant cytoplasmic lysosomal granules.

Osseous or chondroid elements

Metaplastic ossification can occur in scar as well as in benign and malignant neoplasms. In osteosarcoma, osteoid is deposited as trabeculae which may be coarse or delicate and branching. In contrast to metaplastic bone, such malignant osteoid is intimately associated with the neoplastic spindle or round cell population.[15] In classic OssFMT, a peripheral shell of bony trabeculae outlines the well-circumscribed, often lobulated tumor, correlating with its radiographic appearance.

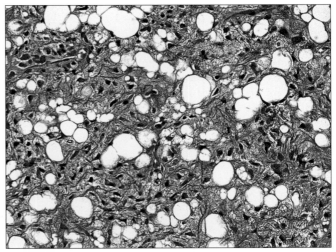

Figure 24.7 Myxoid liposarcoma. Small spindle and stellate cells are haphazardly arranged in a myxoid stroma that contains distinct curvilinear small-caliber vessels. The cytoplasm of some neoplastic cells is filled by large, empty lipid vacuoles that appear to compress the nucleus, producing the scalloped nuclear contour characteristic of 'lipoblasts'. (Image courtesy of Robert Quirey MD, Dallas, TX.)

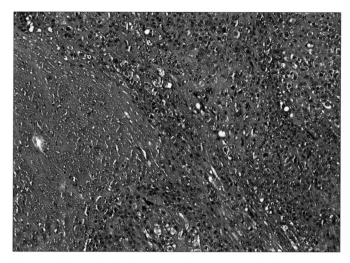

Figure 24.8 Epithelioid sarcoma. Neoplastic cells display the abundant cytoplasm, distinct cell boundaries and cohesive arrangement of epithelioid cells. On low magnification, necrotic foci (such as that on the left) surrounded by an epithelioid cell infiltrate can resemble necrotizing granulomata; however, the nuclei of the epithelioid cells show irregular nuclear contours and coarse chromatin and are therefore distinctly different from the nuclei of epithelioid histiocytes. (Image courtesy of Robert Quirey MD, Dallas, TX.)

Prominent myxoid, fibrous or hyalinized stroma

Myxoid areas are found in a wide variety of malignant and benign soft tissue lesions. Some areas of myxoid DFSP closely simulate neurofibroma. The stroma of OssFMT is myxoid or collagenous and that of para-chordoma varies from hyalinized fibrous to chondroid.

Lipomatous differentiation

Although exceedingly rare, primary cutaneous LPS can manifest any of the histologic subtypes associated with conventional deep (subfascial) LPS. The category of well-differentiated LPS includes adipocytic, spindle cell, sclerosing and inflammatory variants, any of which may be associated with dedifferentiation. Myxoid and round cell types comprise a single category, and pleomorphic LPS yet another. Lipoblasts with scalloped nuclei and vacuolated cytoplasm can be identified, particularly in the dedifferentiated and pleomorphic variants. Unusual features include occasional divergent differentiation such as the presence of smooth muscle elements.

Fine needle aspiration cytology

Notwithstanding the similarities in spindle cell morphology among many cutaneous sarcomas, fine needle aspiration (FNA) cytology can be successfully employed in diagnosis. Thorough knowledge of the classic histopathologic features and of common variant patterns is essential. Aspirates often reveal spindle cells present singly and in aggregates with variable stromal aggregates. Relatively monotonous spindle cells characterize DFSP and fibrosarcomatous transformation of DFSP, whereas nuclear

pleomorphism points to entities such as AFX, MFH and LMS. 'Strap cells' of RMS have abundant eosinophilic cytoplasm and eccentric nuclei. The adipose and fibrovascular elements in aspirates of atypical lipomatous tumor (well-differentiated LPS) contain adipocytes with irregular large nuclei, variable nucleoli and scattered 'lipoblasts' with scalloped nuclei. Fragments of stroma can show fibrous, myxoid or chondroid differentiation. The diagnostic impression gained from cytologic examination of aspirates can be further refined either by immunohistochemistry performed on paraffin embedded cell blocks or by correlation with other modalities. These include cytogenetic studies, *in situ* hybridization to detect tumor-specific transcripts or even conventional radiographic images (e.g. the peripheral rim of ossification of OssFMT).

Immunohistochemistry

Supportive immunohistochemical (IHC) studies are essential in all but the most well differentiated tumors, especially because the differential diagnosis often includes biologically diverse tumors of epithelial, melanocytic and lymphoid differentiation. Almost no IHC marker is entirely sensitive or specific so that it is essential to interpret the results of a well-chosen panel of markers in the context of all available clinical and histopathologic data. IHC profiles are summarized in Table 24.2.

Positivity for vimentin

This marker is positive in all sarcomas as well as several other neoplasms including melanoma. Although not particularly useful in diagnosis, it is useful as an internal control, particularly in cases where initial antibody panels are otherwise negative. Immunoreactivity of either neoplastic cells or non-neoplastic native stromal cells provides evidence of antigen preservation, indicating that negative IHC studies probably represent true negatives in the context of appropriate external positive and negative controls. Weak or negative vimentin staining in the tissue of interest suggests major technical problems, casting doubt on the validity of other IHC studies.

Negativity, in general, for epithelial markers (though with important exceptions)

Cytokeratin expression is found in epithelioid (non-spindle cell) areas of EpS and variably in epithelioid variants of other sarcomas. Epithelial elements of synovial sarcoma are positive for low molecular weight cytokeratins (CK); its glandular nests are additionally positive for high molecular weight CK, display luminal positivity for epithelial membrane antigen and are surrounded by type IV collagen.

Lack of specificity of smooth muscle markers

A number of fibrohistiocytic lesions express smooth muscle actin, so that great care is required in interpreting this marker: attention to the extent and intensity of

Table 24.2   Immunohistochemical profiles

	CD34	Factor XIIIa	S-100 protein	HMB-45	Cytokeratins	EMA	CD68	SMA	MSA (HHF-35)	Calponin	Caldesmon	Desmin	Myoglobin	MyoD1	CD99	NSE	pgp9.5	Osteocalcin
Angiomatoid fibrous histiocytoma							+/-	-/+	-/+	-/+		+/-						
Atypical fibroxanthoma	-	+/-	-	-	-		+/-	-/+	-/+	-/+	-	-/+						
Clear cell sarcoma of soft tissue	-		+	+	-	-		-	-/+		-	-				+/-		-
Dermatofibrosarcoma protuberans	+	-	-		-		-	-	-			-						
FS-DFSP, fibrosarcomatous areas	+/-	-			-	-		-/+	-/+			-					-	
Epithelioid sarcoma	+/-		-	-	+	+		-/+	-/+			-/+						-
Ewing sarcoma			-/+		-/+	-			-			-	-		+	-/+	-/+	-
Fibromatoses, superficial								+/-	+/-									
Fibromyxoid sarcoma, low grade	-/+	-			-/+	+		+/-	+/-			-/+						
Leiomyosarcoma	-/+	-/+	-		-/+	-/+	-/+	+	+	+	+/-	+						
LMS, epithelioid	-/+	-/+	-	-	-			+	+		+/-	+/-						-
Liposarcoma	-	+/-			-			-	-		-	-				-		-
Malignant peripheral nerve sheath tumor			+/-	-		-/+			-			-				+/-	-	
MPNST, epithelioid	-/+		+/-	-	-/+	-/+		-	-/+		-	-/+						-
Myxofibrosarcoma			-	-	-	-		-/+	-/+			-						
Ossifying fibromyxoid tumor of soft parts	-		+	-	-	-		+/-	-/+			+/-				+/-		
Osteosarcoma, extraskeletal			-/+	-	-			-				-				-/+		+
Parachordoma	-		+	+	+			-	-	-		-						
Primitive neuroectodermal tumor			-/+	-	-/+			-	-			-/+	-		+	+	+	-
Plexiform fibrohistiocytic tumor			-	-	-		+	+				-						
Rhabdomyosarcoma, alveolar			-/+	-	-	-		-/+	+			+	-/+	+	-/+	-/+		-
Rhabdomyosarcoma, embryonal			-		-	-		-/+	+			+	-/+	+	-/+	-		-
Synovial sarcoma	-		-/+	-	+	+		-	-		-	-			+/-			-

+, Immunoreactivity in >75%; +/-, Immunoreactivity in approximately 50-75%; -/+, Immunoreactivity in <50%; -, Negative or very rare immunoreactivity (<5%); Blank, Unknown.
The IHC profiles depicted here are a summary of data from primary sources (see References) and from two excellent chapters on the subject (see General References). Because no marker is entirely sensitive or specific, it is important to consider a marker's frequency in a given tumor as well as its expression by other tumors. EMA, epithelial membrane antigen; SMA, smooth muscle actin; MSA, muscle-specific actin; NSE, neuron specific enolase. Tumor abbreviations are listed in Table 24.1. Other abbreviations (e.g. pgp 9.5) are the standard ones used in the literature for IHC markers or the monoclonal antibodies that target them.

staining, judicious choice of additional markers and correlation with routine histologic features are essential (Table 24.2). As one example, AFX exhibits both fibrohistiocytic and myofibroblastic differentiation based on its occasional expression of smooth muscle markers such as desmin, calponin and muscle specific actin.[16]

Utility and limitations of CD34

It is now well established that CD34, while not specific, is invaluable in the diagnosis of DFSP in cases where routine microscopy is inconclusive. One caveat is that CD34 positivity is strongest along the advancing edge of the tumor but may be weak or even negative in nodular portions of the tumor, especially if these are hyalinized or myxoid. Furthermore, foci of fibrosarcomatous transformation may be negative for CD34 at a rate that approaches 50%. The list of CD34-positive neoplasms has grown considerably since the introduction of this marker and CD34-positive spindle cells can be found in EpS and across the spectrum of lipomatous lesions, including strong expression in spindle cell lipoma and by some elements of LPS.

Miscellaneous

Microphthalmia-associated transcription factor is expressed in melanocytic lesions (including melanoma and its spindle cell and desmoplastic variants), in CCS and in so-called PEComas (Perivascular Epithelioid Cell tumors that combine melanocytic and myoid differentiation).

Electron microscopy

Although IHC studies now provide much information regarding cellular differentiation, this was formerly the domain of electron microscopy (a modality which continues to be useful in selected cases). Because it can be impossible to exclude the diagnosis of spindle cell melanoma in the differential diagnosis of MPNST solely on the basis of routine microscopy and immunohistochemistry, failure to demonstrate premelanosomes in a representative ultrastructural study provides evidence in support of MPNST. Also, electron microscopy can confirm diagnostic impressions based on initial histological and immunohistochemical evaluation or provide clues as to the differentiation of very poorly differentiated neoplasms that have lost expected immunohistochemical markers. A full discussion of the ultrastructure of cutaneous sarcomas is beyond the scope of this chapter.

Other advanced techniques: cytogenetics, *in situ* hybridization and PCR

A number of subfascial sarcomas are associated with characteristic cytogenetic abnormalities that are readily identified on G-banded karyotypes prepared from short-term cell cultures. This requires procurement of fresh tissue with prompt transport to a specialized cytogenetics laboratory. Cytogenetic evaluation can be employed with larger cutaneous sarcomas of which a portion of the tumor can be spared and devoted to establishing a cell culture. The characteristic t(17;22) translocation of DFSP has already provided some clues regarding pathophysiology, as noted above. Among the subcutaneous lipomatous tumors, atypical lipomatous tumor, myxoid LPS, spindle cell and pleomorphic lipoma and hibernoma each is associated with particular cytogenetic abnormalities, which could be helpful in the evaluation of unusual or borderline cases. Moreover, atypical lipomatous tumors possessing supernumerary ring or giant marker chromosomes are more likely to recur and to undergo dedifferentiation.

When fresh tissue is not available, *in situ* hybridization techniques can be employed on archival paraffin-embedded tissue to search for marker translocations, such as those involving the *EWS* locus at 22q12 in Ewing family tumors and other deep sarcomas. A majority of CCS (but not melanomas) have been shown by reverse transcriptase polymerase chain reaction or fluorescence *in situ* hybridization to harbor the balanced translocation t(12;22)(q13;q13).

DIFFERENTIAL DIAGNOSIS

Reactive inflammatory simulators of sarcoma

Pleomorphism and hypercellularity are seen in reactive conditions such as nodular fasciitis (NFas), the most common benign soft tissue tumor misdiagnosed as sarcoma; NFas is associated with sudden rapid onset, usually good circumscription, histologic similarity to cells in tissue culture and variably fibrous or myxoid stroma (Fig. 24.9). Nodular lesions of *verruga peruana*, the cutaneous manifestation of *Bartonella bacilliformis* infection, are proliferations of hypercellular epithelioid and spindle cells that sometimes resemble Kaposi's sarcoma, leiomyosarcoma, fibrosarcoma or spindle cell melanoma. Consideration of an infectious rather than a neoplastic etiology is based on the clinical presentation of miliary or nodular angiomatous lesions in a patient from endemic regions of Peru, Ecuador or Colombia.

Benign neoplasms simulating sarcoma

Marked cytologic atypia is neither requisite nor sufficient for the diagnosis of cutaneous sarcoma. Benign simulators include atypical cutaneous leiomyomas that contain large pleomorphic cells. This may represent the cutaneous analog of symplastic uterine leiomyomas. In schwannomas, variable nuclear atypia – even marked pleomorphism – without mitotic activity suggests 'ancient change'. This represents a phenomenon seen in longstanding lesions with other histological signs of degeneration such as hemorrhage, microcyst formation, hyalinization and calcification. Several dermatofibroma (DF) variants enter the differential diagnosis, particularly if the specimen is fragmented or if the characteristic circumscription and peripheral collagen entrapment are not evident. DF with monster cells contains scattered pleomorphic large cells, but mitotic activity is negligible. Cellular DF not uncommonly shows at least focal

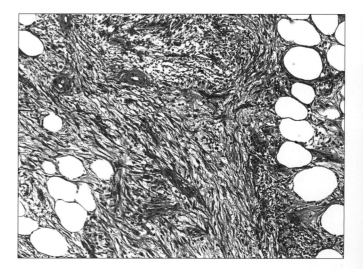

Figure 24.9 Nodular fasciitis. Haphazardly arranged spindle cells have slender nuclei of varying sizes that lack the coarse chromatin, hyperchromasia, irregular nuclear contours and sometimes prominent nucleoli seen in atypical cells of malignant processes. Note also the characteristically loose arrangement of the spindle cells in an edematous matrix that also contains scattered mononuclear inflammatory cells and extravasated erythrocytes. (Image courtesy of Robert Quirey MD, Dallas, TX.)

storiform areas that simulate DFSP. Curiously, cellular, aneurysmal and atypical DF have been reported to metastasize on very rare occasions to regional lymph nodes[17] and lung;[18] understandably, such reports have generated considerable controversy.[19]

Potentially confusing names of different soft tissue lesions

Aneurysmal fibrous histiocytoma (a DF variant – a *benign* entity) can undergo rapid growth due to intralesional hemorrhage, thereby simulating a malignant neoplasm clinically. Careful attention to terminology is necessary to avoid confusion with the unrelated and locally recurrent *angiomatoid* fibrous histiocytoma, which was formerly considered a variant of MFH. This has also been referred to as angiomatoid *malignant* fibrous histiocytoma.

Sarcomatous elements within non-sarcomatous skin tumors

The mere presence of sarcomatous elements does not necessarily point to a diagnosis of sarcoma. Such elements can occur focally in primary cutaneous malignancies such as melanoma, squamous cell carcinoma, Merkel cell carcinoma and adnexal carcinoma. The sarcomatous elements identified in such metaplastic carcinomas include osteosarcoma, chondrosarcoma, LMS and RMS.[20]

Hypercellular pleomorphic pattern

The differential diagnosis of hypercellular and pleomorphic round to spindle cell populations consists of AFX, MFH, LMS, spindle cell melanoma, spindle cell squamous cell carcinoma, poorly differentiated adnexal carcinoma and large cell lymphoma. Less pleomorphic spindle cell sarcomas include the predominantly spindle cell (*fibroma-like*) variant of epithelioid sarcoma, which may lack the more readily recognizable nodular epithelioid areas. Many histological features of MPNST are shared with spindle cell melanoma subtypes (spindle cell, desmoplastic and neurotropic), whether primary or metastatic. Key differences are stronger and more diffuse positivity for S-100 protein, occasional positivity for HMB-45 and negativity for pgp 9.5 in melanoma but not MPNST.

Hypocellular proliferations of small uniform spindle cells with myxoid matrix

The differential diagnosis of myxoid soft tissue tumors includes a broad range of lesions, including benign (e.g. myxoid nodular fasciitis), locally aggressive (low-grade myxofibrosarcoma) and malignant lesions (e.g. myxoid MPNST).[21]

Round cell morphology

A well-chosen panel of immunohistochemical stains is essential in distinguishing among small round blue cell tumors. However, no marker is pathognomonic. Positivity for CD99 (detected using antibodies O13 and 12E7 to the MIC2 gene product) has been reported in a variety of other neoplasms, including Merkel cell carcinoma and small cell carcinoma.

Clear cell neoplasms

The differential diagnosis includes CCS, clear cell variant of AFX, balloon cell melanoma, sebaceous carcinoma, metastatic clear cell carcinoma (especially renal cell carcinoma) and cutaneous LPS.

Epithelioid neoplasms

This differential diagnosis includes other epithelioid mesenchymal tumors such as epithelioid angiosarcoma and epithelioid schwannoma, granulomatous infiltrates with epithelioid macrophages, and melanocytic, lymphoid and epithelial neoplasms. The centrally necrotic aggregates of EpS can be confused with the palisaded granulomas of rheumatoid nodule and granuloma annulare. Even when recognized as frankly malignant, the epithelioid cells of EpS can be mistaken for squamous cell carcinoma.

Granular cell morphology

Benign granular cell tumors are more common than their malignant counterparts, which demonstrate nuclear atypia and mitotic activity. The differential diagnosis of spindle cell proliferations with this peculiar cytoplasmic appearance includes malignant granular cell tumor, granular cell dermatofibroma, and granular cell variants of leiomyosarcoma, angiosarcoma AFX and MFH.

Rhabdoid morphology

Large round eosinophilic intracytoplasmic PAS-positive inclusions with eccentrically displaced atypical nuclei have been described in a variety of neoplasms including squamous cell carcinoma, Merkel cell carcinoma, melanoma and several sarcomas. Therefore, the diagnosis of extrarenal rhabdoid tumor is one of exclusion after thorough histologic, immunohistochemical and ultrastructural evaluation.[22] Rarely, cutaneous nodules have been the sole initial presentation of congenital malignant rhabdoid tumor.

Lipomatous differentiation

When lipomatous differentiation is identified, a number of benign lipomatous tumors must be considered.

Myxoid LPS can rarely affect children, but consideration should be given to the diagnosis of *benign lipoblastoma* (BL), which on low magnification shows lobules of adipose tissue separated by fibrous tissue septa of variable thickness. Unlike BL, myxoid LPS shows at least focal nuclear atypia and the characteristic t(12;16) translocation. *Massive localized lymphedema* is a large mass that occurs on the proximal extremities of morbidly obese individuals and consists of mature adipose tissue with expanded fibrous septa, thereby simulating well-differentiated LPS. However, it lacks the cytologic atypia of LPS and on follow-up has shown local persistence but neither histologic progression nor metastasis.[23] Variants of lipoma that can be mistaken for sarcoma include *spindle cell*, *pleomorphic*, *myxoid* and *chondroid* variants.

Parachordoma

This rare subcutaneous tumor resembles chordoma, extraskeletal myxoid chondrosarcoma (EMC) and soft tissue myoepithelioma. Parachordoma expresses CK 8/18, whereas chordoma expresses CK 1/10 in addition to CK 8/18, while EMC is negative for cytokeratins.

Metastatic sarcoma

Sarcoma in the skin is occasionally metastatic from deeper tumors, such as leiomyosarcoma of the uterus or mesentery, osteosarcoma of bone or rarely extraosseous sites,[24] and LPS of the retroperitoneum.

TREATMENT

Effective treatment is based on correct histopathologic diagnosis as initial misdiagnosis can result in under-treatment, mainly in the form of delayed or inadequate excision. This can set the stage for progression or recurrence, respectively. A high index of suspicion is required in some cases of DFSP and EpS, particularly in the evaluation of small biopsy specimens that do not highlight the classic histopathologic features.

Complete surgical excision – conventional and Mohs techniques

The first step in treatment is to achieve local control by complete excision of the tumor. Mohs micrographic surgery (MMS) has been increasingly used to treat a variety of cutaneous sarcomas – including DFSP, AFX, LMS and MFH.[25] A major challenge in achieving local control is related to the observation that some superficial sarcomas (especially DFSP, EpS and subcutaneous MFH) can extend subclinically for considerable distances along fascial planes. Three-dimensional reconstruction of DFSP has demonstrated infiltrative tentacle-like extensions of tumor.[26] Prior to the widespread use of MMS, excision of DFSP was associated with a recurrence rate exceeding 50% in some series, and even wide surgical excision of DFSP with 30 mm margins was associated with a

recurrence rate of 11%. By MMS or its modified form (i.e. evaluation of permanent tangential margin sections), excision up to 100 mm in some areas beyond the clinically appreciable tumor has been required and the recurrence rate of DFSP has thereby been decreased to approximately 2%.[27] Even for tumors such as AFX that are not generally associated with subclinical extension, excision by MMS results in lower recurrence rates than wide local excision.[28] MMS has been used in treating a wide variety of malignant and benign but locally recurrent tumors including myxoid DFSP, giant cell fibroblastoma, plexiform fibrohistiocytic tumor and infantile digital fibroma.

The increasing morbidity of re-excision and the association of metastasis and death with prior local recurrence emphasize the importance of complete excision. Ensuring histologically negative margins while conserving tissue is critical, especially in esthetically or functionally sensitive areas such as the face or distal extremities. At distal extremity sites, complete excision may leave little local tissue for reconstruction. This may be due to the absence of substantial tissue compartments and the proximity of the skin to critical neurovascular structures and joints. While routinely-stained frozen sections may be adequate at the time of primary excision, difficulty in distinguishing tumor from scar in recurrent lesions excised by MMS can be addressed by the use of immunohistochemical stains.[29]

Closure of surgical defects

Close collaboration of dermatologic Mohs surgeons with plastic-reconstructive surgeons is essential in minimizing the functional and psychological impact of morbid procedures. Immediate free tissue transfer has been employed even in some cases that received post-operative irradiation. Alternatively, split-thickness skin grafts can be used followed by delayed definitive reconstruction. Use of tissue expanders may facilitate reconstruction of especially large defects on the scalp.

Radiotherapy

DFSP is a radioresponsive tumor. Patients with DFSP who were deemed inoperable due to poor health status or unresectability of tumor have in exceptional cases been treated successfully with radiation therapy as the only modality. Radiotherapy has also been used to treat recurrent DFSP and has been advocated as an adjuvant to margin-positive conservative excision for patients in whom more extensive surgery is deemed functionally or cosmetically unacceptable.[30] The radioresponsiveness of less common cutaneous sarcomas has not been established.

Chemotherapy

Metastatic DFSP has been treated with systemic chemo-therapeutic agents such as methotrexate. When confined to an extremity, complete remission of advanced sarcomas, including LMS and EpS, has been achieved by isolated limb perfusion with high-dose tumor necrosis factor-α in combination with melphalan or adriamycin. One patient with metastatic clear cell sarcoma experienced a dramatic response to DAV chemotherapy (dimethyl–triazeno–imidazol–carboxamide, nimustine hydrochloride and vincristine). Recently, imatinib mesylate (STI-571, trade name Gleevec™), a PDGF-receptor antagonist, was used to treat unresectable metastatic FS-DFSP with variable response.[31,32]

Combined modalities

There are case reports documenting long-term disease-free survival of patients with cutaneous sarcomas treated with combined radical surgery, postoperative radiation therapy and adjuvant chemotherapy.

Long-term follow-up

Long-term follow-up is important to detect local recurrence of indolent low-grade tumors[33] and because of the potential for late metastases. Recurrence can still occur after excision by MMS, prompting some to call for a return to wide excision.

FUTURE OUTLOOK

Much of what is known about cutaneous sarcomas is based on case reports and relatively small series. More accurate epidemiological data regarding the incidence and mortality of this category of skin cancer will require greater attention from regional and national cancer registries. A more complete understanding of the natural behavior and a more rigorous assessment of different treatment approaches would probably benefit from cooperative multicenter studies. This would be especially helpful in characterizing the rarest entities.

The advent of modern biological therapies – such as imatinib mesylate (Gleevec™) – holds out the promise of pharmacological agents targeted at specific molecules expressed by tumor cells, and eventually such agents could prove to be useful adjuncts or even primary therapies for these tumors. In the meantime, complete surgical excision, often by MMS, will likely remain the mainstay of therapy.

REFERENCES

1 Fields JP, Helwig EB. Leiomyosarcoma of the skin and subcutaneous tissue. Cancer 1981; 47:156–169.

2 Simon MP, Pedeutour F, Sirvent N, et al. Deregulation of the platelet-derived growth factor β-chain gene via fusion with collagen gene COL1A1 in dermatofibrosarcoma protuberans and giant-cell fibroblastoma. Nat Genet 1997; 15:95–98.

3 Young CR 3rd, Albertini MJ. Atrophic dermatofibrosarcoma protuberans: case report, review, and proposed molecular mechanisms. J Am Acad Derm 2003; 49:761–764.

4 Resnik KS, DiLeonardo M, Hunter CJ. Pedunculated presentation of dermatofibrosarcoma protuberans. J Am Acad Derm 2003; 49:1139–1141.

5 Shmookler BM, Gunther SF. Superficial epithelioid sarcoma: a clinical and histologic stimulant of benign cutaneous disease. J Am Acad Derm 1986; 14:893–898.

6 Wesche WA, Khare VK, Chesney TM, Jenkins JJ. Non-hematopoietic cutaneous metastases in children and adolescents: thirty years experience at St. Jude Children's Research Hospital. J Cutan Pathol 2000; 27:485–492.

7 Godambe SV, Rawal J. Blueberry muffin rash as a presentation of alveolar cell rhabdomyosarcoma in a neonate. Acta Paediatr 2000; 89:115–117.

8 Brecher AR, Reyes-Mugica M, Kamino H, Chang MW. Congenital primary cutaneous rhabdomyosarcoma in a neonate. Pediatr Dermatol 2003; 20:335–338.

9 Dabski C, Reiman HM Jr, Muller SA. Neurofibrosarcoma of skin and subcutaneous tissues. Mayo Clin Proc 1990; 65:164–172.

10 Banerjee SS, Agbamu DA, Eyden BP, Harris M. Clinicopathological characteristics of peripheral primitive neuroectodermal tumour of skin and subcutaneous tissue. Histopathology 1997; 31:355–366.

11 Chow E, Merchant TE, Pappo A, et al. Cutaneous and subcutaneous Ewing's sarcoma: an indolent disease. Int J Radiat Oncol Biol Phys 2000; 46:433–438.

12 Mentzel T, Beham A, Katenkamp D, et al. Fibrosarcomatous ('high-grade') dermatofibrosarcoma protuberans: clinicopathologic and immunohistochemical study of a series of 41 cases with emphasis on prognostic significance. Am J Surg Pathol 1998; 22:576–587.

13 Goldblum JR, Reith JD, Weiss SW. Sarcomas arising in dermatofibrosarcoma protuberans: a reappraisal of biologic behavior in eighteen cases treated by wide local excision with extended clinical follow up. Am J Surg Pathol 2000; 24:1125–1130.

14 Mansoor A, White CR Jr. Myxofibrosarcoma presenting in the skin: clinicopathological features and differential diagnosis with cutaneous myxoid neoplasms. Am J Dermatopathol 2003; 25:281–286.

15 Kuo T-t. Primary osteosarcoma of the skin. J Cutan Pathol 1992; 19:151–155.

16 Sakamoto A, Oda Y, Yamamoto H, et al. Calponin and h-caldesmon expression in atypical fibroxanthoma and superficial leiomyosarcoma. Virchows Arch 2002; 440:404–409.

17 Guillou L, Gebhard S, Salmeron M, Coindre JM. Metastasizing fibrous histiocytoma of the skin: a clinicopathologic and immunohistochemical analysis of three cases. Mod Pathol 2000; 13:654–660.

18 Colome-Grimmer MI, Evans HL. Metastasizing cellular dermatofibroma. A report of two cases. Am J Surg Pathol 1996; 20:1361–1367.

19 Zelger BG, Zelger B. Correspondence re: Guillou L, Gebhard S, Salmeron M, Coindre JM. Metastasizing fibrous histiocytoma of the skin: a clinicopathologic and immunohistochemical analysis of three cases. Mod Pathol 2001; 14:534–536.

20 Patel NK, McKee PH, Smith NP, Fletcher CDM. Primary metaplastic carcinoma (carcinosarcoma) of the skin. A clinicopathologic study of four cases and review of the literature. Am J Dermatopathol 1997; 19:363–372.

21 Graadt van Roggen JF, Hogendoorn PCW, Fletcher CDM. Myxoid tumours of soft tissue. Histopathology 1999; 35:291–312.

22 Parham DM, Weeks DA, Beckwith JB. The clinicopathologic spectrum of putative extrarenal rhabdoid tumors. An analysis of 42 cases studied with immunohistochemistry or electron microscopy. Am J Surg Pathol 1994; 18:1010–1029.

23 Farshid G, Weiss SW. Massive localized lymphedema in the morbidly obese: a histologically distinct reactive lesion simulating liposarcoma. Am J Surg Pathol 1998; 22:1277–1283.

24 Covello SP, Humphreys TR, Lee JB. A case of extraskeletal osteosarcoma with metastasis to the skin. J Am Acad Derm 2003; 49:124–127.

25 Huether MJ, Zitelli JA, Brodland DG. Mohs micrographic surgery for the treatment of spindle cell tumors of the skin. J Am Acad Derm 2001; 44:656–659.

26 Haycox CL, Odland PB, Olbricht SM, Casey B. Dermatofibrosarcoma protuberans (DFSP): growth characteristics based on tumor modeling and a review of cases treated with Mohs micrographic surgery. Ann Plast Surg 1997; 38:246–251.

27 Ratner D, Thomas CO, Johnson TM, et al. Mohs micrographic surgery for the treatment of dermatofibrosarcoma protuberans. Results of a multiinstitutional series with an analysis of the extent of microscopic spread. J Am Acad Derm 1997; 37:600–613.

28 Davis JL, Randle HW, Zalla MJ, et al. A comparison of Mohs micrographic surgery and wide excision for the treatment of atypical fibroxanthoma. (Follow-up data reported by Zalla MJ, Randle HW, Brodland DG, et al. Dermatol Surg 1997; 23:1223–1224.). Dermatol Surg 1997; 23:105–110.

29 Prieto VG, Reed JA, Shea CR. CD34 immunoreactivity distinguishes between scar tissue and residual tumor in re-excisional specimens of dermatofibrosarcoma protuberans. J Cutan Pathol 1994; 21:324–329.

30 Ballo MT, Zagars GK, Pisters P, Pollack A. The role of radiation therapy in the management of dermatofibrosarcoma protuberans. Int J Radiat Oncol Biol Phys 1998; 40:823–827.

31 Maki RG, Awan RA, Dixon RH, et al. Differential sensitivity to imatinib of 2 patients with metastatic sarcoma arising from dermatofibrosarcoma protuberans. Int J Cancer 2002; 100:623–626.

32 Rubin BP, Schuetze SM, Eary JF, et al. Molecular targeting of platelet-derived growth factor β by imatinib mesylate in a patient with metastatic dermatofibrosarcoma protuberans. J Clin Oncol 2002; 20:3586–3591.

33 Orlando R, Lumachi F, Lirussi F. Recurrent dermatofibrosarcoma protuberans sixteen years after radical excition(sic). A case report. Anticancer Res 2003; 23:4233–4234.

General references:

Cerilli LA, Wick MR. Immunohistology of soft tissue and osseous neoplasms. In: Dabbs DJ, ed. Diagnostic Immunohistochemistry. Philadelphia: Churchill Livingstone; 2002:59–112.

Fletcher CDM, Unni KK, Mertens F (eds). World Health Organization Classification of Tumours, Pathology and Genetics of Tumours of Soft Tissue and Bone. Lyon: IARC Press; 2002.

Helm KF. Immunohistochemistry of skin. In: Dabbs DJ, ed. Diagnostic Immunohistochemistry. Philadelphia: Churchill Livingstone; 2002:313–332.

Weiss SW, Goldblum JR. Enzinger and Weiss's soft tissue tumors. 4th edn. St Louis: Mosby; 2001.

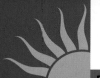
CHAPTER
25 Merkel Cell Carcinoma

Gina Taylor, Darren K Mollick and Edward R Heilman

Key points

- Merkel cell carcinoma is a highly aggressive cutaneous neoplasm, usually of the elderly, exhibiting neuroendocrine differentiation.
- Clinical presentation is nonspecific, with lesions presenting as indolent nodules on sun-damaged skin of the head and neck or upper extremities.
- Diagnosis is made from histopathological examination combined with the use of immunohistochemistry.
- The treatment of choice is surgical removal of the primary tumor with optional sentinel lymph node mapping or elective lymph node dissection.
- Local radiation and/or chemotherapy are frequently employed.
- Prognosis is poor as patients frequently develop regional and distant metastasis.

INTRODUCTION

Merkel cell carcinoma, also known as primary neuro-endocrine carcinoma of the skin, is a rare cutaneous malignancy that has been described as the most virulent of the primary skin tumors. The classically-described clinical presentation is by no means specific for Merkel cell carcinoma and it is frequently mistaken clinically for benign or other malignant neoplasms. The establishment of a high index of suspicion is hindered by the rarity of the entity and by its lack of distinguishing clinical features. However, the very aggressive nature of Merkel cell carcinoma makes prompt diagnosis and adequate treatment essential.

HISTORY

First described in 1972 as trabecular carcinoma of the skin by Toker,[1] Merkel cell carcinoma was initially thought to be an indolent tumor with low malignant potential. Subsequently, with over 800 cases reported in the literature, it is recognized to be a biologically aggressive neoplasm, being associated with a high metastatic rate and a high recurrence rate after excision. It was not until 1978 that the origin of the trabecular carcinoma was associated with the cell first identified in 1875 by Friedrich Sigmund Merkel,[2] a German anatomist and histopathologist. The association between trabecular carcinoma and the Merkel cell was suggested by Tang and Toker,[3] who described the presence of intracellular neurosecretory granules. Since then, several immuno-histochemical and ultrastructural findings, including the presence of cytokeratin 20, have corroborated the notion that the Merkel cell is the precursor cell in Merkel cell carcinoma.

EPIDEMIOLOGY

Merkel cell carcinoma is a rare entity, accounting for far less than 1% of all cutaneous malignancies in the US. However, precise data on international incidence are not available. As previously mentioned, prognosis is relatively poor, with an overall 2-year survival rate of 50–75% and an overall 5-year survival rate reported to be between 30 and 64%.[4]

This is a malignancy of the elderly, typically occurring in the sixth or seventh decades, although it has been reported in patients as young as 15 and as old as 97. Only 5% of cases are diagnosed before age 50. The incidence is approximately equal for men and women but survival appears to be greater in women. There is a 20-fold increased risk in whites relative to blacks.

PATHOGENESIS AND ETIOLOGY

The histogenesis of Merkel cell carcinoma is controversial. Possible cells of origin are the epidermal Merkel cell, a dermal Merkel cell equivalent, a neural crest-derived cell of the amine precursor uptake and decarboxylation (APUD) system, and a residual epidermal stem cell. The controversy stems from the fact that while Merkel cells are primarily located in the epidermis, the cells of Merkel cell carcinoma typically arise intradermally, rarely involving the overlying epidermis. However, Merkel cells have also been found to exist free in the dermis and in association with terminal axons, where they are believed to function as slowly adapting mechanoreceptors. In addition, the tumor cells express the same neuroendocrine markers as epidermal Merkel cells do, namely neuron-specific enolase, chromogranin, synaptophysin and neurofilament proteins, in addition to exhibiting the ultrastructural element, cytokeratin 20.[5]

Cytogenetic abnormalities exist in approximately 40% of investigated cases. Most frequently, there is a loss of heterozygosity due to deletions or translocations involving chromosome 1; in particular, there are two well-defined regions on the short arm (1p36) of chromosome 1 that are implicated in Merkel cell carcinoma.[6] Other abnormalities described include losses in chromosomes 3, 10, 13 and 17 and partial trisomy of chromosomes 1, 3, 5 and 8. Gene amplifications are rare.[6]

An etiologic role of ultraviolet radiation has been proposed due to the greatly increased incidence among whites as compared to blacks and the predominance of tumors on sites of maximal sun exposure, namely the head, neck and distal upper extremities. Other potential risk factors include immunosuppression, erythema ab igne, irradiation, congenital ectodermal dysplasia and Cowden's disease.

CLINICAL FEATURES

Merkel cell carcinoma classically presents as a solitary, painless, smooth, shiny, telangiectatic, non-ulcerated, red-to-violaceous nodule on the sun-damaged skin of the head (Fig. 25.1), neck or extremities (Fig. 25.2) of an elderly white patient. Rarely, there is superficial ulceration. Satellite lesions may be present and rarely there are multifocal or disseminated lesions. It is initially slow-growing and is characterized by a period of more

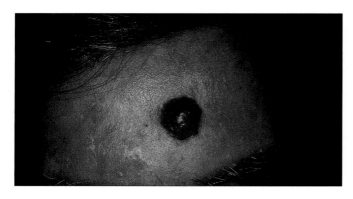

Figure 25.1 Merkel cell carcinoma of the forehead. (Image courtesy of Dr Peter Reisfeld.)

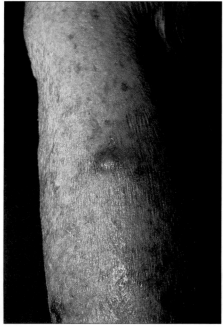

Figure 25.2 Merkel cell carcinoma of the arm. (Image courtesy of Dr Peter Reisfeld.)

rapid growth which prompts the patient to seek medical attention. This tumor has a predilection for the periorbital region (Fig. 25.3). Tumors have been reported on non-sun-exposed areas such as the trunk and the nasal and oral mucosa. About 11–15% of patients present with clinically positive nodes and 50–70% of patients will develop regional lymph node metastases during the course of their disease.[7] Distant metastases develop in up to 50% of patients with the most common sites being distant lymph nodes (e.g. retroperitoneal nodes), liver, bone, brain, lung and skin.

PATIENT EVALUATION, DIAGNOSIS AND DIFFERENTIAL DIAGNOSIS

The non-specific characteristics of the presentation lead to a lengthy differential diagnosis. Most commonly, Merkel cell carcinoma is mistaken clinically for basal cell carcinoma. Also on the differential diagnosis are squamous cell carcinoma, keratoacanthoma, amelanotic melanoma, epidermal cyst, pyogenic granuloma, adnexal tumor, and lymphoma. Consequently, the diagnosis is rarely made before histopathologic evaluation is performed.

Once the diagnosis is suggested by the histology, it is essential to perform radiographic studies to rule out the possibility of metastatic oat cell carcinoma from the lung to the skin, as there are no reliable histologic features to distinguish between this and Merkel cell carcinoma.

The natural history of Merkel cell carcinoma is such that it proceeds in a stepwise fashion – local disease is first followed by regional metastasis to the lymph nodes, then distant metastases.[4] Accordingly, a systematic evaluation must be undertaken in the workup and staging. The staging of Merkel cell carcinoma is important in determining prognosis and treatment options. The most widely used staging system was proposed by Yiengpruksawan et al. in 1991,[4] and is shown in Table 25.1.

Staging of Merkel cell carcinoma

As seen in Table 25.1, a significant proportion of patients present with involvement of the regional nodal basins. Initial workup should include palpation of the lymph nodes, liver and spleen, and liver function tests. Appropriate staging studies should include MRI or CT

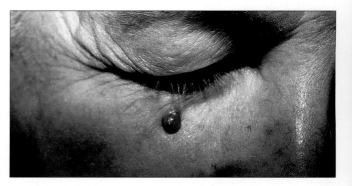

Figure 25.3 Periorbital Merkel cell carcinoma. (Image courtesy of Dr Peter Reisfeld.)

Table 25.1 Staging of Merkel cell carcinoma[4]

Stage	Local disease	Regional nodes	Distant metastasis	Patients at initial presentation (%)	3-year survival (%)
I	+	−	−	60–70	55–73
II	+	+	−	10–40	33
III	+	+	+	<5	

imaging of the head, chest, abdomen and pelvis to assess the possibility of dissemination to lymph nodes and viscera. Fine needle aspiration may also be useful in assessing metastatic spread and octreotide scans may help in evaluating visceral metastases.

In a small study in 2001, Allen *et al.* reported that immunohistochemical analysis of sentinel lymph nodes from patients with Merkel cell carcinoma appears to increase the sensitivity of detecting clinically occult lymph node metastases. This suggested that sentinel lymph node mapping and biopsy may be useful in staging and management of Merkel cell carcinoma.[8]

PATHOLOGY

Diagnosis by light microscopy is often difficult because of the similarity in appearance to many other poorly-differentiated small cell neoplasms. Some 66% of Merkel cell carcinomas are misdiagnosed using light microscopy alone.

On light microscopy, the neoplasm is composed of aggregates of small, closely packed cells with scant cytoplasm and a large nuclear:cytoplasmic ratio infiltrating through the dermis (Figs 25.4, 25.5). It displays a characteristic triad of features: a high mitotic index, apoptosis, and vesicular nuclei with inconspicuous nucleoli (Figs 25.6, 25.7). There is usually sparing of the epidermis with a Grenz zone separating the neoplasm from the epidermis. Lymphocytic infiltrates around the periphery are common. Gould *et al.* described three cellular

patterns in a widely accepted classification of Merkel cell carcinoma.[9]

Trabecular type

Cells are compactly arranged and organized in distinct clusters and trabeculae; individual cells are round to polygonal in shape; cytoplasm of the cells is relatively abundant and well-defined; mitoses are few to moderate in number. The trabecular type pattern is rare and is associated with a less aggressive clinical picture than the other two patterns.

Intermediate type

A solid and diffuse growth pattern with cells more loosely arranged; mitoses and focal necrosis are frequent; these tumors may invade the epidermis. This is the most frequent histologic pattern encountered.

Small-cell type

Solid sheets and clusters of tumor cells; areas of necrosis and 'crush' artifact are frequently seen (Figs 25.8, 25.9); this pattern closely mimics small-cell tumors of other sites. This subtype is associated with the most aggressive biologic behavior.

Merkel cell carcinoma is frequently found in association with other neoplasms, most commonly with

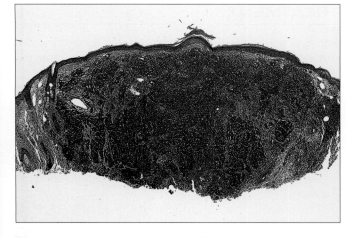

Figure 25.4 Merkel cell carcinoma. The neoplasm is a poorly circumscribed proliferation of densely packed, deeply basophilic staining cells, with an infiltrating pattern. A thin Grenz zone separates the neoplasm from the epidermis.

Figure 25.5 Neoplastic cells densely packed, arranged in sheets and confluent nests.

Figure 25.6 The cells have scant cytoplasm with large vesicular nuclei and inconspicuous nucleoli.

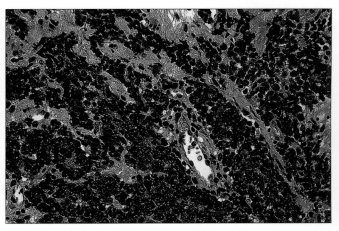

Figure 25.8 Merkel cell carcinoma, small-cell type.

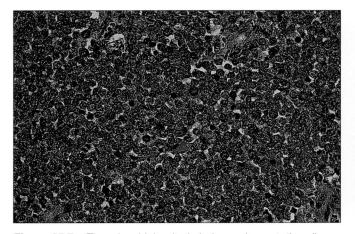

Figure 25.7 There is a high mitotic index and apoptotic cells are numerous.

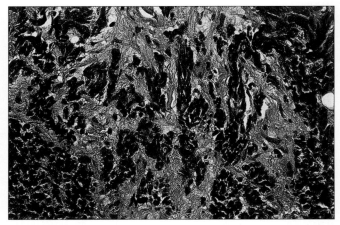

Figure 25.9 'Crush' artifact is a frequent finding in these carcinomas.

squamous cell carcinoma. Other associated neoplasms reported include basal cell carcinoma, Bowen's disease, actinic keratoses and sweat gland neoplasms.

As mentioned previously, immunohistochemistry and ultrastructural studies play a major role in the recognition of Merkel cell carcinoma. The most useful immunohistochemical markers are neuron-specific enolase and cytokeratins, both of which are positive in Merkel cell carcinoma as well as oat cell carcinoma but negative in melanoma, lymphoma and undifferentiated carcinoma. Other markers noted to be variably positive are chromogranin, synaptophysin, adrenocorticotropic hormone, bombesin, calcitonin, gastrin, met-enkephalin, substance P and vasoactive intestinal peptide. The absence of staining for S-100 protein and HMB-45 essentially rules out the diagnosis of malignant melanoma and the absence of staining for leukocyte common antigen rules out cutaneous lymphoma. The presence of a perinuclear dot-like staining pattern for cytokeratin 20 is specific for Merkel cell carcinoma and distinguishes it from oat cell carcinoma (Fig. 25.10).

Although the features on light microscopy are well-documented, examination by electron microscopy can aid in confirming the diagnosis and may be essential if the identity of the tumor is uncertain. Characteristic features on electron microscopy include membrane-bound, dense-core granules 75 to 200 nm in diameter, and perinuclear whorls of intermediate filaments 7–10 nm wide.[10] These findings are not present in any other primary cutaneous neoplasm and essentially confirm the diagnosis of Merkel cell carcinoma.

TREATMENT

There is no standard treatment protocol for Merkel cell carcinoma and therapy is largely dependent upon the presence or absence of metastases.

Wide local excision with 2.5–3 cm margins, whenever possible, is the standard of care for Stage I disease. Margins should be confirmed on frozen section. Mohs' micrographic surgery is reported to compare favorably with wide excision in terms of local recurrence and has been advocated as a tissue-sparing technique, especially in anatomic locations that are not amenable to wide excision.

The orderly 'cascade' pattern of spread of Merkel cell carcinoma combined with the reality that the majority of patients will develop regional lymph node involvement during the course of their disease have led to the suggestion that lymph node dissection may be justified in stage I disease in the absence of clinically positive

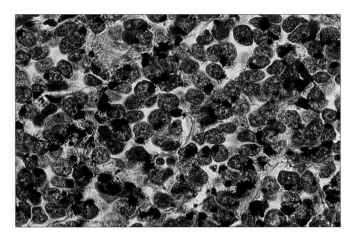

Figure 25.10 Immunohistochemistry staining for cytokeratin 20. The presence of a perinuclear dot staining pattern for cytokeratin 20 is considered specific for Merkel cell carcinoma and distinguishes it from oat cell carcinoma.

nodes. It is uncertain whether elective lymph node dissection (ELND) influences overall survival and it is associated with significant morbidity. ELND is recommended for larger tumors (>2 cm in diameter), tumors with greater than 10 mitoses per high power field, lymphatic or vascular invasion and the small-cell histologic subtypes.[11] Recent studies indicate that negative sentinel lymph node mapping may preclude the need for ELND.

Merkel cell carcinoma is radiosensitive and currently radiation therapy to the primary site and the draining lymph nodes after local excision is used as adjunctive therapy. With the high rates of local recurrence after excision and regional metastasis, radiation therapy is particularly advocated for local recurrence and regional node involvement. However, it is important to note that post-excision irradiation has not been shown to reduce the rates of local or regional recurrence. Goepfert *et al.* proposed that radiation therapy is indicated for: primary tumors >1.5 cm; surgical margins <2 mm; and evidence of lymphatic invasion.[12] Dosing schedules recommended are similar to those for squamous cell carcinoma: 45–50 Gy for 5 weeks, increased to 56–65 Gy for tumors with positive margins.

In Stage II disease, patients conventionally undergo excision of the primary lesion and regional lymph node dissection. Generally, adjuvant radiation therapy is also recommended. Chemotherapy is currently also advocated for Stage II disease. Recommended protocols are similar to those used in the treatment of oat cell carcinoma. Doxorubicin and cyclophosphamide are the most commonly used agents. 5-fluorouracil, bleomycin, cisplatin, etoposide, methotrexate, and vincristine are also used. Merkel cell carcinoma is known to respond to chemotherapeutic agents but remission is usually brief and no chemotherapeutic protocol has been shown to significantly increase overall survival.[13]

Development of distant metastases (Stage III disease) predicts a very poor prognosis with a 5-month life expectancy, on average. As with Stage II disease, a number of chemotherapeutic protocols have been tried without a significant increase in survival. The role of radiation in Stage III disease is palliative.[4,7,14]

Following treatment, patients should be monitored very closely. The recommended follow-up is monthly for 6 months, then every 3 months for the next 2 years. Thereafter, follow-up should occur at 6-month intervals.

FUTURE OUTLOOK

The outlook for having a better understanding of Merkel cell carcinoma in the future remains cloudy. Despite many diagnostic advances, overall prognosis for this aggressive neoplasm remains poor. Due partially to the lack of randomized controlled studies combined with the relative rarity of this entity, optimal treatment modalities remain poorly defined. Current standard treatment centers around wide local excision of the primary lesion. It remains to be seen whether Mohs micrographic surgery versus wide local excision and sentinel lymph node mapping versus ELND will significantly affect overall patient survival.

REFERENCES

1 Toker C. Trabecular carcinoma of the skin. Arch Derm 1972; 105:107.

2 Merkel F. Uiber cie Endigung der sensiblen Nerven in der Haut. Nachr Koniglichen Ges W ss (Gottingen) 1875(5):123.

3 Tang CK, Toker C. Trabecular carcinoma of skin: an ultrastructural study. Cancer 1978; 42:2311–2321.

4 Yiengpruksawan A, Coit DG, Thaler HT, et al. Merkel cell carcinoma. Prognosis and management. Arch Surg 1991; 126(12):1514–1519.

5 Warner TFCS, Uno H, Hafez GR, et al. Merkel cells and Merkel cell tumors: ultrastructure, immunochemistry and review of the literature. Cancer 1983; 52:238–245.

6 Gele M Van, Lecnard JH, Van Roy N, et al. Combined karyotyping, CGH and M-FISH analysis allows detailed characterization of unidentified chromosomal rearrangements in Merkel cell carcinoma. Int J Cancer 2002; 101:137–145.

7 Hitchcock CL, Bland KI, Laney RG 3rd: Neuroendocrine (Merkel cell) carcinoma of the skin. Its natural history, diagnosis, and treatment. Ann Surg 1988; 207(2):201–207.

8 Allen PJ, Zhang Z-F, Coit DG. Surgical management of Merkel cell carcinoma. Ann Surg 1999; 229:97–105.

9 Gould VE, Moll R, Moll I. Neuroendocrine (Merkel) cells of the skin: hyperplasias, dysp asias, and neoplasms. Lab Invest 1985; 52(4):334–353.

10 Reed RJ, Argenyi Z. Tumors of neural tissue. In: Elder D, Elenitsas R, Jaworsky C, et al., eds. Lever's Histopathology of the Skin, 8th edn. Philadelphia, PA: Lippincott-Raven; 1997:977–1009.

11 Silva EG, Mackay B, Goepfert H. Endocrine carcinoma of the skin (Merkel cell carcinoma). Pathol Annu 1984; 19(2):1–30.

12 Goepfert H, Remmler D, Silva E. Merkel cell carcinoma (endocrine carcinoma of the skin) of the head and neck. Arch Otolaryngol 1984; 110(11):707–712.

13 Boyer JD, Zitelli JA, Brodland DG, et al. Local control of primary Merkel cell carcinoma: Review of 45 cases treated with Mohs micrographic surgery with and without adjuvant radiation. J Am Acad Derm 2002; 47:885–892.

14 Haag ML, Glass LF, Fenske NA. Merkel cell carcinoma. Diagnosis and treatment. Derm Surg 1995; 21(8):669–683.

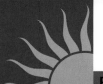

CHAPTER

26 Vascular Neoplasms

Thomas Brenn, Phillip McKee and Martin Mihm

Key points

- Clinical presentation is frequently a red to purple-colored macule, plaque or nodule.
- Helpful diagnostic clues include sharp circumscription versus infiltrative edges of the neoplasm, size, multicentricity, as well as site of involvement, age and other associated disease states such as immunosuppression but biopsy required to confirm diagnosis.
- Conservative excision effective for benign lesions but other extensive treatment modalities may be needed for malignancies.
- High metastatic and mortality rates for vascular malignancies.

INTRODUCTION

Cutaneous vascular lesions are a heterogeneous group of entities ranging from malformations and reactive conditions to benign and malignant endothelial neoplasms. The precise characterization and classification is imperative to predict biological behavior and guide therapy. To date, there is still considerable debate in regard to classification of vascular neoplasms and many vascular tumors defy classification according to currently accepted criteria.

The clinical presentation of these lesions is frequently a purplish discolored macule, plaque or nodule. Helpful diagnostic clues include circumscription versus infiltrative edges of the neoplasm, size, multicentricity as well as site of involvement, age and other associated diseases such as immunosuppression. The precise diagnosis and classification, however, most often requires biopsy and histological examination. Histologically, vascular tumors may be composed of endothelial cells with predominantly spindle or epithelioid morphology or a combination of both with significant variation of obviously vasoformative elements. Those tumors lacking well-differentiated vasoformative areas are histologically easily mistaken for carcinoma, melanoma or non-endothelial mesenchymal neoplasms. Immunohistochemistry is a helpful tool in such circumstances to demonstrate the vascular nature of these tumors. Commonly used endothelial markers include CD31, CD34, Factor VIIIa and the recently described FLI-1. This chapter is not intended to be a complete review of all vascular lesions. It focuses rather on cutaneous vascular neoplasms, which are associated with significant morbidity and mortality.

SPINDLE CELL HEMANGIOMA

INTRODUCTION

Spindle cell hemangioma was first described in 1986 by Weiss and Enzinger[1] as spindle cell hemangioendothelioma. It was, at that time, regarded as a low-grade variant of angiosarcoma. Subsequent studies, however, have demonstrated that it is a benign reactive vascular lesion, and spindle cell hemangioma is the currently preferred terminology.[2,3]

CLINICAL FEATURES

Clinically, spindle cell hemangioma presents as small bluish, sometimes painful nodules with a predilection for the distal extremities. Although it affects a wide age range, the typical presentation is in young adults without gender predominance. Lesions are frequently multicentric (in up to 50% of patients) but tend to affect the same anatomical site and further lesions may develop over an extended time course over a period of decades.[1-3] An association has been identified with Mafucci syndrome (multiple enchondromas and hemangiomas), Klippel–Trenaunay syndrome (soft tissue and bone hypertrophy, nevus flammeus and vascular malformation), lymphedema and vascular malformations.[4] The findings that spindle cell hemangioma may be associated with altered vasculature and blood flow as well as the multicentricity support the reactive nature of this lesion.

PATHOLOGY

Histologically, spindle cell hemangioma is a circumscribed but non-encapsulated nodular lesion based in the dermis or superficial subcutis (Fig. 26.1). It frequently involves a larger pre-existing vessel and about 20–30% are intravascular (Fig. 26.2). It is composed of a solid spindle cell proliferation consisting of an admixture of endothelial cells and pericytes without cytologic atypia and only scarce mitoses (Fig. 26.3). Slit-like spaces are evident. Cytoplasmic vacuolation of endothelial cells may be a prominent feature and is a helpful diagnostic clue. A

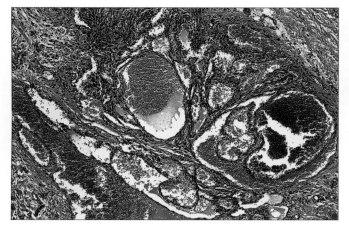

Figure 26.1 Spindle cell hemangioma. This lesion presents as a circumscribed nodular lesion composed of a solid spindle cell component and dilated vascular spaces. (Image courtesy of Mosby, London, UK.)

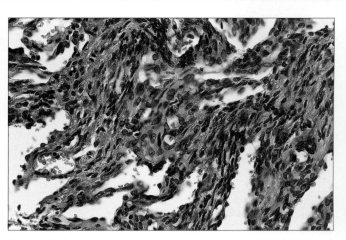

Figure 26.3 Spindle cell hemangioma. A solid spindle cell proliferation is admixed with dilated endothelial lined vascular spaces. Intracellular lumina are present. (Image courtesy of Mosby, London, UK.)

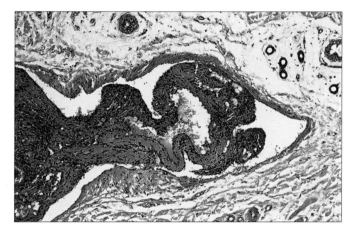

Figure 26.2 Spindle cell hemangioma. Involvement of pre-existing vascular structures may be present. (Image courtesy of Mosby, London, UK.)

second component of this lesion consists of dilated cavernous vascular spaces, which may contain fibrin thrombi or phleboliths. Abnormal thick-walled vessels may be seen in the vicinity of this lesion.[1–3]

PROGNOSIS AND TREATMENT

Despite the initial notion that spindle cell hemangioma may represent a low-grade form of angiosarcoma it is now regarded as a benign reactive vascular lesion. Simple excision is curative in localized lesions. Patients with multiple lesions, however, may develop subsequent lesions in the same anatomic region over a period of decades. True recurrence at a previously biopsied site is rare and no metastases have been reported.

DIFFERENTIAL DIAGNOSIS

Kaposi sarcoma most closely resembles spindle cell hemangioma. It can be separated by its lack of cavernous spaces and vacuolated endothelial cells. The

spindle cell component is more solidly composed of spindled endothelial cells and hyaline globules may be identified. Immunohistochemistry for human herpesvirus-8 is typically positive in Kaposi sarcoma but not in spindle cell hemangioma.

KAPOSI SARCOMA

INTRODUCTION

Kaposi sarcoma (KS) is a locally aggressive predominantly cutaneous vascular lesion first described by Kaposi in 1872. It is associated with human herpes virus-8 infection.[5]

CLINICAL FEATURES

Kaposi sarcoma occurs in distinct clinical and epidemiological settings:

Classic KS

The classic form affects primarily elderly patients from Mediterranean or Eastern European descent. There is a strong male predilection. The lesions of KS predominantly present on the distal extremities as purplish, reddish blue or brown macules, plaques or nodules, which over a period of years progress to affect more proximal sites. It is frequently associated with preexisting lymphedema. Ulceration may be present. The clinical course is indolent and systemic involvement is rare. Classic Kaposi sarcoma may be associated with hematologic malignancies.[5–7]

Endemic KS

This variant occurs in Equatorial Africa and affects middle-aged adults with a male predominance or children without gender predilection. There is no association with HIV-infection. Endemic KS is likely related to chronic immunosuppression. It may present either as progressive cutaneous involvement predominantly involving the distal extremities with rare systemic manifestations or as a rapidly progressive and often lethal lymphadenopathic form in children.[5,7,8]

Iatrogenic KS

This variant is observed in immunosuppressed patients after solid organ transplantation or corticosteroid administration for other diseases. It typically develops several months to years after initiation of immunosuppression. Patients present with cutaneous lesions but visceral involvement may also be seen. The clinical course is mostly indolent and regression of lesions can be noted after withdrawal of immunosuppression. Rarely, this form pursues a clinically aggressive course, especially in patients with visceral involvement.[5,9]

AIDS-related KS

This form of KS occurs in HIV infected patients with a reported relative risk of greater than 10,000 in homo-/bisexual men. It represents the most aggressive form of KS. Cutaneous and mucocutaneous lesions are often disseminated and widespread (Fig. 26.4). Frequently affected sites include face, genitals, oral mucosa and extremities. Involvement of visceral locations such as lymph nodes, gastrointestinal tract and lungs is frequent and may occur without cutaneous involvement. The incidence of AIDS-related KS is decreasing due to the advent of antiretroviral therapy.[5,10]

PATHOGENESIS

In 1994 human herpesvirus-8 was identified as the infectious agent in KS.[11] This virus is present in the spindle cells of all clinical and epidemiological types of KS and may be detected in the peripheral blood even before the development of the disease. The disease results from a complex interaction of the virus with genetic, immunologic and environmental factors.[5]

PATHOLOGY

Pathologically, the cutaneous lesions of all types of KS have similar features including involvement of the reticular dermis. Early *patch stage* lesions show an increase in dermal vascular channels. These channels are oriented parallel to the epidermis and are of irregular shape and often dissect the reticular dermal collagen bundles. They are centered around pre-existing vessels and adnexal structures which may protrude into the lumen of the newly formed vascular spaces ('promontory sign'). Close inspection of vessels in the lower dermis usually reveals a slight proliferation of spindle cells. The endothelial cells show little atypia and no multilayering. Plasma cells, red blood cell extravasation and focal hemosiderin deposition may be additional features.[5-7]

Plaque stage KS is characterized by a more prominent proliferation of spindle cells both centered around pre-existing vessels as well as within reticular dermal collagen (Fig. 26.5). The spindle cells are short with a uniform appearance. The inflammatory component as well as erythrocyte extravasation and hemosiderin deposition are more pronounced than in *patch stage* KS (Fig. 26.6). Hyaline globules, likely representing destroyed

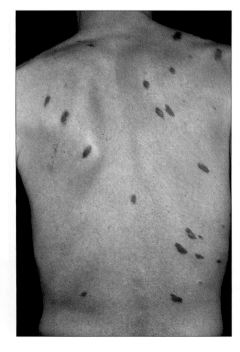
Figure 26.4 Kaposi sarcoma. This HIV-positive patient presents with multiple purplish patches and plaques on the trunk. (Image courtesy of the late Dr NP Smith, Institute of Dermatology, UMDS, London, UK and Mosby, London, UK).

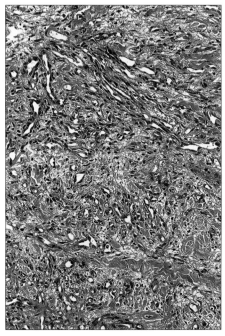
Figure 26.5 Kaposi sarcoma. In plaque stage lesions a proliferation of small dermal vessels is seen accompanied by a spindle cell proliferation.

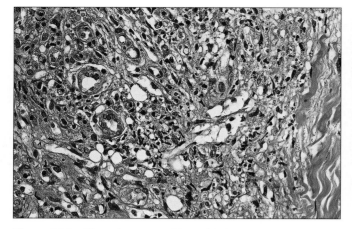

Figure 26.6 Kaposi sarcoma. Hemosiderin deposition and red blood cell extravasation are frequent findings in plaque stage lesions.

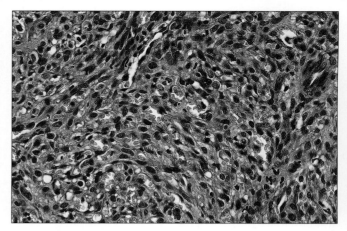

Figure 26.7 Nodular Kaposi sarcoma. Slit-like spaces are noticed within the spindle cell proliferation giving rise to the 'sieve-like appearance'.

erythrocytes, are frequently observed within the slit like spaces and at times in the cytoplasm of the spindle cells.[5–7]

The features of *nodular* KS are those of a well-circumscribed but unencapsulated nodular proliferation of uniform spindle cells arranged in whorls and intersecting fascicles with numerous slit-like spaces containing erythrocytes (Fig. 26.7). The erythrocytes appear similar to rouleaux but with a rectangular morphology leading to the description of 'boxcar' array. Hyaline globules are frequently identified. Mitotic figures may be frequent but cytologic atypia is only minimal. Ectatic vascular channels lined by prominent endothelial cells may be present at the periphery of the lesion.[5–7]

Immunohistochemically, the spindle cells stain positive for endothelial markers and there is intense nuclear positivity for human herpes virus-8.

PROGNOSIS AND TREATMENT

The prognosis of Kaposi sarcoma is dependent on the clinical and epidemiological subtype as outlined earlier. Treatment options include excision for single lesions or resectable recurrences. Radiotherapy administered as a single dose of 8 to 12 Gy is a treatment option for lesions affecting a limited area. Patients with extensive or recurrent disease may benefit from a combination of surgery, radiation and chemotherapy. Chemotherapeutical agents include vinblastine, bleomycin, doxorubicin and dacarbazine as well as intralesional alpha interferon. Patients with visceral involvement often respond poorly.[5]

KAPOSIFORM HEMANGIOENDOTHELIOMA

INTRODUCTION

Kaposiform hemangioendothelioma is a rare, locally aggressive vascular tumor of skin and deep soft tissue frequently associated with the Kasabach–Merritt syndrome, a potentially life threatening coagulopathy.

Approximately 60 cases have been reported in the literature to date.

CLINICAL FEATURES

Kaposiform hemangioendothelioma typically presents in infancy and childhood with an equal sex incidence. Cases occurring in adulthood are increasingly recognized. In children kaposiform hemangioendothelioma predominantly involves the skin and retroperitoneum as well as the deep soft tissue of the trunk and extremities (Fig. 26.8). In adults the lesion more commonly affects the retroperitoneum. Cutaneous lesions present as ill-defined violaceous plaques. These lesions may be a few centimeters in size or may involve an entire limb or a large portion of the trunk (Fig. 26.8). Deep-seated lesions manifest as poorly marginated multinodular and infiltrative masses. An associated consumption coagulopathy (Kasabach–Merritt syndrome) is a frequent finding especially in retroperitoneal tumors. Lymphangiomatosis of the surrounding tissue may be present in up to 20% of patients.[12–14]

PATHOLOGY

Histologically, Kaposiform hemangioendothelioma is characterized by a hypercellular lobular architecture with infiltrative edges. The lobules are separated by fibrous bands and composed of fascicles of uniform spindle cells with pale eosinophilic cytoplasm and elongated nuclei reminiscent of KS (Fig. 26.9). Interspersed capillaries as well as crescent shaped vascular lumina and slit-like spaces frequently containing fibrin are present (Fig. 26.10). Islands of epithelioid appearing cells of endothelial origin are present in the nodules and help to differentiate these lesions from KS (Fig. 26.11). The central proliferative zone is surrounded by ecstatic vessels resembling capillaries. Nuclear atypia or mitoses are inconspicuous. Adjacent areas reminiscent of lymphangiomatosis are often noted and foci of hemorrhage and hemosiderin deposition may be present.[12–14]

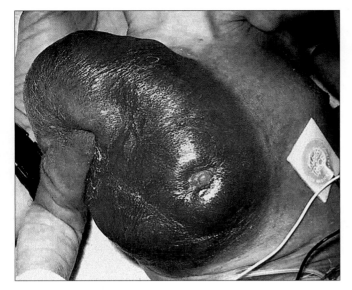

Figure 26.8 Kaposiform hemangioendothelioma. This large lesion was present at birth and was associated with hematochezia due to a very low platelet count. The patient responded to steroids and vincristine therapy. The lesion extended from the shoulder onto the chest wall.

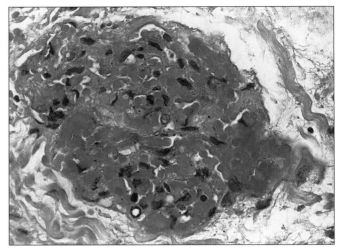

Figure 26.10 Kaposiform hemangioendothelioma. Fibrin/platelet thrombi are characteristically found in the vascular spaces as evidence of platelet trapping leading to thrombocytopenia in affected patients.

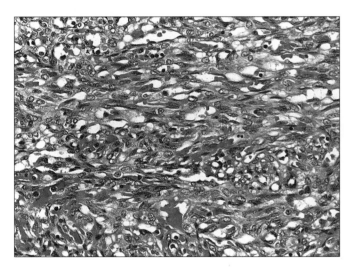

Figure 26.9 Kaposiform hemangioendothelioma. The spindle cells are present in large aggregates and form spaces filled with blood reminiscent of Kaposi sarcoma.

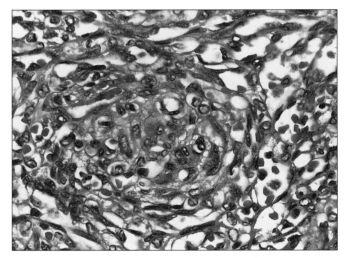

Figure 26.11 Kaposiform hemangioendothelioma. Nodular areas resembling epithelioid cell islands are present throughout the spindle cell areas and are a characteristic feature that helps to distinguish this lesion from Kaposi sarcoma.

PROGNOSIS AND TREATMENT

Kaposiform hemangioendothelioma is a locally infiltrative lesion without tendency for spontaneous regression. No metastases have been reported so far. The prognosis varies depending on tumor size and site and is therefore poor in those tumors occurring in intra-abdominal locations and those complicated by the Kasabach–Merritt syndrome. Treatment in children includes steroids, sometimes requiring doses as high as 5 mg/kg of prednisolone. The next line of therapy is vincristine. Finally, in very refractory cases, alpha interferon may be given. Complete excision should be attempted. Recurrences appear to be rare. However, in previously treated lesions that clinically respond, residua of lesions in apparently normal skin can be found on biopsy.

PAPILLARY INTRALYMPHATIC ANGIOENDOTHELIOMA

INTRODUCTION

This locally aggressive but rarely metastasizing vascular tumor is exceedingly rare with only few reported cases after the original description by Dabska in 1969.[15]

CLINICAL FEATURES

This tumor predominantly affects infants and children but presentation in adults has also been documented. There is no gender predilection and the limbs and trunk are the most frequently affected anatomic sites. The tumors present as slowly enlarging bluish plaques or nodules measuring several centimeters in diameter.[15,16]

PATHOLOGY

Histologically, the lesion presents as an ill-defined dermal and subcutaneous tumor composed of intercommunicating dilated, thin-walled vascular spaces. Prominent intraluminal papillary tufts with hyaline cores lined by 'hobnail' endothelial cells are conspicuous. Basement membrane material is seen within the hyaline cores. Lymphocytes are often noted adjacent and within the vascular channels. A lymphangioma or lymphectasia may accompany this tumor.[15,16]

PROGNOSIS AND TREATMENT

Papillary intralymphatic angioendothelioma was initially reported as a tumor with a tendency for local recurrence and lymph node metastasis and associated mortality. A subsequent report has not confirmed this finding and further studies are necessary to define the biologic behavior of this neoplasm.

If feasible, these tumors should be treated by wide excision.

RETIFORM HEMANGIOENDOTHELIOMA

INTRODUCTION

Retiform hemangioendothelioma is a locally aggressive but rarely metastasizing vascular neoplasm of the skin, first described in 1994 as a distinct clinicopathologic entity by Calonje et al.[17] It is an uncommon neoplasm with only about 20 cases reported in the literature.

CLINICAL FEATURES

Young adults are most frequently affected but the age distribution is wide. There is no gender predilection. Clinically, retiform hemangioendothelioma presents as slowly growing red to bluish plaques or nodules, typically measuring less than 3 cm in maximum dimension. The distal extremities and in particular the lower limbs are predominantly affected. Lesions are usually single although one patient with multiple lesions has been described. Only rarely does this tumor occur in the setting of radiation or lymphedema.[17]

PATHOLOGY

The tumor is located in the dermis with frequent extension into subcutaneous tissue but epidermal involvement is not a feature. It is characterized by a diffuse and infiltrative architecture composed of arborizing, elongated thin-walled blood vessels extending between collagen bundles in a pattern reminiscent of the rete testis (Fig. 26.12). The vascular spaces are lined by a single layer of monomorphic small endothelial cells with prominent rounded, hyperchromatic nuclei protruding into the lumen in a characteristic 'hobnail' appearance (Fig. 26.13). Cytologic atypia and mitotic figures are not seen. Focally, small clusters and aggregates of endothelial cells with more spindle or epithelioid features may be present.

Intraluminal papillary projections with hyalinized collagenous cores reminiscent of those seen in Dabska tumor can sometimes be a feature. The surrounding

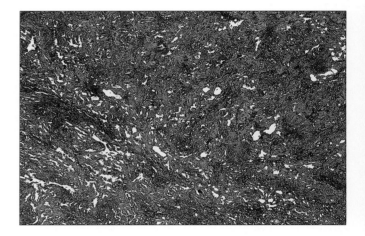

Figure 26.12 Retiform hemangioendothelioma. This vascular tumor is characterized by a branching and arborizing growth pattern of vascular channels reminiscent of rete testis. (Image courtesy of Mosby, London, UK.)

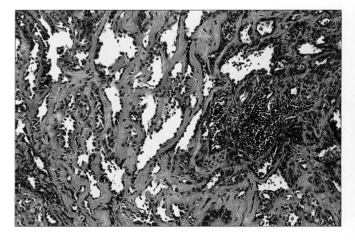

Figure 26.13 Retiform hemangioendothelioma. The vascular channels are lined by prominent 'hobnail' endothelial atypia. Cytologic atypia is minimal. (Image courtesy of Mosby, London, UK.)

stroma is commonly sclerotic. A prominent infiltrate composed of mature lymphocytes is frequently seen in the surrounding stroma as well as within the vascular lumina.[17]

PROGNOSIS AND TREATMENT

Retiform hemangioendothelioma is a locally aggressive but rarely metastasizing vascular neoplasm treated surgically by excision. It is imperative to distinguish retiform hemangioendothelioma from cutaneous angiosarcoma, which has a dismal prognosis and is characterized by high recurrence, metastatic and mortality rates.

COMPOSITE HEMANGIOENDOTHELIOMA

INTRODUCTION

This vascular neoplasm was first described as a distinct entity in 2000 by Nayler et al.[18] and is characterized by an admixture of histologically benign, intermediate and malignant components.

CLINICAL FEATURES

It is an exceedingly rare tumor with less than 10 examples documented in the literature. The age distribution is wide and adults are predominantly affected (median: 40 years). One congenital lesion has also been reported. There appears to be no gender predilection. Clinically, patients present with slowly growing, infiltrative, uni- or multilobular nodules measuring 0.7 to 6 cm and frequently showing red to purple discoloration. There is a strong predilection for the distal extremities and predominantly the hands and feet. One case presenting on the tongue has been reported. The tumors are usually longstanding with a preoperative history ranging from 2 to 10 years. A history of lymphedema of the affected site is identified in 25% of the reported cases.[18]

PATHOLOGY

The diagnosis of composite hemangioendothelioma is based on the histologic appearances from biopsy or excision of these tumors. The lesions are complex, poorly marginated neoplasms that involve the dermis and subcutaneous tissue. There is marked variation in the tumor constituents both from patient to patient as well as within the same patient. The individual components merge imperceptibly and comprise areas reminiscent of epithelioid hemangioendothelioma, retiform hemangioendothelioma, spindle cell hemangioma and well-differentiated angiosarcoma. Rarely, areas resembling arteriovenous malformation and lymphangioma may also be identified. Other findings include large areas of vacuolated endothelial cells with a pseudolipoblast appearance. Stromal lymphoplasmacytic aggregates and surrounding hemosiderin deposition may be present. Changes of the overlying epidermis include hyperplasia and ulceration.[18]

PROGNOSIS AND TREATMENT

Composite hemangioendothelioma is characterized by local recurrence in about 50% of the cases and a single case with lymph node and distant metastasis has been reported. To this date, there is still limited information based on the small number of reported cases but it appears to pursue a clinically more indolent course compared with cutaneous angiosarcoma.

EPITHELIOID HEMANGIOENDOTHELIOMA

INTRODUCTION

Epithelioid hemangioendothelioma is a rare epithelioid vascular tumor morphologically simulating carcinoma, which was first described by Weiss and Enzinger in 1982[19] in soft tissue.

CLINICAL FEATURES

This tumor presents over a wide age range with a peak incidence in the third decade but is very uncommon in childhood. There appears to be no gender predilection. The principal sites of involvement include soft tissue, lung, liver and bone. Presentation in the skin is exceedingly rare and may represent multicentricity of tumor involving bone. There are only about 20 reported cases limited to the skin. Cutaneous tumors present as erythematous painful dermal nodules without predilection for a specific site. No sex predilection has been noted and the median age is 52 years. Tumors have typically been present for a duration of 6 to 12 months when the patient seeks medical advice.[19–21]

PATHOLOGY

Histologically, this vascular neoplasm is well circumscribed with a uni- or multilobular architecture and composed of plump polygonal epithelioid cells with eosinophilic cytoplasm and vesicular nuclei containing prominent eosinophilic nucleoli. The cells are arranged in nests, cords and strands in a myxohyaline matrix (Fig. 26.14). Intracytoplasmic lumina are a frequent finding and mitotic figures are present although generally sparse. Angiocentricity (which is frequently noted in tumors located in soft tissue) is not a prominent finding in dermal tumors. Immunohistochemistry for endothelial markers is positive.[19–21]

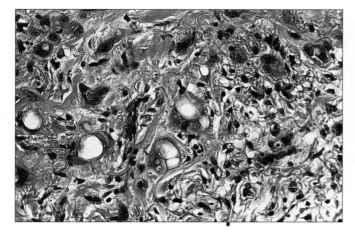

Figure 26.14 Epithelioid hemangioendothelioma. Epithelioid endothelial cells are arranged in cords and strands in a myxohyaline stroma. Intracytoplasmic lumina are easily identified.

PROGNOSIS AND TREATMENT

While epithelioid hemangioendothelioma is regarded as a malignant vascular tumor with a local recurrence rate of around 10% and metastatic and mortality rates of approximately 20%, purely cutaneous tumors do not appear to recur or metastasize. Treatment of cutaneous lesions should therefore consist of complete excision and work up for systemic disease, especially bone involvement.

CUTANEOUS ANGIOSARCOMA

INTRODUCTION

Angiosarcoma is a frankly malignant endothelial neo-plasm occurring in skin, soft tissue and visceral locations.

CLINICAL FEATURES

Cutaneous angiosarcoma typically occurs in specific clinical settings including:

Idiopathic cutaneous angiosarcoma

This form was described by Wilson-Jones in 1964[22] and affects the head and neck area of the elderly with a male predilection. It presents as single or multiple ill-defined bluish to violaceous bruise-like patches in sun-exposed areas of the head and neck region (Fig. 26.15). More advanced lesions may present as indurated plaques or nodules and occasionally ulceration and satellite nodules may be evident.

Cutaneous angiosarcoma arising in chronic lymphedema

Cutaneous angiosarcoma arising in the setting of chronic lymphedema was initially reported by Stewart and

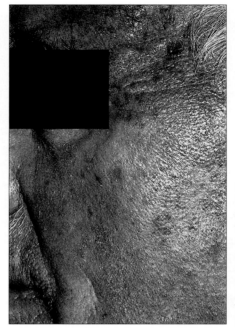

Figure 26.15 Cutaneous angiosarcoma. This tumor presents as a violaceous patch on sun exposed skin of the head. (Image courtesy of D Burrows, Royal Victoria Hospital, Belfast, N Ireland.)

Treves in 1948[23] as postmastectomy lymphangiosarcoma. The interval between mastectomy and the development of angiosarcoma ranges from 1 to 30 years with an average of approximately 12 years. These lesions present as bruise-like areas on an edematous limb. Other causes of lymphedema such as surgery other than mastectomy, congenital lymphedema, chronic venous stasis, chronic filarial lymphedema and lymphedema due to malignancies have also been recognized more recently to be associated with the development of angiosarcoma.

Radiation associated cutaneous angiosarcoma

Cutaneous angiosarcoma may also arise at the site of previous radiation therapy for various benign as well as malignant conditions. It typically arises several years after radiation treatment.[24,25] Clinically, it presents as infiltrative patches or plaques at the site or in the vicinity of prior radiation.

PATHOLOGY

Pathologically, the appearances of cutaneous angiosarcoma are identical irrespective of the underlying etiology and there is considerable variation in the appearances even within the same lesion in regard to cellularity and vasoformative elements. Better differentiated areas are characterized by irregular vascular channels infiltrating and dissecting dermal collagen bundles in a complex anastomosing fashion. Vascular channels are lined by endothelial cells showing varying degrees of cytologic atypia, pleomorphism and mitotic activity as well as endothelial multilayering with papillary tufts (Fig. 26.16). The lesions may infiltrate into deep dermis and sub-cutaneous tissue. Less differentiated areas show increased

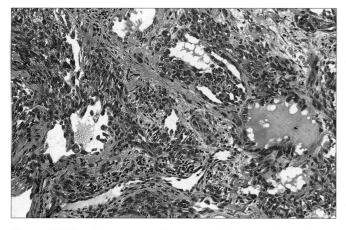

Figure 26.16 Cutaneous angiosarcoma. Vascular channels are lined by atypical endothelial cells showing multilayering and papillary tufts.

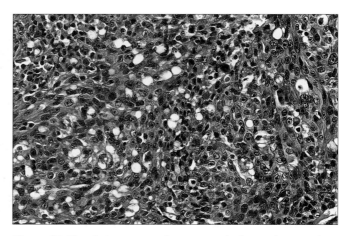

Figure 26.18 Cutaneous angiosarcoma. A clue to the vascular nature of this tumor are multiple intracytoplasmic lumina.

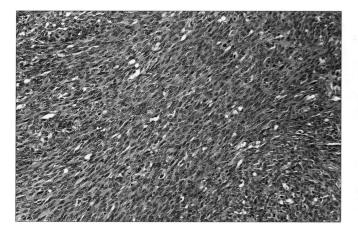

Figure 26.17 Cutaneous angiosarcoma. This poorly differentiated area consists of a solid and sheet-like proliferation of cytologically atypical spindle cells.

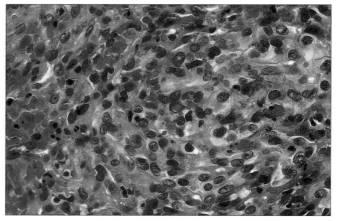

Figure 26.19 Epithelioid angiosarcoma. This variant of angiosarcoma is characterized by cytologically atypical epithelioid cells with early intracytoplasmic lumina formation.

cellularity and the cells are more closely packed and often spindle shaped resulting in a solid sheet-like growth pattern with loss of obvious vasoformative elements (Fig. 26.17). Intracytoplasmic lumina may be identified and are a helpful diagnostic clue (Fig. 26.18). There may be marked cytological atypia and frequent mitotic figures.[26] The diagnosis in these examples is based on the identification of better-differentiated areas with more obvious vasoformative elements in addition to immuno-histochemistry, which displays positivity for endothelial markers.

PROGNOSIS AND TREATMENT

The clinical outcome in patients with cutaneous angiosarcoma is generally poor and does not correlate with histological differentiation. There is a high rate of distant metastasis and mortality. Primary metastatic sites include skin, soft tissue, lymph nodes, lung, liver and bone and the overall 5-year survival is estimated at around 15% irrespective of the underlying etiology or treatment. Primary treatment consists of surgical excision. Those

lesions not accessible to surgery may be treated with chemotherapy or radiation but the overall prognosis is dismal.

EPITHELIOID ANGIOSARCOMA

A rare, but highly aggressive variant of angiosarcoma is *epithelioid angiosarcoma*. This most often affects young to middle aged adults with a male predominance. The clinical presentation is identical to other forms of cutaneous angiosarcoma. Histologically this angio-sarcoma unit is characterized by a solid and sheet-like proliferation of large polygonal epithelioid cells containing pale eosinophilic cytoplasm and vesicular nuclei with prominent eosinophilic nucleoli[27] (Fig. 26.19). Mitotic figures are conspicuous and an attempt of early vasoformation in the form of intracytoplasmic lumina (sometimes containing erythrocytes) can be identified (Fig. 26.19). An overt vasoformative element in the form of vascular channels may also be present. This neoplasm closely resembles truly epithelial tumors or melanoma, for which it may easily be mistaken.

Immunohistochemistry for endothelial markers reveals the vascular nature of this tumor.

FUTURE OUTLOOK

Vascular neoplasms of the skin span the spectrum from benign to highly malignant. Current classification systems may need to be revised to include immunohistochemical and genetic markers to better assess prognosis and enhance our understanding of these tumors.

REFERENCES

1 Weiss SW, Enzinger FM. Spindle cell hemangioendothelioma, a low-grade angiosarcoma resembling a cavernous hemangioma and Kaposi's sarcoma. Am J Surg Pathol 1986; 10:521–530.

2 Perkins P, Weiss SW. Spindle cell hemangioendothelioma. An analysis of 78 cases with reassessment of its pathogenesis and biologic behavior. Am J Surg Pathol 1996; 20:1196–1204.

3 Fletcher CD, Beham A, Schmid C, et al. Spindle cell hemangioendothelioma: a clinicopathological and immunohistochemical study indicative of a non-neoplastic lesion. Histopathology 1991; 18:291–301.

4 Fanburg JC, Meis Kindblom JM, Rosenberg AE, et al. Multiple enchondromas associated with spindle cell hemangioendotheliomas. An overlooked variant of Maffucci's syndrome. Am J Surg Pathol 1995; 19:1029–1038.

5 Antman K, Chang Y. Kaposi's sarcoma. N Engl J Med 2000; 342:1027–1038.

6 Chor PJ, Santa Cruz DJ. Kaposi's sarcoma. A clinicopathologic review and differential diagnosis. J Cutan Pathol 1992; 19:6–20.

7 Tappero JW, Connant MA, Wolfe SF, et al. Kaposi's sarcoma. Epidemiology, pathogenesis, histology, clinical spectrum, staging criteria and therapy. J Am Acad Derm 1993; 28:371–395.

8 Dorfman RF. Kaposi's sarcoma. With special reference to its manifestations in infants and children and to the concepts of Arthur Purdy Stout. Am J Surg Pathol 1986; 10:68–77.

9 Trattner A, Hodak E, David M, et al. The appearance of Kaposi sarcoma during corticosteroid therapy. Cancer 1993; 72:1779–1783.

10 Gottlieb GJ, Ackerman AB. Kaposi's sarcoma: an extensively disseminated form in young homosexual men. Hum Pathol 1982; 13:882–892.

11 Moore PS, Chang Y. Detection of herpesvirus-like DNA sequences Kaposi's sarcoma in patients with and without HIV infection. N Engl J Med 1995; 332:1181–1185.

12 Mentzel T, Mazzoleni G, Dei Tos AP, et al. Kaposiform hemangioendothelioma in adults: clinicopathologic and immunohistochemical analysis of three cases. Am J Clin Pathol 1997; 108:450–455.

13 Zukerberg LR, Nickoloff BJ, Weiss SW. Kaposiform hemangioendothelioma of infancy and childhood. An aggressive neoplasm associated with Kasabach–Merritt syndrome and lymphangiomatosis. Am J Surg Pathol 2001; 17:321–328.

14 Mac-Moune Lai F, Fai To K, Choi PCL, et al. Kaposiform hemangioendothelioma: five patients with cutaneous lesion and long follow-up. Mod Pathol 2001; 14:1087–1092.

15 Dabska M. Malignant endovascular papillary angioendothelioma of the skin in childhood. Cancer 1969; 24:503–510.

16 Fanburg-Smith JC, Michal M, Partanen TA, et al. Papillary intralymphatic angioendothelioma (PILA). A report of twelve cases of a distinctive vascular tumor with phenotypic features of lymphatic vessels. Am J Surg Pathol 1999; 23:1004–1010.

17 Calonje E, Fletcher CDM, Wilson-Jones E, et al. Retiform hemangioendothelioma. A distinctive form of low-grade angiosarcoma delineated in a series of 15 cases. Am J Surg Pathol 1994; 18:115–125.

18 Nayler SJ, Rubin BP, Calonje E, et al. Composite hemangioendothelioma. A complex, low-grade vascular lesion mimicking angiosarcoma. Am J Surg Pathol 2000; 24:352–361.

19 Weiss SW, Enzinger FM. Epithelioid hemangioendothelioma: a vascular tumor often mistaken for a carcinoma. Cancer 1982; 50:970–981.

20 Mentzel T, Beham A, Calonje E, et al. Epithelioid hemangioendothelioma of skin and soft tissues: clinicopathologic and immunohistochemical study of 30 cases. Am J Surg Pathol 1997; 21(4):363–374.

21 Quante M, Patel NK, Hill S, et al. Epithelioid hemangioendothelioma presenting in the skin. A clinicopathologic study of eight cases. Am J Derm 1998; 20:541–546.

22 Wilson Jones E. Malignant angioendothelioma of skin. Br J Derm 1964; 76:21–39.

23 Stewart FW, Treves N. Lymphangiosarcoma in postmastectomy lymphedema. A report of six cases in elephantiasis chirurgica. Cancer 1948; 1:64–81.

24 Fineberg S, Rosen PP. Cutaneous angiosarcoma and atypical vascular lesions of the skin and breast after radiation therapy for breast carcinoma. Am J Clin Pathol 1994; 102:757–763.

25 Goette DK, Detlefs RL. Postirradiation angiosarcoma. J Am Acad Derm 1985; 12:922–926.

26 Meis-Kindblom JM, Kindblom LG. Angiosarcoma of soft tissue: a study of 80 cases. Am J Surg Pathol 1998; 22:683–697.

27 Fletcher CD, Beham A, Bekir S, et al. Epithelioid angiosarcoma of deep soft tissue: a distinctive tumor readily mistaken for an epithelial neoplasm. Am J Surg Pathol 1991; 15:915–924.

CHAPTER

27

Neoplastic Disorders in HIV Infected Patients

Alvin E Friedman-Kien and Clay J Cockerell

Key points

- Cutaneous neoplasms are common in HIV infected patients. As these individuals are now living longer as a consequence of administration of HAART, these are becoming a more important ongoing problem in neoplasm management.
- The most common cancers seen are epithelial and are similar to those seen in immunocompetent patients such as basal cell carcinoma and squamous cell carcinoma.
- HPV-associated neoplasms such as Bowenoid papulosis and anorectal carcinoma are seen more commonly in this patient population.
- Several unusual neoplasms such as certain lymphomas may occasionally be encountered, especially in patients who are immunocompromised. Certain common lesions may demonstrate unusual histologic features that may cause difficulty in diagnosis.
- Treatment may need to be more aggressive than in non-HIV infected counterparts.
- The incidence of Kaposi's sarcoma has declined with the advent of HAART.

INTRODUCTION

Cutaneous neoplasms are common problems in individuals infected with the human immunodeficiency virus (HIV). When patients are immunocompromised, malignancies can be severe and life threatening. With the advent of highly active antiretroviral therapy (HAART), these individuals now live for longer periods of time and may be immunocompetent for many months or even years. As such, they are at risk to develop cutaneous malignancies in patterns similar to non-HIV infected persons. On the other hand, some neoplasms such as Kaposi's sarcoma have a tendency to undergo remission when immunity is reconstituted. In this chapter, lesions that arise in both immunocompromised and immunocompetent patients will be discussed.

CUTANEOUS EPITHELIAL NEOPLASMS IN HIV PATIENTS

DEFINITION

Epithelial neoplasms are growths that differentiate towards an epithelial structure. Some of those that may develop in HIV-seropositive patients include neoplasms of the anorectal area such as anal intraepithelial neoplasia, squamous cell carcinoma *in situ*, fully developed squamous cell carcinoma and cloacogenic carcinoma; cervical intraepithelial neoplasia and fully developed cervical carcinoma in HIV-infected women; Bowenoid papulosis; basal cell carcinoma (multiple, primary and metastatic); multiple cutaneous squamous cell carcinomas associated with epidermodysplasia verruciformis; and multiple sebaceous gland tumors.

EPIDEMIOLOGY

There is an increased incidence of epithelial neoplasms in patients infected with HIV, most commonly involving oral, cervical and anorectal sites. Women with AIDS have been found to have a two-fold increased risk for the development of cervical cancer as compared to the general population.[1,2] American patients with AIDS have been shown to have a greater than 40-fold increased risk for the development of anal cancer and anal intraepithelial neoplasia has been found in a high percentage of patients with AIDS.[3] Bowenoid papulosis as well as cloacogenic carcinoma are also increased in incidence in these patients. Both of these neoplasms as well as carcinoma of the cervix are closely associated with human papilloma virus (HPV) infection. Transitional cell carcinoma has been reported on occasion, also linked to HPV infection. Patients with anal carcinoma have a much higher incidence of venereal warts when compared with patients with carcinoma of the colon and rectum.

The incidence of intraepithelial neoplasia of both the uterine cervix in women and the anorectal mucosa in homosexual men is markedly increased in HIV-infected individuals.[1,3] In one study, HPV DNA was detected in 54% of HIV-infected male homosexuals.[4] Cytologic specimens from 39% of the subjects demonstrated abnormalities ranging from atypia in 19% to fully developed anal intraepithelial neoplasia in 15%. HIV-infected women have been shown to have cervical dysplasia rates 5 to 10 times higher than that of non-HIV-infected women, i.e. up to 33%.[5] In a study of HIV-infected women, 74% had vulvar HPV infection, 47% had condylomata acuminata and 26% had vulvar intraepithelial neoplasia.[5] Cytologic techniques used in cervical pap smears applied to smears obtained from the anorectal junction in HIV-infected homosexual men indicate an HPV infection rate greater than 50%.[3] The incidence of anal intraepithelial neoplasia rises to up to 11% in patients with CD4+ counts lower than 50.[3,6] Although it was predicted that invasive squamous cell carcinoma arising in HPV-induced anal intraepithelial neoplasia or cervical intraepithelial neoplasia would become a major clinical problem as patients survived longer with HIV infection, fortunately because of close monitoring and immune reconstitution, this has not proven to be a significant problem.[6]

Cutaneous epithelial malignancies, while occasionally reported in association with HIV infection, have not been shown to be present in significant numbers. In a recent study of HIV-infected individuals in a military setting, it was found that basal cell and squamous cell carcinoma developed in less than 5% of patients.[7] It is yet to be seen whether this will hold as patients live for significantly longer time periods as a consequence of administration of HAART, however.

PATHOGENESIS

The most important predisposing factor in the development of epithelial neoplasms in HIV infected patients is infection with HPV. It has been demonstrated that HIV tat protein up-regulates the expression of human papillomavirus in tissue. This finding would be expected to lead to exaggerated expression of HPV-induced lesions especially in the context of immunocompromise.[8] Furthermore, the E6 protein derived from HPV-16 interacts with p53 tumor suppressor gene product causing its inactivation which may promote the development of neoplasms.[9]

Although HPV infection is prevalent in these patients, only certain types are oncogenic. HPV-16, 18, 31 and 33 are associated with malignant potential on mucosal sites, while HPV-5 and 8 are found in association with epidermodysplasia verruciformis. Even HPV types not usually associated with intraepithelial neoplasia and invasive squamous cell carcinoma have been detected in invasive squamous cell carcinoma of the penis.[10]

CLINICAL MANIFESTATIONS

Anal intraepithelial neoplasia and cervical intraepithelial neoplasia clinically are asymptomatic and may have no visible findings. Evidence that these conditions exist are found only by microscopic evaluation of biopsy specimens or exfoliative cytology. Cervical carcinoma initially appears as a red friable area that mimics chronic cervicitis and can only be detected by colposcopically directed biopsy or exfoliative cytology. Similar findings are noted in anal squamous cell carcinoma *in situ*. Over the course of time, invasive squamous cell carcinoma may occur either in the cervix or in the anorectal area. These are manifested as thickened indurated cauliflower-like areas that may be deeply infiltrating. Lesions may ulcerate, necrose and become painful if nerves are involved. Cloacogenic carcinoma has a similar clinical appearance.

Bowenoid papulosis is generally manifested as brown flat-topped papules on the labia or penile skin. (Fig. 27.1) Lesions are often hyperpigmented but in some cases, they appear identical to condylomata acuminata. Rarely, brownish macules may be the only manifestation of the disease. Epidermodysplasia verruciformis has a

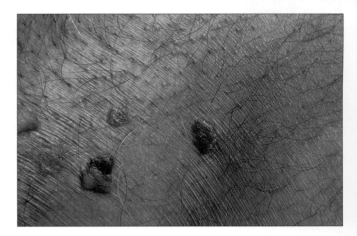

Figure 27.1 Bowenoid papulosis. These brownish warty lesions in the groin, with features similar to those seen in condyloma acuminata, were demonstrated to represent Bowenoid papulosis, a form of squamous cell carcinoma *in situ*, when examined microscopically.

clinical appearance of widespread warty papules that may be reddish. In some cases, diffuse erythematous pruritic areas of the skin may be seen.[11] Biopsies are necessary to establish the diagnosis.

Basal cell carcinomas that have been reported have had clinical appearances similar to those seen in immunocompetent hosts although multiple primary nodular and superficial basal cell carcinomas may develop (Figs 27.2, 27.3). Rarely, basal cell carcinoma may metastasize, usually always in the setting of neglected lesions and in immunocompromise.[12] Most metastases have been to draining lymph nodes and the lung. Squamous cell carcinoma appears identical to that seen in immunocompetent patients and usually arises from solar keratoses (Figs 27.4, 27.5).

HISTOPATHOLOGY

The histopathologic findings of lesions in the spectrum of squamous cell carcinoma in HIV patients range from subtle atypical intraepithelial proliferations within stratified squamous epithelium to extensive full-thickness involvement of the epithelium and underlying structures. As lesions progress, epithelial retia become expanded and replaced by atypical cells, many of which are pleomorphic and in mitosis. In time, bulbous aggregations of atypical cells extend from the epithelium into the underlying lamina propria and reticular dermis. Deeper involvement as well as involvement of nerves and blood vessels may develop in due course. Lesions are often digitated, verrucous and may be associated with necrosis.

Bowenoid papulosis is manifested histologically by similar cytologic features except that lesions have a histologic architectural pattern similar to that of condyloma acuminatum. Epidermodysplasia verruciformis is characterized by a diffuse infiltrate of bluish-purple pale-appearing cells in the epidermis. There is also dyskeratosis and characteristic 'corps rond-like' structures in the stratum corneum.[13] Basal cell carcinoma has a

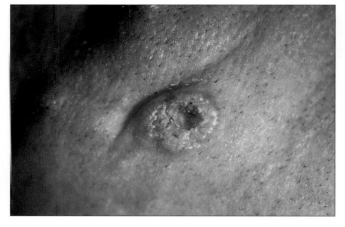

Figure 27.2 Basal cell carcinoma. This lesion developed in a patient with molluscum contagiosum. Note the translucent appearance that simulates molluscum contagiosum.

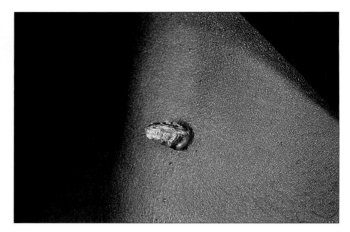

Figure 27.4 Squamous cell carcinoma with cutaneous horn. There is a verrucous papule with a horny excrescence that on biopsy proved to represent squamous cell carcinoma.

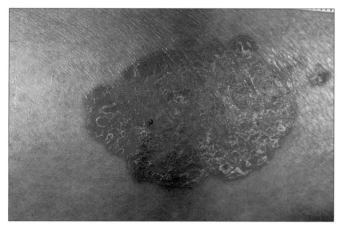

Figure 27.3 Superficial multicentric basal cell carcinoma. This scaly red plaque has features simulating an inflammatory skin disease such as psoriasis.

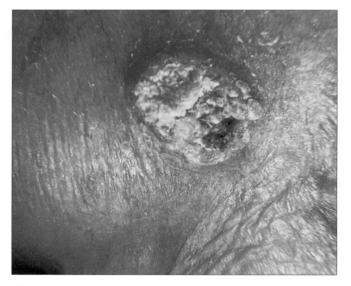

Figure 27.5 Solar induced squamous cell carcinoma. As patients with HIV infection survive longer, the risk for the development of cutaneous epithelial neoplasms such as squamous cell carcinoma increases.

histologic appearance that is identical to that seen in immunocompetent hosts.

LABORATORY FINDINGS

No specific abnormalities are found in the blood that relate directly to these neoplasms except for the fact that CD4+ counts are often well below 500 cells/mm^3 at the time of diagnosis. Immunoperoxidase staining for human papillomavirus is usually strongly positive, as is the polymerase chain reaction, which demonstrates the presence of HPV genomes within infected cells.

DIFFERENTIAL DIAGNOSIS

Bowenoid papulosis clinically may appear quite similar or identical to condyloma acuminata. Biopsies are necessary to establish the diagnosis. Squamous cell carcinoma may have clinical and histologic features similar to pseudocarcinomatous hyperplasia, including that induced by infectious agents. Giant HPV-induced verrucous carcinoma may have histologic features similar to giant condylomata. Epidermodysplasia verruciformis may clinically simulate widespread warts or, in some cases, other forms of erythroderma or widespread red scaly dermatoses. Basal cell carcinoma may mimic molluscum contagiosum as well as nondescript papular lesions of opportunistic infections.

DIAGNOSIS

Diagnosis is established primarily on the basis of clinical appearance and skin biopsy. Exfoliative cytology is generally used to determine the presence of intraepithelial neoplasia of the cervix and anal areas although this technique has a high rate of false negatives when compared with colposcopically or sigmoidoscopically directed tissue biopsies.[14]

341

TREATMENT

Treatment of squamous cell carcinoma in HIV patients generally requires excision or aggressive destructive measures. Cryotherapy, generally used for the management of cervical intraepithelial neoplasia, has been shown in one study to have an overall efficacy of 25%, significantly below that observed in HIV-seronegative patients.[15] Carbon dioxide laser destruction may be more effective in this setting. Bowenoid papulosis, while generally effectively treated with simple cryosurgical destruction, topical application of 5-fluorouracil or imiquimod, should be treated with either electro-desiccation and curettage or other surgical destructive measures with biopsy confirmation of removal rather than by conservative topical measures in immuno-compromised hosts. Basal cell carcinoma also should be treated aggressively with destructive measures such as excision as there is the potential for recurrence and (rarely) metastasis. Epidermodysplasia verruciformis is refractory to all forms of therapy. Any neoplasms that develop should be destroyed or excised. Systemic administration of retinoids such as etretinate or 13,cis-retinoic acid at doses of 1–2 mg/kg may be effective in preventing development of carcinomata.

LYMPHORETICULAR MALIGNANCIES

DEFINITION

Lymphoreticular malignancies of both B- and T-cell lineage may develop in patients with HIV infection. The majority of these involve lymph nodes and the reticulo-endothelial system although the skin may be involved either primarily or secondarily. Non-Hodgkin's lymphoma, mostly high grade (small non-cleaved cell and large cell immunoblastic) and intermediate grade (diffuse large cell) B cell lymphomas are seen most commonly although cutaneous T-cell lymphomas, Hodgkin's disease, lymphomatoid granulomatous (angiocentric peripheral T-cell lymphoma) and adult T-cell leukemia-lymphoma caused by HTLV-1 have been reported.

INCIDENCE

Non-Hodgkin's lymphomas have increased in the greatest proportion in patients with HIV infection. The incidence of non-Hodgkin's lymphoma in never-married men in the Los Angeles area is nearly twice that of married men aged 15–54.[16] In San Francisco, the rate of non-Hodgkin's lymphoma is five times greater in patients with HIV infection than in non-HIV-infected individuals.[17] HIV associated Hodgkin's disease is less well appreciated but several studies have demonstrated a statistically significant increase in the incidence of this neoplasm as well. Other lymphomas such as cutaneous T-cell lymphoma have been reported sporadically.

PATHOGENESIS

Approximately 25% of AIDS patients with non-Hodgkin's lymphoma have had a prior history of generalized lymphadenopathy with histologic findings of follicular hyperplasia observed on biopsy. These lymph nodes contain polyclonal proliferations of B lymphocytes, a finding similar to what is seen in African children with endemic Burkitt's lymphoma as well as in iatrogenically immunosuppressed patients.[18] Polyclonal B-cell proliferation is thought to be caused directly by viral infection or as a consequence of loss of T-cell immunoregulation. Clonal immunoglobulin heavy chain rearrangements, however, have been found in HIV-associated lymph node hyperplasia suggesting a premalignant nature. In most cases, lymphomas associated with HIV infection are monoclonal in nature although on occasion more than one neoplastic clone may be demonstrated.

Chromosomal abnormalities are also well documented in patients with HIV-related lymphoma with translocations between chromosomes 8 and 14 being found in the majority of endemic and nonendemic Burkitt's lymphoma-like lesions.[19] The translocation breakpoint in chromosome 8 is near the c-myc proto-oncogene region which suggests that rearrangements of the c-myc oncogene may be related to malignant transformation in these patients. Juxtaposition of this gene to important regulatory regions may cause unregulated transcriptional activation and monoclonal proliferation of tumor cells. Other chromosomal abnormalities include duplications and deletions of chromosomes 1, 7, 9 and 12.[19]

Epstein–Barr virus infection is another factor of importance in the pathogenesis of HIV-related lymphoma. Activation of the B-cell arm of the immune system develops in HIV infected patients as a consequence of constant stimulation by foreign antigens. Concomitant infection by EBV may lead to immortalization of infected lymphocytes resulting in uncontrolled lymphoproliferation and eventually in malignancy.

CLINICAL MANIFESTATIONS

Most cases of lymphoma in HIV-infected patients involve visceral sites. When the skin is affected by non-Hodgkin's lymphoma, it is usually manifested as pink to purplish papules or nodules (Fig. 27.6). Any site may be involved including the head and neck, trunk or extremities. Deeply seated soft tissue involvement may expand superficially forming dome-shaped nodules that often ulcerate.

Cutaneous Hodgkin's disease is extremely rare and usually is a consequence of direct extension from underlying nodal disease. When it is encountered, it usually appears similar to non-Hodgkin's lymphoma, either as diffuse nodular lesions or as a 'panniculitis.' HIV-related cutaneous T-cell lymphoma may have a clinical appearance similar to mycosis fungoides manifest as widespread plaques that may progress to erythroderma.[20] HTLV-1-associated lymphoma may also resemble mycosis fungoides although it may have a

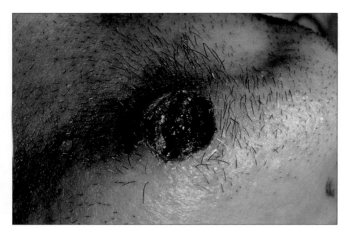

Figure 27.6 Cutaneous B-cell lymphoma. Patients who have infection are prone to develop lymphoreticular malignancies, some of which may affect the skin as in this case.

abundant circulating atypical lymphocytes that may number up to 600,000 cells/mm³ in Sézary's syndrome and in adult T-cell lymphoma/leukemia. In contrast, when hemophagocytosis or extensive bone marrow involvement supervenes, there may be profound anemia and pancytopenia.

DIFFERENTIAL DIAGNOSIS

The differential diagnosis of malignant lymphoma in the skin includes other lymphoid infiltrates such as inflammatory pseudolymphoma and other malignant neoplasms that may spread to the skin. Cutaneous T-cell lymphoma may mimic inflammatory dermatoses including psoriasis, atopic dermatitis and other forms of erythroderma. Ulcerated nodules of lymphoma may be nondescript and may simulate any cause of cutaneous ulceration in the skin ranging from infection to trauma.

DIAGNOSIS

The routine diagnosis of these neoplasms is based on the characteristic clinical appearance taken in the context of histopathologic features. In many cases, gene rearrangement studies, flow cytometric immunologic analysis and the use of DNA probes are necessary to further characterize and subtype the neoplasm. Immunophenotyping of mycosis fungoides-like CTCL in HIV patients may be characterized by an infiltrate of CD8+ lymphocytes in some cases.[21] HTLV-1-associated leukemia/lymphoma is characterized by an infiltrate of CD4+ cells with absent CD2+ and CD7+ antigens.[22]

TREATMENT

Treatment consists of the usual therapy for systemic lymphoma. Some of the regimens utilized include methotrexate, prednisone, bleomycin, adriamycin, cyclophosphamide and vincristine. Cutaneous T-cell lymphoma may respond to psoralen and ultraviolet A therapy, total body electron beam and topical nitrogen mustard. As expected, these lymphomas tend to be more aggressive than in patients who are immunocompetent.[21] As patients are already immuno-compromised, administration of many of these agents may cause profound immunocompromise with acceleration of death.

KAPOSI'S SARCOMA

DEFINITION

Kaposi's sarcoma (KS) is a vascular neoplastic disorder that prior to the onset of the AIDS pandemic was observed only in a very small select subset of individuals. It was first described by Moritz Kaposi in 1872 and is the most frequent neoplastic disorder to develop in patients with AIDS.[23]

clinical picture of an acute viral exanthem with an eruption of morbilliform papules and small fine vesicles.

HISTOPATHOLOGY

When the skin is involved by lymphoma, there is generally a diffuse infiltrate of atypical lymphoid cells that are generally monomorphous in appearance. Many of the cells are large, pleomorphic and in mitosis. The infiltrate tends to be deeply situated involving the lower portions of the dermis and subcutaneous fat and there is often extensive necrosis as well as obliteration of pre-existing adnexal structures. Hodgkin's disease may have an appearance similar to an inflammatory infiltrate in the skin although the diffuse nature of the infiltrate as well as the presence of large, atypical cells having a Reed–Sternberg-like morphology generally aid in making the diagnosis.

Cutaneous T-cell lymphoma is usually manifested histologically by psoriasiform hyperplasia of the epidermis with a band-like infiltrate of atypical lymphocytes, many having convoluted nuclei with a cerebriform appearance. These cells are also present in the epidermis where they often form small collections. In some cases, minimal epidermotropism is noted but the atypical nature of the cells allows the diagnosis to be made. In cases of HTLV-1-associated lymphoma, neoplastic lymphocytes are often extremely large and multilobulated having a 'clover leaf' appearance. There is also usually prominent exocytosis and, in that there is an associated leukemia, atypical lymphoid cells are often seen in blood vessels and lymphatics.

LABORATORY FINDINGS

In HIV patients with systemic lymphoma, no specific laboratory findings are noted, although patients generally have CD4+ counts less than 250 cells/mm³ when the diagnosis of lymphoma is made. Patients may have

EPIDEMIOLOGY

Shortly after the beginning of the AIDS epidemic, KS was observed in approximately 50% of the male homosexual AIDS patients in San Francisco.[24] This incidence has dropped significantly and is now reported in only 15% of HIV-seropositive patients, almost all of them homosexual men. The reason for this is thought to be related to the assumption of more safe sexual practices in the homosexual community with decreased transmission of HHV-8, the causative agent.

The disorder is far less common among intravenous drug users and is rare in women, hemophiliacs and their sexual partners. In some regions of Africa, however, the incidence of KS in women is much greater and is responsible for up to 40% of the total number of KS cases related to HIV infection.[23] In addition to HIV positive homosexual men, KS has been reported in a group of homosexual men with no HIV infection yet with risk factors for such. In these patients KS tends to have a more indolent course similar to that observed in elderly Italian and Jewish men.[25]

PATHOGENESIS

The pathogenesis of KS has now been defined and it is known to be caused by Human Herpesvirus Type 8 (HHV-8) or Kaposi's sarcoma-associated herpesvirus (KS-HV).[26] This virus has been shown to be transmitted sexually which explains the epidemiology of the lesion being seen predominantly in homosexual men in the US and around the world among heterosexual black men and women in Africa. Remarkably, KS has not been seen among homosexual men with AIDS in Thailand or China. It also explains why KS is rare among hemophiliacs and intravenous drug users. Nevertheless, genetic and hormonal factors may also play a role in the development of KS as HLA DR5 is associated with both classical and HIV-related KS. Furthermore, HIV infection may cause release of cytokines such as IL-6 and fibroblast growth factor that act as stimuli for vascular proliferation.[27] Kaposi's sarcoma-like proliferations have been shown to develop when mesenchymal cells are placed in tissue culture media and produce cell lines termed KS-like cells.[28] These cells have autocrine and paracrine activity as a consequence of production of growth factors such as basic fibroblast growth factor and interleukin-1. In addition, HIV *tat* protein can stimulate the growth of AIDS-associated KS cells *in vitro*. This can be blocked by anti-*tat* antibody, additional evidence for an indirect role of HIV in the induction of KS.[29]

CLINICAL MANIFESTATIONS

Clinically, KS skin lesions may be pink, red, brown or purple macules, patches or plaques. Purplish to brown-black nodules and tumors may also develop (Figs 27.7, 27.8). Early lesions are commonly mistaken for bruises, purpura or nevi and may have a yellow-green bruise-like appearance at their periphery. They may be symmetrical

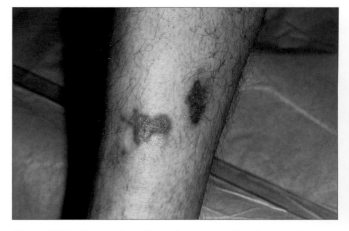

Figure 27.7 Plaque-stage Kaposi's sarcoma. Note the purplish plaques present on the lower extremity of this individual. These lesions have been found to be caused by Human Herpesvirus type 8.

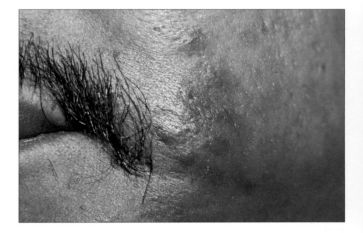

Figure 27.8 Plaques and early nodules of Kaposi's sarcoma on the face. These lesions may be associated with swelling and discoloration as is evident in this case.

with smooth borders or asymmetrical with jagged edges and may be oriented along skin lines.[30] In time, lesions darken and become scaly and may develop into raised plaques, papules or nodules. Lesions may spread locally in areas of trauma such as at sites of venipuncture, BCG injection, cutaneous abscesses or contusions.[31]

About one-third to one-half of patients have lesions on the legs and feet, which is a similar distribution to that seen in the classic form of KS not associated with HIV infection.[32] Lesions commonly develop on other sites, however, including the mucous membranes, the trunk and the scalp (Fig. 27.9). The hard palate, gums and lips are commonly involved, as is the nose. Skin lesions occur singly or in groups and they may coalesce to form large confluent plaques or aggregations of nodules and tumors. When pressure-bearing areas such as the soles are involved, severe pain may supervene especially when they become ulcerated (Fig. 27.10). Internal organ involvement is common and, as a general rule, one internal lesion develops for every five skin

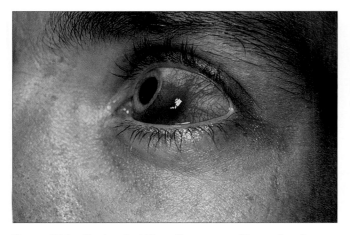

Figure 27.9 Conjunctival Kaposi's sarcoma. The conjunctiva as well as other mucosal surfaces are common sites of involvement.

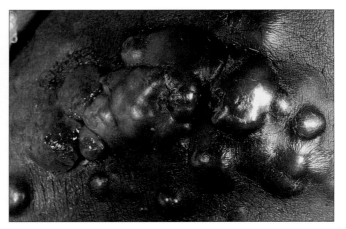

Figure 27.10 Multiple erosive nodules of Kaposi's sarcoma. When present in multiplicity, these may be debilitating and deforming.

lesions.[35] Involvement of the gastrointestinal tract may be dangerous if it causes blockage or hemorrhage. When tumors involve the lymphatics, marked edema may develop leading to diffuse areas such as the lower extremities or the head and neck that may give an appearance similar to that seen with a superior vena cava syndrome. Lesions tend to begin as pink macules and patches that develop into plaques to form nodules and tumors in time.

HISTOPATHOLOGY

The histopathologic findings of Kaposi's sarcoma vary with the stage of the lesion. Early patch lesions appear simply as proliferations of spindle-shaped endothelial cells surrounding preexisting blood vessels forming small jagged vascular slits. Scattered siderophages, extravasated erythrocytes and a few plasma cells may be noted. Plaque-stage lesions are characterized by a more diffuse interstitial proliferation of jagged, irregular slit-like spaces associated with extravasated erythrocytes, hemosiderin deposition and an infiltrate of plasma cells. Small, pink, hyaline globules that represent breakdown products of erythrocytes are characteristically seen. Nodules and tumors appear as diffuse fascicles of spindle-shaped cells with atypical cytologic features and mitoses. Small vascular slits and extravasated erythrocytes may be observed with careful inspection. Resolved Kaposi's sarcoma appears as a diffuse infiltrate of siderophages with few if any residual vascular slits.

A variant of KS that may be difficult to diagnose histologically is the so-called angiomatous variant characterized by a proliferation of larger dilated vascular spaces with only slightly irregular features. The presence of spindle-shaped cells in association with blood vessels that vary in size and shape and are filled with sludged erythrocytes aid in making this diagnosis although a search for more characteristic plaque or nodular areas is important. Immunoperoxidase stains for Factor VIII antigen and other vascular markers such as CD31 and CD34 demonstrate strong positivity of the neoplastic cells in most cases although Factor XIIIa, a marker of dermal dendritic cells, is also positive in some foci.[34]

LABORATORY FINDINGS

No specific laboratory findings are seen in patients with AIDS-related KS. Although many patients do have CD4+ cell counts that are quite low, the neoplasm may develop at any point in the course of HIV infection and its development or extent is not strictly correlated with the degree of immunosuppression. In general, however, more extensive disease is seen in patients with CD4+ cell counts below 200 cells/mm^3.

DIFFERENTIAL DIAGNOSIS

A number of different cutaneous disorders, both inflammatory and neoplastic, may simulate Kaposi's sarcoma. Purpura, hemangiomata, bacillary angiomatosis, dermatofibromata, lichen planus, pityriasis rosea, mycosis fungoides, nevi, malignant melanoma, cutaneous lymphoma and secondary syphilis have all been reported as simulators of Kaposi's sarcoma. In many cases, biopsies are required to establish the diagnosis. Histologically, there are a number of KS simulators as well. Some of these include microvenular hemangioma, targetoid hemosiderotic hemangioma, proliferative angiomata, severe stasis dermatitis, granuloma annulare and dermatofibroma. Clinical correlation is generally required in difficult cases to render an unequivocal diagnosis.

DIAGNOSIS

Diagnosis is generally based on the characteristic clinical features of purplish skin lesions in the appropriate clinical setting in conjunction with histopathologic findings. The diagnosis of HIV-related Kaposi's sarcoma should be made with caution in women and children from the United States as the neoplasm occurs only rarely in these patient populations.

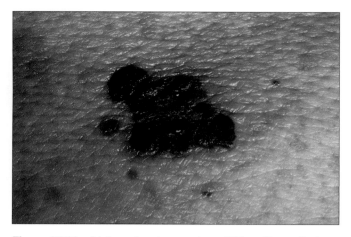

Figure 27.11 Malignant melanoma in an HIV positive patient. While relatively rare, occasionally melanoma may develop in these individuals. They may behave more aggressively in immunocompromised patients.

TREATMENT

As KS lesions often resolve as the immune system of HIV infected patients improves with HAART, it is often recommended that no treatment be undertaken until these agents have been administered for several months. Local destructive measures are generally effective for isolated or sporadic lesions. Liquid nitrogen cryotherapy is usually the first therapeutic option although radiation treatment and electron beam therapy may be used in selected cases. Radiotherapy is quite effective for painful lesions of the palms and soles although it is not used for oral ulcers as AIDS patients are more likely to develop severe radiation-associated mucosal ulcers and stomatitis. Intralesional injections of vinblastine sulfate at a concentration of 0.2–0.4 mg/cc at biweekly intervals is quite effective, especially if the patient has only a few small lesions. The method is quick but often associated with pain on injection. Interferon alpha 2B has also been used in this way to treat Kaposi's sarcoma. Systemic therapy with interferon and liposomally encapsulated doxorubicin and daunorubicin are also quite effective.[35]

OTHER CUTANEOUS NEOPLASMS

In addition to the aforementioned, other cutaneous malignancies have been reported in HIV-seropositive patients. Cases of malignant melanoma have been described many of which have been quite aggressive, even with Breslow thicknesses of 0.6–1.4 mm (Fig. 27.11). These developed in patients with CD4+ cell numbers ranging from 27 to 350 cells/mm^3.[36] In all cases lymphocytic infiltrates were quite sparse. We have observed several patients with amelanotic malignant melanoma, one that clinically mimicked molluscum contagiosum. In addition to melanoma, multiple dysplastic nevi have been observed in these individuals in some cases, in eruptive fashion.[37]

Smooth muscle tumors including leiomyoma, leiomyosarcoma and nodal myofibroblastoma have been described in children with HIV infection having CD4+ cell numbers less than 75 cells/mm^3.[38,39] The development of these tumors in this age group is extremely rare so that the association with HIV infection is likely important although the number of such case reports is small. The presence of HIV infection may play a direct or indirect role in formation of these lesions as evidenced by the synchronous development of multiple tumors.

Multiple tumors of sebaceous gland origin were described in a patient with AIDS. Three different primary sebaceous carcinomata developed over the course of several months although no evidence of metastatic spread was noted.[40]

FUTURE OUTLOOK

Cutaneous-related neoplastic disorders are important sources of morbidity in patients with HIV infection. Fortunately, patients with HIV infection today live much longer than they did at the advent of the HIV pandemic. As patients live longer, they may be prone to acquire the more common neoplasms that develop in immunocompetent hosts. Clinicians need to remain vigilant to detect such lesions at the earliest stages of evolution and to treat them appropriately.

Patients are becoming better educated about skin disorders and the effects of immunocompromise on the development of cutaneous neoplasia. As such, it is expected that although this population is still at risk for the development of skin cancer, the incidence of these neoplasms may fall and lesions will be detected earlier. In fact, many of the unusual neoplasms that were seen in severely immunocompromised patients early in the AIDS epidemic have already decreased in incidence.

As future generations of therapeutic regimens and vaccines for HIV are developed, it is hoped that factors leading to immunocompromised status will be able to be kept in check and that individuals with HIV will demonstrate biologic behavior similar to that of immunocompetent counterparts.

REFERENCES

1 Nelson AM, Mvula M, St. Louis M, et al. Increased rates of cervical dysplasia associated with clinical and immunological evidence of immunodeficiency. Poster presentation, VIII International Conference on AIDS, Amsterdam, 19–24 July 1992.

2 Galfetti M, Irion O, Beguin F. Vulvar and cervical pathologies in HIV-seropositive (HIV+) women followed in a colposcopy outpatient clinic, Abstract, Vol II, VI International Conference on AIDS, San Francisco, California, 20–24 June 1990.

3 Palefsky JM, Gonzales J, Greenblatt RM, Ahn DK, Hollander K. Anal intraepithelial neoplasia and anal papillomavirus infection among homosexual males with group IV HIV disease. JAMA 1990; 263:2911–2916.

4 Beck DE, Jaso RF, Zajac RA. Surgical management of anal condylomata in the HIV-positive patient. Dis Col Rect 1990; 33:180–183.

5 Marte C, Cohen M, Fruchter R, et al. Pap test and STD findings in HIV positive women at ambulatory care sites, Abstract, Vol I, VI International Conference on AIDS, San Francisco, California, 20–24 June 1990.

6 Goedert JJ, Caussy D, Palefsky J, et al. Interaction of HIV and papillomaviruses: association with anal intraepithelial abnormality in homosexual men, Abstract, Vol I, VI International Conference on AIDS, San Francisco, California, 20–24 June 1990.

7 Smith KJ, Skelton HG, Yeager J, et al. Cutaneous neoplasms in a military population of HIV-1-positive patients. J Am Acad Derm 1993; 29:400–406.

8 Tornesello ML, Buonaguro FM, Galloway DA, Beth-Giraldo E, Giraldo G. HIV and HPV interaction: Transactivation of HPV long control region by HIV-tat protein. Poster presentation, VIII International Conference on AIDS, Amsterdam, 19–24 July 1992.

9 Yabe Y, Tanimura Y, Sakai A, Hitsumoto T, Nohara N. Molecular characteristics and physical state of human papillomavirus DNA change with progressing malignancy: studies in a patient with epidermodysplasia verruciformis. Int J Cancer 1989; 43:1022–1028.

10 Rosemberg SK. Subclinical papilloviral infection of male genitalia. Urology 1985; 26:552–557.

11 Pandya AG and Cockerell CJ. Personal observation, 1993.

12 Sitz KV, Keppen M. Metastatic basal cell carcinoma in acquired immunodeficiency syndrome-related complex. JAMA 1987; 257:340–343.

13 Berger TG, Sawchuk WS, Leonardi C, Langenberg A, Tappero J, LeBoit PE. Epidermodysplasia verruciformis-associated papillomavirus infection complicating human immunodeficiency virus disease. Br J Derm 1991; 126:79–83.

14 Fink MJ, Fretcher R, Mamand M, et al. Cytology, colposcopy and histology in HIV-positive women. Poster Presentation, IX International Conference on AIDS, Berlin, Germany, 6–12 June 1993.

15 Guinness K, LaGuardia K. Cryotherapy in the management of cervical dysplasia in HIV-infected women. Poster Presentation, IX International Conference on AIDS, Berlin, Germany, 6–12 June 1993.

16 Bernstein L, Levin D, Minck H, Ross RK. AIDS-related secular trends in Los Angeles county men: a comparison by marital status. Cancer Ref 1989; 49:466–470.

17 Harnley MS, Swann SH, Holley EA, et al. Temporal trends in the incidence of non-Hodgkin's lymphoma and selected malignancies in a population with a high incidence of acquired immunodeficiency syndrome (AIDS). Am J Epidemiol 1988; 128:261–267.

18 Chadbourne A, Metroka C, Nmuradian J. Progressive lymph node histology and its prognostic value in patients with acquired immunodeficiency syndrome and AIDS-related complex. Hum Pathol 1989; 20:579–587.

19 Bernheim A, Berger R. Cytogenic studies of Burkitt's lymphoma/leukemia in patients with acquired immunodeficiency syndrome. Cancer Genet Cytogenet 1988; 32:67–74.

20 Parker SC, Fenton DA, McGibbon DH. L'homme rouge and the acquired immunodeficiency syndrome. N Engl J Med 1989; 321:906–907.

21 Knowles DM, Chamulak G, Subar M, et al. Clinical pathologic immunophenotypic and molecular genetic analysis of AIDS-associated lymphoid neoplasia: clinical and biologic implications. Pathol Ann 1988; 23:33–67.

22 Nagatani T, Miyazawa T, Matsuzaki T, et al. Adult T-cell leukemia/lymphoma (ATL) – Clinical, histopathological, immunological and immunohistochemical characteristics. Exp Derm 1992; 1:248–252.

23 Friedman-Kien AE, Saltzman BR. Clinical manifestations of classical endemic African and epidemic AIDS-associated Kaposi's sarcoma. J Am Acad Derm 1990; 22:1237–1250.

24 Rutherford GW, Payne SF, Lemp GF. The epidemiology of AIDS-related Kaposi's sarcoma in San Francisco. J Acq Immun Def Syndr 1990; 3(suppl)(1):S4–S7.

25 Friedman-Kien AE, Saltzman BR, Cao YZ, et al. Kaposi's sarcoma in HIV-negative homosexual men. Lancet 1990; 335:168–169.

26 Moore PS, Chang Y. Detection of herpesvirus-like DNA sequences in Kaposi's sarcoma patients with and without HIV infection. N Engl J Med 1995; 332:1181–1185.

27 Martinez-Masa O, Durato I, Kishimoto T, et al. Elevated serum IL-6 levels are associated with the development of AIDS-related Kaposi's sarcoma. Poster Presentation, IX International Conference on AIDS, Berlin, Germany, 6–12 June 1993.

28 Salahuddin SZ, Nakamura S, Biberfield P, et al. Angiogenic properties of Kaposi's sarcoma-derived cells after long term culture in vitro. Science 1988; 242:430–433.

29 Rusnati M, Presta M. HIV-1 Tat protein and endothelium: from protein cell interaction to AIDS-associated pathologies. Angiogenesis 2002; 5:141–151.

30 Rendon MI, Roberts LJ, Tharp MD. Linear cutaneous lesions of Kaposi's sarcoma: A clinical clue to the diagnosis of AIDS. J Am Acad Derm 1988; 19:327–329.

31 Janier M, Moral P, Civatte J. The Koebner phenomenon in AIDS-related Kaposi's sarcoma. J Am Acad Derm 1990; 22:125–126.

32 Krigel RL, Friedman-Kien AE. Epidemic Kaposi's sarcoma. Semin Oncol 1990; 17:350–360.

33 Safai B, Johnson KG, Myskowski PL, et al. The natural history of Kaposi's sarcoma in the acquired immunodeficiency syndrome. Ann Int Med 1985; 103:744–750.

34 Massarelli G, Scott CA, Ibba M, Tanda F, Cossu A. Immunocytochemical profile of Kaposi's sarcoma cells: their reactivity to a panel of antibodies directed against different tissue cell markers. App Path 1989; 7(1):34–41.

35 Simpson JK, Cottrell CP, Miller RF, Spitel MF. Liposomal doxorubicin: initial experience of a major London center. Poster Presentation, IX International Conference on AIDS, Berlin, Germany, 6–12 June 1993.

36 Tindall B, Finlayson R, Moltimer K, Billson FA, Monro VF, Cooper DA. Malignant melanoma associated with human immunodeficiency virus infection in three homosexual men. J Am Acad Derm 1989; 20:587–591.

37 Duvic M, Lowe L, Rapini RP, Rodriguez S, Levi ML. Eruptive dysplastic nevi associated with the human immunodeficiency virus infection. Arch Derm 1989; 125:397–401.

38 Orlow SJ, Kamino H, Lawrence RL. Multiple subcutaneous leiomyosarcomas in an adolescent with AIDS. Am J Ped Hemat Oncol 1992; 14:265–268.

39 Badochio S, Churiko E, Marocolo D, et al. Nodal myofibroblastoma in an AIDS patient with disseminated Kaposi's sarcoma. Poster Presentation, IX International Conference on AIDS, Berlin, Germany, 6–12 June 1993.

40 Hennessey NP, Armington KG. Multiple tumors of sebaceous gland origin in an AIDS patient. Poster Presentation, IX International Conference on AIDS, Berlin, Germany, 6–12 June 1993.

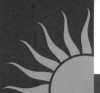

Cutaneous T-cell Lymphoma: Mycosis Fungoides and Sézary Syndrome

Kenneth B Hymes

Key points

- The most common cutaneous T-cell lymphomas (CTCL) are mycosis fungoides and Sézary syndrome.
- CTCL is caused by clonal proliferation of cells.
- Mycosis fungoides is manifested by chronic patches, plaques and tumors on skin that progress slowly.
- Sézary syndrome is manifested by erythroderma and abnormal T-cells in the blood and progresses more rapidly.
- CTCL therapy is based on stage of disease.

INTRODUCTION

Cutaneous T-cell lymphoma is a chronic lymphocytic malignancy of the skin which may also involve the blood, lymph nodes and visceral organs. Its precise diagnosis is important since it simulates many other lymphocytic cutaneous infiltrates and requires specific therapy for long-term control.

The most common T-cell lymphomas of the skin are mycosis fungoides and Sézary syndrome (MF/SS). Other cutaneous lymphomas including panniculitic T-cell lymphoma, NK lymphoma of the skin, peripheral T-cell lymphomas and adult T-cell leukemia/lymphoma are less common. This chapter will concentrate on the clinical and pathological features of MF/SS.

HISTORY

Mycosis fungoides was first described by Alibert in 1806 who published series of patients with mushroom-like cutaneous lesions.[1] The term mycosis fungoides was used to describe the appearance of the lesions and not to suggest the etiology, since the association of fungal infections with human diseases was not made until late nineteenth century. Darier in 1890 described the intra epidermal collections of leukocytes in patients with mycosis fungoides and this observation was popularized by Pautrier whose name was given to the histologic lesion of mycosis fungoides.[2,3] In 1936, Sézary described a patient with erythroderma, leukocytosis and lymphadenopathy. This patient had atypical cerebriform lymphocytes in the peripheral blood leading to the association of his name with this presentation of cutaneous lymphoma.[4]

Progress in immunopathology over the last 20 years has permitted the identification of the intra-epidermal lymphocytic cells in MF and the cerebriform cells of SS as CD4 positive lymphocytes. Molecular biology techniques have demonstrated rearrangement of T-cell receptor genes of lymphoid cells from patients with MF/SS, thus establishing these disorders as clonal T-cell proliferations.[5,6]

EPIDEMIOLOGY

MF/SS is a rare disorder with an annual incidence between 0.2–0.4 cases per 100,000. Epidemiologic data accumulated between 1973 and 1984 appeared to show an increase in the incidence of this disease.[7] Subsequent data has shown a stabilization of the rate of new cases suggesting that the apparent increase was due to better diagnosis and more accurate reporting.[8] Despite its low incidence, many patients with MF/SS have a prolonged survival thus contributing to measurable prevalence of the disease.

The male:female ratio of MF/SS is 2.1:1 and MF/SS is twice as common in African Americans as in Caucasians. The incidence of the disease in the Asian population is 0.6:1 compared with the Caucasian population. The disease occurs most commonly in the fourth and fifth decade of life. However, MF/SS has been described in patients of all ages.[9]

PATHOGENESIS AND ETIOLOGY

The proliferation of clonal T lymphocytes MF/SS has been ascribed to chronic antigenic stimulation, viral infection, failure of apoptosis, over expression of oncogenes, chromosomal deletions or inversions, or environmental toxins. The observation that cutaneous lymphomas may progress from polyclonal to oligoclonal to monoclonal populations of T-cells suggests that chronic exposure to an agent causing proliferation and selection of the T-cells is important in the pathogenesis of these diseases.

Bacterial antigens have been extensively studied as a source of chronic antigenic stimulation of skin-associated lymphocytes. Stimulation of lymphocyte proliferation and cytokine secretion has been implicated in flares of the activity of SS. Treatment of bacterial infections, particularly *Staphylococcus aureus*, has been associated with significant clinical improvement even in the absence of definitive anti-neoplastic therapy. Clonal T-cells reactive to Staphylococcal antigens have also been demonstrated in the skin and in the blood of patients with MF/SS.[10–11]

Infection with viruses including herpesviruses and retroviruses has also been implicated. Serologic testing for herpes simplex types 1, 2 and 6 yielded inconsistent results in large clinical studies.[12–14] A recent study by Herne *et al.* showed a high rate of cytomegalovirus (CMV) seropositivity in a large cohort of MF/SS patients. This report, however, did not identify T-cell clones, which were reactive to CMV antigens in either blood or skin samples.[15]

Retroviruses have been identified as the cause of acute T-cell leukemia/lymphoma.[16] Zucker–Franklin *et al.*[17] have identified retroviral particles in cultures of peripheral blood obtained from patients with MF/SS. These investigators have also described tax-like cDNA sequences[18] and tax proteins[19] in the blood and skin of patients with MF/SS. Antibodies to tax proteins have also been described in patients with MF/SS as well as normal blood donors.[20] These studies have not been confirmed by other groups. Thus, the role of HTLV-I like retroviruses in cutaneous T-cell lymphomas remains controversial.[21,22]

Epidemiologic studies have attempted to demonstrate an association between chemical exposure and cutaneous T-cell lymphomas. To date, no convincing association exists.

Multiple cytogenetic abnormalities have been described in tumor specimens from patients with MF/SS. The most common abnormalities are found in the 1q 32 region of chromosome 1.[23] An oncogene, Lyt-10, resides in this location, but overexpression of its products has not been demonstrated.[24] Abnormalities of chromosome 9 in MF/SS tumors have been found to have aberrant expression or regulation of the tumor suppressor proteins p15 and p16.[25] Other tumor suppressor genes such as p53 or the retinoblastoma gene do not appear to be involved in the pathogenesis of MF/SS.

The malignant lymphocytes in MF/SS have a TH2 cytokine profile and are deficient in the production of IL-2 and IL-12.[26] Soluble IL-2 receptor is increased with advanced stages of the disease and decreases with effective treatment.[27] There is a modest overproduction of IL-15 and an increase in proliferation in response to IL-7.[28,29] These observations suggest that chronic inflammation might provide a cytokine environment favorable for the proliferation of malignant T-cells and that recombinant cytokines (particularly IL-2 and IL-12) might have a therapeutic role in MF/SS.

Other mechanisms contribute to the unique biologic behavior of MF/SS. The modulation of the processes may provide novel therapeutic approaches to the disease. Homing of the malignant lymphoid cells to dermal endothelial cells is mediated via the binding of T-cell molecules CLA-1 and integrin to their receptors E-selectin, ICAM-1 and E-selectin and interruption of these interactions may provide specific therapies for MF/SS.[26]

CLINICAL FEATURES

Patients with MF/SS may have a long prodromal phase before the diagnosis is established. They may present with refractory, scaly, patches or plaques, which are initially diagnosed as psoriasis, eczema or atopic dermatitis and transient responses to topical corticosteroids may confuse or delay the diagnosis. Often, suspicious skin lesions yield non-diagnostic results. Should the patient have persistent lesions, repeated biopsies are essential, since the interval between the appearance of the skin lesion and the definitive diagnosis of MS/SS can be as long as 7 years.

The cutaneous lesions of MF/SS are described as patches, plaques, tumors and erythroderma. The precise definition of these lesions is important since they are the most important determinants of stage and therapy.

Patch lesions (Fig. 28.1) are flat salmon-colored lesions, which are minimally elevated above the plane of the skin. They are often pruritic and occur most commonly in non-sun exposed areas of the skin in the so-called 'bathing suit' distribution.

Plaque lesions (Fig. 28.2) are raised pinkish lesions, which follow the skin cleavage plane. Scaling and pruritus are common and there may be atrophy of the surrounding skin resulting in a 'cigarette paper' appearance.

Cutaneous tumors (Fig. 28.3) are nodules elevated >1 cm above the surrounding skin and may be associated with ulceration, pain and infection. Unlike patch and plaque lesions, tumors may be seen in areas exposed to the sun.

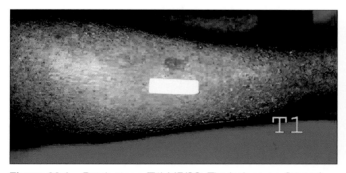

Figure 28.1   Patch stage (T1) MF/SS. The lesions are flat and salmon colored with irregular margins and are minimally elevated above the plane of the skin.

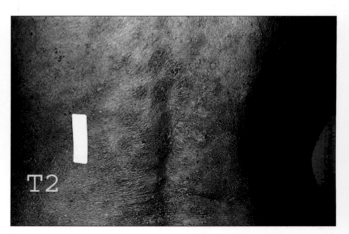

Figure 28.2   Plaque stage (T2) MF/SS. The lesions are raised and pinkish and follow the skin cleavage plane. Scaling and pruritus are common.

The erythroderma associated with SS (Fig. 28.4) is characterized by a brawny edema of the skin and a color ranging from light pink to violaceous. The histopathology of the lesions does not show dense infiltration with lymphoma cells and the erythroderma is due to vaso-dilatation. Consequently there may be variation in the intensity of the erythroderma probably as a result of variations in cytokine secretion by the lymphoma cells.

Although many patients progress from patch to plaque to tumor stage over a period of several years, some patients may have tumors as their initial presentation. This variant (described as the D'emblee presentation by Bazin in 1876[30]) indicates a biologically aggressive variant of MF/SS and a worse prognosis.

Several variations of the skin disease seen in MF/SS have also been described including granulomatous slack skin (GSS), large plaque parapsoriasis en plaque (LPP) and follicular mucinosis (FM). These lesions can all be shown to contain T-cells bearing the immunophenotypic and molecular characteristics of MF/SS. It is not clear if these lesions represent variations in the histopathology or MF/SS or are pre-malignant conditions.

GSS presents as large indurated plaques that progress to erythematous nodules and loss of skin elasticity. The lesions typically cause redundant skin folds in the axillary and inguinal regions. Biopsies of GSS show a CD4 positive clonal T-cell infiltrate of the skin. In addition, zones of granulomatous inflammation, degenerated connective tissue and multinucleated giant cells are observed. Patients with GSS may have other lymphoproliferative diseases including MF/SS and Hodgkin's disease.

LPP (Fig. 28.5) is characterized by large (>6 cm) scaly, erythremic or brown atrophic patches usually over buttocks, inguinal and axillary regions. Biopsies of the lesions show a hyperkeratosis, acanthosis and patchy parakeratosis. A scattered perivascular infiltrate may be present and in thicker lesions epidermotropism can be identified. The T-cell receptor gene rearrangements are seen in approximately half of the cases and there is a 10% incidence of transformation to MF/SS.

FM (Fig. 28.6), also called alopecia mucinosa, presents with thickened papules usually on the face, scalp and neck although lesions may be seen anywhere on the

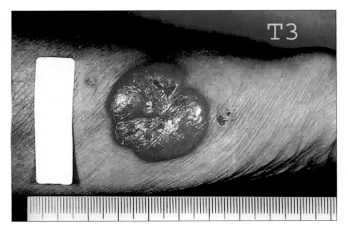

Figure 28.3 Tumor stage (T3) MF/SS. The nodules are elevated >1 cm above the surrounding skin and may be associated with ulceration, pain and infection.

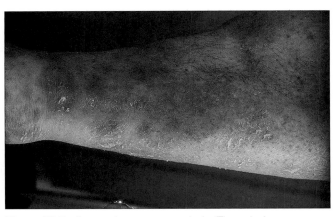

Figure 28.5 Large plaque parapsoriasis. These lesions are characterized by large (>6 cm) scaly, erythremic or brown atrophic patches usually over buttocks, inguinal and axillary regions. Biopsies of the lesions show a hyperkeratosis, acanthosis and patchy parakeratosis.

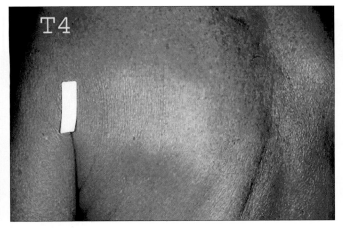

Figure 28.4 Erythrodermic (T4) SS. This manifestation is characterized by edema of the skin and a color ranging from light pink to purple. There may be variation in the intensity of the erythroderma probably as a result of variations in cytokine secretion by the lymphoma cells.

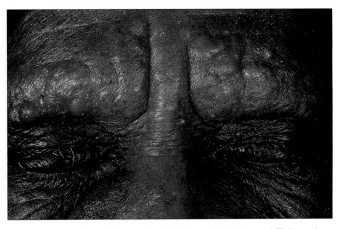

Figure 28.6 Follicular mucinosis. The skin lesions of FM can be located anywhere on the body, but most commonly on the face, scalp and neck. The lesions are indurated and involve the hair follicles and sebaceous glands resulting in hair loss. This lesion may coexist with other forms of MF/SS.

integument. The papules are associated with alopecia of the scalp and eyebrows and biopsy reveals a lymphocytic infiltrate of the skin adnexal structures. Mucinous degeneration of the hair follicles and sebaceous glands is present. CD4 positive cells with T-cell receptor gene rearrangement are present in the infiltrate and this lesion may coexist with more typical patches, plaques and tumors of MF/SS.

The extracutaneous manifestations of MF/SS include involvement of the peripheral blood, lymphoid nodes, liver, spleen, lungs and central nervous system. In SS the peripheral blood contains atypical lymphocytes with convoluted or cerebriform nuclei (Fig. 28.7). These cells may be observed in the peripheral blood of patients with any stage of MF/SS, however, when they exceed 10–20% of the circulating lymphoid cells there is a worse prognosis than expected for any stage of skin disease. The presence of large numbers of Sézary cells may also imply bone marrow involvement, although sensitive immunopathologic or molecular studies may be necessary to document this involvement.

Lymphadenopathy is usually restricted to the superficial lymph node bearing areas. Aspiration or biopsy of those these lymph nodes is an important staging tool, since it will distinguish between dermatopathic lymphadenopathy and true infiltration of the nodes by lymphoma.

Infectious complications of MF/SS

Patients with cutaneous T-cell lymphoma are at increased risk for infections both because of the disruption of the normal integument as a barrier to microorganisms and due to the immunosuppressive effects of many therapeutic modalities. Patients with advanced patch and plaque stage disease, as well as those with erythroderma, are particularly prone to develop spontaneous bacterial sepsis.

They may present with low-grade fevers, chills and hypotension as symptoms and positive blood cultures for *Staphylococcus aureus* are often recovered. It is important that patients with this presentation be rapidly treated with intravenous antibiotics providing adequate Staphylococcal coverage to prevent septic shock.

Patients with extensive ulcerative tumors may also develop a necrotic eschar covering open areas of the wound. This is often due to superinfection of skin with Enterococcus. Specific anti-Enterococcal antibiotic therapy is necessary to prevent dissemination of this infection.[31]

PATIENT EVALUATION, DIAGNOSIS AND DIFFERENTIAL DIAGNOSIS

The clinical staging of MF/SS is based on the 1979 TNM classification.[32] This system (Table 28.1) classifies the skin lesions as patches (T1), plaques (T2), tumors (T3) and erythroderma (T4) (Figs 28.1–28.4). Lymph nodes are classified as either being non-palpable (N0) or palpable (N1, N3) and have been either involved (N2, N3) or uninvolved (N0, N1) with lymphoma (Table 28.1). The clinical staging data is combined to yield a clinical stage (Table 28.2) and this clinical stage can predict overall survival (Table 28.3).[33]

The prognosis of MF/SS can also be estimated from the appearance of the skin lesions (the T stage) alone. Zackheim *et al.* have published a retrospective analysis of 486 patients with MF/SS and determined 10 year survival for patients grouped only by the stage of their skin disease.[34] Patients with early-stage disease had a 10-year survival, which was comparable with age and sex matched controls, while patients with T2, T3, or T4 disease had a statistically significant inferior survival (Table 28.4).

Based upon these data, the recommended staging evaluation for a newly diagnosed patient with MF/SS includes a history and physical examination with attention to symptoms of disseminated malignancy (fevers, chills, night sweats, or weight loss), the extent of the skin lesions and the presence or absence of peripheral lymphadenopathy or palpable enlargement of the liver or spleen (Table 28.5). Laboratory studies should include a

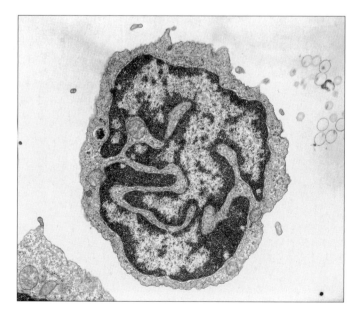

Figure 28.7 *Sézary cell.* This electron micrograph of a Sézary cell demonstrates the nuclear convolutions that create the 'cerebriform' morphology. (Image courtesy of Dr Dorothea Zucker-Franklin, New York University Medical Center.)

Table 28.1	TNM staging of MF/SS	
Tumor (Skin)	T1	Limited plaques (10% of BSA)
	T2	Generalized plaques
	T3	Cutaneous tumors
	T4	Generalized erythroderma
Lymph nodes	N0	No adenopathy, histology negative
	N1	Adenopathy, histology negative
	N2	No adenopathy, histology positive
	N3	Adenopathy, histology positive
Metastasis (visceral organs)	M0	No involvement
	M1	Visceral Involvement
Adapted from Diamandou et al.[33]		

complete blood count, liver function tests, serum lactate dehydrogenase and a HTLV-1 antibody assay. If lymph node enlargement is present, a lymph node aspiration for both cytologic and flow cytometric examination or an excisional lymph node biopsy should be performed. A chest X-ray should also be performed. However, CT scans of the chest, abdomen and pelvis should be reserved for those patients with stage IIB disease or higher, patients with biologically active disease suggested by an elevation in the lactate dehydrogenase, or patients with a rapidly progressive clinical course. Flow cytometry of the peripheral blood is a useful test for identifying circulating MF/SS cells even in the absence of a typical Sézary cell morphology. T-cell receptor gene rearrangement studies of peripheral blood or skin biopsies may be helpful in distinguishing between clonal and non-clonal lymphocytic processes. Patients who have abnormal peripheral blood counts should have a bone marrow aspiration and biopsy. Patients may rarely present with cranial nerve palsies or signs of a thoracic or lumbar radiculopathy. In those cases, imaging studies of the central nervous system and lumbar puncture are recommended, as the results of these studies will alter the choice of therapy offered to the patient.[35]

Table 28.2 Stage groupings for MF/SS based upon the TNM system[32]

Stage	Definition
IA	Patches or plaques <10% of BSA; no enlarged or pathologically involved lymph nodes, no metastases (T1N0M0)
IB	Patches or plaques >10% of BSA; no enlarged or pathologically involved lymph nodes, no metastases (T2N0M0)
IIA	Limited or generalized patches or plaques with adenopathy (T1–2N1M0)
IIB	Cutaneous tumors; with or without enlarged or pathologically uninvolved lymph nodes, no metastases (T3N1–2M0)
IIIA	Generalized erythroderma without adenopathy or metastases (T4N0M0)
IIIB	Generalized erythroderma with adenopathy but without metastases (T4N0-1M0)
IVA	Any skin lesion; histologic involvement of lymph nodes (T1–4N2–3M0)
IVB	Any skin lesion; histologic involvement of visceral organ (T1–4N0–3M1)

Table 28.3 5-year survival based on stage determined by TNM grouping[32]

Stage	5-year survival (%)
I	80–90
II	60–70
III	40–50
IV	25–35

Differential diagnosis

Other clinical conditions may simulate MF/SS including cutaneous pseudo T-cell lymphoma, large plaque parapsoriasis, lymphomatoid papulosis, poikiloderma atrophicans vasculare, pagetoid reticulosis, primary cutaneous T-cell lymphoma of the skin (CD30 positive), NK lymphoma of the skin and HTLV-I associated acute T-cell leukemia/lymphoma. In addition, morphologic variants of MF/SS including granulomatous lack skin disease and follicular mucinosis may complicate the differential diagnosis.

Cutaneous pseudo T-cell lymphoma usually presents as solitary lesions and may be associated with drug ingestion particularly anticonvulsants. There is spontaneous resolution of the lesion upon withdrawal of the offending drug. Histopathologically the lesion is in the band-like T-cell infiltrate without formation of Pautrier's abscesses or epidermotropism of the lymphocytic infiltrate. The infiltrate may be nodular or diffuse and express CD2, 3, 4 and 5. The lesions are usually CD30 negative, however T-cell receptor beta gene rearrangement may be present.

Lymphomatoid papulosis (Fig. 28.8) is an eruption of papules, nodules and erythematous plaques which resolve spontaneously occasionally leaving hyperpigmentation and scarring. The histopathology of these lesions is indistinguishable from an anaplastic large cell lymphoma. Immunopathologic studies identify large, atypical CD4 positive and CD30 positive lymphoid cells and molecular studies show T-cell receptor gene rearrangement. Unlike

Table 28.4 10-year survival of patients with MF/SS correlated with tumor stage alone (Note the excellent survival for patients with T1 lesions)

Tumor stage at diagnosis	10-year relative survival (%)	P value vs controls
T1	100	NS
T2	67	0.002
T3	39	<0.001
T4	41	<0.001

Table 28.5 Staging procedures for patients with newly diagnosed MF/Sézary syndrome

History + physical exam, with particular attention to lymphadenopathy and enlargement of liver and spleen
Laboratory tests (CBC, LFT, LDH, HTLV-1 antibody)
Chest X-ray
CT of chest, abdomen, pelvis in stage IIB or higher disease, elevated LDH, or rapidly progressive disease
Node biopsy for cytology and flow cytometry, if nodes clinically enlarged
Bone marrow biopsy if CBC is abnormal
T-cell receptor gene rearrangement of peripheral blood or skin biopsies to distinguish between clonal and non-clonal proliferations

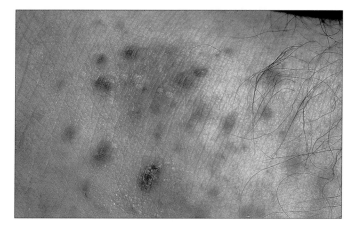

Figure 28.8 Lymphomatoid papulosis. These lesions are papular and pruritic. They may undergo central umbilication and necrosis and they may cause scarring of the skin. Although these lesions have histologic and molecular biologic features of malignancy, they resolve spontaneously.

a true CD30 positive T-cell lymphoma of the skin these lesions spontaneously remit. Patients with lymphomatoid papulosis have a 10–25% risk for developing lymphoma with the most common histologic types being MF/SS, Hodgkin's disease, anaplastic large cell lymphoma of the skin and T-cell immunoblastic lymphoma.

Poikiloderma atrophicans vasculare presents as reticulate hyperpigmentation of the skin with telangiectasia and skin atrophy. The skin biopsy shows vacuolization of the basal layer of the epidermis and Pautrier's abscesses are not present. A small percentage of patients with this disorder may develop papules and plaques and ultimately transform to MF/SS.

Pagetoid reticulosis is a T-cell lymphoma of the skin, however, it is not part of the spectrum of mycosis fungoides. This lesion has two forms, the localized, benign (Woringer–Kolopp) and the disseminated aggressive (Ketron–Goodman) variants. The localized form presents with solitary hyperpigmented plaques, while the aggressive form presents with erythematous psoriasiform patches as well as nodules and tumors. The skin biopsy shows epidermal infiltration with large atypical mononuclear cells. The immunopathologic studies identify these cells as CD3 positive and CD4 negative; the cells may be either CD8 positive or negative and molecular studies identify a rearranged T-cell receptor.

Mycosis fungoides and Sézary syndrome are members of the larger class of peripheral T-cell lymphomas. Other lymphomas of this group include angioimmunoblastic T-cell lymphomas, angiocentric T-cell lymphomas and the adult T-cell leukemia/lymphoma. The angioimmunoblastic lymphomas present with peripheral lymphadenopathy, fevers, chills, night sweats and weight loss as well as pleural effusions and ascites. Their clinical course is similar to intermediate grade B-cell lymphomas. Although skin lesions may occasionally be seen, epidermotropism is usually not present.

Angiocentric T-cell lymphomas present with symptoms of vascular occlusion due to the proliferation and homing of the malignant cells to the vascular endothelium. These disorders may appear as a vasculitis with waxing and waning skin lesions, pulmonary infiltrates and central nervous system symptoms. The skin biopsies show intravascular collections of the malignant cells without epidermotropism or Pautrier's abscesses.

Adult T-cell leukemia/lymphoma is a high-grade CD4 positive lymphoproliferative disorder associated with infection with HTLV-I. Infection with HTLV-I is more frequent in Japan and the Caribbean and can be seen in immigrants from these regions. Since the virus can be transmitted vertically, descendants of immigrants from these areas may also present with this form of lymphoma. The cutaneous manifestations of this disorder include patches, plaques and tumors, although the cells infiltrating in dermis and epidermis are larger and more atypical than those usually seen in MF/SS. Peripheral blood involvement is common and large atypical lymphoid cells are seen in the circulation. The nuclei of these cells have a characteristic 'floral' or 'clover leaf' morphology, which is distinguishable from the 'cerebriform' nuclear morphology of the circulating cells in SS (Fig. 28.9). The extracutaneous manifestations of this disease include hypercalcemia, bone lesions, lymphadenopathy, splenomegaly, pulmonary infiltrates and opportunistic infections. Despite treatment with both chemotherapy and antiretroviral medications the prognosis for this disorder is poor.

Primary cutaneous T-cell lymphoma of the skin (CD30 positive) is a histologically high-grade but biologically low-grade malignancy (Fig. 28.10). This lymphoma usually presents as solitary nodules, often on the extremities and on biopsy large anaplastic lymphoid cells are observed. The cells are CD4 and CD30 positive, however unlike lymphomatoid papulosis, these lesions do not spontaneously regress. In most patients, staging studies do not identify disease outside of the skin and local radiation therapy can provide long-term remissions or cures.

The natural killer cell lymphomas of the skin are aggressive subcutaneous lymphoma usually presenting as hemorrhagic or ecchymotic nodules over the trunk and extremities. On biopsy, these cells are shown to be large anaplastic CD4 positive CD56 positive cells. This disease usually pursues its aggressive course and often terminates in bone marrow involvement with infiltration of CD34 positive cells simulating an acute myeloid leukemia. The prognosis for this disorder is extremely poor, despite progressive chemotherapy.

Subcutaneous (panniculitic) CD8 positive lymphoma is a unique entity presenting with painful, ulcerative subcutaneous nodules (Fig. 28.11). On biopsy, atypical lymphocytes are seen infiltrating along the septae of the subcutaneous fat. Systemic symptoms including fevers and weight loss are common and laboratory abnormalities include anemia, abnormal liver function tests and elevations of lactate dehydrogenase. This lymphoma is poorly responsive to chemotherapy and radiation therapy. In the terminal stages of the disease patients may develop an erythrophagocytic syndrome.

PATHOLOGY

The skin biopsy in patch and plaque lesions of MF/SS shows prominent epidermotropism of atypical mono-

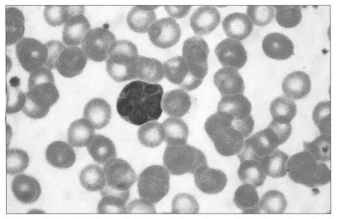

Figure 28.9 Adult T-cell leukemia/lymphoma, This is a cloverleaf or floral cell seen in the peripheral blood of patients with ATLL. Its nuclear convolutions are different than those seen in Sézary cells. (Image ccurtesy of Drs S Ibrahim and R Persad, New York University Medical Center.)

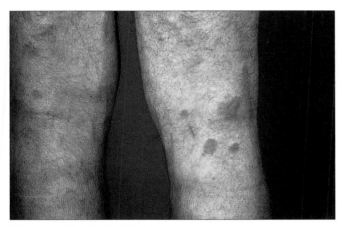

Figure 28.10 CD30 (Ki-1) lymphoma. This lymphoma presents as solitary nodules, often on the extremities. Unlike lymphomatoid papulosis, it does not undergo spontaneous regression. Systemic dissemination is rare and local radiation is often curative.

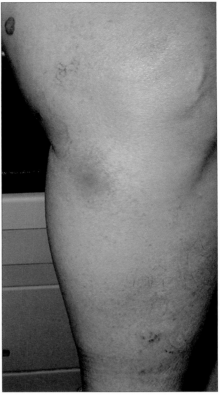

Figure 28.11 Panniculitic (CD8 positive) subcutaneous lymphoma. These lesions are indurated, erythremic nodules which may progress to painful ulceration. Systemic symptoms, including fever and weight loss are common.

nuclear cells and formation of intraepidermal collections recognized as Pautrier's microabscesses. In addition, there is a band-like infiltrate of the papillary dermis composed of mononuclear cells with variable size.[36] The cells may have complex, convoluted nuclei and minimal spongiosis is present (Fig. 28.12). An inflammatory cell infiltrate may be present which makes identification of the characteristic lymphoma cells more difficult. In more advanced lesions, dermal extension is present and epidermotropism may be lost.[36]

Immunohistochemical studies show the lymphocytic infiltrates express the pan-T cell antigens CD2, CD3 and CD5. In addition CD4 and CD45RO are also expressed indicating that these cells are derived from the memory T-cell population. Loss of the CD7 and CD26 antigens is typical of MF/SS cells.[37]

The clonal nature of the lymphocytic infiltrates can be further established by demonstration of rearrangement of the TCR beta gene by Southern blot analysis or polymerase chain reaction amplification of cDNA of the TCR gamma gene. The demonstration of the clonal T-cell population by either of these techniques is not proof of

malignancy as oligoclonal or clonal T-cell populations may be observed in inflammatory conditions.[38]

TREATMENT

Cutaneous T-cell lymphoma is responsive to many radiation and pharmacologic modalities. The localization of the lymphoma to this skin and the trafficking of lymphoma cells between blood, bone marrow, lymph node and skin enable the use of topical or skin directed therapy to achieve systemic effects. Despite the large number of treatments available, this malignancy remains chronic and incurable. This fact needs to be recognized when therapy is chosen since aggressive application of radiation or chemotherapy in patients with early-stage disease will not prolong survival and may introduce life-threatening complications.

The treatment of cutaneous T-cell lymphoma can be divided into skin directed and systemic therapies (Table 28.6). Skin directed therapies include topical nitrogen mustard, ultraviolet B irradiation (UVB), psoralen plus ultraviolet a (PUVA), topical steroids, topical retinoid analogs, total skin electron beam therapy and conventional radiation therapy. Options for systemic therapy include retinoid analogs, interferon, interleukins, single agent chemotherapy, combination chemotherapy, targeted immunotherapy and bone marrow transplantation.

Topical corticosteroids

Treatment with topical steroids is often the first modality employed. Topical steroids with or without occlusion

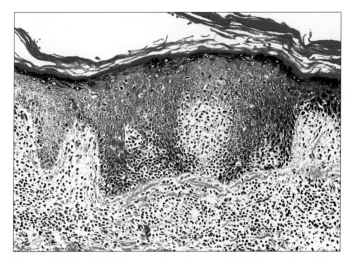

Figure 28.12 Skin biopsy of patch stage MF. This is a band-like infiltrate of the dermis consisting of pleomorphic mononuclear cells as well as the intra-epithelial collections of similar cells forming Pautrier's 'abscesses'.

Table 28.6   Therapeutic options for MF/Sézary syndrome

Type of therapy	Therapy	Response rate
Topical	Topical steroids	Up to 60% complete responses
	Topical nitrogen mustard	30–60% complete responses
	Narrow band UVB irradiation	up to 75% complete responses
	PUVA	up to 58%
	Topical retinoids	20% complete responses
	Total skin electron beam	up to 98%
Systemic	Extracorporeal photopheresis	50–75%
	Retinoids (bexarotene)	up to 67%
	Interferon-α	up to 55%
	IL-2	up to 60%
	Chemotherapy	30–40%
	Denileukin diftitox	10%

have been shown to have overall response rates of over 90%, with ~60% complete response rates in early-stage disease. Complications of this treatment include skin atrophy and the potential for suppression of the pituitary adrenal axis by systemic absorption of steroids.[39]

Topical nitrogen mustard: Mechlorethamine (HN2)

Topical HN2 has been extensively studied in early-stage CTCL. The treatment consists of application of 10 mg of HN2 and 50–60 ml of water to the entire skin surface with the exception of the eyelids, lips, rectal and vaginal orifices. This treatment is repeated daily for 6–12 months and has produced complete response rates between 30–60%.[40]

The most common complication of this treatment is a hypersensitivity reaction presenting as erythema following application of the drug. Treatment can be briefly interrupted and then re-instituted using a more dilute solution (10 mg in 500 ml of water). The concentration of the HN2 can then be slowly increased over a period of several months.[41] Patients who experience this form of hypersensitivity reaction often have an excellent clinical response to treatment following this desensitization regimen. This skin reaction has to be distinguished from an urticarial allergic response to the HN2. In this event, treatment should be discontinued and other treatment initiated. HN2 can also be applied in an Aquaphor base and it is the opinion of some clinicians that this preparation causes less hypersensitivity.

Since HN2 is a carcinogen there is a potential for exposure of household contacts to the drug or its adducts. For practical purposes, the aqueous solution is easier to manage and tends not to migrate through the household as might occur with an ointment-based treatment. Once the patient has achieved a complete remission the frequency of treatments can be tapered from daily applications to a less frequent schedule. The rate of tapering varies widely in the literature and no schedule has demonstrated superiority.

Toxicities of HN2 include the potential for myelo-suppression, reduced or abnormal spermatogenesis, teratogenicity and secondary skin cancers (basal and squamous cell carcinomas). Monitoring for patients on this treatment includes regular complete blood counts and counseling the patients to use an effective form of barrier contraception.

Topical retinoids

The synthetic retinoid X agonist bexarotene has recently been approved for the treatment of MF/SS as a topical and systemic agent. In a phase I/II study of safety and efficacy of bexarotene gel, 61 patients with early stage CTCL (61% IA, 30% IB, 8% IIA, 1% IIB) were treated with escalating concentrations from 0.1–1% and increasing frequency from QD to QID. Complete responses of treated lesions were observed in 21% of patients and partial responses of treated lesions were seen in 42% of patients (ORR 63%). In a phase III trial, topical bexarotene was applied to all lesions in patients with early stage refractory or resistant CTCL. The overall response rate in this group of patients was 44%. Common toxicities included erythema, pruritus and pain at the site of application.[42] Maintenance therapy with this drug is necessary, as interruption of treatment almost always leads to recurrence of skin lesions.

Phototherapy

UVB phototherapy is an effective modality in early-stage CTCL. Complete response rates in patients treated with narrow band (311 nm) UV light are as high as 75% with durable responses.[43] Narrow band UVB is equally effective in patients with fair or dark skin and may have the advantage of a lower risk of secondary skin cancers compared with broader band UVB irradiation.[44] Disadvantages of this therapy include the necessity of prolonged treatment (up to 5 months to achieve a complete response in most studies), the necessity of multiple treatments per week and the unavailability of UVB in some communities.

PUVA phototherapy consists of the administration of 8-methoxypsoralen (8-MOP) at a dose of 0.6 mg/kg 2 h before exposure to UVA radiation (330–340 nm). The treatment is initiated in a three-day per week schedule, with gradual escalation of the UVA exposure. The 8-MOP binds to the DNA and forms bifunctional thymidine adducts leading to DNA strand breakage, apoptosis and cell death. Response rates from PUVA alone can be as high as 58% in patients with stage I and II disease.[44] Once the patient has achieved a maximal response to this treatment maintenance therapy is usually required. Toxicities of PUVA include cutaneous erythema and increased frequency of melanoma, non-melanoma skin cancers and cataracts. Protection of the eyes with ultraviolet light absorbing goggles is necessary for 24 hrs following the ingestion of 8-MOP.[45,46] Systemic effects of PUVA include lymphopenia and the theoretical concern over reduced or abnormal spermatogenesis in men and teratogenic effects in pregnancy. Consequently, patients should be practicing effective birth control while receiving this treatment.

Total skin electron beam therapy

Total skin electron beam (TSEB) therapy takes advantage of the limited penetration of 4–9 MeV electrons through the skin. The radiation energy of these particles is restricted to 1–2 cm and can be used to irradiate the skin with sparing of deeper parenchymal structures. Usually patients are treated with 3600 cGy administered by the dual fixed angle 6-field method over a period of 8–10 weeks.[47] Response rates for limited plaque stage disease are as high as 98% and proportionately lower for erythrodermic and tumor stage disease. Over 50% of the patients achieving major responses with TSEB remain in remission for over three years. Toxicities of this treatment include erythema, telangiectasia, xerosis, desquamation and secondary malignancies. In addition, patients experience at least a temporary loss of the adnexal skin structures including hair follicles and sweat glands.[48]

Extracorporeal photopheresis

Extracorporeal photopheresis is a novel therapy in which peripheral blood is removed, separated by continuous centrifugation into red blood cells, plasma and leukocytes. The leukocytes are isolated and exposed to ultraviolet light in the UVB spectrum. The patient ingests 8-MOP either 2 hrs before the procedure, or the drug is directly instilled into the leukocytes following their separation. This procedure is performed on two successive days every 4 weeks and has achieved overall response rates of 50–75% in patients with stage I to III CTCL.[49] Patients with Sézary syndrome have higher response rates than other manifestations of CTCL. In addition to the direct cytotoxic action of 8-MOP and UVB on the malignant lymphocytes, it has been proposed that injury induced by the process causes *in vivo* immunization and recruits CD8 cytotoxic T-cells to provide additional anti-tumor effect.[50] This hypothesis is supported by the observation that patients with that area near the function and higher native CD8 positive cell populations have the highest response rates of those patients treated with extracorporeal photopheresis.[51] Whether these advantages are restricted to this form of photochemotherapy or can also be achieved with standard PUVA has not been rigorously tested. Toxicities of this therapy include leukopenia, sepsis due to the requirement for large bore catheters for vascular access and iron deficiency anemia due to chronic blood loss from repeated apheresis treatments.

Retinoids

Retinoids have long been used in the treatment of cutaneous T-cell lymphoma as they reduce proliferation and cause apoptosis and differentiation. The retinoic acid receptor agonists, isotretinoin, etretinate and acitretin are able to induce response rates in patients with early stage CTCL of ~50% with complete responses occurring in 20% of patients. The duration of these responses is brief, usually lasting <1 year.[52]

Bexarotene is a synthetic retinoid X receptor agonist, which also demonstrates pro-apoptotic and anti-proliferative effects in both CTCL and other cancer cell lines *in vitro*. In both phase I and II/III studies of this drug high response rates were observed in all stages of CTCL despite extensive treatments with other modalities.[53,54]

Overall response rates (ORR) in patients receiving bexarotene at doses of 6.5, 300 or >300 mg/m^2 or greater for the early stage protocol were 20, 54 and 67%, respectively. For the late stage protocol patients receiving 300 or >300 mg/m^2 had overall response rates of 45 and 55%, respectively. Late stage patients treated at the 300 mg/m^2 dose had a duration of response of 42.7 weeks. Responses were evenly distributed across all disease stages; responses in tumor stage disease (IIB) and Sézary syndrome (III) were frequent.

Treatment-related toxicity included hypertriglyceridemia (79%), hypercholesterolemia (62%) and hypothyroidism (53%). Hyperlipidemia was managed by sequential dose reduction in decrements of 100 mg/m^2 and by treatment with atorvastatin and fenofibrate. Monitoring of potential hepatic and skeletal muscle toxicity of this combination of medications is essential. Assays for thyroid and liver function, creatine kinase, cholesterol and triglycerides should be repeated monthly during treatment. In some patients sustained release niacin was necessary to control the hypertriglyceridemia. Treatment with gemfibrozil was avoided due to pharmacokinetic evidence that this drug increased plasma levels of bexarotene. Leukopenia was noted in 47% of patients, however, no episodes of neutropenic fever were noted and no patient required treatment with G or GM-CSF.[53,54]

Interferons

Interferons are a family of naturally occurring proteins with anti-viral, proinflammatory and anti-tumor effects. The genes for alpha, beta and gamma interferon have been cloned and expressed and are available as pharmaceutical products. Alpha interferon has been used for the treatment of cutaneous T-cell lymphoma for almost 20 years.[55] The overall response rates in patients with early stage cutaneous lymphoma are as high as 55% with close to 20% of patients achieving a complete remission. Patients with newly diagnosed disease and less advanced stages have the best response. Toxicities of this treatment include fever, chills, weight loss, hair loss and thyroiditis leading to either hyper or hypothyroidism.

Alpha interferon has been the predominant form of interferon used for the treatment of CTCL. Early clinical studies of systemically administered gamma interferon showed only partial responses, although isolated case reports describe long-term remissions.[56] A higher complete response rate has been achieved with both intra-lesional and systemic administration of gamma interferon, however the toxicities are greater than with alpha interferon. Treatment with beta interferon has shown little efficacy in the treatment of CTCL.[57]

Interleukins

The malignant lymphocytes of CTCL have a TH2 cytokine profile loss and are deficient in the secretion of IL-2 and IL-12. Thus, there is a rationale for the use of these cytokines in this disorder. Administration of IL-2 in patients with advanced malignancies has been postulated to induce proliferation and recruitment of cytotoxic T-lymphocytes to induce an anti-tumor response. Administration of IL-2 to seven patients with advanced stage CTCL induced a complete response in three and partial response in two. The responses in two of the five responding patients persisted for as long as 5 years.[58] The toxicity of IL-2 therapy includes fever, chills, nausea, vomiting, diarrhea, weight gain, anemia, thrombocytopenia and hypotension.[58]

A phase I trial of subcutaneous and intra-lesional IL-12 was associated with an overall 56% response rate and a complete response rate of 22%. A somewhat lower response rate was reported in a subsequent trial. The toxicities of IL-12 include low-grade fever, headache and depression.[59]

CHEMOTHERAPY

Cytotoxic chemotherapy has been widely used in the treatment of cutaneous T-cell lymphoma. Alkylating agents such as cyclophosphamide, BCNU and chlorambucil are able to achieve a response rate of 62% overall and complete response rates as high as 32%. Unfortunately

the duration of these responses are brief with the median duration of responses between 3 and 22 months. In addition, these drugs are myelosuppressive and immunosuppressive and repeated cycles of treatment may increase the already high risk of infection in patients with CTCL.[60]

Methotrexate, as a single agent, has overall response rates of 58% and had a complete response rate of 41%, with less severe myelosuppression and immunosuppression, particularly when combined with leucovorin rescue. Other toxicities include hepatic fibrosis, pulmonary fibrosis, and mucositis. This favorable toxicity profile makes the use of methotrexate an attractive alternative to other cytotoxic drugs as a single agent.[61]

Recent studies of purine analogs including pentostatin, fludarabine and chloro-deoxyadenosine have shown both overall and complete response rates comparable with combination chemotherapy regimens. As with combination chemotherapy, the duration of these responses are brief and prolonged myelosuppression and immunosuppression are common. The severe T-cell in the dysfunction induced by drugs of this class requires prophylactic treatment with trimethoprim/sulfamethoxazole for prophylaxis against *Pneumocystis carinii* pneumonia and acyclovir for prophylaxis against Herpes zoster.[62–64]

Newer chemotherapeutic agents including pegylated liposomal doxorubicin and gemcitabine are currently under study. Their advantage over currently available chemotherapy remains to be established.[65]

Combination chemotherapy using cyclophosphamide, doxorubicin, vincristine, prednisone and etoposide is capable of achieving response rates of >80% with approximately 40% with a complete response. Again, the median duration of responses is brief, ranging from 5 to 41 months and not associated with improvement of overall survival. These combinations are myelosuppressive and immunosuppressive and have the risk of chronic bone marrow injury leading to myelodysplasia or acute leukemia. Consequently, these treatments are best reserved for patients with advanced stage disease who have proven to be refractory to other modalities.[66]

Denileukin diftitox

Denileukin diftitox has recently been approved by the FDA for the treatment of refractory cutaneous T-cell lymphoma. This drug is a fusion of proteins containing interleukin-2 and the diphtheria toxin A chain. The molecule can bind to the IL-2 receptor of the T-cell lymphoma cell, be internalized with the receptor and the diphtheria toxin cleaved from the fusion proteins. A single molecule of diphtheria toxin is capable of killing a cell thus providing a novel targeted immunotherapy for this disease. The molecule can bind any of the IL-2 receptors, although CD25 is the only receptor whose presence can be determined on routine clinical immunopathology laboratory studies. Consequently, it is possible that CD25 negative lymphoma cells may still be killed by this drug.[67,68]

CTCL patients receiving either a low dose (9 mg/kg per day) or high dose (18 mg/kg per day) of denileukin diftitox for 5 days on a 21-day cycle achieved a 30% overall response rate and a 10% complete response rate. The median duration of the response was 4.4 months from the time of first response or 6.9 months from the time of first dose. Responses were seen in all stages of CTCL although the drugs seem to be particularly effective in patients with stage IIB disease. Toxicities of this treatment include infusion related hypotension, fever, transient cutaneous erythema and the capillary leak syndrome. These toxicities can be ameliorated by pretreatment with glucocorticoids, acetaminophen and antihistamines.[69,70]

Monoclonal antibodies

Although chimeric, humanized and radiolabeled monoclonal antibodies have demonstrated significant therapeutic effect in B-cell malignancies treatment with anti-CD5 monoclonal antibodies either as native, chimeric, or radiolabeled antibodies have been disappointing in the treatment of CTCL.[71] Similarly, a chimeric anti-CD4 antibody showed limited therapeutic benefit in CTCL.[72]

Lundin et al.[73] recently reported treatment of 22 patients with a chimeric anti-CD52 monoclonal antibody (alemtuzumab, CAMPATH-1H). These patients had stage III and IV disease and achieved an overall response rate of 55% and a complete response rate of 32%. Responses with reduction in erythroderma, pruritus and Sézary cell counts were more frequent than reductions in plaques or tumors. The median duration of response was 12 months. The treatment was complicated by CMV, herpes simplex and mycobacterial infections.

External beam radiation therapy

MF/SS is an extremely radiosensitive tumor. Doses as low as 2000–3000 cGy can produce rapid resolution of cutaneous tumors. This treatment however has limited utility since conventional orthovoltage radiation has sufficient tissue penetration both to cause radiation dermatitis and to affect parenchymal structures beneath the skin. Consequently, this therapy is best reserved as a palliative measure for relieving pain or discomfort secondary to large tumors.

Treatment by stage

The treatment of cutaneous T-cell lymphoma depends not only upon the correct histologic diagnosis and the stage of the disease but also upon the biological aggressiveness of the process. In addition, complexity of the treatment may compromise the patient's ability to comply with therapy and economic, geographic and socioeconomic considerations must also be taken into account (Table 28.7).

In patients with limited patches or plaques (stage IA or IB) treatment with narrow band UVB or topical HN2 may provide long-term remissions with minimal toxicities. The choice between these approaches is affected by the availability of a UVB treatment facility, the patient's

Table 28.7   Therapy by stage of disease

Stage	Therapy
IA–IB	• Topical steroids • Topical nitrogen mustard • Narrow band UVB • Total skin electron beam
IIA	• Same as IA–IB • PUVA
IIB	• Combination topical and systemic Rx • Interferon-α + PUVA • Retinoids
III	• Interferon-α + PUVA • Photophoresis
IV	• Retinoids • Chemotherapy

willingness to learn to apply HN2 on a daily basis and the availability of HN2 (as there are periodic shortages due to variations in manufacturing schedules). Other therapeutic modalities, including TSEB therapy have been advocated for the treatment of early-stage MS/SS. The rationale behind this recommendation is that a fraction of patients treated with therapy may achieve complete remission 'cure'. Unfortunately, many patients receiving TSEB will experience long-term radiodermatitis, hair loss and potential for secondary skin malignancies. Since patients with early-stage MS/SS can be expected to live many years these complications may have a significant impact on quality of life.

In patients with stage IIA disease both HN2 and UVB therapy may be appropriate, however, these patients tend to biologically more aggressive disease and in addition to the previously mentioned therapies PUVA is necessary for adequate disease control.

Patients with stage IIB disease require a combination of systemic and topical therapies. The highest response rates have been achieved by the combination of alpha interferon and PUVA phototherapy. This combination has a high response rate and a long median duration of response. The majority of patients with this stage of MS/SS will require other systemic modalities. Bexarotene has a 50% response rate in previously treated patients with acceptable toxicity. Patients who fail to have an adequate response to this drug will require systemic chemotherapy either as single agent methotrexate or combinations of cyclophosphamide, doxorubicin, vincristine, prednisone and etoposide.

Patients with Sézary syndrome will require treatment with PUVA and interferon as initial therapy. When available, extracorporeal photopheresis is an effective treatment. As with patients with stage IIB disease, relapses following responses are common and salvage therapy with bexarotene or chemotherapy will be required.

Patients with stage IV disease will require systemic therapy in addition to symptomatic treatment of painful or disfiguring skin lesions. Initial choices for systemic therapy include bexarotene as this drug maintains its 50% response rate even in patients with high stage MF/SS. Although transient responses in this group of patients can be achieved with combination chemo-therapy, more aggressive modalities such as allogeneic bone marrow transplantation should be considered in patients of the appropriate age, performance status and who have a suitable bone marrow or peripheral blood stem cell donor.[74–78]

FUTURE OUTLOOK

Interest in CTCL is increasing as more is understood about this disease. However, actual etiologic and prognostic factors need to be determined to better assess the efficacy of current and future management strategies. Future studies will hopefully unlock the mysteries associated with CTCL to facilitate the development of effective therapy.

REFERENCES

1 Alibert JLM. Tableau de plan fongoide: Description des maladies de la peau observe a l'hopital St. Louis et exposition des meilleures methods suivies pour leur traitment. Paris, France: Barior l'Aine et Files; 1806.

2 Hallopeau H. Sur une lymphodermie scarlatiniforme, début probable d'un mycosis fongoïde atypique. In: Dr Henri Feulard, ed. Congrès international de Dermatologie et de Syphiligraphie tenu à Paris en 1889. Paris: Masson; 1890:525–538.

3 Pautrier LM. Erythrodermie quasi-généralisée, mais respectant des ilôts de peau saine, avec petites tumeurs à formule histologique de mycosis fongoïde. Bull Soc Derm Syphil 1937; 44:1307–1319.

4 Sézary A, Bouvrain Y. Erythrodermie avec présence de cellules monstrueuses dans le derme et le sang circulant. Bull Soc Derm Syphil 1938; 45:254–260.

5 Michie SA, Abel EA, Hoppe RT, et al. Expression of T-cell receptor antigens in mycosis fungoides and inflammatory skin lesions. J Invest Derm 1989; 93:116–121.

6 Weiss LM, Hu E, Wood GS, et al. Clonal rearrangements of T cell receptor genes in mycosis fungoides and dermatopathic lymphadenopathy. N Eng J Med 1985; 313:539–544.

7 Weinstock MA, Horn JW. Mycosis fungoides in the United States – Increasing incidence and descriptive epidemiology. JAMA 1988; 260:42–46.

8 Whittemore AS, Holly EA, Lee IM, et al. Mycosis fungoides in relation to environmental exposures and immune response: A case–control study. J Natl Cancer Inst 1989; 81:1560–1567.

9 Tuyp E, Burgoyne A, Aitchison T, et al. A case–control study of possible causative factors in mycosis fungoides. Arch Derm 1987; 123:196–200.

10 Jackow CM, Cather JC, Hearne V, et al. Association of erythrodermic cutaneous T-cell lymphoma, superantigen-positive Staphylococcus aureus and oligoclonal T-cell receptor Vb gene expansion. Blood 1997; 89:32–39.

11 Tokura Y, Heald PW, Yan SL, Edelson RL. Stimulation of cutaneous T-cell lymphoma cells with superantigenic staphylococcal toxins. J Invest Derm 1992; 98:33–38.

12 Lee LA, Huff JC, Edmond BJ, et al. Identification of herpes simplex virus antigens and DNA in lesions of mycosis fungoides. J Invest Derm 1983; 80:333–339.

13 Duvic M, Magee K, Storthz KA. In situ hybridization for herpes simplex virus in mycosis fungoides and alopecia areata. J Invest Derm 1989; 92:423–429.

14 Brice SL, Jester JD, Friednash M, et al. Examination of cutaneous T-cell lymphoma for human herpesvirus by using the polymerase chain reaction. J Cutan Pathol 1993; 20:304–307.

15 Herne KL, Rakhshandra T, Breuer-McHam J, et al. Cytomegalovirus seropositivity is significantly associated with mycosis fungoides and Sézary syndrome. Blood 2003; 101:2132–2135.

16 Poiesz BJ, Ruscetti FW, Gazdar AF, et al. Detection and isolation of type C retrovirus particles from a patient with cutaneous T-cell lymphoma. Proc Natl Acad Sci 1980; 77:7415–7419.

17 Zucker-Franklin D, Coutavas EE, Rush MG, et al. Detection of HTLV-like microparticles in cultures of peripheral blood lymphocytes from patients with mycosis fungoides. Proc Natl Acad Sci USA 1991; 88:7630–7634.

18 Pancake BA, Zucker-Franklin D, Coutavas EE, et al. The cutaneous T-cell lymphoma, mycosis fungoides is a human T-cell lymphotrophic virus-associated disease. J Clin Invest 1995; 95:547–554.

19 Zucker-Franklin D, Pancake BA. Demonstration of antibodies to HTLV-I tax in patients with the cutaneous T-cell lymphoma, mycosis fungoides who are seronegative for the structural proteins of the virus. Blood 1996; 88:3004–3009.

20 Zucker-Franklin D, Pancake BA. Human T-cell lymphotrophic virus type I (HTLV-I) tax among American blood donors. Clin Diagn Lab Immunol 1998; 5:831–835.

21 Kikuchi A, Nishikawa T, Ikeda Y, et al. Absence of human T-lymphotropic virus type I in Japanese patients with cutaneous T-cell lymphoma. Blood 1997; 89:1529–1532.

22 Wood GS, Schaffer JM, Boni R, et al. No evidence of HTLV-I proviral integration in lymphoproliferative disorders associated with cutaneous T-cell lymphoma. Am J Pathol 1997; 150:667–673.

23 Mao X, Lillington D, Scarisbrick JJ, et al. Molecular cytogenetic analysis of cutaneous T-cell lymphomas: identification of common genetic alterations in Sézary syndrome and mycosis fungoides. Br J Dermatol 2002; 147:464–475.

24 Garatti SA, Roscetti E, Trecca D, et al. bcl-1, bcl-2, p53, c-myc and lyt-10 analysis in cutaneous lymphomas. Recent Results Cancer Res 1995; 139:249–261.

25 Scarisbrick JJ, Wooford AJ, Calonje E, et al. Frequent abnormalities of the P15 and P16 genes in mycosis fungoides and the Sézary syndrome. J Invest Derm 2002; 118:493–499.

26 Rook AH, Heald P. The immunopathogenesis of cutaneous T-cell lymphoma. Hematol Oncol Clin North Am 1995; 9:997–1010.

27 Zachariae C, Larsen CS, Kaltoft K, et al. Soluble IL2 receptor serum levels and epidermal cytokines in mycosis fungoides and related disorders. Acta Derm Venereol 1991; 71:465.

28 Dalloul A, Laroche L, Bagot M, et al. Interleukin-7 is a growth factor for Sézary lymphoma cells. J Clin Invest 1992; 90:1054–1060.

29 Leroy S, Dubois S, Tenaud I, et al. Interleukin-15 expression in cutaneous T-cell lymphoma (mycosis fungoides and Sézary syndrome). Brit J Derm 2001; 144:1016–1023.

30 Duvic M, Feasel AM, Schwartz CA, et al. Enterococcal eschars in cutaneous T-cell lymphoma tumors: a distinct clinical entity. Clin Lymphoma 2000; 1:141–145.

31 Bazin PAE. Maladies de la peau. Observees a l'Hopital St Louis, Paris, France 1876

32 Minna JD, Roenigh HH Jr, Glatstein E. Report of the committee on therapy for mycosis fungoides and Sézary syndrome. Cancer Treat Rep 1979; 63:729–736.

33 Diamandidou E, Cohen PR, Kurzrock R. Mycosis fungoides and Sézary syndrome. Blood 1996; 88:2385–2406.

34 Zackheim HS, Amin S, Kashani-Sabet M, et al. Prognosis in cutaneous T-cell lymphoma by skin stage: Long-term survival in 489 patients. J Am Acad Derm 1999; 40:418–425.

35 Zonenshayn M, Sharma S, Hymes K, et al. Mycosis fungoides metastasizing to the brain parenchyma: case report. Neurosurgery 1988; 42:933–937.

35 Harris NL, Jaffe ES, Stein H, et al. A revised European-American classification of lymphoid neoplasms: A proposal from the International Lymphoma Study Group. Blood 1994; 84:1361–1392.

37 Jones D, Dang NH, Duvic M, et al. Absence of CD26 expression is a useful marker for diagnosis of T-cell lymphoma in peripheral blood. Am J Clin Pathol 2001; 115:885–892.

38 Duncan KO, Heald PW. T-cell technology in the diagnosis and management of cutaneous T-cell lymphoma. Comp Ther 1998; 24:117–122.

39 Zackheim HS, Kashani-Sabet M, Amin S. Topical corticosteroids for mycosis fungoides: experience in 79 patients. Arch Derm 1988; 134:949–954.

40 Ramsay DL, Meller JA, Zackheim HS. Topical treatment of early cutaneous T-cell lymphoma. Hematol Oncol Clin North Am 1995; 9:1031–1055.

41 Ramsay DL, Halperin PS, Zeleniuch-Jacquotte A. Topical mechlorethamine therapy for early stage mycosis fungoides J Am Acad Derm 1988; 19:684–691.

42 Breneman D, Duvic M, Kuzel T, et al. Phase I–II trial of bexarotene gel for the skin-directed treatment of patients with cutaneous T-cell lymphoma. Arch Derm 2002; 138:325–332.

43 Ramsay DL, Lish KM, Yalowitz CB, et al. Ultraviolet-B phototherapy for early stage cutaneous T-cell lymphoma. Arch Derm 1992; 128:931–933.

44 Clark C, Dawe RS, Evas AT, et al. Narrowband TL-01 phototherapy for patch-stage mycosis fungoides. Arch Derm 2000; 136:748–752.

45 Molin L, Thomsen K, Volden G, et al. Photochemotherapy (PUVA) in the pretumor stage of mycosis fungoides: A report from the Scandinavian Mycosis Fungoides Study Group. Acta Derm Venereol 1980; 61:47–51.

46 Hermann JJ, Roenigk HH Jr, Honigsmann H. Ultraviolet radiation for treatment of cutaneous T-cell lymphoma. Hematol Oncol Clin North Am 1995; 9:1077–1088.

47 Reddy S, Parker CM, Shidnia H, et al. Total skin electron beam radiation therapy for mycosis fungoides. Am J Clin Oncol 1992; 15:119–124.

48 Hoppe RT, Cox RS, Fuks Z, et al. Electron-beam therapy for mycosis fungoides: The Stanford University experience. Cancer Treat Rep 1979; 63:691–700.

49 Edelson R, Berger C, Gasparro F, et al. Treatment of cutaneous T-cell lymphoma by extracorporeal photochemotherapy. N Engl J Med 1987; 316:297–303.

50 Edelson R, Heald P, Perez M, et al. Photopheresis update. Prog Derm 1991; 25:1–6.

51 Fraser-Andrews E, Seed P, Whittaker S, et al. Extracorporeal photopheresis in Sézary syndrome: No significant effect in the survival of 44 patients with a peripheral blood T-cell clone. Arch Derm 1998; 134:1001–1005.

52 Kessler JF, Jones SE, Levine N, et al. Isotretinoin and cutaneous helper T-cell lymphoma (mycosis fungoides). Arch Derm 1987; 123:201–204.

53 Duvic M, Hymes K, Heald P, et al. Bexarotene is effective and safe for treatment of refractory advanced-stage cutaneous T-cell lymphoma: multinational phase II–III trial results. J Clin Oncol 2001; 19:2456–2471.

54 Duvic M, Martin AG, Kim Y, et al. Phase 2 and 3 clinical trial of oral bexarotene (Targretin capsules) for the treatment of refractory or persistent early-stage cutaneous T-cell lymphoma. Arch Dermatol 2001; 137:581–593.

55 Olsen EA, Rosen ST, Vollmer RT, et al. Interferon alfa-2a in the treatment of cutaneous T-cell lymphoma. J Am Acad Derm 1989; 20:395–407.

56 Kaplan EH, Rosen ST, Norris DB, et al. Phase II study of recombinant human interferon gamma for treatment of cutaneous T cell lymphoma. J Natl Cancer Inst 1990; 82:208–212.

57 Zinzani PL, Mazza P, Tura S. Beta interferon in the treatment of mycosis fungoides (letter). Haematologica 1988; 73:547–548.

58 Marolleau JP, Baccard M, Flageul B, et al. High-dose recombinant interleukin-2 in advanced cutaneous T-cell lymphoma. Arch Derm 1995; 131:574–579.

59 Rook AH, Vowels BR, Jaworsky C, et al. The immunopathogenesis of cutaneous T-cell lymphoma. Arch Derm 1993; 129:486–489.

60 Bunn PA Jr, Hoffman SJ, Norris D, et al. Systemic therapy of cutaneous T-cell lymphomas (mycosis fungoides and Sézary syndrome). Ann Intern Med 1994; 121:592–602.

61 Zackheim HS, Kashani-Sabet M, Hwang ST. Low-dose methotrexate to treat erythrodermic cutaneous T-cell lymphoma: results in twenty-nine patients. J Am Acad Derm 1996; 34:626–631.

62 Kurzrock R, Pilat S, Duvic M. Pentostatin therapy of T-cell lymphomas with cutaneous manifestations. J Clin Oncol 1999; 17:3117–3121.

63 Foss F, Ihde D, Linnoila IR, et al. Phase II study of fludarabine phosphate and interferon alfa-2a in advanced mycosis fungoides/Sézary syndrome. J Clin Oncol 1994; 12:2051–2059.

64 Kuzel TM, Hurria A, Samuelson E, et al. Phase II trial of 2-chlorodeoxyadenosine for the treatment of cutaneous T-cell lymphoma. Blood 1996; 87:906–911.

65 Wollina U. Pegylated doxorubicin for primary cutaneous T-cell lymphoma: a report on ten patients with follow-up. J Cancer Res Clin Oncol 2001; 127:128–134.

66 Rosen ST, Foss FM. Chemotherapy for mycosis fungoides and the Sézary syndrome. Hematol Oncol Clin North Am 1995; 9:1109–1116.

67 LeMaistre CF, Meneghetti C, Rosenblum M, et al. Phase I trial of an interleukin-2 (IL-2) fusion toxin (DAB486IL-2) in hematologic malignancies expressing the IL-2 receptor. Blood 1992; 79:2547–2554.

68 Foss FM, Borkowski TA, Gilliom M, et al. Chimeric fusion protein DAB486IL-2 in advanced mycosis fungoides and the Sézary syndrome: correlation of activity and interleukin-2 receptor expression in a phase II study. Blood 1994; 84:1765–1774.

69 Saleh MN, LeMaistre CF, Kuzel TM, et al. Antitumor activity of DAB389IL-2 fusion toxin in mycosis fungoides. J Am Acad Derm 1998; 39:63–73.

70 Foss FM, Bacha P, Kuzel TM. Biological correlates of acute hypersensitivity events with DAB389IL-2 (denileukin diftitox, ONTAK) in cutaneous T-cell lymphoma: decreased frequency and severity with steroid premedication Clin Lymphoma 2001; 1:298–302.

71 Bertram JH, Gill PS, Levine AM, et al. Monoclonal antibody T101 in T cell malignancies: a clinical pharmacokinetic and immunologic correlation. Blood 1986; 68:752–761.

72 Knox S, Hoppe RT, Maloney D, et al. Treatment of cutaneous T-cell lymphoma with chimeric anti-CD4 monoclonal antibody. Blood 1996; 87:893–899.

73 Lundin J, Hagberg H, Repp R, et al. Phase II study of alemtuzumab (anti-CD52 monoclonal antibody, Campath-1H) in patients with advanced mycosis fungoides/Sézary syndrome. Blood 2003; 101(11):4267–4272.

74 Guitart J, Wickless SC, Oyama Y, et al. Long-term remission after allogeneic hematopoietic stem cell transplantation for refractory cutaneous T-cell lymphoma. Arch Dermatol 2002; 138(10):1359–1365.

75 Masood N, Russell KJ, Olerud JE, et al. Induction of complete remission of advanced stage mycosis fungoides by allogeneic hematopoietic stem cell transplantation. J Am Acad Dermatol 2002; 47(1):140–145.

76 Russell-Jones R, Child F, Olavarria E, et al. Autologous peripheral blood stem cell transplantation in tumor-stage mycosis fungoides: predictors of disease-free survival. Ann N Y Acad Sci 2001; 941:147–154.

77 Olavarria E, Child F, Woolford A, et al. T-cell depletion and autologous stem cell transplantation in the management of tumour stage mycosis fungoides with peripheral blood involvement. Br J Haematol 2001; 114(3):624–631.

78 Burt RK, Guitart J, Traynor A, et al. Allogeneic hematopoietic stem cell transplantation for advanced mycosis fungoides: evidence of a graft-versus-tumor effect. Bone Marrow Transplant 2000; 25(1):111–113.

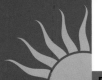

CHAPTER
29

Genetic Disorders Predisposing to Cutaneous Malignancy

Karina Gritsenko, Marsha Gordon and Mark Lebwohl

Key points

- Genetic disorders can manifest a wide range of clinical presentations.
- Genetic problems are often associated with increased susceptibility to malignancy.
- Basal cell nevus syndrome (BCNS), an autosomal dominant disorder, affects a tumor suppressor gene involved in growth control and regulation of development. It exhibits a wide range of manifestations and phenotypes.
- Xeroderma pigmentosa (XP) is an autosomal recessive disorder with multiple mutations, caused by a deficiency of DNA endonuclease, which increases susceptibility to sunlight via impaired base excision repair of DNA.
- Both autosomal dominant and recessive forms of dystrophic epidermolysis bullosa (DEB) are associated with defects in the dermal–epidermal basement membrane region and anchoring complexes in the sublaminar densa.
- Deletions, nonsense mutations, mutations of splice sites (XP), chromosomal mutations (DEB), or abnormal protein cascades (BCNS) may be seen in genetic disorders predisposing to malignancies.
- Often a diagnosis can be established upon clinical presentation and history. For more specific testing, complement studies, biopsy and histological analysis and immunochemical mapping can be used.
- Treatment of genetic disorders of the skin is directed towards the clinical symptoms as they arise.
- Treatment can be preventative (as in XP), surgical (excision of lesions (BCNS, XP); surgical manipulation of digits (DEB)), or drugs and vitamin supplements to counteract the mechanism or effects of disease.

GENERAL INTRODUCTION

Genetic disorders predisposing to cutaneous malignancy are uncommon. However, they are of interest because their cutaneous manifestations may be the primary indicator reflecting the underlying systemic illness. In some cases, histopathology is not specific because basal cell carcinoma (BCC) and squamous cell carcinoma (SCC) also occur in the general population, emphasizing the need for correlation between histopathology and clinical features for diagnosis of some genetic disorders[1].

BASAL CELL NEVUS SYNDROME

INTRODUCTION

Basal cell nevus syndrome (BCNS) (also known as nevoid basal cell carcinoma syndrome, Gorlin syndrome) is a rare autosomal dominant disorder.

Salient features of the disease include multiple basal cell carcinomas, palmar and/or plantar pits, odontogenic keratocysts, skeletal and developmental anomalies and ectopic calcification. Also related are internal tumors, both malignant and benign, including ovarian fibromas and medulloblastomas.

With the discovery and classification of the BCNS, there have been major breakthroughs in identifying abnormal gene sequences that allow significant insight into cancer pathways.

The current information allows for BCNS and other genodermatoses to be better understood and diagnosed earlier, allowing for the earlier detection of malignancies. At the same time, knowledge of the actual site of the genetic lesion is crucial in gaining insight to the genetic basis of this disease and may increase development of better remedies and treatments.

HISTORY

In 1960, two American physicians, Robert James Gorlin and William Goltz, defined this syndrome, after seeing a patient in January 1958. Their curiosity, coupled with a literature search, led Gorlin and Goltz to stumble onto a disorder that would have serious implications with regards to identifying genetic sequences and relations to cancer pathways. The discovery of this genetic disease provided one template to understand genodermatoses leading to skin cancer.

EPIDEMIOLOGY

BCNS has a prevalence in the US population of 1:56,000.[2] Patients tend to present at an early age with a variety of clinical symptoms.

Although all races and ethnicities can be affected, basal cell skin cancer develops most often in fair-skinned patients living in warm climates with significant sun exposure and sun-damaged skin.[3] Black-skinned patients with BCNS have fewer BCCs and skin cancer than white patients of the same age. Australians have been found to have more lesions than those in less sunny climates. About 10% of BCNS patients have no BCCs.[4]

PATHOGENESIS AND ETIOLOGY

BCNS is an autosomal dominant genetic disorder and can exhibit extensive interfamilial and intrafamilial variability with respect both to manifestation and severity of the phenotype. The basic pathology of the disease lies in a mutation of the PATCHED (PTCH) gene, located on chromosome 9q21–23. This mutation involves a tumor suppressor gene affecting growth control. A relationship exists between the human PTCH gene and the patched gene in drosophila. The function of the gene in drosophila is to affect growth and regulation of segmental development. This function can correlate with the developmental and tumor abnormalities in the human disorder. The patched gene is important in cell division and differentiation but also is thought to be important in skin and tooth development.[2]

The patched protein is a cell surface receptor for the hedgehog protein and is involved with the hedgehog (Hh) signaling pathway that affects growth and development.[5] The PTCH protein is thought to be involved with inhibition of the hedgehog signaling pathway. With mutation of the PTCH gene, the amount of patch protein available to bind to the hedgehog protein is diminished, causing a release of smoothened (SMO) protein from its normally suppressed state.[5,6] The release of smoothened protein initiates a signaling cascade leading to activation of Gli transcription factors for proteins involved in cell growth and differentiation. This signaling pathway creates a negative feedback loop: with insufficient PTCH protein function, the pathway is activated and produces more PTCH mRNA and protein, which then blocks the pathway.[6]

In addition to homologous mutations found in tumors, heterozygous PTCH mutations have also been located in basal cell carcinomas. These mutations have occurred on multiple sites indicating that it is the mutation of the hedgehog pathway and not specifically the location of the mutation that may be important. This constant upregulation of the synthesis of PTCH mRNA may be important in the development and maintenance of BCCs.[6]

Recent studies with odontogenic keratocysts (OKC) have shown BCNS to be directly related to Knudson's two hit hypothesis through a comparison between inherited (BCNS) cysts and sporadic cysts. The first 'hit' is located in the PTCH gene mutation found in BCNS patients. This second 'hit', a random mutation, leads to PTCH gene insufficiency or absence of normal patched protein, which is thought to result in malignancies associated with the clinical syndrome.[5] In other words, patients with the inherited tumor are born with the first hit, whereas individuals with sporadic tumors are not born with the hit. Therefore, inherited tumors often occur earlier and are often multiple because the body has a genetic predisposition (i.e. the inherited hit). With a second hit, a tumor will develop.[2]

It has been estimated that approximately 80% of the PTCH gene mutations result in a variation within the production of the patched protein, such as premature translation of the protein resulting in frame shift mutations and development of mutated alleles.[7] Normally, the PTCH gene has 22 exons.[5] Each and every mutation of the gene allows for variation within clinical expression of the disease.

CLINICAL FEATURES

BCNS often presents in patients at an early age with cutaneous findings including palmar and plantar pits. However, this finding does not ensure a BCNS diagnosis. Ensuing development of many basal cell carcinomas provides more evidence but it is the occurrence of multiple characteristics that allows for a definitive diagnosis.

Clinical features of the disease include developmental anomalies such as cysts of the jaw, pits of the palms and soles, congenital skeletal abnormalities including ectopic calcification (especially of the falx cerebri), as well as rib and spinal malformations. Postnatal characteristics include tumor development; especially prevalent are basal cell carcinomas. Other characteristics include ocular defects, cleft lip and palate, as well as possible cataracts, coloboma and even mental retardation.

The most notable characteristic of BCNS seems to be the hundreds of basal cell carcinomas that develop, leading patients to require frequent dermatological care (Fig. 29.1). These tumors generally appear between puberty and age 35, but can be seen as early as birth to 6 years of age.[8] Multiple epidermoid cysts measuring 1–2 cm on the limbs and trunk can be seen in more than half of patients.[8,9]

Problems with dentitia can be seen with the development of cysts, which continue to develop throughout the patient's life. If left untreated, they can expand and cause further damage to underlying soft tissue.[8] Odontogenic keratocysts have been found in 70–80% of BCNS cases, including the first case assessed by Dr Gorlin.[9]

Pits of the palmar region and the soles are also a significant clinical feature of the disease (Fig. 29.2). The pits range in size from 1–4 mm and look erythematous when large.[8] Though the histology of the skin is normal, there is an absence of keratin which constitutes the pit itself. Tumors rarely develop from the pit itself.[8]

Ovarian fibromas occur in 75% of female patients with BCNS and recurrence rarely has been reported in literature.[10] Fibromas left undetected can cause infertility and have a slight chance of degenerating into ovarian fibrosarcoma.[5]

It has been cited that 5% of patients with basal cell nevus syndrome develop medulloblastoma.[5]

PATIENT EVALUATION, DIAGNOSIS AND DIFFERENTIATION

The diagnosis of BCNS can be difficult because abnormalities may vary with individuals and many of the

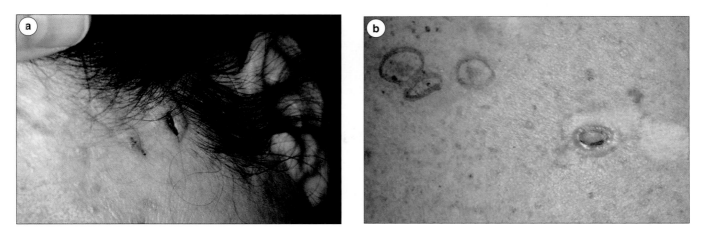

Figure 29.1 Basal cell nevus syndrome. (a) Patient with basal cell nevus syndrome. Note basal cell cancer on the face. (b) Same patient as in (a). Note the circled multiple basal cell carcinomas on the back. (Image courtesy of Mount Sinai Slide Collection.)

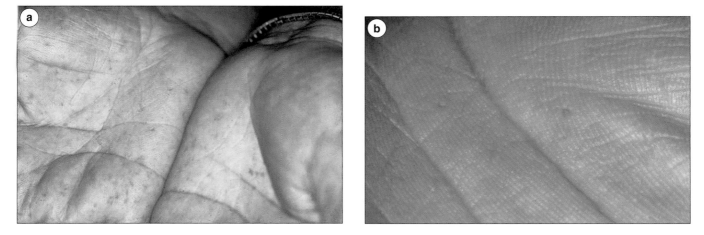

Figure 29.2 Basal cell nevus syndrome. (a) Palmer pits in patient with basal cell nevus syndrome. (b) Close up view. (Image courtesy of Mount Sinai Slide Collection.)

symptoms can be associated with other diseases. The diagnosis is made most easily in patients with multiple symptoms occurring in unexpectedly large numbers at an early age.

Guidelines for diagnosis include a family history, oral and skin examinations, chest and skull radiography, panoramic X-ray imaging of the jaw, magnetic resonance imaging of the brain and pelvic ultrasound in female patients. Attention should be given to inheritance by asking about family members with disease characteristics (although 25–30% of patients have no affected ancestors). Checking for abnormalities of the ribs, spine and phalanges (each of which are present in one third to one half of BCNS patients) may be helpful.[6]

While many of the aforementioned examinations are useful, clinical examinations including assessment of palmar and plantar pits or BCC identification are less reliable strategies of diagnosis than actual examination of the PTCH gene. Detection of mutation involves screening of the entire PTCH gene for mutations.[5]

PATHOLOGY

Histological examination and analysis cannot differentiate between abnormalities associated with BCNS and other diseases.

TREATMENT

Treatment of BCNS is directed to the symptoms of the disease at the sites of individual lesions as they arise. Frequent examination and monitoring are important in order to prevent tumor progression. As multiple skin neoplasms and their surgical removal may cause aesthetic issues, emotional support may be part of the patient's overall therapeutic protocol.

In >50% of BCNS in all ethnicities and climates, patients exhibit basal cell carcinomas.[11] These lesions should be removed and followed up. Small BCC lesions can be removed by cryotherapy and curettage with electrodesiccation with an effort to prevent as much scarring as possible. X-irradiation of BCCs should be avoided if possible in order to avoid radiation-induced carcinogenesis. Radiation therapy in BCNS patients can increase the prevalence and speed of tumor recurrence. In BCNS patients treated with radiation, BCC development can ensue within 6 months to 3 years as opposed to the typical 20–30 year lag period seen in patients with sporadic BCC.[11]

In order to avoid further potential BCC development from repetitive sunlight exposure, precautions should be taken to avoid exposure to the sun.[11] Surgical treatment of the BCCs has a cure rate of 95–99%.[11] Surgical treatment also is suitable for the removal of the ovarian fibromas.[10] Topical imiquimod, an immune response modifier that has been used in a variety of dermatological disorders, can significantly reduce and even clear basal cell carcinoma lesions. One may extrapolate that this treatment could be useful in patients with BCNS as well. Genetic counseling and prenatal diagnosis are appropriate for the sake of progeny, given that 50% of children of affected individuals are expected to develop BCNS.[6]

XERODERMA PIGMENTOSUM

INTRODUCTION

Xeroderma pigmentosum (XP) is an autosomal recessive disease characterized by its increased susceptibility to DNA damage. This damage is brought on by UV radiation, as well as by other carcinogens in some cases and is attributed to abnormal DNA repair. The disease is characterized by elevated sensitivity to sunlight, multiple epidermal skin cancers in childhood and early adulthood and an increased risk of malignant melanoma.

In the last 35 years, developments in the field of genetics have allowed XP to be characterized not only by clinical analysis but also by its specific genetic mutation. Eight genetic sub-types of the disease have been described.

Both excision repair and post-replication repair are important in preventing radiation-induced carcinogenesis. The various subtypes of XP exhibit defects in each of these repair mechanisms.[8] Damaged DNA that is repaired in a defective manner may result in mutagenesis, which may be an important step in carcinogenesis.

HISTORY

The term xeroderma pigmentosum ('pigmented dry skin') was coined in 1870 by Moritz Kaposi to describe the characteristic dry, dyspigmented skin that is the first permanent cutaneous change that is observed with the disease. Since then, XP has become a particularly well studied example of a disease in which early onset of malignancy is related to unrepaired DNA lesions, mutations and/or chromosomal modifications.

EPIDEMIOLOGY

Photoaging changes in XP (except solar elastosis) begin in childhood. Sun induced neoplasms, including actinic (solar) keratoses, keratoacanthomas, squamous cell carcinomas and melanomas, often ensue in large numbers with time.

Estimated frequency of XP in the US is 1:1,000,000. The condition is more common in Japan. Patients have been reported in diverse racial groups including whites, Asians, blacks and Native Americans.[12] There seemingly is no correlation with gender, age of onset, blood groups, or number of siblings affected in a family.[8] A high frequency of cases of XP appear to be centered in Egypt and the Near East, where consanguinity is common.[8] The type one subcategory of the disease, XPA, accounts for most Japanese patients and also is the most common type of XP in Egypt.[5]

PATHOGENESIS AND ETIOLOGY

In 1968, studies by Cleaver revealed the etiology of cultured XP cell hypersensitivity to UV light to be the result of defective DNA repair. Studies conducted with cultures of fibroblasts from xeroderma pigmentosum patients in various geographic areas displayed a wide range in the ability of fibroblasts to undergo base excision repair of UV damaged DNA. Through further hybridization experiments with the fusion of fibroblasts from different XP patients, it was determined that there are eight repair-deficient complementation groups of the disease (XPA through to XPH). They included seven excision repair defective forms of various DNA repair problems post radiation and an additional variant group with normal excision repair post radiation and a defect in post-replication repair.[8,12] Each genetic subset of the overall syndrome has a different location of a mutated chromosome which correlates to a form of base excision repair. These differences can be related to the idea that each group has its own variation of clinical characteristics and symptoms (see clinical features). The actual XP genes have been localized, as shown in Table 29.1. XP variant is caused by mutations in POLH (actual location unknown) which codes for DNA polymerase.[5]

With the exception of the variant type of XP, cells in tissue culture show a marked decrease in the ability to conduct base excision repair in which single strand areas of DNA are excised and replaced with a new set of bases after sunlight induced damage. On the other hand, in the variant form of XP there is a problem with the second DNA repair mechanism. Here, a post-transcriptional problem causes a delay in the rate of newly replicating DNA.[12] This problem is intensified with exposure to caffeine.

Genetic abnormalities responsible for defective base excision repair are caused by a variety of problems, including small deletions, missense and nonsense mutations and mutations affecting splice sites. The XPC category has been noted to have large deletions with the

Table 29.1   Localization of xeroderma pigmentosa genes[5]

Gene	XP subset
9q22.3	XPA
2q21	XPB
3p25	XPC
19q13.2	XPD
11p12	XPE
16p13.3	XPF
13q13	XPG

involvement of Arg(788)Trp in ERCC4.[5] The XP variant (POLH) mutation has deletions and mutations causing the truncation of proteins.[5]

The defect in the process lies in a deficiency of DNA endonuclease which initiates the excision process.[13] Studies have shown a range of 0–90% base pair excision function. Affected siblings usually have the same level of function.[13] A defect in DNA repair mechanisms can result in increased risk of UV light induced neoplasms. This was shown experimentally using narrow wavebands of ultraviolet, ranging between 290 and 320 nm. Following exposure to UV light, XP patients develop increased numbers of squamous cell and basal cell cancers.

In addition to human studies, similar studies have been carried out on tissue culture. Without UV radiation, cells of XP patients have a normal karyotype without excessive chromosome breakage or increased sister chromatid exchanges.[12] Yet, with UV radiation, abnormally large increases have been documented.

CLINICAL FEATURES

Cutaneous symptoms of XP begin at an early age with the median age of presentation being 1–2 years.[12] Scaling and small areas of hyper-pigmentation, resembling freckles are primary characteristics. Following initial scaling, skin becomes atrophied, pigmentation is mottled and telangiectases, similar to chronic radiodermatitis, appear. Solar keratoses in the areas of scaling ensue. By 2 or 3 years of age, senile skin and tumors begin to appear, including squamous cell carcinoma, basal cell carcinoma and, more infrequently, fibrosarcoma. Some 3% of patients can develop malignant melanomas, which in some patients show no tendency to metastasize, whereas others metastasize rapidly.[13]

In contrast, skin that has not been exposed to UV light, such as skin of the buttocks and axillae, remains unaffected. Usually one can see a sharp contrast between areas that are exposed to UV light and areas of the body that are habitually covered and not exposed to the sun. In children with XP, the development of erythema, freckling and increased pigmentation occur from initial exposure to sunlight. Common features that follow include drying, scaling and atrophy of the skin with fine

telangiectasia.[8] Skin rapidly degenerates on exposure to sunlight, simulating generalized radiodermatitis in appearance. By 3 or 4 years of age, patients may have multiple skin cancers: squamous cell, basal cell tumors and melanomas.[8]

It has been reported that patients under 20 years of age have a greater than 1000-fold increase in risk for BCC, SCC, or melanoma.[12] XP is associated with squamous cell carcinoma of the lip, tip of the tongue and anterior oral cavity (the most UV accessible area of the mouth). Various other forms of cancer including medulloblastomas, sarcomas, lung, uterine, breast, pancreatic, gastric, renal, testicular and leukemia have been reported in a multitude of XP patients.[12]

Photophobia, keratitis and ectropion in association with corneal opacities and loss of vision are common, as well as epidermoid carcinoma and malignant melanoma arising from cornea and limbus. There can also be increased pigmentation of the lids and loss of eyelashes. Atrophy of the skin of the lid may lead to ectropion and/or complete loss of the lids. Papillomas or conjunctival inflammation of the lids may occur. Epitheliomata, SCC and melanoma of the eye commonly occur.[12] Posterior portions of the eye, which are shielded by the anterior portion and thus sheltered from UV radiation, remain unaffected.

In the variant form of XP, further findings include developmental and neurological disorders. The most severe form of this subset is De Sanctis Cacchione syndrome. Characteristics include: microcephaly, degenerative mental deficiency, spastic paralysis, deafness, choreoathetosis, ataxia, Achilles tendon shortening eventually leading to quadriparesis, dwarfism, delay in bone maturation and gonadal underdevelopment.[8,12]

PATIENT EVALUATION, DIAGNOSIS AND DIFFERENTIATION

The diagnosis can be made prenatally by analysis of the amniotic cells and trophoblasts for the ability to perform base excision repair on damaged DNA.[12] Postnatally, base excision repair tests can be done on fibroblasts. In addition, analysis of reactions to UV light are conducted. Development of many skin lesions can be avoided if diagnosis is made early on. (Only the XP patients with the XP variant mutation type cannot be determined by this technique.)[8]

A presumptive initial diagnosis may be made upon finding the characteristic dry, dyspigmented skin, analysis of sun sensitivity and presence of cancerous and pre-cancerous lesions in sun-exposed areas at an early age. In order to differentiate between the specific subsets of the disease, complement studies can be conducted. Heterozygous carriers also can be identified via direct mutation analysis of a specific XP gene. This technique is also useful in XP identification for prenatal diagnosis.[5] In patients with XP variant, deep tendon reflex testing and routine audiometry can be used as a screen for the presence of neurological deficiency in association with XP.

PATHOLOGY

Generally, the pathology of a squamous cell or basal cell of an XP patient is no different from that of a sporadic patient. In the XP variant form of the disease, one can see a histological differentiation in patients who have involvement of the central nervous system in their disease. Neuronal loss or deficiency is indicated by a diminution of neural fibers in the tissue preparations.

TREATMENT

Because of the early onset and life-threatening aspects of the disease, treatment must be conducted vigorously if the patient is to survive beyond childhood. Management includes the avoidance of sun exposure and the surgical removal of cancerous and pre-cancerous skin, ocular and oral lesions as they develop.

Much of the protective measures require common sense. The effects of the disease can be cumulative. Therefore, the patient must wear protective clothing, sunglasses, sunscreens with high SPFs and partake in a lifestyle that avoids sun exposure (i.e. sitting away from windows, maintaining protection during outdoor activities, etc.). Patients with XP variant should avoid high levels of caffeine, smoking or exposure to second-hand smoke and general exposure to toxic fumes and carcinogens. Agents that are presumed to induce DNA damage within nonfunctional repair zones in XP patients include: drugs (psoralens, chlorpromazine), cancer chemo-therapeutic agents (cisplatin, carmustine) and chemical carcinogens (benzo(a)pyrene derivatives).[12]

Cancerous and precancerous lesions must be assessed in terms of multitude as well as level of malignancy. Some lesions can be removed with liquid nitrogen, 5-fluorouracil, dermatological shaving and/or curettage. The surgical procedure chosen varies depending on the number and severity of the lesions because additional lesions can occur in the same locations in the future. The margins of the actual excision should vary based on the severity of the lesion.[14] In some severe cases, tumor growth is so widespread that skin grafting may be a necessary means of treatment. Recent studies using isotretinoin, a vitamin A derivative, have shown evidence of a preventative effect against skin cancer.[15]

DYSTROPHIC EPIDERMOLYSIS BULLOSA

INTRODUCTION

Epidermolysis bullosa (EB) is a family of genetic skin disorders marked by skin fragility in which minor trauma can lead to massive blistering. The disease is divided into three categories based on the location of the tissue separation within the skin. In the simplex form, the blister forms in basal keratinocytes. In the junctional (atrophicans) form of the disease, the split occurs in the lamina lucida of the basement membrane. In dystrophic EB (the most severe group), blisters form in the sublamina densa, below the basement membrane at the level of the anchoring fibers, which are composed of type VII collagen.

Through new advances in the understanding of pathophysiology on a molecular level, there is much to hope in terms of protein and gene therapy for this genetic disease.

EPIDEMIOLOGY

Data from the National EB Registry collected between 1986–1990 estimates the total incidence of EB to be 19.6 live births per million births in the US. The estimates for dystrophic (dermolytic) EB was 4.9.[16] There is no race or cultural limitation. Onset is worldwide. The age of onset for the dominant form varies between birth and adolescence. The recessive form develops at birth or during early infancy.

Multiple dominant and recessive forms of the disease with similar clinical characteristics exist so that distinguishing between them can be a challenge. Therefore, as accuracy in the genetic typing of EB improves, the accuracy of current statistical data will be improved.

PATHOGENESIS AND ETIOLOGY

Dystrophic EB includes both autosomal dominant and recessive inherited forms. The basis for the dysfunction is a genetic mutation in the COL7A1 gene located on chromosome 3p21, which encodes for type VII collagen. This genetic mutation is associated with defects of the dermal–epidermal basement membrane region and the anchoring complexes present in the sublamina densa.

Nearly all dominant mutations are associated with a defective replacement of a glycine residue for some other amino acid. The presence of a replacement amino acid affects the stability of the type VII collagen helix, causing a reduction and thinning of the anchoring filaments. Recessive mutations have multiple causes including premature cut of the codon, missense, or inframe deletions in one or both alleles.[5]

Under electron microscopy, a cleavage of the basement membrane is visible. The extent and location of cleavage of the basement membrane vary in each form of EB. In dystrophic EB, the cleavage is located between the lamina densa and the sparse ill-formed anchoring fibrils.

Changes in the anchoring fibrils can be subtle. In the dominant forms of the disease there is a decrease of anchoring filaments whereas in the recessive form the anchoring fibrils are absent altogether.

CLINICAL FEATURES

Dominant form (DDEB)

The dominant form of EB has many variants. Characteristic features of the disease include vesicles and bullae most pronounced over areas of tension: knuckles, knees, fingers, toes, etc. Often in adolescence, spontaneous appearance of flesh-colored, scar-like lesions (albopapuloid lesions) may appear with no traumatic exposure. Healing of lesions usually occurs with scarring and atrophy. Epidermal cysts are common on extremities.

In addition, mucosal involvement includes bullae, vesicles and general erosions in the oral cavity, tongue, esophagus, pharynx and larynx. Scarring is common, creating difficulty in eating. Severe oral involvement can lead to esophageal stenoses. The teeth are usually normal. Other changes include nail dystrophy, absence of body hair, dwarfism, development of pseudosyndactyly with mitten-like hands and atrophy of phalangeal bones.

Histologically, a subepidermal bulla is present. By electron micrograph: the cleavage develops beneath the basal lamina and anchoring fibers are reduced in numbers.

Recessive form (RDEB)

There are multiple forms of RDEB ranging in severity from moderate to life threatening. Generalized RDEB forms mild blisters limited primarily to the extremities. The more severe variety begins at birth and has generalized cutaneous and mucosal blistering.

The most severe form of the recessive disorder is characterized by digital fusion forming a mitten like encasement of fingers and toes in scar tissue. This deformity occurs in approximately 90% of patients with severe RDEB by age 25.[17] In addition, dental complications include caries and microstomia. Esophageal stricture is common. Patients have difficulty with swallowing and eating. Malnutrition becomes a serious problem. Anemia and growth retardation are characteristic. Of greatest concern is the high likelihood of squamous cell carcinomas developing in scarred areas which can metastasize (Fig. 29.3). Death usually occurs within the first three decades of life.[18]

PATIENT EVALUATION, DIAGNOSIS AND DIFFERENTIATION

During clinical examination, there may be confusion in the differentiation between dominant and recessive forms, particularly in the first days of life. Therefore, it is beneficial to obtain a biopsy for electron microscopy to gain a more definitive classification. Patient and family history can be helpful, especially if there is evidence of a familial dominant variety.

On skin biopsy, histopathology may not be able to differentiate between EB types. Electron microscopy will be able to localize and differentiate between blisters of junctional and dystrophic diseases. Electron microcopy can also show anchoring fibril defects. Another method, immunohistochemical mapping, may show the presence or absence of specific basement membrane components and the level of cleavage. Genetic studies are also used but can be expensive. PCR amplification of exons from genomic DNA, followed by heteroduplex analysis are used.[5] Prenatal diagnosis can be provided via a chorionic villus sampling as early as 8–10 weeks into a pregnancy or by amniocentesis in the second trimester.[16]

TREATMENT

Treatment of EB is supportive. Avoidance of trauma, treatment of infections and nutritional well-being are all essential components of health preservation. Minimizing trauma may include protective foam pads, various non-adhesive dressings and the avoidance of high trauma risk activities.

Avoidance of wound infections also is important to avoid sepsis, as well as possible mortality. Both topical and systemic antibiotics are used, but topical treatments should be rotated to avoid resistance and systemic antibiotics should not be used for long periods of time.[19]

EB can cause esophageal erosions, leading to chewing and swallowing difficulties with esophageal strictures, as well as mineral/nutrient deficiencies and malnutrition. Daily multivitamins, zinc supplements and other forms of maintenance of nutritional balance are essential to compensate for these deficiencies and to encourage growth and faster healing of skin lesions. Iron supplementation and erythropoietin are also suggested when anemia occurs.

For more severe EB, surgical treatment to release the fused digits is a therapeutic option. However, the therapy may require periodic repetition.[16] Studies have now begun to consider skin grafts, including split thickness skin grafts, allogeneic and autogeneic cultured

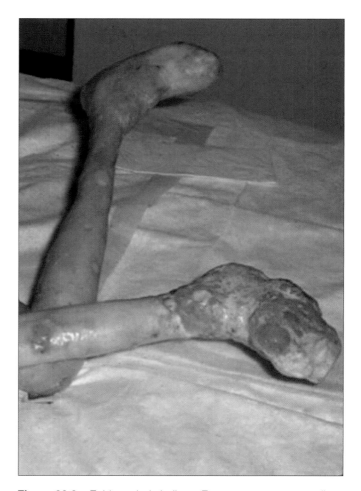

Figure 29.3 Epidermolysis bullosa. Enormous squamous cell carcinoma in patient with RDEB. Patient went on to die of metastasis. (Image courtesy of Mount Sinai Slide Collection.)

keratinocytes and cryopreserved acellular human dermis, to treat the actual lesions as a more proactive form of care.[19]

FUTURE OUTLOOK

The diseases discussed in this chapter serve to provide examples of genetic disorders predisposing to cutaneous malignancies, their clinical manifestations, diagnosis and possible methods of treatment. These patients need to be carefully monitored and early diagnosis is crucial. Though these disorders are uncommon, their clinical manifestations can be clear markers for illness, even before any chromosomal or genetic testing is conducted. Diagnosis provides an impetus for initiating prophylaxis and supportive treatment in all three diseases mentioned. Genetic disorders progressing to malignancy may be deadly.

Individuals at high genetic risk should be conscious of their predetermined risk and be wary of any environmental agonists that could exacerbate the disease. In addition, as a cure has not been found for these genetic diseases, all attempts should be made to minimize painful clinical symptoms and prevent progression of any disease.

At this time, in each of the genetic diseases/syndromes described above, treatment mainly is directed towards the symptoms of the diseases rather than the diseases themselves. In the future, a deeper understanding of the genetic and molecular bases for these disorders may lead to more effective prophylaxis and therapy.

REFERENCES

1 Kemft W, Burg G. Tumors of the epidermis. In: Burg G, ed. Atlas of Cancer of the Skin. New York: Churchill Livingstone; 2000:4–20.

2 Kim Y, Donoff RB, Wong DT, Todd R. The nucleotide: DNA sequencing and its clinical applications. J Oral Maxillofac Surg 2002; 60(8):924–930.

3 Anderson PC, Malaker KS. Managing Skin Diseases. Philadelphia: Williams and Williams; 1999.

4 Burgdorf W. Cancer Associated Genodermatoses. In: Burg G, ed. Atlas of Cancer of the Skin. New York: Churchill Livingstone; 2000:198–202.

5 Bale SJ. Genetics for Dermatologists: the Molecular Genetic Basis of Dermatological Disorders. London: ReMedica Publishing; 2000.

6 Epstein E Jr. Genetic determinants of basal cell carcinoma risk. Med Pediatr Oncol 2001; 36(5):555–558.

7 Tate G, Li M, Suzuki T, et al. A new germline mutation of the PTCH gene in a Japanese patient with nevoid basal cell carcinoma syndrome associated with meningioma. Jpn J Clin Oncol 2003; 33(1):47–50.

8 Braverman IM. Skin Signs of Systemic Disease, 3rd edn. Philadelphia, PA: WB Saunders; 1998.

9 Gorlin RJ. Living history-biography: from oral pathology to craniofacial genetics. Am J Med Genet 1993; 46(3):317–334.

10 Seracchioli R, Bagnoli A, Colombo FM, et al. Conservative treatment of recurrent ovarian fibromas in a young patient affected by Gorlin syndrome. Hum Reprod 2001; 16(6):1261–1263.

11 Byrd KM and Peck GL. Nevoid basal cell carcinoma. In: Lebwohl M, Heymann WR, Berth-Jones J, et al., eds. Treatment of Skin Disease: Comprehensive Therapeutic Strategies. New York: Mosby; 2002:422–425.

12 Kraemer KH. Heritable diseases with increased sensitivity to cellular injury. In: Freedberg IM, Eisen AZ, Wolff K, et al., eds. Fitzpatrick's Dermatology in General Medicine, 5th edn., Vol. 2. New York, NY: McGraw-Hill; 1999:1848–1862.

13 Johnson B Jr, Honig P. Congenital diseases (genodermatoses). In: Elder D, Elenitsas R, Jaworsky C, et al., eds. Lever's Histopathology of the Skin, 8th edn. New York: Lippincott-Raven; 1997:124.

14 Lambert WC, Gagna CE, Centurion SA, et al. Xeroderma pigmentosum. In: Lebwohl M, Heymann WR, Berth-Jones J, et al., eds. Treatment of Skin Disease: Comprehensive Therapeutic Strategies. New York: Mosby; 2002:660–664.

15 Anolik JH, Di Giovanna JJ, Gaspari AA. Effect of isotretinoin therapy on natural kill cell activity in patients with xeroderma pigmentosum. Br J Derm 1998; 138(2):236–241.

16 Marinkovich MP, Herron GS, Khavari, et al. Hereditary epidermolysis bullosa. In: Freedberg IM, Eisen AZ, Wolff K, et al., eds. Fitzpatrick's Dermatology in General Medicine, 5th edn, Vol 1. New York, NY: McGraw-Hill; 1999:690–702.

17 Odom RB. Andrews' Diseases of the Skin: Clinical Dermatology, 9th edn. Philadelphia, PA: Saunders; 2000.

18 Bauer EA, Briggaman RA. Hereditary epidermolysis bullosa. In: Fitzpatrick TB, Eisen AZ, Wolff K, et al., eds. Dermatology in General Medicine, 4th edn., Vol. 1. New York, NY: McGraw-Hill; 1993:654–669.

19 Bello YM, Falabella AF, Schachner LA. Epidermolysis bullosa. In: Lebwohl M, Heymann WR, Berth-Jones J, et al., eds. Treatment of Skin Disease: Comprehensive Therapeutic Strategies. New York: Mosby; 2002:182–184.

CHAPTER
30

Dermatologic Manifestations of Internal Malignancy

Bruce H Thiers, Jeffrey P Callen and Leander Cannick

Key points

- Internal malignancy can involve the skin either directly or indirectly.
- Direct involvement is defined as tumor metastatic to the skin.
- Indirect involvement refers to changes in the skin that suggest the possibility of an underlying malignancy.
- Patients with direct involvement should be assumed to have an underlying neoplasm and must be evaluated accordingly.
- Patients with indirect involvement may not have an underlying neoplasm when first evaluated, but must be monitored for its possible future development.

INTRODUCTION

The skin, the largest organ in the body, often mirrors changes occurring within the organism it envelops. A wide spectrum of inflammatory, proliferative, metabolic and neoplastic diseases may affect the skin in association with an underlying malignancy. This chapter will focus on these changes, known collectively as the skin signs of internal malignancy.

Internal cancer may affect the skin both directly and indirectly.[1] Direct involvement may be defined as the actual presence of malignant cells within the skin and includes neoplasms that often first become manifested in the skin, but eventually affect internal organs (such as mycosis fungoides), visceral neoplasms metastatic to the skin (such as the Sister Joseph nodule of gastric carcinoma) and tumors arising within or below the skin that ultimately spread to the cutaneous surface (such as Paget's disease of the nipple). Indirect involvement of the skin in cancer patients implies the absence of tumor cells within the skin. Inherited syndromes associated with skin manifestations and an increased incidence of systemic neoplasia are included in this group, as are cutaneous changes resulting from hormone secretion by tumors and a wide spectrum of proliferative and inflammatory disorders occurring in conjunction with internal malignancy (Table 30.1). This chapter will focus on these indirect effects.

HISTORY

In the original text *Cancer of the Skin*, Curth outlined a set of criteria that could be used to analyze the relationship between an internal malignancy and a cutaneous disorder.[2] Curth's postulates, as Callen has subsequently labeled them, consist of five characteristics: (1) a concurrent onset – the malignancy is discovered when the skin disease occurs; (2) a parallel course – if the malignancy is removed or successfully treated, the skin disease remits and when the malignancy recurs, the cutaneous disease also recurs; (3) a uniform malignancy – there is a specific tumor cell type or site associated with the skin disease; (4) a statistical association – based on sound case–control studies there is a significantly more frequent occurrence of malignancy in a patient with a cutaneous disease; and (5) a genetic association. These criteria are extremely useful and must be satisfied before a link between an internal neoplasm and a specific skin change can be assumed.

DESCRIPTION

Inherited syndromes associated with internal malignancy

Cowden's disease (multiple hamartoma syndrome) occurs more often in women than in men. The disorder, which is inherited as an autosomal dominant trait, displays a variety of cutaneous and mucosal manifestations that can occur at any time from childhood to middle age.[3] Small (1–4 mm) flesh-colored papules are found mainly on the head and neck and may assume a wart-like appearance (Fig. 30.1); the lesions are characterized histologically as trichilemmomas. Similar papules may coalesce and produce a cobblestone appearance on the gums. Flat wart-like papules have been noted on the dorsum of the hands and feet and keratosis punctata may be present on the soles, sides of the feet and palms. Lipomas and hemangiomas may also be found.

Internal manifestations are variable. Almost all affected women have fibrocystic disease of the breasts; many of them ultimately develop breast cancer, often bilaterally. Thyroid tumors, both benign and malignant, are frequent (75%). Cancers of the lung and colon have also been

Table 30.1 Cutaneous manifestations of internal malignancy
Inherited syndromes   • Cowden's disease (multiple hamartoma syndrome)   • Gardner's syndrome   • Peutz–Jegher's syndrome   • Cronkhite–Canada syndrome   • Muir–Torre syndrome   • Howel–Evans syndrome (tylosis)   • Birt–Hogg–Dubé syndrome   • Multiple leiomyomas syndrome   • Multiple mucosal neuromas syndrome   • Von Recklinghausen's disease (type 1 neurofibromatosis)   • Immunodeficiency syndromes
Hormone-secreting tumors   • Ectopic ACTH syndrome   • Carcinoid syndrome   • Glucagonoma syndrome
Proliferative and inflammatory dermatoses   • Hypertrichosis lanuginosa   • Acanthosis nigricans   • Leser–Trelat sign   • Skin tags   • Bazex syndrome   • Punctate palmar keratoses   • Bowen's disease   • Primary amyloidosis   • Scleromyxedema   • Kaposi's sarcoma   • Sweet's syndrome   • Pyoderma gangrenosum   • Blistering diseases   • Dermatomyositis   • Digital clubbing   • Vasculitis   • Coagulopathies   • Figurate erythemas   • Eczematous and ichthyotic disorders   • Infectious disorders

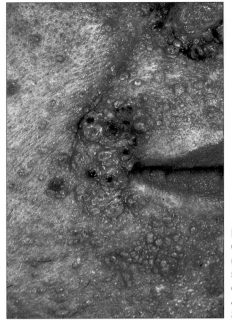

Figure 30.1
Cowden's disease (multiple hamartoma syndrome) (Image courtesy of Dr Joseph Bikowski, Sewickley, PA.)

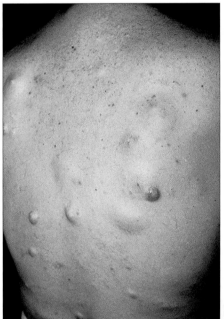

Figure 30.2
Gardner's syndrome.

reported. Hamartomatous polyps of the gastrointestinal tract occur in one-third of patients and are generally benign. The significance of Cowden's disease lies in its value as a marker for the eventual development of thyroid or breast disease. A mutation in the PTEN tumor suppressor gene is thought to play a role in the susceptibility to cancer in this condition.[4,5]

Extensive polyps of the gastrointestinal tract, especially the colon and rectum, also occur in *Gardner's syndrome*, another autosomal dominant disorder.[6] In Gardner's syndrome, however, the polyps are adenomatous and thus the potential for malignant degeneration is high (approaching 100%); therefore, prophylactic colectomy may be indicated for patients demonstrating multiple polyps on radiologic examination. Skin lesions include large, deforming epidermoid cysts (Fig. 30.2), fibromas, lipomas, leiomyomas, trichoepitheliomas and neurofibromas. Osteomas involving the membranous bones of the face and head occur in about 50% of affected patients.[7] Congenital hypertrophy of the retinal pigment epithelium has also been associated with Gardner's syndrome.[8]

Peutz–Jegher's syndrome is characterized by extensive hamartomatous polyps throughout the gastrointestinal tract. This syndrome is also inherited in an autosomal dominant manner. Bleeding and abdominal pain caused by intussusception are the most common gastrointestinal manifestations.[9] The incidence of malignant change in these polyps is controversial but is certainly much less than in Gardner's syndrome.[10] In addition, breast and gynecologic cancers may be found more frequently in Peutz–Jeghers syndrome and in patients with sporadically occurring Peutz–Jeghers-like mucocutaneous pigmentation than in the general population.[11–13] This characteristic feature of the condition appears as freckle-like pigmented macules on the lips (Fig. 30.3), nose, buccal mucosa, fingertips and under the nails.

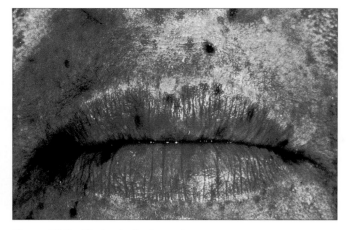

Figure 30.3 Peutz–Jegher's syndrome.

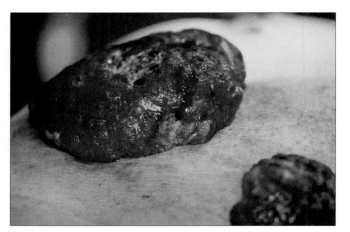

Figure 30.4 Muir–Torre syndrome.

Cutaneous and, rarely, mucosal hyperpigmentation may also occur in the *Cronkhite–Canada syndrome*; other cutaneous features include onychodystrophy and alopecia.[14] Hamartomatous polyps occur throughout the stomach and intestines and the incidence of gastrointestinal cancer is approximately 15%. The disease does not appear to be heritable.

In the *Muir–Torre syndrome* (also known as *Torre syndrome*), multiple carcinomas, usually of the gastrointestinal tract, are associated with numerous sebaceous gland tumors (both benign and malignant), primarily on the trunk (Fig. 30.4);[15] other visceral cancers and keratoacanthomas have also been reported.[16] In contrast, solitary sebaceous gland tumors are not genetically determined, occur most often on the head and neck and are not associated with visceral malignancy. The diagnosis of gastrointestinal cancer usually precedes the recognition of the cutaneous lesions. The cutaneous tumors do not behave in an aggressive manner even if histologically malignant. Similarly, the gastrointestinal cancers often behave as low-grade malignancies. Muir–Torre syndrome appears to be inherited as an autosomal dominant trait.

An association between diffuse palmoplantar hyperkeratosis (tylosis) and esophageal cancer (*Howel–Evans syndrome*) has been noted in two English families. The keratoderma usually develops during childhood and is accentuated over pressure sites. Onset of the esophageal carcinoma is delayed until middle age. A genetic locus on chromosome 17q25 that appears to be associated with this syndrome is frequently deleted in sporadic esophageal squamous cell carcinoma as well.[17]

Two syndromes with skin manifestations and an apparent predisposition to renal cancer have been described.[18] The *Birt–Hogg–Dubé syndrome* is an autosomal dominant condition characterized by skin tags and benign hair follicle tumors (fibrofolliculomas and trichodiscomas) of the head and neck (Fig. 30.5).[19] The incidence of spontaneous pneumothorax as well as chromophobe renal carcinoma, an uncommon type of renal cancer, is increased, although a proposed association with colon cancer has not been confirmed.[20] Multiple cutaneous leiomyomas may also be inherited and are associated with uterine leiomyomas as well as papillary renal cell carcinoma.[21]

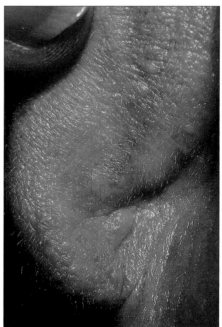

Figure 30.5
Birt–Hogg–Dubé syndrome. (Image courtesy of Dr Maria Turner, Bethesda, MD.)

Patients with the rare autosomal dominant disorder *multiple mucosal neuromas syndrome* display a constellation of abnormalities, including medullary carcinoma of the thyroid, pheochromocytoma, parathyroid hyperplasia or adenomas and intestinal ganglioneuromatosis; the latter may give rise to persistent diarrhea.[22] Multiple neuromas appear as whitish nodules mainly on the lips and anterior one third of the tongue (Fig. 30.6) but also may be noted on the buccal mucosa, gingivae, palate, pharynx, conjunctivae and cornea. Affected individuals have characteristic facies, with thick, protuberant, bumpy lips; the eyelids may be thickened and slightly everted. Many patients have a 'marfanoid' habitus with long, slender extremities, poor muscle development, sparse body fat, laxity of joints, pectus excavatum and dorsal kyphosis. Although multiple mucosal neuromas syndrome is classified as one of the three familial syndromes of multiple endocrine neoplasia (see below), many sporadic cases have been reported.

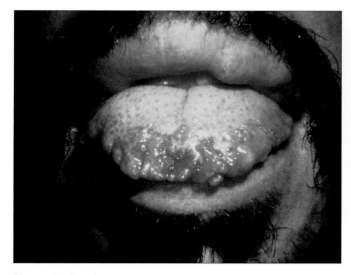

Figure 30.6 Multiple mucosal neuromas syndrome.

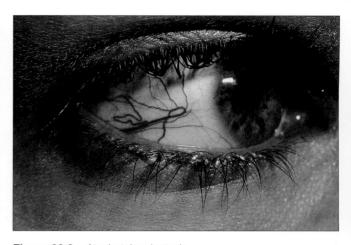

Figure 30.8 Ataxia-telangiectasia.

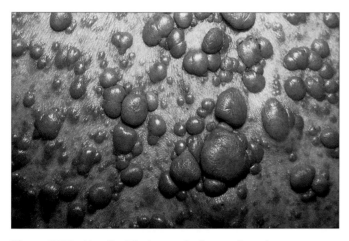

Figure 30.7 Von Recklinghausen's disease (type 1 neurofibromatosis).

In *type 1 neurofibromatosis (von Recklinghausen's disease)* (Fig. 30.7), multiple Schwann cell tumors, malignant degeneration of neurofibromas and pheochromocytomas (often bilateral) may complicate the clinical course. Gastrointestinal stromal tumors have also been reported.[23] The salient features of this disorder have received extensive review in the recent medical literature.[24,25] It, like multiple mucosal neuromas syndrome, may be classified among the APUDomas (see below).

Internal malignancy can occur in patients with inherited immunodeficiency disorders, including *ataxia-telangiectasia* (Fig. 30.8) and the *Wiskott–Aldrich syndrome*.[26] Most tumors are of lymphoreticular origin and may be associated with Epstein–Barr virus infection.[27]

Skin changes resulting from hormone-secreting tumors

Ectopic humoral syndromes are best understood in context of the APUD cell system (i.e. cells with a capacity for *A*mino *P*recursor *U*ptake and *D*ecarboxylation).[28,29] These cells, which may have a common origin from the neural crest, can secrete a variety of biologically active amines and polypeptide hormones. Neoplastic proliferation of these cells may result in characteristic symptom complexes associated with specific cutaneous changes.

Ectopic ACTH-producing tumors cause many of the typical signs and symptoms of Cushing's syndrome. Intense hyperpigmentation (Fig. 30.9), present in only 6 to 10% of patients with Cushing's disease, is especially common in association with ectopic ACTH production and should alert the clinician to the possibility of a hormone-secreting tumor.[30] Although the cause of the hyperpigmentation is unclear, it may be related to tumor production of the peptide beta-lipotropin, which contains within its sequence of 91 amino acids the 22 amino acid sequence of beta-MSH. A myasthenia gravis-like syndrome including profound proximal muscle weakness may be a striking clinical feature and may reflect either underlying hypokalemia or polymyositis. Oat cell carcinoma of the lung is the tumor most often associated with ectopic ACTH production, although other malignancies have been reported.

The *carcinoid syndrome* is a second example of a humoral syndrome associated with a non-endocrine tumor.[31] The disorder is probably most often caused by the release of the enzyme kallikrein from tumor cells with subsequent conversion of kininogen to vasoactive kinin peptides, including bradykinin; in addition, increased blood levels of histamine may be important in the rare metastatic gastric carcinoid. The most striking cutaneous manifestations are episodes of flushing, initially lasting 10 to 30 min and involving only the upper half of the body; as the flush resolves, gyrate and serpiginous patterns may be noted. With successive attacks more extensive areas may be affected and the redness takes on a cyanotic quality, eventually leading to a more permanent facial cyanotic flush with associated telangiectasia, resembling rosacea (Fig. 30.10). Persistent edema and erythema of the face may result in leonine facies. A pellagra-like picture, as has been noted in some patients, may be due to abnormal tryptophan metabolism. Systemic symptoms associated with cutaneous flushing include abdominal pain with explosive watery diarrhea, shortness of breath and hypertension.

Carcinoid tumors are usually found in the appendix or small intestine; extraintestinal carcinoids may arise in the bile ducts, pancreas, stomach, ovaries, or bronchi. The carcinoid syndrome occurs primarily with intestinal carcinoids metastatic to the liver or with extraintestinal tumors; flushing attacks can be provoked by palpation of hepatic or abdominal metastases or by alcohol ingestion, enemas, emotional stress, or sudden changes in body temperature. When the syndrome is associated with bronchial adenomas of the carcinoid variety, the flushing is more prolonged and often associated with fever, marked anxiety, disorientation, sweating, salivation and lacrimation.

The three clinical patterns of familial *multiple endocrine neoplasia* (MEN types 1,2 and 3) are examples of polyglandular endocrine disorders involving the APUD cell system. A carcinoid-like syndrome has been described in MEN 2 (Sipple's syndrome);[32] otherwise, mucocutaneous lesions occur only in MEN 3 (multiple mucosal neuromas syndrome), which has already been discussed.

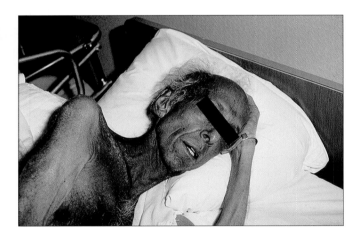

Figure 30.9 Ectopic ACTH syndrome. (Image courtesy of Dr Donald Lookingbill, Jacksonville, FL.)

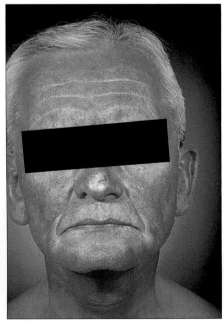

Figure 30.10 Carcinoid syndrome. (Image courtesy of Dr Walter Lobitz, Portland, OR.)

The *glucagonoma syndrome* is associated with an APUDoma involving the glucagon-secreting alpha cell of the pancreas.[33] The characteristic cutaneous eruption, necrolytic migratory erythema, usually occurs on the abdomen, perineum, thighs, buttocks and groin. The perioral region and the distal extremities are often affected. Patches of intense erythema with irregular outlines expand and coalesce resulting in circinate or polycyclic configurations (Fig. 30.11). Superficial vesicles on the surface rupture quickly to form crusts, but new vesicles may continue to develop along the active margins. An eczema craquelé-like appearance may be noted. Pressure or trauma may initiate or aggravate the eruption, which seems to share features of staphylococcal scalded skin syndrome and acrodermatitis enteropathica. Like the latter disorder, necrolytic migratory erythema sometimes responds to diiodohydroxyquin; however, zinc levels are normal and zinc treatment is ineffective. Complete surgical resection is the only curative treatment for the tumor, as chemotherapy yields only modest benefit.[34]

Neurofibromatosis, discussed earlier, may be classified as an APUDoma. Malignant melanoma is a non-hormone-secreting APUDoma. Patients with widespread metastases can develop diffuse gray to blue-black hyperpigmentation of the skin and mucous membranes.

Proliferative and inflammatory dermatoses associated with cancer

Many of the conditions discussed in this section are nonspecific and have been reported both in association with and in the absence of underlying malignant disease. Malignancy is most often only one of a number of possible provoking factors.

The association of acquired *hypertrichosis lanuginosa* (malignant down) with cancer is among the most

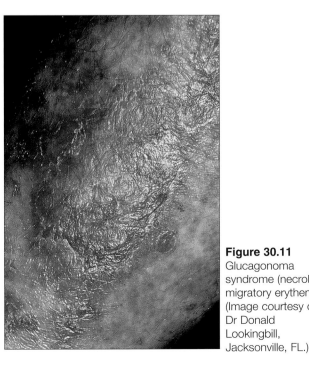

Figure 30.11 Glucagonoma syndrome (necrolytic migratory erythema). (Image courtesy of Dr Donald Lookingbill, Jacksonville, FL.)

consistent.[35] The extensive growth of silky, nonpigmented lanugo hair on the face, neck, trunk and sometimes the extremities may antedate discovery of the malignancy, which usually involves the gastrointestinal tract (Fig. 30.12). Other causes of hypertrichosis, such as porphyria cutanea tarda and endocrinopathies, must be ruled out. A painful glossitis and swollen red fungiform papillae on the anterior half of the tongue may accompany the cutaneous changes.

Acanthosis nigricans is perhaps the best known of the cutaneous markers of internal malignancy.[36] Flexural areas, especially the axillae, groin and neck, are most often involved; the skin has a hyperpigmented velvety appearance and in severe cases can become quite verrucous (Fig. 30.13). Papillomatous changes may be noted in the oral cavity and hyperkeratosis in a rugose pattern may develop on the palms and dorsal surfaces of large joints.[37,38] The cutaneous changes can occur before, coincident with, or after the discovery of the underlying malignancy, which most often is an adenocarcinoma, commonly of the stomach, but almost always in the abdominal cavity. Because acanthosis nigricans can also occur in association with a variety of benign conditions, e.g. as a familial lesion, at puberty, or in association with endocrine disease and obesity, a detailed history must

be included in the evaluation of all affected patients.[39,40] The possibility of underlying cancer should be strongly considered in any non-obese adult who develops acanthosis nigricans in the absence of a recognizable endocrinopathy. This individual should have an extensive gastrointestinal evaluation.

The *sign of Leser–Trelat*, the sudden appearance and/or rapid increase in size of multiple seborrheic keratoses (Fig. 30.14), may be associated with carcinoma of the gastrointestinal tract or female reproductive system.[41] Because most of these patients have coexistent acanthosis nigricans and the malignancy is often an adenocarcinoma of gastrointestinal origin, some clinicians believe that this condition may represent a generalized variant of acanthosis nigricans.

A relationship between *skin tags*, colonic polyps and internal malignancy has been suggested but never proven.[42] Skin tags are commonly seen by dermatologists in otherwise healthy patients. Although the purported association is of interest, proof awaits a prospective evaluation of adults with skin tags.

Patients with *Bazex syndrome (acrokeratosis paraneoplastica)* develop a psoriasiform eruption primarily on the face and extremities (Fig. 30.15).[43,44] The ears, nose, cheeks, hands, feet and knees are most often affected; the nails are dystrophic and the palms are hyperkeratotic. The disorder is associated with carcinomas of the upper respiratory and digestive tracts (larynx, pharynx, trachea, bronchus and/or upper esophagus).

The significance of *punctate palmar keratoses* as a sign of internal malignancy is controversial,[45] although they have been reported in Cowden's syndrome. Similarly, the purported relationship between Bowen's disease (intraepidermal squamous cell carcinoma) and systemic cancer has been disputed.[46]

Patients with *primary systemic amyloidosis* almost always have an underlying plasma cell dyscrasia, usually

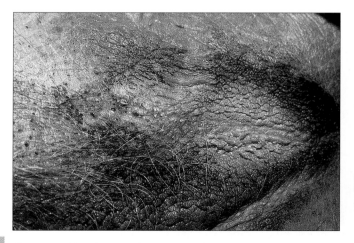

Figure 30.12 Acquired hypertrichosis lanuginosa.

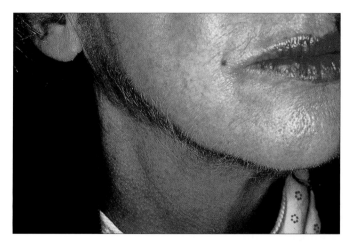

Figure 30.13 Acanthosis nigricans. (Image courtesy of Dr Frederic Stearns, Tulsa, OK.)

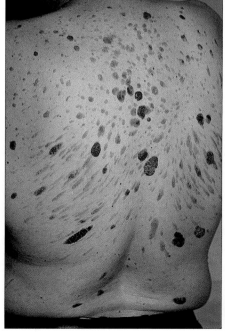

Figure 30.14 Leser–Trelat sign.

multiple myeloma.[47] The skin takes on a generalized waxy appearance and bleeds easily when traumatized ('pinch purpura') (Fig. 30.16). Hemorrhagic lesions are especially common around the eyes. Macroglossia is an associated finding (Fig. 30.17). Skin lesions are not seen in secondary amyloidosis.

Scleromyxedema, a cutaneous mucinosis representing the generalized variant of *lichen myxedematosus*, has been associated with a peculiar serum monoclonal paraprotein.[48–50] The paraprotein is a basic, electrophoretically homogenous 7S gamma globulin, usually of the IgG class, that almost always possesses light chains of the lambda type. Clinically, the disorder appears as a generalized eruption of 2–3-mm waxy lichenoid papules, often in a linear arrangement (Fig. 30.18); lesions are most common on the hands, elbows, forearms, upper trunk, face and neck but may be found anywhere. Induration of the underlying tissue may produce a resemblance to scleroderma; mucin deposition in forehead skin may be disfiguring and lead to longitudinal furrowing

somewhat reminiscent of leonine facies. No correlation appears to exist between levels of the paraprotein and the extent or progression of the skin disease. Indeed, the serum monoclonal paraprotein is an inconsistent finding and only a minority of patients have overt myeloma or a detectable plasma cell dyscrasia. Thus, the role of plasma cells or the paraprotein in the pathogenesis of scleromyxedema remains unclear. Nevertheless, affected patients should have a serum protein electrophoresis, immunoelectrophoresis and measurement of immunoglobulin levels; these tests should be repeated every six months.

The well-documented association of *Kaposi's sarcoma* (Fig. 30.19) with states of altered immunity, such as the acquired immunodeficiency syndrome (AIDS)[51,52] or pharmacologic immunosuppression necessitated by renal transplantation,[53] may explain the increased incidence of lymphoreticular neoplasms in patients with that disorder. Infection with human herpesvirus-8 (HHV-8) appears to be the unifying provoking factor.[54] The most commonly

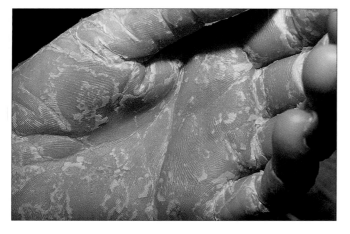

Figure 30.15 Bazex syndrome. (Image courtesy of Dr Joseph Bikowski, Sewickley, PA.)

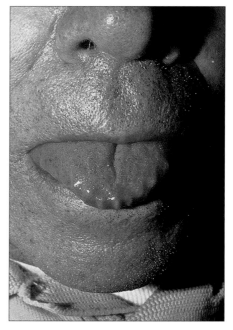

Figure 30.17 Primary amyloidosis.

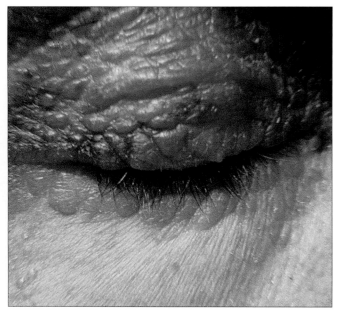

Figure 30.16 Primary amyloidosis.

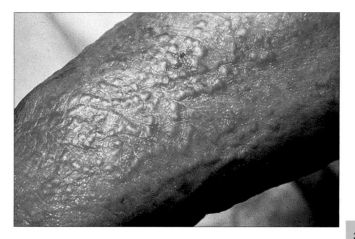

Figure 30.18 Lichen myxedematosus (scleromyxedema).

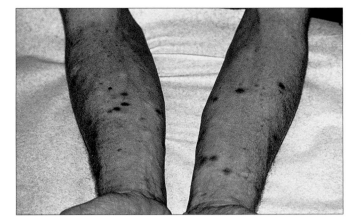

Figure 30.19   Kaposi's sarcoma.

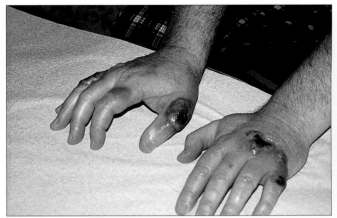

Figure 30.20   Sweet's syndrome.

reported lymphoproliferative disorders have been Hodgkin's disease and non-Hodgkin's lymphoma, but multiple myeloma, hairy cell leukemia and angioimmuno-blastic lymphadenopathy have also occurred. Nevertheless, unless dictated by findings on physical examination or routine screening laboratory tests, an exhaustive workup for myeloproliferative disease is unnecessary in patients with Kaposi's sarcoma.

Sweet's syndrome (acute febrile neutrophilic dermatosis) may occasionally be associated with leukemia, particularly the acute myeloid or myelomonocytic varieties.[55,56] Red, tender, sometimes vesicular or pustular papules, plaques, or nodules appear suddenly on the face, extremities and upper trunk (Fig. 30.20). Fever, malaise and neutrophilia accompany the cutaneous eruption, which histologically shows a dense dermal neutrophilic infiltrate. The presence of moderate to severe anemia may be helpful in distinguishing Sweet's syndrome associated with myeloproliferative disease from the idiopathic variant. Patients with Sweet's syndrome and anemia should have a bone marrow biopsy as part of their overall systemic evaluation.

Pyoderma gangrenosum is a neutrophilic ulcerative dermatosis. Its superficial form, known as atypical or bullous pyoderma gangrenosum, often occurs on the head and neck and has been associated with hematologic malignancy (Fig. 30.21).[57] Most often the association is with acute myelogenous leukemia, but several cases of chronic myelogenous leukemia, acute lymphoblastic leukemia and preleukemic states such as myelofibrosis or agnogenic myeloid metaplasia have also been reported. The skin and blood disease often present concurrently and run a parallel course. There has been some suggestion that pyoderma gangrenosum may be related to Sweet's syndrome. As with Sweet's syndrome, affected patients should have a careful hematologic evaluation including a bone marrow biopsy when indicated.

In addition to its more familiar nonneoplastic associations, classic pyoderma gangrenosum (Fig. 30.22) has been associated with a monoclonal gammopathy (and, occasionally, myeloma), with several solid tumors and with non-Hodgkin's lymphoma. The gammopathy, which has been noted in up to 20% of patients with pyoderma gangrenosum, results from an IgA paraprotein. However, in patients with coexistent pyoderma gangrenosum and

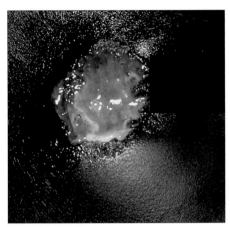

Figure 30.21
Pyoderma
gangrenosum.

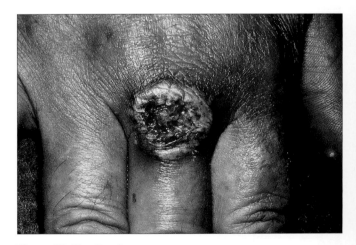

Figure 30.22   Pyoderma gangrenosum.

IgA paraproteinemia or myeloma, there is no information to suggest a parallel course.

Blistering diseases have been reported in patients with cancer. Various forms of pemphigus have been associated with thymoma. The occurrence of paraneoplastic pemphigus in patients with cancer, especially lymphoreticular malignancy, is well documented.[58–60] The proposed association of bullous pemphigoid with malignancy probably reflects the tendency of both of these conditions to occur in the elderly rather than any true association. An increased incidence of malignancy has also been reported in the anti-epiligrin variant of cicatricial pemphigoid (Fig. 30.23).[61] Individuals with dermatitis herpetiformis may have an increased relative risk of intestinal lymphoma similar to that noted in patients with celiac disease sprue.[62] Epidermolysis bullosa acquisita has also very rarely been reported in patients with lymphoreticular tumors.

Approximately 10 to 30% of adult patients with *dermatomyositis* have an associated malignancy.[63,64] The neoplasm may occur before, during, or after the diagnosis of dermatomyositis. An awareness of this potential should alert the physician to carefully evaluate all dermatomyositis patients for malignancy. Pathognomonic clinical manifestations include an edematous, violaceous eruption of the upper eyelids (heliotrope rash) (Fig. 30.24) and atrophic scaly papules over bony prominences (Gottron's papules) (Fig. 30.25); photosensitivity, malar erythema, poikiloderma and periungual telangiectasias are important, although less specific, findings. Dermatomyositis is not specific for any particular site or cell type of cancer; however, in Western countries, ovarian and breast carcinoma in women and lung and prostate carcinoma in men are especially frequent. The risk of developing cancer is highest the first 2 years after the diagnosis of dermatomyositis.[65] Raynaud's phenomenon or sclerodermatous changes in an adult with dermatomyositis suggests an overlap syndrome; this variant is rarely associated with malignant disease. Childhood dermatomyositis is not associated with malignancy.

A number of musculoskeletal disorders have been reported in patients with cancer. Clubbing is noted in about 10% of individuals with lung cancer and tumors metastatic to the lung (Fig. 30.26).[66] Subperiosteal new bone formation in patients with clubbing (hypertrophic osteoarthropathy) occurs most commonly along the shaft of the phalanges but may affect other bones as well.[67] Joint swelling, synovitis, periarticular swelling, hyperhidrosis and palmar erythema may be pronounced and create a picture similar to early rheumatoid arthritis. Hypertrophic osteoarthropathy associated with acromegaloid features (pachydermoperiostosis) can occur either in association with lung cancer or as a genetic disease unassociated with malignancy.

Polyarthritis simulating rheumatoid arthritis (in the absence of hypertrophic osteoarthropathy), tenosynovitis and fibrositis have also been reported in association with cancer. The predisposition of rheumatoid arthritis patients to lymphoma is well known.[68]

A purported association between *cutaneous leukocytoclastic vasculitis* and cancer has never been proven, although numerous individual case reports have related various vasculitic syndromes to malignancy, including solid tumors and lymphoproliferative disorders. Interestingly, both cutaneous leukocytoclastic vasculitis and systemic necrotizing vasculitis have been observed in patients with hairy cell leukemia (leukemic reticuloendotheliosis). Often, the patient with coexistent neoplastic disease has the malignancy at the time of diagnosis of the vasculitis. In other cases, release of tumor antigens into the circulation, such as after radiation therapy or chemotherapy, may be the inciting event. A parallel course between the tumor and the vasculitis has not been evident except in a few instances.

Internal malignancy, especially lymphoproliferative disease, may be heralded by a number of disorders that probably represent variants of *disseminated intravascular coagulation*.[69] In purpura fulminans, thrombosis and hemorrhage occur simultaneously (Fig. 30.27); purpura

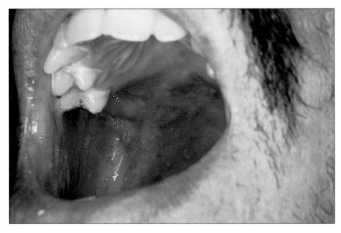

Figure 30.23 Anti-epiligrin bullous pemphigoid. (Image courtesy of Dr Kim Yancey, Milwaukee, WI.)

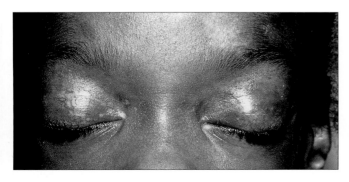

Figure 30.24 Dermatomyositis.

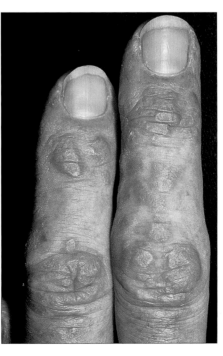

Figure 30.25 Dermatomyositis. (Image courtesy of Dr William James, Philadelphia, PA.)

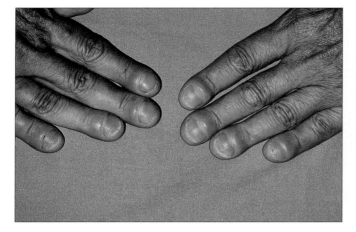

Figure 30.26 Digital clubbing.

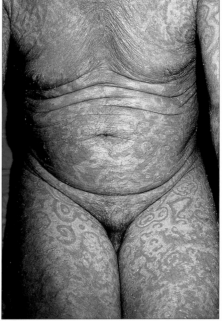

Figure 30.28
Erythema gyratum
repens. (Image
courtesy of
Dr Donald
Lookingbill,
Jacksonville, FL.)

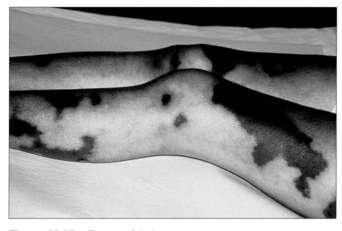

Figure 30.27 Purpura fulminans.

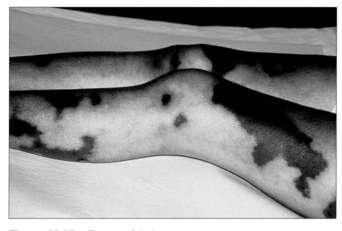

Figure 30.29
Acquired ichthyosis.

fulminans in adults with malignancy usually runs a chronic, less fulminant course than the post-infectious disorder of the same name, although digital gangrene has been reported. A defibrination syndrome, characterized by easy bruising, purpura and a bleeding diathesis, may also be a feature of internal malignancy.

Migratory superficial thrombophlebitis and *multiple deep venous thromboses* have been noted in cancer patients, especially those with tumors arising in the pancreas, lung, stomach, prostate or hematopoietic system.[70] The neck, chest, abdominal wall, pelvis and limbs are most frequently affected.

The *figurate erythemas* may be divided into at least three groups. Erythema chronicum migrans follows a tick bite and may be associated with Lyme disease. Erythema annulare centrifugum may be secondary to a variety of causative factors including, rarely, malignancy. Erythema gyratum repens (Fig. 30.28) is almost always associated with cancer,[71] although no one tumor type or site seems to predominate. Multiple wavy urticarial bands with a fine scale migrate over the cutaneous surface, giving it an appearance similar to the grain of wood. The eruption usually occurs within a few months before or after the diagnosis of cancer.

Urticaria is very rarely a manifestation of internal malignancy. *Erythema multiforme*, also an uncommon

sign of visceral cancer, occurs most often after deep X-ray therapy, presumably as a hypersensitivity response to tumor antigens released from necrotic tumor tissue.

Generalized pruritus, ichthyosis and *exfoliative dermatitis* are seen as non-specific features of lymphoproliferative disorders (Fig. 30.29);[72] uncommonly, they may be associated with solid tumors. *Pityriasis rotunda* may be a variant of acquired ichthyosis; the eruption consists of geometrically perfect, circular patches of scales. The disease was first reported in the Japanese, South African blacks and West Indian blacks, in whom an associated neoplasm was occasionally described.[35] A familial variant has been recognized in Europe that does not appear to be associated with cancer.[73] Although the exact status of pityriasis rotunda as a paraneoplastic

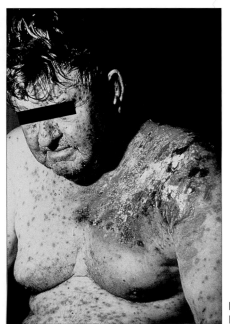

Figure 30.30
Disseminated zoster.

condition remains to be delineated, it seems prudent to rule out concurrent malignancy in affected patients.

Infectious disorders are frequent in cancer patients and may either be directly related to depressed cell-mediated immunity associated with the neoplasm or secondary to pharmacologic immunosuppression. The increased incidence of herpes zoster (Fig. 30.30), either localized or disseminated, in patients with leukemia and lymphoma has been appreciated for years, although such infection usually develops during the course of the illness rather than as a presenting sign.[74] Rarely, herpes zoster may be associated with an underlying carcinoma.

FUTURE OUTLOOK

The dermatologist can play an integral role in cancer diagnosis by recognizing cutaneous manifestations of internal malignancy. The better recognition of these signs may lead to enhanced future diagnosis.

REFERENCES

1 Thiers BH. Dermatologic manifestations of internal cancer. CA Cancer J Clin 1986; 36(3):130–148.

2 Curth HO. Skin lesions and internal carcinoma. In: Andrade R, Gumport SL and Popkin GL, eds. Cancer of the Skin. Philadelphia, PA: WB Saunders; 1976:1308–1309.

3 Hildenbrand C, Burgdorf WH, Lautenschlager S. Cowden syndrome – diagnostic skin signs (Review). Dermatology 2001; 202(4):362–366.

4 Waite KA, Eng C. Protean PTEN: form and function (Review). Am J Hum Genet 2002; 70(4):829–844.

5 Zhou XP, Hampel H, Roggenbuck J, Saba N, Prior TW, Eng C. A 39-bp deletion polymorphism in PTEN in African American individuals: implications for molecular diagnostic testing. J Mol Diagn 2002; 4(2):114–117.

6 Parks ET, Caldemeyer KS, Mirowski GW. Gardner syndrome. J Am Acad Derm 2001; 45(6):940–942.

7 Sayan NB, Ucok C, Karasu HA, Gunhan O. Peripheral osteoma of the oral and maxillofacial region: a study of 35 new cases. J Oral Maxillofac Surg 2002; 60(11):1299–1301.

8 Parks ET, Caldemeyer KS, Mirowski GW. Gardner syndrome. J Am Acad Derm 2001; 45(6):940–942.

9 Marschall J, Hayes P. Intussusceptions in a man with Peutz–Jeghers syndrome. CMAJ 2003; 168(3):315–316.

10 Boardman LA. Heritable colorectal cancer syndromes: recognition and preventive management. Gastroenterol Clin North Am 2002; 31(4):1107–1131.

11 Boardman LA, Pittelkow MR, Couch FJ, et al. Association of Peutz–Jeghers-like mucocutaneous pigmentation with breast and gynecologic carcinomas in women. Medicine (Baltimore) 2000; 79(5):293–298.

12 Boardman LA, Thibodeau SN, Schaid DJ, et al. Increased risk for cancer in patients with the Peutz–Jeghers syndrome. Ann Intern Med 1998; 128(11):896–899.

13 Papageorgiou T, Stratakis CA. Ovarian tumors associated with multiple endocrine neoplasias and related syndromes (Carney complex, Peutz–Jeghers syndrome, von Hippel–Lindau disease, Cowden's disease). Int J Gynecol Cancer 2002; 12(4):337–347.

14 Ward EM, Wolfsen HC. Review article: the non-inherited gastrointestinal polyposis syndromes. Aliment Pharm Ther 2002; 16(3):333–342.

15 Alessi E, Brambilla L, Luporini G, Mosca L, Bevilacqua G. Multiple sebaceous tumors and carcinomas of the colon. Torre syndrome. Cancer 1985; 55(11):2566–2574.

16 Southey MC, Young MA, Whitty J, et al. Molecular pathologic analysis enhances the diagnosis and management of Muir–Torre syndrome and gives insight into its underlying molecular pathogenesis. Am J Surg Pathol 2001; 25(7):936–941.

17 Risk JM, Evans KE, Jones J, et al. Characterization of a 500 kb region on 17q25 and the exclusion of candidate genes as the familial Tylosis Oesophageal Cancer (TOC) locus. Oncogene 2002; 21(41):6395–6402.

18 Choyke PL, Glenn GM, Walther MM, Zbar B, Linehan WM. Hereditary renal cancers. Radiology 2003; 226(1):33–46.

19 Collins GL, Somach S, Morgan MB. Histomorphologic and immuno-phenotypic analysis of fibrofolliculomas and trichodiscomas in Birt–Hogg–Dubé syndrome and sporadic disease. J Cutan Pathol 2002; 29(9):529–533.

20 Zbar B, Alvord WG, Glenn G, et al. Risk of renal and colonic neoplasms and spontaneous pneumothorax in the Birt-Hogg-Dube syndrome. Cancer Epidemiol Biomarkers Prev 2002; 11(4):393–400.

21 Launonen V, Vierimaa O, Kiuru M, et al. Inherited susceptibility to uterine leiomyomas and renal cell cancer. Proc Natl Acad Sci USA 2001; 98(6):3387–3392.

22 Morrison PJ, Nevin NC. Multiple endocrine neoplasia type 2B (mucosal neuroma syndrome, Wagenmann–Froboese syndrome). J Med Genet 1996; 33(9):779–782.

23 Giuly JA, Picand R, Giuly D, Monges B, Nguyen-Cat R. Von Recklinghausen disease and gastrointestinal stromal tumors. Am J Surg 2003; 185(1):86–87.

24 Khosrotehrani K, Bastuji-Garin S, Zeller J, Revuz J, Wolkenstein P. Clinical risk factors for mortality in patients with neurofibromatosis 1: a cohort study of 378 patients. Arch Derm 2003; 139(2):187–191.

25 Lynch TM, Gutmann DH. Neurofibromatosis 1. Neurol Clin 2002; 20(3):841–865.

26 Sandoval C, Swift M. Hodgkin disease in ataxia-telangiectasia patients with poor outcomes. Med Pediatr Oncol 2003; 40(3):162–166.

27 Okano M, Gross TG. A review of Epstein–Barr virus infection in patients with immunodeficiency disorders. Am J Med Sci 2000; 319(6):392–396.

28 DeLellis RA. The neuroendocrine system and its tumors: an overview. Am J Clin Pathol 2001; 115 (Suppl):S5–S16.

29 Day R, Salzet M. The neuroendocrine phenotype, cellular plasticity and the search for genetic switches: redefining the diffuse neuroendocrine system. Neuroendocrinol Lett 2002; 23(5/6):447–451.

30 Torpy DJ, Mullen N, Ilias I, Nieman LK. Association of hypertension and hypokalemia with Cushing's syndrome caused by ectopic ACTH secretion: a series of 58 cases. Ann N Y Acad Sci 2002; 970:134–144.

31 McStay MK, Caplin ME. Carcinoid tumour. Minerva Med 2002; 93(5):389–401.

32 Kousseff BG. Multiple endocrine neoplasia 2 (MEN 2)/MEN 2A (Sipple syndrome). Derm Clin 1995; 13(1):91–97.

33 Zeng J, Wang B, Ma D, Li F. Glucagonoma syndrome: diagnosis and treatment. J Am Acad Derm 2003; 48(2):297–298.

34 Brentjens R, Saltz L. Islet cell tumors of the pancreas: the medical oncologist's perspective. Surg Clin North Am 2001; 81(3):527–542.

35 Kurzrock R, Cohen PR. Cutaneous paraneoplastic syndromes in solid tumors. Am J Med 1995; 99(6):662–671.

36 Anderson SH, Hudson-Peacock M, Muller AF. Malignant acanthosis nigricans: potential role of chemotherapy. Br J Derm 1999; 141(4):714–716.

37 Ramirez-Amador V, Esquivel-Pedraza L, Caballero-Mendoza E, Berumen-Campos J, Orozco-Topete R, Angeles-Angeles A. Oral manifestations as a hallmark of malignant acanthosis nigricans. Oral Pathol Med 1999; 28(6):278–281.

38 Mekhail TM, Markman M. Acanthosis nigricans with endometrial carcinoma: case report and review of the literature. Gynecol Oncol 2002; 84(2):332–334.

39 Torley D, Bellus GA, Munro CS. Genes, growth factors and acanthosis nigricans. Br J Derm 2002; 147(6):1096–1101.

40 Garcia Hidalgo L. Dermatological complications of obesity. Am J Clin Derm 2002; 3(7):497–506.

41 Schwartz RA. Sign of Leser–Trelat. J Am Acad Derm 1996; 35(1):88–95.

42 Radack K, Park S. Is there a valid association between skin tags and colonic polyps: insights from a quantitative and methodologic analysis of the literature. J Gen Intern Med 1993; 8(8):413–421.

43 Bolognia JL, Brewer YP, Cooper DL. Bazex syndrome (acrokeratosis paraneoplastica). An analytic review. Medicine (Baltimore) 1991; 70(4):269–280.

44 Buxtorf K, Hubscher E, Panizzon R. Bazex syndrome. Dermatology 2001; 202(4):350–352.

45 Cuzick J, Babiker A, Stavola BL De, McCance D, Cartwright R, Glashan RW. Palmar keratoses in family members of individuals with bladder cancer. J Clin Epidemiol 1990; 43(12):1421–1426.

46 Rho NK, Choi SJ, Lee ES. A case of multiple Bowen's disease with squamous cell carcinoma of the larynx and adenocarcinoma of the prostate. J Derm 2002; 29(8):516–521.

47 Daoud MS, Lust JA, Kyle RA, Pittelkow MR. Monoclonal gammopathies and associated skin disorders. J Am Acad Derm 1999; 40(4):507–535.

48 Pomann JJ, Rudner EJ. Scleromyxedema revisited. Int J Derm 2003; 42(1):31–35.

49 Jackson EM. English JC 3rd. Diffuse cutaneous mucinoses. Derm Clin 2002; 20(3):493–501.

50 Mori Y, Kahari VM, Varga J. Scleroderma-like cutaneous syndromes. Curr Rheumatol Rep 2002; 4(2):113–122.

51 Eltom MA, Jemal A, Mbulaiteye SM, Devesa SS, Biggar RJ. Trends in Kaposi's sarcoma and non-Hodgkin's lymphoma incidence in the United States from 1973 through 1998. J Natl Cancer Inst 2002; 94(16):1204–1210.

52 Carrieri MP, Pradier C, Piselli P, et al. Reduced incidence of Kaposi's sarcoma and of systemic non-Hodgkin's lymphoma in HIV-infected individuals treated with highly active antiretroviral therapy. Int J Cancer 2003; 103(1):142–144.

53 Rubel JR, Milford EL, Abdi R. Cutaneous neoplasms in renal transplant recipients. Eur J Derm 2002; 12(6):532–535.

54 Geraminejad P, Memar O, Aronson I, Rady PL, Hengge U, Tyring SK. Kaposi's sarcoma and other manifestations of human herpesvirus 8. J Am Acad Derm 2002; 47(5):641–655.

55 Avivi I, Rosenbaum H, Levy Y, Rowe J. Myelodysplastic syndrome and associated skin lesions: a review of the literature. Leuk Res 1999; 23(4):323–330.

56 Cho KH, Han KH, Kim SW, Youn SW, Youn JI, Kim BK. Neutrophilic dermatoses associated with myeloid malignancy. Clin Exp Derm 1997; 22(6):269–273.

57 Rogalski C, Paasch U, Glander HJ, Haustein UF. Bullous pyoderma gangrenosum complicated by disseminated intravascular coagulation with subsequent myelodysplastic syndrome (chronic myelomonocytic leukemia). J Derm 2003; 30(1):59–63.

58 Nguyen VT, Ndoye A, Bassler KD, et al. Classification, clinical manifestations and immunopathological mechanisms of the epithelial variant of paraneoplastic autoimmune multiorgan syndrome: a reappraisal of paraneoplastic pemphigus. Arch Dermatol 2001; 137:193–206.

59 Joly P, Richard C, Gilbert D, et al. Sensitivity and specificity of clinical, histologic and immunologic features in the diagnosis of paraneoplastic pemphigus. J Am Acad Derm 2000; 43(4):619–626.

60 Allen CM, Camisa C. Paraneoplastic pemphigus: a review of the literature. Oral Dis 2000; 6(4):208–214.

61 Egan CA, Lazarova Z, Darling TN, Yee C, Yancey KB. Anti-epiligrin cicatricial pemphigoid: clinical findings, immunopathogenesis and significant associations. Medicine (Baltimore) 2003; 82(3):177–186.

62 Askling J, Linet M, Gridley G, Halstensen TS, Ekstrom K, Ekbom A. Cancer incidence in a population-based cohort of individuals hospitalized with celiac disease or dermatitis herpetiformis. Gastroenterology 2002; 123(5):1428–1435.

63 Chen YJ, Wu CY, Shen JL. Predicting factors of malignancy in dermatomyositis and polymyositis: a case–control study. Br J Derm 2001; 144(4):825–831.

64 Hill CL, Zhang Y, Sigurgeirsson B, et al. Frequency of specific cancer types in dermatomyositis and polymyositis: a population-based study. Lancet 2001; 357(9250):96–100.

65 Stockton D, Doherty VR, Brewster DH. Risk of cancer in patients with dermatomyositis or polymyositis and follow-up implications: a Scottish population-based cohort study. Br J Cancer 2001; 85(1):41–45.

66 Myers KA, Farquhar DR. The rational clinical examination. Does this patient have clubbing? JAMA 2001; 286(3):341–347.

67 Kishi K, Nakamura H, Sudo A, et al. Tumor debulking by radiofrequency ablation in hypertrophic pulmonary osteoarthropathy associated with pulmonary carcinoma. Lung Cancer 2002; 38(3):317–320.

68 Brown SL, Greene MH, Gershon SK, Edwards ET, Braun MM. Tumor necrosis factor antagonist therapy and lymphoma development: twenty-six cases reported to the Food and Drug Administration. Arthritis Rheum 2002; 46(12):3151–3158.

69 Takahashi N, Chubachi A, Kume M, et al. A clinical analysis of 52 adult patients with hemophagocytic syndrome: the prognostic significance of the underlying diseases. Int J Hematol 2001; 74(2):209–213.

70 Naschitz JE, Kovaleva J, Shaviv N, Rennert G, Yeshurun D. Vascular disorders preceding diagnosis of cancer: distinguishing the causal relationship based on Bradford–Hill guidelines. Angiology 2003; 54(1):11–17.

71 Eubanks LE, McBurney E, Reed R. Erythema gyratum repens. Am J Med Sci 2001; 321(5):302–305.

72 Callen JP, Bernarci DM, Clark RA, Weber DA. Adult-onset recalcitrant eczema: a marker of noncutaneous lymphoma or leukemia. J Am Acad Derm 2000; 43(2):207–210.

73 Aste N, Pau M, Aste N, Biggio P. Pityriasis rotunda: a survey of 42 cases observed in Sardinia, Italy. Dermatology 1997; 194(1):32–35.

74 Egerer G, Hensel M, Ho AD. Infectious complications in chronic lymphoid malignancy. Curr Treat Options Oncol 2001; 2(3):237–244.

CHAPTER
31 **Spitz Nevus**

Les Rosen

Key points

- Spitz nevi are clinically and histopathologically differentiated from malignant melanomas.
- Spitz nevi are predominantly seen in children and young adults.
- Spitz nevi are classically solitary, well circumscribed pink papules.
- Spitz nevi can be junctional, compound and dermal and composed of epithelioid and/or spindled melanocytes.
- Kamino bodies can be seen in Spitz nevi but are neither pathognomonic nor diagnostic.

INTRODUCTION

The inclusion of Spitz nevus in a book entitled *Cancer of the Skin* is obviously problematic, since, by definition, a melanocytic nevus is benign. However, Spitz nevi at times are difficult to differentiate histopathologically from Spitzoid malignant melanomas and for this reason alone are presented and discussed in this chapter. Spitz nevus is a benign melanocytic nevus that clinically and histopathologically differs from other types of melanocytic nevi and malignant melanoma. Clinically, Spitz nevi present predominantly in children as a solitary pink, red or brown papule. Histopathologically, they are usually small (less than 6.0 mm), well circumscribed, symmetrical and are composed of epithelioid and/or spindled melanocytes. The difficulty in diagnosing Spitz nevi histopathologically is often secondary to the biopsy technique. The lesion submitted may have been shaved, punched or curetted and the histopathologist is unable to ascertain size, circumscription, symmetry and maturation of melanocytes with progressive descent into the dermis. A surgically excised Spitz nevus usually allows for an accurate diagnosis.

HISTORY

Spitz nevi are melanocytic nevi that were initially described by Sophie Spitz in 1948 in her landmark paper titled 'Melanomas of childhood'.[1] The detailed clinical and histopathologic descriptions of childhood or juvenile melanomas that behaved in a biologically benign fashion were discussed. Prior to 1948 other authors had recognized this clinicopathologic conundrum of childhood malignant melanomas that behaved in a totally benign fashion and designated the terms 'juvenile melanomas' and prepubertal melanomas.[2] In 1953, Allen and Spitz reported that adults could also have these same lesions and referred to them as 'postpubertal juvenile melanomas'.[3] The long-term follow-up of these patients proved without a doubt the benign nature of this lesion and supported the histopathologic entity which eponymically is now regarded as a Spitz nevus.

EPIDEMIOLOGY

Prevalence

The prevalence of Spitz nevi is unknown in the general population. However, they occur much less commonly than other melanocytic nevi, including congenital and acquired melanocytic nevi. Furthermore, the prevalence decreases with increasing age and is highly unusual in the elderly population, especially on severely sun-damaged skin.

Incidence

The incidence of Spitz nevi in the general population is less than 0.2%.[4] There were 430 Spitz nevi diagnosed over 10 years at Florida Pathology Associates in Miami Beach, Florida, USA out of 302,148 specimens, representing 0.14% of submitted specimens. However, the incidence among children is higher. In a series of surgically removed melanocytic nevi in children it was shown that Spitz nevi represented approximately 1% of the nevi.

Age

Spitz nevi occur predominantly in children during the first two decades of life with about 42% occurring before age 20. Some 61% occur before age 30. Only about 11% of Spitz nevi occur in patients older than 50 years of age. Spitz nevi have been reported from birth to over 80 years of age (Table 31.1).[5] Most of the Spitz nevi are acquired with few reports of congenital Spitz nevi.

Sex

There is no true sex predilection for Spitz nevi, although there may be a slight predominance in women. There

385

Table 31.1	Spitz nevi occurrence[5]	
Age (years)	Female	Male
<1	2	0
1–10	34	35
11–20	69	40
21–30	49	32
31–40	48	25
41–50	28	20
51–60	16	9
61–70	7	7
71–80	5	3
>80	1	0
Total	259	171

were 60% females and 40% males out of the 430 Spitz nevi compiled from Florida Pathology Associates, Miami Beach, Florida, USA.

Race

Spitz nevi occur predominantly in Caucasians with a few case reports in Asians and Africans.

Hereditary factors

There is no known pattern of hereditary or familial transmission.

CLINICAL FEATURES

There are many different clinical variations of Spitz nevi (Figs 31.1–31.9). The classical presentation of a Spitz nevus is a child with an acquired, well circumscribed, solitary, pink papule on the face.

Duration and growth

Congenital Spitz nevi are present at birth and therefore are recognized immediately as congenital nevi and managed according to the size, shape and location. When a patient presents to their clinician the usual duration of an acquired Spitz nevus is historically reported to be present for less than 6 months. Reported durations of Spitz nevi range from 1 month to more than 36 years.[5] Usually, there is a history of a change in size, shape or color of the lesion.

Symptoms and signs

Spitz nevi are usually asymptomatic but can be traumatized resulting in erosion, ulceration and bleeding with the development of a scale crust and secondary bacterial infection.

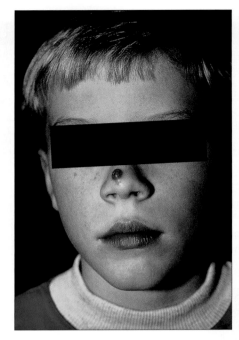

Figure 31.1 Solitary red brown papule on the nose. (Image courtesy of New York University Department of Dermatology.)

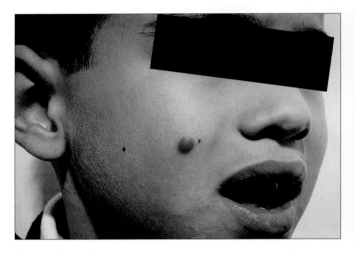

Figure 31.2 Solitary red brown papule on the cheek. (Image courtesy of Alfred Kopf MD, New York University Department of Dermatology.)

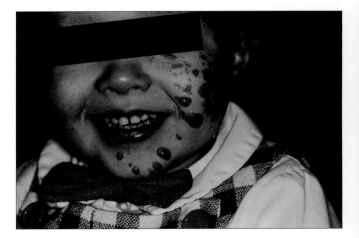

Figure 31.3 Multiple agminated red brown papules on the face. (Image courtesy of New York University Department of Dermatology.)

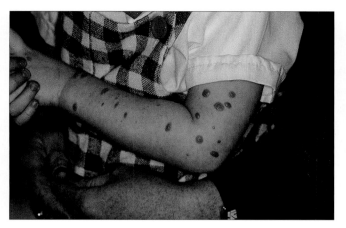

Figure 31.4 Multiple agminated red papules and nodules on the arm. (Image courtesy of New York University Department of Dermatology.)

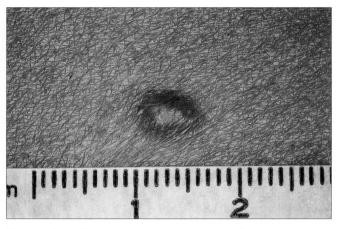

Figure 31.7 Solitary tan papule on the back. (Image courtesy of New York University Department of Dermatology.)

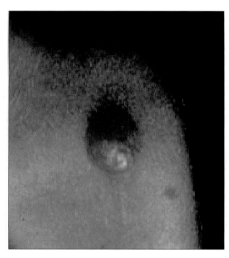

Figure 31.5 Solitary red brown nodule on the shoulder. (Image courtesy of New York University Department of Dermatology.)

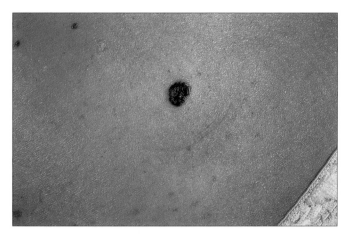

Figure 31.8 Sclitary brown papule on the back. (Image courtesy of Harold Rabinovitz MD.)

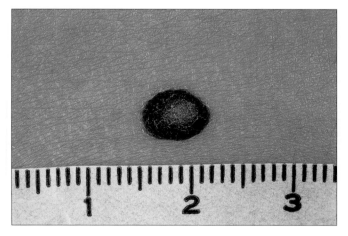

Figure 31.6 Solitary brown papule on the leg. (Image courtesy of New York University Department of Dermatology.)

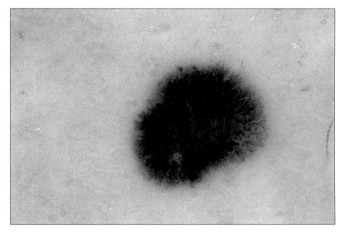

Figure 31.9 Dermoscopy of solitary brown papule. Central bluish-white color with a negative pigment network extending almost to the periphery of the lesion. (Image courtesy of Harold Rabinovitz MD.)

Location

Spitz nevi occur approximately 16% on the head and neck, 28% on the lower extremities, 37% on the trunk and 19% on the upper extremities. Spitz nevi have been reported involving the mucosal surface, tongue, conjunctiva, genitalia and volar skin[6] (Table 31.2).

Multiplicity

Spitz nevi are usually solitary papules. Occasionally they can be multiple, widespread, grouped, agminated or eruptive.

Size

Spitz nevi are usually less than 1.0 cm in diameter with the majority less than 0.6 cm in diameter. They can range in size from 0.1 cm to 3.0 cm.

Color and consistency

Spitz nevi are usually pink to red but can range in color from flesh colored to tan, dark brown and black depending on the amount of melanin present and vascularity of the lesion. The consistency ranges from soft to firm. The surrounding skin can be hyperpigmented or hypopigmented resulting in a halo phenomenon.

Morphology

Spitz nevi are usually smooth, sessile, dome shaped papules or less commonly nodules; however, they can be macular and plaque-like. Occasionally Spitz nevi can be polypoid and have a verrucous surface.

Classification of clinical forms

There are four clinical types of Spitz nevi described with transitions among them.[2] The clinical types include:

- The light colored soft form, which is pink to light tan, smooth, and flattens with diascopy.

- The light colored hard form, which appears like a dermatofibroma or keloid and may have a halo of fine telangiectases.

- The dark form, which is variably pigmented and smooth.

- The multiple form, which includes the agminated and widespread, disseminated, eruptive lesions.

CLINICAL DIFFERENTIAL DIAGNOSES

A Spitz nevus can clinically resemble a banal acquired melanocytic nevus, dysplastic melanocytic nevus (Clark's nevus), congenital melanocytic nevus, blue nevus, pyogenic granuloma, dermatofibroma, hemangioma, angiofibroma, scar, keloid, fibroma, xanthogranuloma, verruca vulgaris, molluscum contagiosum, epidermal nevus, histiocytoma, xanthoma, arthropod bite reaction, hypertrophic lichen planus, lupus vulgaris, granuloma faciale, eosinophilic granuloma (histiocytosis), pseudolymphoma, seborrheic keratosis, chondrodermatitis nodularis helicis, actinic keratosis, pale cell acanthoma, granular cell tumor, leiomyoma, glomus tumor, squamous cell carcinoma, basal cell carcinoma, Kaposi's sarcoma and angiosarcoma.

HISTOPATHOLOGIC FEATURES

Spitz nevi are melanocytic nevi that are junctional, compound and dermal in distribution (Figs 31.10–31.17). The majority of Spitz nevi are compound (66%), with the remainder junctional (16%) and dermal (18%). (Compiled data from Florida Pathology Associates, Miami Beach, Florida, USA.) Furthermore, Spitz nevi are symmetrical, well circumscribed, and composed of epithelioid or large spindled melanocytes arranged in nests and as solitary units, predominantly along the dermal–epidermal junction with extension into the dermis. Clefting between nests of melanocytes and the epidermis is often seen. Maturation of melanocytes with progressive descent into the dermis, dull pink globules (Kamino bodies), uniform melanin distribution, telangiectases and a sparse perivascular lymphocytic infiltrate are also seen.

Architecture

At scanning magnification the majority of Spitz nevi are dome shaped papules, symmetric and well circumscribed when junctional and compound in distribution. The Spitz nevi that are dermal in distribution are dome shaped and symmetrical; however they may not be well circumscribed. The spindled and/or epithelioid melanocytes in dermal Spitz nevi are often seen between and among collagen bundles throughout the dermis. The majority of melanocytes in Spitz nevi are present within the dermis with extension into the subcutis in about 5% of the cases.

Table 31.2	Anatomic sites of Spitz nevi[5]			
Site	*n*	(%)	Female	Male
Head and neck	70	16	36	34
Upper extremities	82	19	51	31
Trunk	159	37	81	78
Lower extremities	119	28	91	28
Total	430		259	171

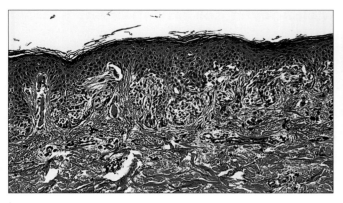

Figure 31.10 Junctional Spitz nevus, medium power. Well circumscribed with acanthosis and clefting.

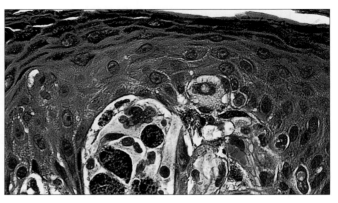

Figure 31.13 Compound Spitz nevus, high power. Hypergranulosis and acanthosis.

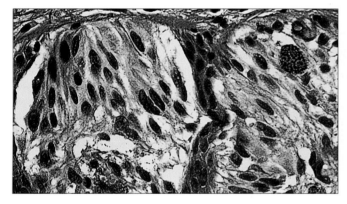

Figure 31.11 Junctional Spitz nevus, high power. Spindle cells in nests.

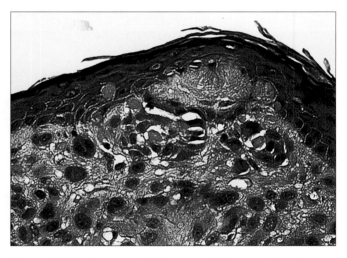

Figure 31.14 Compound Spitz nevus, high power. Kamino bodies (dull pink globules).

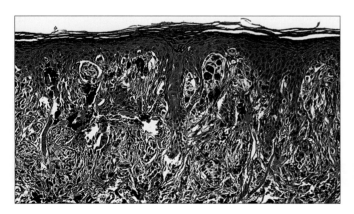

Figure 31.12 Compound Spitz nevus, medium power. Acanthosis with abundant melanin.

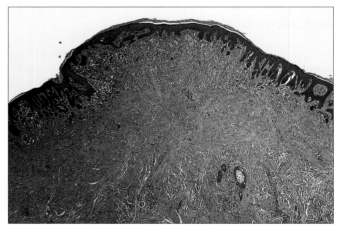

Figure 31.15 Dermal Spitz nevus, low power. Symmetrical papule.

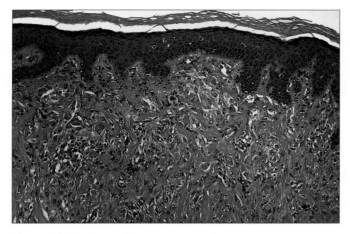

Figure 31.16 Dermal Spitz nevus, medium power.

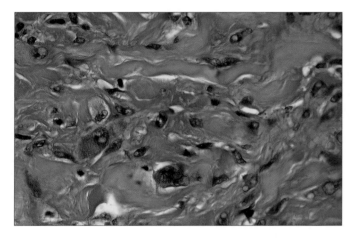

Figure 31.17 Dermal Spitz nevus, high power. Epithelioid melanocytes with abundant cytoplasm.

Melanocytic cell types

Spitz nevi are composed of essentially two distinct types of melanocytes: large epithelioid cells and large spindle cells. Spitz nevi can contain both types of cells and are sometimes classified according to the predominant melanocytic cell type. Spitz nevi composed of predominantly spindle cells are the most common type seen in approximately 60% of cases, followed by a roughly equal combination of mixed spindle and epithelioid melanocytes in slightly more than 20% of cases with epithelioid cell predominant Spitz nevi composing slightly less than 20% of cases. (Compiled data from Florida Pathology Associates, Miami Beach, Florida, USA.) Spitz nevi can also be combined with other types of melanocytic cells, including small round, large round, oval, dendritic, Pagetoid, multinucleated and ballooned. These other types of melanocytic cells can be distributed in a regular or irregular pattern among and between the spindle and epithelioid cells or can be arranged in large distinct aggregates and adjacent to the predominant spindle cells or epithelioid cells of a Spitz nevus.

Melanocytic cell arrangement

The melanocytic cell arrangement of a Spitz nevus is usually consistent within the nevus. The melanocytes when spindle in shape tend to occur in elongated nests within the epidermis and as fascicles throughout the dermis. These fascicles may show a parallel or whorled pattern with separation of these fascicles by bands of collagen. When the melanocytic cells are predominantly epithelioid they occur more often in small round and/or oval nests.[7] Solitary epithelioid melanocytes can be distributed throughout the dermis between and among thick collagen bundles. The junctional component of a Spitz nevus is usually well circumscribed, composed of spindle or epithelioid cells as solitary units and in nests along the dermal–epidermal junction and at times above the dermal–epidermal junction into the stratum granulosum and stratum corneum. Pagetoid cells are not seen within the epidermis of a Spitz nevus. The extension of epithelioid melanocytes above the dermal–epidermal junction in a Pagetoid pattern should not be confused with the Pagetoid melanocyte, which is a melanocyte with a round nucleus and abundant cytoplasm containing dusty melanin. Solitary epithelioid melanocytes may predominate in evolving junctional Spitz nevi. When the melanocytes have formed nests, these nests may demonstrate clefting from the surrounding epithelium of the epidermis. Most of the Spitz nevi, when compound, show maturation of melanocytes with progressive descent into the dermis.[7] Maturation is present when the cells and/or nuclei get smaller as they get deeper into the dermis.

MELANOCYTIC NEVUS CELL CYTOLOGY

The spindle cells of a Spitz nevus may vary in size and shape and are large fusiform cells that are uniform throughout the lesion. The spindle cells may have abundant eosinophilic cytoplasm with distinct borders. Melanin, when present, may be fine and granular and evenly distributed throughout the cytoplasm. The nuclei are large round to oval and have a thin nuclear membrane with folds and indentations. The nuclear chromatin is fine and stippled with small round conspicuous basophilic nucleoli. Intranuclear pseudo-inclusions are often present. These pseudo-inclusions represent invaginations of cytoplasm into the nucleus.[7]

The epithelioid cells of a Spitz nevus also may vary in size and shape and are large polygonal or round cells that are uniform throughout the lesion. The epithelioid cells have abundant eosinophilic or amphophilic cytoplasm with distinct borders. Melanin, when present, may be fine and granular and evenly distributed throughout the cytoplasm. The nuclei are large round to oval and have a thin nuclear membrane. The nuclear chromatin is vesicular with large round conspicuous eosinophilic nucleoli.[8]

The epithelioid cells and spindle cells of a Spitz nevus may be combined with other types of melanocytes including small round, large round, oval, dendritic, multinucleated, ballooned, and Pagetoid melanocytes. This combination of cells will result in a diagnosis of a combined Spitz nevus, which as a rule is asymmetrical.

Mitoses

Mitotic figures are usually not present in Spitz nevi. However, when mitotic figures are present they are typical, and present in the upper half of the lesion. Mitotic figures are more commonly seen in lesions biopsied during puberty or in children that are rapidly growing. Atypical mitotic figures and mitotic figures in the lower half of a lesion are unusual.[7]

Pigment

Spitz nevi are usually amelanotic or contain minimal fine dusty melanin. When present, melanin is usually more pronounced superficially and can be found in the cytoplasm of melanocytes, keratinocytes, histiocytes (melanophages) and extracellularly in the dermis. There are Spitz nevi that can be heavily pigmented, obscuring the spindle and epithelioid cells, requiring bleaching of the melanin to visualize the cells. The pigmented spindle cell tumor described by Reed in 1975 is an example of a heavily pigmented junctional Spitz nevus of spindled cells that is most often seen on the proximal extremities of young adults.[9]

Epidermal changes

There is usually hyperorthokeratosis, hypergranulosis, and irregular epidermal hyperplasia present. Focal parakeratosis can be seen.[10,11] Ulceration and erosions are usually secondary to excoriations and other forms of trauma. The epidermal changes can mimic the histologic changes seen in prurigo nodularis and when extensive can resemble pseudoepitheliomatous hyperplasia. Conversely, epidermal atrophy can occur but usually this is focal and associated with epidermal hyperplasia. Spongiosis and microvesicle formation can also occur and usually is secondary to a contactant or trauma.

Intraepidermal dull pink globules (Kamino bodies) occur in many Spitz nevi.[12] They are located within the epidermis or along the dermal–epidermal junction in a suprapapillary location. These Kamino bodies range in diameter from about 5 to 10 mm in coalesced aggregates with scalloped borders. Kamino bodies represent extracellular matrix composed of fibronectin, neutral mucopolysaccharides, glycoproteins, collagen, basal lamina and unidentified fibrillar and granular material.[12,13]

Kamino bodies are neither pathognomonic for, nor diagnostic of, Spitz nevi since they can be seen in other melanocytic nevi and malignant melanomas. Kamino bodies are seen more frequently in Spitz nevi that are compound or junctional and rarely in the dermal variant, and occur rarely in other melanocytic nevi and malignant melanoma.

Dermal changes

Spitz nevi characteristically exhibit telangiectases, edema of the papillary dermis and a superficial perivascular lymphocytic infiltrate. Dermal fibrosis and sclerosis can occur. Adnexal structures are usually intact and not obliterated.

Telangiectases or vascular ectasia is often seen in the suprapapillary dermis along with edema. The vascular ectasia may be due to dilated venules, capillaries, arterioles and lymphatic vessels. Cavernous dilatation occurs occasionally. The vascular ectasia can be seen in the deep portion of the reticular dermis along with a proliferation of vessels.

The edema of the papillary dermis can be minimal or extensive. When the edema is extensive the individual, nested, fascicles or aggregates of spindle or epithelioid melanocytes appear to be floating in the markedly edematous stroma of the papillary dermis.

The inflammatory infiltrate is usually a superficial perivascular infiltrate composed of lymphocytes, histiocytes, mast cells and occasional plasma cells. This inflammatory infiltrate can also be scattered around the periphery of the lesion, along the base of the lesion, scattered throughout the lesion and as a lichenoid infiltrate along the dermal–epidermal junction.[7,10] If secondary changes of an ulceration or erosion are present then the inflammatory infiltrate can include neutrophils and eosinophils. If a halo phenomenon is present then a dense, diffuse infiltrate of lymphocytes, histiocytes and melanophages is present.

Dermal fibrosis and sclerosis can occur making it difficult to distinguish spindle and dendritic melanocytes from fibroblasts. This differentiation can be accomplished with the use of immunoperoxidase stains for S-100 protein and Melan-A since melanocytes will be positive and fibroblasts will be negative for these antigens.

HISTOLOGIC DIFFERENTIAL DIAGNOSIS

The diagnosis of a Spitz nevus is usually not difficult when the biopsy is adequate and the characteristic histopathologic criteria are present. The difficulty in making an accurate diagnosis of Spitz nevus is often secondary to an inadequate biopsy. Spitz nevi and Spitzoid malignant melanomas share many histopathologic features and occasionally some lesions are diagnostic dilemmas. The histopathologic differential diagnosis of Spitz nevus is almost always that of a malignant melanoma.

The histopathology of malignant melanoma is discussed in Chapter 18. However, the histopathologic criteria that favor a diagnosis of malignant melanoma include: (1) asymmetry; (2) poor circumscription; (3) lack of maturation of melanocytes with progressive descent into the dermis; (4) numerous melanocytes as solitary units and in nests above the dermal–epidermal junction throughout all layers of the epidermis and extending down epithelial structures of adnexae; (5) Pagetoid cells within the epidermis; (6) mitotic figures, some atypical, throughout the lesion; and (7) ulceration.

The Spitz nevus that is composed predominantly of spindle cells must also be differentiated from spindle cell malignant melanoma, spindle cell basal cell carcinoma, spindle cell squamous cell carcinoma, common and cellular blue nevi, dermatofibrosarcoma protuberans and malignant nerve sheath tumors.

ULTRASTRUCTURE

Electron microscopic examination of the melanocytes of a Spitz nevus reveals the same subcellular structure and organelles of melanocytes as an intradermal melanocytic nevus with the exception of less melanization of premelanosomes. The Golgi apparatus, mitochondria, endoplasmic reticulum and ribosomes are identical. In the region of the Golgi apparatus, the melanocytes of a Spitz nevus have numerous pigment organelles, which range from small vesicles to mature melanosomes. Melanization of the premelanosomes is incomplete and there is lysosomal degradation of melanosome complexes and low dispersion of premelanosomes, which elucidate the scant pigmentation of some Spitz nevi. There are fewer premelanosomes with maturation of melanocytes.[14]

Melanosomes of Spitz nevus cells located along the dermal–epidermal junction are ovoid to spindle-shaped and have a maximum dimension of 150×450 nm. In contrast, melanosomes in dermal Spitz nevus cells are more spherical to ovoid and are about 180×190 nm in maximum dimension.[14]

Intraepidermal Spitz nevus cells are in immediate contact with adjacent keratinocytes, whereas nevus cells in the dermis are separated from the dermal connective tissue by a basement membrane. The clefts that are present around the nests of melanocytes in a Spitz nevus and the surrounding keratinocytes are artifacts caused by cellular shrinkage. Both intranuclear inclusions and pseudoinclusions are seen.

The Kamino bodies are composed of interlacing thick and thin, long wavy extracellular fibrils, which have a regular periodicity of 51 nm. The thin fibrils are 8.1–13.2 nm in diameter and resemble colloid bodies or apoptotic keratinocytes. The thick fibrils are 23.1–34.7 nm in diameter and resemble immature or altered collagen.[12]

Amyloid can be seen in Spitz nevi as with other melanocytic nevi along with benign and malignant neoplasms. There is no associated serum protein abnormality. The amyloid may be present within the parenchyma of the Spitz nevus or in the surrounding stroma.

IMMUNOHISTOCHEMICAL AND SPECIAL STUDIES

Presently there is no one immunohistochemical study that would help diagnose and differentiate Spitz nevi from malignant melanoma with specificity. The MIB-1 monoclonal antibody recognizes the Ki-67 antigen and has been studied as an adjunctive tool in the differential diagnoses of Spitz nevus and malignant melanoma. A total of 25 compound Spitz nevi, 27 malignant melanomas and 26 banal (non-dysplastic) melanocytic nevi were stained with the MIB-1 antibody.[15] This study revealed that

the mean MIB-1 counts were significantly lower in the Spitz nevi and banal melanocytic nevi when compared with the malignant melanomas. Additionally, Spitz nevi may express components of the plasminogen activation system.[16] The plasminogen activation system facilitates the invasion and metastases of malignant neoplasms. The components of the plasminogen activation system include: (1) urokinase; (2) tissue-type plasminogen activator; (3) plasminogen activation inhibitor types 1 and 2; (4) receptor for urokinase. In one study the expression of the components of the plasminogen activation system were compared in Spitz nevi, banal melanocytic nevi, dysplastic melanocytic nevi and malignant melanomas. It was demonstrated that Spitz nevi express tissue-type plasminogen activator, inhibitors and the receptor for urokinase in a much smaller proportion than in malignant melanomas, while there is no expression of urokinase. Conversely, some of the malignant melanomas express urokinase.

Although not widely available at this time, molecular pathology may prove to be an invaluable technique to aid in the differential diagnosis of Spitz nevi and malignant melanomas. The role of comparative genomic hybridization and interphase fluorescence *in situ* hybridization in diagnosis and prognosis of difficult melanocytic neoplasms is still evolving.[17] Nine persistent (recurrent) Spitz nevi were evaluated using comparative genomic hybridization yielding results consistent with Spitz nevi in eight cases. The remaining case showed a comparative genomic hybridization profile more typical of a malignant melanoma. Spitz nevi were compared to malignant melanomas using interphase fluorescence *in situ* hybridization.[18] This comparison showed significant differences involving chromosome 9 signal indices, which were higher in the malignant melanomas when compared to the Spitz nevi.

TREATMENT AND RECURRENCE

Spitz nevi are benign neoplasms that theoretically need no further treatment. However, there is no consensus on the management of Spitz nevi. This lack of uniformity in treating Spitz nevi is due to the difficulty of differentiating histopathologically a Spitz nevus from a Spitzoid malignant melanoma. In a recent study at the pigmented-lesion clinic of the New York University Skin and Cancer Unit, the recommendation was to completely excise Spitz nevi because of the concern for misdiagnosing a malignant melanoma as a Spitz nevus.[19]

FUTURE OUTLOOK

The ability to diagnose Spitz nevi with 100% specificity and sensitivity is the future goal for all histopathologists. However, there are limitations with the use of conventional light microscopy, and therefore adjunctive techniques, procedures and methodologies need to be developed. A specific and sensitive monoclonal antibody, flow cytometry, fluorescent *in situ* hybridization and comparative genomic hybridization may eventually prove effective in diagnosing Spitz nevi with 100% accuracy.

REFERENCES

1 Spitz S. Melanomas of childhood. Am J Pathol 1948; 24:591.

2 Kopf AW, Andrade R. Benign juvenile melanoma. In: Kopf AW, Andrade R, eds. The Year Book of Dermatology (1965–1966 Series). Chicago: Year Book Medical Publishers Inc.; 1966:7–52.

3 Allen AC, Spitz S. Malignant melanoma: A clinicopathological analysis of the criteria for diagnosis and prognosis. Cancer 1953; 6:1.

4 Weedon D, Little JH. Spindle and epithelioid cell nevi in children and adults. Cancer 1977; 40:217–225.

5 Coskey RJ, Mehregan A. Spindle cell nevi in adults and children. Arch Derm 1973; 108:535–536.

6 Dorji T, Cavazza A, Nappi O, et al. Spitz nevus of the tongue with pseudoepitheliomatous hyperplasia: report of three cases of a pseudomalignant condition. Am J Surg Pathol 2002; 26(6):774–777.

7 Kernen JA, Ackerman LV. Spindle cell nevi and epithelioid cell nevi (so-called juvenile melanomas) in children and adults: A clinicopathological study of 27 cases. Cancer 1960; 13:612–625.

8 Echevarria R, Ackerman LV. Spindle and epithelioid cell nevi in the adult. Cancer 1967; 20:175–189.

9 Reed RJ, Ichinose H, Clark WH, et al. Common and uncommon melanocytic nevi and borderline melanomas. Semin Oncol 1975; 2:119–147.

10 Allen AC. Juvenile melanomas of children and adults and melanocarcinomas of children. Arch Derm 1960; 82:325–335.

11 Allen AC. Juvenile melanomas. Ann NY Acad Sci 1963; 100:29–48.

12 Kamino H, Misheloff E, Ackerman AB, et al. Eosinophilic globules in Spitz's nevi. New findings and a diagnostic sign. Am J Derm 1979; 1:319.

13 Kamino H, Jagirdar J. Fibronectin in eosinophilic globules of Spitz's nevi. Am J Derm 1984; 6 (Suppl)(1):313.

14 Mishima Y. Melanotic tumors. In: Zelickson AS, ed. Ultrastructure of Normal and Abnormal Skin. Philadelphia, PA: Lea & Febiger; 1967:388–424.

15 Bergman R, Malkin L, Sbo E, et al. MIB-1 monoclonal antibody to determine proliferative activity of Ki-67 antigen as an adjunct to the histopathologic differential diagnosis of Spitz nevi. Am Acad Derm 2001; 44(3):500–504.

16 Ferrier CM, Gelocf WL Van, Straatman H, et al. Spitz naevi may express components of the plasminogen activation system. J Pathol 2002; 198(1):92–99.

17 Harvell JD, Bastian BC, LeBoit PE. Persistent (recurrent) Spitz nevi: a histopathologic, immunohistochemical, and molecular pathologic study of 22 cases. Am J Surg Pathol 2002; 26(5):654–661.

18 Wettengel GV, Draeger J, Kiesewetter F. Differentiation between Spitz nevi and malignant melanomas by interphase fluorescence in situ hybridization. Int J Oncol 1999; 14(6):1177–1183.

19 Gelbard SN, Tripp JM, Marghoob AA, et al. Management of Spitz nevi: a survey of dermatologists in the United States. J Am Acad Derm 2002; 47(2):224–230.

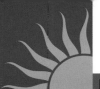
Keratoacanthoma

Molly Chartier, Marti Jill Rothe and Jane M Grant-Kels

Key points

- Keratoacanthoma is a lesion that usually undergoes three phases: rapid growth, maturation and regression.
- There are several forms of solitary keratoacanthomas as well as syndromes involving multiple lesions. Some of these syndromes are familial.
- The specific etiology of keratoacanthoma formation and regression, including the potential role of infectious, environmental and genetic factors, is not yet known.
- The major risk factor for developing this lesion is sun exposure.
- Keratoacanthoma shares several histological features of squamous cell carcinoma. There are features that usually distinguish keratoacanthoma from squamous cell carcinoma; however, no one architectural or histopathological marker clearly delineates between the two.
- Keratoacanthoma may be a variant of squamous cell carcinoma, which can metastasize (although this is a rare occurrence) and should be treated accordingly. There are both surgical and chemotherapeutic treatment options.

INTRODUCTION

Keratoacanthoma (KA) is a neoplasm of the skin and mucous membranes that exhibits rapid growth, maturation and regression. It occurs most often on the sun-exposed areas of fair-skinned adults and is thought to arise from cells in the hair follicle.[1] Much of this lesion's etiology, pathophysiology and even true prevalence remain unknown in spite of ongoing research in these areas. The level of malignant potential in KA is a long-debated issue, leading to various classifications including benign, pre-malignant, pseudomalignant and malignant. An illustration of this point is the multitude of names given to the lesion, including: crateriform ulcer of the face, molluscum sebaceum, *kyste sébacé atypique*, *molluscum pseudocarcinomatum*, *verrucome avec adénite*, multiple self-healing epithelioma, self-healing primary squamous cell carcinoma, tumor-like keratosis, idiopathic cutaneous pseudoepitheliomatous hyperplasia, keratocarcinoma, familial primary self-healing squamous epithelioma of the skin and, most recently, squamous cell carcinoma, keratoacanthoma-type.[2–5]

KA is now recognized as a lesion with low, but not negligible, metastatic potential that often causes sig-nificant local tissue destruction or scarring. Although KA exhibits a unique clinical and pathologic profile, the lesion also shares several characteristics of squamous cell carcinoma (SCC) and is now considered by many dermatologists to be a subset of squamous cell carcinoma.[6]

HISTORY

In 1889, Sir Jonathan Hutchinson first described a lesion that Freudenthal is later credited with naming 'keratoacanthoma'.[2,7] The lesion has several forms, which were elucidated over the next several decades (Table 32.1). Ferguson and Smith described a case of multiple familial KA in 1934 and Grzybowski described an eruptive form of multiple KA in 1950.[8,9] Miedzinski and Kozakiewicz described the KA centrifugum form in 1962, Stevanovic the agglomerate or multinodular form in 1965, and Webb and Ghadially described giant KA in 1966.[10–12]

EPIDEMIOLOGY

Solitary: The incidence of solitary KA is highest in fair-skinned individuals and the majority of lesions occur on sun-exposed areas of the body. In 1963, Ghadially documented that KA occurs twice as often in men than women and that the most frequently afflicted age group was 60–65, while the average age was 56. From this group, 90% of the lesions were on sun-exposed skin, with the cheeks, nose and dorsa of hands being most commonly affected.[13] In 1984, Kligman and Callen noted that the majority of the lesions occurred on sun-exposed skin and were accompanied by 'actinic damage ... including a 'leathered' aged appearance, actinic keratosis, other cutaneous neoplasms, solar lentigines, poikilodermas, or a combination of these findings'.[14]

The incidence of KA is difficult to accurately assess because the lesion usually regresses on its own or may be mistaken for a benign or malignant neoplasm. The incidence of Japanese Hawaiians seeking care for KA between 1983 and 1987 was 22.1/100,000, while the incidence in white Hawaiians was 104/100,000 and the incidence in Japanese residing in Japan was approximately 0.1/100,000.[15,16] While the rate in Japan was an estimate, it still demonstrates the marked increase of KA in the lower latitude regions. The group studying KA in Hawaii also noted that the male:female ratio of KA in Japanese Hawaiians was 1:3 (the inverse of relationships previously reported) and hypothesized this could be due

Table 32.1   Keratoacanthoma and associated types

Solitary	• Giant • Aggressive • Verrucous • Multinodular • Centrifugum • Subungual • Dyskeratoticum and segregans
Multiple	• Multiple persistent • Ferguson-Smith • Witten-Zack • Generalized eruptive of Grzybowski
Associations	• Muir–Torre syndrome • Xeroderma pigmentosum • Florid cutaneous papillomatosis • Nevus sebaceous

to cultural differences in which Japanese Hawaiian women were more likely than their male counterparts to engage in outdoor activities such as gardening. Additionally, Dufresne et al. in Rhode Island, an area with marked seasonal variation in temperature and daylight hours, noted a statistically significant increase in the presentation of KA during the summer months.[17] While there are case reports of KA in patients with brown and black skin, the lesion is rare in darkly pigmented populations.

Variant forms: Multiple keratoacanthomas of Ferguson-Smith is an autosomal dominant disorder in which lesions may be numerous (up to hundreds) and both men and women are equally affected. Although lesions can begin as early as infancy, the mean age of onset is 25.5 years for women and 26.9 years for men.[5]

PATHOGENESIS AND ETIOLOGY

A single cause for KA is unknown. The lesion occurs most often on hair bearing, sun exposed skin, but can occur on non-hair-bearing, sun-protected skin as well. For instance, KA has been reported on the hard palate, tongue, gingiva, lip, nasal mucosa, conjunctiva, anal mucosa, vulva, palms and soles.[18–21] Because no one specific etiology is common to all KA types, a discussion of several proposed mechanisms is offered here.

Sun exposure

The observed facts that most KAs occur on sun-exposed skin and occur more often in individuals who spend more time in the sun imply a connection between solar radiation and the lesion's pathogenesis. The specific mechanism is unclear. However, Filipowicz et al. have demonstrated that the apoptotic mediator CD95 (Fas) is down regulated in two-thirds of KA lesions developing on sun-exposed skin.[22] This data suggests that loss of the protective apoptotic mechanism may be one path to KA formation. A similar down regulation of CD95 was also

seen in other lesions such as actinic keratosis, SCC and BCC and indeed these lesions have been described as occurring in the same patients and the same sun-exposed areas of skin as KA.[14]

Other radiation forms

There have been case reports of KA occurring after cutaneous exposure to radiation therapy. Shaw et al. described the development of several KAs on the face of a woman shortly after radiation therapy to her sinuses for a squamous cell carcinoma.[23] Baer and Kopf described KA formation on skin sites treated with radiation for basal cell epitheliomas.[24] There have also been case reports of psoralen and ultraviolet A (PUVA) therapy inducing KA.[25] It is unclear whether these forms of radiation themselves induce the formation of KAs or whether the lesion is a reaction to the skin damage or the skin's repair mechanisms.

Trauma

There have been numerous reports of KA developing at sites of skin trauma. Several specific case reports describe KA formation at the margins of excisions and skin grafts. KAs have also developed at the site of thermal burns and CO_2 laser resurfacing.[26] Beyond these reports, patients often recall minor trauma to the area near the lesion such as insect bites, scratches, thorn punctures and excoriations.[27] However, the skin is subject to minor trauma on a daily basis and there may be recall bias for any area that develops a lesion. Therefore, the reported history of trauma associated with KA development may be incidental. A mechanism explaining cause and effect has yet to be elucidated. It is possible that trauma in combination with other inherent or environmental factors leads to formation of the lesion.

Carcinogens

KAs are known to occur in conjunction with certain chemical and carcinogen exposures. Ghadially et al. have documented induction of KA in experimental animals (such as rabbit, mouse, hamster and chicken) using topical carcinogen exposure.[28–31] In 1963, Ghadially et al. noted an increased incidence of KA in smokers, suggesting that there may be a topical effect of cigarette smoke carcinogens.[13] El-Hakim and Ethman also reported on a KA of the lip developing in a 'Goza' tobacco smoker. The authors suggest that carcinogenic effects may act in combination with other local factors (such as 'mechanical trauma and irritation by the bamboo or plastic tubes used in the mouthpiece, the heat generated by the smoke and the possible chronic infections that might be contagious from the use of one "Goza" by several individuals') to cause KA formation on the lip.[32] There is also a correlation with pitch and tar workers and KA. Letzel and Drexler documented that 19% of workers in a tar refinery developed KAs, with lesions occurring usually on the face, hands and forearms.[33]

Viral

The idea that KA may stem from a viral etiology began from work by Ereaux et al. who reported papillomatous growth with virus-like particles in chick embryos inoculated with KA cell culture.[34] Zelickson and Lynch and later, Preito et al., also reported on these intranuclear virus-like inclusion bodies.[35,36] However, Fisher et al. observed that similar intranuclear inclusion bodies were seen in a variety of processes including normal cells.[37] Thus the significance of these particles remains unknown.

Because of this early work and similarities of KA with virally mediated lesions such as verrucae, many researchers have continued to study the possible role of viral infection in KA formation. Specifically, HPV DNA has been demonstrated in several KAs by various techniques including *in situ* hybridization and PCR. There have been conflicting reports on the prevalence of HPV DNA in KAs developing in both immunosuppressed and non-immunosuppressed patient populations. Stockfleth et al. suggested that HPV infection does not cause KA formation in all people, but may be one predisposing factor in some patients and a cofactor for malignant transformation.[38]

Hair follicle cycling

Whiteley documented that experimental animals were likely to develop KAs from topical carcinogen exposure during certain phases of the hair cycle.[31] Ghadially later proposed pathways by which KAs develop from cells in the hair follicle; delineating specific forms of KA depending on the follicular cells of origin. In this nomenclature, type I KAs arise from cells in the distal hair follicle, are superficially placed and 'bud shaped', while type II lesions arise from cells in the deeper hair germ, invade more deeply into the skin and are 'dome-shaped or berry-shaped'.[3]

The cyclic nature of hair growth – anagen (growth phase), catagen (regression phase) and telogen (resting phase) – offers a similarity to the rapid growth, maturation and regression of most KAs. The mechanism of formation of lesions on mucosa and other non-hair-bearing skin is not known, but an origin in glandular cells has been proposed. It is also interesting to note that KAs arising in the subungual area may arise from cells in the nail bed which grow constantly and do not cycle. Since the nail bed cells do not cycle, it follows logically that KAs arising in this area would rarely show spontaneous regression. In fact KAs of the subungual area often continue to grow, without regression, causing severe local tissue and bone destruction.

Immune factors

There are conflicting reports on the level of immune involvement in KA regression. Ramselaar and van der Meer concluded that KAs regress via pathways that are not immune mediated.[39] More recently Patel et al. demonstrated significant differences in the profiles of immune cells invading KAs and squamous cell carcinomas. The infiltrates of KAs were demonstrated to be higher in CD3+ and CD4+ cells as well as cells expressing the interleukin-2 receptor and the adhesion molecule, CD-36.[40] In a small study of 25 patients, Gualde et al. documented that patients with KAs were more likely to express HLA-Bw35 than a control population, but the difference was not statistically significant.[41] Additionally, KAs develop more frequently in immunosuppressed patients and the lesions tend to be more locally aggressive in this population. These differences suggest that there is an immunologic role in KA regression, although a specific mechanism has not been elucidated.

Genetics

Several forms of KA express specific genetic patterns. KAs are found in conjunction with sebaceous skin tumors and internal malignancies in Muir–Torre syndrome. This syndrome is a variant of the hereditary non-polyposis colon cancer (HNPCC) syndrome and is inherited in an autosomal dominant pattern. Patients with Muir–Torre syndrome have germline mutations in their DNA mismatch repair genes. Several researchers have utilized microsatellite instability to document mutations in MSH-2 and MLH-1 mismatch repair genes in lesions from patients with both Muir–Torre syndrome and HNPCC.[42]

On the other hand, microsatellite instability and loss of heterozygosity in mismatch repair genes does not seem to be important in spontaneous KA formation.[43] DNA repair defects do characterize xeroderma pigmentosum, a syndrome in which KAs are seen with basal cell carcinomas, squamous cell carcinomas and melanomas on sun-exposed skin. Ferguson-Smith KAs also demonstrate an autosomal dominant pattern of inheritance and KAs of the Witten-Zak type have been reported in families. It is possible that undetected infection or other environmental agents cause the familial pattern of these lesions, but genetic inheritance remains a likely mechanism.

Activated ras genes have been detected in several tumors including KA. Ras is a family of proteins, involved in cell signal transduction, that normally cycle between active and inactive states. Mutations in the ras gene can lead to proteins that are disproportionately active and thus tumorigenic. In a study by Peng et al., rabbits were altered to express human EJras, a ras mutant, and all of these transgenic rabbits developed KAs at approximately 3 days after birth. Additionally, nearly all of these lesions spontaneously regressed. Some 18% of the transgenic rabbits went on to develop SCCs at about 5 months after birth.[44] Clearly, mutation in this family of ras proteins has the potential to explain KA formation in humans. Additionally mutations in p53, a tumor suppressor gene involved in many cancers, may play a role in KA formation. p53 mutations are often seen in KA, but this mutation alone is not sufficient to cause the tumor formation; therefore p53 mutation may act in conjunction with other genetic alterations or environmental factors.[44] A study by Hu et al. demonstrated that p27[kip], a cyclin dependent kinase inhibitor, is expressed in regressing KAs more than in expanding KAs and may be a therapeutic target for upregulation.[45]

Associations with other dermatoses and neoplasms

KA has been documented in association with several dermatoses. It is not known whether these are chance associations, or whether the presence of these dermatoses predisposes the adjacent skin to KA formation via trauma or some other mechanism. Dermatoses that have been noted in conjunction with KAs include atopic dermatitis, seborrheic dermatitis, stasis dermatitis, psoriasis, linear epidermal nevus, lichen planus and hypertrophic lichen planus, rosacea, folliculitis, drug eruptions, acne congoblata, nevus sebaceus, herpes simplex, radiation dermatitis, lichen simplex chronicus, insect and tick bites, venipuncture and vaccination sites, thermal burns, nitrogen mustard patch testing, erythema multiforme, epidermolysis bullosa dystrophica, pemphigus foliaceus, discoid lupus erythematosus and lepromatous leprosy.[4,5] KAs have also been documented in conjunction with other neoplasms and neoplastic syndromes such as Muir–Torre syndrome, xeroderma pigmentosum, in nevus sebaceous and in florid cutaneous papillomatosis.

CLINICAL FEATURES

KA is a lesion that undergoes three phases: proliferation, maturation and regression. These phases correlate with both its clinical and histological appearance. As is the case with most neoplasms, the KA starts as a macule but soon evolves into a papule and nodule. In the early proliferative phase, KA appears as a flesh-toned to pink bud, dome, or berry-shaped papule that grows rapidly over the course of several weeks into a firm nodule that often has scale on its top. During maturation phase, a central, firmly embedded keratin plug develops. This plug may appear verrucous, may grow to resemble a cutaneous horn, or may become more darkly pigmented with the appearance of a necrotic center. The firmly embedded keratinous plug cannot be dislodged with ease. Often there is bilateral cutaneous lipping around the horn that may be erythematous and/or display telangiectasias. The periphery of the lesion may also be erythematous and slopes down to merge with the surrounding normal skin.

The tumor is usually not fixed to deeper structures (Figs 32.1, 32.2). In the regression phase, the lesion involutes and eventually expels its keratinous center (Fig. 32.3a, b). During this phase the plug often appears as a blackish keratinous crust. Regression usually results initially in a saucer-shaped depression when the plug is dislodged; this evolves into an atrophic, hypopigmented, depressed scar (Fig. 32.4). Although a KA may persist for years, it often traverses its entire lifecycle within 2–6 months. For a synopsis of the clinical characteristics and time-line, see Table 32.2. Although KA has many forms, they are all variations on this template of growth characteristics and clinical appearance.

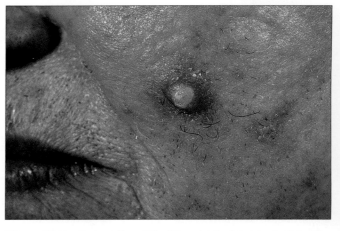

Figure 32.1 Early solitary KA of the cheek. (Image courtesy of New York University Department of Dermatology.)

Solitary keratoacanthoma

Solitary KA (Figs 32.1–32.4) is the most common form of this tumor. It occurs most often on the sun-exposed, hair-bearing skin, especially the face and dorsal hands, of adults with fair complexion. Solitary KA has the classic appearance (described above) of a rapidly growing hemispheric nodule with central keratin filled crater that spontaneously regresses over a period of months. It most commonly occurs as a single lesion but there can be several lesions or additional lesion formation over the course of the patient's lifetime. These lesions are usually asymptomatic, although local pruritus and pain have been reported.[46] The appearance of multiple KAs should trigger an investigation into one of the syndromes described below.

Giant keratoacanthoma

A KA is considered giant if it grows larger than 3 cm in diameter (Fig. 32.5a, b). Giant KA may grow to 10 cm while retaining the proportions of its smaller, solitary cousin. This giant nodule is a clinically impressive tumor whose height may be several centimeters from the plane of surrounding skin. Giant KA may be locally invasive and disfiguring or may remain superficially situated. In spite of its size, giant KA can still demonstrate complete, spontaneous regression.

Keratoacanthoma centrifugum

Keratoacanthoma centrifugum, also called keratoacanthoma centrifugum marginatum, is a rare, large lesion demonstrating a plaque-like appearance with central clearing and scarring. The diameter is similar to or larger than a giant KA, but the proportions have changed so that the lesion is flat and atrophic in the center with a raised rim that grows outwards and demonstrates keratin production. There are reports of lesions greater than 20 cm in diameter at time of excision.[47] KA centrifugum

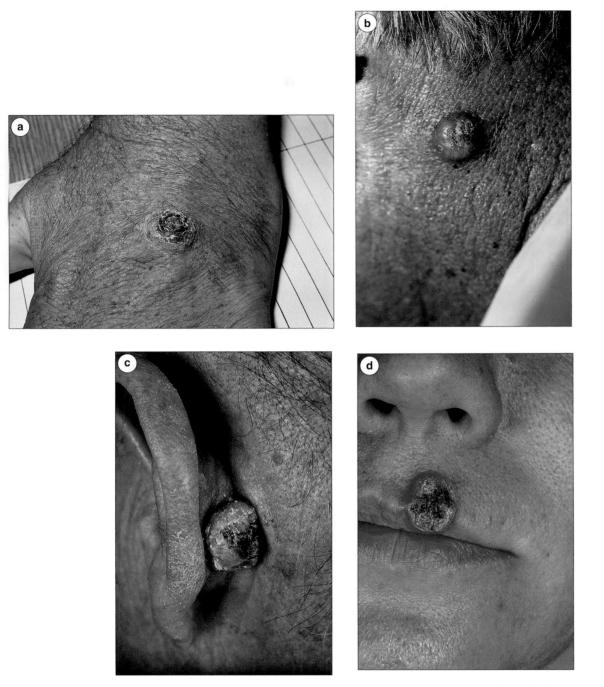

Figure 32.2 (a) Fully developed solitary KA of the dorsal hand. (Image courtesy of James Rosokoff MD.) (b) Fully developed solitary KA of the posterior neck. (Image courtesy of James Rosokoff MD.) (c) Fully developed solitary KA of the dorsal ear. (d) Fully developed solitary KA of the upper lip. (Image courtesy of New York University Department of Dermatology.)

often do not regress and can pose a significant therapeutic challenge.

Multinodular keratoacanthoma

Multinodular KA (Fig. 32.6) is an expanding plaque with several overlapping foci of KA at the periphery. Like keratoacanthoma centrifugum, this lesion can have central atrophic clearing and is unlikely to spontaneously regress. Unlike keratoacanthoma centrifugum, the advancing

peripheral border is composed of individual nodules of KA instead of one annular lesion.[48]

Subungual keratoacanthoma and distal digital keratoacanthoma

Subungual KA is a rare tumor derived from the nail bed. Unlike solitary KA, which usually regresses and remains superficially situated, subungual KAs cause significant tissue destruction and do not regress. These lesions

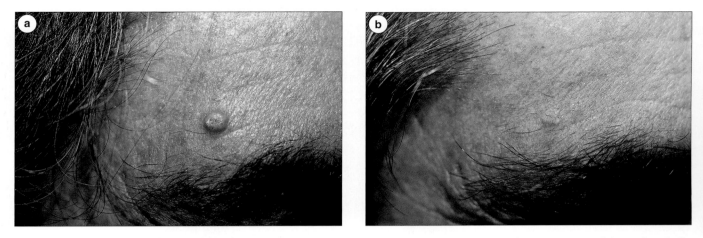

Figure 32.3 (a) Evolving KA of the forehead and (b) resolving KA of the forehead several months later. (Image courtesy of James Rosokoff MD.)

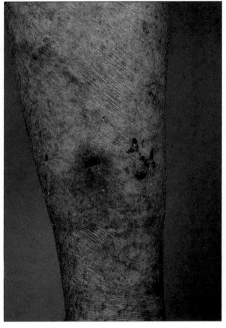

Figure 32.4 Almost completely spontaneously resolved KA of the leg. (Image courtesy of New York University Department of Dermatology.)

classically cause cup-shaped osteolysis without periosteal reaction in the underlying distal phalanx due to pressure erosion. Other symptoms include local swelling, erythema, pain, nail bed deformity and in some cases, drainage or bacterial superinfection.[49] These lesions may occur on the proximal nail fold and may involve nails of the fingers or toes, although they are seen most often on the thumb, index and middle fingers of patients in the third through seventh decades.[5] Distal digital KAs (Fig. 32.7) that do not involve the nail plate may still demonstrate local tissue destruction possibly because of the limited area for tumor growth.

Keratoacanthoma dyskeratoticum and segrecans

Clinically, keratoacanthoma dyskeratoticum and segrecans may only be differentiated by a serous exudate from the central keratin plug or moistening of the central plug, which is usually dry in solitary KA. This variant is distinguished histologically by the presence of significant dyskeratosis and acantholysis, features that mimic adenoid SCC.

Aggressive keratoacanthoma

In certain locations, such as the nose, lips, ears and eyelids, the KA can be destructive both during its proliferative phase as well as during regression (Figs 32.2d, 32.6, 32.7). In immunosuppressed patients, the natural course of KA has also been reported to lead to significant morbidity and destruction of normal tissue. KAs that occur on the distal digits are usually so destructive they are considered as a distinct subtype of KA.

Verrucous keratoacanthoma

Some KAs have a verrucous surface and lack the more common cup-shaped central invagination. There is still overlying keratotic material. This type of verrucous KA may be more common in multiple KA syndromes.

Multiple keratoacanthoma syndromes

Multiple persistent keratoacanthomas
In this non-familial presentation, several KAs may be present simultaneously and the lesions are slow to heal. In a lifetime, the patient may develop several outbreaks of these slow-healing lesions (Fig. 32.8).

Ferguson-Smith type keratoacanthomas
Multiple KA of Ferguson-Smith is an autosomal dominant disorder seen mostly in males (3:1 predominance) with an onset in the second and third decades of life. The lesions occur first in small crops and are self-healing with scar formation. The lesions tend to reoccur periodically throughout life and later developing lesions have a lower tendency to spontaneously regress.

Table 32.2   Growth characteristics for solitary keratoacanthoma

Stage	Time-frame	Size	Morphology
Rapid growth	2–8 weeks	10–25 mm	Macule evolves to firm, smooth papule then forms central keratinous core
Maturation	2–8 weeks	10–25 mm diameter × 5–10 mm in height	Skin-toned to erythematous, hemispheric nodule with firmly embedded keratin plug
Resolution	2–8 weeks, although some lesions persist for years	Diminishing	Expulsion of keratin plug and resorption of tumor, leaving atrophic scar

Adapted from Straka and Grant-Kels.[4]

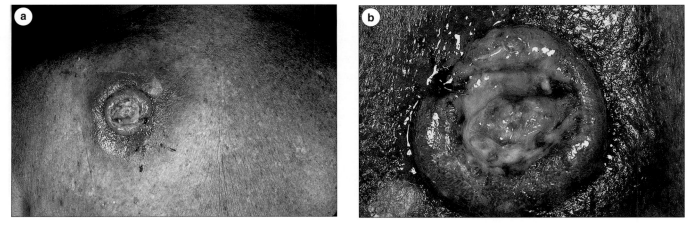

Figure 32.5   (a–b) Giant KA of the upper back. (Images courtesy of New York University Department of Dermatology.)

Generalized eruptive keratoacanthomas of Grzybowski

Grzybowski first described a form of eruptive KAs in which thousands of small, 1–5 mm KAs appear simultaneously or progressively. The lesions are more concentrated on sun-exposed skin but also involve the oral mucosa, larynx and intertriginous areas.[50] The lesions can appear in groups or clusters and demonstrate koebnerization. Because of severe facial involvement and resultant scarring, patients exhibit masked facies and ectropion. This variant has been reported in white, Asian and black patients with equal incidence in men and women.

Witten and Zak type keratoacanthomas

In Witten and Zak type KAs, there is a combination of both Ferguson-Smith type lesions and the smaller, eruptive Grzybowski type lesions. This variant has been reported in multiple siblings of the same family.

PATIENT EVALUATION, DIAGNOSIS AND DIFFERENTIAL DIAGNOSIS

The approach to the patient begins with obtaining a complete medical history. The patient's overall health, timing of lesion development, sun exposure, family history of similar lesions and possible carcinogen exposure should be evaluated. The physical examination should include a careful investigation of the lesion as well as a full skin and mucosal examination to look for other lesions and palpation of regional lymph nodes. A biopsy is warranted, especially if the lesion does not have a classic appearance. Clinical differential diagnosis for solitary KA includes SCC (Table 32.3), cancer metastasis, verruca, any cutaneous horn, amelanotic melanoma and a giant molluscum contagiosum, while KA centrifugum may resemble granuloma annulare, hypertrophic lichen planus, or porokeratosis Mibelli and multiple KAs may rarely resemble atypical molluscum contagiosum. Incisional, excisional, or deep shave saucerization biopsy usually establishes the correct diagnosis. Once the lesion has been identified, the goal is eradication. If multiple lesions are present, or systemic therapy anticipated, then baseline lab work is appropriate. If there is no clinical evidence of metastasis, then a metastatic work-up is not indicated.

KAs rarely metastasize. However, when they do, the most common site of involvement is regional lymph nodes. Lymph node biopsies of metastatic KA have sometimes demonstrated preservation of a KA's architectural pattern in the metastasis and sometimes met criteria for squamous cell carcinoma. Other sites of metastasis include the lungs and mediastinum.[51] At least one death has been attributed solely to metastatic KA.[6]

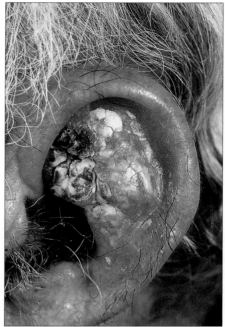

Figure 32.6
Multinodular KA of
the ear. (Image
courtesy of New
York University
Department of
Dermatology.)

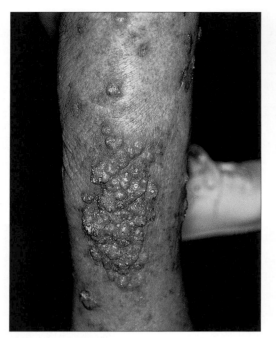

Figure 32.8 Multiple persistent KAs. (Image courtesy of Yale Dermatology Residency Collection.)

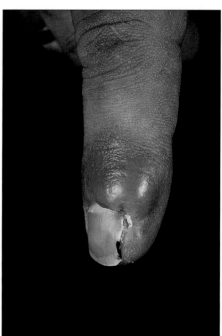

Figure 32.7
Subungual KA.

PATHOLOGY

The histologic diagnosis, similar to the clinical diagnosis of KA, is based on the architectural pattern of the lesion, which is best evaluated at scanning magnification. This is true at each stage of the lesion's evolution.

An early evolving papule of KA (Fig. 32.9) will usually demonstrate dome-shaped epidermal hyperplasia with a suggestion of a crater filled with ortho-keratotic and parakeratotic cells. Beneath this plugging there is endophytic and exophytic, often slightly papillated, epithelial hyperplasia that frequently resembles contiguous follicular infundibular hyperplasia. Mitotic figures are usually numerous. Within the sur-

rounding dermis there is a predominantly lymphocytic infiltrate.

Fully developed nodular lesions of KA (Fig. 32.10) demonstrate a unique architecture. The heart-shaped exophytic and endophytic lesion has a central horn-filled crater surrounded by bilateral epithelial lipping, beneath which is atypical pale staining epithelial hyperplasia. The crater is predominantly filled with cornified cells.

The squamous epithelium is composed of cells with large, hyperchromatic, pleomorphic nuclei with abundant pale staining cytoplasm. Marked cytologic atypia is common. Mitotic figures (typical and even atypical), multinucleated keratinocytes, necrotic and dyskeratotic keratinocytes and acantholytic keratinocytes are prominent. Abscesses of neutrophils often admixed with eosinophils are noted within the hyperplastic epidermis; these abscesses are often associated with acantholytic keratinocytes. At the sides and even base of the lesion there are frequently tongues of atypical squamous epithelium extending between collagen bundles. The surrounding dermis has a moderately dense mixed inflammatory cell infiltrate composed of lymphocytes, histiocytes, neutrophils, eosinophils and plasma cells.

Late, or resolving lesions of KA (Fig. 32.11) can clinically appear as horny lesions overlying a scar. The histologic counterpart to this cutaneous horn is the central horn filled crater now protruding about the skin surface. Remnants of epithelial lipping may still be identified to either side of this cornified cell mass. The underlying epidermis however is now usually atrophic with effacement of the normal rete ridge – dermal papillae pattern. Granulation tissue beneath the lesion ultimately is replaced with fibrosis.

There are no histologic findings that have been proven to predict biologic behavior. Numbers of mitotic figures, atypical mitotic figures, perineural invasion and

Table 32.3   Clinical features of keratoacanthoma and squamous cell carcinoma

Attribute	Keratoacanthoma	SCC
Growth pattern	Rapid growth followed by stationary phase	Slower growth that occurs indefinitely
Regression	Usually	No
Shape	Crateriform	Irregular
Border	Well-circumscribed	Ill-defined
Central portion	Keratotic plug	Necrosis and/or ulceration
Average age of onset	55	70
Adapted from Straka and Grant-Kels.[4]		

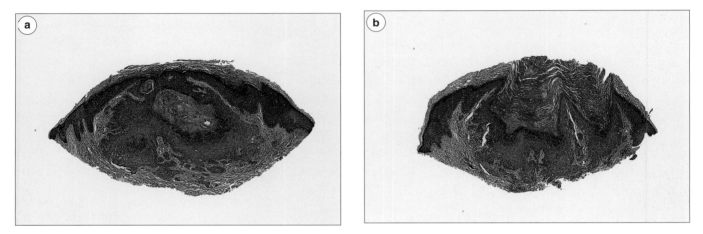

Figure 32.9   (a–b) Scanning magnification of an early evolving KA (×2.5; H&E).

extension into subcutaneous tissue do not appear to differentiate between those lesions that will involve spontaneously and those that will persist.

Some reported metastases of KA to the lymph node have retained the architectural and cytologic features of the primary fully developed lesion.[52]

DIFFERENTIAL DIAGNOSIS: SCC

The differentiation of KA from SCC (Table 32.4) has undergone a great deal of study. A study by Cribier *et al.* looked at 296 cases of either KA or SCC and concluded that even architectural patterns cannot always differentiate between these two lesions. In that study, criteria with the greatest significance were 'epithelial lip and sharp outline between tumor and stoma' favoring KA; 'ulceration, numerous mitoses and marked pleomorphism/anaplasia' favored SCC; while intra-epithelial microabscesses, extension more lateral than downward, parakeratosis and dyskeratosis and elastic fibers were not useful in differentiating.[53] The volume of experiments conducted in the area of marker studies precludes an in-depth discussion of each individual paper. Unfortunately, there is no single diagnostic marker study to date that can reliably differentiate KA from SCC (Table 32.5).[54–79]

TREATMENT

At one time, KA was considered a benign lesion that could be allowed to run its natural course to regression. It is now known that KA, while usually demonstrating a benign course, does have a limited tendency to metastasize and can additionally exhibit significant local tissue destruction. KAs also have a tendency to reoccur which is lessened with therapeutic intervention.[4] For all of these reasons, it is therefore recommended that KAs be treated. Preferred treatment options for KA vary with both the size and location of the lesion. Many treatments have been tried and reported. However, the lesion's tendency to spontaneously involute makes the comparative efficacy of treatment to placebo difficult to quantify.

Surgery

Excision of a KA allows for a controlled cosmetic outcome and is the treatment of choice. While there is a small risk of a new lesion developing in the scar, surgery limits the progression and invasion of the lesion and allows for definitive diagnosis. Mohs micrographic surgery has also met with good success in removal of lesions from the head and neck and of recurrent lesions.

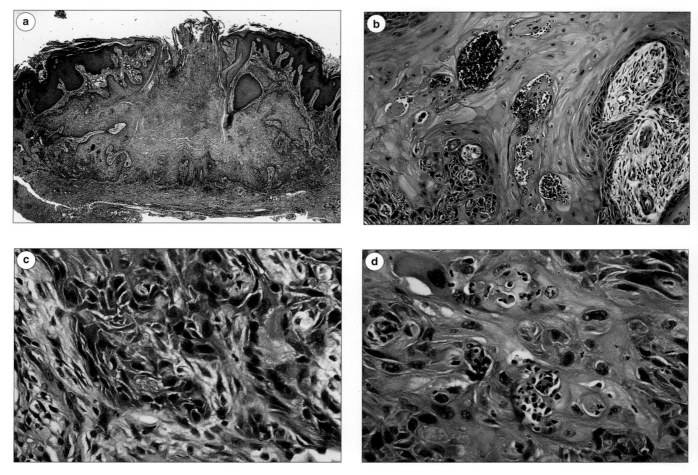

Figure 32.10 (a) Scanning magnification of a fully developed KA (×25; H&E). (b) Hyperplastic pale staining eosinophilic keratinocytes with intraepidermal abscesses (×25; H&E). (c) Tongues of atypical squamous epithelium between collagen bundles (×62.5; H&E). (d) Marked cytologic atypia and intraepidermal abscess (×62.5; H&E).

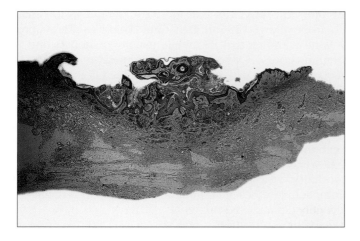

Figure 32.11 Scanning magnification of a resolving KA (×1; H&E).

Additionally, Mohs has been combined with topical or intralesional 5-fluorouracil (described below). Large lesions require surgical skill and possible skin grafting and multiple lesions may not be amenable to a surgical option.

Electrodesiccation and curettage

This modality of treatment has been used successfully, but it has two main drawbacks: (1) inadequate removal of tissue leads to reoccurrence up to 8% of the time[80] and (2) the resultant hypopigmented and depressed scar may be prominent.

Radiation therapy and topical photodynamic therapy

KAs are sensitive to radiation therapy, which is a viable treatment option. Additionally topical photodynamic therapy with delta aminolevulinic acid has been successful for solitary and giant KAs.[81]

Chemotherapy

Chemotherapeutic agents offer a convenient form of treatment and are an option for lesions too large or numerous for surgery. A disadvantage of chemotherapy,

Table 32.4 Histopathologic features of keratoacanthoma *vs* squamous cell carcinoma

Attribute	Keratoacanthoma	SCC
Growth pattern	Exophytic and endophytic	Endophytic predominantly
Shape	Central crater with surrounding lips of epithelium	Irregular
Central portion	Keratotic horn	Necrosis often with ulceration
Keratinization	Abundant pale staining keratinocytes	Keratinization and differentiation variable
Intraepidermal abscesses	Common within neoplasm	Rare
Acantholysis	Present in association with neutrophils and within intraepidermal abscesses	Present without neutrophils
Inflammation	Polymorphous inflammatory infiltrate with eosinophils and neutrophils; histiocytes and multinucleated histiocytes later	Lymphocytes and plasma cells predominate
Fibrosis beneath resolving lesions	Fibrosis beneath resolving lesions	Desmoplastic variant with thickened collagen bundles around tumor aggregates reported; fibrosis beneath lesion not usually noted

Adapted from Straka and Grant-Kels.[4]

shared by all modalities except excision, is that a definitive diagnosis cannot be made without additional biopsy.

5-Fluorouracil: Successful treatment with both intra-lesional and topical 5-fluorouracil (5-FU) is well established. Topical application is reported both with and without occlusion. Gray and Meland recommend that if daily application of 5% 5-FU cream is used, any lesion that does not respond to treatment in 3 weeks or resolve by 8 weeks should be excised. They also recommend that after involution, a 3-mm punch biopsy of the remaining base be taken to rule out residual squamous cell carcinoma.[81]

Methotrexate: Intralesional and oral methotrexate are reported and appear to be most efficacious if utilized during the growing phase of the KA.[82] Additionally, intramuscular methotrexate in conjunction with intramuscular triamcinolone acetonide has been reported.[83] Pancytopenia is a rare adverse reaction that can occur with even intralesional methotrexate and the incidence of hematologic reactions with low-dose systemic treatment is approximately 1.5–3.0%.[84]

Bleomycin: Intralesional bleomycin can be used, but pain has been associated with this treatment.[85]

Steroids: Intralesional hydrocortisone, triamcinolone and prednisolone are reported, with 70% of lesions regressing after 2–3 treatments in one study. Systemic steroid therapy is additionally reported with varying degrees of success.[85]

Interferon-alpha: Somlai and Hollo described intra- and peri-lesional INF-α, administered as a weekly 3 million IU dose, as effective treatment in a 6–15 week period.[86]

Podophyllin: Podophyllin has been reported as a single therapy and in conjunction with radiation therapy and cautery with curettage. It has several side effects including local effects of pain, swelling, conjunctivitis with chemosis and corneal ulceration (with eye contact) and contact dermatitis and systemic effects of fever, neurologic symptoms, sensitization and urticaria.[87]

Retinoids: Both etretinate and isotretinoin in oral doses of 1 mg/kg/day have been reported with good outcome in treatment of recurrent and multiple KA syndromes.[88] Maintenance oral therapy is also reported.

Imiquimod: There is limited data on the use of imiquimod for KAs. Dendrofer *et al.* have recently reported on four patients with solitary KAs of the face, all successfully treated with topical 5% imiquimod cream qod for 4–12 weeks.[89]

Subungual keratoacanthoma

Subungual and distal digital KA show less tendency to regress and often demonstrate significant local soft-tissue and bone involvement. For this reason, these lesions should be surgically removed when possible. There has also been a report of a patient with several KAs of the digits, successfully treated with systemic methotrexate.[49]

FUTURE OUTLOOK

KA remains a fascinating lesion. It shares many attributes of other skin cancers, such as increased incidence on sun exposed and elderly skin, while being unique both in its clinical appearance and its usual course of growth, cessation and spontaneous involution. Future research on genetic and environmental risk factors may uncover the pathway that leads not only to KA formation, but also the trigger for its regression. Perhaps further biochemical marker studies will also elucidate the relationship between KA and squamous cell carcinoma. Understanding the critical pathway steps leading to either resolution or to metastasis may uncover treatment options, perhaps even prophylactic treatment, for these and other malignant lesions.

Table 32.5   Marker studies comparing keratoacanthoma and squamous cell carcinoma

Marker	Findings	Author/Reference
Proliferating cell nuclear antigen (PCNA)	KAs demonstrated PCNA staining around the periphery of squamous nests, while SCCs had diffuse staining throughout the squamous nests	Phillips and Helm[54]
P53 and Ki-67	80% of both mature and regressing KAs were positive for p53; while 60% of the SCCs were also positive, differences in Ki-67 staining was not statistically significant	Kerschmann et al.[55]
Bcl-2	Proliferating KAs demonstrated weak basal layer staining for bcl-2, while involuting KAs had only rare basal cells staining positive and well-differentiated squamous cell carcinomas (WDSCC) showed diffuse, moderate staining	Sleater et al.[56]
Aneuploidy and p53	Aneuploidy found in 1/24 KAs and 12/21 SCCs; over-expression of p53 found in 14/24 KAs and 16/21 SCCs	Pilch et al.[57]
Trisomy 7	Trisomy 7 was found in 1/6 KAs, 1/8 squamous cell carcinomas with KA-like features (SCC-KA) and 2/7 well-differentiated squamous cell carcinomas (WDSCC)	Cheville et al.[58]
p53 protein and proliferating cell nuclear antigen (PCNA)	KAs had PCNA staining in basal cell layers, while WDSCC had a diffuse staining pattern and SCC-KA had an overlap of both patterns; p53 had basal, patchy and diffuse patterns in all groups	Cain et al.[59]
Desmoglein/Dsg	35/38 KAs positively stained in an extensive pericellular pattern, 5/38 stained in a focal pericellular pattern, 20/62 SCCs stained in a focal pericellular pattern, 31/62 had juxtanuclear staining and 11/62 had no staining	Krunic et al.[60]
c-erbB-2	1/5 KAs had few weakly positive cells, 4/5 did not stain, 20/24 SCCs stained positively	Ahmed et al.[61]
Collagenase-3 (MMP-13)	In 3/5 KAs a few individual cells at the edge of the lesions stained positively, while in 7/8 SCCs there were focal areas of positive staining, also at the tumor edge	Airola et al.[62]
Bcl-2 antagonist bak protein	All specimens of KAs and SCCs stained positively	Tomkova et al.[63]
Vinculin	5/5 KAs had intense, uniform, labeling; 5/6 SCC in situ had intense labeling, while 1/6 had weak labeling; 5/15 invasive SCC had no labeling, 6/15 had weak labeling and 4/15 had intense labeling; the pattern in SCCs was sometimes sporadic and sometimes uniform	Lifschitz-Mercer et al.[64]
Proliferating cell nuclear antigen (PCNA) and Le^Y	KAs showed variation in location and intensity of both PCNA and Le^Y expression depending on their stage of progression, while SCCs showed strong PCNA and Le^Y expression diffusely except for lack of PCNA in the horny layer and Le^Y in the basal layer	Tsuji[65]
Dsg	12/12 KAs demonstrated uniform pericellular staining, 5/24 SCCs had focal pericellular staining, 12/24 had weak juxtanuclear staining and 7/24 had no Dsg staining	Krunic et al.[66]
Volume-weighted mean nuclear volume	The volume-weighted nuclear volume of 18 KAs was 704.5±170.5 while that of 19 SCCs was 533.9±164.9	Binder et al.[67]
Ki-67 and mean nuclear volume	21/21 KAs demonstrated nuclear Ki-67 staining at the periphery of the squamous cells, while 21/21 SCCs demonstrated stained nuclei in a diffuse pattern; there was no statistically significant difference in mean nuclear volume	Sagol et al.[68]
HLA-A, B and DR	No difference in expression of HLA-A, B, or DR in 11 patients with KA and 9 patients with SCC	Lowes et al.[69]
Cytokine mRNA	KAs had increased IL-10 and decreased GM-CSF compared with SCCs; there was no difference in lymphotoxin-alpha, IL-2, IFN-gamma, IL-13, TGF-beta, IL-8, or TNF-alpha	Lowes et al.[70]
Sialyl-Tn/STn	16/27 KA basaloid tumor cells were at least weakly positive for STn, while only 3/29 SCCs were positive in the same cell areas; also keratinized, differentiated tumor cells were positive in 89% of KAs and only 31% of SCCs	Lensen et al.[71]
Stromelysin 3	22% of KAs, 47% of SCCs and 70% of metastatic SCCs were positive in the fibroblastic cells surrounding the tumor cells, without a differentiating staining pattern between the two lesions	Asch et al.[72]
Oncostatin M (OSM)	OSM expression in 20/21 (95%) of mature KAs, 4/7 (53%) of regressing KAs and 17/27 (63%) SCCs. OSM labeled macrophages in 4 per 3 high-power fields in KA and 7 per 3 high-power fields in SCC	Tran et al.[73]

Table 32.5   Marker studies comparing keratoacanthoma and squamous cell carcinoma—cont'd

Marker	Findings	Author/Reference
Small proline rich proteins SPRR-1,-2,-3	6/6 KAs and 4/4 SCCs were positive for all SPRR-1, -2, and -3; 11/11 SCCs *in situ* were positive for SPRR 1 and 2, while 6/11 were positive for SPRR 3	De Heller-Milev *et al.*[74]
Angiotensin type-1 receptor	77% of KAs and 8% of SCCs showed a 'negative periphery' pattern of staining for ATI receptor	Takeda and Kondo[75]
E-cadherin and α-, β-, and γ-catenin	'Classical' KAs demonstrated normal staining for these markers in 79–86% of cases and a pattern similar to well-differentiated SCC in the rest; 'borderline' KAs demonstrated abnormal staining in all cases, similar to poorly-differentiated SCC	Papadavid *et al.*[76]
Syndecan-1	Syndecan-1 expression was moderate to strong in all KAs, which mirrored adjacent epidermis and SCC *in situ*	Mukunyadzi *et al.*[77]
CD-95 (Fas)	2/2 keratoacanthomas and 6/8 SCCs demonstrated CD95 positivity at interfaces with lymphocytes	Filipowicz *et al.*[22]
Lamins A/C, B1 and B2	A/C antibody expressed in KA and well-differentiated SCC, A/C antibody expression diminished in poorly differentiated SCC; B-type lamins expressed at borders of KA in a few layers of cells while B-type lamin expressed in dispersed cells of well-differentiated SCC	Oguchi *et al.*[78]
Chromosomal aberrations via CGH	Genetic aberrations found in 25/70 (35.7%) KAs and 7/10 (70%) of SCCs	Clausen *et al.*[79]

REFERENCES

1 Ghadially FN. The role of hair follicle in origin and evolution of some cutaneous neoplasms in man and experimental animals. Cancer 1961; 14:801–816.

2 Hutchinson J. Morbid growths and tumors. 1. The crateriform ulcer of the face, a form of acute epithelial cancer. Trans Path Soc Lond 1989(40):275–281.

3 Ghadially R, Ghadially FN. Keratoacanthoma. In: Fitzpatrick TB, Eisen AZ, Wolff K et al. eds. Fitzpatrick's Dermatology in General Medicine, 5th edn. New York, NY: McGraw-Hill; 1999:865–871.

4 Straka BF, Grant-Kels JM. Keratoacanthoma. In: Friedman RJ, Rigel DS, Kopf AW, et al., eds. Cancer of the Skin. Philadelphia, PA: WB Saunders; 1991:390–407.

5 Schwartz RA. Keratoacanthoma. J Am Acad Derm 1994; 30:1–19.

6 Hodak E, Jones RE, Ackerman AB. Solitary keratoacanthoma is a squamous cell carcinoma: three examples with metastases. Am J Derm 1993; 15(4):332–342.

7 Rook A, Whimster I. Keratoacanthoma – a 30 year retrospect. Br J Derm 1979; 100:41–47.

8 Ferguson-Smith J. A case of primary squamous cell carcinoma of the skin in a young man with spontaneous healing. Br J Derm 1934; 46:267–313.

9 Gryzbowski M. A case of peculiar generalized epithelial tumours of the skin. Br J Derm Syph 1950; 62:310–313.

10 Miedzinski F, Kozakiewicz J. Das Keratoacanthoma centrifugum – eine besondere Varietät des Keratoacanthoms. Hauzarzt 1962; 13:348–352.

11 Stevanovic DV. Keratoacanthoma dyskeratoticum and segrecans. Arch Derm 1965; 170:666–669.

12 Webb AJ, Ghadially FN. Massive or giant keratoacanthoma. J Pathol Bacterio 1966; 91:505–509.

13 Ghadially FN, Barton BW, Kerridge DF. The etiology of keratoacanthoma. Cancer 1963; 16:603–611.

14 Kligman J, Callen JP. Keratoacanthoma: a clinical study. Arch Derm 1984; 120:736–740.

15 Chuang T, Reizner GT, Elpern DJ, et al. Keratoacanthoma in Kauai, Hawaii. Arch Derm 1993; 129:317–319.

16 Reizner GT, Chuang T, Elpern DJ, et al. Keratoacanthoma in Japanese Hawaiians in Kauai, Hawaii. Int J Derm 1995; 34:851–853.

17 Dufresne RG, Marrero MG, Robinson-Bostom L. Seasonal presentation of keratoacanthomas in Rhode Island. Br J Derm 1997; 36:227–229.

18 Kopf AW. Keratoacanthoma. In: Andrade R, Gumport SL, Popkin GL, et al., eds. Cancer of the Skin. Philadelphia: WB Saunders; 1976:755–781.

19 Tulvatana W, Pisarnkorskul P, Wanakrairot P. Solitary keratoacanthoma of the conjunctiva: report of a case. J Med Assoc Thai 2001; 84(7):1059–1064.

20 Gilbey S, Moore DH, Look KY, et al. Vulvar keratoacanthoma. Obstet Gynecol 1997; 89(5):848–850.

21 Silberg I, Kopf AW, Baer RL. Recurrent keratoacanthoma of the lip. Arch Derm 1962; 86:44–53.

22 Filipowicz E, Adegboyega P, Sanchez RL, et al. Expression of CD95 (Fas) in sun-exposed human skin and cutaneous carcinomas. Cancer 2002; 94(3):814–819.

23 Shaw JC, Storrs FJ, Everts E. Multiple keratoacanthomas after megavoltage radiation therapy. J Am Acad Derm 1990; 23:1009–1011.

24 Baer RL, Kopf AW. Complications of therapy of basal cell epitheliomas. In:Yearbook in Dermatology, 1964–1965. Chicago: Year Book Medical; 1965:7–25.

25 Sina B, Adrian RM. Multiple keratoacanthomas possibly induced by psoralens and ultraviolet A photochemotherapy. J Am Acad Derm 1983; 9:686–688.

26 Gwertzman A, Meirson DH, Rabinovitz H. Eruptive keratoacanthomas following carbon dioxide laser resurfacing. Derm Surg 1999; 25(8):666–668.

27 Pattee S, Silvis NG. Keratoacanthoma developing in sites of previous trauma: a report of two cases and review of the literature. J Am Acad Derm 2003; 48:S35–S38.

28 Ghadially FN. A comparative morphologic study of the keratoacanthoma of man and similar experimentally produced lesions in the rabbit. J Pathol Bacteriol 1958; 75:441–453.

29 Ghadially FN. The experimental production of keratoacanthomas in the hamster and mouse. J Pathol Bacteriol 1959; 77:277–282.

30 Ridgon RH. Keratoacanthoma experimentally produced with methylcholanthrene in the chicken. Arch Derm 1959; 79:139–147.

31 Whiteley HJ. The effect of the hair growth cycle on experimental skin carcinogenesis in the rabbit. Br J Cancer 1957; 11:196–205.

32 El-Hakim IE, Uthman MAE. Squamous cell carcinoma and keratoacanthoma of the lower lip associated with 'Goza' and 'Shisa' smoking. Int J Derm 1999; 38:108–110.

33 Letzel S, Drexler H. Occupationally related tumors in tar refinery workers. J Am Acad Derm 1998; 39(5):712–720.

34 Ereaux LP, Schopflocher P, Fournier CJ. Keratoacanthomata. Arch Derm 1955; 71:73–83.

35 Zelickson AS, Lynch FW. Electron microscopy of virus-like particles in keratoacanthoma. J Invest Derm 1961; 37:79–83.

36 Gay Preito J, Perez PR, Huertos MR, et al. On the virus etiology of keratoacanthoma. Acta Derm Venereol (Stockh) 1964; 44:180.

37 Fisher ER, McCoy MM, Wechsler HL. Analysis of histopathologic and electron microscopic determinants of keratoacanthoma and squamous cell carcinoma. Cancer 1972; 29:1387–1397.

38 Stockfleth E, Meinke B, Arndt R, et al. Identification of DNA sequences of both genital and cutaneous HPV types in a small number of keratoacanthoma of nonimmunosuppressed patients. Dermatology 1999; 198:122–123.

39 Ramselaar CG, Meer JB van der. The spontaneous regression of keratoacanthoma in man. Acta Derm Venereol (Stockh) 1976; 56:245–251.

40 Patel A, Halliday GM, Cooke BE, et al. Evidence that regression in keratoacanthoma is immunologically mediated: a comparison with squamous cell carcinoma. Br J Derm 1994; 131:789–798.

41 Gualde N, Bonnetblanc JM, Malinvand G. HLA antigens and keratoacanthoma. Tissue Antigens 1981; 17:349–350.

42 Machin P, Catasus L, Pons C, et al. Microsatellite instability and immunostaining for MSH-2 and MLH-1 in cutaneous and internal tumors from patient with Muir–Torre syndrome. J Cutan Pathol 2002; 29(7):415–420.

43 Langenbach N, Kroiss MM, Rüschoff J, et al. Assessment of microsatellite instability and loss of heterozygosity in sporadic keratoacanthomas. Arch Derm Res 1999; 291(1):1–5.

44 Peng X, Griffith JW, Han R, et al. Development of keratoacanthomas and squamous cell carcinomas in transgenic rabbits with targeted expression of EJras oncogene in epidermis. Am J Pathol 1999; 155(1):315–324.

45 Hu W, Cook T, Oh WC, et al. Expression of the cyclin-dependent kinase inhibitor p27 in keratoacanthoma. J Am Acad Derm 2000; 42:473–475.

46 Frank TL, Maguire HC Jr, Greenbaum SS. Multiple painful keratoacanthomas. Int J Derm 1996; 35(9):648–650.

47 Weedon D, Barnetti L. Keratoacanthoma centrifugum marginatum. Arch Derm 1975; 111:1024–1026.

48 Sardana K, Sarkar R, Kumar V, et al. Multinodular keratoacanthoma: a rare but definite entity. Int J Derm 2002; 41:905–907.

49 Baran R, Goettmann S. Distal digital keratoacanthoma: a report of 12 cases and review of the literature. Br J Derm 1998; 139(3):512–515.

50 Consigli JE, González ME, Morsino R, et al. Generalized eruptive keratoacanthoma (Grzybowski variant). Br J Derm 2000; 142:800–803.

51 Alyahya GA, Heegaard S, Prause JU. Malignant changes in a giant orbital keratoacanthoma developing over 25 years. Acta Ophthalmol Scand 2000; 78:223–225.

52 Piscioli F, Boi S, Zumiani G, et al. A gigantic metastasizing keratoacanthoma. Am J Derm 1984; 6:123–129.

53 Cribier B, Asch P, Grosshans E. Differentiating squamous cell carcinoma from keratoacanthoma using histopathological criteria. Is it possible? A study of 296 cases. Dermatology 1999; 199(3):208–212.

54 Phillips P, Helm KF. Proliferating cell nuclear antigen distribution in keratoacanthoma and squamous cell carcinoma. J Cutan Pathol 1993; 20:424–428.

55 Kerschmann RL, McCalmont TH, LeBoit PE. p53 oncoprotein expression and proliferation index in keratoacanthoma and squamous cell carcinoma. Arch Derm 1994; 130:181–186.

56 Sleater JP, Beers BB, Stephens CA, et al. Keratoacanthoma: a deficient squamous cell carcinoma? Study of bcl-2 expression. J Cutan Pathol 1994; 21:514–519.

57 Pilch H, Weiss J, Heubner C, et al. Differential diagnosis of keratoacanthomas and squamous cell carcinomas: diagnostic value of DNA image cytometry and p53 expression. J Cutan Pathol 1994; 21:507–513.

58 Cheville JC, Bromley C, Argenyi ZB. Trisomy 7 in keratoacanthoma and squamous cell carcinoma detected by fluorescence in-situ hybridization. J Cutan Pathol 1995; 22:546–550.

59 Cain CT, Niemann TH, Zrgenyi ZB. Keratoacanthoma versus squamous cell carcinoma: an immunohistochemical reappraisal of p53 protein and proliferating cell nuclear antigen expression in keratoacanthoma-like tumors. Am J Derm 1995; 17(4):324–331.

60 Krunic AL, Garrod DR, Smith NP, et al. Differential expression of desmosomal glycoproteins in keratoacanthoma and squamous cell carcinoma of the skin: an immunohistochemical aid to diagnosis. Acta Derm Venereol 1996; 76(5):394–398.

61 Ahmed NU, Ueda M, Ichihashi M. Increased level of c-erbB-2/neu/HER-2 protein in cutaneous squamous cell carcinoma. Br J Derm 1997; 136(6):908–912.

62 Airola K, Johansson N, Kariniemi AL, et al. Human collagenase-3 is expressed in malignant squamous epithelium of the skin. J Invest Derm 1997; 109(2):225–231.

63 Tomkova H, Fujimoto W, Arata J. Expression of bcl-2 antagonist bak in inflammatory and neoplastic skin diseases. Br J Derm 1997; 137(5):703–708.

64 Lifschitz-Mercer B, Czernobilsky B, Feldberg E, et al. Expression of the adherens junction protein vinculin in human basal and squamous cell tumors: relationship to invasiveness and metastatic potential. Hum Pathol 1997; 28(11):1230–1236.

65 Tsuji T. Keratoacanthoma and squamous cell carcinoma: study of PCNA and LeY expression. J Cutan Pathol 1997; 24:409–415.

66 Krunic AL, Garrod DR, Madani S, et al. Immunohistochemical staining for desmogleins 1 and 2 in keratinocytic neoplasms with squamous phenotype: actinic keratosis, keratoacanthoma and squamous cell carcinoma of the skin. Br J Cancer 1998; 77(8):1275–1279.

67 Binder M, Steiner A, Mossbacher U, et al. Estimation of volume-weighted mean nuclear volume discriminates keratoacanthoma from squamous cell carcinoma. Am J Derm 1998; 20(5):453–458.

68 Sagol Ö, Kurtoglu B, Özer E, et al. Stereological estimation of mean nuclear volume and staining pattern of Ki-67 antigen in keratoacanthomas and squamous cell carcinomas. Gen Diagn Pathol 1997; 98(143):305–309.

69 Lowes MA, Dunckley H, Watson N, et al. Regression of melanoma, but not keratoacanthoma, is associated with increased HLA-B22 and decreased HLA-B27 and HLA-DR1. Melanoma Res 1999; 9:539–544.

70 Lowes MA, Bishop GA, Cooke BE, et al. Keratoacanthomas have an immunosuppressive cytokine environment of increased IL-10 and decreased GM-CSF compared to squamous cell carcinomas. Br J Cancer 1999; 80(10):1501–1505.

71 Jensen P, Clausen OPF, Bryne M. Differences in sialyl-Tn antigen expression between keratoacanthomas and cutaneous squamous cell carcinomas. J Cutan Pathol 1999; 26:183–189.

72 Asch PH, Basset P, Roos M, et al. Expression of stromelysin 3 in keratoacanthoma and squamous cell carcinoma. Am J Derm 1999; 21(2):146–150.

73 Tran TA, Ross JS, Shehan CE, et al. Comparison of oncostatin M expression in keratoacanthoma and squamous cell carcinoma. Mod Pathol 2000; 13(4):427–432.

74 Heller-Milev M De, Huber M, Panizzon R, et al. Expression of small proline rich proteins in neoplastic and inflammatory skin diseases. Br J Derm 2000; 143(4):733–740.

75 Takeda H, Kondo S. Differences between squamous cell carcinoma and keratoacanthoma in angiotensin type-1 receptor expression. Am J Pathol 2001; 158(5):1633–1637.

76 Papadavid E, Pignatelli M, Zakynthinos S, et al. The potential role of abnormal E-cadherin and alpha-, beta- and gamma-catenin immunoreactivity in determination of the biological behaviour of keratoacanthoma. Br J Derm 2001; 145(4):582–589.

77 Mukunyadzi P, Sanderson RD, Fan CY, et al. The level of syndecan-1 expression is a distinguishing feature in behavior between keratoacanthoma and invasive cutaneous squamous cell carcinoma. Mod Pathol 2002; 15(1):45–49.

78 Oguchi M, Sagara J, Matsumoto K, et al. Expression of lamins depends on epidermal differentiation and transformation. Br J Derm 2002; 147(5):853–858.

79 Clausen O, Beigi M, Bolund L, et al. Keratoacanthomas frequently show chromosomal aberrations as assessed by comparative genomic hybridization. J Invest Derm 2002; 119(6):1367–1372.

80 Gray RJ, Meland NB. Topical 5-fluorouracil as primary therapy for keratoacanthoma. Ann Plast Surg 2000; 44(1):82–85.

81 Radakovic-Fijan S, Honigsmann H, Tanew A. Efficacy of topical photodynamic therapy of a giant keratoacanthoma demonstrated by partial irradiation. Br J Derm 1999; 141(5):936–938.

82 Spieth K, Gille J, Kaufmann R. Intralesional methotrexate as effective treatment in solitary giant keratoacanthoma of the lower lip. Dermatology 2000; 200:317–319.

83 Santoso-Pham JC, Shelley ED, Shelley WB. Aggressive giant keratoacanthoma of the face treated with intramuscular methotrexate and triamcinolone acetonide (abstract). Cutis 1997; 59(6):329–332.

84 Goebeler M, Lurz C, Kolve-Goebeler ME, Brocker EB. Pancytopenia after treatment of keratoacanthoma by single lesional methotrexate infiltration. Arch Derm 2001; 137(8):1104–1105.

85 Sanders S, Busam KJ, Halpern AC, et al. Intralesional corticosteroid treatment of multiple eruptive keratoacanthomas: case report and review of a controversial therapy. Derm Surg 2002; 28(10):954–958.

86 Somlai B, Hollo P. Use of interferon-alpha (IFN-alpha) in the treatment of keratoacanthoma (abstract). Hautarzt 2000; 51(3):173–175.

87 Cipollaro VA. The use of podophyllin in the treatment of keratoacanthoma. Int J Derm 1983; 22:436–440.

88 Ogasawara Y, Kinoshita E, Ishida T, et al. A case of multiple keratoacanthoma centrifugum marginatum: response to oral etretinate. J Am Acad Derm 2003; 48:282–285.

89 Dendorfer M, Oppel T, Wollenberg A, et al. Topical treatment with imiquimod may induce regression of facial keratoacanthoma. Eur J Derm 2003; 13(1):80–82.

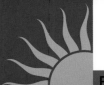

CHAPTER

33 Pseudolymphomas of the Skin

Helmut Kerl and Lorenzo Cerroni

Key points

- Cutaneous pseudolymphomas are benign inflammatory skin diseases that mimic malignant lymphomas either clinically, histopathologically, or both.
- Many disorders included in the past among the cutaneous pseudolymphomas represent in reality examples of low-grade malignant cutaneous lymphomas.
- Integration of clinical, histopathologic, immunophenotypic and molecular genetic features is crucial for the diagnosis of cutaneous pseudolymphomas.
- Cutaneous pseudolymphomas should be classified precisely according to specific clinicopathologic entities.

INTRODUCTION

Pseudolymphomas of the skin are benign lymphocytic proliferations that simulate cutaneous malignant lymphomas clinically and/or histopathologically.[1] The term pseudolymphoma is not specific but is merely descriptive. It does not refer to any particular disease but rather to a heterogeneous group of inflammatory conditions and benign 'tumors' of diverse causes. For proper treatment it is important to identify these lesions more precisely and specifically.

HISTORY: CLASSIFICATION

Cutaneous pseudolymphomas have been known for a long time.[2,3] The prototype of these lesions represents so-called lymphocytoma/lymphadenosis benigna cutis, which is a benign cutaneous infiltration of B-lymphocytes that can arise in reaction to several antigenic stimuli. In recent years, many inflammatory skin diseases have been added to the group of the cutaneous pseudolymphomas, mainly because of the presence of histopathologic features similar to those observed in malignant lymphomas of the skin.[1,4] On the other hand, 'transformation' of cutaneous pseudolymphomas into overt malignant lymphomas has been described in several instances as well, casting doubts as to the exact nature of at least some of these disorders.

In fact, several entities classified in the past as cutaneous pseudolymphoma have been re-classified as low-grade malignant lymphomas based on clinico-pathologic and genetic features, as well as on follow-up data. For example, lymphomatoid papulosis, which was listed as cutaneous pseudolymphomas in the past, has been now included in the group of primary cutaneous T-cell lymphomas proposed by the European Organization for Research and Treatment of Cancer (EORTC) as well as in the classification of hematological malignancies published by the World Health Organization (WHO). Likewise, one of the patients depicted in Kerl and Smolle[5] as representing an example of 'lymphadenosis benigna cutis' (Fig. 33.1) was later found to have in reality a cutaneous marginal zone B-cell lymphoma with a specific chromosomal translocation (14;18)(q32;q21). Nonetheless, most of the diseases reported as 'pseudolymphoma' in the past do represent benign reactive skin disorders and they need to be clearly separated from cutaneous malignant lymphomas.

Table 33.1 shows a modern clinicopathologic classification of conditions that are currently viewed as cutaneous pseudolymphomas.

EPIDEMIOLOGY

There are no exact data concerning the incidence, prevalence and geographic distribution of cutaneous pseudolymphomas. Cutaneous pseudolymphomas induced by

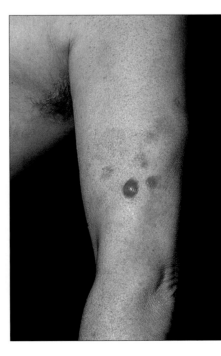

Figure 33.1
Cutaneous marginal zone B-cell lymphoma.

Table 33.1   Classification of cutaneous pseudolymphomas

Simulated malignant lymphoma	Clinicopathologic entity
Mycosis fungoides/Sézary syndrome	• Actinic reticuloid • Lymphomatoid contact dermatitis • Lymphomatoid drug reaction, T-cell type • Solitary T-cell pseudolymphoma ('unilesional mycosis fungoides') • Lichenoid ('lymphomatoid') keratosis • Lichenoid pigmented purpuric dermatitis (including lichen aureus) • Lichen sclerosus et atrophicus
Lymphomatoid papulosis/Anaplastic large cell lymphoma – CD30+	• Atypical lymphoid infiltrates (CD30+) associated with: – Orf–Milker's nodule – Herpes simplex/Zoster – Molluscum contagiosum – Arthropod reactions including nodular scabies
Subcutaneous T-cell lymphoma	• Lupus panniculiti
Follicle center cell lymphoma Marginal zone B-cell lymphoma Diffuse large B-cell lymphoma	• Lymphocytoma cutis
Follicle center cell lymphoma	• Lymphomatoid drug reaction, B-cell type
Marginal zone B-cell lymphoma	• Pseudolymphoma after vaccination • Pseudolymphoma in tattoos • Pseudolymphoma caused by *Hirudo medicinalis* therapy
Marginal zone B-cell lymphoma	• Morphea, inflammatory stage • Syphilis (secondary)
Chronic lymphocytic leukemia, B-cell type	• Lymphocytic infiltration Jessner–Kanof
Plasmacytoma	• Inflammatory pseudotumor
Marginal zone B-cell lymphoma	• 'Acral pseudolymphomatous angiokeratoma' (small papular pseudolymphoma)

the spirochetal microorganism *Borrelia burgdorferi* (i.e. *Borrelia* lymphocytoma) commonly arise in regions with endemic *Borrelia burgdorferi* infection. However, there is an increasing number of tourism-associated diseases and typical lesions of *Borrelia* lymphocytoma can be observed also in countries where *Borrelia* species are absent, in patients returning from travels in endemic regions.

PATIENT EVALUATION, DIAGNOSIS AND DIFFERENTIAL DIAGNOSIS

The clinical manifestations of cutaneous pseudolymphomas are variable (Table 33.2). The lesions are often solitary, but they may be regionally clustered or generalized in distribution. Usually nodules or tumors are present, but there may be macules, miliary papules, or plaques. They frequently reveal a smooth surface and vary in color from pink to deeper hues of red, including plum; some may be red-brown. Cutaneous pseudolymphomas may also show the features of generalized erythroderma. The course of pseudolymphomas varies considerably. The lesions may persist for weeks, months, or even years; they may resolve spontaneously and they may recur unpredictably.

For the histologic diagnosis of cutaneous pseudolymphomas it is necessary to have criteria of proven accuracy in order to avoid overdiagnosis of pseudolymphoma and

underdiagnosis of malignant lymphoma. Histologic diagnosis of cutaneous pseudolymphomas depends upon two considerations: (1) the architectural patterns of the infiltrates, which can be studied only in adequate biopsy specimens, and (2) the cellular composition of those infiltrates, which frequently shows a mixed character. Histologic features should be integrated by phenotypic data that can be obtained on routinely-fixed, paraffin-embedded sections of tissue.[6]

The recent introduction of polymerase chain reaction analysis of the T-cell receptor and immunoglobulin heavy chain (IgH) genes allows checking of the clonality of cutaneous T- and B-cell infiltrates, respectively.[7] Malignant lymphomas reveal a monoclonal population of lymphocytes, whereas pseudolymphomas show a polyclonal infiltrate. In this context, it must be underlined that differentiation of benign from malignant lymphoid infiltrates of the skin is possible only upon careful synthesis and integration of clinical features with histopathologic, immunophenotypic and molecular data. In some cases follow-up is an essential diagnostic guiding principle for patients with such lesions.

Cutaneous T-cell lymphoma *vs* T-cell pseudolymphoma

Mycosis fungoides, the most frequent type of cutaneous lymphoma, must be differentiated from benign inflam-

Table 33.2 Criteria for the diagnosis of cutaneous B-cell pseudolymphomas

Clinical features	• Papules, plaques or nodules • Usually solitary (sometimes multiple, example: lymphomatoid drug reaction) • Smooth surface, ulceration rare • Favored sites: face (nose, earlobe), mammary region, scrotum, arms • Recurrences: rarely • Extracutaneous involvement: absent • Prognosis: excellent
Histopathology	• Symmetrical, wedge-shaped dense nodular or diffuse infiltrates • Mixed cellular infiltrates (including plasma cells, histiocytes, and eosinophils) • Germinal centers frequently present: zonal architecture of germinal centers, regular shapes, marginated sharply by surrounding mantle zone lymphocytes, presence of tingible body macrophages
Immunohistology	• Immunoglobulin light chains: polyclonal pattern • Germinal centers: high proliferation rate (Ki-67/MIB-1) • Bcl-2 negative, MT-2 negative • Bcl-6/CD-10 positive cells not outside of follicles • Regular pattern of CD21-positive dendritic cells
Genotype	• Immunoglobulin heavy chain gene rearrangement: absent in most cases

matory conditions that may simulate it either clinically, histologically, or both. The diagnosis of mycosis fungoides in early stages and differentiation from benign reactive infiltrates often cannot be achieved without correlation of the histologic features with the clinical picture. Clinical features that are helpful in the differential diagnosis of mycosis fungoides from benign inflammatory dermatoses are location on sun-protected areas such as the buttocks, presence of lesions with different morphological aspects and history of long-standing lesions that do not tend to regress without treatment. The main histopathologic criteria for diagnosis of early lesions of mycosis fungoides include the following:[4] band-like or patchy lichenoid infiltrate of lymphocytes in the papillary dermis; thickened, fibrotic papillary dermis; coarse bundles of collagen in the papillary dermis; epidermotropic T-lymphocytes with nuclei that are larger than those of T-lymphocytes in the dermis; epidermotropic T-lymphocytes aligned along the basal layer of the epidermis; and intraepidermal collections of T-lymphocytes (so-called Pautrier's microabscesses). It must be underlined, however, that Pautrier's microabscesses are rare in early lesions of mycosis fungoides.

Most cases of mycosis fungoides show in the early phases a T-helper phenotype indistinguishable from that seen in benign chronic inflammatory dermatoses. Only a minority exhibit a T-suppressor lineage. It has been suggested that in early stages of mycosis fungoides, in

contrast to benign (inflammatory) cutaneous infiltrates of T-lymphocytes, there is a loss of expression of the T-cell-associated antigen CD7. However, this finding has not been confirmed by other studies showing normal CD7+ populations in early mycosis fungoides. In addition, T-lymphocytes in some cases of benign inflammatory dermatosis can also show partial loss of CD7. Therefore, the value of CD7 staining in the differential diagnosis of cutaneous T-cell infiltrates is still unclear.

Molecular analysis of T-cell receptor gene rearrangement is a further criterion helpful in the differentiation of MF from benign skin conditions.[8] However, it must be underlined that early lesions of MF reveal a monoclonal rearrangement only in about 50% of the cases and that several benign dermatoses have been shown to harbor a monoclonal population of T-lymphocytes (e.g. lichen planus, lichen sclerosus). Thus, as a rule the presence or absence of a monoclonal pattern of T-cell receptor gene rearrangement cannot be considered as a crucial criterion in the differentiation of mycosis fungoides from its simulators.

Cutaneous B-cell lymphoma *vs* B-cell pseudolymphoma

Most of the cutaneous B-cell lymphomas arising primary in the skin belong to the group of follicle center cell lymphoma and marginal zone B-cell lymphoma.[4] It may be difficult to differentiate them from benign infiltrates of B-lymphocytes. Clinical features that favor a diagnosis of cutaneous B-cell lymphoma are the presence of clusters of irregularly shaped reddish papules and nodules surrounded by erythematous patches and plaques. Typical locations are the head and neck and the trunk ('Crosti's reticulohistiocytoma of the back'). B-cell pseudolymphomas, in contrast, present commonly with solitary lesions, but exceptions to this rule are well known (i.e. drug-induced B-cell pseudolymphoma).

In lesions showing a follicular pattern, histopathologic features that suggest a diagnosis of cutaneous B-cell lymphoma are the monomorphism of the follicles, the lack of a well-formed mantle zone and the absence of tingible body macrophages.[9] It must be underlined that many cutaneous B-cell lymphomas, especially marginal zone B-cell lymphomas, reveal a mixed cell infiltrate with presence of plasma cells, eosinophils and sometimes small granulomas and that differentiation from reactive conditions can be very difficult on histopathologic grounds alone.

Immunohistochemical criteria for differentiation of benign from malignant infiltrates rely upon the analysis of the immunoglobulin light chains (κ and λ), which can be studied on routinely fixed, paraffin-embedded biopsy specimens.[6] Malignant cell populations of B-lymphocytes usually show a monoclonal restriction to either κ or λ light chain, whereas benign infiltrates exhibit a polyclonal pattern with expression of both light chains. Unfortunately, however, there are several cases of B-cell lymphoproliferative disorders, both benign and malignant, in which the cells do not express immunoglobulins.

A useful immunohistochemical criterion in malignant lymphoid infiltrates with a follicular pattern is the presence of CD10+ and/or Bcl-6+ clusters of cells outside the follicles.[6,9] In contrast, B-cell pseudolymphomas with a follicular pattern reveal a population of CD10+/Bcl-6+ cells confined to reactive germinal centers. Another important clue for the diagnosis of follicle center cell lymphoma with follicular growth pattern is the diminished proliferation activity of malignant germinal center cells as outlined by the Ki67/MIB-1 antibody. Reactive germinal centers show a high proliferation, whereas malignant ones often are characterized by a much lesser degree of positivity.

Molecular analysis of cutaneous B-cell lymphomas often reveals a monoclonal rearrangement of immunoglobulin heavy and light chain genes. However, it is not unusual that in cases of follicle center cell lymphoma a monoclonal rearrangement cannot be demonstrated. One possible explanation resides in the high number of somatic hypermutations found in these cases that may render the annealing of DNA primers impossible. Monoclonality of B-lymphocytes in B-cell pseudolymphomas is infrequent, but rare cases of otherwise typical *Borrelia burgdorferi*-associated lymphocytoma cutis with monoclonal rearrangement of the IgH gene have been observed. Recently, a chromosomal translocation (14;18) (q32;q21) involving *IGH* and *MALT1* has been detected in a subset of primary cutaneous marginal zone B-cell lymphomas.[10]

About 80–85% of follicular lymphomas and 15–30% of high-grade malignant non-Hodgkin's lymphomas in the lymph nodes are characterized by the t(14;18), which results in the production of higher amounts of *bcl-2* protein. Using the anti-*bcl-2* protein antibody 85% to 100% of the follicular lymphomas in the lymph nodes stain positive and negativity is considered as a diagnostic criterion of benign follicular hyperplasia rather than follicular lymphoma in the lymph nodes. Investigation of cutaneous cases demonstrated that the t(14;18) is rare in primary cutaneous B-cell lymphomas and that the majority of cutaneous follicle center cell lymphoma do not show expression of *bcl-2* protein by neoplastic cells.[9] Thus, although positivity of germinal center lymphocytes for *bcl-2* protein is synonymous with malignancy, in the skin *bcl-2* protein expression is less useful than other morphologic and immunophenotypic criteria for differentiation of follicle center cell lymphoma from B-pseudolymphoma with a follicular pattern.

The salient features of cutaneous B-cell pseudolymphomas are listed in Table 33.2.

SPECIFIC CLINICOPATHOLOGIC ENTITIES

Actinic reticuloid

The concept of chronic actinic dermatitis encompasses four chronic photodermatoses: persistent light reactivity, photosensitivity dermatitis, photosensitive eczema and actinic reticuloid.[11,12] Actinic reticuloid (Table 33.3) is a severe persistent photodermatitis that usually affects older men. The disease is characterized by extreme photosensitivity to a broad spectrum of UV radiation. Clinically and histologically it has many features of cutaneous

Table 33.3	Criteria for the diagnosis of actinic reticuloid
Clinical features	• Erythemas, lichenoid papules, and scaly plaques on uncovered skin • Erythroderma • Pruritus
Histopathology	• Band-like or patchy infiltrates of lymphocytes (often CD8-positive T-lymphocytes), histiocytes, and eosinophils • Atypical cells • Fibrosis
Pathogenesis	• Ultraviolet radiation

T-cell lymphoma. The patients present in the early stages erythemas on the face and neck and on dorsa of the hands. As the eruption progresses, it becomes lichenified and reddish-purple (Fig. 33.2). Sometimes scaly plaques develop on sites exposed to sunlight. In some areas the lesions may consist of lichenoid papules. The course may be characterized by recurrent erythroderma. The patient's face may have a leonine appearance with deep furrowing of markedly thickened skin. Diffuse alopecia can also be seen. Pruritus is generally severe and intractable. Frequently a history of eczema is present. The disease is chronic and shows no tendency to spontaneous remission.[13]

Histologic examinations reveal dense, band-like or patchy, mixed-cell infiltrates of lymphocytes, histiocytes, plasma cells and eosinophils as well as some atypical mononuclear cells with hyperchromatic lobulated nuclei in the upper part of the dermis (Fig. 33.3). The papillary dermis is usually thickened; stellate and multinucleated fibroblasts are present. Lymphocytes can be found in the hyperplastic epidermis. Immunohistology is characterized by predominance of T-helper cells, often also CD8-positive T-lymphocytes and the presence of Langerhans cells.

The clinical differentiation of actinic reticuloid from cutaneous T-cell lymphomas (mycosis fungoides and Sézary's syndrome) can be difficult because circulating Sézary cells may be found in the peripheral blood of patients with actinic reticuloid. The histologic changes of actinic reticuloid are usually distinguishable from those of mycosis fungoides. The former has features of lichen simplex chronicus superimposed upon an inflammatory process (similar to a persistent light eruption) whereas the latter is an epidermotropic form of malignant lymphoma.

On phototesting, patients with chronic actinic dermatitis were found to be sensitive to UV-B, UV-A and, in most instances, to visible light. Fluorescent light is said to lead sometimes to exacerbation of the disease. The minimal erythema dose is lower than normal in patients with actinic reticuloid. There is some evidence that the photosensitivity in actinic reticuloid is related to oleoresins from Compositae plants and weeds or to fragrances. In rare instances, exposure to halogenated salicylanilides has been demonstrated. Some investigators believe that progression to malignant lymphoma can occasionally occur, although this remains controversial.

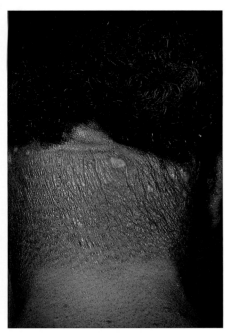

Figure 33.2
Actinic reticuloid.
Thickened and
furrowed skin on the
neck.

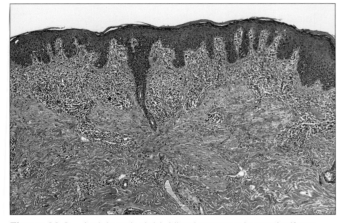

Figure 33.3 Actinic reticuloid. Histology reveals psoriasiform epidermal hyperplasia and a patchy band-like inflammatory infiltrate resembling mycosis fungoides.

Treatment of chronic actinic dermatitis is difficult and numerous therapeutic approaches have been proposed. Photoprotection is most important. Any relevant associated contact or photocontact allergens have to be identified and avoided. Some patients have been reported to respond to corticosteroids, photochemotherapy with PUVA, alpha-interferon, or to a combination treatment with azathioprine, hydroxychloroquine and prednisone. Cyclosporine A (sometimes combined with bath-PUVA) or topical tacrolimus ointment (especially for facial lesions) appear also to be effective.[14]

Lymphomatoid contact dermatitis

The term lymphomatoid contact dermatitis (Table 33.4) was coined by Gomez Orbaneja *et al*.[15] These authors described four patients with persistent allergic contact dermatitis proved by patch tests. The clinical picture

Table 33.4 Criteria for the diagnosis of lymphomatoid contact dermatitis

Clinical features	• Multiple reddish papules and plaques • Erythroderma
Histopathology	• Simulator of mycosis fungoides • Band-like or patchy lymphocytic infiltrates in the papillary dermis • Spongiotic foci and few lymphocytes in the epidermis
Genetics	• No monoclonal rearrangement of the T-cell receptor genes
Etiology	• Allergic contact dermatitis should be proven by positive patch test

and histologic features in their patients were highly suggestive of mycosis fungoides. Clinically, lymphomatoid contact dermatitis is characterized by pruritic erythematous plaques (Fig. 33.4a, b). The lesions grow progressively and generalized reddish papules and scaly eczematous plaques that may become confluent as well as exfoliative erythroderma can be observed. The lesions undergo phases of exacerbation and remission.

Histologically, lymphomatoid contact dermatitis resembles mycosis fungoides ('spongiotic simulator of cutaneous T cell lymphoma') (Fig. 33.5). The differentiation from mycosis fungoides is usually done on the basis of changes within the epidermis. In lymphomatoid contact dermatitis, there are usually only a few atypical lymphocytes in the epidermis that have no tendency to form collections of Pautrier's microabscesses there. Ultrastructural studies of the dermal infiltrate in lymphomatoid contact dermatitis have revealed atypical lymphocytes with cerebriform nuclei resembling those of Lutzner cells in mycosis fungoides.

Patch tests to a variety of common antigens, such as ethylenediamine dihydrochloride, can give a positive reaction. Although lymphomatoid contact dermatitis has been reported to evolve into true malignant lymphoma, it is more likely that such patients had malignant lymphoma from the outset. The diagnosis lymphomatoid contact dermatitis should be reserved for patients in whom the lymphomatoid skin lesions are due to a positively reacting antigen. For the management of patients, a thorough search for antigens is necessary in order to interrupt the process. When contact with the responsible allergens is avoided, the lesions heal in a relatively short time.

Lymphomatoid drug reactions

A large number of drugs may induce lymphoid infiltrates in the skin that simulate malignant lymphoma[16,17] (Table 33.5 and Fig. 33.6a–c). A number of anticonvulsants, particularly hydantoin derivatives, have been shown to cause a pseudolymphoma syndrome characterized by generalized lymphadenopathy, hepatosplenomegaly, leucocytosis, fever, malaise, arthralgia, severe edema of the face and cutaneous lesions such as erythematous pruritic macules and reddish papules and nodules.

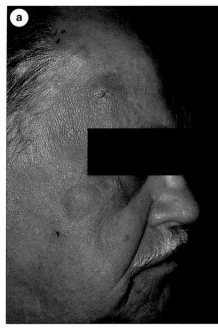

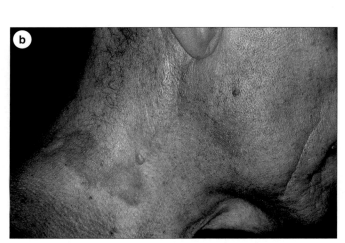

Figure 33.4 (a) Lymphomatoid contact dermatitis. Eczematous papules and plaques on the cheek and forehead. (b) Mycosis fungoides. Patches and plaques involving the neck and cheek.

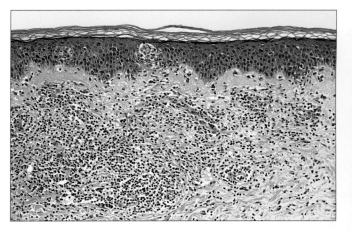

Figure 33.5 Lymphomatoid contact dermatitis. Dense band-like infiltrate in the superficial dermis. Note the small intraepidermal collection of cells representing a 'Pautrier's microabscess'-like cluster of Langerhans cells and lymphocytes.

Table 33.5 Criteria for the diagnosis of lymphomatoid drug reactions

Clinical features	• Multiple erythematous patches, papules, and small nodules • Erythroderma • T- or B-cell pattern simulating either mycosis fungoides or cutaneous B-cell lymphoma • Dense band-like, nodular or diffuse infiltrates, sometimes atypical cells
Genetics	• Usually no clonally rearranged T-cell receptor or immunoglobulin genes present
Etiology	• Frequently anticonvulsants and antidepressants responsible

Table 33.6 illustrates important preparations, which can produce generalized macules, papules, plaques, or nodules and even erythroderma. The external use of etheric plant oils may also cause lymphoproliferative reactions that mimic malignant lymphomas, clinically and histologically.

Histologically, pseudolymphomatous drug eruptions are characterized by dense band-like or nodular and diffuse infiltrates of sometimes atypical lymphocytes revealing T- (mycosis fungoides-like) or B-cell (marginal zone lymphoma-like) patterns (Fig. 33.7). Eosinophils may or may not be present.

Lymphomatoid drug reactions invariably regress when the drug is withdrawn.

CD30+ (T-cell-) pseudolymphomas

An important group of cutaneous T-cell lymphomas, including anaplastic large cell lymphoma and lym-phomatoid papulosis, is characterized by the expression of the CD30 antigen by large, atypical neoplastic cells. It is crucial to underline that CD30-positivity alone does not imply a diagnosis of lymphomatoid papulosis or cutaneous anaplastic large cell lymphoma. In fact, CD30+ large blasts have been observed in the skin in several reactive conditions including various viral infections (Orf, milker's nodule, molluscum contagiosum, herpes simplex, herpes zoster), arthropod reactions, scabies and drug eruptions among others.[18–20]

Besides the presence of large, atypical CD30+ cells, histology reveals the typical changes of the specific underlying disorder. Moreover, in these reactive conditions CD30+ lymphocytes are present in small numbers scattered throughout the infiltrate and are usually not arranged in clusters or sheets as observed in lym-phomatoid papulosis or anaplastic large cell lymphoma. However, in given cases differentiation may be very difficult or even impossible on histologic and immunohistochemical grounds alone. Unlike the situation in lymphomatoid papulosis and anaplastic large cell lymphoma, gene rearrangement studies in CD30+ pseudolymphomas reveal the presence of a polyclonal population of T lymphocytes.

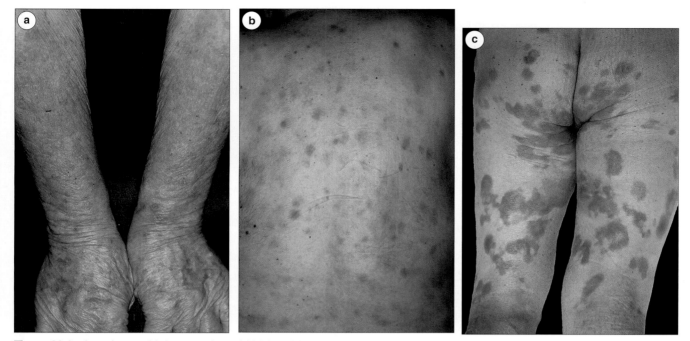

Figure 33.6 Lymphomatoid drug reactions. (a) Lichenoid papules and plaques on the arms simulating cutaneous T-cell lymphoma. (b) Generalized papules and small nodules on the back simulating cutaneous B-cell lymphoma. (c) Malignant diffuse large B-cell lymphoma. Generalized macules, papules, plaques and nodules.

The treatment of CD30+ pseudolymphomas depends on the specific diagnosis.

Persistent nodular arthropod bite reactions

The most typical example of this group of lymphomatoid infiltrates (Table 33.7) is nodular scabies.[4] Clinically, elevated round or oval bright red to brownish red papules and nodules occur most frequently on the genitalia, elbows and in the axillae (Fig. 33.8). The lesions are found in about 7% of patients with scabies. The nodules are very pruritic and may persist for many months or even years.

The mite and its parts are seldom identified in longstanding papules or nodules of scabies. The clinical differential diagnosis includes prurigo nodularis and malignant lymphoma; some lesions of secondary syphilis may be diagnosed incorrectly as pseudolymphoma of this type.

Histologically, dense superficial and deep perivascular predominantly lymphohistiocytic infiltrates with plasma cells and varying numbers of eosinophils are seen (Fig. 33.9). Eosinophils are also scattered among collagen bundles. Prominent vessels with thickened walls lined by plump endothelial cells are sometimes found. The epidermis may be slightly spongiotic, hyperplastic and hyperkeratotic. The histologic features of nodular scabies may sometimes mimic those of mycosis fungoides and Hodgkin's disease.

Immunohistologic investigations reveal T lymphocytes as the predominant cells of nodular scabies. In some cases positivity of large lymphoid cells for the CD30 antigen may simulate the immunophenotypic pattern of lymphomatoid papulosis. Occasionally a B-cell pattern analogous to lymphocytoma cutis can be recognized in persistent nodular arthropod bite reactions.

Antiscabietic therapy is usually ineffective. Intralesional injection of corticosteroids in larger nodules may be helpful. Spontaneous resolution in time is the rule.

Lupus panniculitis

Recently, a cutaneous T-cell lymphoma with predominant involvement of the subcutaneous fat tissue has been recognized (so-called subcutaneous panniculitis-like T-cell lymphoma), which may mimic lupus profundus (lupus panniculitis) both clinically and histologically. Subcutaneous panniculitis-like T-cell lymphoma presents histologically with prominent involvement of the fat lobules, often simulating a lobular panniculitis. Neoplastic cells usually reveal a CD3+, CD4–, CD8+, CD56–, α/β phenotype.

Lupus panniculitis reveals clinically subcutaneous plaques and indurations, mostly located on the extremities.[21] Anti-nuclear antibodies and other markers of systemic lupus erythematosus may be absent in some cases. Histology shows a lobular panniculitis, often with concomitant presence of broadened, fibrotic septa. A useful feature for differentiation of subcutaneous panniculitis-like T-cell lymphoma from lupus panniculitis is the presence in the former of so-called 'rimming' of fat cells by pleomorphic, atypical T-lymphocytes that are positive for proliferation markers. However, rimming of fat lobuli by lymphocytes is not a diagnostic feature *per se*, as it can be observed in several benign and malignant lymphoid infiltrates with involvement of the fat lobules. In contrast to subcutaneous panniculitis-like T-cell lymphoma, B-cells, plasma cells and germinal

Table 33.6 Important drugs involved in pseudolymphomas	
Category	**Drug**
Anticonvulsant	Carbamazepine Clonazepam Lamotrigine Phenytoin
Antidepressant	Amitriptyline Desipramine Doxepin Fluoxetine Lithium
Antipsychotic	Chlorpromazine Perphenazine Thioridazine
Anxiolytic tranquilizer	Alprazolam Lorazepam
Uricosuric	Allopurinol
Diuretic	Furosemide Hydrochlorothiazide
Beta-adrenergic blocker, antihypertensive, antianginal	Atenolol
Antihypertensive	Clonidine Losartan
Calcium channel blocker	Diltiazem
Cephalosporic antibiotic	Cefixime
Macrolide antibiotic	Clarithromycin
Urinary tract antibiotic	Nitrofurantoin
Sulfonamide	Sulfasalazine
Antibacterial	Co-trimoxazole Sulfamethoxazole
H_2-receptor antihistamine	Cimetidine Nizatidine Ranitidine
H_1-receptor antihistamine	Terfenadine
Antineoplastic, anti-inflammatory	Methotrexate
Immunosuppressant	Cyclosporine
Antiarthritic	Gold/gold compounds
Antihyperlipidemic	Gemfibrozil

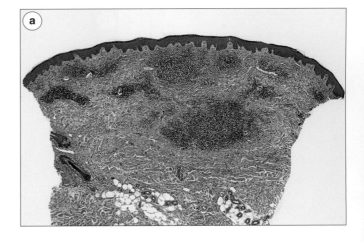

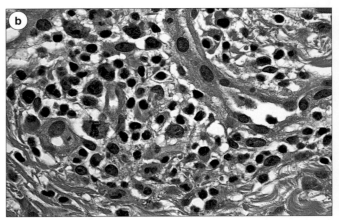

Figure 33.7 Lymphomatoid drug reaction. (a) Dense nodular dermal infiltrates of lymphocytes and histiocytes. (b) Note large atypical cells.

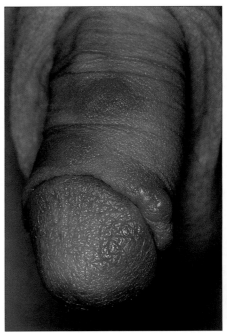

Figure 33.8 Nodular lesions of scabies on genital skin.

centers are commonly a prominent feature in lupus panniculitis. Moreover, the dermo-epidermal junction may show features of lupus erythematosus (interface dermatitis). Analysis of T-cell receptor gene rearrangement reveals polyclonal populations of T- and B-lymphocytes in lupus panniculitis, in contrast to subcutaneous panniculitis-like T-cell lymphoma, where monoclonality of T-lymphocytes is found as a rule.

Treatment of lupus panniculitis is similar to treatment of other variants of lupus erythematosus. Lesions respond well to systemic steroids, but recurrences are the rule.

Lymphocytoma cutis

Several synonyms have been used for lymphocytoma cutis including lymphadenosis benigna cutis, cutaneous

Table 33.7   Criteria for the diagnosis of persistent nodular arthropod bite reactions – example: nodular scabies

Clinical features	• Erythematous to brownish-red, itching papules and nodules, often located on the genitalia and in the axillae
Histopathology	• Superficial and deep perivascular, sometimes lichenoid dermatitis • The dense infiltrates consist of lymphocytes, histiocytes, plasma cells, and eosinophils

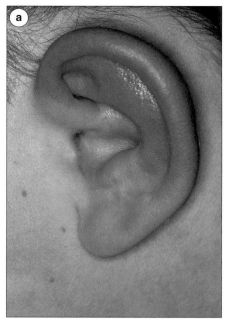

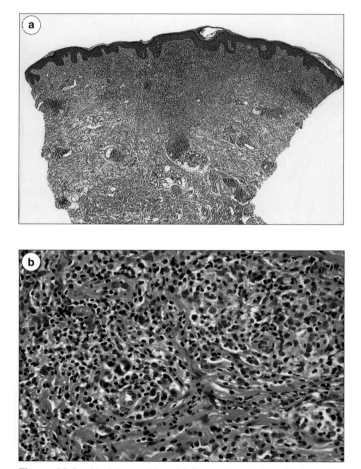

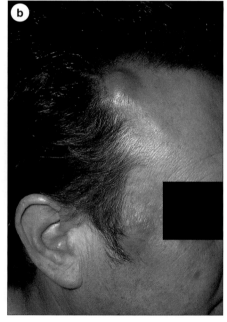

Figure 33.9   Nodular scabies. (a) Dense lymphoid infiltrates with a 'top-heavy' arrangement. Note a cuniculus within the horny layer. (b) The inflammatory infiltrate is composed of lymphocytes, histiocytes, plasma cells and eosinophils.

Figure 33.10   (a) Lymphocytoma cutis. Involvement of the ear as a manifestation of borreliosis. (b) Malignant cutaneous lymphoma, follicle center cell type. Nodules on the face and forehead.

lymphoplasia, cutaneous lymphoid hyperplasia and pseudolymphoma of Spiegler-Fendt. Various stimuli can induce lesions of lymphocytoma cutis: insect bites, drugs, vaccinations,[22] acupuncture, wearing of gold pierced earrings, medicinal leech therapy,[23] and tattoos among others. One of the most common associations is found with the spirochetes *Borrelia burgdorferi*.

There are numerous clinical presentations of lymphocytoma cutis.[4] Frequently, a firm solitary lesion can be observed. However, lesions may be clustered in a region or, rarely, may be scattered widely. There is

usually a nodule or tumor, but there may be papules or plaques present. The color varies from reddish-brown to reddish-purple. Scaling and ulceration are absent. Favored sites of involvement are the face, chest (mamillary area) and genital area. Involvement of special body sites (earlobe, nipple, scrotum) is almost pathognomonic of *Borrelia burgdorferi*-associated lymphocytoma cutis (Fig. 33.10a). Women are affected more commonly than men. The *Borrelia burgdorferi*-associated type of lymphocytoma cutis often occurs in children. Clinically, lymphocytoma cutis must be

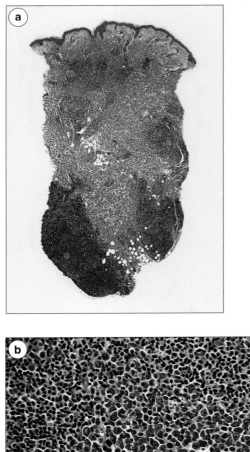

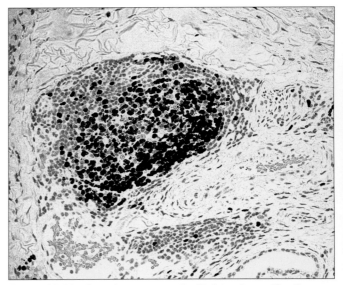

Figure 33.12 Lymphocytoma cutis. Staining for proliferating cells (MIB-1/Ki67) reveals high proliferation within a reactive germinal center.

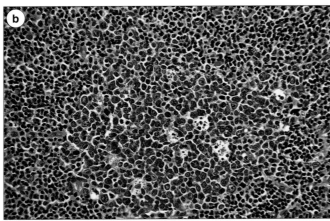

Figure 33.11 Lymphocytoma cutis. (a) Nodular lymphoid infiltrates with reactive germinal centers. (b) Germinal center with centroblasts, centrocytes and 'tingible body'-macrophages. This case, located on the nipple, was due to infection with *Borrelia burgdorferi*.

differentiated from malignant lymphoma (Fig. 33.10b), granuloma faciale, angiolymphoid hyperplasia with eosinophilia, nodular secondary syphilis, Merkel cell tumor and primary or metastatic carcinoma.

Histologic examination shows dense, nodular, mixed-cell infiltrates, often with formation of lymphoid follicles (Fig. 33.11). Although the infiltrates may be 'top-heavy', in lymphocytoma cutis there may be dense diffuse lymphoid infiltrates simulating the histopathologic picture of a B-cell lymphoma.

Differentiation of lymphocytoma cutis from malignant lymphoma may be extremely difficult or even impossible on histologic grounds alone. Reactive lymphoid follicles are frequently found in both, lymphocytoma cutis and marginal zone B-cell lymphoma. The histopathologic, immunophenotypic (Fig. 33.12) and molecular criteria discussed above (Table 33.2) are crucial in distinguishing lesions of lymphocytoma cutis from those of cutaneous B-cell lymphomas.[6]

Lymphocytoma cutis may resolve spontaneously in several months or years. Small nodules can be removed by surgical excision and local injection of corticosteroids or interferon-α may result in regression. Patients with lesions of lymphocytoma cutis and detection by ELISA of immunoglobulins in serum specific for *Borrelia burgdorferi* or detection of *Borrelia* DNA by polymerase chain reaction on tissue sections can be treated with tetracycline, penicillin or cephalosporins. A very effective treatment method is radiotherapy.

Other pseudolymphomas

Several other inflammatory disorders may mimic the clinical and/or histopathologic picture of cutaneous lymphoma:

Solitary erythematous patches, papules, nodules or plaques with histopathologic features of mycosis fungoides represent distinct entities which have been referred to as 'unlesional mycosis fungoides' or 'solitary T-cell pseudolymphoma'. In several patients a monoclonal rearrangement of the T-cell receptor genes has been reported. These lesions are frequently located on the breast of women.[24]

Lichenoid (lymphomatoid) keratosis, lichenoid pigmented purpuric dermatitis (including lichen aureus) and lichen sclerosus on genital skin can also be added to the list of cutaneous T-cell pseudolymphomas.[25,26] The histopathological features with dense band-like inflammatory lymphoid infiltrates and often epidermotropism of lymphocytes may be indistinguishable from those of mycosis fungoides. Moreover, T-lymphocyte clonality can be sometimes found in these diseases. Accurate clinico-pathological correlation is crucial to establish a correct diagnosis.

Reactions to tattoos (Fig. 33.13) may sometimes reveal lymphoid follicular structures or a mycosis fungoides-like pattern.[27] Red tattoo pigment (cinnabar) is most frequently responsible for the lymphomatoid infiltrate.

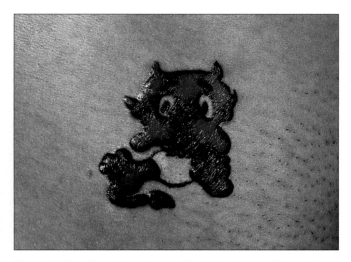

Figure 33.13 Pseudolymphoma. Reddish plaques within a tattoo.

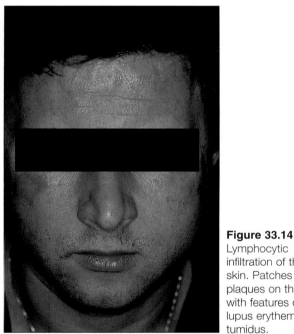

Figure 33.14 Lymphocytic infiltration of the skin. Patches and plaques on the face with features of lupus erythematosus tumidus.

The presence of pigment suggests the correct diagnosis; however, one well documented case of cutaneous lymphoma arising in a tattoo has been reported and follow-up should be performed very carefully.

Localized scleroderma/morphea (inflammatory stage) and secondary syphilis may simulate cutaneous lymphomas, especially marginal zone B-cell lymphoma, histopathologically. A polyclonal pattern of immunoglobulin light chain expression (and serologic tests for syphilis) favors a diagnosis of an inflammatory process.

Lymphocytic infiltration of the skin (Jessner-Kanof) can be confused with B-chronic lymphocytic leukemia, B-type (Fig. 33.14). The expression of B-cell markers and CD5 on the B-cells of chronic lymphocytic leukemia will help to distinguish both diseases. It has been recently proposed that lymphocytic infiltration of the skin represents lupus erythematosus tumidus.[28]

Cutaneous inflammatory pseudotumors present clini-

cally as firm dermal-subcutaneous nodules.[29] On histopathological examination circumscribed nodules with thick hyalinized collagen bundles and an inflammatory infiltrate with lymphocytes, plasma cells (polyclonal) and occasionally germinal centers can be observed. Some cases represent in our opinion postinfective reactions (EBV, *Borrelia*, mycobacteria, HHV-8).

Acral pseudolymphomatous angiokeratoma is characterized by unilateral clustered red-violaceous papules and small nodules, usually located on the hands and feet of children. Histopathologic investigations reveal a dense nodular lymphoid infiltrate with occasional plasma cells and eosinophils. Proliferation of capillaries can be observed. The term angiokeratoma is misleading and based on the distinctive clinicopathologic features the designation 'small papular pseudolymphoma' has been suggested for this benign lymphoproliferative disease.[30]

FUTURE OUTLOOK

The field of cutaneous lymphoid infiltrates is in continuous evolution. Benign and malignant diseases are better characterized and re-defined as a consequence of our expanding knowledge. Pseudolymphoma of the skin is a convenient term for a group of disorders that demonstrate the same problem, namely, differentiation from malignant lymphomas. Until better differentiation methods are developed, these entities should be classified precisely according to specific etiologic, genetic and pathogenesis factors.

REFERENCES

1 Kerl H, Ackerman AB. Inflammatory diseases that simulate lymphomas: Cutaneous pseudolymphomas. In: Fitzpatrick TB, Wolff K, Eisen AZ et al., eds. Dermatology in General Medicine, 4th edn. New York, NY: McGraw-Hill; 1993:1315–1327.

2 Caro WA, Helwig EB. Cutaneous lymphoid hyperplasia. Cancer 1969; 24:487–502.

3 Clark WH, Mihm MC, Reed RJ, Ainsworth AM. The lymphocytic infiltrates of the skin. Hum Pathol 1974; 5:25–43.

4 Cerroni L, Gatter K, Kerl H. An illustrated guide to skin lymphomas. Oxford: Blackwell Science; 2004.

5 Kerl H, Smolle J. Pseudolymphomas of the skin. In: Friedman RJ, Rigel DS, Kopf A et al., eds. Cancer of the Skin. Philadelphia, PA: WB Saunders; 1991:409.

6 Cerroni L, Kerl H. Diagnostic immunohistology: cutaneous lymphomas and pseudolymphomas. Semin Cut Med Surg 1999; 18:64–70.

7 Wood GS. T-cell receptor and immunoglobulin gene rearrangements in diagnosing skin disease. Arch Derm 2001; 137:1503–1506.

8 Nihal M, Mikkola D, Horvath N, et al. Cutaneous lymphoid hyperplasia: a lymphoproliferative continuum with lymphomatous potential. Hum Pathol 2003; 34:617–622.

9 Cerroni L, Arzberger E, Pütz B, et al. Primary cutaneous follicle center cell lymphoma with follicular growth pattern. Blood 2000; 95:3922–3928.

10 Streubel B, Lamprecht A, Dierlamm J, et al. T(14;18)(q32;q21) involving IGH and MALT1 is a frequent chromosomal aberration in MALT lymphoma. Blood 2003; 101:2335–2339.

11 Ive FA, Magnus IA, Warin RP, Wilson Jones E. Actinic reticuloid: A chronic dermatosis associated with severe photosensitivity and the histological resemblance to lymphoma. Br J Derm 1969; 81:469–485.

12 Norris PG, Hawk JLM. Chronic actinic dermatitis: a unifying concept. Arch Derm 1990; 126:376–378.

13 Dawe RS, Crombie IK, Ferguson J. The natural history of chronic actinic dermatitis. Arch Derm 2000; 136:1215–1220.

14 Uetsu N, Okamoto H, Fujii K, Doi R, Horio T. Treatment of chronic actinic dermatitis with tacrolimus ointment. J Am Acad Derm 2002; 47:881–884.

15 Gomez Orbaneja J, Iglesias Diez L, Sanchez Lozano JL, Conde Salazar L. Lymphomatoid contact dermatitis. Contact Dermatitis 1976; 2:139–143.

16 Magro CM, Crowson AN, Kovatich AJ, Burns F. Drug-induced reversible lymphoid dyscrasia: a clonal lymphomatoid dermatitis of memory and activated T cells. Hum Pathol 2003; 34:119–129.

17 Ploysangam T, Breneman DL, Mutasim DF. Cutaneous pseudolymphomas. J Am Acad Derm 1998; 38:877–905.

18 Gallardo F, Barranco C, Toll A, Pujol RM. CD30 antigen expression in cutaneous inflammatory infiltrates of scabies: a dynamic immunophenotypic pattern that should be distinguished from lymphomatoid papulosis. J Cutan Pathol 2002; 29:368–373.

19 Nathan DL, Belsito DV. Carbamazepine-induced pseudolymphoma with CD-30 positive cells. J Am Acad Derm 1998; 38:806–809.

20 Rose C, Starostik P, Bröcker EB. Infection with parapoxvirus induces CD30-positive cutaneous infiltrates in humans. J Cutan Pathol 1999; 26:520–522.

21 Magro CM, Crowson AN, Kovatich AJ, Burns F. Lupus profundus, indeterminate lymphocytic lobular panniculitis and subcutaneous T-cell lymphoma: a spectrum of subcuticular T-cell lymphoid dyscrasia. J Cutan Pathol 2001; 28:235–247.

22 Stavrianeas NG, Katoulis AC, Kanelleas A, Hatziolou E, Georgala S. Papulonodular lichenoid and pseudolymphomatous reaction at the injection site of hepatitis B virus vaccination. Dermatology 2002; 205:166–168.

23 Smolle J, Cerroni L, Kerl H. Multiple pseudolymphomas caused by *Hirudo medicinalis* therapy. J Am Acad Derm 2000; 43:867–869.

24 Cerroni L, Fink-Puches R, El-Shabrawi-Caelen L, Soyer HP, LeBoit PE, Kerl H. Solitary skin lesions with histopathologic features of early mycosis fungoides. Am J Dermatopathol 1999; 21:518–524.

25 Al-Hoqail I, Crawford RI. Benign lichenoid keratoses with histologic features of mycosis fungoides: clinicopathologic description of a clinically significant histologic pattern. J Cutan Pathol 2002; 29:291–294.

26 Crowson AN, Magro CM, Zahorchak R. Atypical pigmentary purpura: a clinical, histopathologic and genotypic study. Hum Pathol 1999; 30:1004–1012.

27 Kahofer P, El-Shabrawi-Caelen L, Horn M, Kern T, Smolle J. Pseudolymphoma occurring in a tattoo. Eur J Dermatol 2003; 13:209–212.

28 Weber F, Schmuth M, Fritsch P, Sepp N. Lymphocytic infiltration of the skin is a photosensitive variant of lupus erythematosus: evidence by phototesting. Br J Derm 2001; 144:292–296.

29 Hurt MA, Santa Cruz DJ. Cutaneous inflammatory pseudotumor. Lesions resembling inflammatory pseudotumors or plasma cell granulomas of extracutaneous sites. Am J Surg Pathol 1990; 14:764–773.

30 Kaddu S, Cerroni L, Pilatti A, Soyer HP, Kerl H. Acral pseudolymphomatous angiokeratoma. Am J Dermatopathol 1994; 16:130–133.

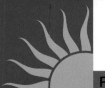

CHAPTER
34

Cutaneous Carcinogenesis Related to Dermatologic Therapy

Eric Berkowitz and Mark Lebwohl

Key points

- Risks and benefits of all forms of therapy should be discussed with patients.
- When prescribing a medication that confers carcinogenic potential, screening exams should be performed.
- Beware of a synergistic response related to cancer risk when prescribing multiple medications.

INTRODUCTION

Systemic therapies utilized in dermatology have typically been developed for use in other specialties. Therefore, dermatologists must take greater precautions when prescribing systemic drug therapy. The clinician in any field is obligated to avoid creating a greater risk with the drug therapy than the risk of the underlying illness that is already present. Regardless of how careful a physician is, adverse effects will inevitably occur given the imperfect nature of the medical risk reduction system and the unpredictability of the human body. Therefore, special effort must be taken to increase knowledge of certain associations so that adverse reactions are minimized.

POTENTIAL MECHANISMS OF DRUG-RELATED CARCINOGENESIS

Physiologic balances are properly maintained in tissues and among cells in circulation. Normal cells function under the control of their environment. However, cancer is a disease of cells whose growth and function is 'out of control'. Cells communicate via signal transduction pathways through which cascades of chemical interactions lead to the activation or deactivation of certain cellular processes. Additionally, internal cellular signaling pathways exist for further control of the functioning of individual cells. Cell proliferation and terminal differentiation are regulated by these internal and external signaling pathways. Cancer appears to result from the disturbances in a combination of these growth-controlling pathways. These cells lose their original confinement, invade and disrupt the surrounding tissues.

Six alterations in cell physiology have been proposed to define malignant growth: Self-sufficiency in growth signals; insensitivity to growth-inhibitory signal's evasion

of programmed cell death (apoptosis); limitless replicative potential; sustained angiogenesis; and tissue invasion/ metastasis. Each of these physiologic changes represents a breaching of an anticancer defense mechanism.[1]

Many issues affect the signaling pathways. Environmental factors may evoke certain expected proper responses while toxic agents may adversely disturb the growth controlling pathways. Multiple occurrences may, therefore, enhance or inhibit carcinogenic progression acting as either a promoter or a suppressor. However, a permanent disturbance in a signaling pathway may be introduced by damaging a gene that codes for a protein in a specific pathway. This genetic alteration will then be passed on to daughter cells and then the altered signal transduction will propagate.

Skin cancers are the most common human tumors and their frequencies have increased regularly over the past decades. There are several causes that can initiate skin cancer and ultraviolet (UV) is the most common. UVB irradiation induces bulky DNA lesions between two adjacent pyrimidines, and oxidizes bases, and single strands break via the UVA spectrum. The nucleotide excision repair pathway repairs the former types of lesions, and the latter are repaired primarily by the base excision repair system.

The *p53* tumor suppressor gene is mutated in many human cancers. This gene plays an important role in several signaling pathways related to DNA damage and the expression of oncogenes.[2] It is normally quiescent. However, nuclear *p53* expression is found to be elevated after UV irradiation and after a genotoxic insult helping to orchestrate cell cycle arrest and apoptosis.

Studies have demonstrated the existence of three independent pathways through which the *p53* system is initiated. The first pathway is triggered by ionizing radiation, activating two protein kinases (ATM, for ataxia-telangiectasia mutated, and Chk2).[3] The second pathway is triggered by aberrant growth signals such as those from the expression of RAS and bcl-2.[4,5] A wide range of chemotherapeutic drugs, ultraviolet light, and protein kinase inhibitors induces the third pathway. It is distinguished from the other mechanisms because it is not dependent on intact ATM, Chk2 or p14.

The vast majority of *p53* mutations are base pair substitutions located on DNA binding sites. These 'hot spots' correspond to sequences that are more often mutated. There are five major hot spots and all correspond to sequences that are composed of a C-C-G where the 3'C is methylated. This methyl cytosine produces a less stable base that can easily be deaminated, giving rise to a T and also able to induce a C to T transition in the absence of a full repair.[6] Mutations in *p53* are present in about 56% of human BCCs[7] and 40–60% of SCCs and 10% of MMs.[6]

Another significant factor is the hedgehog pathway. The pathway begins with the patched-smoothened (Ptc-Smo) membrane receptor complex, where Ptc prevents Smo from functioning. However, when hedgehog (Hh) binds Ptc, the Ptc-Smo inhibition stops allowing Smo to then signal and 'turn on' Gli protein function. There are three known possible actions of the Hh-Gli complex: proliferation, differentiation, and growth. The two actions are clearly evident in embryogenesis and demonstrate the relationship between Hh and cell-cycle regulations. Finally, its role in growth may provide clues to its role in cancer.[8] It has been found that Hh augments the cell's capacity for long-term growth. This combined with the ability of Hh to induce Bcl-2, potentially resisting apoptosis are important milestones in carcinogenesis.[9] However, recent data demonstrate that the expression of Gli1 in basal cells are predicted to induce basal cell carcinoma (BCC) formation.[10] There is emerging evidence that the PTCh gene is mutated in squamous cell carcinoma (SCC).[11]

There are also some familial cutaneous melanomas (MM) that are linked to chromosome 9 which lead to the identification of the multiple tumor suppressor gene (MTS1). The locus is named INK4α, which then becomes associated with a cyclin dependent kinase and acts to inhibit CDK4 and CDK6. The exact mechanism and extent to which environmental factors trigger this pathway is still yet to be elucidated but thought to be triggered by UVB irradiation.[12]

The understanding of the mechanisms of carcinogenesis, the molecular mechanisms and signal pathways is rapidly growing. Hopefully, with future advances it will be possible to correct these genetic defects and correct them before progressing to cancer. However, now that some mechanisms of cancer pathogenesis are known, we can apply risk assessment and predict with some certainty the cancer risk associated with a certain treatment. Therefore, knowledge of the full range of therapies that can cause DNA damage and cancer is important both for proper risk assessment and for further health surveillance.

THERAPIES ASSOCIATED WITH INCREASED SKIN CANCER RISK

Multiple therapies advocated for other medical disorders have been linked to increased risk of skin cancer. These treatments and their associated skin cancer risks are reviewed in Table 34.1.

Therapeutic Radiation

PUVA photochemotherapy is the photochemical interaction between psoralen and ultraviolet A radiation (320 nm to 400 nm). Psoralens are naturally occurring compounds that lead to a phytophotodermatitis when exposed to sunlight. PUVA therapy is thought to be therapeutic via different mechanisms. It is thought that PUVA therapy suppresses gene transcription impairing

cell replication; inhibits the regulation of ICAM, a surface molecule that functions in inflammatory dermatoses; decreases the expression of the inflammatory cytokines; and stimulates melanocytes.[13,14]

PUVA has a beneficial effect in the treatment of psoriasis, vitiligo, certain neoplastic dermatoses, pruritic dermatoses, and many papulosquamous dermatoses, to name a few. Many clinical follow-up studies have revealed that high dose exposure to PUVA increases the risk of SCC.[15,16] Another study evaluating patients receiving PUVA therapy in Sweden demonstrated that exposure to PUVA increased the risk for cutaneous SCC but not for MM.[17] However, another study indicated that there is an increase in both SCC and BCC even at low cumulative doses of PUVA[18] (Fig. 34.1). Recent data suggests that the mechanism of PUVA induced carcinogenesis acts by mutating p-53 and Ha-ras.[19,20] The data suggests that PUVA may play a role in the development of MM (Fig. 34.2). There have been many studies addressing this exact issue, but epidemiologic studies are inconclusive. There was a 16 center US cooperative study that observed an increased incidence of MM in PUVA treated patients who had received more than 250 PUVA exposures[21] and multiple reports of patients in Austria who developed MM after PUVA exposure (none of the patients had any co-carcinogenic treatments).[22] PUVA co-carcinogens include: episodes of prior ionizing radiation, arsenic treatment, xeroderma pigmentosum, and a history of skin cancers (methotrexate is not contraindicated, however, caution should be exercised if both therapies are co-administered).[18] Noteworthy, is the observation that there is a dose related increase in the risk of genital tumors in men treated with PUVA despite the decreased PUVA administration and increased genital shielding.[23]

Narrowband UVB is another newer phototherapeutic treatment that has been developed for the treatment of psoriasis, vitiligo, small plaque parapsoriasis, mycosis

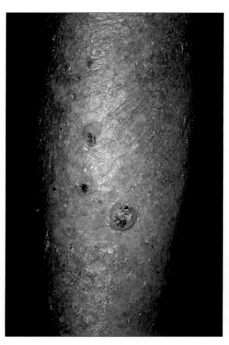

Figure 34.1
Keratoacanthoma and squamous cell carcinomas in a patient treated with PUVA.

fungoides and atopic dermatitis to name a few. The desire to use narrowband UVB is justified because it has an efficacy profile superior to that of broadband UVB and a theoretical superior safety profile.[24] However, broadband UVB has a long history of safety based on many years of experience. The safety profile for narrowband UVB will not be fully known for years, yet animal studies have demonstrated that UVB administered to animals resulted in the development of MM[25] and that suberythemal UVB therapy can lead to changes in melanocytic nevi detectable by dermoscopy.[26]

Ionizing radiation has been observed to increase the risk of skin cancer. Initial evidence for this was observed in uranium miners, radiologists and survivors from

Table 34.1   Therapeutic carcinogenic risks

Therapy	SCC	BCC	MM	Other
PUVA	+ (Stern,[15] Stern,[16] Lindelof,[17] Studinberg,[18] Kreimer-Erlacher[20])	+ (Studinberg[18])	– (Lindelof[17]) + (Stern,[19] Stern,[21] Kreimer-Erlacher,[20] Wolf[22])	Increased genital tumours (Stern[23])
UVB (Narrowband)	Undetermined	Undetermined	+ (Robinson,[25] note: studies were performed in animals)	
Ionizing radiation	+ (Lichter[27]) – (Karagas[28])	+ (Lichter,[27] Karagas,[28] Shore[29])	– (Shore[29])	
Methotrexate				Increased risk of lymphoma found to have associated + EBV (Paul,[30] Theate,[31] Tournadre,[32] and Abdel Baki[33])
Cyclosporine	+ (Paul[36] and Marcil[37] but patients in study were on concurrent PUVA)			Increased risk of lymphoma (Kirby[34] and Koo[35])
Mycophenolate Mofetil	+(Silverman-Kitchin[38]) – (Epinette[39])			
Azathioprine	+ (Bottomley[40] and Nachbar[41])			+ Kaposi's sarcoma (Vandercam[42] and Halpern[43]) + Lymphoma (Ehrenfeld[44]) + Merkel cell tumour (Gooptu[45])
Hydroxyurea	+ (Aste,[46] de Simone,[47] Najean[48])	+ (Aste,[46] de Simone,[47] Najean[48])		
Nitrogen mustard	+ (Smith[50] of note patient underwent treatment with other modalities as well, i.e. PUVA)			
Arsenic	+ (Germolac[54])	+ (Boonchai[55])		+ Dermatofibrosarcoma Pertuberans (Schneidman[56])
Tar or 'Tar like' substances Tacrolimus/ Pimecrolimus Corticosteroids	+ (Letzel[57]) – (Arnold[58]) – (Duncan,[66] Reitamo[67] and Wahn[68]) + (Karagas[59])	+ (Karagas[59])		+ Keratoacanthoma (Letzel[57]) + Kaposi's sarcoma (Trattner[60])
Biological agents Etanercept Infliximab Efalizumab	+(Smith[62], however, patients in study were on other immunosuppressants) – (Fleishmann[61]) – (Lebwohl[64] and Weinberg[65])			+ Lymphoma (Brown[63]) + Lymphoma (Brown[63])

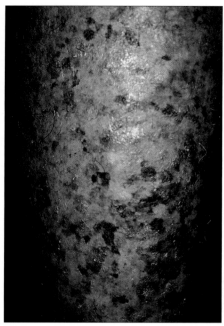

Figure 34.2 PUVA lentigenes: an increase in skin pigmentation caused by PUVA.

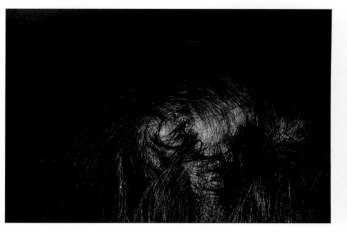

Figure 34.3 BCC at site of ionizing radiation therapy that occurred 20 years earlier.

Hiroshima and Nagasaki. However, it is not clear whether therapeutic ionizing radiation is a cause of skin cancer. Disorders for which ionizing radiation therapy is implicated are: inflammatory dermatoses (eczema, atopic dermatitis, psoriasis, and tinea capitis – although this is purely mentioned for historical completeness) and malignancy. Other pathologies employing ionizing radiation treatment include goiters, acute lymphocytic leukemia and astrocytoma to name a few. It has been observed that ionizing radiation causes an increased risk of SCC and BCC, primarily in the areas of the body that were exposed to the radiotherapy (Fig. 34.3), and that risk increases with younger age of onset of treatment.[27] Another report indicates an increase in BCC but not an increase in SCC[28] and a follow-up study, looking at children who were treated with ionizing radiation for tinea capitis found an increased risk of BCC and no association between ionizing radiation and MM.[29]

Chemotherapy and immunosuppressive agents

Methotrexate (MTX), a folic acid antagonist, potently irreversibly inhibits the enzyme dihydrofolate reductase. Thus, the overall effect of MTX is an inhibition of cell division being specific for the S phase of the normal cell cycle. The beneficial effect of MTX in dermatology is thought to be due to the suppression of hyper-proliferation of keratinocytes and the immunosuppressant effects that occur when inhibiting DNA synthesis in immunologically competent cells. Dermatologic therapeutic uses of MTX include: psoriasis, Sézary syndrome, proliferative dermatoses, pityriasis rubra pilaris, PLEVA, Behçet's disease, pyoderma gangrenosum, atopic dermatitis, sarcoid, lymphomatoid papulosis, mycosis fungoides and autoimmune diseases. The long-term effects of MTX are well known because of its general wide use and its particular use in collagen vascular diseases. A number of patients treated with MTX for different dermatological disorders were reported to have developed lymphomas. Of note, many of the patients that developed lymphoma were found to have Epstein–Barr virus within the neoplasm. This association was also found in psoriasis,[30] sarcoid[31] and dermatomyositis.[32] Another study of patients who had mycosis fungoides concurrently treated with MTX were found to have an increased transformation to large cell lymphoma, a malignancy that confers a worse prognosis.[33]

Cyclosporine (CsA), a neutral cyclic peptide composed of 11 amino acids, was discovered from a soil fungus in 1970. CsA's mechanism of action is thought to be mediated through its effects on T lymphocytes by inhibiting interleukin-2 reducing the number of activated CD4 and CD8 cells which subsequently reduce their secretion of proinflammatory cytokines (like IFN-γ). CsA has found many uses in dermatology: psoriasis, atopic dermatitis, lichen planus, bullous dermatoses, autoimmune connective tissue disease, neoplastic disorders, graft versus host, keratinization disorders, and alopecia.

The use of CsA carries some concerns regarding the development of lymphoproliferative disorders and non-melanoma skin cancers. There are a few reports of patients developing lymphoma while on low dose CsA. In one case, when the treatment was stopped, the lymphoma regressed and resolved.[34] However, there is another case reported that reveals a man who was treated with CsA and reportedly developed a lymphoma 7 months later and died from it.[35] In a 5-year cohort study looking at the relationship between CsA and cancer it was observed that the risk of malignancy, primarily SCC, was increased when used with a cumulative dose of more than two years.[36] Additionally, concurrent use of CsA and PUVA or other therapies reportedly increases the risk of SCC, and therefore, must be balanced against its efficacy.[37]

Mycophenolate mofetil (MMF), a weak organic acid, acts by inhibiting de novo purine synthesis by non-competitively inhibiting inosine monophosphate dehydrogenase, an important step in proliferating responses of B and T cells. MMF has been reported to be successful for the treatment of pyoderma gangrenosum, blistering disorders, psoriasis, dishydrotic eczema and metastatic

Crohn's disease. There is evidence for and against the development of cancer secondary to MMF. In a study where patients with psoriasis were treated with MMF there were three patients who developed cancer (however, on further review the patients who developed cancer had other co-morbidities).[38] However, in a study of longer duration, it was concluded that there was no increase in cancer incidence in patients treated with MMF.[39]

Azathioprine was initially synthesized from its parent compound in 1959. It was found to have both immunosuppressive and anti-inflammatory properties and, thus, became useful to dermatologists. There are three mechanisms through which azathioprine's first metabolite is metabolized further: anabolized to its active form, a purine analog by hypoxanthine-guanine phosphoribosyltransferase (HGPRT); catabolized by TPMT to inactive metabolites; or catabolized by xanthine oxidase to inactive metabolites. The anabolic pathway ultimately leads to purine analogs that interfere with DNA and RNA synthesis. However, if inactive the catabolic pathways will shift more 6-MP to the anabolic pathway potentially leading to more immunosuppression. The two pathways in the catabolic pathway have demonstrated genetic variation or pharmacologic variability that can lead to decreased levels of the enzymes.

Azathioprine's active metabolite is a purine analog that inhibits DNA/ RNA synthesis that ultimately leads to the depression of T-cell activity and decreased B-cell production. It has found use, for example, in psoriasis, atopic dermatitis, bullous disorders, vasculitides, sarcoid, connective tissue disorders, lichen planus and pyoderma gangrenosum.

There are limited studies indicating the incidence of cancers secondary to azathioprine's use in dermatology. However, the cases described in these studies were highly aggressive. Two studies demonstrated a relationship between azathioprine and SCC. One study had three patients who were all reported to develop aggressive SCCs (although there were additional excessive co-morbidities thought to be secondary to PUVA).[40] The other study revealed an aggressive anaplastic SCC 10 years after being treated with azathioprine for localized scleroderma.[41] Two other case reports were of HIV negative patients treated with azathioprine for atopic dermatitis and bullous pemphigoid who developed Kaposi's sarcoma (Fig. 34.4).[42,43]

With the lower dosing used in dermatology there are no cases of lymphoproliferative diseases attributed to azathioprine reported in the literature. However, there are significant numbers of cases of lymphoma and Merkel cell tumors reported in patients with rheumatoid arthritis or transplant patients treated with azathioprine.[44,45]

Hydroxyurea was first synthesized in the mid-1800s and was first used in dermatology in 1969. Hydroxyurea affects DNA synthesis, repair and gene regulation. It primarily functions through the inhibition of ribonucleotide reductase, a rate-limiting enzyme in DNA synthesis. Hydroxyurea has been used to treat SCC, MM, psoriasis, polycythemia vera, cryoglobulinemia, pyoderma gangrenosum and others. There are many reports of squamous cell cancer and basal cell cancer related to hydroxyurea therapy used for the treatment of leukemias and poly-

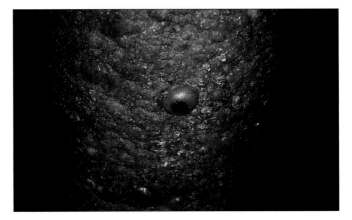

Figure 34.4 Kaposi's sarcoma: ecchymotic-like macules that evolve into papules, nodules and tumors that are violaceous, red, pink or tan can occur in patients on immunosuppressive medications.

cythemia vera.[46–48] Noteworthy, in the studies mentioned, the patients had significant amounts of sun exposure and were subjected to other chemotherapeutic agents perhaps weakening their immune systems and leading to increased numbers of cancers. Regardless, frequent skin checks for cancer should be performed for those patients placed on hydroxyurea therapy.

Nitrogen mustard, a topical medicine used first in the 1950s to treat cutaneous T-cell lymphoma (CTCL), exerts its antineoplastic effects by means of alkylation, in which an alkyl group becomes covalently linked to cellular components primarily inhibiting DNA replication. These effects are mutagenic, carcinogenic as well as cytotoxic. A study that examined biopsy specimens of mycosis fungoides treated with topical nitrogen for a period of 10–76 months after/during treatment. The findings demonstrated epidermal hyperplasia with foci of flat rete ridges, atypical keratinocytes with large nuclei, suprabasal mitotic figures, some dyskeratotic cells, increased numbers of enlarged junctional melanocytes, atypical endothelial cells and large fibroblasts with atypical nuclei.[49]

There is also evidence of some interaction of nitrogen mustard with the epidermal cell–Langerhans cell–T cell axis. Topical nitrogen is used primarily for the treatment of CTCL, but has also been used to treat Langerhans histiocytosis, psoriasis, alopecia areata, and pyoderma gangrenosum.

The risk of secondary malignancy has been documented, but needs to be put into perspective with regard to treatment and the stage of the CTCL. There are some case reports that show very aggressive cancers secondary to treatment with topical nitrogen mustard. One such report describes a male who developed squamous cell cancers after treatment with topical nitrogen mustard for CTCL and who was later treated with PUVA after the topical nitrogen mustard was stopped. During his next year, he developed many squamous cell carcinomas.[50] In a recent study, it was found that when topical nitrogen mustard was used as monotherapy the risk of secondary carcinogenesis was low and only occurred in 1% of patients. However, secondary cancers including SCC and MM were more common in patients who received other therapies, i.e. PUVA or electron beam therapy in addition to the topical nitrogen mustard (9%).[51]

Arsenic is a natural element that has been used in the past for various therapeutic approaches. Inorganic arsenic is much more toxic than the organic type. Its proposed mechanism of action is thought to bind sulfhydryls resulting in protein denaturation and the subsequent inhibition of enzyme activity, which exerts both cytotoxic and genotoxic effects. Arsenic was used in the treatment of CTCL in a formulation that was known as Fowler's solution. It currently is still used and is finding new uses in the treatment of African trypanosomiasis[52] and in leukemia and lymphoma.[53]

Arsenic contamination of water supplies is also a significant health concern that has led to an increased incidence of skin cancers in Asia, Europe, the Western United States, and Central and South America. Arsenic functions to cause low level chronic stimulation of keratinocyte growth factor, induces ornithine decarboxylase activity, and alters DNA binding sites in the AP-1 and AP-2 transcription factors, all of which are associated with proliferation and increased incidence of SCC (Fig. 34.5).[54] Genetic studies have indicated there are alterations in methylation patterns caused by arsenic that may lead to altered gene expression and, thus, a decrease of the *p53* tumor suppressor gene leading to increased BCC in the skin.[55] Additionally there is a reported case that documents the development of dermatofibrosarcoma protuberans after exposure to arsenic.[56]

The use of 'tar-like' substances in the treatment of dermatological disorders was first described nearly two thousand years ago. Tar is prepared via a process called destructive distillation, a process that heats organic materials in the absence of oxygen. Tar has demonstrated antimitotic and anti-inflammatory effects but the precise mechanisms are unknown. Tar preparations are useful topical therapy in the management of inflammatory skin diseases, especially psoriasis, atopic dermatitis and seborrheic dermatitis, tinea versicolor and pruritus. The safety of tar has been a matter of debate. The data from a study comprised of 606 workers with tar-induced dermatosis in a German tar refinery found a reversal of the ratio of SCC to BCC thereby demonstrating an increased incidence of SCC. Additionally, an increased incidence of keratoacanthomas was found (Fig. 34.6).[57] However, conclusive evidence for the carcinogenicity of tar in dermatologic practice is lacking. While the tar products are demonstrated in urine and blood none of the evaluated studies demonstrated an increased incidence in skin cancer.[58]

Anti-inflammatory therapies

Corticosteroids were first described in 1935 and first used in inflammatory dermatoses in the early 1950s. Corticosteroids have both anti-inflammatory and immuno-suppressive effects. The anti-inflammatory effects are: inhibition of NF-κB and AP-1 resulting in decreased amounts of certain cytokines; induction of lymphocyte and eosinophil apoptosis; inhibition of phospholipase A2, eicosanoids and COX-2. The immunosuppressive effects act to decrease the amount of B cells, T cells, PMNs, mast cells, monocytes/macrophages, Langerhans cells, and eosinophils. Dermatologic uses for corticosteroids are: Bullous dermatoses, autoimmune disorders, neutrophilic dermatoses, vasculitis, sarcoid, contact dermatitis, atopic dermatitis, and lichen planus, for example.

There is debate as to whether patients taking corticosteroids are at an increased risk of cutaneous malignancy. In a retrospective case–control study, the use of oral steroids was thought to lead to an increase of both SCC and BCC. For SCC the risk was elevated more than two-fold and for BCC the risk was modestly, but not clearly, elevated.[59] Another study reported 10 patients who were treated with corticosteroids for autoimmune disease, lymphoproliferative disorders and other diseases unrelated to the immune system. During the course of their treatment, these patients developed

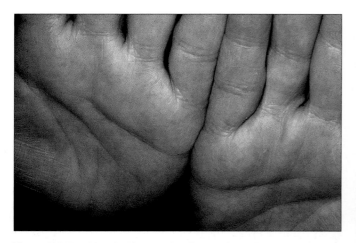

Figure 34.5 Arsenical keratosis: discrete hyperkeratotic papules that occur in the palmer creases associated with malignancy and arsenic exposure.

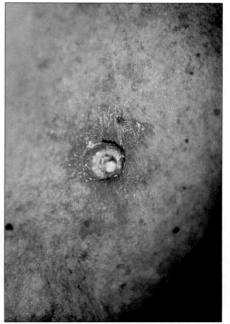

Figure 34.6 Keratoacanthoma: dome-shaped nodule often with central keratotic plug following years of PUVA therapy or tar therapy.

Kaposi's sarcoma that was thought to be associated to their immunosuppressive treatment.[60]

Biologic agents

Over the last few years, new biologic agents have been in development. Most of these agents target the activity of T lymphocytes and cytokines responsible for the inflammatory response. Weak associations with some of these agents and skin cancer have been reported.

There are four biologic agents that are at the forefront; infliximab, etanercept, efalizumab, and alefacept. Infliximab is a chimeric (mouse-human) IgG1 monoclonal antibody that binds to tumor necrosis factor-α (TNF-α) and inhibits the production of proinflammatory cytokines. It is currently used for rheumatoid arthritis and Crohn's disease and is currently undergoing phase II trials for use for psoriasis. The risk of malignancy is yet to be determined. Etanercept is a human TNF-receptor made from the fusion of two naturally occurring TNF receptors allowing it to bind to TNF with greater affinity resulting in a reduction in inflammatory activity. It is currently approved for the treatment of rheumatoid arthritis (RA) and psoriatic arthritis and has proven beneficial in the treatment of pustular psoriasis and atopic dermatitis. Etanercept has been used safely for the past few years in patients with RA and thus has a very safe track record. There is evidence to demonstrate that there is no increase in malignancy with etanercept[61] even though another study reported several SCCs. Many of the patients that developed the cancer in this study already had a history of skin cancer before starting treatment with etanercept and had been treated with other immunomodulating agents (like MTX).[62] Additionally, it has been observed that there is an increase in lymphoproliferative disease in patients who receive TNF-α therapy, perhaps secondary to the immunosuppressive effects of the medicine, the natural pathogenesis of the disease or because of the relationship between lymphomas and Epstein–Barr virus (EBV). Although it was found that there was an increase in the incidence of lymphoma (94 reported cases: 47 due to infliximab; and 47 due to etanercept) the exact mechanism has not been elucidated.[63] Efalizumab is a humanized monoclonal antibody against CD11a, a molecule that serves an important role in T-cell activation, migration and cytotoxic T-cell activation. Efalizumab has been used safely in nearly 2000 patients.[64] Alefacept is a recombinant protein that binds CD2 on memory effector T lymphocytes inhibiting their activation. To date, no increase in malignancy has been observed.[65]

FUTURE OUTLOOK

The advent of new medical therapies will continue to lead to new potential adverse effects. Some of these will include associated skin cancer. Physicians must be alert to these issues, carefully analyzing the events that lead to skin cancer complications and learning how to minimize the likelihood of similar events in the future.

REFERENCES

1 Hanahan D, Weinberg RA. The hallmarks of cancer. Cell 2000; 100:57–70.

2 Vogelstein B, Lane D, Levine AJ. Surfing the p53 network. Nature 2000; 408:307–310.

3 Carr AM. Piecing together the p53 puzzle. Science 2000; 287:1765–1766.

4 de Gruijl FR, van Kranen HJ, Mullenders LH. UV-induced DNA damage, repair, mutations and oncogenic pathways in skin cancer. J Photochem Photobiol B: Biology 2001; 63:19–27.

5 Wikonkal NM, Berg RJ, van Haselen CW, et al. Bcl-2 vs. p53 protein expression and apoptotic rate in human nonmelanoma skin cancers. Arch Derm 1997; 133(5):599–602.

6 Sarasin A, Giglia-Mari G. P53 gene mutations in human skin cancers. Exp Dermatol 2002; 11(1):44–47.

7 Lacour JP. Carcinogenesis of basal cell carcinoma: genetics and molecular mechanisms. Br J Dermatol 2002; 146(61):17–19.

8 Ruiz I, Altaba A. Gli proteins and hedgehog signaling: development and cancer. Trends Genet 1999; 15(10):418–425.

9 Fan H and Khavari PA. Sonic hedgehog opposes epithelial cell cycle arrest. Cell Biol 1999; 147(1):71–76.

10 Dahmane N, Lee J, Robins P, Heller P, Ruiz I, Altaba A. Activation of the transcription factor Gli1 and the sonic hedgehog signaling pathway in skin tumours. Nature 1997; 389:876–881.

11 Ping XL, Ratner D, Zhang H, et al. PTCH mutations in squamous cell carcinoma of the skin. J Invest Derm 2001; 116:614–616.

12 Piepkorn M. The expression of p16ink4a, the product of a tumor suppressor gene for melanoma, is upregulated in human melanocytes by UVB irradiation. J Am Acad Derm 2000; 42:741–745.

13 Beissert S, Schwarz T. Role of immunomodulation in diseases responsive to phototherapy. Methods 2002; 28:138–144.

14 Clingen PH, Berneburg M, Petit-Frere C, et al. Contrasting effects of an ultraviolet B and an ultraviolet A tanning lamp on interleukin-6, tumor necrosis factor-α and intercellular adhesion molecule-1 expression. Br J Dermatol 2001; 145:54–62.

15 Stern RS, Lunder EJ. Risk of squamous cell carcinoma and methoxsalen (pscralen) and UV-A radiation (PUVA). Arch Dermatol 1998; 134; 1582–1585.

16 Stern RS, Liebman EJ, Vakeva L. Oral psoralen and ultraviolet-A light (PUVA) treatment of psoriasis and persistent risk of nonmelanoma skin cancer. J Natl Cancer Inst 1998; 90(17):1278–1284.

17 Lindelof B, Sigurgeirsson B, Tegner E, et al. Puva and cancer risk: the Swedish follow-up study. Br J Dermatol 1999; 141:108–112.

18 Studniberg HM and Weller P. PUVA, UVB, psoriasis, and nonmelanoma skin cancer. J Am Acad Derm 1993; 29:1013–1022.

19 Stern RS, Bolshakov S, Nataraj AJ, Ananthaswamy HN. P53 Mutations in nonmelanoma skin cancers occurring in psoralen ultraviolet A-treated patients: evidence for heterogeneity and field cancerization. J Invest Derm 2002; 119:522–526.

20 Kreimer-Erlacher H, Seidl H, Back B, Kerl H, Wolf P. High mutation frequency at Ha-ras exons 1–4 in squamous cell carcinoma from PUVA-treated psoriasis patients. Photochem Photobiol 2001; 74(2):323–330.

21 Stern RS, Nichols KT, Vakeva LH. Malignant melanoma in patients treated for psoriasis with methoxsalen (psoralen) and ultraviolet A radiation (PUVA). N Engl J Med 1997; 336:1041–1045.

22 Wolf P, Schollnast R, Hofer A, Smolle J, Kerl H. Malignant melanoma after psoralen and ultraviolet A (PUVA) therapy. Br J Dermatol 1998; 138(6):1100–1102.

23 Stern RS, Bagheri S, Nichols K. The persistent risk of genital tumors among men treated with psoralen plus ultraviolet A (PUVA) for psoriasis. J Am Acad Derm 2002; 47(1):33–39.

24 Lebwohl M. Should we switch from combination UVA/UVB phototherapy units to narrowband UVB? Photodermatol Photoimmunol Photomed 2002; 18:44–46.

25 Robinson ES, Hubbard GB, Dooley TP. Metastatic melanoma in an adult opossum (monodelphis domestica) after short-term intermittent UVB exposure. Arch Derm Res 2000; 292:469–471.

26 Hofmann-Wellenhof R, Wolf P, Smolle J, Reimann-Weber A, Soyer HP, Kerl H. Influence of UVB therapy on dermascopic features of acquired melanocytic nevi. J Am Acad Derm 1997; 37:559–563.

27 Lichter MD, Karagas MR, Mott LA, Spencer SK, Stukel TA, Greenberg ER. Therapeutic ionizing radiation and the incidence of basal cell carcinoma and squamous cell carcinoma. Arch Derm 2000; 136:1007–1011.

28 Karagas MR, McDonald JA, Greenberg ER, et al. Risk of basal cell and squamous cell skin cancers after ionizing radiation therapy. For the skin cancer prevention study group. J Natl Cancer Inst 1996; 88(24):1848–1853.

29 Shore RE, Moseson M, Xue X, Tse Y, Harley N, Pasternack BS. Skin cancer after X-ray treatment for scalp ringworm. Radiat Res 2002; 157:410–418.

30 Paul C, Le Tourneau A, Cayuela JM, et al. Epstein–Barr virus-associated lymphoproliferative disease during methotrexate therapy for psoriasis. Arch Derm 1997; 133(7):867–871.

31 Theate I, Michaux L, Dardenne S, et al. Epstein–Barr virus-associated lymphoproliferative disease occurring in a patient with sarcoidosis treated by methotrexate and methylprednisolone. Eur J Haematol 2002; 69(4):248–253.

32 Tournadre A, D'Incan M, Dubost JJ, et al. Cutaneous lymphoma associated with Epstein–Barr virus infection in 2 patients treated with methotrexate. Mayo Clin Proc 2001; 76(8):845–848.

33 Abd-el-Baki J, Demierre MF, Li N, et al. Transformation in mycosis fungoides: the role of methotrexate. J Cutan Med Surg 2002; 6(2):109–116.

34 Kirby B, Owen CM, Blewitt RW, Yates VM. Cutaneous T-cell lymphoma developing in a patient on cyclosporin therapy. J Am Acad Derm 2002; 47:S165–S167.

35 Koo J, Kadonaga JN, Wintroub BV, Lozada-Nur FI. The development of B-cell lymphoma in a patient with psoriasis treated with cyclosporine. J Am Acad Derm 1992; 26(5):836–840.

36 Paul CF, Ho VC, McGeown C, et al. Risk of malignancies in psoriasis patients treated with cyclosporine: a 5y cohort study. J Invest Derm 2003; 120:211–216.

37 Marcil I, Stern RS. Squamous cell cancer of the skin in patients given PUVA and ciclosporin: nested cohort crossover study. Lancet 2001; 358:1042–1045.

38 Kitchin JE, Pomeranz MK, Pak G, Washenik K, Shupack JL. Rediscovering mycophenolic acid: a review of its mechanism, side effects, and potential uses. J Am Acad Derm 1997; 37(3):445–449.

39 Epinette WW, Parker CM, Jones EL, Greist MC. Mycophenolic acid for psoriasis. A review of pharmacology, long-term efficacy, and safety. J Am Acad Derm 1987; 17(6):962–971.

40 Bottomley WW, Ford G, Cunliffe WJ, Cotterill JA. Aggressive squamous cell cancer developing in patients receiving long term azathioprine. Br J Dermatol 1995; 133(3):460–462.

41 Nachbar F, Stolz W, Volkenandt M, Meurer M. Squamous cell carcinoma in localized scleroderma following immunosuppressive therapy with azathioprine. Acta Derm Venereol 1993; 73(3):217–219.

42 Vandercam B, Lachapelle JM, Janssens P, Tennstedt D, Lambert M. Kaposis sarcoma during immunosuppressive therapy for atopic dermatitis. Dermatology 1997; 194(2):180–182.

43 Halpern SM, Parslew R, Cerio R, Kirby JT, Sharpe G. Kaposis sarcoma associated with immunosuppression for bullous pemphigoid. Br J Dermatol 1997; 137(1):140–143.

44 Ehrenfeld M, Abu-Shakra M, Buskila D, Shoenfeld Y. The dual association between lymphoma and autoimmunity. Blood Cells Mol Dis 2001; 27(4):750–756.

45 Gooptu C, Woollons A, Ross J, et al. Merkel cell carcinoma arising after therapeutic immunosuppression. Br J Derm 2001; 137(4):637–641.

46 Aste N, Fumo G, Biggio P. Multiple squamous epitheliomas during long term treatment with hydroxyurea. J Eur Acad Dermatol Venereol 2001; 15(1):89–90.

47 De Simone C, Guerriero C, Guidi B, Rotoli M, Venier A, Tartaglione R. Multiple squamous cell carcinomas of the skin during long term treatment with hydroxyurea. Eur J Dermatol 1998; 8(2):114–115.

48 Najean Y, Rain JD. Treatment of polycythemia vera: the use of hydroxyurea and pipobroman in 292 patients under the age of 65 years. Blood 1997; 90(9):3370–3377.

49 Reddy VB, Ramsay D, Garcia JA, Kamino H. Atypical cutaneous changes after topical treatment with nitrogen mustard in patients with mycosis fungoides. Am J Derm 1996; 18(1):19–23.

50 Smith SP, Konnikov N. Eruptive epidermal cysts and multiple squamous cell carcinomas after therapy for cutaneous T-cell lymphoma. J Am Acad Derm 1991; 25(5):940–943.

51 Kim YH, Martinez G, Varghese A, Hoppe RT. Topical nitrogen mustard in the management of mycosis fungoides. Arch Derm 2003; 139:165–173.

52 Burri C, Nkunku S, Merolle A, Smith T, Blum J, Brun R. Efficacy of new, concise schedule for melarsoprol in treatment of sleeping sickness caused by *Trypanosoma brucei gambiense*: a randomized trial. Lancet 2000; 355:1419–1425.

53 Novick SC, Warrell RP Jr. Arsenicals in hematological cancers. Semin Oncol 2000; 27(5):495–501.

54 Germolec DR, Spalding J, Yu HS, et al. Arsenic enhancement of skin neoplasia by chronic stimulation of growth factors. Am J Pathol 1998; 153(6):1775–1785.

55 Boonchai W, Walsh M, Cummings M, Chenevix-Trench G. Expression of *P53* in arsenic-related and sporadic basal cell carcinoma. Arch Derm 2000; 136:195–198.

56 Shneidman D, Belizaire R. Arsenic exposure followed by the development of dermatofibrosarcoma protuberans. Cancer 1986; 58(7):1585–1587.

57 Letzel S, Drexler H. Occupationally related tumors in tar refinery workers. J Am Acad Derm 1998; 39:712–720.

58 Arnold WP. Tar. Clin Dermatol 1997; 15:739–744.

59 Karagas MR, Cushing GL Jr, Greenberg ER, Mott LA, Spencer SK, Nierenberg DW. Non-melanoma skin cancers and glucocorticoid therapy. Br J Cancer 2001; 85(5):683–686.

60 Trattner A, Hodak E, David M, Sandbank M. The appearance of Kaposi sarcoma during corticosteroid therapy. Cancer 1993; 72(5):1779–1783.

61 Fleischmann R, Iqbal I, Nandeshwar P, Quiceno A. Safety and efficacy of disease-modifying anti-rheumatic agents: focus on the benefits and risks of etanercept. Drug Saf 2002; 25(3):173–197.

62 Smith KJ, Skelton HG. Rapid onset of cutaneous squamous cell carcinoma in patients with rheumatoid arthritis after starting tumor necrosis factor α receptor IgG1-Fc fusion complex therapy. J Am Acad Derm 2001; 45:953–956.

63 Brown SL, Greene MH, Gershon SK, Edwards ET, Braun MM. Tumor necrosis factor antagonist therapy and lymphoma development. Arthritis Rheum 2002; 46(12):3151–3158.

64 Lebwohl M. New developments in the treatment of psoriasis. Arch Derm 2002; 138:686–688.

65 Weinberg JM, Saini R, Tutrone WD. Biologic therapy for psoriasis – The first wave: Infliximab, Etanercept, Efalizumab, and Alefacept. J Drugs Derm 2002; 3:303–310.

66 Duncan JI. Differential inhibition of cutaneous T-cell mediated reactions and epidermal cell proliferation by cyclosporin A, FK506, and rapamycin. J Invest Derm 1994; 102:84–88.

67 Reitamo S, Wollenberg A, Schopf E, et al. Safety and efficacy of 1 year of tacrolimus ointment monotherapy in adults with atopic dermatitis. Arch Derm 2000; 136:999–1005.

68 Wahn U, Bos JD, Goodfield M et al. Efficacy and safety of pimecrolimus cream in long-term management of atopic dermatitis in children. Pediatrics 2002; 110:E2.

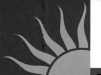

CHAPTER
35

The Use of Dermoscopy in the Diagnosis of Skin Cancer

Robert H Johr, Giuseppe Argenziano and Iris Zalaudek

Key points

- With training and experience, dermoscopy has been shown to increase the accuracy of the clinical diagnosis of melanoma.
- Pattern analysis, the ABCD rule of dermatoscopy, Argenziano's 7-point checklist and Menzies 11-point checklist are the established algorithms used to evaluate melanocytic lesions.
- If the diagnosis of a lesion by dermoscopy is not definitive, the lesion should be biopsied for histopathological examination.

INTRODUCTION

Dermoscopy is an *in vivo*, non-invasive technique that magnifies the skin in such a way that color and structure in the epidermis, dermo-epidermal junction and papillary dermis becomes visible. Dermoscopy is also known as dermatoscopy, skin surface microscopy and epiluminescence microscopy (ELM). The term 'dermoscopy' first used by Friedman *et al.* in 1991 currently enjoys the greatest international consensus.[1] This technique allows for the structures and colors that cannot be seen with the naked eye or with the typical magnification lenses clinicians use to be visualized. An entirely new series of subsurface features have been identified, which can be integrated into the diagnostic evaluation of skin lesions.[2]

With training and experience,[3] dermoscopy has been shown to significantly improve the clinical diagnosis of melanocytic, non-melanocytic, benign and malignant pigmented skin lesions and thus melanoma.[4–7] Patients with all skin phototypes benefit from the technique.

The criteria derived from dermoscopy should be added to the patient's personal and family history and the history and appearance of a lesion and/or lesions before a decision for or against excision or follow-up is made. The technique is not 100% diagnostic of any specific pathology whether benign or malignant. However, it has many advantages over clinical evaluation by other methods currently used (Table 35.1).[8,9]

In 1995, a nation-wide dermoscopy survey of dermatologists discovered that only 5% of those surveyed used the technique. In a more recent survey in 2002, it was estimated that 23% of US dermatologists now use dermoscopy.[10] Dermoscopy is the standard of care in many countries around the world and is becoming more popular in the United States, not only with dermatologists,

but with oncologists, surgeons, pediatricians and general physicians.[11]

Readily available instrumentation includes two options: (1) relatively inexpensive hand held dermascopes (i.e. Dermatoscope, Dermlite, Episcope) and (2) expensive computer systems (i.e. MoleMaxII, Dermogenius). With the dermatoscope (×10 magnification), some type of oil or fluid (mineral oil, immersion oil, K-Y jelly, alcohol or water) is placed on the lesion to be examined. The liquid eliminates surface light reflection and renders the stratum corneum transparent allowing visualization of subsurface colors and structures. The dermatoscope is then placed directly on the lesion. The Dermlite utilizes a polarizing system and fluid is no longer needed, which is very practical if many lesions are being evaluated. These hand-held instruments clearly demonstrate all of the dermoscopic features that are present in a lesion. Digital computer systems are also available. Some of the advantages of computer systems over hand-held instruments are listed in Table 35.2.

Recent articles in the literature present objective data that support the use of dermoscopy over clinical evaluation alone, to examine certain pigmented skin lesions. In one study where dermoscopy was not used, only 9 out of 199 atypically pigmented skin lesions (using ABCD clinical criteria) in children younger than 18 years of age were found to be histologically dysplastic.[12] It may not be appropriate for a patient in that age group to have a pigmented skin lesion excised before examining it with dermoscopy, because the chance of having high risk pathology is not great and unnecessary scarring surgery and concern can be avoided. In a study of 2731 excised pigmented skin lesions (using ABCDE clinical criteria),[13] it was found that dermoscopy was extremely effective in improving the clinical diagnosis of benign and malignant pigmented skin lesions and determining which ones to biopsy. A total of 165 new melanomas were identified with the technique and 24 were *in-situ* lesions that were not identified with clinical examination alone. Most recently, a meta-analysis of the literature clearly demonstrated the diagnostic benefits of dermoscopy.[9]

TECHNIQUE

Examining pigmented skin lesions with dermoscopy is a two-step process.[11,14–16] The process begins by determining if the lesion is melanocytic or non-melanocytic. If any of the following criteria can be found; pigment network, branched streaks (which are thickened and branched pigment network anywhere in the lesion),

Table 35.1 Benefits of dermoscopy

Differentiation of melanocytic from non-melanocytic skin lesions
Differentiation of benign from malignant skin lesions
Protect you from inexperienced pathologists (dermoscopic clinico-pathologic correlation)
Helps to plan surgery
Avoidance of unnecessary surgery
Follow patients with dysplastic nevi
Patient reassurance

Table 35.2 Advantages of digital technology

Greater magnification
Captures and stores images in the patient's database
Side-by-side comparison of old and new digital dermoscopy images on a computer monitor.
'Mole Mapping' with side-by-side comparison of old and new gross images on a computer monitor. New or changing lesions can be detected
Automatic image analysis
An archived history of individual lesions
Electronic enhancement of images
Teleconsulting with centers of excellence
Patients take part in the examination by viewing their lesions on the computer monitor which offers another visual way of patient education

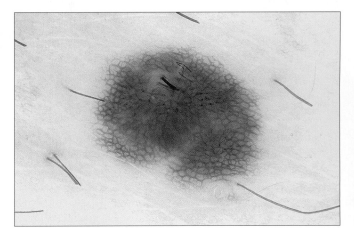

Figure 35.1 Dots and globules plus pigment network identify this as a melanocytic lesion.

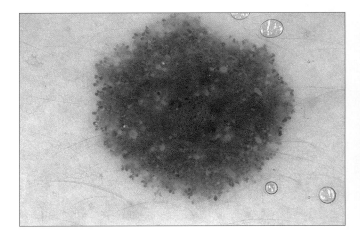

Figure 35.2 Even though there is no pigment network, dots and globules identify this as a melanocytic lesion.

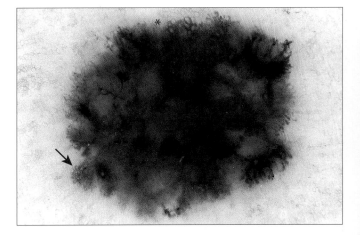

Figure 35.3 Melanocytic, non-melanocytic, benign and malignant lesions can all have intense black color. The presence of branched streaks (asterisk), dots and globules plus a subtle pigment network (arrow) identify this as a melanocytic lesion. Any of the reviewed algorithms will diagnose this as melanoma.

dots/globules, homogeneous or parallel global patterns then, by definition, the lesion is melanocytic (Figs 35.1–35.3). A lesion should also be considered melanocytic by default, if the criteria required to diagnose a melanocytic lesion, seborrheic keratosis, basal cell carcinoma, hemangioma or dermatofibroma are not identified (Table 35.3[17–22] and Figs 35.4–35.11). The histologic correlates of the dermoscopic findings are helpful in appreciating their significance in diagnosis (Table 35.4).[15,23–25]

After determining that a lesion is melanocytic, the next step is to determine if it is benign or malignant. Several different dermoscopic methods have been developed to accomplish this.

DERMOSCOPIC DIAGNOSTIC ALGORITHIMS

Various pattern-oriented diagnostic algorithms have been used in dermoscopy. In an attempt to evaluate these approaches and to select the best one, the Second Consensus Meeting on Dermoscopy was held over the Internet in 2000.[11] Experts from around the world were asked to evaluate melanocytic, non-melanocytic, benign and malignant skin lesions using pattern analysis, the ABCD rule of dermatoscopy, Menzies' 11-point scoring method and the 7-point checklist. One of the main con-

Table 35.3	Primary dermoscopic criteria

Criteria for a melanocytic lesion
- Pigment network
- Dots/globules
- Branched streaks (thickened branched pigment network)
- Homogenous and parallel global patterns

Criteria for seborrheic keratosis[17,18]
- Milia-like cysts
- Comedo-like openings
- Brain-like pattern (ridges and furrows)
- Finger-print pattern

Criteria for basal cell carcinoma[19,20]
- Absence criteria for melanocytic lesion
- Arborizing blood vessels
- Structureless areas of pigmentation
- Spoke-wheel structures

Criteria for vascular lesion[21,22]
- Red lacunas
- Red-bluish homogeneous areas

Criteria for dermatofibroma
- Central white patch

If none of the above criteria are present, evaluate as a melanocytic lesion

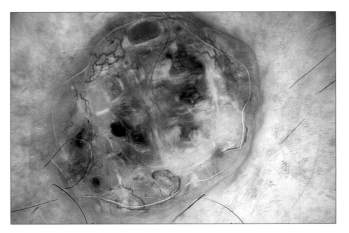

Figure 35.5 Stereotypical dermoscopic image of basal cell carcinoma. There is an absence of criteria to diagnose a melanocytic lesion plus large branching (arborizing) blood vessels. There are many variations of structureless pigmentation seen in basal cell carcinomas. In this case, a large bluish-white ovoid area can be seen.

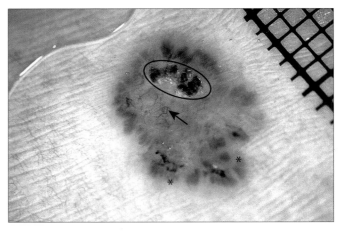

Figure 35.6 There are many variations of morphology seen with basal cell carcinomas. This lesion demonstrates ulceration (circle) and a few branching blood vessels (arrow). It might be difficult for the novice dermoscopist to determine if the pigmentation seen at the periphery (asterisks) represents globules, blotches or streaks. It is important to develop a dermoscopic differential diagnose when evaluating difficult cases. Here it is basal cell carcinoma vs. melanoma.

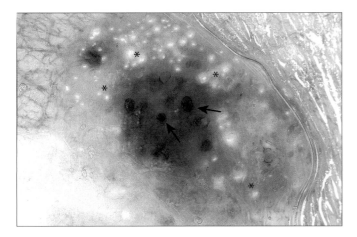

Figure 35.4 There is an absence of criteria used to diagnose a melanocytic lesion. The presence of multiple milia-like cysts (asterisks) and follicular openings (arrows) diagnose a stereotypical seborrheic keratosis. Do not confuse the pigmented follicular openings with globules seen in melanocytic lesions.

clusions from the consensus meeting was that the four melanocytic algorithms studied were all valid ways to evaluate pigmented skin lesions with dermoscopy.[23]

PATTERN ANALYSIS

The majority of the members of the International Internet Consensus Group (IICG) use pattern analysis. With pattern analysis, one has to identify all of the criteria found in a lesion and the criteria identified are then put into patterns (Table 35.5).[14–16,23,26,27] Patterns correlate with specific pathology. There are patterns

of criteria suggestive of different types of melanoma (superficial spreading, nodular, lentigo maligna, lentigo maligna melanoma, and amelanotic melanoma), different types of melanocytic nevi (junctional, compound, dermal, combined, blue, dysplastic and Spitz), and other types of skin lesions such as collision lesions which are made of two completely different pathologies adjacent to each other or mucosal melanotic macules.

It is important to identify and analyze as many criteria as possible in a lesion before making a dermoscopic diagnosis. No criterion by itself is 100% diagnostic of melanoma, however, there are *melanoma specific criteria*. These are criteria that can be seen in both benign and malignant lesions, but are more specifically seen in high-risk dysplastic nevi or melanoma. When several melanoma

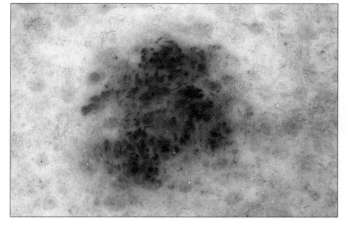

Figure 35.7 Dermoscopic image of a hemangioma. At times these lesions can be very dark and dermoscopy will make the diagnosis. This lesion has well demarcated reddish dots and globules. Not uncommonly, hemangiomas have a diffuse whitish color.

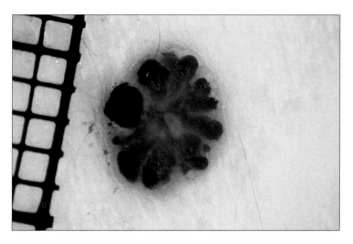

Figure 35.8 This is a variation of the morphology seen in hemangiomas. The dark blotches represent thrombosis in the vessels. (Reproduced with permission from Johr R *et al*. Dermoscopy: The Essentials. Philadelphia: Elsevier; 2004.)

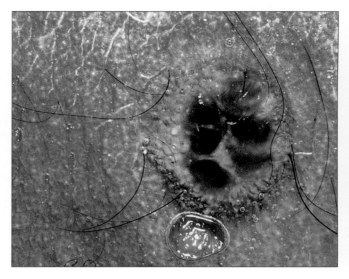

Figure 35.9 A dermatology resident was planning to treat this angiokeratoma destructively making the clinical diagnosis of a wart. Dermoscopic examination identified this as a vascular lesion thus avoiding unnecessary and inappropriate destructive therapy in a child.

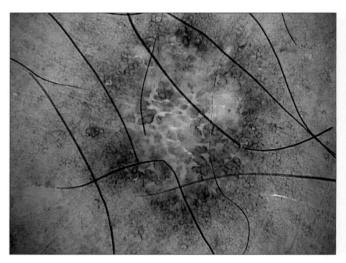

Figure 35.10 The bone-white central patch and surrounding delicate pigment network are diagnostic of a dermatofibroma. Dermatofibromas are one of the few non-melanocytic lesions that can have a pigment network.

specific criteria are identified, the lesion should be considered for excision (Table 35.6). For the novice dermoscopist, if a lesion demonstrates even one well-defined melanoma specific criteria, it is better to error on the side of conservatism and biopsy the lesion for a histopathologic diagnosis.

If a pigment network is identified, it then must be determined if it is regular or irregular, prominent or subtle, and whether it thins out gradually at the periphery or ends abruptly. The more prominent and irregular the pigment network is, the greater the chance that the lesion is malignant. If dots and/or globules of any color other than red (pink to red dots and globules represent a vascular pattern) are present, it is necessary to determine whether they are regular, or irregular in size, shape and distribution in the lesion.

Symmetrical and uniform criteria favor a benign diagnosis, while irregular criteria are suggestive of dysplastic nevi or melanoma. All of the potentially identifiable criteria should be analyzed in this way to come up with a pattern analysis dermoscopic diagnosis (Figs 35.12 and 35.13).

THE ABCD RULE OF DERMATOSCOPY

The ABCD rule of dermatoscopy was the first attempt to simplify the diagnostic process.[14,15,23,28–30] After a multivariate analysis of 31 dermoscopic criteria, four criteria were found to be significant cofactors for diagnosing melanoma. The key factors were determined to be asymmetry (A), borders (B), colors (C) and different structural components (D). These four criteria are defined as follows:

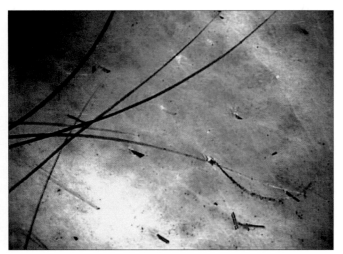

Figure 35.11 A 1 cm flat pink lesion on a very hairy patient. There is an absence of criteria to diagnose a melanocytic lesion, seborrheic keratosis, basal cell carcinoma, hemangioma, or dermatofibroma. By default, this should now be considered melanocytic. It is a featureless pink lesion. Only a high index of suspicion led to the diagnosis of this *in-situ* amelanotic melanoma.

Table 35.4 Dermoscopic criteria, histopathologic correlates and diagnostic significance of melanocytic and non-melanocytic skin lesions

Criterion	Morphological description	Histopathological correlate	Diagnosis
Pigment network	Network of brownish lines over a diffuse tan background	Pigmented rete ridges	Melanocytic lesion
Regular network	Brown pigmented, regularly meshed and narrowly spaced network	Regular and elongated rete ridges	Benign melanocytic lesion
Irregular network	Black, brown, or gray network with irregular holes and thick lines	Irregular and broadened rete ridges	Melanoma
Dots/globules	Black, brown and/or gray round to oval, variously sized structures regularly or irregularly distributed within the lesion	Pigment aggregates within stratum corneum, epidermis, dermoepidermal junction, or papillary dermis	If regular, benign melanocytic lesion; if irregular, melanoma
Streaks	Irregular, linear structures not clearly combined with pigment network lines at the margins	Confluent junctional nests of melanocytes	Melanoma Spitz nevi
Blue-white veil	Irregular, confluent, gray-blue to whitish-blue diffuse pigmentation. Can have a 'ground glass' appearance	Acanthotic epidermis with focal hypergranulosis above sheets of heavily pigmented melanocytes and/or melanophages in the dermis	Melanoma Spitz nevi
Regression structures	White (scar-like) areas, blue (pepper-like) areas, or combination of both	Thickened papillary dermis with fibrosis and/or variable amounts of melanophages	Melanoma
Starburst pattern	Pigmented radial linear structures at the edge of the lesion	Discrete junctional nests of spindle-shaped melanocytes at the periphery	Spitz nevi Dysplastic nevi Melanoma
Central white patch with delicate network	Delicate network of brownish lines surrounding a central white area	A variable amount of fibrosis in the papillary dermis immediately beneath the epidermis	Dermatofibroma
Milia-like cysts	White-yellowish, roundish dots	Intraepidermal horn globules, also called horn pseudocysts	Seborrheic keratosis
Comedo-like openings	Brown-yellowish, round to oval or irregularly shaped, sharply circumscribed structures	Keratin plugs situated within dilated follicular openings	Seborrheic keratosis
Leaf-like areas	Brown-gray to gray-black patches revealing a leaf-like configuration	Pigmented, solid aggregations of basaloid cells in the papillary dermis	Basal cell carcinoma
Red-blue lacunas	Sharply demarcated, round to oval areas with a reddish, red-bluish, or red-black coloration	Dilated vascular spaces situated in the upper dermis	Vascular lesion

Table 35.5 Pattern analysis criteria

Global patterns (reticular, globular, cobblestone, homogeneous, parallel, starburst, multicomponent, non-specific)
Pigment network
Blotches (structureless pigmentation)
Dots/globules
Streaks (pseudopods/radial streaming)
Blue-white structures (blue-white veil and/or depigmentation)[a]
Vascular structures

[a]At times, it is not possible to differentiate the white color of regression and the blue-white veil. You can consider these criteria together and call them blue-white structures. Whatever variation you see, they are high risk and often seen in melanomas.

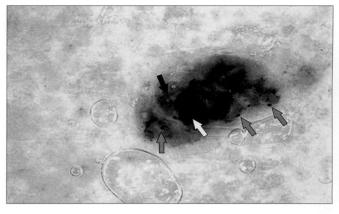

Figure 35.12 This 5 mm diameter thin superficial spreading melanoma was surrounded by similar appearing seborrheic keratosis. Dots and globules identify it as a melanocytic lesion. There is asymmetry of color and structure, irregular dots and globules (yellow arrows), a blue white structure (blue arrow) and an irregular black blotch (white arrow). This pattern of criteria suggests melanoma until proven otherwise.

Table 35.6 Melanoma specific criteria with pattern analysis (trunk and extremities)

Asymmetry of color and structure
Multicomponent global pattern (3 different dermoscopic areas in a lesion)
Non-specific global pattern
Irregular pigment network
Irregular dots/globules
Irregular streaks (pseudopods/radial streaming)
Irregular blotches
Blue-white structures
5–6 colors
Atypical vascular pattern
Milky-red areas

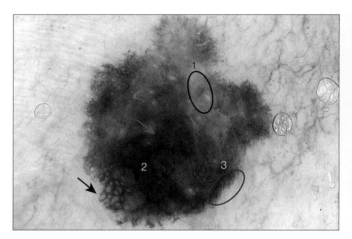

Figure 35.13 This superficial spreading melanoma with regression has a multicomponent global pattern [1, 2, 3] and significant asymmetry of color and structure. Other melanoma-specific criteria include an irregular pigment network (black arrow), subtle streaks (red circle), and blue-white structures (green arrow and black circle).

Asymmetry (A)

To determine the asymmetry score, the lesion is visually divided into two 90 degree right angle axes, then assigned a score ranging from zero for a lesion that is completely symmetrical in contour, color or structure to one point for a lesion that is asymmetrical in one axis and a maximum of two points for a lesion that is asymmetrical in both axes. When the axes are created visually in your mind, it should be done with the idea of creating the lowest possible asymmetry score.

One simple way to determine the symmetry of a lesion is to see if each side of the axis is a mirror image of the other for any of the criteria (contour, color or structure). If it is not symmetrical in appearance for any or all of the criteria, it would then be considered asymmetrical in that axis and receive one point. Dysplastic nevi and early melanomas can appear symmetrical when examined with the naked eye. However, the same lesions often demonstrate asymmetry of contour, color, and/or structure if dermoscopy is used.

Borders (B)

To determine the border score, the lesion is visually divided into eight pie-shaped segments or 'eights', and then the number of segments is counted in which there is an abrupt cut-off at the margins of *the pigment pattern*. That could be pigment network, branched streaks, dots, globules or diffuse pigmentation. It is not simply a well-demarcated lesion that gets border points. The score can range from zero to eight.

Colors (C)

Colors to look for include red, white, light and dark brown, blue-gray and black. In general, different shades of colors have no differential diagnostic importance, however, the number of colors does. White should be counted only if it is lighter than the surrounding skin, and should not be confused with hypopigmentation that is commonly seen in all types of melanocytic lesions. Each color gets a point, and the total score ranges from one to six. A lesion with five or six bright and distinct colors is a significant clue that it might be a melanoma.

The colors seen dermoscopically depend on the location of melanin in the skin. Black means that the melanin is high in the epidermis, and this is not always an ominous sign because many benign or dysplastic nevi often have black color. If melanin is at the level of the dermoepidermal junction it appears light or dark brown. Gray indicates that melanin is in the papillary dermis, which can be seen with melanophages. Melanophages are a pattern recognition diagnosis with distinct appearing brown, gray, or bluish-gray dots (granules) that are irregular in size and shape, often described as 'pepper like'. Melanophages are commonly seen in regressing melanomas (Fig. 35.14). As you get deeper into the dermis, the colors appear steel gray or dark bluish. White color can represent hyperkeratosis or the scarring seen with regression. Yellow can be caused by hyperkeratosis and red indicates an inflammatory process that is commonly seen in dysplastic nevi or melanomas.

Identifying colors can have practical clinical applications. If a flat black lesion contains black and/or dark brown colors and structures with dermoscopy, there is a good chance if it is a melanoma it will be an *in-situ* or early invasive lesion. If colors indicating deeper involvement are identified, the prognosis is potentially more ominous.[31–33]

Different structural components (D)

Look for a pigment network, branched streaks (thickened and branched pigment network anywhere in the lesion not only at the borders), structureless or homogeneous areas (color, but no structures such as pigment network, branched streaks, dots or globules), dots and globules. To be counted, structureless or homogeneous areas should be larger than 10% of the lesion. Branched streaks, dots and globules are counted only when more than two are clearly seen. The total different structural component score ranges from one to five.

CALCULATING THE TOTAL DERMATOSCOPY SCORE (TDS)

The ABCD rule applies the above criteria in an algorithm using a semi-quantitative mathematical approach that gives points for the criteria identified in a lesion and a formula to determine the total dermatoscopy score (TDS) for each lesion. Each of the ABCD features identified are quantified and then the TDS is calculated by multiplying the points by conversion factors (A × 1.3 + B × 0.1 + C × 0.5 + D × 0.5 = TDS) (Fig. 35.15 and Table 35.7). In most cases, an experienced clinician can calculate the TDS relatively easily and rapidly.[34]

A TDS less than 4.75 in most cases would indicate a lesion that is benign. A TDS of 4.80 to 5.45 is suggestive, but not diagnostic, of melanoma. A lesion with a score in this range can either be excised or followed. A TDS greater than 5.45 is highly suspicious but not 100% diagnostic of melanoma. It is not uncommon to get a false high total dermatoscopy score (TDS) with benign lesions (Table 35.8). With the development of digital systems, a database of lesions that a clinician wishes to follow can now be created. Side-by-side computer monitor comparisons of the baseline and follow-up images can then be made to look for significant dermoscopic changes over time (Fig. 35.16).[35–39]

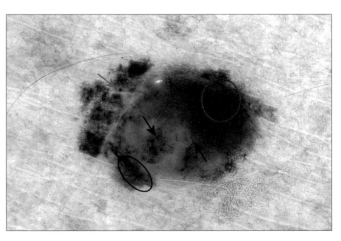

Figure 35.15 This superficial spreading melanoma with regression has a well-developed atypical vascular pattern (black arrows). It is easily diagnosed as a melanoma with the ABCD rule of dermatoscopy.
A = 2×1.3 = 2.6
B = 6×0.1 = 0.6
C = 5×0.5 = 2.5 (light and dark brown, blue-gray, black, white)
D = 5×0.5 = 2.5 (network (black circle), structureless areas (red circle), dots and globules (green arrow)

A + B + C + D = TDS of 8.2

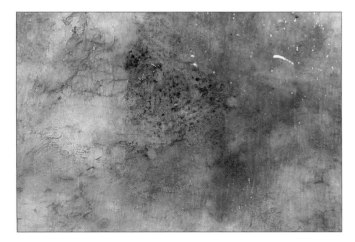

Figure 35.14 Melanophages have a characteristic dermoscopic appearance. In many cases, a suspicious lesion turns out to only have melanophages, which points to a diagnosis of post-inflammatory hyperpigmentation like in this case.

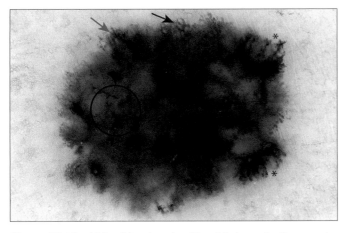

Figure 35.19 Using Menzies algorithm this is easily diagnosed as a melanoma. There is asymmetry, more than one color and four positive features. Blue-white veil (circle), brown dots (asterisks), streaks (green arrow) and a broadened network (black arrow).

Broadened network

Localized pigment network in which the line segments are thickened and irregular.

With Menzies' algorithm, there is an 8% false negative melanoma diagnosis rate. Problems can involve *in-situ*, early invasive and hypomelanotic melanomas. With all of their 'featureless' melanomas Menzies' patients had a history of recent change that they felt would help increase the index of suspicion of a potentially high-risk lesion although with the authors' experience, patients with featureless, hypomelanotic or pink melanomas were not aware that their lesions had changed clinically or even existed.[41,48,49] One study has demonstrated that Menzies' 11-point checklist could be easily taught to non-expert primary care physicians.[50]

THE 7-POINT CHECKLIST

This dermoscopic method is another variation of pattern analysis, but also incorporating a point system.[14,15,23,30,51] There are fewer criteria to identify and analyze than in pattern analysis and the point system is less complicated than in the ABCD rule of dermatoscopy.

Major criteria

Atypical pigment network

Black, brown or gray thickened and irregular line segments anywhere in a lesion.

Blue-white veil

Irregular, confluent, gray-blue to whitish-blue diffuse pigmentation that can be associated with pigment network alterations, dots, globules or streaks. This differs from Menzies' definition in which the blue color should be featureless.

Atypical vascular pattern

Linear irregular and/or dotted red vessels not seen in regression areas.

Minor criteria

Irregular streaks

Pseudopods or radial streaming asymmetrically seen at the periphery.

Irregular pigmentation (blotches)

Black, brown or gray featureless areas with irregular shape and/or distribution.

Irregular dots/globules

Black, brown or gray round to oval variously sized structures irregularly distributed in the lesion.

Regression structures

White scar-like areas, and/or bluish-white areas that can be homogeneous or contain multiple blue-gray dots. Not uncommonly, melanomas can have both color patterns of regression in a lesion.

Major and minor criteria

Major and minor criteria in a lesion must be identified. Major criteria receive two points each and minor criteria receive one point. A score of three or greater has a 95% sensitivity of being melanoma (Fig. 35.20). The 7-point checklist does not include criteria not associated with melanoma, or include criteria used to diagnose pigmented skin lesions that are not melanocytic such as seborrheic keratoses, or basal cell carcinoma (Table 35.10).

3-POINT CHECKLIST

Results of the Second Consensus Meeting on Dermoscopy discovered that asymmetry of color and structure, atypicality or irregularity of pigment network and the presence of blue-white structures were especially important criteria in helping to diagnose melanoma. The presence of any two of the criteria indicated a high likelihood of melanoma. A preliminary clinical study[52,53] was undertaken to see if the 3-point checklist could be used as a screening algorithm for non-expert dermoscopists. After a 1 hr lecture, six non-experts were asked to evaluate 231 clinically suspicious pigmented skin lesions. Using this method, the group was able to correctly diagnose melanoma 96.3% of the time. One-third of the lesions were also correctly diagnosed as banal nevi with this simplified algorithm.

OTHER CONSIDERATIONS

Dysplastic nevi

Some dysplastic nevi also share the same clinical features of melanoma and the ABCD clinical criteria can not always perfectly differentiate between them. A similar problem exists when using dermoscopy to diagnose dysplastic nevi. Whichever dermoscopic method is used, both melanoma and dysplastic nevi can share the same criteria. The intensity and number of criteria do not always correlate with the histology (Figs 35.21 and 35.22).

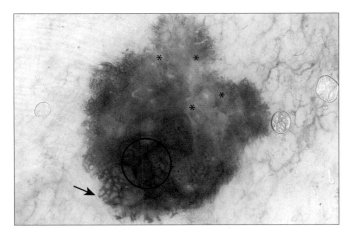

Figure 35.20 Using the 7-point checklist, the major criteria found in this lesion include an atypical pigment network (arrow) and a blue-white structure (circle). With 4 points this is already in the melanoma range. It also has one minor criteria, a regression area (enclosed by asterisks) which adds another point. This melanoma has a 7-point checklist score of 5.

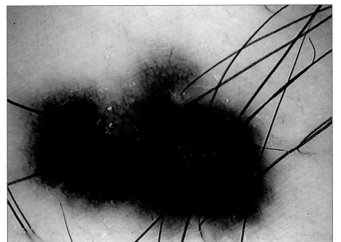

Figure 35.21 Black is not always an ominous sign. Tape stripping can often remove some of the black color and uncover hidden criteria. The presence of black blotches and an irregular network can be enough to warrant a histopathologic diagnosis. The differential diagnosis for this lesion is dysplastic nevus vs *in-situ* melanoma. In this case it was only a mildly dysplastic nevus.

Table 35.10 7-point checklist	
	Points
Major criteria	
Atypical pigment network	2
Atypical vascular pattern	2
Blue-white veil	2
Minor criteria	
Irregular streaks	1
Irregular pigmentation (blotch)	1
Irregular dots/globules	1
Regression areas	1
7-point total score	
<3 Non-melanoma	
≥3 Melanoma	

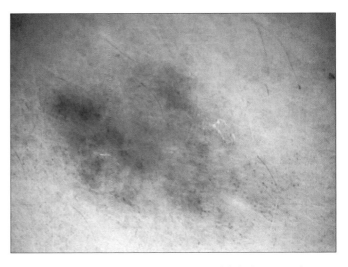

Figure 35.22 This relatively featureless pink lesion turned out to be a severely dysplastic nevus.

When using pattern analysis to diagnose melanoma, a finding of asymmetry of color and structure, a multi-component global pattern and melanoma specific criteria, such as an irregular pigment network, irregular dots and globules or streaks, is helpful. However, these features can also be seen in dysplastic and congenital nevi (Fig. 35.23).

Not uncommonly, a lesion that looks high risk with dermoscopy may not be histopathologically, and relatively featureless lesions turn out to be severely dysplastic nevi. Multifocal hypopigmentation and variations of an irregular pigment network may often be seen in dysplastic nevi (Fig. 35.24).[54,55]

The 'ugly duckling' approach as a tool for melanoma screening is also useful when evaluating multiple pigmented skin lesions with dermoscopy.[56] Lesions that stand out dermoscopically would be the ones to sample to make a dermoscopic clinicopathologic correlation. More research is needed to identify criteria and patterns that can more specifically diagnose high-risk dysplastic nevi. Experience and gut feelings are two very important factors when evaluating patients with dysplastic nevi. It has been the authors' experience that unnecessary surgery can often be avoided and high-risk lesions can be identified in this subset of patients when evaluated with dermoscopy.

Congenital melanocytic nevi

Dermoscopy may be especially helpful to evaluate congenital melanocytic nevi of any size, often avoiding unnecessary surgery in the newborn period and with young children.[57] The technique is not as effective for thick, dark lesions where the local dermoscopic features cannot be evaluated.

Several global patterns are commonly seen in congenital melanocytic nevi. These lesions can have diffuse

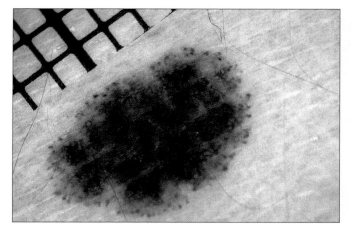

Figure 35.23 Dots and globules at the periphery of this dysplastic nevus are a sign of an actively changing lesion, which can be seen in benign and malignant lesions. That pattern would be an important indication for an excision.

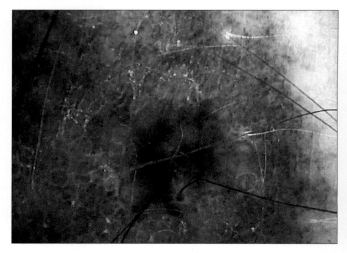

Figure 35.25 The black blotch and blue-white structure were biopsied and found to be severe cellular atypia in a congenital melanocytic nevus. The patient was a 17 year old with 30 similar appearing lesions both clinically and with dermoscopy all having a globular pattern without black blotches. The black blotch was the 'ugly duckling' that led to a biopsy.

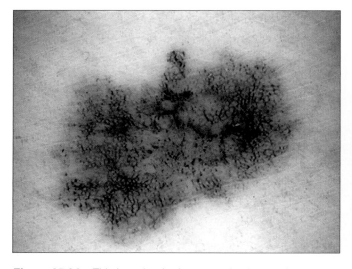

Figure 35.24 This is a classic dermoscopic picture of a dysplastic nevus with multifocal hypopigmentation, irregular pigment network and irregular dots and globules. If the patient has one lesion, consider excision. If there are multiple similar appearing lesions, excise one to make a dermoscopic clinicopathologic correlation.

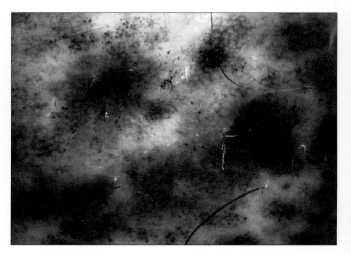

Figure 35.26 Superficial spreading melanoma arising in a medium sized congenital melanocytic nevus. It has the pattern of islands of normal skin and islands containing criteria. In this case the criteria were irregular which led to a biopsy.

pigmentation (a homogeneous global pattern), dots and globules (globular or cobblestone patterns), pigment network (reticular pattern), a multicomponent pattern with three or more distinct areas or a non-specific pattern. Coarse hairs are commonly found in these lesions and are an important differential diagnostic point.

Another very common dermoscopic pattern found in congenital nevi consists of islands of normal skin or hypopigmentation and islands with criteria. Diagnostic criteria could include pigment network, dots and globules or blotches of diffuse pigmentation. Any area that stands out from the uniform pattern should be considered for biopsy (Fig. 35.25). Due to irregularities of the pigment network and nests of melanocytes plus melanin at different levels in the skin creating a multivariate color

scheme, banal pathology in these nevi can look very worrisome with dermoscopy (Fig. 35.26). When in doubt, biopsy the lesion.

Site specific dermoscopic criteria

There are anatomic site-specific dermoscopic criteria that exist and it is important to be aware of this and learn them so that a correct dermoscopic diagnosis is made. These would include lesions on the palms, soles, nail beds, head and neck.

There are ridges and furrows in the skin on the palms and soles, and melanocytic skin lesions should have what is referred to as parallel pattern of the pigment network.[58] If this is not seen, a potentially high-risk lesion should be considered as the diagnosis (dysplastic nevi *vs* melanoma).

There are two parallel patterns that can be seen. The parallel-ridge pattern can be seen *in situ* in early invasive melanoma and the parallel-furrow pattern, the most common one seen in benign acral melanocytic nevi (Figs 35.27 and 35.28). At times, it is difficult to tell them apart. Pigmentation can also be seen at right and oblique angles to the ridges and furrows creating two other benign patterns, the lattice-like (ladder-like) and fibrillar patterns. If the lines forming the fibrillar pattern are dark and thickened, this can be seen in melanoma.

The parallel-ridge pattern often has thicker areas of pigmentation that contain rows of sweat gland ostia. They appear as white dots like a 'string of pearls'. The ostia are not always identifiable in the ridges. Other melanoma specific criteria for acral pigmented skin lesions includes irregular dots and/or globules, irregular blotches of pigmentation and blue/white structures.

It may be difficult on the head or neck to differentiate between solar lentigenes or seborrheic keratoses and lentigo maligna or lentigo maligna melanoma. A serious dermoscopic misdiagnosis can be made on these lesions if the concept of differentiating the pseudonetwork of melanocytic lesions is not made from the milia-like cysts seen in seborrheic keratoses.[17,18,59,60] Both can appear as yellowish dots or hypo-pigmented round to oval areas of different sizes and shapes. At times this differentiation is not possible (Fig. 35.29).

Melanoma specific criteria for head and neck lesions includes asymmetrically pigmented follicles (irregular pigmentation around ostia), annular-granular structures (multiple blue-gray or brown dots surrounding follicular ostia), gray pseudonetwork (formed by confluent annular-granular areas), rhomboid structures (gray-brown or black pigmentation surrounding the follicular ostia with a rhomboidal shape. A rhomboid is a parallelogram with unequal angles and sides), irregular dots and/or globules, irregular pigmentation and blue-white structures (Fig. 35.30). At times, lentigo-maligna can be featureless with dermoscopy, and it is important to look carefully at the lesion clinically for other clues to suggest the correct diagnosis.

Dermoscopic evaluation of nail-apparatus pigmentation

Nail apparatus melanoma (NAM) is a rare tumor, accounting for 1–2% of all melanomas in the light skinned population, and 15–20% of melanomas in people of color. Commonly at presentation, the melanoma has reached Clark's level IV or V. The differential diagnosis of NAM is extensive including both benign and malignant tumors. Making the diagnosis more difficult is the fact that up to 30% of these tumors are amelanotic.

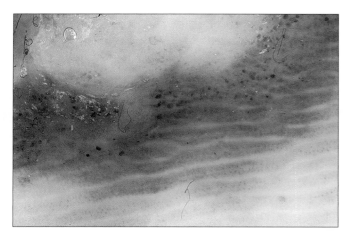

Figure 35.27 This is the parallel-ridge pattern. The 'string of pearls' is not seen in this case. Add the irregular dots and globules and it spells melanoma until proven otherwise.

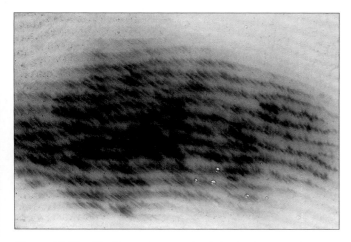

Figure 35.28 The linear pigmentation is in the furrows of the skin. The classic benign parallel-furrow pattern. If in doubt do not hesitate to make a histopathologic diagnosis.

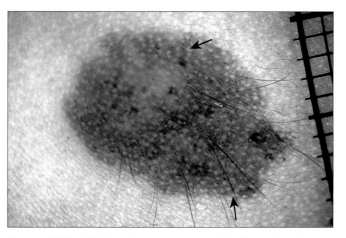

Figure 35.29 This is a benign melanocytic lesion on the face. The hairs point to a congenital lesion. It has a pseudonetwork composed of follicular ostia (arrows) and pigmentation forming a honeycomb like picture. The pigment network seen on the trunk and the extremities has a similar dermoscopic appearance but is related to elongated pigmented rete ridges. It is important to differentiate the ostia from milia-like cysts seen in seborrheic keratosis.

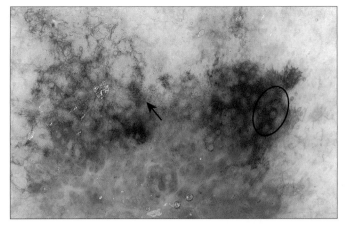

Figure 35.30 This lentigo-maligna has several site-specific and melanoma-specific criteria: Asymmetrically pigmented follicles (green arrow), annular-granular structures (black arrow), well-developed rhomboid structures (circle) and pink color.

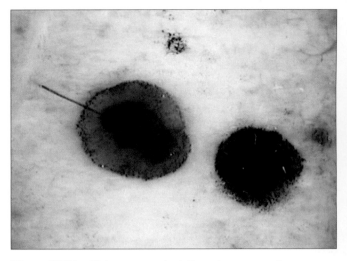

Figure 35.31 Cutaneous metastatic melanoma can have many morphologic dermoscopic variants. They can be pigmented and amelanotic without distinguishing features.

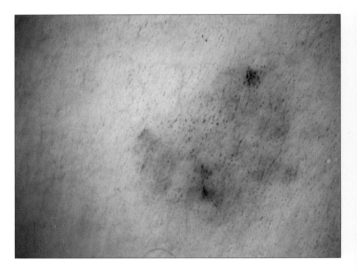

Figure 35.32 This relatively featureless small pink macule is an in-situ amelanotic melanoma arising in a dysplastic nevus. There are no clues to the seriousness of this lesion.

To biopsy or not to biopsy is often the question. Blanket statements that any pigmentation of the nail apparatus should be biopsied are no longer so absolute, especially in pediatric patients where studies indicate that melanoma would be extremely rare in this age group.

The clinical appearance of the nail apparatus is made clearer with dermoscopy.[61,62] Potentially high-risk criteria suggestive of nail apparatus melanoma includes an overall picture of asymmetry of color and structure, irregular pigmented bands, irregular diffuse pigmentation, the presence of multiple colors, irregular dots and globules and a Hutchinson's sign.

One potential caveat would be the presence of blood in the dermatoscopic image. This can usually be easily recognized as amorphous purple color, with some purple dots and globules. Blood can also be seen in NAM and, when found, indicates that it would be prudent to make a careful search for other high-risk criteria.

FUTURE OUTLOOK

Dermoscopy is an extremely useful readily available tool to evaluate pigmented skin lesions. However, there are limitations to the technique's effectiveness. It may not be helpful to make a specific diagnosis with lightly or heavily pigmented lesions, when the pathology is located deep in the dermis, for cutaneous metastatic melanoma (Fig. 35.31), amelanotic melanoma or small pink lesions. The most innocuous appearing small pink macule or papule could be an *in-situ* or invasive amelanotic melanoma (Fig. 35.32).[41] A very important dermoscopic principle that is fundamental, especially for the novice, is whenever in doubt consider biopsying the lesion for histopathological evaluation.

Whatever the dermoscopic diagnostic algorithm chosen, dermoscopy opens up a world of colors and structures that cannot be seen with the naked eye. For those clinicians that keep up with the literature and use the technique, one point has proven to be consistently true.[63] Even though dermoscopy is not 100% diagnostic

of pigmented skin lesions, it significantly improves the clinical diagnosis of melanocytic, non-melanocytic, benign, and malignant skin lesions and thus melanoma. The integration of digital image analysis and computer-aided diagnosis with dermoscopy will enhance its effectiveness in the future. With one person dying from melanoma every hour in the US, dermoscopy may become the standard of care not only in the US, but in all countries where melanoma leads to significant morbidity and mortality. Any clinician that sees patients with pigmented skin lesions should consider using dermoscopy.

REFERENCES

1 Friedman RJ, Rigel DS, Silverman MK, et al. Malignant melanoma in the 1990s: The continued importance of early detection and the role of

physician examination and self-examination of the skin. CA Cancer J Clin 1991; 41:201–226.

2 Johr R, Izakovic J. Should you be using epiluminescence microscopy? Skin Aging 2000; 28–38.

3 Binder M, Schwartz M, Steiner A, et al. Epiluminescence microscopy of small pigmented skin lesions: short-term formal training improves the diagnostic performance of dermatologists. J Am Acad Derm 1997; 37:197–202.

4 Pehamberger H, Binder M, Steiner A, Wolff K. In vivo epiluminescence microscopy: improvement of early diagnosis of melanoma. J Invest Derm 1993; 100(Suppl):356–625.

5 Argenziano G, Soyer HP. Dermoscopy of pigmented skin lesions: a valuable tool for early diagnosis of melanoma. Lancet Oncol 2001; 2:443–449.

6 Argenziano G, Soyer HP, Chimenti S, Ruocco V. Impact of dermoscopy on the clinical management of pigmented skin lesions. Clin Derm 2002; 20:200–202.

7 Wolff K. Why is epiluminescence microscopy important? Recent Results Cancer Res 2002; 160:125–132.

8 Menzies SW, Ingvar C, McCarthy WH. A sensitivity and specificity analysis of the surface microscopy features of invasive melanoma. Melanoma Res 1996; 6:55–62.

9 Kittler H, Pehamberger H, Wolff K, et al. Diagnostic accuracy of dermoscopy. Lancet Oncol 2002; 3:159–165.

10 Tripp JM, Kopf AW, Marghoob AA, et al. Management of dysplastic nevi: A survey of fellows of the American Academy of Dermatology. J Am Acad Derm 2002; 46:674–682.

11 Argenziano G, Soyer HP, Chimenti S, et al. Dermoscopy of pigmented skin lesions: Results of a consensus meeting via the Internet. J Am Acad Derm 2003; 48:679–693.

12 Haley JC, Hood AF, Chuang TY, et al. The frequency of histologically dysplastic nevi in 199 pediatric patients. Pediatr Dermatol 2000; 17(4):266–269.

13 Ascierto PA, Palmieri G, Celentanoe, et al. Sensitivity and specificity of epiluminescence microscopy: evaluation on a sample of 2731 excised cutaneous pigmented lesions. Br J Derm 2000; 142:893–898.

14 IICG. Consensus Net Meeting on Dermoscopy. Unifying Concepts of Dermoscopy, www.dermoscopy.org; 2000.

15 Argenziano G, Soyer HP, DeGiorgi V, et al. Interactive atlas of dermoscopy: a tutorial. Milan: EDRA Medical Publishing and New Media; 2000.

16 Rabinovitz H, Kopf A, Katz B. Dermoscopy: A Practical Guide. MMM A Worldwide Group Inc.; 1999.

17 Braun RP, Rabinovitz H, Kopf AW, et al. Dermoscopic diagnosis of seborrheic keratosis. Clin Dermatol 2002; 20:270–272.

18 Argenziano G, Rossiello L, Staibano S, et al. Melanoma simulating seborrheic keratosis: a major dermoscopy pitfall. Arch Derm 2003; 139:389–391.

19 Menzies SW, Westerhoff K, Rabinovitz H, et al. Surface microscopy of pigmented basal cell carcinoma. Arch Derm 2000; 136:1012–1016.

20 Menzies SW. Dermoscopy of pigmented basal cell carcinoma. Clin Dermatol 2002; 20 268–269.

21 Wolf I. Dermoscopic diagnosis of vascular lesions. Clin Dermatol 2002; 20:273–275.

22 Kreusch JF. Vascular patterns in skin tumors. Clin Dermatol 2002; 20:248–254.

23 Soyer HP, Argenziano G, Chimenti S, et al. Dermoscopy of pigmented skin lesions: an atlas based on the Consensus Net Meeting on Dermoscopy 2000. Milan: EDRA Medical Publishing and New Media; 2001.

24 Bauer J, Metzler G, Rassner G, et al. Dermatoscopy turns histopathologists attention to the suspicious area in melanocytic lesions. Arch Derm 2001; 137:1338–1340.

25 Ferrara G, Argenziano G, Soyer HP, et al. Dermoscopic-pathologic correlation: an atlas of 15 cases. Clin Dermatol 2002; 20:228–235.

26 Steiner A, Binder M, Schemper M, et al. Statistical evaluation of epiluminescence microscopic criteria for melanocytic pigmented skin lesions. J Am Acad Derm 1993; 29:581.

27 Braun RP, Rabinovitz HS, Kopf AW, et al. Pattern analysis: A two-step procedure for the dermoscopic diagnosis of melanoma. Clin Dermatol 2002; 20:236–239.

28 Nachbar F, Stolz W, Merkel T, et al. The ABCD rule of dermatoscopy: high prospective value in the diagnosis of doubtful melanocytic skin lesions. J Am Acad Derm 1994; 30:551–559.

29 Stolz W, Braun-Falco O, Bilek P, et al. Color atlas of dermatoscopy, 2nd edn. Oxford: Blackwell Science; 2002.

30 Johr RH. Dermoscopy: Alternative melanocytic algorithms – The ABCD rule of dermatoscopy, Menzies Scoring method, and 7-point checklist. Clin Dermatol 2002; 20:240–247.

31 Argenziano G, Fabbrocini G, Carli P, et al. Epiluminescence microscopy: Criteria of cutaneous melanoma progression. J Am Acad Derm 1997; 37:68–74.

32 Argenziano G, Fabbrocini G, Carli P, et al. Clinical and dermatoscopic criteria for the preoperative evaluation of cutaneous melanoma thickness. J Am Acad Derm 1999; 40:61–68.

33 Carli P, DeGiorgi V, Palli D, et al. Preoperative assessment of melanoma thickness by ABCD score of dermatoscopy. J Am Acad Derm 2000; 43:459–466.

34 Binder M, Kittler H, Steiner A, et al. Reevaluation of the ABCD rule for epiluminescence microscopy. J Am Acad Derm 199(40):171–176.

35 Kittler H, Pehamberger H, Wolff K, et al. Follow up with melanocytic skin lesions with digital epiluminescence microscopy: patterns of modifications observed in early melanoma, atypical nevi, and common nevi. J Am Acad Derm 2000; 43:467–476.

36 Johr RH, Schachner LA, Izakovic J. Lesson on dermoscopy, No. 8. Derm Surg 2000; 26(9):893–894.

37 Menzies S, Gutenev A, Avramidis M, et al. Short-term digital surface microscopic monitoring of atypical or changing melanocytic lesions. Arch Derm 2001; 137:1583–1589.

38 Kittler H, Seltenheim M, Dawid M, et al. Frequency and characteristics of enlarging common melanocytic nevi. Arch Derm 2000; 136:316–320.

39 Kittler H, Binder M. Follow-up of melanocytic skin lesions with digital dermoscopy: risks and benefits. Arch Derm 2002; 138:1379.

40 Johr RH, Stolz W. Lesions in dermoscopy 'milky-red' areas. Derm Surg 2002; 28:299–300.

41 Johr RH. Pink lesions. Clin Dermatol 2002; 20:189–296.

42 Feldmann R, Fellenz C, Gschnait F. The ABCD rule in dermatoscopy: analysis of 500 melanocytic lesions. Hautarzt 1998; 49:473–476.

43 Lorentzen HF, Weismann K, Secher L, et al. The dermatoscopic ABCD rule does not improve diagnostic accuracy of malignant melanoma. Acta Derm Venereol 2000; 80:223.

44 Pizzichetta MA, Talamini R, Piccolo D, et al. The ABCD rule of dermatoscopy does not apply to small melanocytic skin lesions. Arch Derm 2001; 137:1376–1378.

447

45 Lorentzen HF, Weismann K, Larsen FG. Structural asymmetry as a dermatoscopic indicator of malignant melanoma: a latent class analysis of sensitivity and classification errors. Melanoma Res 2001; 11:495–501.

46 Menzies SW. A method for the diagnosis of primary cutaneous melanoma using surface microscopy. Derm Clin 2001; 19:299–305.

47 Menzies SW, Crotty KA, Ingvar C, McCarthy WM. An atlas of surface microscopy of pigmented skin lesions: dermoscopy. New York, NY: McGraw-Hill; 2003.

48 Menzies SW, Ingvar C, Crotty KA, et al. Frequency and morphologic characteristics of invasive melanomas lacking specific surface microscopic features. Arch Derm 1996; 132:1178–1182.

49 Carli P, Massi D, DeGiorgi V, Giannotti B. Clinically and dermoscopically featureless melanoma: When prevention fails. J Am Acad Derm 2002; 46:957–959.

50 Westerhoff K, McCarthy WH, Menzies SW. Increase in the sensitivity for melanoma diagnosis by primary care physicians using skin surface microscopy. Br J Derm 2000; 143:1016–1020.

51 Argenziano G, Fabbrocini G, Carli P, et al. Epiluminescence microscopy for the diagnosis of doubtful melanocytic skin lesion: comparison of the ABCD rule of dermatoscopy and a new 7-point checklist based on pattern analysis. Arch Derm 1998; 134:1563–1570.

52 Soyer HP, Argenziano G, Zalaudek I, et al. 3-Point Checklist of Dermoscopy: A new screening method for early detection of melanoma. Dermatology 2004; 208: 27–31.

53 Johr R, Soyer HP, Argenziano G. Dermoscopy: The Essentials. Philadelphia: Elsevier, 2004.

54 Salopek TG, Kopf AW, Stetanoto CM, et al. Differentiation of atypical moles (dysplastic nevi) from early melanoma by dermoscopy. Derm Clin 2001; 19:337–345.

55 Hofmann-Wellenhof R, Blum A, Wolf IH, et al. Dermoscopic classification of Clark's nevi (atypical melanocytic nevi). Clin Dermatol 2002; 20:255–258.

56 Grob JJ, Bonerandi JJ. The 'ugly duckling' sign: identification of the common characteristics of nevi in an individual as a basis for melanoma screening. Arch Derm 1998; 134:103–104.

57 Seidenari S, Pellacani G. Surface microscopy features of congenital nevi. Clin Dermatol 2002; 20:263–267.

58 Saida T, Oguchi S, Miyazaki A. Dermoscopy for acral-pigmented skin lesions. Clin Dermatol 2002; 20:279–285.

59 Johr RH, Stolz W. Lentigo maligna and lentigo maligna melanoma. J Am Acad Derm 1997; 37:512.

60 Stolz W, Schiffner R, Burgdorf W. Dermatoscopy for facial pigmented lesions. Clin Dermatol 2002; 20:274–278.

61 Johr RH, Izakovic J. Dermatoscopy/ELM for the evaluation of nail-apparatus pigmentation. Derm Surg 2001; 27:315–322.

62 Ronger S, Touzet S, Ligeron C, et al. Dermoscopic examination of nail pigmentation. Arch Derm 2002; 138:1327–1333.

63 Johr RH. You cannot use what you do not know. Arch Dermatol 2003; 139(6):810–811.

Computer Aided Diagnosis for Cutaneous Melanoma

Steven Q Wang, Harold Rabinovitz and Margaret Oliviero

Key points

- Computer aided diagnosis for cutaneous melanoma is an emerging but promising field of research that has the potential to help physicians to improve diagnostic accuracy.
- The combination of rising incidence of melanomas and the need to improve diagnostic accuracy have spurred the research in this field.
- Sequential steps are involved in creating a computer-assisted analysis system. These include image acquisition, lesions segmentation, feature extraction and lesion classification. For each step, there are a number of obstacles that must be resolved.
- There is not yet an optimal approach to computer-aided diagnosis and current computer-assisted analysis systems use differing algorithms and specifications.
- Comparison of studies and diagnostic accuracy from the different imaging analysis systems is difficult and caution is needed in interpreting the results of these studies.

INTRODUCTION

The rising incidence of cutaneous malignant melanoma has reached an epidemic proportion in the past decade.[1,2] Currently, there is no cure for advanced cutaneous melanoma. Only early diagnosis followed by prompt excision ensures a good prognosis. Various diagnostic arsenals are currently available to clinicians, including the ABCD clinical rule,[3] following patients with total cutaneous photography,[4] and the use of dermoscopy.[5–10]

To further improve the diagnostic accuracy various research groups[11–26] in the world have been engaged in developing equipment and analysis software that can provide objective evaluations and diagnosis of pigmented skin lesions (Table 36.1). For many researchers, it is the ultimate objective to develop an end-to-end, fully automated, diagnostic instrument with the capability of diagnosing pigmented skin lesions without the intervention and assistance from expert dermatologists. In this review, we will introduce the concept and process of these approaches, update the progress and highlight the difficulties in this research arena.

CONCEPTS AND PROCESS

The sequential steps involved in computer-assisted analysis include image acquisition, lesion segmentation, feature extraction and lesion classification. Initially, the lesion must be acquired. Both the clinical and dermatoscopic images of lesions can be used for analysis. Currently, most researchers rely on dermatoscopic images.

Initially, images that were analyzed were acquired by digitizing 35 mm Kodachrome slides. As optical equipment improved along with the availability of inexpensive electronic cameras, current research has focused on the direct digital acquisition of images. Most researchers have opted to use calibrated three CCDs (charge-coupled device) video cameras to take dermatoscopic images of pigmented skin lesions (Fig. 36.1). The advantage of using the three CCDs camera permits the three bands of color (red, green and blue) to be separately recorded. Amount of illumination and the spectrum of waveband are important factors in the overall quality of the image.

The imaging acquisition technique from the MelaFind[24] and SIAscope[27] are slightly different from the others described above. Both systems employ multispectral narrow band ranging from 400 to 1000 nm. For each lesion, the MelaFind™ imaging system obtains images from each of 10 spectral bands between 430 and 950 nm. The SIAscope® captures the images of a single lesion using eight narrow bands between 400 and 1000 nm. Regardless of the method of image acquisition, the final digitized images are stored in computer hardware or copied onto CDs for analysis.

The lesion in the image must be separated from normal surrounding skin using the process of segmentation. Mathematical algorithms capable of differentiating and demarcating the border between the lesion and surrounding skin achieve this process. To obtain the most optimal segmentation, hairs on and surrounding the lesion are often trimmed before the images are taken. This process can be very challenging when dealing with a collision lesion, a lesion with regression, or a lesion on sun damaged skin. Many of the image systems allow the physicians to reject the segmentation automatically provided by the computer, or allow the physicians to modify the actual border of the lesion to provide for a more accurate analysis.

Once the lesion is properly segmented, lesion features that have the potential for differentiating benign

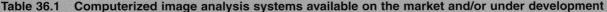

Table 36.1 Computerized image analysis systems available on the market and/or under development

Device names	Company	Website	Reference
DermoGenius Ultra	LINOS Photonics Inc.	www.dermogenius.de	37
MelaFind	Electro-Optical Sciences, Inc.	www.melafind.com	27,31,32
SIAscope	Astron Clinica	www.astronclinica.com	30
MoleMax II	Derma Instruments L.P.	www.derma.co.at/molemax.htm	
MicroDerm	VisioMED	www.zn-ag.com	
NevusScan	Romedix	www.romedix.com	
Solarscan	Polartechnics Limited	www.polartechnics.com.au	36
FotoFinder Derma	Edge Systems Corp.	www.edgesystem.net	
DBDermo-Mips	University of Siena	www.skinlesions.net	26,28,33–35

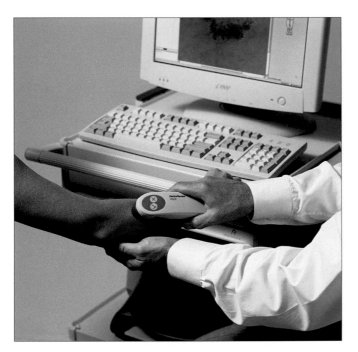

Figure 36.1 Cutaneous pigmented lesion on forearm being captured by a physician using video device (DermoGenius® system).

vs malignant pigmented cutaneous lesions are identified. These features are objective and mathematically characteristic of lesion morphology (e.g. asymmetry, blotchiness, color variation, dermatoscopic structures) converting the qualitative interpretation of dermatoscopic structures and patterns into quantitative values, thus providing the objectivity of analysis. Although a large number of features are often identified, only a small subset are incorporated into the final classifier.

Combining a subset of features creates the classifier or neural network that can best differentiate benign vs. malignant lesions. Since histopathology is still the 'gold standard' for diagnosis, the results of the initial evaluations of these systems are tested against a series of lesions with known histological diagnoses. To test the performance of the classifier, an independent lesion set is preferably employed. More often, the same lesion set used for training or building the classifier is used and the performance of the classifier is then cross-validated by using substitution or 'leave-one-out' techniques.

The diagnostic performance of the classifier can be improved by increasing the number of lesions in the database for training. By 'showing' the computer a vast number of lesions, the system can identify more robust and reliable features to be incorporated into the classifier to determine whether lesions should or should not be biopsied. In addition, as the training process proceeds with additional lesions, features in the old classifier may become obsolete or irrelevant as the diagnostic algorithms are updated and newer features replace them.

COMPUTER ANALYSIS SYSTEMS

Many of the currently developed computer-aided diagnosis systems rely on dermoscopy for image and data input. Dermoscopy is a non-invasive diagnostic tool that allows the physicians to inspect structures under the skin surface that are normally not visible to the naked eye exam. In the hand of experienced users, dermoscopy has been reported to improve diagnostic accuracy by five, to 30%.[5,7–9,28] Despite its clinical efficacy, dermoscopy has a few shortcomings. Interpretation and analysis of lesions with dermoscopy is a qualitative process that is complex and subjective. There is a steep learning curve to master the use of this diagnostic tool. The diagnostic accuracy is heavily dependent on operators' experience. Binder *et al.*[29] has shown that the diagnostic accuracy actually decreases for non-experienced users. Dermoscopy is reviewed in further depth in Chapter 35. At time of writing, only 23% of US dermatologists use dermoscopy in their clinical practice.[30] The use of a computer system to analyze the dermatoscopic data may lead to more consistent diagnostic results.

The MelaFind 100™[24,31] (Electric Optical Sciences Inc. NY, USA) was developed using a dermoscopy base. MelaFind is an end-to-end, fully automatic analysis system with a capacity to acquire the images, perform segmentation and classify lesions as benign or malignant. An imaging probe employing ten distinct spectral bands, from 430 to 950 nm, is used to capture a sequence of ten images of each lesion (Fig. 36.2). The deeper penetration of the longer wavelengths results in different imaging depths being obtained (Fig 36.3).

The imaging process takes less than five seconds to complete. The system has demonstrated high precision and repeatability in measuring and computing the feature parameters.[32] In a multicenter study,[24] 63 melanomas (33 invasive and 30 *in situ*) and 183 melanocytic nevi (of which 111 were dysplastic) were

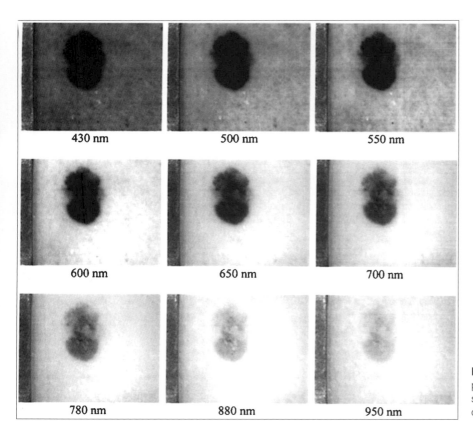

430 nm 500 nm 550 nm

600 nm 650 nm 700 nm

780 nm 880 nm 950 nm

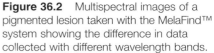

Figure 36.2 Multispectral images of a pigmented lesion taken with the MelaFind™ system showing the difference in data collected with different wavelength bands.

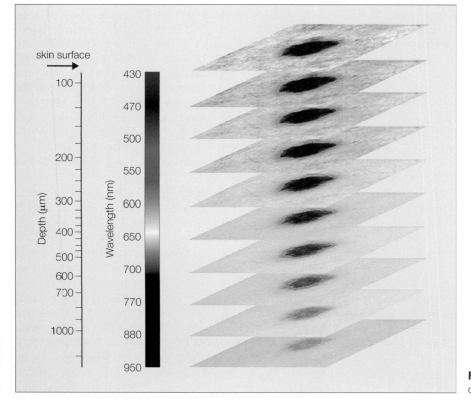

Figure 36.3 Image acquisition using different wavelengths varies by depth.

examined. After segmentation, 822 candidate features or parameters were identified. Both linear and non-linear classifiers were created. In the linear classifier, only 13 parameters were chosen to achieve a sensitivity of 100% with specificity of 85%. In the non-linear classifier, 12 parameters were selected and a sensitivity of 100% with a specificity of 73% was reached. This study demonstrated the feasibility of the MelaFind™ in differentiating melanomas from benign melanocytic lesions.

Currently, system development researchers are conducting a 20-center study testing the MelaFind 100™ system. A hand-held probe with a size slightly larger than a telephone receiver captures the lesion images. In the commercial models, the probe will contain the software for lesion segmentation and features extraction. The quantitative information of the selected features will be transmitted to a central server via Internet or telephone line. At the server, a classifier will determine whether the lesion has the score in the range of a benign vs malignant lesion. The score will then be transmitted back to the clinician and will help the physicians decide whether a lesion should or should not biopsied.

The DBDermo-Mips system™[23,25,33–35] (Burroni-Dell'Eva Biomedical Engineering Group, Siena, Italy) uses a similar approach. The hardware consists of a 3CCD PAL Broadcast video camera with 730 lines of imaging resolution. The camera is connected to a hand-held microscope with magnification from 6× to 40×. The field of view ranges from 6 mm to 4 cm. Light is provided by a 150 W source. Video signals from the lesions are connected to a frame-grabber interfaced with a personal computer. The analysis software (DBDermo-Mips) is operated in Microsoft Windows environment. The system operates in real-time and provides an end-to-end analysis at a fast rate. It has the capacity to make 25 diagnoses in one second. To make the diagnosis, the system separates the lesion from surrounding skin based on a Laplacian filter and zero-crossing algorithm. Important features are identified; these belong to four categories: geometries, colors, textures and islands of colors. A single-layered perceptron artificial neural network (ANN) is used for classifying the lesions.

In 2002, researchers examined a series of 217 melanomas (60 *in situ*) and 371 benign melanocytic nevi (including 137 atypical nevi).[35] A preliminary 48 critical differentiating features or parameters were identified. Only 13 features were needed by the ANN to differentiate malignant from benign lesions. The ANN was able to achieve a diagnostic accuracy of 94%.

SolarScan® (Fig. 36.4) is a system developed by Polartechnics Limited (Sydney, Australia). The system also uses a 3-CCD camera to capture dermatoscopic images of lesions. In a study[36] using an earlier version of the system, a sensitivity of 89% and a specificity of 80% were achieved in classifying 45 invasive melanomas (median Breslow thickness of 0.62 mm) from 176 benign pigmented skin lesions. Currently, the group is engaged in a multicenter trial in Australia and the US.

FotoFinder Derma™ is a system developed in Griesbach, Germany. The system was initially designed for monitoring pigmented skin lesions using digitized dermatoscopic images and currently research is under-

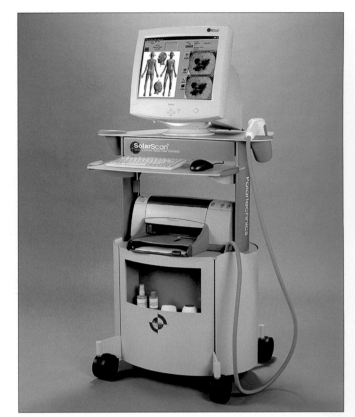

Figure 36.4   SolarScan® system.

way to provide the option for automatic diagnosis. From a database of 84 melanomas and 753 benign pigmented skin lesions, a preliminary classifier was able to achieve a sensitivity of 88% with a specificity of 86%.

SIAscope® (Astron Clinica, Cambridge, UK), like MelaFind, employs an imaging probe that takes multispectral images of lesions illuminated in the range of 400 to 1000 nm wavelength. Eight narrow bands spectrally filtered images of the skin are obtained with a probe that has a field of view 24 × 24 mm. This system (Fig. 36.5) takes approximately five seconds to acquire the images and an additional 10 seconds to process the data and return the images as visual information. SIAscope permits the examination of distribution, positions and quantity of melanin, blood and collagen within the papillary dermis and the position of melanin relative to the dermoepidermal junction. However, unlike other systems mentioned above, SIAscope does not have the analysis software that automatically identifies the features and build classifiers to identify benign vs. malignant diagnoses. Instead, a clinician needs to recognize and interpret the important diagnostic features. In comparison to interpretation of traditional dermatoscopic features, researchers contend that SIAscopy® features are relatively easy to identify.[27]

In 2002, the above group examined 52 melanomas (six *in situ*) and 296 benign pigmented lesions (including seven dysplastic nevi). A total of nine SIAscopy features were identified: melanin globules, blood globules, blood displacement, erythematous blush, dermal melanin, dermal melanin globules, collagen holes, biaxial symmetry and asymmetry. When combined with

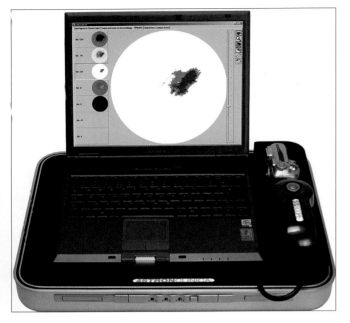

Figure 36.5 SIAscope® system.

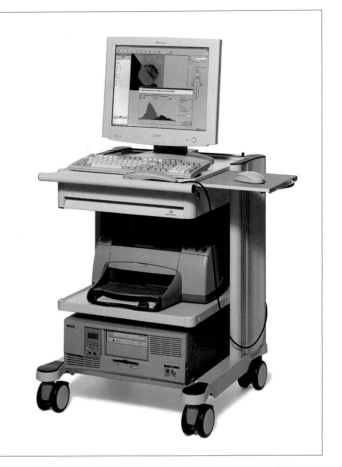

Figure 36.6 DermoGenius® system. (Image courtesy of Canfield Scientific.)

clinical information (i.e. lesion greater than 6 mm in size) and with two features (i.e. dermal melanin and blood blush/displacement), the researchers achieved sensitivity of 82% and specificity of 80% in separating benign vs malignant lesions.[27]

The DermoGenius® system (Fig. 36.6) (Rodenstock Prazisionsoptik, Munich, Germany) uses hardware consisting of a hand-held digital dermatoscope attached to a 3-CCD video camera with a horizontal resolution of more than 700 lines. The system incorporates a wide field of view of 11 × 11 mm and the imaging system has a 20× magnification. The captured digital images of pigmented skin lesions are stored in the computer database, automatically segmented and analyzed using a classifier based on the ABCD dermoscopy system.[10] The automated classifier has been further validated based on 749 histologically confirmed pigmented lesions (including 189 melanomas). Each lesion is assigned with a score between –2.5 and 6. Lesions with high scores are at high risk for being melanomas. In 2003, using this imaging analysis system, Jamora *et al.*[37] demonstrated that this computerized image analysis system could identify early melanomas or atypical nevi with moderate to severe atypia that can appear clinically benign.

Aside from the above-mentioned systems, NevusScan® (Romedix, Rehovot, Israel), MoleMax II™ (Derma Instruments) and microDerm® (VisioMED) are working in developing similar computer aided analysis systems. To date, the data from these groups are not yet available in the published literature.

OBSTACLES

The research in the computer-aided diagnosis of cutaneous melanoma is both exciting and promising. In a recent meta-analysis reviewing 30 studies, Rosado *et al.*[38] have shown that computer-aided diagnosis of melanoma is reliable and comparable to the diagnostic accuracy achieved by human specialists. However, the authors concluded that a comparison of different studies is difficult and that caution is needed in interpreting results. Some of the same sentiments have also been expressed by Menzies[39] and Elbaum.[31]

Currently, most of the clinical researchers who are involved in the development of computer-assisted systems are specialists in using dermoscopy and in managing patients with pigmented skin lesions. They tend to select difficult lesions for biopsies, i.e. early invasive and *in situ* melanomas and atypical nevi with severe cytological atypia. Therefore, some common benign lesions that may not be biopsied are then excluded from the studies because there is no histopathology. Algorithms based on a database of clinically difficult lesions may not readily recognize benign lesions such as pigmented seborrheic keratosis and common nevi that are frequently encountered in general practice. Hence, it is important that future studies include not only difficult lesions that may stumble experts, but also the common benign lesions that are necessary to train computer algorithms. However, it may be unethical to biopsy lesions for such research when they are known for certain to be benign. An alternative to histopathology in these cases may be a concordant diagnosis from two expert dermatoscopists for these analyses.

As previously noted, computer based diagnostic classifiers rely on histopathology as the 'gold' standard for determining whether a lesion should or should not be biopsied. However, even the gold standard may sometimes be 'tainted'. For example, there is a considerable inter-observer difference in the histologic diagnosis of atypical nevi. In addition, oftentimes it is very difficult to differentiate early invasive and *in situ* melanomas from severe atypical nevi and Spitz nevi. In these cases, the accuracy and validity of the histopathologic diagnosis limit the computer systems' ability to determine whether lesions should or should not be biopsied.

The small field of view in most imaging systems may also pose a problem in diagnosing some clinical lesions. Currently, lesions that are larger than the designated field of view are excluded from analysis largely because it is not possible to segment these lesions. Thus, many large melanocytic nevi, congenital nevi and lentigo malignas cannot yet be analyzed. In addition, certain anatomic locations of lesions, such as the ear concha or medial canthus, may preclude the use of these diagnostic devices.

It is difficult to compare the diagnostic accuracies of the available systems. The technology, both hardware and software, employed in each system is unique. More importantly, the classifier in each system is trained by its own set of lesions database. Since each contains differing numbers of melanomas, atypical nevi and other pigmented skin lesions, this may lead to differing results. For instance, a classifier trained with a database with a large number of deep invasive melanomas may not achieve the same diagnostic accuracy in differentiating early invasive and *in situ* melanomas from benign lesions when compared to one that used thinner melanomas in classifier development. Ideally, to compare the sensitivity and specificity of each system, all systems need to be tested on the same blind set of pigmented skin lesions.

FUTURE OUTLOOK

The future of computer-aided diagnosis is promising. It is very probable that such 'machine vision' instruments can act as adjuvant to clinical and dermatoscopic examinations to aid the clinician in the proper *in vivo* diagnosis of melanocytic neoplasms. With continual advancement in computer processing power and speed, researchers can search for a larger database of lesions features that have the potential to differentiate benign vs malignant melanocytic lesions. This will shorten the time needed to develop more robust classifiers with higher diagnostic accuracy. As the ever-rapid pace of innovation in electro-optical technology continues, designers will have more options and resources to miniaturize diagnostic hardware, thus making it more user-friendly and easily portable. In addition, the time needed to acquire and process the images in real time will be shortened which will save valuable time for clinicians in a busy practice setting.

Currently, only dermatologists in academic centers who have keen interests in pigmented skin lesions typically use computer-aided diagnostic systems for diagnosing pigmented lesions and melanoma. It is foreseeable that, as the cost of these 'machine vision' systems declines and diagnostic accuracy increases, practitioners in other settings (especially those in rural areas where access to a dermatologist is difficult) will wish to incorporate this technology in their practices to screen, monitor and ultimately aid in the diagnosis of pigmented neoplasms.

REFERENCES

1 Koh HK. Cutaneous melanoma. N Engl J Med 1991; 325:171–182.

2 Ernstoff MS. Melanoma. Screening and education. Clin Plast Surg 2000; 27:vii, 317–322.

3 Friedman RJ, Rigel DS, Kopf AW. Early detection of malignant melanoma: the role of physician examination and self-examination of the skin. CA Cancer J Clin 1985; 35:130–151.

4 Slue W, Kopf AW, Rivers JK. Total-body photographs of dysplastic nevi. Arch Derm 1988; 124:1239–1243.

5 Pehamberger H, Steiner A, Wolff K. In vivo epiluminescence microscopy of pigmented skin lesions. I. Pattern analysis of pigmented skin lesions. J Am Acad Derm 1987; 17:571–583.

6 Steiner A, Pehamberger H, Wolff K. In vivo epiluminescence microscopy of pigmented skin lesions. II. Diagnosis of small pigmented skin lesions and early detection of malignant melanoma. J Am Acad Derm 1987; 17:584–591.

7 Soyer HP, Smolle J, Kerl H, Stettner H. Early diagnosis of malignant melanoma by surface microscopy. Lancet 1987; 2:803.

8 Menzies SW. Surface microscopy of pigmented skin tumours. Australas J Derm 1997; 38(Suppl 1):S40–S43.

9 Argenziano G, Fabbrocini G, Carli P, Giorgi V De, Delfino M. Clinical and dermatoscopic criteria for the preoperative evaluation of cutaneous melanoma thickness. J Am Acad Derm 1999; 40:61–68.

10 Nachbar F, Stolz W, Merkle T, et al. The ABCD rule of dermatoscopy. High prospective value in the diagnosis of doubtful melanocytic skin lesions. J Am Acad Derm 1994; 30:551–559.

11 Green A, Martin N, McKenzie G, et al. Computer image analysis of pigmented skin lesions. Melanoma Res 1991; 1:231–236.

12 Green A, Martin N, Pfitzner J, O'Rourke M, Knight N. Computer image analysis in the diagnosis of melanoma. J Am Acad Derm 1994; 31:958–964.

13 Cascinelli N, Ferrario M, Bufalino R, et al. Results obtained by using a computerized image analysis system designed as an aid to diagnosis of cutaneous melanoma. Melanoma Res 1992; 2:163–170.

14 Schindewolf T, Stolz W, Albert R, Abmayr W, Harms H. Classification of melanocytic lesions with color and texture analysis using digital image processing. Anal Quant Cytol Histol 1993; 15:1–11.

15 Schindewolf T, Schiffner R, Stolz W, et al. Evaluation of different image acquisition techniques for a computer vision system in the diagnosis of malignant melanoma. J Am Acad Derm 1994; 31:33–41.

16 Horsch A, Stolz W, Neiss A, et al. Improving early recognition of malignant melanomas by digital image analysis in dermatoscopy. Stud Health Technol Inform 1997; 43:531–535.

17 Seidenari S, Pellacani G, Pepe P. Digital videomicroscopy improves diagnostic accuracy for melanoma. J Am Acad Derm 1998; 39:175–181.

18 Binder M, Kittler H, Seeber A, et al. Epiluminescence microscopy-based classification of pigmented skin lesions using computerized image analysis and an artificial neural network. Melanoma Res 1998; 8:261–266.

19 Binder M, Kittler H, Dreiseitl S, et al. Computer-aided epiluminescence microscopy of pigmented skin lesions: the value of clinical data for the classification process. Melanoma Res 2000; 10:556–561.

20 Andreassi L, Perotti R, Rubegni P, et al. Digital dermoscopy analysis for the differentiation of atypical nevi and early melanoma: a new quantitative semiology. Arch Derm 1999; 135:1459–1465.

21 Seidenari S, Pellacani G, Giannetti A. Digital videomicroscopy and image analysis with automatic classification for detection of thin melanomas. Melanoma Res 1999; 9:163–171.

22 Smith Y, Weinberg A, Klauss S, Soffer D, Ingber A. Improving screening for melanoma by measuring similarity to pre-classified images. Melanoma Res 2000; 10:265–272.

23 Bauer P, Cristofolini P, Boi S, et al. Digital epiluminescence microscopy: usefulness in the differential diagnosis of cutaneous pigmentary lesions. A statistical comparison between visual and computer inspection. Melanoma Res 2000; 10:345–349.

24 Elbaum M, Kopf AW, Rabinovitz HS Jr, et al. Automatic differentiation of melanoma from melanocytic nevi with multispectral digital dermoscopy: a feasibility study. J Am Acad Derm 2001; 44:207–218.

25 Rubegni P, Ferrari A, Cevenini G, et al. Differentiation between pigmented Spitz naevus and melanoma by digital dermoscopy and stepwise logistic discriminant analysis. Melanoma Res 2001; 11:37–44.

26 Kahofer P, Hofmann-Wellenhof R, Smolle J. Tissue counter analysis of dermatoscopic images of melanocytic skin tumours: preliminary findings. Melanoma Res 2002; 12:71–75.

27 Moncrieff M, Cotton S, Claridge E, Hall P. Spectrophotometric intracutaneous analysis: a new technique for imaging pigmented skin lesions. Br J Derm 2002; 146:448–457.

28 Ascierto PA, Palmieri G, Celentano E, et al. Sensitivity and specificity of epiluminescence microscopy: evaluation on a sample of 2731 excised cutaneous pigmented lesions. Melanoma Coop Study. Br J Derm 2000; 142:893–898.

29 Binder M, Schwarz M, Winkler A, et al. Epiluminescence microscopy. A useful tool for the diagnosis of pigmented skin lesions for formally trained dermatologists. Arch Derm 1995; 131:286–291.

30 Tripp JM, Kopf AW, Marghoob AA, Bart RS. Management of dysplastic nevi: a survey of fellows of the American Academy of Dermatology. J Am Acad Derm 2002; 46:674–682.

31 Elbaum M. Computer-aided melanoma diagnosis. Derm Clin 2002; 20:x–xi, 735–747.

32 Gutkowicz-Krusin D, Elbaum M, Jacobs A, et al. Precision of automatic measurements of pigmented skin lesion parameters with a MelaFind(TM) multispectral digital dermoscope. Melanoma Res 2000; 10:563–570.

33 Rubegni P, Burroni M, Dell'eva G, Andreassi L. Digital dermoscopy analysis for automated diagnosis of pigmented skin lesions. Clin Derm 2002; 20:309–312.

34 Rubegni P, Burroni M, Cevenini G, et al. Digital dermoscopy analysis and artificial neural network for the differentiation of clinically atypical pigmented skin lesions: a retrospective study. J Invest Derm 2002; 119:471–474.

35 Rubegni P, Cevenini G, Burroni M, et al. Automated diagnosis of pigmented skin lesions. Int J Cancer 2002; 101:576–580.

36 Menzies S, Bischof L, Peden G, et al. Automated instrumentation for the diagnosis of invasive melanoma [abstract]. Skin Res Technol 1997; 3:200.

37 Jamora MJ, Wainwright BD, Meehan SA, Bystryn JC. Improved identification of potentially dangerous pigmented skin lesions by computerized image analysis. Arch Derm 2003; 139:195–198.

38 Rosado B, Menzies S, Harbauer A, et al. Accuracy of computer diagnosis of melanoma: a quantitative meta-analysis. Arch Derm 2003; 139:361–367.

39 Menzies SW. Automated epiluminescence microscopy: human vs machine in the diagnosis of melanoma. Arch Derm 1999; 135:1538–1540.

Confocal Microscopy in Skin Cancer

Salvador González, Agnieszka Niemeyer and Abel Torres

Key points

- Reflectance confocal microscopy is a non-invasive way to image skin similar in principle to ultrasonography but utilizing reflected light from a laser as opposed to ultrasound.
- Reflectance confocal microscopy allows for static and dynamic imaging of the skin portending the use of a modality to diagnose disease based on morphology as well as disease activity.
- Reflectance confocal microscopy has shown promise as a diagnostic tool, as an adjunct to surgery and for monitoring invasive and non-invasive treatment of skin conditions.

INTRODUCTION

The diagnosis of skin cancer usually depends on the histopathological microscopic analysis of excised and processed tissue. The latter provides high-resolution cellular and sub-cellular tissue detail. However, it requires an invasive sampling of skin tissue (biopsy), which can be time-consuming, painful, costly and carries the risk of scarring and infection. In addition a biopsy provides information only on the excised tissue and involves processing and staining of the specimen, which may induce artifacts.

Recent advances in non-invasive high-resolution skin imaging *in vivo* may help to overcome some of the limitations of biopsies. These developments include optical coherence tomography (OCT),[1] high frequency ultrasound (HFU),[2] magnetic resonance imaging (MRI),[3] and reflectance confocal microscopy (RCM).[4–6] Of these, RCM offers high resolution imaging comparable to routine histology.

PRINCIPLES OF REFLECTANCE CONFOCAL LASER MICROSCOPY

The confocal scanning microscope was invented by Marvin Minsky at Harvard in 1955 while working as a post-doctoral fellow.[7] Yet, tissue imaging *in vivo* was not possible until the development of light source and computerization technologies. Since the 1980s, several research groups have demonstrated the use of tandem scanning confocal microscopy for imaging human and animal tissue *in vivo*.[8–11] In 1995, confocal scanning laser microscopy for imaging human skin *in vivo* was first reported.[6] *In vivo* RCM offers important advantages over conventional histology in that imaging is non-invasive, causes no tissue injury, is painless and the tissue is not altered by processing, minimizing artifact. The data is collected in real time which is faster than routine histology and the skin site can be repeatedly imaged to evaluate dynamic changes such as response to therapy.[12–16]

Reflectance confocal microscopy involves the use of a point source of light to illuminate a small spot within tissue. The reflected light (reflectance) is then imaged onto a detector after passing through a small pinhole (microscopy). The pinhole minimizes out of focus light reaching the detector and only the region of the specimen that is in focus (confocal) is detected (Fig. 37.1). To image the entire horizontal axis of a sample being studied, the point source beam is scanned. This results in 'virtual sectioning' of a thin horizontal tissue plane (microscopy) *in vivo* similar to the horizontal sections produced in Mohs surgery or similar to X-ray tomograms.

The resolution for RCM is influenced by the wavelength used, the pinhole size and the numerical aperture of the objective lens. Lasers of different wavelengths may be used as a light source for RCM with longer wavelengths penetrating deeper into the skin but providing less lateral resolution. Due to local variations of the refractive index in tissue as well as light scatter when a structure has a size similar to the illuminating wavelength, back-scattering of light occurs. Despite melanin absorption at near-infrared wavelengths (800–1064 nm) there is strong back-scattering from melanosomes, because they have a high refractive index relative to the surrounding epidermis and a structure size similar to the illuminating wavelength. Thus, cells containing melanin, such as basal keratinocytes and melanocytes, image brightly and more contrast is obtained where the skin being imaged has a darker color or is a pigmented lesion.

The commercially available RCM made by Lucid, Inc. has a wavelength of 830 nm and 30× objective lens of NA 0.9 which provides an axial resolution (section thickness) of 3–5 µm and a lateral resolution of approximately 1 µm. Thus, the section thickness is comparable with the thickness of sections one can obtain with routine histology. This system allows for the imaging of normal skin to a depth of 200–250 µm, which is sufficient for imaging epidermis, papillary dermis and upper reticular dermis. Imaging deeper layers in the skin can

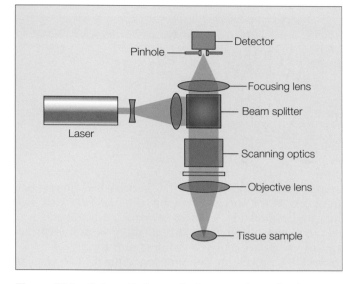

Figure 37.1 Schematic for a reflectance mode confocal microscope illustrating non-invasive imaging of a thin plane of skin. Back-scattered light rather than transmitted light is collected by a detector. The small aperture (pinhole) in front of the detector controls the amount of light collected that is in focus, rejecting light that is out of focus.

be achieved by utilizing laser power, greater than the 30 mW used in the commercially available device. However, the 30 mW power causes no tissue or eye injury while higher power settings hold the potential for causing tissue damage.

Deeper layers can also be imaged if one removes the more superficial layers such as the stratum corneum through techniques such as tape stripping. Since the refractive index of water (1.33) is close to that of epidermis (1.34) water immersion lenses are used to minimize spherical aberrations caused by the light passing through the tissue air interface. When imaging a scaly or hyperkeratotic lesion it is also possible to use water-based gels as immersion media, since the gel settles between disrupted corneocytes and reduces refraction irregularities.[12] Gels are also useful for imaging skin sites that are not flat, since the gel does not run off of the skin in the same way as water.

To reduce motion artifact during imaging and contain the water or gel interface, a concave metal ring is fixed to the patient's skin with adhesive and is coupled to the microscope housing with a magnet.[12] By moving the objective lens in the z (vertical) axis with respect to the skin, the focal plane (point) can be progressively moved deeper. It is then possible to image at different horizontal levels within the tissue providing tomogram like images. Images can be 'captured' to produce static horizontal skin section images or recorded on videotape (20–30 Hz) to produce movies that demonstrate dynamic events such as blood flow.[6,12–16]

Unlike routine histology the images obtained are horizontal or *en face*, rather than the vertical sections that are traditionally obtained with routine histology. Unlike traditional histology the images lack color and instead are gray-scale images similar to radiographs. The field of view with RCM varies with the microscope, but

is generally 250–500 μm across. The level being imaged can be ascertained by measuring the depth of the section using a micrometer attached to the z stage of the objective lens or by interpretation of the morphological appearance of tissue to establish a given depth.

REFLECTANCE CONFOCAL MICROSCOPY OF NORMAL SKIN

When imaging the skin (Fig. 37.2a) starting from the surface, the first skin images (layer) obtained are of the superficial stratum corneum. This produces a very bright (almost whitewashed) image, since the refractive difference at the interface between the stratum corneum (1.54) and the immersion medium water (1.33) results in a large amount of back-scattered light. Lowering the laser fluence can minimize the whitewashing brightness. The morphology seen consists of anucleated polygonal keratinocytes measuring between 10–30 μm in size and grouped in 'islands' separated by dark appearing skin folds (Fig. 37.2b).

As one continues to image from the surface in a progressively deeper fashion, the next layer (section) visualized is the stratum granulosum consisting of 2 to 4 layers of cells measuring between 25–35 μm in size. The cells appear as nuclei, which look like dark central ovals within the cell surrounded by a bright grainy cytoplasm. The architectural pattern resembles that of a honeycomb or chicken wire like pattern (Fig. 37.2c). Progressing deeper below the stratum granulosum one can next visualize the stratum spinosum, which usually is imaged 20–100 μm beneath the stratum corneum. The architectural honeycomb or chicken wire like pattern is preserved but appears tighter (more compact) consisting of smaller cells measuring between 15–25 μm in size with well-demarcated cell borders (Fig. 37.2d).

The next layer to be visualized is the deepest layer of epidermis, the basal layer. The honeycomb/chicken wire pattern is preserved but is even tighter (more compact) appearing as clusters of cells measuring between 7–10 μm. This honeycombing appears to correlate with progressive normal differentiation of epidermal cells, which are small at the basal layer and enlarge and flatten as they differentiate upwards.

When imaging progressively deeper, the supra-papillary epidermal plate at the dermo-epidermal junction is apparent as bright rings surrounding a dark central area. The brightness is presumably due to the increased melanin, thus increased refraction present in the cells at the basal cell layer. The bright rings represent the stacking of these more refractile cells in the rete ridges that surround the less cellular and less refractile dermal papillae. That the darker oval zone within the bright rings represents the dermal papillae is supported by the fact that often one can visualize in these areas a central area of increased refractility that appears as a bright single round and oval cells moving in a flowing manner in small caliber tortuous cylinders consistent with small papillary dermal vascular loops (Fig. 37.2e).

Imaging deeper still, the deeper papillary and reticular dermis can be seen to consist of a fine network of more refractile strands, which we interpret as collagen

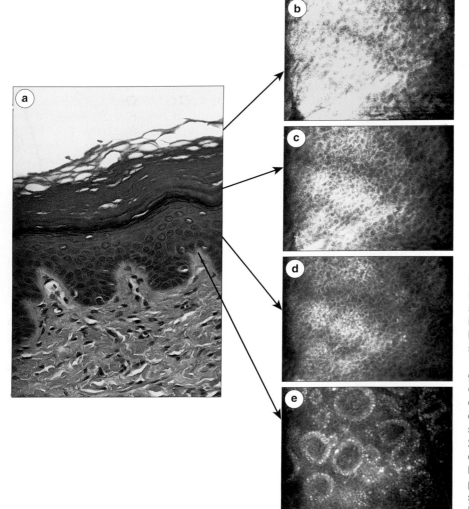

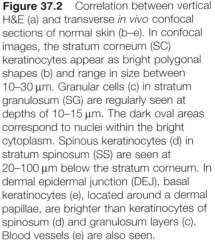

Figure 37.2 Correlation between vertical H&E (a) and transverse *in vivo* confocal sections of normal skin (b–e). In confocal images, the stratum corneum (SC) keratinocytes appear as bright polygonal shapes (b) and range in size between 10–30 μm. Granular cells (c) in stratum granulosum (SG) are regularly seen at depths of 10–15 μm. The dark oval areas correspond to nuclei within the bright cytoplasm. Spinous keratinocytes (d) in stratum spinosum (SS) are seen at 20–100 μm below the stratum corneum. In dermal epidermal junction (DEJ), basal keratinocytes (e), located around a dermal papillae, are brighter than keratinocytes of spinosum (d) and granulosum layers (c). Blood vessels (e) are also seen.

fibers. These strands/fibers are interspersed in a lace-like reticulated pattern interspersed with darker nondescript areas that correlate to the spaces seen between collagen bundles and are ascribed to ground substance in routine hematoxylin and eosin stained slides (Fig. 37.3). Often larger caliber blood vessels characterized by larger diameter less tortuous dark cylinders with increased flow of round bright cells can be visualized at this level but the caliber of the vessels is usually much smaller and with less flow than that seen with neoplastic lesions.

Other features, which can be observed in normal skin, include eccrine/sweat ducts, which appear as bright centrally hollow structures that spiral through the epidermis and dermis (Fig. 37.4). Hair follicles present with similar but non-spiraling whorled centrally hollow structures and elliptical elongated cell layers at the circumference with a central refractile long cylindrical tube (hair shaft) often connected to highly refractile clusters of cells consistent with pilosebaceous units (Fig. 37.5).

The above-described confocal images demonstrate consistent reproducible patterns, which we refer to as the normal architecture and cell morphology of the skin. However the appearance of normal skin will vary according to the skin site and skin color being imaged, degree of sun damage present and the location of

the skin.[17] Skin from sun-exposed or darkly pigmented sites generally is more refractile and thus brighter because of what appears to be more pigment in the cytoplasm at the basilar layer. Sun-exposed skin also demonstrates thicker and more fissured stratum corneum with more randomly arranged and irregularly shaped dermal papillae and clumping of the dermal reticulated pattern, consistent with increased elastotic fibers. Variation in the density of keratinocytes is often seen directly related to the degree of sun exposure with sun-protected sites appearing as having a greater cellular density than sun-exposed sites. On the other hand, the sun-exposed sites tend to show more pleomorphism of the morphology of the cells and more disorganization of the normal honeycomb architecture.

REFLECTANCE CONFOCAL MICROSCOPY OF NEOPLASTIC SKIN LESIONS

Basal cell carcinoma

The reflectance confocal microscopy morphological characteristics of basal cell carcinoma have recently been

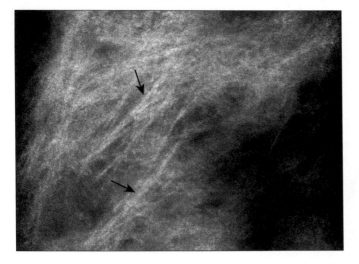

Figure 37.3 Collagen strands (arrows) interspersed in a lace-like reticulated pattern interspersed with darker nondescript areas that correlate to the spaces seen between collagen bundles and ascribed to ground substance in routine hematoxylin and eosin.

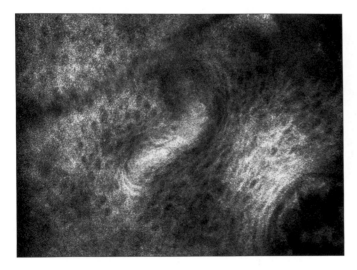

Figure 37.4 Spiral eccrine duct.

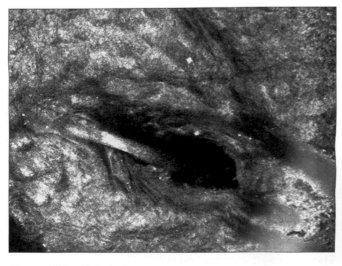

Figure 37.5 Hair shaft.

defined in a previous study that investigated the major histological features for diagnosing BCC *in vivo*.[18] A set of five major confocal imaging criteria was established using biopsy-correlated confocal images. These criteria were: presence of monomorphic tumor cells with elongated nuclei (Fig. 37.6a); orientation of these nuclei along the same axis, producing a polarized appearance (Fig. 37.6a); pleomorphism of the overlying and adjacent epidermal cells indicative of actinic damage (Fig. 37.6a); increased vasculature with pronounced superficial blood vessel prominence, dilation, tortuosity (Fig. 37.6b) and a prominent inflammatory infiltrate among the tumor cells often with associated slowing of the flow of some of the intravascular cells, with what appears to be the adhesion and rolling of leukocytes along the endothelial wall (Fig. 37.6c). This polarized cell pattern persists throughout the thickness of the lesion with loss of the normal progressive size difference of differentiating epidermal cells and thus, loss of the normal architectural honeycomb pattern. In addition, there is a loss of dermal papillae architecture, follicular and eccrine duct architecture (Fig. 37.6d). All of these changes are consistent with destruction and replacement of normal epidermis and dermis by the basal cell carcinoma and can be used to differentiate normal skin from tumor (Table 37.1).

The authors have been participating in a large study evaluating the sensitivity and specificity of RCM features for accurately diagnosing BCC *in vivo*.[19] A retrospective study of images from 152 skin lesions with a variety of benign and malignant diagnoses were imaged with RCM under IRB-approved studies at four different institutions. All 152 lesions had confirmed diagnoses based on either clinical examination or biopsy and of the 152 lesions, 83 were BCC. Using the five criteria for diagnosis of BCC described previously, a blinded retrospective analysis of the images from all 152 lesions was carried out to determine the sensitivity (ability of the five criteria to correctly detect the presence of BCC) and specificity (ability of the five criteria to correctly identify the absence of BCC) of RCM for diagnosing BCC. The results showed that the presence of two or more criteria is 100% sensitive for the diagnosis of BCC. As the number of criteria increased, the specificity increased, so that with four or more criteria present, the sensitivity was 82.9% and specificity was 95.7%. The most sensitive and specific criterion was the presence of polarized and monomorphic nuclei, with a sensitivity of 91.6% and specificity of 97% (Table 37.2). These results were found to have little variability across study sites and across BCC subtypes. The combination of RCM with photography-based predictions of clinical probability of BCC *significantly* improved the accuracy for non-invasive diagnosis of BCC.

In another *study, the authors* further investigated the use of RCM to non-invasively monitor the response to imiquimod, a topical immunomodulatory agent.[20] That study evaluated the negative predictive value (NPV) (ability of RCM to correctly identify the absence of BCC) and positive predictive value (PPV) (ability of RCM to correctly identify presence of tumor) in 24 patients treated with the non-invasive treatment of BCC with immune response modifier imiquimod for 6 weeks. patients underwent a biopsy pre-treatment to identify

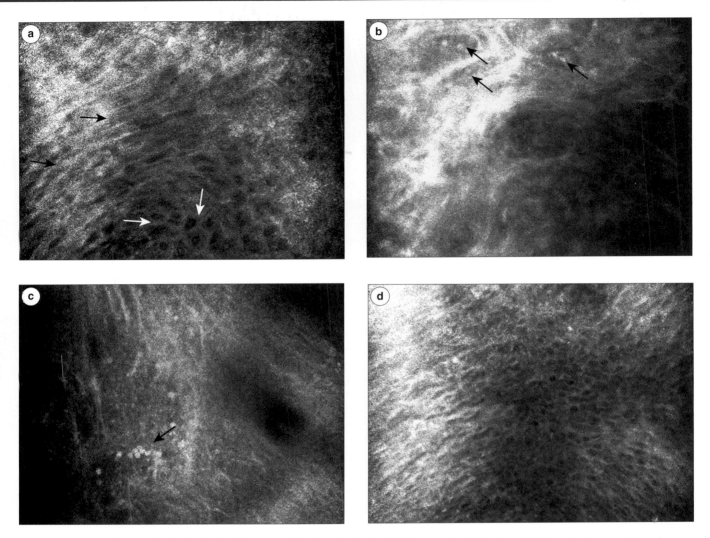

Figure 37.6 (a) RCM morphologic criteria: Monomorphic elongated cells (black arrows), polarization of cells and pleomorphism of adjacent epidermis (white arrows). (b) RCM morphologic criteria: Increased vascularity of BCC visualized as multiple tortuous vessels in superficial papillary dermis (arrow). (c) RCM morphologic criteria: Increased inflammation and WBC rolling (arrow). (d) Loss of normal differentiation of epidermis and loss of dermal papillae pattern.

presence of tumor and Mohs surgery 2 weeks after treatment to identify the clearance or persistence of BCC. All RCM images regardless of their quality were evaluated for NPV and PPV. The results were a NPV of 70% and PPV of 84.6%. However, if all poor quality RCM images were excluded, the correlation between the ability of RCM to accurately predict the presence or absence of BCC before, during and after treatment was 100%. This indicates that RCM holds the potential to become a useful tool for the diagnosis and non-invasive monitoring of treatment of BCC.

Actinic keratoses and squamous cell carcinomas

The key RCM histopathological features of actinic keratoses have been previously reported by Gonzalez et al.[21] These features include epidermal cell nuclear enlargement with pleomorphism and parakeratosis in a pattern of architectural disarray (Fig. 37.7). Similar to

routine hematoxylin and eosin stained histology slides of actinic keratosis the cellular changes seen in actinic keratoses with RCM tend not to involve the full thickness of the epidermis but rather mainly the dermo-epidermal junction. Observation of full thickness dysplastic features on RCM is suggestive of squamous cell carcinoma (Fig. 37.8) Other changes suggesting squamous cell carcinoma (SCC) such as vascular patterns, are currently being evaluated but not yet firmly established. The shallow penetration of the RCM illuminating wavelengths prevents accurate visualization at the dermo-epidermal junction in particularly hyperkeratotic lesions. This, together with the current dearth of criteria for distinguishing SCC from AK, currently restricts the potential of this tool for accurate differentiation of actinic keratoses vs squamous cell carcinomas. However, since the criteria for normal skin have been well established as described above, RCM holds the potential to be useful in monitoring the response to treatment of actinic keratosis and squamous cell carcinoma. Currently, a study examining the response of actinic keratoses to photodynamic therapy

Table 37.1   Criteria for RCM of normal skin vs BCC

	Normal skin	BCC
Morphology	Honeycomb cell arrangement	Elongated and polarized cell
Differentiation of cells	Surface large to basilarsmall	No differentiation
Structural pattern	Normal structures (reteridges, papillae)	Lack of structures
Vascular structures	Small capillary loops	Large vascular highway
Dermal layer	Reticulated pattern	Amorphous pattern
Inflammatory cells	No WBC activity	Rolling of WBC

Table 37.2   Sensitivity and specificity of major criteria of RCM for BCC

Criteria	Sensitivity (%)	Specificity (%)
Polarized nuclei	92	97
Elongated monomorphic nuclei	100	71
Increased vascularity	88	54
Pleomorphism	64	64
Inflammatory infiltrate	83	55
2 or more criteria	100	54
3 or more criteria	94	78
4 or more criteria	83	96

over time is ongoing and has initially demonstrated progressive normalization of architecture in successfully treated lesions.[22]

PIGMENTED SKIN LESIONS

Melanocytic nevi

Melanocytic lesions are well imaged by RCM since the melanin they possess provides good contrast. The RCM features of common melanocytic nevi are the presence of small monomorphous round or oval cells with brightly refractile cytoplasm with nuclei, which when visualized, are centrally positioned.[23,24] In junctional nevi, these cells are seen clustered in the epidermis usually surrounding dermal papillae at the dermo-epidermal junction (Fig. 37.9). In compound nevi, the rounded clusters of cells can be seen both at the dermo-epidermal junction and in the superficial dermis. In both of these nevus types, the normal RCM architecture of the stratum corneum, granulosum, spinosum and basal cell layer is visualized and remains unchanged. By contrast, dysplastic nevi show focal loss of the cell–cell keratinocyte borders at the dermo-epidermal junction, greater variety in nevomelanocyte size and shape though cells still tend

to be rounded or oval and fine bright granules within the epidermis that probably represent melanin bodies. Dysplastic nevi also show a greater variety in nevomelanocyte size and shape though cells still tend to be rounded or oval rather than dendritic.

Malignant melanoma

Melanomas imaged with RCM commonly show the presence of pleomorphic bright cells within the epidermis and dermis, often stellate in shape and possessing coarse branching dendritic processes with eccentrically placed large nuclei (Fig. 37.10).[25] The stratum spinosum tends to exhibit indistinct cell borders with bright grainy particles disrupting the usual normal epidermal honeycomb architectural pattern. It currently appears that it is not difficult to distinguish between benign nevi *vs* atypical or malignant melanocytic lesions but accurate differentiating criteria need to be further characterized and tested. It remains to be seen whether malignant cells with small amounts of pigment can be accurately identified although two cases of clinically amelanotic tumor have been reported in the literature to have detectable melanocytes, presumably because of the presence of some melanin.[26]

USE OF REFLECTANCE CONFOCAL MICROSCOPY AS AN ADJUNCT TO SURGERY

Margin assessment

RCM has the potential to help delineate lesion margins before or during surgical therapy. This could be particularly helpful in margin assessment of tumors that are difficult to delineate clinically such as lentigo maligna, amelanotic melanomas and sclerosing basal cell carcinomas. However, the RCMs' limited penetration depth, makes accurate imaging at depths below the superficial dermis difficult. Lack of endogenous contrast such as melanosomes in some lesions can also make imaging difficult. However, the use of 5% acetic acid *ex vivo* and aluminum chloride 20% or less *in vivo* may compensate for lack of endogenous contrast as described below.[27,28] Despite these limitations, RCM may help identify atypical lesions in need of a biopsy even if it cannot be used to delineate their margins.

RCM holds the potential to be useful for rapidly establishing tumor margins in excised specimens. Using 5% acetic acid to enhance contrast and cross-polarized illumination with RCM of *ex vivo* unprocessed tissue, it is possible to detect neoplastic cells, which appear as bright nuclei against a dark surrounding dermis.[27] It is also possible to examine *ex vivo*, non-melanoma skin cancer tissue during Mohs' micrographic surgery without frozen sections providing good and potentially more rapid visualization of margins as compared to permanent sectioning with the added capability of being able to perform special stains on the very same excised tissue.

We have also used RCM effectively *in vivo* during Mohs surgery to help locate BCC and melanoma but poor visualization of convex or concave wound surfaces,

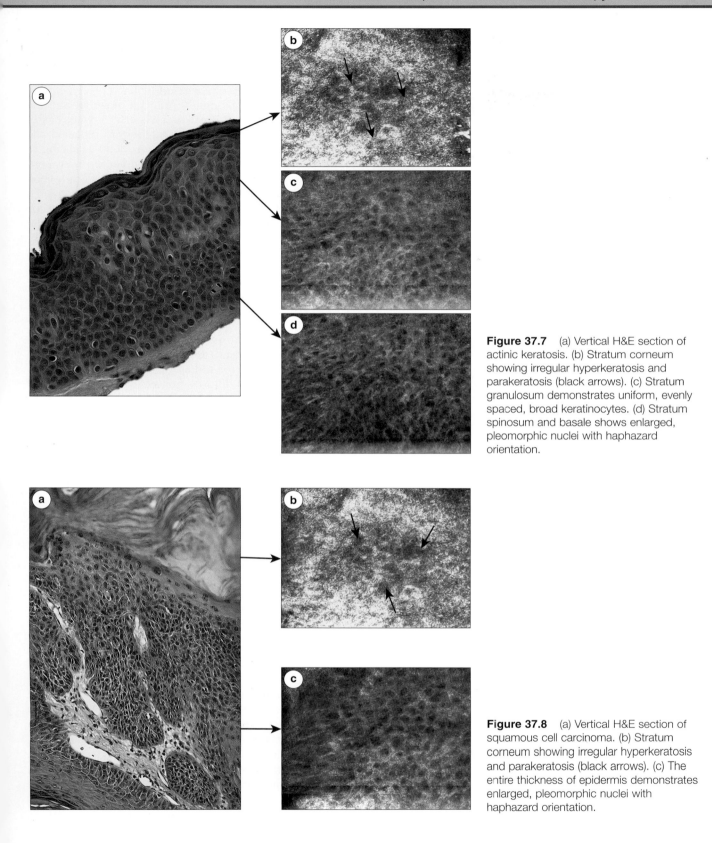

Figure 37.7 (a) Vertical H&E section of actinic keratosis. (b) Stratum corneum showing irregular hyperkeratosis and parakeratosis (black arrows). (c) Stratum granulosum demonstrates uniform, evenly spaced, broad keratinocytes. (d) Stratum spinosum and basale shows enlarged, pleomorphic nuclei with haphazard orientation.

Figure 37.8 (a) Vertical H&E section of squamous cell carcinoma. (b) Stratum corneum showing irregular hyperkeratosis and parakeratosis (black arrows). (c) The entire thickness of epidermis demonstrates enlarged, pleomorphic nuclei with haphazard orientation.

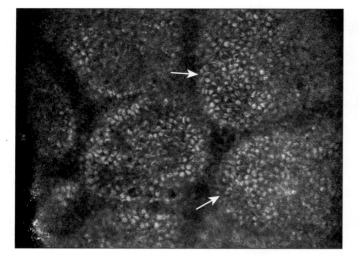

Figure 37.9 Confocal image of benign nevus. This *en face* section at the basal layer demonstrates bright monomorphic cells in uniform nests (arrows).

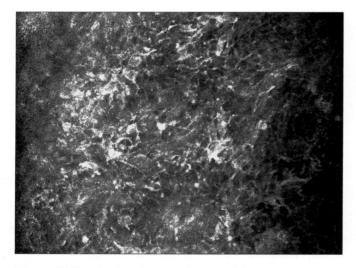

Figure 37.10 Confocal images of a superficial spreading malignant melanoma. This *en face* image demonstrates pleomorphic cells with 'stellate morphology', eccentric nuclei and dendritic branches. Overall there is a loss of keratinocyte cell border definition and 'dust-like' granular appearance as well as pigment globules.

wound fluid interference and limited wavelength penetration make it impractical at this time to use RCM *in vivo* for Mohs surgery.[28] Yet, our recent observation that aluminum chloride solution enhances visualization *in vivo* of malignant BCC cells together with other technical refinements in RCM may make *in vivo* margin assessment more practical.[28]

USE OF CONFOCAL REFLECTANCE MICROSCOPY FOR EVALUATING RESPONSE TO NON-INVASIVE TOPICAL THERAPY

Unlike a biopsy, it is possible to repeat RCM on the same skin site repeatedly. This permits evaluation of the same

area indefinitely and evaluation of dynamic processes such as response to therapy. RCM monitoring of the response to laser treatment of cherry angiomata has shown that after treatment with a pulsed dye laser, blood flow within the lesions ceased with replacement by amorphous cords of brightly refractile material and the development of new small vessels. By 3 weeks after treatment, normal epidermis and dermis replaced the lesion.[15] On the other hand, RCM enabled visualizing of the krypton laser was different, with no amorphous cord development but only dark spaces, as an early event, with healing and normalization of architecture seen 4 weeks after treatment. Likewise, RCM has proven to be accurate in establishing the presence of BCC prior to treatment and responsiveness of the BCCs to a treatment regimen with the non-invasive immunomodulator imiquimod.[20]

FUTURE OUTLOOK

Reflectance confocal microscopy (RCM) promises to be useful as a diagnostic tool, adjunct modality to skin cancer surgery and for monitoring non-invasive therapy results. Since RCM allows for static interpretation of morphology and dynamic imaging of disease activity of the skin it may help accomplish these future tasks by opening a new medical era whereby the physician can make decisions based on clinically non-perceptible changes in disease activity as well as the traditional morphologic parameters.

There are many potential benefits to using RCM, but there are also some current limitations that need to be overcome. The current RCM microscopes come with a learning curve for operating and interpreting images, are costly and cumbersome and have a limited depth of penetration particularly when lesions are hyperkeratotic. This should improve with different immersion media and illumination sources. The current contact device is also cumbersome and difficult to use on a non-flat surface. However, a smaller more user friendly RCM version is due to be available soon with a portable prototype being developed and work is ongoing to facilitate vertical and 3-dimensional sections.

RCM is in its infancy with similarities to early X-ray imaging and ultrasound. It remains to be seen if the technical challenges can be overcome although with today's technological advances this seems very likely. A bigger hurdle may be procuring the type of funding that a start up technology such as this one requires. In today's economic climate the prospects are worrisome. Yet the potential benefit is enormous.

In research, *in vivo* RCM can be used to study normal or pathophysiologic processes non-invasively, to establish the occurrence of a dynamic immunologic event or guide tissue sampling. *Ex vivo* RCM allows multiple testing and evaluation on the same exact tissue site. Clinically, *ex vivo* tissue can first be evaluated with RCM and when necessary a specific finding can be confirmed on the same exact tissue using appropriate markers or stains. Likewise, with the advent of non-invasive therapies such as immunomodulators, non-invasive RCM can be used to establish timing and dosing responses to therapy as well as to establish the effectiveness of therapy in a non-invasive manner.

The potential of RCM is enormous. The hope is that the fantasy of 'Star Trek' medicine may not be so far fetched, in that with a little portable instrument, skin lesions could be non-invasively diagnosed and new minimally invasive topical therapies could be monitored.

The reflectance confocal microscope is already available in a smaller more user friendly machine and may soon be available in a more portable hand held version, which should open up more possibilities as to its use. If it does not become a useful tool for skin cancer care, the reason may have more to do with the economics of developing new technologies than the merits of this new technology.

REFERENCES

1 Tearney GT, Brezinski ME, Southern JF, Bouma BE, Hee MR, Fujimoto JG. Determination of the refractive index of highly scattering human tissue by optical coherence tomography. Opt Lett 1995; 20:2258–2260.

2 Mansotti L. Basic principles and advanced technical aspects of ultrasound imaging. In: Guzzardi R, ed. Physics and Engineering of Medical Imaging. Boston: Martinus Nijhoff; 1987:263–317.

3 Markisz JA, Aquilia MG. Technical magnetic resonance Imaging. Stanford, Stamford, CN: Appleton and Lange; 1996.

4 New KC, Petroll WM, Boyde A et al. In vivo imaging of human teeth and skin using real-time confocal microscopy. Scanning 1991; 13:369–372.

5 Corcuff P, Leveque JL. In vivo vision of the human skin with the Tandem scanning microscope. Dermatology 1993; 186:50–54.

6 Rajadhyaksha M, Grossman M, Esterowitz D, Webb RH, Anderson RR. In vivo confocal scanning laser microscopy of human skin: melanin provides strong contrast. J Invest Derm 1995; 104:946–952.

7 Minsky M. Microscopy apparatus. US Patent No. 3013467, 7 November, 1957.

8 Cavanagh HD, Jester JV, Essepian J, Shields W, Lemp MA. Confocal microscopy of the living eye. CLAO J 1990; 16(1):65–73.

9 Jester JV, Andrews PM, Petroll WM, Lemp MA, Cavanagh HD. In vivo, real-time confocal imaging. J Electron Microsc Tech 1991; 18(1):50–60.

10 Andrews PM, Petroll WM, Cavanagh HD, Jester JV. Tandem scanning confocal microscopy (TSCM) of normal and ischemic living kidneys. Am J Anat 1991; 191(1):95–102.

11 Masters BR, Thaer AA. In vivo human corneal confocal microscopy of identical fields of subepithelial nerve plexus, basal epithelial and wing cells at different times. Microsc Res Tech 1994; 29(5):350–356.

12 Rajadhyaksha M, González S, Zavislan J, Anderson RR, Webb RH. In vivo confocal scanning laser microscopy of human skin II: Advances in instrumentation and comparison to histology. J Invest Derm 1999; 113:293–303.

13 González S, White WM, Rajadhyaksha M, Anderson RR, González E. Confocal imaging of sebaceous gland hyperplasia in vivo to assess efficacy and mechanism of pulsed dye laser treatment. Lasers Surg Med 1999; 25(1):8–12.

14 González S, Sackstein R, Anderson RR, Rajadhyaksha M. Real-time evidence of in vivo leukocyte trafficking in human skin by reflectance confocal microscopy. J Invest Derm 2001; 117(2):384–386.

15 Agasshi D, Anderson RR, González S. Time-sequence histologic imaging of laser-treated cherry angiomas using in vivo confocal microscopy. J Am Acad Derm 2000; 43:37–41.

16 Agasshi D, González E, Anderson RR, Rajadhyaksha RR, González S. Elucidating the pulsed dye laser treatment of sebaceous hyperplasia in vivo using real-time confocal scanning laser microscopy. J Am Acad Derm 2000; 43:49–53.

17 Huzaira M, Rius F, Rajadhyaksha M, Anderson RR, González S. Topographic variations in normal skin histology, as viewed by in vivo confocal microscopy. J Invest Derm 2001; 116(6):846–852.

18 González S, Tannous Z. Real-time in vivo confocal reflectance microscopy of basal cell carcinoma. J Am Acad Derm 2002; 47(6):869–874.

19 Nori S, Swindells K, Rius Diaz F, et al. Sensitivity and specificity of near infrared reflectance confocal scanning laser microscopy for in vivo diagnosis of basal cell carcinoma – A multi-center clinical trial (Abstract). Soc Invest Derm 2002

20 Torres A, Schanbacher C, Marra D, González S. Imiquimod 5% cream preceding surgery for BCC monitoring with confocal microscopy (Abstract). 20th World Congress of Dermatology.

21 Agasshi D, Anderson RR, González S. Confocal laser microscopic imaging of actinic keratoses in vivo: a preliminary report. J Am Acad Derm 2000; 43:42–48.

22 Trehan M, Swindells K, Taylor CR, Racette AL, Gonzalez S. Confocal microscopy imaging of actinic keratoses post-photodynamic therapy with 5-ALA (Abstract). 20th World Congress of Dermatology.

23 Langley RGB, Rajadhyaksha M, Dwyer PJ, Sober AJ, Flotte TJ, Anderson RR. Confocal scanning laser microscopy of benign and malignant melanocytic skin lesions in vivo. J Am Acad Derm 2001; 45:365–376.

24 Busam KJ, Charles C, Lee G, Halpern AC. Morphologic features of melanocytes, pigmented keratinocytes and melanophages by in vivo confocal scanning laser microscopy. Mod Pathol 2001; 14(9):862–868.

25 Tannous Z, Mihnn M, Flotte T, González S. In vivo examination of lentigo maligna, in situ malignant melanoma, lentigo maligna type by near-infrared confocal microscopy: Comparison of confocal images with histologic sections. J Am Acad Derm 2002; 46:260–263.

26 Busam KJ, Hester K, Charles C, Sachs DL, Antonescu C, González S, Halpern A. Detection of clinically amelanotic malignant melanoma and assessment of its margins by in vivo confocal scanning laser microscopy. Arch Derm 2001; 137(7):923–929.

27 Rajadhyaksha M, Menaker G, Flotte T, Dwyer P, González S. Confocal examination of non-melanoma cancers in skin excisions to potentially guide Mohs micrographic surgery without histopathology. J Invest Dermatol 2001; 117(5):1137–1143.

28 Tannous Z, Torres A, González S. Real-time, in-vivo confocal reflectance microscopy, a surgical guide for Mohs micrographic surgery (Abstract). 20th World Congress of Dermatology.

CHAPTER

38 Biopsy Techniques

Ken K Lee, Annalisa Gorman and Neil A Swanson

Key points

- Proper biopsy is critical in the diagnosis and management of skin cancers.
- Melanocytic lesions should be removed with an excisional biopsy in order to obtain the most accurate diagnosis and prognostic factors although there is no evidence that an incisional biopsy adversely effects prognosis.
- Non-melanocytic lesions can be removed with a shave biopsy or other incisional techniques.

INTRODUCTION

The biopsy is a critical start to the diagnosis of skin cancer. Generally defined, it is 'the process of removing tissue from patients for diagnostic examination'.[1] Fortunately, the skin is easily accessible, making this process simple relative to other organ systems. Skin cancers are often identifiable visually by an experienced clinician. Nevertheless, a properly performed biopsy is paramount to the diagnosis and eventual management of the skin cancer. There are numerous biopsy techniques including excisional, incisional, shave, saucerization and punch. Each of these techniques serves a different purpose and clinicians managing skin cancers should understand and master all of them. This is exemplified by the increasing importance for correctly biopsied pigmented lesions, as there are significant ramifications beyond the initial diagnosis of melanoma. Factors such as depth of invasion, ulceration, microsatellitosis, angiolymphatic invasion and mitotic index can impact prognosis and proper management. The decision to implement new techniques such as sentinel lymph node biopsy and systemic adjuvant therapies is often determined by the results from the initial biopsy. It is, therefore, critical that an adequate specimen be presented to the dermatopathologist assuring that a correct and complete diagnosis can be made. Furthermore, as many biopsied lesions are benign, it is also important, whenever possible, to create the best aesthetic results. This chapter reviews the decision-making process and discusses in detail the biopsy techniques and rationales for their use.

DECISION-MAKING PROCESS – SELECTING THE APPROPRIATE TECHNIQUE

There are many different types of skin cancers that are frequently divided into two categories: melanoma and non melanoma skin cancers. The reason for this division relates to the relative difficulty and controversy surrounding the histologic diagnosis of melanoma. The controversy arises as similar appearing melanocytes, the pigment forming cells of the skin, can be seen in a benign nevus, atypical or dysplastic nevus, and invasive melanoma. Furthermore, since the prognosis and management of melanoma is based primarily on the Breslow depth of invasion, an adequate deep margin is necessary in the diagnosis. Thus, a proper initial biopsy is critical toward achieving a correct diagnosis and to characterize melanoma. This type of information is best obtained in the initial biopsy. There is more flexibility in the type of biopsy technique used to diagnose non melanoma skin cancers, with location, appearance, and size of the lesion each serving as important factors

An *excisional biopsy* refers to *en toto* removal of a suspicious lesion. This is performed with a margin (as defined below) of clinically normal tissue. It is the preferred method of removing a pigmented lesion for histologic interpretation.

An *incisional biopsy* is used to sample only a part of a suspicious lesion for histologic evaluation. It is an appropriate method to biopsy a suspicious non-melanoma skin cancer.

Shave biopsy refers to a shallow removal of a lesion at a depth confined to the dermis. It can be performed by a scalpel, a dermablade, a razor blade, or scissors.

A *saucerization* is a biopsy which occurs through viable dermis into subcutaneous fat. It is performed by angling a scalpel at approximately 45 degrees to the skin and removing a disc of tissue, including all or part of the suspicious lesion, well into the subcutaneous fat.

Punch biopsy refers to the use of a sharp circular instrument to remove tissue well into the subcutaneous fat. It is usually sutured.

Fusiform ellipse allows for full thickness removal of the suspicious lesion, as well as a margin of surrounding skin. It is sutured.

The *margin* removed by a biopsy is defined as the area of normal appearing tissue surrounding the lesion to be removed and has two components. The *peripheral margin* is the area of normal skin extending radially from the clinically suspicious lesion while the *deep margin* is the depth to which skin and subcutaneous tissue is entered and removed during the biopsy.

Equipment

The equipment needed for biopsies need not be elaborate, but should be of good quality. The equipment should be properly maintained and sterilized prior to each use.

Following is a list of commonly used equipment (Figs 38.1 and 38.2):

- Scalpel: 15 blade is the most often used
- Needle holder: Webster
- Forceps: Adson type with teeth
- Scissors: Iris and Metzenbaum
- Skin hook: single or double prong

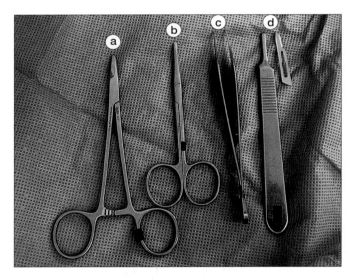

Figure 38.1 Biopsy equipment. Some of the commonly used equipment listed from left to right. (a) Webster needle holder, (b) small Metzenbaum scissors, (c) Adson forceps with teeth, (d) scalpel handle and 15-blade.

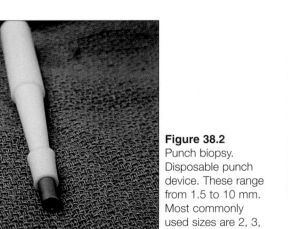

Figure 38.2 Punch biopsy. Disposable punch device. These range from 1.5 to 10 mm. Most commonly used sizes are 2, 3, 4, 6 and 8 mm.

- Dermablade or Gillette blue blade
- Punch: 2, 3, 4, 5, 6, 8 mm
- Suture
- Aluminum chloride: 35%
- Electrocautery
- Gauze
- Cotton tipped applicator.

When performing a biopsy, a tray should be prepared with all the equipment that is needed for that particular procedure. *On or near the tray should be the formalin containing specimen bottle(s) with the patient's identifying information* (Fig. 38.3). This cannot be overemphasized, as there have been unfortunate cases of mislabeled specimen bottles and/or lost specimens that were left on the tray intended for subsequent transfer. Sterile surgical gloves are generally not necessary for biopsies with the exception of excisional and incisional biopsies needing buried absorbable sutures to close the biopsied site.

Anesthesia

Lidocaine 1% mixed with epinephrine at 1:100,000 is typically used for local anesthesia. The onset of action is almost immediate with local injection and the duration of action is 1–2 hrs,[2] thus making Lidocaine 1% with epinephrine ideal for short biopsy procedures. However, it is optimal to wait 7–10 min following local infiltration to optimize the full vasoconstrictive effects of the epinephrine. Lidocaine and epinephrine mix can be obtained as a premixed formula or can be freshly mixed on a daily basis. Premixed lidocaine with epinephrine contains preservatives and has a low pH of 3.3–5.5. This low pH causes an increased amount of pain upon injection. Freshly mixed solution is desirable as it has a more neutral pH of 6.5–6.8, thus minimizing the pain from local infiltration. Sodium bicarbonate can be mixed to buffer stock (premixed) lidocaine by the addition of 1 cc $NaHCO_3$ to every 10 cc of lidocaine to neutralize the pH and decrease the pain of injection.[3]

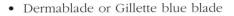

Figure 38.3 Biopsy tray. A labeled specimen bottle should always be set out prior to the biopsy.

Patients can give a history of heart palpitations and tremors with local anesthesia, leading them to report this as an allergy. Very few patients are truly allergic to lidocaine and most often these symptoms are due to the systemic adrenergic effects of epinephrine. The history should be carefully assessed and the epinephrine diluted or eliminated accordingly. The most frequent side effect encountered is a vasovagal reaction manifested by hypotension and bradycardia. Amide anesthetics do not cross-react with other drugs and true allergic reactions are extremely rare. If a true allergy to lidocaine (in the amide family of anesthetics) is documented, an anesthetic from the ester family such as procainamide can be used. However, it is more likely to have an allergy to the esters as these can cross-react with para-amino benzoic acid, sulfonamides and thiazides among others. Lastly, diphenhydramine solution (12.5–25 mg/kg) or normal saline can be used as local anesthesia for smaller lesions.[4] When the medical history is unclear, an evaluation by an allergist to determine a safe local anesthetic is critical.

The local anesthetic is injected intradermally using a 30 gauge needle (Fig. 38.4). Rapid needle insertion through the skin and slower infiltration of anesthetic agent causes less discomfort. Furthermore, it often eases anxiety to prepare the patient by discussing the technique prior to injection. In children and very anxious adults, a topical anesthetic cream can be applied 30 min to 2 hrs prior to injection to reduce the pain of needle insertion and injection pain.[5]

Contraindications to biopsy

There are no absolute contraindications to a skin biopsy. The main relative contraindication is the potential for bleeding. Many patients requiring skin biopsies are older and are on blood thinners. Although, there may be an elevated risk of postoperative bleeding, medications such as warfarin or aspirin are not contraindications for these smaller biopsy procedures. Extra measures such as electrocoagulation and pressure dressings may be needed for enhanced hemostasis in these cases. In patients on

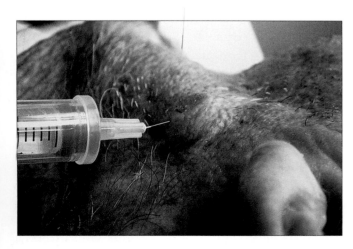

Figure 38.4 Anesthesia injection. 1% lidocaine with epinephrine is most commonly used for local anesthesia. A 30-gauge needle is used to infiltrate slowly into the dermis.

chemotherapy or with diseases which affect platelets, it is best if the platelet count is above 10,000.

BIOPSY TECHNIQUES ILLUSTRATED

Punch biopsy

Punches are available in sizes ranging from 1.5 mm to 1.0 cm and may be used for excisional or incisional biopsies. When performing a punch biopsy, one must first select the proper size. Selection of proper size is determined by whether an incisional or excisional biopsy is indicated. For an excisional biopsy, the punch should be 1.0 to 1.5 mm greater in diameter than the lesion. For an incisional biopsy, a 4 mm punch is commonly used. After adequate anesthesia, traction is placed across the skin tension lines converting a circular region into an elliptical shape (Fig. 38.5). When the traction is released the resultant elliptical defect allows for an easier and aesthetically superior closure. The punch is rotated back and forth on the skin with constant pressure through the full thickness of the dermis. A characteristic 'give' is felt when the subcutaneous fat is reached. The specimen should be carefully grasped on one edge only to minimize crush artifact on histologic examination. The base of the specimen is cut at the level of the subcutaneous fat. Hemostasis is usually achieved with pressure and suture closure. Rarely, electrocauterization may be needed. Punch biopsies, with rare exception, are closed with simple interrupted or vertical mattress stitches for wound edge eversion to obtain the best cosmetic result.

Shave biopsy

Shave biopsy is used to remove the superficial component of a lesion that is raised above the level of the surrounding skin. The level at which the shave is performed is either at the level of the surrounding skin or slightly deeper. The intent is usually not to remove the entire neoplasm but rather to obtain a representative sample for histopathologic examination. The shave biopsy needs to be performed both for accurate sampling as well as cosmetic outcome, especially considering that many biopsied lesions are benign. The infiltration of anesthesia in the mid-dermis will provide a rigid plane and squeezing the surrounding skin will provide an elevated plane for shave biopsy. Using a 15 blade scalpel, Dermblade®, or razor blade, a shallow horizontal incision is made through the lesion at the level of the surrounding skin or slightly below. Forceps can also be used for countertraction (Fig. 38.6). A Dermablade® or a razor blade also allows for a precise shave biopsy. The blade is flexed to match the size of the lesion and is slid back and forth through the lesion until the entire lesion is removed (Fig. 38.7). Hemostasis is obtained with aluminum chloride 35%. The resultant scar is circular and approximates the size of the initial lesion. There may be a subtle indentation if the incision was made in a deeper plane.

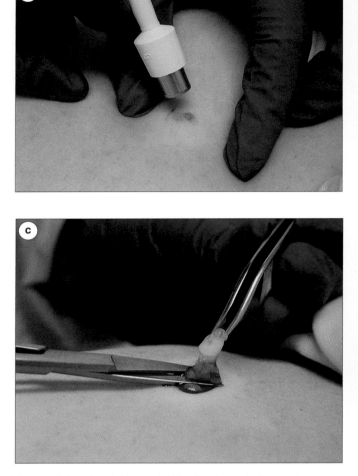

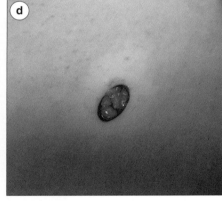

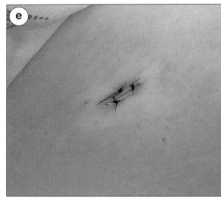

Figure 38.5 Punch biopsy. (a) Traction is applied using two fingers perpendicular to the relaxed skin tension lines providing a rigid surface for the cutting edge of the punch device. (b) The punch is then pushed through skin while applying a circular back and forth motion. (c) The specimen is gently grasped on one edge and transected at the level of the subcutaneous fat. (d) The resultant defect is elliptical because the circular biopsy was done under traction. This allows for an easier linear closure. (e) After closure with cuticular sutures.

Saucerization

A saucerization provides an excisional specimen for the dermatopathologist. This technique is easy to perform, time effective, and often preferred by patients and physicians in areas of the body where it is difficult to create an elegant scar. These areas include the upper back, shoulders, upper arms, and anterior chest where scars often spread and/or become hypertrophic. Occasionally saucerizations are also used to biopsy lesions on the lower extremities and ears. The key is to perform true saucerization, i.e. a biopsy into subcutaneous fat. With saucerization a smaller, rounder, and more cosmetically acceptable scar will replace a longer, linear spread excisional scar while providing adequate tissue for histologic interpretation. A 15-blade scalpel is placed

approximately 45 degrees to the skin surface. The incision is made around a 1–2 mm peripheral margin of the lesion then angled tangentially deeper through dermis to the level of the subcutaneous fat. This generates a disc or saucer shaped piece of tissue that contains the entire lesion (Fig. 38.8). The defect then heals by second intent without the need for sutures.

Fusiform ellipse

The fusiform elliptical excision is the cornerstone of cutaneous surgery. It is easy to perform, gives excellent cosmetic results, and provides enough tissue of sufficient depth to aid in an accurate diagnosis by the dermatopathologist.[6] In designing the ellipse, the long

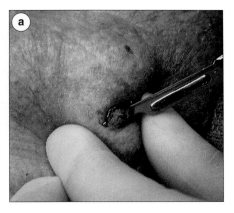

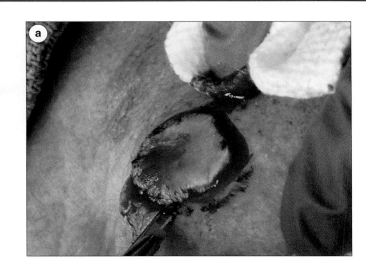

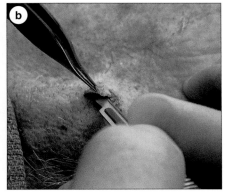

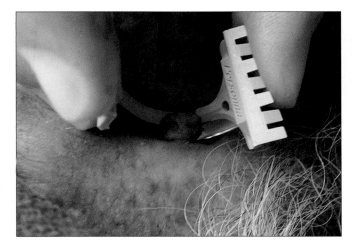

Figure 38.6
Shave biopsy. A 15-blade scalpel is used to shave the raised component of the suspected cancer. (a) The surrounding skin is squeezed together to provide an elevated and rigid plane or (b) forceps are used for counter traction.

Figure 38.7 Shave biopsy. Dermablade® is flexed to fit the lesion and is slid side to side through the lesion.

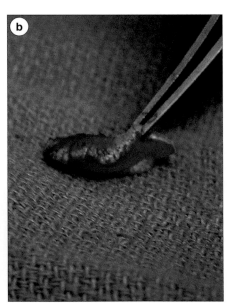

Figure 38.8
Saucerization. (a) The scalpel blade is angled at 45 degrees. The incision is made tangentially to create a disc shaped specimen. (b) The specimen is removed at the level of the fat.

wound eversion. After adequate hemostasis is achieved, the wound is carefully reapproximated using an absorbable buried dermal interrupted suture. The initial needle insertion should be from the deep aspect as this will place the knot deeply and lessen the chances of a spitting suture. The superficial or cuticular layer is generally closed with a non-absorbable monofilament suture (Fig. 38.10).

DIAGNOSIS OF MELANOMA

When examining a patient with one or several suspicious pigmented lesions, the question often arises, 'Do I need to perform a biopsy, and if so, which technique do I choose?' There are patients with specific risk factors as well as characteristics of individual lesions which portend higher risk to develop melanoma. Patient risk factors include any of the following: a personal or family history of melanoma, a fair complexion, the presence of multiple nevi or atypical (dysplastic) nevus syndrome, a history of numerous or severe sunburns, and an advanced age, to name a few. Risk factors for

axis should generally be oriented along the relaxed skin tension lines and the draining lymphatics for that site. The length is approximately three times the width, but this can vary from site to site. The ideal angle of the elliptical ends is 30 degrees in order to minimize puckering of redundant skin. The 15-blade scalpel is angled perpendicular to the skin surface and the incision is carried through the skin into the subcutaneous fat. The specimen is removed in its entirety maintaining a flat bottomed surface (Fig. 38.9).

The fusiform ellipse is usually closed in linear layered fashion. The defect is undermined at the level of the subcutaneous fat to alleviate tension and to promote

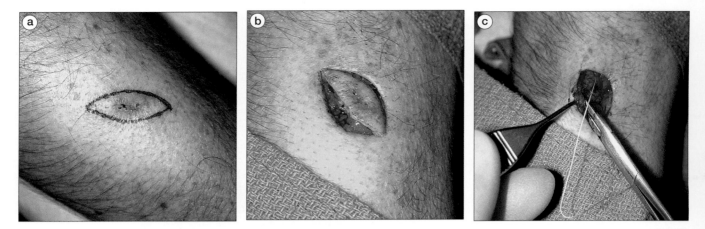

Figure 38.9 Fusiform elliptical excision. (a) 1–2 mm margin is delineated around the lesion and oriented along the relaxed skin tension lines and/or direction of lymphatic drainage. (b) Incision is made through the dermis into the fat. (c) Defect is ready for layered closure.

individual lesions include: appearance *de novo*, a change in size, texture or shape, the ABCD criteria, and the symptom of pruritus. Clinically asymptomatic nevi which begin to itch should alert both patient and physician to pay closer attention to that particular lesion. A clinician must also listen to the patient. If they sense that there is something changing or different in a particular lesion, it is often best to biopsy that lesion. Experienced clinicians have many anecdotes of clinically benign lesions removed purely based on patient request which turn out to be melanoma despite lacking clinical features of melanoma. Lastly, a clinician must weigh the given risks of a particular lesion with the patient or family concern (in the case of children) for scarring, inherent in all biopsy procedures.[7]

There are several tools available which can help to decide whether or not to biopsy a particular pigmented lesion. These include dermoscopy, precise photography, 'mole mapping' by computer, as well as others in developmental stages. As clinicians, we develop expertise to determine which group of patients and which particular lesions are concerns for the development of melanoma. If our suspicion is moderate or high, we will routinely remove the pigmented lesion and submit it for histologic analysis by a dermatopathologist. This is both reassuring to the patient as well as clinician and frequently leads to a diagnosis of melanoma in its earlier, less advanced stage.

The excisional biopsy is the preferred method of removing a clinically suspicious pigmented lesion. It provides the dermatopathologist with the maximal opportunity to diagnose a melanoma in a given biopsy sample. If present, the maximum depth of invasion of the melanoma (Breslow level) can be measured as well as other histologic criteria of importance, which helps define the extent of further necessary surgery.

When performing an excisional biopsy, the clinician should first examine the lymph nodes in the suspected draining basin(s) from the lesion in question. If the lesion turns out to be a melanoma, inflammation from the biopsy procedure can result in a false positive 'dermatopathic' node. A Wood's light is helpful to assess the complete margin, sometimes extending beyond the obvious clinical appearance of the lesion. A 1.0 mm to 1.5 mm margin is marked around the lesion and removed at the level of the subcutaneous fat.[8,9] When possible, the biopsy is aligned along relaxed skin tension lines and along the draining lymphatics from that site. The former allows for an easier and more cosmetically acceptable procedure if the lesion is a melanoma and requires re-excision. The latter allows for a more accurate sentinel lymph node biopsy if indicated.

The excisional biopsy can be performed with either a punch or a fusiform (elliptical) excision. Choosing a punch 1.0 mm to 1.5 mm greater in diameter than the lesion to be biopsied assures a full-thickness removal of the entire lesion that is easy and quick to perform with a cosmetically acceptable scar. If the lesion is larger and/or in a cosmetically sensitive area such as the head and neck, a fusiform (elliptical) excision with full thickness closure provides adequate tissue for the pathologist and an excellent cosmetic result if the pigmented lesion is benign.

A saucerization biopsy can also be used to provide an excisional specimen for the dermatopathologist. Again, the key is to make sure this is a saucerization, i.e. a biopsy into fatty tissue as the depth of the melanoma is critical for staging purposes. Because, in areas such as those described previously, scars often spread and/or become hypertrophic, a saucerization is often the biopsy method of choice. Superficial shave biopsies should not be used for pigmented lesions, especially if one is ruling out melanoma. The transection of the specimen base will lead to an uninterpretable Breslow level.

An incisional biopsy can be used to diagnose melanoma in a worrisome pigmented lesion. However, because it does not sample the entire lesion in question, incisional biopsies are not as accurate diagnostically or prognostically as their excisional counterpart. Incisional biopsies can be performed on very large lesions and/or in cosmetically sensitive regions (Fig. 38.11). The darkest pigmented and/or raised area of the lesion should be biopsied. This can be performed using a punch biopsy, small fusiform ellipse or a saucerization down to the level of the

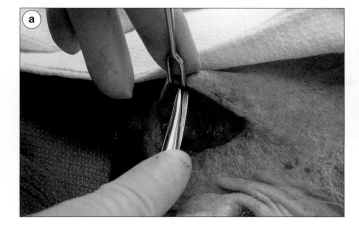

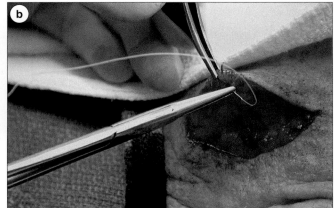

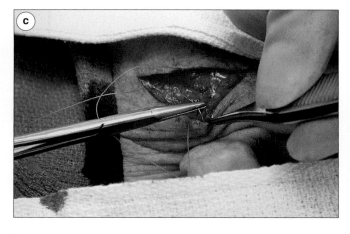

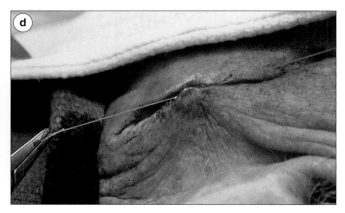

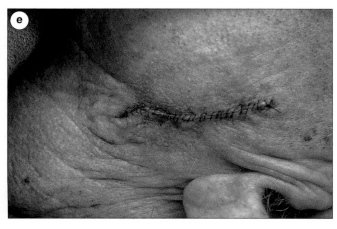

Figure 38.10 Fusiform elliptical excision – closure. (a) Wound is undermined using a skin hook and Metzenbaum scissors. (b) Dermal suture is inserted from the deep aspect of the wound, then (c) passed superficial to deep on the other side and (d) knotted to create an everted wound. (e) Final appearance.

subcutaneous fat. Although most clinicians feel that an incisional biopsy does not 'spread' tumor or influence survival,[10] there still exists a theoretical risk that cutting through the tumor may lead to local spread of the melanoma. Studies indicate that performing an incisional biopsy does not influence prognosis.[11–14] Others have shown that an incisional biopsy, especially of a deeper melanoma, may negatively influence local recurrence and/or survival.[15,16]

When performed, the incisional biopsy specimen should be cut and processed along the longitudinal axis to maximize the cross section area available histologi-cally for the dermatopathologist. It is helpful to actually draw this schematic on the pathology requisition slip.

DIAGNOSIS OF NON-MELANOMA SKIN CANCER

Non-melanoma skin cancers encompass a large number of heterogeneous cancers. The two most prevalent in this category are basal cell carcinoma (BCC) and squamous cell carcinoma (SCC). These cancers number 1 million and 250,000 per year, respectively, in the US.[17]

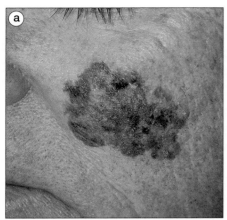

Figure 38.11
Incisional biopsy. (a) A large and ill-defined pigmented lesion on the cheek, with variegate pigmentation. Punch biopsies can be taken from the darker areas or (b) an incisional ellipse is made through the most suspicious area. The lines demonstrate the axis of sectioning in order to maximize the cross section seen by the dermatopathologist.

Given these large numbers, clinically recognizing and obtaining a biopsy diagnosis is very important. Careful inspection and examination of the pertinent lymph nodes should be performed routinely in all patients with skin cancers.

Morphologically, skin cancers can be exophytic, macular, or ulcerated. They can be pinpoint in size, or consume large parts of a face, trunk, or extremity. These differences impact the choice of biopsy. An excisional biopsy is rarely needed for non-melanoma skin cancers.

An exophytic lesion such as a nodular BCC, or a hyperkeratotic SCC can be biopsied using the shave technique. Near complete removal of the surface component usually results in an adequate tissue sample for an accurate diagnosis. One must be cautious, however, of lesions that have a significant hyperkeratotic component (e.g. cutaneous horn). A shave through only the hyperkeratotic component may not remove the full epidermis, necessary to distinguish a SCC from an actinic keratosis. Occasionally, amelanotic melanoma can present as a skin colored papule or nodule. If there is any concern that a lesion is something other than a clinically routine BCC or SCC, a deeper biopsy should be considered.

Basal cell carcinomas can present as different histologic subtypes. Sclerosing (morpheaform) and infiltrative types of BCC typically have a significant component that is below the level of the skin surface and can be clinically subtle or in apparent (subclinical extension). When there is minimal or no raised component, a deeper biopsy is indicated and a punch biopsy usually results in an accurate diagnosis. Sometimes, however, multiple punch biopsies may need to be performed on the same lesion especially when the cancer is recurrent and is adjacent to or part of a prior surgical scar.

Many different malignant and non-malignant skin conditions can present as an ulcer. Due to the dense inflammation invariably present in the ulcer bed, the biopsy should be taken from the edges in order to obtain proper diagnosis. As most ulcers are not cancerous, all longstanding ulcers without obvious cause should raise the concern of possible malignancy.

POST BIOPSY CARE

Biopsy sites that are healing by second intent need to be cleaned daily with soap and water. They should heal under moist conditions and therefore need to be covered with an antibiotic ointment and non-adherent bandage. Sutured wounds need less daily care but should be kept clean. Fusiform excisions closed with a layered closure should have a pressure bandage placed for 24 hrs postoperatively. Postoperative pain is usually managed effectively with acetaminophen. Nonsteroidal anti-inflammatories and aspirin are not recommended as these can increase the risk for postoperative bleeding.

CONCLUSIONS

Choosing the appropriate biopsy technique for a suspicious cutaneous lesion is critical in establishing a correct and complete diagnosis and in the case of melanoma to gauge maximum depth of invasion and other diagnostic criteria. This, in turn, influences the extent of further necessary surgery and/or other adjuvant therapy. The clinician must also consider the cosmetic result although not at the expense of a proper diagnosis. Excisional biopsies should extend to the subcutaneous fat by means of a punch biopsy, a fusiform ellipse, or a saucerization. Incisional biopsies are appropriate for non-melanoma skin cancers and can be performed in limited circumstances for pigmented lesions, but should be done so with caution as sampling error may lead to missed diagnosis or inaccurate histologic criterion, such as depth.

FUTURE OUTLOOK

Today, a definitive diagnosis can only be obtained through invasive biopsies. In the future, new technologies may allow the use of a non-invasive 'biopsy.' Optical imaging techniques are under current development and hold an exciting potential for the future in this area.

REFERENCES

1 Stedman's Medical Dictionary, 24th edn. Baltimore, MD: Williams & Wilkins; 1982.

2 Norris RL Jr. Local anesthetics. Emerg Med Clin North Am 1992; 10(4):707–718.

3 Stewart JH, Chinn SE, Cole GW, Klein JA. Neutralized lidocaine with epinephrine for local anesthesia. J Derm Surg Oncol 1990; 16(9):842–845.

4 Dire DJ, Hogan DE. Double-blinded comparison of diphenhydramine versus lidocaine as a local anesthetic. Ann Emerg Med 1993; 22(9):1419–1422.

5 Raveh T, Weinberg A, Sibirsky O, Caspi R, Alfie M, Moor EV, et al. Efficacy of the topical anesthetic cream, EMLA, in alleviating both needle insertion and injection pain. Ann Plast Surg 1995; 35(6):576–579.

6 Swanson NA. Atlas of Cutaneous Surgery. Boston/Toronto: Little, Brown; 1987.

7 Swanson NA, Lee KK, Gorman A, Lee HN. Biopsy techniques – diagnosis of melanoma. Derm Clin 2002; 20:677–680.

8 Brown MD, Johnson TM, Swanson NA. Changing trends in melanoma treatment and the expanding role of the dermatologist. Derm Clin 1991; 9:657–637.

9 Holmstrom H. Surgical management of primary melanoma. Semin Surg Oncol 1992; 8:366–369.

10 Penneys NS. Excision of melanoma after initial biopsy. J Am Acad Derm 1985; 13:995–998.

11 Eldh J. Excisional biopsy and delayed wide excision versus primary wide excision of malignant melanoma. Scand J Plast Reconstr Surg 1979; 13:341–345.

12 Drzewiecki KT, Ladefoged C, Christensen HE. Biopsy and prognosis for cutaneous malignant melanomas in clinical stage I. Scand J Plast Reconstr Surg 1980; 14:141–144.

13 Lederman JS, Sober AJ. Does wide excision as the initial diagnostic procedure improve prognosis in patients with cutaneous melanoma? J Derm Surg Oncol 1986; 12:697–699.

14 Epstein E, Bragg K, Linden G. Biopsy and prognosis of malignant melanoma. JAMA 1969; 208:1369–1371.

15 Lees VC, Briggs JC. Effect of initial biopsy procedure on prognosis in stage 1 invasive cutaneous malignant melanoma: review of 1086 patients. Br J Surg 1991; 78:1108–1110.

16 Lederman JS, Sober AJ. Does biopsy type influence survival in clinical Stage I cutaneous melanoma? J Am Acad Derm 1985; 13:983–987.

17 Miller DL, Weinstock MA. Nonmelanoma skin cancer in the United States: incidence. J Am Acad Dermatol 1994; 30(5):774–778.

CHAPTER

39

Curettage and Electrodesiccation

Glenn Goldman

Key points

- Curettage and electrodesiccation (CE) is an expedient method of treating many non-melanoma skin cancers (NMSC).
- Cure rates and cosmetic outcome for CE of NMSC are site and lesion dependent.
- The most important aspect of CE is choosing the correct lesion to treat.
- Models exist to predict where cure is likely and where treatment failure may occur.
- Careful incorporation of proper lesion selection and good technique make CE a valuable therapeutic technique in the treatment of uncomplicated NMSC.

INTRODUCTION

Curettage and electrodesiccation (CE) is a technique employed by many dermatologists to destroy benign skin lesions and selected non-melanoma skin cancers (NMSC). General surgeons usually excise malignant lesions. The use of CE for the treatment of NMSC has been both widely extolled and also fervently criticized and clearly CE has both virtues and shortcomings. In order to appropriately utilize CE to treat NMSC it is essential to learn the basis for CE, the proper technique, the likely cure rates for given lesions and the expected level of cosmesis.

Formerly the dermatologists' treatment of choice for many skin cancers, CE is now only one method in an increasing therapeutic armamentarium. To utilize CE most judiciously, it is valuable to examine this technique in depth and to come to some thoughtful conclusions about its use for patients with skin cancer. In 2000, Sheridan and Dauber published a remarkably complete, favorable review of curettage, electrosurgery and skin cancer.[1] For anyone performing curettage this article is a must read. However, many of the truisms that dermatologists have promulgated about CE need to be carefully examined and the limitations of this technique need to be comprehensively evaluated in order to best utilize its strengths.

HISTORY OF CE AND REPORTED CURE RATES

Historically, most malignant skin lesions were excised. High cure rates have been reported throughout the dermatology and surgery literatures for excision of NMSC with standard permanent section margins. In the largest series reported for standard excision, Lauritzen *et al.* reported a 96.6% 10-year cure rate for the standard excision of BCC, although the verification of patient follow-up in this series is not clear.[2]

Electrodesiccation of skin lesions was first established in 1911 by William Clark, who noted superficial tissue drying or desiccation when he applied a high voltage, low current to the skin, through a monoterminal electrode. Clark reported the treatment of a variety of skin lesions including some basal cell carcinomas with electrodesiccation alone. Most lesions were clinically cured over a 1 to 2 year follow-up and he reported one recurrence.[3] The technique of electrodesiccation became available to the office practitioner through the development of instrumentation such as the original Hyfrecator units produced by the Birtcher Corporation.

The literature surrounding the original implementation of curettage is actually quite sparse. Use of the dermal curette was reported in 1870 by Dr Henry Piffard.[4] Several years later Dr Edward Wigglesworth used the dermal curette to treat a variety of skin lesions including psoriasis and syphilitic condylomata.[5] In 1902, Dr George Fox introduced the Fox model curette, which has remained the most popular type of curette to this day.[6] As dermatology evolved in the 1950s and 1960s, an increasing number of epithelial tumors were primarily treated by CE or by curettage alone. At this time, many dermatologists received little training in surgery and most large lesions were handled either through excision by general surgeons or plastic surgeons or by radiation therapy. As dermatologists explored avenues for office-based treatment of cutaneous tumors the technique of CE was embraced as an efficient method for the removal of benign lesions and NMSC.

In the 1960s and early 1970s, a number of large series reported cure rates for the treatment of NMSC by CE. In 1960, Knox *et al.* reported a cure rate of 96–98% for 765 BCC and SCC treated by CE,[7] and in 1966, he reported a cure rate of 98–99% for CE in 1493 tumors.[8] In the 1960s and 1970s numerous other authors reported large series with cure rates ranging from 88% to 100% for CE of NMSC.[9–15] These studies have formed the basis for CE as a treatment regimen, but they have been rightly criticized for selection bias and a lack of long-term follow-up. In the early to mid 1970s, Reymann reported cure rates of 92–98% in the three separate publications of separate series for the treatment of BCC by curettage alone.[16–18] Using similar technique, McDaniel reported two series with cure rates of 92–93%.[19,20] Notably, in a subsequent study with longer followup, Reymann reported cure rates of 87–90% for the same study groups.[21] The latter article sheds light on what many in the surgical community have long believed; that, given adequate followup, the recurrence rate following removal of NMSC is substantially higher than that routinely reported with a 2–5 year series.

TECHNIQUE FOR CE OF NON-MELANOMA SKIN CANCER

The premise behind CE is that using a curette the clinician can distinguish precisely between disease (tumor) and a normal dermis. Most nodular and superficial BCC and some SCC have a less cohesive texture than normal epidermis and dermis and are thus delineated from healthy tissue by curettage. Sturm and Leider noted that 'solid cutaneous malignancies are felt to the hand that wields the curette as soft, yielding and easily dislodged whereas healthy fibrous tissue is hard, unyielding and almost impossible to dislodge except by cutting, which the curette does not really do'.[22] While this is true for the majority of nodular BCC, many superficial SCC are firm and keratotic. While treatable by curettage, such lesions have the tendency to be removed as chunks that tear away from the underlying dermis and peripheral epidermal tissues.

A large or medium curette is used to remove the bulk of the tumor and residual foci are removed and the defect sculpted with a fine curette. Most authors who are proponents of CE recommend vigorous and precise curettage prior to electrodesiccation. The lesion has been fully removed when a flat off white dermis with regularly spaced hair follicles, pinpoint bleeding and no intervening epidermal tissue is seen.

While there are many types of curettes (Fig. 39.1), most clinicians use a combination of standard round and oval head Fox curettes or oval Cannon curettes with or without delicate angle. The standard Fox round head curette has a rectangular handle with a tapered cylindrical extension to the head, which is round with a thicker dull side and a thin sharp side. The Fox oval curette has the same handle, but the head is oval with its longest axis along the length of the curette. The Cannon angled oval curette has a more delicate (thinner) handle and the head is tilted at a slight angle to facilitate curettage. Curettes are labeled by size from 0 to 8, based on the approximate diameter of the longest axis in mm. There are some specialty sizes and the size of a 'given size' curette may vary from vendor to vendor and should be checked. A typical setup for CE is illustrated in Figure 39.2.

Two curettage techniques may be employed and these methods have been reviewed in a detailed fashion.[23] In the pen technique, the curette is held like a pencil in the dominant hand and the lesion is stabilized with the nondominant hand. Most clinicians use this technique. In the potato peeler technique, which has been touted for larger tumors, the curette is held in the distal interdigital joint of the index, middle finger, ring finger and pinky. Using the thumb to brace against the tissue the lesion is then peeled from the dermis. It is essential that the area

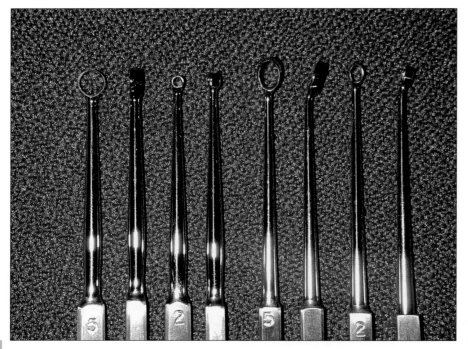

Figure 39.1 Fox (straight) curettes (left) and Cannon (oval, angled) curettes (right).

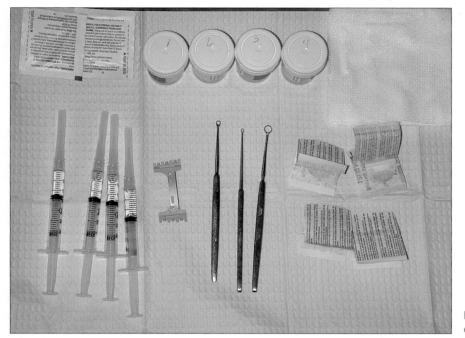

Figure 39.2 Setup for biopsy and curettage of several lesions.

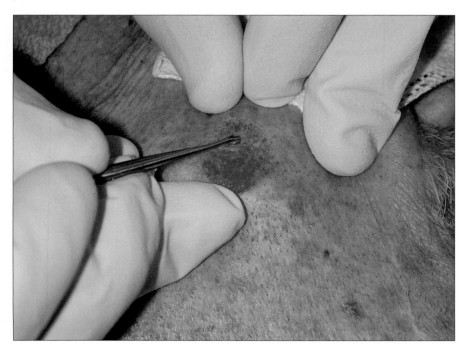

Figure 39.3 Pen CE technique for removal of SCC *in situ* on the cheek.

to be treated is braced firmly to provide a taught surface for the curette. With either method, curettage is performed vigorously until all tumor is removed by tactile feel and until a firm dermis with pinpoint bleeding is observed (Fig. 39.3).

A great deal has been written about the feel of curettage, its relative under appreciation and even its superiority to surgical margins. In their 2000 review of CE, Sheridan and Dawber note that 'this feel is both undeniably and readily learnt'. On the other hand, Salsche has definitively demonstrated that even in highly experienced hands tumor is left behind by curettage in 12–30% of

facial BCC. Clearly the 'feel' is far more reliable on the trunk and proximal extremities where the dermis is thick and taut and the recurrence rate for NMSC following CE is much lower at these locations. 'Feel' is at its weakest on the eyelid, medial cheek and eyelid, which 'float' during the curettage procedure and on the nose where follicular BCC is beyond the feel of the curette.[24]

Some authors believe that electrodesiccation and subsequent curettage of the char effects a higher cure rate,[1] but the data to support this assertion is weak. Likewise it is not clear that performing three cycles of CE is statistically more effective than one. It is clear that those who have reported the highest cure rates always destroy a substantial peripheral margin around the initial curettage. This is accomplished most readily by electro-desiccation and then curettage of a rim of 2 mm, to as much as 8 mm of tissue around the initial defect.[7,13] Several authors comment further that any undermined epidermis at the periphery of the curettage site should be trimmed away with scissors.[25]

CURE RATES

Various authors report highly disparate cure rates for CE of NMSC. As noted earlier, all of the large series from the 1960s and 1970s report cure rates for CE well over 90%. These articles paint a glowing testimonial of the technique, extolling high cure rates and superior cosmesis. Reading these articles and taking the reported cure rates at face value one would be inclined to treat almost all NMSC with CE. Most of these series, however, suffer from selection bias and inadequate follow-up. In 1971, Crissey analyzed the 13 prior available studies for CE and compiled a cumulative 92.6% cure rate, additionally commenting that certain lesions responded poorly to CE. Specifically, he noted that CE was usually unsuitable for large cutaneous carcinomas, lesions of the nose greater than 1 cm, lesions of the margin of the eyelid and the vermillion border of the lip, lesions involving cartilage and sclerosing epitheliomas.[26]

In 1977, Kopf *et al.* published an exhaustive review of data compiled at New York University. Depending on the setting, private office *vs* academic setting, NYU physicians compiled cure rates for CE of BCC ranging from 81.8% to 94.2%.[27] In a multivariate analysis of the same data, the 5-year CE recurrence rate for BCC between 1955 and 1969 was 26%, as opposed to a 9.6% recurrence rate for BCC treated by surgical excision or radiation.[28] Salasche commented on the importance of this study in terms of defining realistic recurrence rates for CE, stating that 'Foremost in this regard is the almost wishful expectation of a 95% 5-year cure rate following C&D'.[29]

In 1991, Silverman *et al.* reported a detailed review of cure rates following CE over nearly 30 years at the New York University Skin and Cancer Unit.[30] Multivariate analysis identified low, intermediate and high-risk sites for recurrence following CE of primary BCC. The neck, trunk and extremities were considered low risk sites with a five-year recurrence rate of 8.6%. The scalp, forehead and temples were of intermediate risk with a 12.9% recurrence rate. High-risk sites such as the nose, eyelids, chin, jaw and ear had a recurrence rate of 17.5%. The authors noted that to achieve a 95% cure rate for CE at middle risk sites, lesions should measure less than 1 cm in diameter and that, in high risk areas, a 95% cure rate for CE may be achieved by selecting lesions less than 6 mm in diameter. Although others have continued to report much higher cure rates for CE,[25] most in the dermatologic surgery community feel that the NYU data reflects the reality of CE in daily practice quite accurately and that their high, intermediate and low risk stratification is valuable in planning appropriate care for a given tumor (Figs 39.4, 39.5 and Table 39.1[31]).

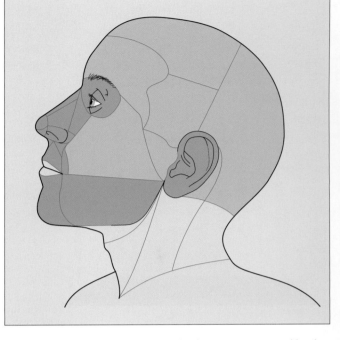

Figure 39.4 The high-risk anatomic sites are represented by the darkest areas. The middle-risk sites by the intermediate areas and the low-risk sites by the lightest areas. Included in the low-risk sites are the trunk and extremities.

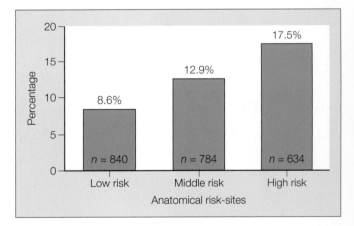

Figure 39.5 5-year recurrence rates by anatomic risk sites for BCCs treated from 1955 to 1982 ($P < 0.001$). *n* refers to the number of BCCs. (*Note:* 56 lesions in which the anatomic site was not recorded are excluded.)[31]

CE FOLLOWED BY EXCISION – EFFECTIVENESS IN ERADICATING TUMOR AT GIVEN SITES

Any oncologic surgeon will stress that complete tumor extirpation is essential to effect cure. Historically, the gold standard for removal of a skin cancer has been, and remains, complete excision with reliable negative margins. In the favorable curettage literature the 'feel' of a negative margin has been stressed as equal to surgical margin control and it has been noted that 'simple curettage has a certain surety'.[22] In order to test the veracity of such statements, several excellent studies have been performed to assess the presence of residual

Table 39.1 Cure rates reported for curettage of basal cell carcinoma and squamous carcinoma

Author	Tumor	Method	Lesions treated (n)	Peripheral margin destroyed (mm)	Reported cure rate (%)	5-year follow-up (%)
Knox et al.[7]	BCC	CE × 2	450	2–4	97	12
Knox et al.[8]	SCC	CE × 2	315	2–4	97	12
Freeman et al.[31]	BCC	CE × 2	540	2–4	97–100	22
	SCC	CE × 2	407	2–4	96–100	14
Sweet et al.[11]	BCC	CE × 1, thorough char	497	2–4	88	47
Wheelan et al.[13]	BCC	Electrocoagulation followed by curettage (several cycles)	114	3–8	94	Unknown
Honeycutt et al.[14]	SCC	CE × 2	281	2–4	99	Unknown
Reymann[18]	BCC	Curettage alone	397	NA	90	Unknown
McDaniel[20]	BCC	Curettage alone	644	NA	92	51
Spiller et al.[25]	BCC	CE × 1–3	233	3–6	97	100
Kopf et al.[27]	BCC	CE (technique not clarified)		NA		Life table method
		Unsupervised trainees	597		81	
		Supervised trainees	91		90	
		Private attendings	210		94	
Dubin et al.[28]	BCC	CE (trainees)	758	NA	74	Life table
Silverman et al.[30]	BCC	CE	2314	NA		Life table method
		High risk sites			83	
		Medium risk sites			87	
		Low risk sites			91	

tumor following seemingly definitive curettage and/or CE. In 1983, Salasche performed CE (three cycles) on selected BCC and subsequently excised the defect with a 1 mm margin. This tissue was then analyzed for the persistence of tumor nests using Mohs surgery. Residual BCC was identified in 12% of extra-nasal lesions and in 30% of nasal and paranasal lesions.[24] Shortly thereafter, Edens et al. published a similar study in which tumor persisted in 37–45% of cases following CE of either one or three cycles respectively.[32] Suhge d'Aubermont and Bennett reiterated these findings with a similar study that demonstrated persistent tumor in 46.6% of BCC on the head treated by CE, but in only 8.3% of truncal lesions treated by CE.[33]

Numerous authors have acknowledged the persistence of tumor following CE but point to a higher clinical cure rate than that which might be expected when tumor is left behind. A postulate long referred to by those who write favorably about CE is that due to inflammation and scar formation in the maturation process of the curettage site residual basal cell carcinoma is destroyed and this leads to an augmented cure rate. Two recent studies have demonstrated that over a 1–3 month period persistent BCC is in fact not eradicated but remains present at the site of CE.[34,35] Even in the face of what should be considered relatively overwhelming evidence to the contrary, some prominent dermatologists continue to suggest that tumor will regress when present in scar tissue following a destructive procedure. In reconciling tumor persistence with clinical cure rates, it is more likely that many individuals are simply living with residual tumor. Incidentally, such tumor may be very difficult to detect clinically, particularly when it is at the base of a curettage scar. It is reasonably clear that a fair number of individuals die with undetected or undiagnosed persistent BCC.

RECURRENCE FOLLOWING CE

All dermatologists, particularly dermatologic surgeons, are well acquainted with the recurrent NMSC. In practice, the majority of recurrent NMSC were originally treated as primary lesions by CE. Despite frequent recurrences, particularly on the nose, lip and ear and despite literature evidence to the contrary, many dermatologists persist in quoting a cure rate of 95% across the board for CE for facial BCC. There is also a tendency of some physician authors to minimize the implications of recurrent NMSC. For example, in their 1972 paper Whelan and Deckers noted that 'when there is a recurrence after electrocoagulation, it occurs on the surface of the scar, is quickly detected and may be expeditiously recoagulated'.[13] This is clearly true for some cases of small superficial NMSC on the trunk and extremities. However, recurrence on the head and neck is frequently either infiltrative at a peripheral or deep margin, is often overlooked as scarring for years and can have devastating consequences. Spencer et al. have recognized that 'a relatively benign primary BCC can become an aggressive, invasive, destructive recurrence that is much more difficult to treat'.[35] In addition, recurrence is often multifocal, thus necessitating removal of the entire prior treated site in order to achieve an adequate cure rate.[36] Even most physicians who recognize CE as a valuable primary treatment modality for NMSC recognize the ineffectiveness of CE for the treatment of recurrent lesions.[1] Fundamentally, the practicing dermatologist should choose a procedure that offers a high cure rate, particularly when the implication of recurrence is significant (Fig. 39.6).

HISTOLOGIC SUBTYPES *VS* EFFECTIVENESS

It is widely agreed that infiltrative (morpheaform and micronodular) basal cell carcinomas are not readily treated by CE and are therefore best treated by excisional means.[1] Many physicians will therefore biopsy lesions and treat them subsequently by various methods depending on the histologic subtype of tumor identified by the biopsy specimen. Other physicians will biopsy and destroy multiple lesions and will then re-treat by excisional means any tumors that are found to be infiltrative on histology. The problem with these treatment models lies in the fact that the histopathology of NMSC is heterogeneous in a given lesion. Maloney has reported that 40% of BCC are composed of more than one histologic subtype and that 13% of tumors classified on biopsy as nodular BCC in fact have a component of infiltrative BCC.[37] However, even given the limitations that are imposed by a partial biopsy, it is clearly reasonable to base treatment decisions at least in part on histologic subtype. For example, while a reading of nodular BCC does not guarantee that a lesion is amenable to curettage at an appropriate location, a reading of infiltrative BCC would strongly discourage this form of treatment.

COSMESIS

In 1963, Sweet wrote that the cosmetic results from curettage and electrodesiccation were 'so astoundingly good that I think they would justify this form of treatment even if the recurrence rate were far higher'.[11]

Subsequent authors who have promoted the technique of CE or curettage alone have extolled the cosmetic virtues of curettage over surgical excision. With regard to curettage alone, Reymann noted that 'it must be emphasized that after treatment solely with curettage, the cicatrices are much more satisfactory than those resulting from any other type of therapy'.[17] In contrast, Epstein noted in 1977 that 'surgical excision produces cosmetic results clearly superior to CE' and that 'the dermatology profession should stop trying to justify the second-rate cosmetic results obtainable by CE and abandon the technique in treating BCC'.[38] To this date there have been no blinded studies of the cosmetic outcome of CE *vs* excision.

Clearly the cosmetic result following both CE and excision is site dependent. On the trunk and extremities CE often leads to a flat, white macule or patch, but may lead to a raised or depressed oval scar, or occasionally a longstanding Keloidal scar. Even if the eventual result is satisfactory, often CE sites remain pink and elevated for a period of months before improving. Surgical excision at these sites frequently leads to a fine line but can produce either a spread scar or a keloidal scar. On the face CE may heal with a fine white patch or macule. However, despite many claims to the contrary, healed CE sites on the face are often depressed, sometimes markedly so, often retract free margins as they heal and can produce a firm rope-like scar due to wound contraction. It is important to note that a skillfully performed surgical excision on the face often leads to a scar that is almost imperceptible even on close inspection, while CE can never do this. In general it is the author's feeling that excision or Mohs surgery followed by proper repair more often leads to a better aesthetic scar than does CE (Figs 39.7–39.10).

INDICATIONS AND CONTRAINDICATIONS

It is important to incorporate many factors in developing a formula to select the most appropriate therapy for

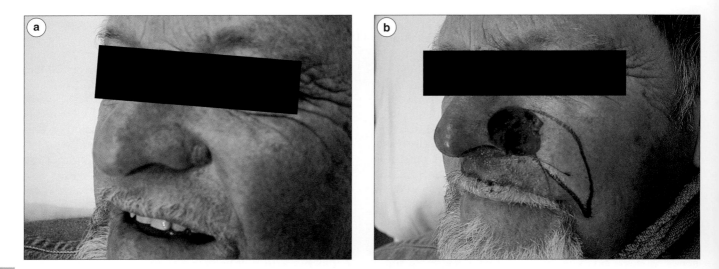

Figure 39.6   Recurrent BCC following CE at high-risk site. Note the larger defect size needed for removal by Mohs surgery vs minimal size of tumor.

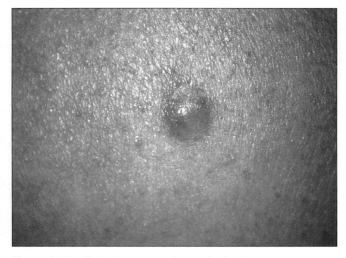

Figure 39.7 Typical curettage site on the back at two months. Note pink color and elevation. Frequently the site is pruritic.

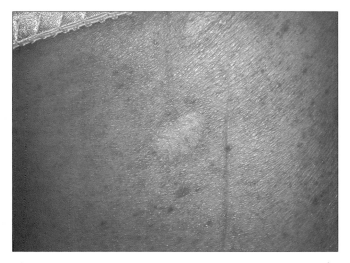

Figure 39.8 Well-healed curettage site at 1 year. Note flat, white, soft, supple scar. This is an excellent result and in this case is likely superior to the result that would have been achieved surgically.

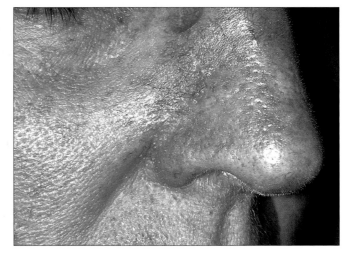

Figure 39.9 One month following surgical excision and linear repair of 1.5 by 1.5 cm BCC in nasofacial sulcus. This cosmetic result could not be duplicated by CE at this location. Also, cure rate would be much lower. Note small retained suture at junction of cheek and nose.

NMSC. CE is an expedient and suitable form of treatment for selected NMSC and can be widely utilized within a set of defined guidelines. Except in the isolated case of a long-term patient with many skin cancers, it is advisable to biopsy lesions first and to treat on a subsequent visit. Even to the relatively skilled eye, some lesions that appear to be nodular or superficial BCC or superficial SCC can prove on histology to be something else (i.e. amelanotic melanoma). Since CE can complicate further care by 'enlarging' the primary lesion, it is rational to postpone further care pending the biopsy result. All biopsies to diagnose NMSC should be superficial or mid-dermal shave biopsies, in order to avoid disturbing the underlying deep dermis. Curettage specimens are inherently inferior due to fragmentation and crush artifact. Punch biopsies, which poke through to the subcutis and simulate deep tumor extension, make subsequent CE difficult. If a punch biopsy has been performed prior to surgical treatment, it is reasonable to avoid CE. Histology

that supports the use of CE as primary treatment includes nodular and/or superficial basal cell carcinoma, hypertrophic actinic keratoses, *in situ* squamous carcinomas without deep follicular involvement and superficially invasive squamous carcinomas in select locations. Infiltrative and micronodular BCC are not amenable to curettage, nor are deeply-invasive SCC.

On the face, CE should be employed only for lesions that are under 1 cm in diameter and CE should be employed with caution for all NMSC of the nose, ear, lip, eyelid, or hair-bearing scalp. On the trunk and proximal extremities many lesions are amenable to treatment by CE. Truncal lesions that are readily treated by CE include superficial or nodular BCC, SCC *in situ* and small invasive SCC. The highest cure rates are seen in those lesions less than 1 cm in diameter. Lesions greater than 2 cm in diameter should generally be treated with surgery.

In considering when to treat a given lesion by CE, it is crucial to make an assessment of lesion depth, the character and thickness of the underlying dermis and the lack or abundance of deeply-seated hair follicles. Relatively broad and superficial lesions which are located in areas with thick dermis (particularly the trunk and extremities) are well suited to CE. On the trunk and extremities superficial lesions tend to just wipe off of the thick underlying dermis and are also in general quite well defined on clinical examination. At such sites, the procedure of CE is also much less invasive than a surgical excision, requires minimal wound care effort and leads to a very high cure rate. On the other hand, CE may best be avoided for deeper lesions on the trunk and extremities. The reasons for this are several. First, a deep CE treatment site may take many weeks to heal and often leads to a substantial depression or paradoxically elevated firm scar. Second, it is substantially more difficult to determine the depth of a deep lesion by use of the curette. It has been widely stated that if, during curettage, the curette pokes through to fat the procedure should be abandoned in favor of excision. In fact, one

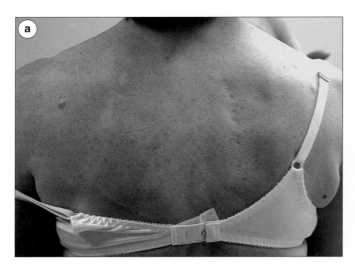

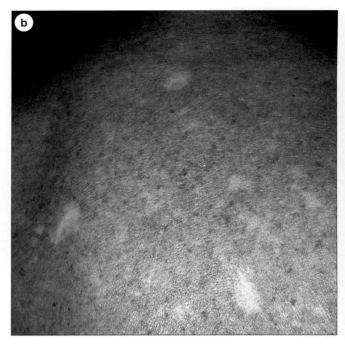

Figure 39.10 Multiple curettage sites at various stages of healing. Note well-healed flat white scars, somewhat newer flat pink scars and several fresh elevated pink scars (scapular regions). Also note long linear repair from much larger infiltrative tumor.

should generally avoid starting curettage when there is any realistic chance of extension into the subcutis. It is not usually difficult to make this decision prior to tumor removal and deep nodular lesions on the trunk and extremities are often best removed by excision.

SCC treated by CE should be well differentiated, only superficially invasive and in general should be located in an area with a thick firm dermis such as the back or proximal extremity. SCC *in situ* is often optimally treated by CE. However, evidence of deep follicular extension on pretreatment biopsy should prompt treatment by excisional means. Not all in situ lesions are alike. Many *in situ* SCC on the balding scalp, forehead, trunk and extremities affect only the interfollicular epithelium and are readily destroyed by CE. On the other hand, SCC *in situ* on the distal nose may burrow far down hair follicles requiring Mohs surgery or at least full thickness excision to effect cure.

For facial NMSC, the decision to treat by CE must always be considered a judgment call. Many authors note that small lesions on the face are amenable to curettage. This clearly is true. However, these lesions are also extremely easy to excise, with minimal impact and a faster healing course since the small wound has been sutured. Nonetheless, CE of selected lesions on the face can be extremely valuable. Very superficial BCC and *in situ* SCC without follicular involvement can simply be peeled from the underlying dermis and are readily cured. Since the depth of curettage in these cases is so minimal, the procedure has an extremely low morbidity.

Some clinicians feel comfortable treating somewhat larger more invasive nodular NMSC by CE. The literature does support this as being within the standard of care so long as the procedure is done within appropriate guidelines as above enumerated. However, as dermatologists become more facile and experienced with surgical excision, they often find themselves utilizing this technique more often than CE. Contrary to the criticisms of some physicians that this is for financial gain, on a minute for minute and expense for expense basis, excision is in fact less productive financially than CE. While excision does have a higher overall cost than CE, the higher cure afforded by a well-planned surgical excision can cut back on the expenditures for future tumor recurrence.

FUTURE OUTLOOK

When treating NMSC, it is our goal to effect a cure rate of at least 90% on the trunk and extremities and a cure rate of 95% on the face. With the increased availability of excision and Mohs surgery and with a true paradigm shift in the treatment of NMSC, we have witnessed a dramatic reduction in the number of recurrences. We continue to utilize the time-honored technique of CE for selected tumors and effect a high cure rate in these cases.

CE will remain a workhorse in practice, where appropriate, for years to come. However, the era of CE as the most utilized primary treatment for NMSC in dermatology may have passed. As dermatology continues to refine and improve upon its surgical skills, the treatment of NMSC will continue to evolve. It will be important to continue to utilize older techniques where valuable. However, it will be equally important to define and recognize the limitations of our older therapies and move forward by incorporating new available treatment modalities.

REFERENCES

1 Sheridan AT, Dawber RPR. Curettage, electrosurgery and skin cancer. Australas J Derm 2000; 41:19–30.

2 Lauritzen RT, Johnson RE, Spratt JS. Pattern of recurrence in basal cell carcinoma. Surgery 1965; 57:813–816.

3 Clark WM. Oscillatory desiccation in the treatment of accessible malignant growths and minor surgical conditions. J Adv Ther 1911; 29:169–183.

4 Pifard HG. Histological contribution. Am J Syph Derm 1870(1):217.

5 Wigglesworth E. The curette in dermal therapeutics. Boston Med Surg J 1876(94):143.

6 Fox GH. Photographic atlas of the diseases of the skin in four volumes. New York: Kettles Publishing Co; 1905:19.

7 Knox JM, Lyles TW, Shapiro EM, et al. Curettage and electrodesiccation in the treatment of skin cancer. Arch Derm 1960; 82:197–203.

8 Knox JM, Freeman RG, Duncan WC, et al. Treatment of skin cancer. South Med J 1967; 60:241–246.

9 Williamson GS, Jackson R. The treatment of basal cell carcinoma by electrodesiccation and curettage. Can Med J 1962; 86:855.

10 Williamson GS, Jackson R. Treatment of squamous cell carcinoma of the skin by electrodesiccation and curettage. Can Med J 1964; 90:408–413.

11 Sweet RD. The treatment of basal cell carcinoma by curettage. Brit J Derm 1963; 75:137–148.

12 Popkin GL. Curettage and electrodesiccation. NY State J Med 1968; 866–868.

13 Whelan CS, Deckers PJ. Electrocoagulation and curettage for carcinoma involving the skin of the face, nose, eyelids and ears. Cancer 1973; 31:159–164.

14 Honeycutt WM, Jansen GT. Treatment of squamous cell carcinoma of the skin. Arch Derm 1973; 108:670–672.

15 Chernosky ME. Squamous cell and basal cell carcinomas: Preliminary study of 3817 primary skin cancers. South Med J 1978; 71:802–803.

16 Reymann F. Treatment of basal cell carcinoma of the skin with curettage. Arch Derm 1971; 103:623–627.

17 Reymann F. Treatment of basal cell carcinoma of the skin with curettage. A follow-up study. Arch Derm 1973; 108:528–531.

18 Reymann F. Multiple basal cell carcinomas of the skin. Treatment with curettage. Arch Derm 1975; 111:877–879.

19 McDaniel WE. Surgical therapy for basal cell epitheliomas by curettage only. Arch Derm 1978; 114:1491–1492.

20 McDaniel WE. Therapy for basal cell epitheliomas by curettage only. Further study. Arch Derm 1983; 119:901–903.

21 Reymann F. 15 years' experience with treatment of basal cell carcinomas of the skin with curettage. Acta Derm 1985; 120:56–59.

22 Sturm HM, Leider M. An editorial on curettage. J Derm Surg Oncol 1979; 5:532–533.

23 Adam JE. The technic of curettage surgery. J Am Acad Derm 1986; 15:697–702.

24 Salasche SJ. Curettage and electrodesiccation in the treatment of midfacial basal cell epithelioma. J Am Acad Derm 1983; 8:496–503.

25 Spiller WF, Spiller RF. Treatment of basal cell epithelioma by curettage and electrodesiccation. J Am Acad Derm 1984; 11:808–814.

26 Crissey JT. Curettage and electrodesiccation as a method of treatment for epitheliomas of the skin. J Surg Oncol 1971; 3:287–290.

27 Kopf AW, Bart RS, Schrager D. Curettage-electrodesiccation treatment of basal cell carcinomas. Arch Derm 1977; 113:439–443.

28 Dubin N, Kopf A. Multivariate risk scores for recurrences of cutaneous basal cell carcinomas. Arch Derm 1983; 119:373–377.

29 Salasche SJ. Status of curettage and electrodesiccation in the treatment of primary basal cell carcinoma. J Am Acad Derm 1984; 10:285–287.

30 Silverman MK, Kopf AW, Grin CM, et al. Recurrence rates of treated basal cell carcinomas. Part 2: Curettage-electrodesiccation. J Derm Surg Oncol 1991; 17:720–726.

31 Freeman RG, Knox JM, Heaton CL. The treatment of skin cancer. Cancer 1964; 17:535–538.

32 Edens BL, Bartlow GA, Haghighi P, et al. Effectiveness of curettage and electrodesiccation in the removal of basal cell carcinoma. J Am Acad Derm 1983; 9:383–388.

33 Suhge d'Aubermont PC, Bennett RG. Failure of curettage and electrodesiccation for removal of basal cell carcinoma. Arch Derm 1984; 120:1456–1460.

34 Spencer JM, Tannenbaum A, Sloan L, et al. Does inflammation contribute to the eradication of basal cell carcinoma following curettage and electrodesiccation? Derm Surg 1997; 23:625–631.

35 Nouri K, Spencer JM, Taylor R, et al. Does wound healing contribute to the eradication of basal cell carcinoma following curettage and electrodesiccation. Derm Surg 1999; 25:183–188.

36 Wagner RF, Cottel WI. Multifocal recurrent basal cell carcinoma following primary treatment by electrodesiccation and curettage. J Am Acad Derm 1987; 17:1047–1049.

37 Jones MS, Maloney ME, Billingsly EM. The heterogeneous nature of in vivo basal cell carcinoma. Derm Surg 1998; 24:881–884.

38 Epstein E. Curettage-electrodesiccation vs surgical excision. Arch Derm 1977; 113:1729.

CHAPTER

40 Cryosurgery

Gloria F Graham and Christopher M Scott

Key points

- Cryosurgery: A century old procedure
- Cryogen of choice: Liquid nitrogen
- Thermocouple monitoring to –50°C
- Fast freeze, slow thaw important
- Cosmetic result generally good
- Cure rate 97–98% for selected lesions.

INTRODUCTION

When choosing definitive treatment for skin tumors, the initial dichotomy exists between excision and local destruction. Many factors, such as the general health of the patient, cost, patient expectations and tumor characteristics, help define the appropriate course of action. The most common technique for ablation of benign skin tumors is cryosurgery. This techique is characterized by the introduction of an element which depresses the temperature of the targeted tissue below its cold-resistance threshold. This modality induces localized frostbite, producing necrosis and tissue destruction. With the introduction of accurate monitoring techniques, cryosurgery has gained further utility in treating malignant skin tumors. Basal cell carcinoma, squamous cell carcinoma, Bowen's disease (squamous cell carcinoma *in situ*), lentigo maligna and Kaposi's sarcoma may be treated by cryosurgery. Cryogen application may be used for palliation in metastatic melanoma. Cryosurgery has been recognized as the treatment of choice for many cutaneous conditions and has supplemented the use of various other modalities, such as excision, curettage, electrosurgery, chemosurgery, laser surgery and radiation therapy. Benefits of cryosurgery include cost effectiveness, good cosmetic results and high cure rates.[1] Cryosurgery seems to fit into the gap where other procedures have shortcomings.

HISTORY

The first recorded application of medical cryogens described Egyptians using cold temperatures for topical anesthesia over 4000 years ago. Palliative treatment of cancerous tumors was first performed by James Arnott in 1855. Arnott used a brine solution as his cryogen, achieving freezing temperatures around –24°C.[2] In the earliest part of the twentieth century, Campbell White used cotton swab application of liquid air to treat various skin conditions, and W.A. Pusey used carbon dioxide to treat acne and nevi.[3,4] In 1907, Whitehouse engineered the first spray device to deliver cryogen.[5] Cryosurgery has been in continuous use since that time. Some 50 years later, H.T. Brodthagen demonstrated the utility of barometer-thermocouple measurements, improving the precision of cryosurgical methods.[6]

In the mid-1960s, modern cutaneous cryosurgery was pioneered by Douglas Torre and Setrag Zacarian. Their cryosurgical innovations facilitated ease of use and effective cryogen delivery. Zacarian designed a method of indirectly administering liquid nitrogen by cooling copper cylinders. Torre developed the first reliable liquid nitrogen spraying system.[7] Later, Zacarian in conjunction with Michael Bryne, engineered a small hand-held device for spraying liquid nitrogen on the skin.[8] These advances enabled cryosurgery to become widely used and recognized as an effective and inexpensive surgical modality.

DESCRIPTION OF PROCEDURE/THERAPY

Physiology of cryosurgery

Heat flows from a warm object to a cold object. Heat can be withdrawn from tissues by placing a cold object onto a warm target. The ability to draw heat from a tissue depends on the target size, composition and temperature difference. Conductivity of cold temperatures is facilitated by formation of an ice-ball. Within the resultant ice-ball, thermal gradients develop which promote tissue freezing. Destructive effects are determined by the rate of temperature fall, the rate of rewarming, solute concentration, the duration of freeze and the coldest temperature reached in the target tissue. These factors are important to consider when treating malignancies, since the goal is complete cryoablation of the target tissue (Fig. 40.1).

The motto 'freeze fast, thaw slow' summarizes the practical elements of cryosurgery. The rate of tissue cooling is one of the most important factors. Rapidly cooling the target tissue produces intracellular ice crystals, where slowly freezing produces extracellular ice crystals. When intracellular water freezes, solutes concentrate within the tissue. Intracellular ice crystals are much more destructive, which is beneficial in treating malignancies.

If frozen tissue is allowed to thaw slowly, solute gradients form within the tissue. These chemical concentrations further damage the target tissue, augmenting the potency of ice crystal formation. Electrolyte concentrations promote recrystallization and grain growth, producing maximum damage to cells.

In treating malignancies, maximum destruction is achieved by generating minimum temperatures of −40° to −60°C as confirmed by electrical impedence.[9] Although capable of achieving this extent of freezing, helium is not readily accessible. The only routinely available cryogen able to accomplish this significant depth of freezing is liquid nitrogen (Table 40.1). Since cryosurgery is a field therapy, surgical precision requires generation of objective end-point criteria. It is critical that depth of freezing and freezing temperature are quantified. One method is thermo-coupling, where the temperature at a given depth may be measured. The standard instrument-aided assessment involves one or more thermocouples attached to a pyrometer (Fig. 40.2). Thermocouple needles may be inserted at the borders or underneath the tumor (Fig. 40.1). Proper placement of thermocouple needles is required (Fig. 40.3–40.6). Therefore, lack of clinical

expertise allows room for error so a clinical standard of adequate treatment cannot be disregarded.

A more common, clinical assessment is the lateral extent of freezing and duration of thaw, primarily devised by Torre.[10] When treating a lesion centrally, the freezing will spread peripherally. An ice halo may be observed around the frozen tumor. The lateral progression of the halo correlates to the freezing depth (Fig. 40.1). In practical terms, a 6 mm diameter spread on the surface roughly indicates freezing depth of 6 mm. Cryosurgery for benign lesions or pre-malignancies should attain a 1–2 mm halo, where a 5 mm halo is more indicative of adequate treatment when freezing malignancies (Fig. 40.4). Large, superficial basal cell carcinomas may require treatment in sections over several applications.

Another measure of success in treating malignancies is halo thaw time (HTT), which should be achieved between 60 and 90 seconds. When HTT is in under 30 seconds, the freeze may not be adequate and will need repeating. If using double-freeze technique, it is important to allow both the halo and the tumor to completely thaw before the second cryogen exposure. It is critical that enough cryogen is delivered, without excess freezing (Table 40.2).

Remember, 'Freeze fast, thaw slow'. Effective cryosurgery will rapidly freeze the tumor and thaw-time will require the longer portion of the procedure.[11]

Equipment

The most elemental components of cryosurgery are the cryogen and the delivery vehicle. In the most basic form, cryosurgery may be performed with liquid nitrogen in a Styrofoam cup and a cotton swab (Fig. 40.7). As discussed earlier, the preferred cryogen is liquid nitrogen due to availability, cost, and its temperature (Table 40.1). Liquid nitrogen is available from most welding supply companies.

Stainless steel probes and spray attachments direct the cryogen appropriately toward the target tissue (Fig. 40.7). Two commonly used spray devices are the hand-held Cry-Ac from Brymill Corporation and the NitroSpray Plus from Premier Medical Products (Fig. 40.5). Many

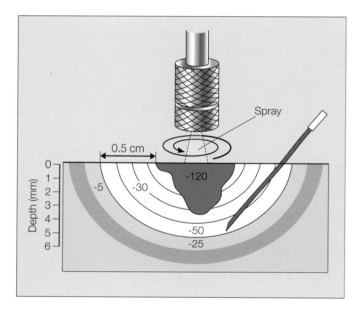

Figure 40.1 Development of isotherms in the cryosurgical site. A halo of 0.5 cm is needed beyond the tumor margins. The ice ball should include the −50°C isotherm and the thermocouple needle should register −50°C. The freeze time is around 1 min and the thaw time 1–1.5 min. The complete thaw is 3–5 min.

Table 40.1	Cryogens historically used in cutaneous surgery
Agent	**Temperature (°C)**
Solid CO_2	−79.0
Liquid N_2O	−88.5
He	−185
Liquid N_2	−195.8

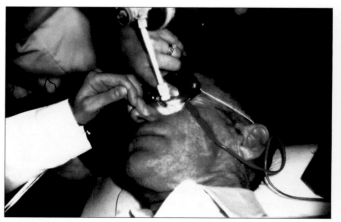

Figure 40.2 Thermocouple needle is inserted beneath the tumor. It is attached to a pyrometer for reading the temperature.

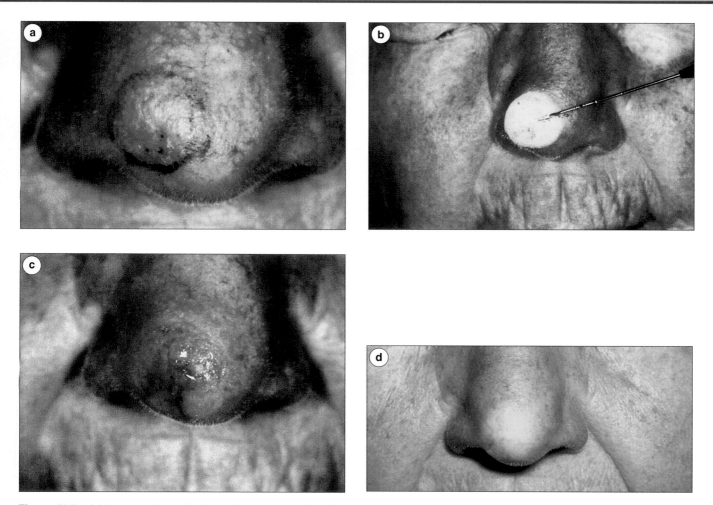

Figure 40.3 (a) A recurrent basal cell carcinoma on the tip of the nose of a 73 year old woman who has multiple health problems. Patient chose to have cryosurgery after careful considerations of her options. (b) Thermocouple needle is implanted to the cartilage and double freeze-thaw cycles to –50°C. Freeze time was about 1 min and halo thaw 1.5 min. (c) Typical edema, erythema and vesiculation is noted a few minutes after freezing. (d) The site is well-healed 21 months after freezing. Hypopigmentation is observed. (Reproduced with permission from Graham GF. Cryosurgery in the management of cutaneous malignancies. Clin Dermatol 2001; 19:321–327.)

types of cryoprobes and spray attachments are currently commercially available (Fig. 40.6).

Insulated cones direct cooling deeper into the target tissue, while sparing lateral tissues. In addition, cones may reduce inadvertent spraying into the eyes, nose, or ears. The cryoplate has conical openings of 5, 8, 10 mm (Fig. 40.7).

Protective equipment, such as eye shields, may be required in sensitive areas. A simple tongue blade or cotton gauze may serve as adequate protection. It is advisable to use a plastic Jaegher retractor when treating tumors on the eyelid margins.

If a malignant lesion is suspected, a preliminary biopsy is recommended. Biopsy is also advisable when the diagnosis is in question. Cryosurgery should be delayed if the diagnosis is in doubt until the biopsy has been examined by a dermatopathologist.

Thermocoupling devices improve efficacy of cryo-surgery for deeper tumors, especially malignancies (Fig. 40.8). Operator skill is important, since needle place-ment will determine accuracy of the monitoring. Inexperience necessitates thermocouple monitoring. In large tumors, multiple needles may be required to accurately assess freezing. Ultrasound use has increased the accuracy of needle placement, since the full depth of the solid tumor may be grossly visualized. Freezing is continued until the needle registers –50°C (Fig. 40.1).

Clinical techniques

Three main methods are used to apply liquid nitrogen: cotton-swab, spray and probe (Fig. 40.7). Using a cotton-swab is sufficient to treat pre-malignant conditions and benign skin tumors, which are superficial. 'Dipstick' techniques freeze only 2–3 mm deep. Cotton swabs may allow virus transmission between patients, since viruses can survive in liquid nitrogen.[12,13] It is recommended that cryogen should be dispensed individually, and discarded after each patient. Very sensitive areas may be accurately targeted with forceps dipped in cryogen, minimizing collateral damage.[14] Once again, the depth of freeze will be limited, precluding use of this technique in treating malignancies.

Spray application of cryogen may be used for all tumors, including malignancies, since depth of penetration is adequate. Cryogen is propelled from a reservoir, through an aperture selected for the target tissue. Liquid nitrogen is delivered directly to the tumor (Fig. 40.3b). Distribution patterns include a direct spray for tumors less than 6 mm, spiral pattern for 5 to 10 mm and a side to side 'paint-brush' pattern for larger or irregularly-shaped lesions. Intermittent spray is more effective than continuous application. An insulating cone may focus the cryogen, resulting in deeper freezing, which is preferred when treating malignancies (Fig. 40.7a). Cones may consist of either neoprene or plastic, but metal cones should be avoided.

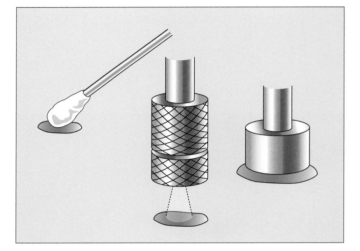

Figure 40.4 Three different freezing methods: cotton swab, spray and probe.

Table 40.2 Approximate freeze times for common benign and malignant lesions[a]	
Lesions	Freeze times (s)
Verruca plana	2–5
Lentigo	2–5
Actinic keratosis	5–10
Molluscum contagiosum	5–10
Sebaceous adenoma	5–10
Seborrheic keratosis	10–15
Verruca vulgaris	10–15
Prurigo nodularis	15–20
Leukoplakia	15–30
Keloid	30
Dermatofibroma	30–45
Basal cell carcinoma	60–120[b]
Squamous cell carcinoma	60–120[b]
Lentigo maligna	60–120[b]

[a]Using Brymill Cry-AC with a B tip. Various factors alter freeze times.
[b]Double freeze if over 3 mm in depth.

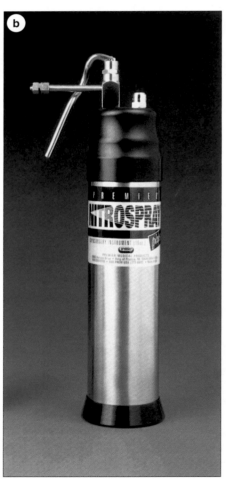

Figure 40.5 (a) (Image courtesy of Brymill Cryogenic Systems, Ellington, CT.) (b) NitroSpray Plus. (Image courtesy of Premier Medical Products, Plymouth Meeting, PA.)

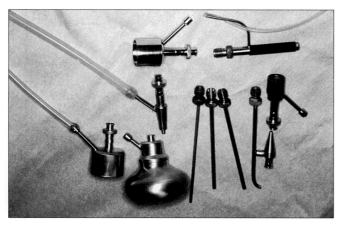

Figure 40.6 Probe and spray attachments. (Reproduced with permission from Wheeland RG, ed: Cutaneous Surgery. Philadelphia: Saunders; 1993.)

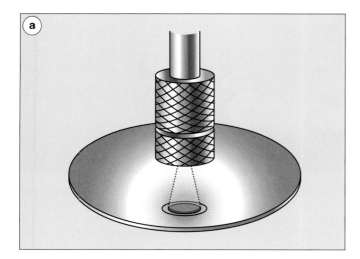

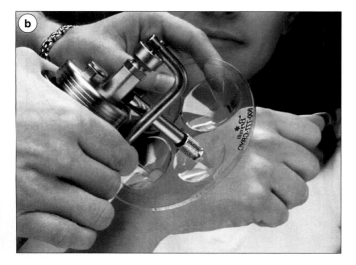

Figure 40.7 (a) Insulated cone will direct spray more precisely on the lesion and decreases spray time by a few seconds. (b) Cryoplate by Brymill Cryogenic Systems has openings of 3, 5, 8 and 10 mm. (Image courtesy of Brymill Cryogenic Systems, Ellington, CT.)

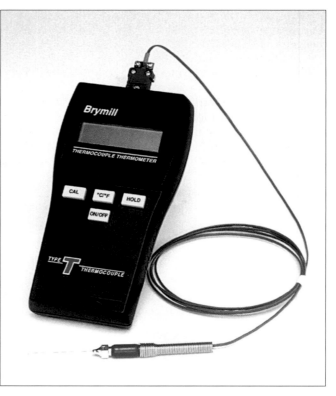

Figure 40.8 Tissue temperature monitor with thermocouple needles. (Image courtesy of Brymill Cryogenic Systems, Ellington, CT.)

Although probe freezing takes more time than cryosurgery with sprays, the probe possesses a deeper depth-of-freeze to lateral spread ratio.[15,16] Probes are cooled by circulating liquid nitrogen through the hollow center, indirectly exposing the target tissue to cryogen. The tumor dictates the probe size and shape to be used.

The most effective technique is double-freeze cryosurgery, preceded by curettage or deep shave excision (Fig. 40.9). Single-freeze treatment is sufficient for actinic keratoses, and tumors 2–3 mm deep; those greater are best treated with two cycles of freezing. The double-freeze, or freeze-thaw-freeze, cryosurgical technique facilitates tumor destruction by direct freezing and by reperfusion injury via inflammatory cytokines. Preliminary debulking of the tumor effectively reduces tumor depth. Cryosurgery may then target lower regions of the initial tumor. In addition, curettage may better elucidate the lateral extent of the tumor (Fig. 40.9c). Another benefit of shaving the tumor is acquisition of a specimen for pathologic evaluation (Fig. 40.9b). Freezing may immediately follow debulking, since re-epithelialization and dermal fibrosis in the healing biopsy site may impair future treatment (Fig. 40.9d).

Local anesthesia is beneficial when treating malignancies. Vasoconstriction caused by anesthetic with epinephrine will lengthen the thaw time, and perhaps result in higher cure rates. Anesthesia should be used in debulking or biopsying the tumor, which may be immediately followed by cryosurgery if the diagnosis is certain.

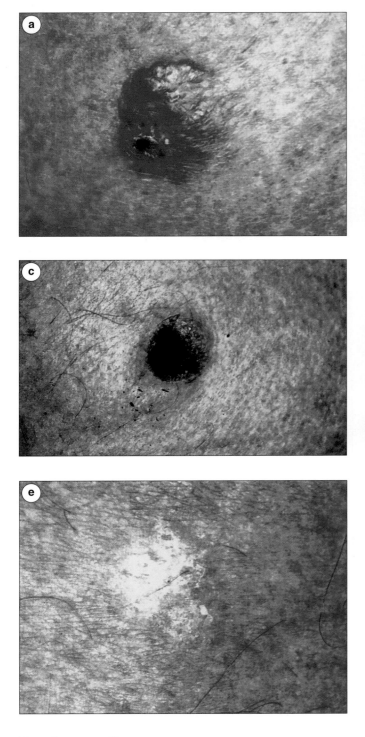

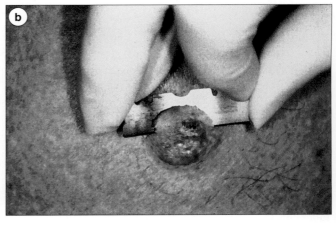

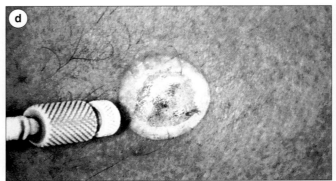

Figure 40.9 (a) Basal cell carcinoma on the back. (b) Tangential shave excision of the exophytic portion of the tumor. (c) Basal cell carcinoma site following shave and curettage. Monsel's solution applied. (d) Freeze until a 0.5 cm halo. (e) Hypopigmentation is noted 1 month later. (Reproduced with permission from Graham GF, Barham K. Cryosurgery. Curr Probl Dermatol, in press.)

Postoperative care

Patients should be instructed to cleanse the surgical site daily with soap and water. After the initial bulla resolves, a natural biologic dressing will remain, reducing the likelihood of infection. The resulting eschar will separate naturally within 3–6 weeks. If trauma causes earlier removal of the eschar, topical antibiotics may be applied.

Cure rates

Overall cure rates for skin cancers treated by cryosurgery are reported in the range of 94–99%.[17–20] As mentioned above, the best cure rates are achieved when curettage or deep shave excision is followed by double-freeze cryosurgery. Treatment of periauricular tumors with combined curettage-cryosurgery was studied by Nordin and Stenquist. Of 100 non-melanoma skin cancers treated, only one tumor exhibited recurrence during 5 years of follow-up.[21] Careful patient selection is critical. Recurrent or histologically very aggressive tumors should be treated with another modality. To maximize cure, it is important to know the limits of cryosurgery before attempting to freeze. Important variables which determine cure rates include appropriate patient selection, experience of the health care provider, cryosurgical modality, single- versus double-freeze techniques, use of monitoring devices, use of cones to direct freezing, and preliminary assessment for tumor depth.

Considering tumors that are responsive to cryosurgery, the most critical variable in determining success is tumor depth. Most tumors, up to 5 mm in depth, are considered in the domain of cryosurgery. Tumor depth dictates the freezing time required. Interestingly, the best cure rates for basal cell carcinomas and squamous cell carcinomas have been observed in large tumors (>24 mm). The superficial nature of large tumors is probably responsible for their high cure rate, which have been reported to be greater than 97.8%. Tumors up to 5 mm diameter showed a 96.6% cure rate, while tumors ranging 6–12 mm exhibit a 97.1% cure rate. The lowest cure rates were associated with tumors 13–24 mm across (94.1% cure rate). New follow-up data has been obtained and further analysis will be published.

INDICATIONS AND CONTRAINDICATIONS

Advantages of cryosurgery

Benefits of cryosurgery include cost effectiveness, good cosmetic results and high cure rates. Tumor selection is important. Cryosurgery is best suited for tumors involving infected sites, tumors of the chest and back, and multiple or superficial tumors. As long as the tumor depth is 4–5 mm, cryosurgery can be quite accurate. Freezing tumors overlying cartilage may be preferable to excision since cartilage is tolerant of freezing. Also, if demonstrating well-defined margins, select tumors of the tip of the nose, eyelid or ear may be treated by cryosurgery (Fig. 40.10). There is preservation of the lacrimal duct, even with freezing to –70°C.

Patient selection is extremely important in any surgical procedure. Quite often, patients who are poor candidates for another surgical modality will be well-suited for cryosurgery (Fig. 40.3). Complex medical patients, such as those with congestive heart failure or kidney disease, may be at poor risk for excisional procedures. Even those who have been heavy smokers heal well following freezing. Patients receiving anticoagulation therapy or with a history of poor wound healing after standard cutaneous surgery do not have increased risk of morbidity with cryosurgery. Cryosurgery has a role in palliation for inoperable lesions. If poor compliance or loss to follow-up is anticipated, cryosurgery is advantageous since minimal postoperative care is required. Follow-up at 3- and 6-month intervals is recommended.

Elderly patients usually tolerate cryosurgery without difficulty. Relatively few complications are associated with cryosurgery.

Contraindications

Cryosurgery is not the preferred treatment modality if the tumor is deeply invasive or fixed to underlying structures. It is strongly recommended that these cases be handled by Mohs micrographic surgery or wide excisional surgery. Mohs surgery is ideal for histologically aggressive tumors, or those in an area of high-risk recurrent carcinoma, if deep to the central area of the original tumor. However, marginal recurrences may be treated with cryosurgery.

Patients with tumors such as large morpheaform basal cell carcinoma, metatypical basal cell carcinoma, and *de novo* squamous cell carcinoma are not ideal cryosurgical candidates. Morpheaform basal cell carcinoma has a fibrous component that limits adequate curettage. Each of these tumors responds to freezing when smaller than 2 cm, but Mohs surgery is the preferred technique for the larger tumors.

Indefinite margins are considered a contraindication to cryosurgery. However, some tumor margins may be delineated by careful curettage.

If large areas are to be treated, cryosurgery should not be used in patients with severe cold-intolerance, such as Raynaud's syndrome, cryoglobulinemia and cryofibrinogenemia. Excision is the preferred treatment of melanoma. However, freezing is very effective in lentigo maligna, especially for larger lesions in elderly patients.

Tumor site also determines the utility versus potential harm of cryosurgery. Since a common side-effect of cryosurgery is alopecia, tumors on the scalp may be best treated by excision. Extreme care should be taken when freezing tumors on the eyelid, but this site may be treated with cryosurgery. There are numerous published studies of the effectiveness of freezing eyelid and periocular tumors with well-defined margins.

SIDE-EFFECTS AND COMPLICATIONS

While cryosurgery is considered quite safe, several well-defined complications have been linked to cutaneous freezing. In many instances, complications are extensions or accentuations of normal physiologic events. Knowledge of these effects serves not only to assure that cryosurgical procedures proceed correctly, but is also necessary to be able to interpret complications from normal expectations.

Immediate clinical effects

After cryosurgery, it is common to acutely experience pain and edema. Less common immediate effects include hemorrhage, nitrogen gas insufflation and syncope.

Within a few minutes, erythema and urtication are observed (Fig. 40.3c), followed by edema. If freezing is superficial, vesicles or bullae develop. Deeper freezing, as used in treatment of malignancies, may not elicit bullae formation. Stromal elements are more resistant to freezing than cellular elements.

While freezing benign and pre-cancerous lesions is relatively painless, malignancies require deeper freezing, resulting in more intense discomfort. A burning sensation may be experienced during treatment, exaggerated during the thaw period. Immediate intense pain usually remits after the first 20–30 min. Since treatment of cutaneous malignancies may be augmented by initially debulking the tumor, local anesthetic is often used prior

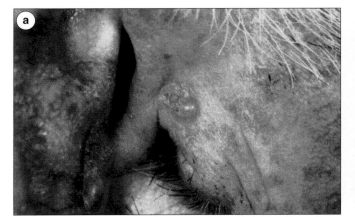

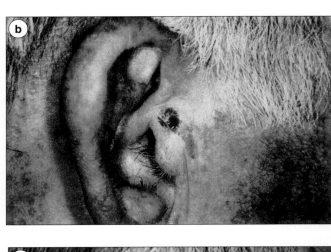

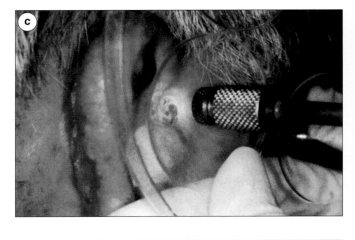

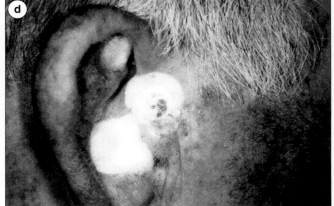

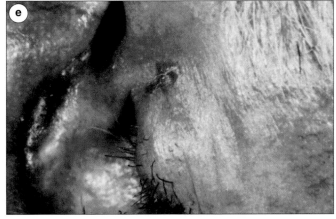

Figure 40.10 (a) Well-defined basal cell carcinoma in the preaurical area in a 66-year-old man. (b) After shave and curettage. (c) Cone surrounds tumor and cotton protects ear canal. (d) Double freeze thaw cycles used of about 1 min each. Halo thaw time was 4 min and complete thaw over 5 min. (e) Pseudoepitheliomatous hyperplasia noted at 1 month and cleared by 3 months. (Reproduced with permission from Graham GF. Cryosurgery in the management of cutaneous malignancies. Clin Dermatol 2001; 19:321–327.)

to incision and cryosurgery. It is advisable to pre-treat these patients with acetaminophen or aspirin, continuing analgesic use up to 24–48 hrs postoperatively. Be aware that mucous membranes, the forehead, temporal areas, distal fingers and distal nose are more susceptible to pain. A migraine-type headache may result from freezing preauricular tumors, as well as lesions involving the forehead or temples.

Edema is observed after almost every cryosurgery (Fig. 40.3c). The patient's normal response to cold temperatures, the duration of cryogen application, the cryosurgical modality and the location of the lesion, may help predict the severity of resultant edema. Swelling may persist for 5–7 days. Edema is more pronounced after freezing loose skin, such as periorbital tumors, the forehead, the

mandibular area and around the ears. Periorbital edema may be prolonged, up to 5 days, but systemic steroids tend to suppress this edema. However, delayed wound healing may result from steroid use.[22] Cold water compresses are sufficient for symptomatic relief.

Hemorrhage may occur if a biopsy is performed in conjunction with freezing. Ulcerated or edematous tumors also may bleed after cryogen delivery. Therefore, adequate hemostasis prior to cryosurgery is important. Aluminum chloride or electrosurgery provides improved hemostasis after debulking malignancies or biopsy acquisition. Anti-inflammatory drugs, which inhibit cyclo-oxygenase, increase the likelihood of acute hemorrhage, but rarely necessitate drug discontinuation. If incidentally frozen, large blood vessels would rarely rupture.

Frozen tissues may also be traumatized by withdrawing the adherent probe tip from the cryosurgical site. This risk is diminished by preliminary application of lubricating jelly to the probe tip or by pre-chilling the probe.

When cryogen spray enters an opening in the skin surface, the surgical site may immediately distend as gas separates tissue planes. *Nitrogen gas insufflation* is a rare occurrence. Biopsy predisposes the patient to insufflation. Loose tissues, such as the periorbital area and the dorsal hand, can facilitate this complication. The site should be manipulated, expelling nitrogen gas from the wound manually. If the surgical site involves a natural or created skin opening, risk of insufflation is minimized by utilizing pressure rings, or a cone placed with moderate pressure. It may be advisable to use the cryo-probe (Fig. 40.4), rather than spray, after biopsy or tumor debulking. Swelling resolves spontaneously within a few hours, up to 24 hrs.

Syncope may occur during or immediately after cryosurgery. Special consideration should be given to elderly patients or when freezing is especially uncomfortable. Patients should remain seated or supine postoperatively. Cryosurgical syncope is likely a vasovagal response. Deeper freezing may cause more intense pain, increasing the probability of a vasovagal reaction. Local anesthesia is more often used in these instances. Place these patients in a supine or Trendelenburg's position for recovery.

Short-term reactions

In the days and weeks following cryosurgery, the surgical site continues to change. It may be difficult to distinguish between normal evolution and pathologic conditions. Changes to the frozen tissue may include bullae formation, infection, hemorrhage, appearance of pyogenic granuloma and systemic reactions.

Superficial cryogen application causes *bullae formation* by separation of the dermo-epidermal junction. Bullae indicate successful treatment of superficial epidermal lesions. Since malignancies require deeper freezing, it is less likely that a vesiculobullous reaction will occur. If painful due to large size or hemorrhage, a bulla may require evacuation. Otherwise, bullae resolve spontaneously and serve as a sterile dressing. Topical anti-biotics may be indicated after penetrating the barrier to infection.

Thick crusts and delayed wound healing promote *infection*. Venous stasis or diabetes mellitus are associated with poor wound healing, so lower extremity cryosurgery should be cautiously approached in these patients. If immunocompromised or at high risk for infections, prophylactic systemic antibiotics may be indicated. Most patients only require antibiotics if symptomatic. Culture may be required to discern whether fluid accumulation is due to normal exudation or infection. Topical antibiotic ointments may also be used if bullae or eschar is inadvertently removed.

As the tissue at the surgical site evolves, necrosis may lead to *hemorrhage* on rare occasions. The friable, damaged tumor may have an underlying persistent vascular supply or vascular infiltration that is revealed as the mass breaks away. Application of manual pressure to the surgical site for several minutes is usually adequate to achieve hemostasis. A pressure dressing or suture may be required in extreme cases.

Pyogenic granulomas, which are benign vascular tumors, occasionally arise at cryosurgical sites, several weeks postoperatively. This tumor has been described after combined cryoablation and salicylic acid treatment of verruca vulgaris[23] and with cryosurgery alone.[24] In addition, this uncommon complication was noted to appear after cryogen was applied to a venous lake.[25] Treatment is required to promote site healing. Either electrodesiccation and curettage, application of aluminum chloride, or curettage and silver nitrate therapy should adequately treat the pyogenic granuloma.

If the patient receives cryogen applied to an especially large lesion or multiple treatments during one session, there is an increased risk of developing a *systemic, febrile reaction* within a few hours. The patient may experience flu-like symptoms or a fever, which usually resolves within 24 hrs. Antipyretics may be used for relief.

Long-term reactions

After the surgical site has healed, several reactions may affect the patient's view of treatment success. Pigmentation changes are very common and should be considered in all patients. Concerns regarding alopecia or scar formation may dictate body areas where another treatment modality should be considered. Other less common side effects of cryosurgery include pseudo-epitheliomatous hyperplasia, milia, and nerve damage.

Both *hyperpigmentation* and *hypopigmentation* may be caused by cryosurgery (Fig. 40.3d). Pigment changes at the surgical site are frequently described as central hypopigmentation with peripheral hyperpigmentation. Post-inflammatory hyperpigmentation usually resolves over time, but may persist more than 12 months. Metal cones should not be used since they promote peripheral hyperpigmentation.

Melanocytes are more sensitive to cold temperatures than keratinocytes. Pigment-producing cells do not survive below −4 to −7°C.[26] Treatment of malignant tumors demands freezing of tissues to −40 to −60°C. Therefore, some degree of hypopigmentation is observed universally in cryosurgery for cutaneous malignancies. Patients should be advised of likely pigment changes, especially dark-skinned individuals, or patients with freckles or telangiectasias involved in the cryosurgical site. The distal nose, the trunk, and the helix are regions that demonstrate a greater predilection toward hypopigmentation. Pigment will advance from the periphery and areas within the surgical site, including hair follicles. However, hypopigmentation may be permanent (Fig. 40.3d). Malignancies require freezing for more than 30 seconds and several deep freeze-thaw cycles. Better cosmetic results may be appreciated with multiple brief freeze-thaw applications.[27] These are not sufficient for cancer therapy. Be aware that brief treatments do not eliminate the possibility of local hypopigmentation, which may even be observed with freezing times of 5–10 seconds.

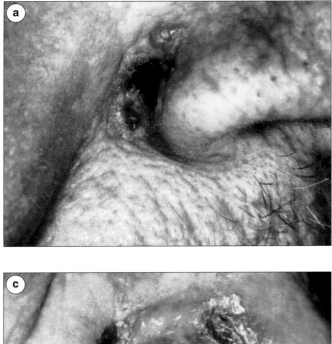

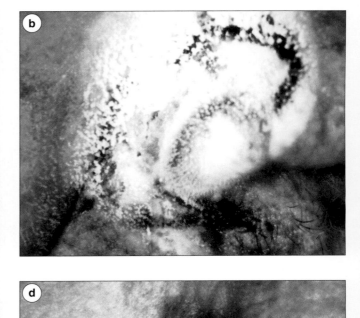

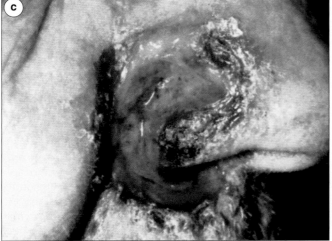

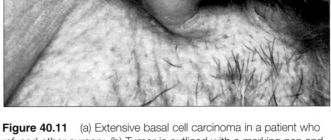

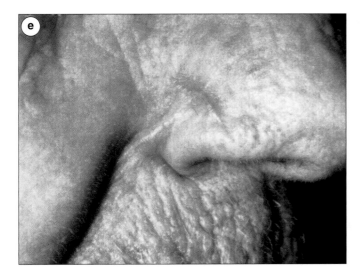

Figure 40.11 (a) Extensive basal cell carcinoma in a patient who refused other surgery. (b) Tumor is outlined with a marking pen and frozen for 1 min using a circular pattern until 5 mm halo is obtained. A double freeze thaw-cycle is used. (c) Extensive exudative reaction noted one week later. Soap and water used for cleansing the area. (d) At 1 month, there is some pseudoepitheliomatous hyperplasia. (e) Approximately 6 months later, the site is well-healed.

Pseudoepitheliomatous hyperplasia is an inflammatory reaction, which is difficult to distinguish from a persistent neoplasm (Fig. 40.11d). It represents a self-limited reaction that follows cryosurgery after 3–6 weeks. The hyperplasia mimics tumor recurrence, but no treatment is required since improvement is usually noted within 3 months.

Milia, or subepidermal keratin cysts, may be transiently observed after cryosurgery for malignancies. Since the cone spray technique directs deeper freezing, cone use has been reported to promote milia formation.[28] Milia develop around the periphery of the lesion, after the surgical site has healed. These cysts may be simply unroofed. Patients may be concerned about recurrence of the primary tumor, so reassurance should be conveyed to the patient.

Superficial nerves may be affected during cryosurgery. Unmyelinated nerves, or c fibers, are most often affected. Permanent nerve dysfunction is rare, especially regarding indirect cooling from cutaneous cryosurgery. However, permanent neural loss has been reported. Most often, sensation is depressed temporarily and returns to normal or near-normal after several months. Extra care should be taken when treating pre- and post-auricular areas, fingers, lateral regions of the tongue, and the ulnar fossa since nerves are more superficial in these locations. As long as the neural sheath is not damaged extensively, the neural function may be spared. When treating cutaneous tumors with known underlying nerves such as the ulnar fossa, either manipulate loose skin to isolate the cryosurgical field from subcutaneous nerves, or inject local anesthetic or saline beneath the target tissue to elevate the cryosurgical field. The latter described technique is called 'ballooning'.

Any hair-bearing region is susceptible to *alopecia* if cryogen destroys the hair follicles. Fifteen to 20 seconds of treatment may lead to local permanent alopecia. Malignancies require >30 seconds of freezing and the tumor may extend into the hair follicle. Therefore, local hair loss is a common complication of treating cutaneous malignancies. The likelihood of hair loss may prompt the patient to consider an alternative therapy.

As freezing depth increases, the risk of *scar formation* increases. Some atrophy will be observed in the healed cryosurgical site. Over-treating a cutaneous tumor destroys the dermal fibrous network, resulting in greater atrophy and less desirable cosmetic results. It is critical that the extent of freezing is appropriately monitored, whether by time or thermo-coupling devices. Also, regions, such as helix of the ear and the rim of the ala nasi, are more sensitive to cryosurgery and demonstrate an increased tendency toward atrophy.

Malignancies frequently occur over nasal and otic cartilage (Fig. 40.10a). Cartilage necrosis, notching, and perforation may be caused by full-thickness freezing. Perforation is rare and resulted in one case when a basal cell carcinoma was treated on the anterior pinna and a squamous cell carcinoma was frozen on the opposing posterior pinna. This treatment was performed at the patient's insistence that they be done concomitantly. Nonetheless, this patient was satisfied with the therapeutic outcome and demonstrated no recurrence over many years of follow-up.

A central, linear scar within the cryosurgical site may represent *hypertrophic scarring*. This cosmetic complication develops four to six weeks post-surgery. Hypertrophic scaring occurs more often on the back, chest, side of the nose and upper lip. These scars improve with time, so treatment is rarely required. Intralesional steroid injections may be considered if still present after 6–9 months.

FUTURE OUTLOOK

Cryosurgery has a century-long record of successful use in treating skin cancer. With the development of superior instruments that preserve and apply liquid nitrogen for a day, the use of cryosurgery has spread worldwide. Measuring tumor depth with ultrasound allows for better placement of the thermocouple needle and is an asset to those surgeons who have this available.

The perfect procedure to effectively treat skin cancer has not yet been developed. The use of imiquimod and other similar topicals may prove to fill the niche for the more superficial tumors, and Mohs surgery is undoubtedly the best technique for ill-defined, deep and aggressive tumors. However, general dermatologists and some well-trained primary care physicians will continue to care for the remainder of the skin cancers, quite often using cryosurgery due to its remarkable safety and efficacy profile. Until the perfect cure for skin cancer is found, cryosurgery will remain a treatment that fits into a niche between topical therapies of the future and proven excisional techniques, as it is used to effectively and inexpensively treat tumors.

Kuflik's recently published cure rates in 4406 new and recurrent basal and squamous carcinomas in 2932 patients showed an overall 30-year cure rate of 98.6%.[29] He also reported a 5-year cure rate of 99%. These along with other series show a high cure rate for cryosurgery and confirm its usefulness in the management of skin cancers.

REFERENCES

1 Graham GF. Chair's summary: Cryosurgery. Dermatology: Progress and Perspectives, 18th World Congress of Dermatology, New York, 12–18 June 1992.

2 Arnott J. On the treatment of cancers by regulated application of an anaesthetic temperature. Edinburgh, UK: Churchill Livingstone; 1955.

3 White AC. Liquid air in medicine and surgery. Med Rec 56 1899:109–112.

4 Pusey WA. The use of carbon dioxide snow in the treatment of nevi and other lesions of the skin. JAMA 1907; 49:1354–1356.

5 Whitehouse HH. Liquid air in dermatology: its indications and limitations. JAMA 1907; 49:371–377.

6 Brodthagen HT. Local freezing of the skin by carbon dioxide snow. Acta Derm Venereol 1961; 41:9.

7 Torre D. Cradle of cryosurgery. NY State J Med 1967; 67:465–467.

8 Zacarian SA. Cryogenics: The cryolesion and the pathogenesis of cryonecrosis. In: Zacarian SA, ed. Cryosurgery for Skin Cancer and Cutaneous Disorders. St. Louis: CV Mosby; 1985:2–3.

9 Le Pivert P. Predictability of cryonecrosis by tissue impedancemetry. Low Temp Med 1977; 4:129–138.

10 Torre D. Cryosurgical instrumentation and depth dose monitoring. In: Breitbart E, Dachow-Siwiec E, eds. Clinics in Dermatology: Advances in Cryosurgery. New York, NY: Elsevier Science; 1990:59.

11 Torre D. Cryosurgery of basal cell carcinoma. J Am Acad Dermatol 1986; 15:917–929.

12 Burke WA, Baden TJ, Wheeler CE, Bowdre JH. Survival of herpes simplex virus during cryosurgery with liquid nitrogen. J Derm Surg Oncol 1986; 12(10):1033–1035.

13 Jones SK, Darville JM. Transmission of virus by cryotherapy and multi-use caustic pencils: a problem for dermatologists? Br J Derm 1989; 12:481–486.

14 Biro L. Pediatric cryosurgery. Syllabus for basic cryosurgery course. Evanston, IL: American Academy of Dermatology; 1990:21.

15 Grimmett R. Liquid nitrogen therapy: histologic observations. Arch Derm 1961; 83:563–567.

16 Torre D, Lubritz RR, Kuflik EG. Cryobiology. In: Torre D, Lubritz RR, Kuflik EG, eds. Practical Cutaneous Cryosurgery. Norwalk, CT: Appleton and Lange; 1988:17.

17 Graham GF, Clark LC. Statistical update in cryosurgery for cancers of the skin. In: Zacarian SA, ed. Cryosurgery for Skin Cancer and Cutaneous Disorders. St. Louis: CV Mosby; 1985:298–305.

18 Graham GF, Clark LC. Statistical analysis in cryosurgery of skin cancer. In: Breitbart E, Dachow-Siwiec E, eds. Clinics in Dermatology. Advances in Cryosurgery. New York, NY: Elsevier Science; 1990:101–107.

19 Kuflik EG, Gage AA. The five-year cure rate achieved by cryosurgery for skin cancer. J Am Acad Dermatol 1991; 24:1002–1004.

20 Holt PSA. Cryotherapy for skin cancer: results over a five-year period using liquid nitrogen spray. Cryosurgery 1988; 119:231–240.

21 Nordin P, Stenquist B. Five-year results of curettage-cryosurgery for 100 consecutive auricular non-melanoma skin cancers. J Laryngol Otol 2002; 116:893–898.

22 Kuflik EG, Webb W. Effects of systemic corticosteroids on post-surgical edema and other manifestations of the inflammatory response. J Dermatol Surg Oncol 1985; 11:464.

23 Kolbusz RV, O'Donoghue MN. Pyogenic granuloma following treatment of verruca vulgaris with cryotherapy and Duoplant. Cutis 1991; 47:204.

24 Greer KE, Bishop GE. Pyogenic granuloma as a complication of cutaneous cryosurgery. Arch Derm 1975; 111:1536–1537.

25 Cecchi R, Giomi A. Pyogenic granuloma as a complication of cryosurgery for venous lake. Br J Derm 1999; 140(2):373–374.

26 Gage AA, Meenaghan MA, Natiella JR, Greene GW Jr. Sensitivity of pigmented mucosa and skin to freezing injury. Cryobiology 1979; 16(4):348–361.

27 Lubritz RR. Cryosurgical approach to benign and precancerous tumors of the skin. In: Zacarian SA, ed. Cryosurgery for Skin Cancer and Cutaneous Disorders. St. Louis: Mosby; 1985:44–48.

28 Zacarian SA. Cryosurgery for cancer of the skin. In: Zacarian SA, ed. Cryosurgery for Skin Cancer and Cutaneous Disorders. St. Louis: CV Mosby; 1985:96–162.

29 Kuflik EG. Cryosurgery for skin cancer: 30-year experience and cure rates. Dermatol Surg 2004; 30:297–300.

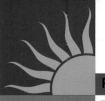

CHAPTER
41

Immune Response Modulators in the Treatment of Skin Cancer

Brian Berman and Adriana M Villa

Key points

- Interferons have antiproliferative, antiangiogenic and immunomodulatory properties that can be used to treat skin cancer including malignant melanoma, Kaposi's sarcoma, basal cell carcinoma and cutaneous T-cell lymphoma (CTCL).
- An immune response modifier stimulates both innate and acquired immune responses, including induction of interferons, interleukin-12 (IL-12), and tumor necrosis factor-α (TNF-α).
- A topical immune response modifier (Imiquimod) is now being used for the treatment of actinic keratoses, superficial basal cell carcinoma and lentigo maligna.
- Interleukin-2 is being used in clinical trials as an adjuvant therapy for metastatic melanoma and advanced CTCL.
- Other immune-related medical agents are being investigated for their potential efficacy in skin cancer therapy.

Table 41.1 Antitumor mechanisms of the immune system

Effector T cells: Recognize an antigen presented in the context of class I and II major histocompatibility complex (MHC) molecules.
Natural killer (NK) cells: Lyse tumor cells in a non-MHC-restricted manner.
Tumor-associated macrophages: Stimulate CD4+ helper cells at the tumor site by expressing high levels of MHC class II antigens. Tumor killing mechanisms include secretion of cytotoxic cytokines, such as tumor necrosis factor-alpha (TNF-alpha) interleukin-1 (IL-1), nitric oxide, proteases and reactive oxygen intermediates.
Co-stimulatory signals after antigen-specific stimulation: B7-1 and B7-2 are capable of stimulating T-cell growth.
Cytokines: Interleukin-2 (IL-2) activates NK cells. Interleukin-12 (IL-12) stimulates Th1 responses, exerting a direct effect on T cells, inducing interferon-gamma (IFN-gamma) production by NK cells, and augmenting the cytotoxic capacity of both NK and cytotoxic T cells. Interferons have antiproliferative and immunomodulatory properties.
Apoptosis is a key factor in keratinocyte homeostasis.

INTRODUCTION

The immune system possesses different effective mechanisms responsible for the surveillance, detection and elimination of cancer cells (Table 41.1). The importance of this role is appreciated *in vivo* by the generation of *de novo* skin cancer after long-term immunosuppression following transplantation. Immuno-suppression in these patients is associated with a dramatically increased risk of malignancy, most frequently non-Hodgkin's lymphoma and skin cancer. Approximately 40% of transplant recipients experience pre-malignant skin tumors and squamous and basal cell carcinomas within the first 5 years of suppressive therapy.[1] On the other hand, cancer does not present solely in immunocompromised hosts, implying that tumor cells somehow manage to escape from this immune surveillance. The possible mechanisms implicated in tumoral evasion from the immune system are listed in Table 41.2.[2–5]

Based on the importance of the role that the immune system has in controlling the growth and metastatic spread of tumors, immunotherapy has been used in the past decades as a tool in the treatment of cancer. Surgery is the cornerstone of therapy for melanoma and non-melanoma skin cancer. However, in patients with multiple or extensive lesions, tumors in critical locations, or with certain genodermatoses or immunosuppressed states, surgical treatment may not be the first option. Immunotherapy is a promising modality for the treatment of skin cancer in immunocompetent, immuno-compromised and immunosuppressed patients.

Historically, interferons were the first immunotherapy used in the treatment of cancer. Currently, therapeutic interventions to augment tumor antigenicity or increase the host's immune response against cancer cells include recombinant cytokines, immune modulators, vaccination with tumor antigens, T-cell-based immunotherapy and gene therapy. This chapter focuses on the use of immune modulators in the therapy of skin cancer. The role of retinoids, which have been suggested to possess immunomodulatory activities in the prophylaxis and treatment of cutaneous cancers is addressed elsewhere in this text.

Table 41.2 Tumoral evasion of the immune system

Secondary to tumor activity

Tumor antigens may be weakly expressed, may be recognized as 'self' antigens, or mutate.

MHC class I (or II in the case of melanoma), may not be expressed by tumor cells.

Tumor cells can secrete immune effector suppressors.

Tumor-induced immunosuppression over lymphocytes: recent studies imply that reactive oxygen species, produced by tumor-infiltrating monocyte/macrophages, may contribute to the state of lymphocyte inhibition in neoplastic tissue.[2]

Resistance of cancer cells to lysis mediated by homologous complement.[3]

Release of transforming growth factor-B1 (TGF-B1) can reduce dendritic cell (DC) migration and reduce their ability to mature into potent antigen presenting cells (APC).[4]

Expression of Fas ligand molecules on tumor cells interacting with Fas receptors on T cells, resulting in T-cell death.[5]

Secondary to faulty immune system

Lack of tumor-reactive T cells.

Incomplete antigen processing.

Interleukin-10 (IL-10) may contribute to the development of skin squamous cell carcinomas after renal transplantation.[6]

INTERFERONS

Introduction

Interferons (IFNs) are a family of naturally occurring glycoproteins that have antiproliferative, antiviral and immunomodulatory properties. These properties, along with their availability in sufficient quantities utilizing recombinant DNA techniques, have favored their use in different clinical disorders, including skin cancer. Depending upon cellular source and mode of induction, human cells produce three antigenically distinct forms of human IFNs, originally described as leukocyte (α), fibroblast (β), and immune (γ).

Mechanism of action

In order to be active, IFN requires binding to specific receptors on the surface of target cells. The intracellular events following receptor binding leading to gene expression are unclear.

The main mechanisms involved in the ability of IFNs to treat skin cancer successfully are (Fig. 41.1):

- Anti-proliferative effects: IFNs affect all phases of the cell cycle. The mechanisms may involve IFN

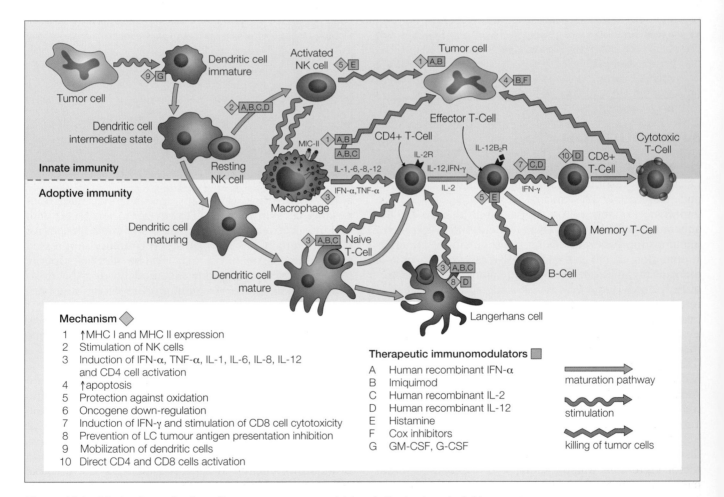

Figure 41.1   Mechanisms of action of immune response modulators in the treatment of skin cancer.

induction of 2′–5′A synthetase with its products, inhibiting mitosis and growth factors, the down-regulation of c-myc, c-fos and certain c-ras oncogenes, as well as IFNs' ability to induce expression of *p53* tumor suppressor gene and to enhance apoptosis.

- Up-regulation of skin immune system: IFN-α and IFN-β are generally less potent stimulators of major histocompatibility complex (MHC) antigens required for cellular immune reactions when compared with IFN-γ. IFNs-α and -β are capable of enhancing/inducing the expression of class I and/or II (MHC) antigens on immunocompetent cells and tumor cells. There is an increase in natural killer (NK) cell numbers and activity following exposure to IFN, also leading to an enhanced immune status.

Indications

Melanoma

The use of IFN-α2b for the treatment of patients with high-risk melanoma is FDA-approved. This includes patients with melanomas thicker than 4 mm and patients with lymph node metastasis. Statistically significant increases in the median overall survival by 1.04 and 1.6 years in IFN-α2b-treated patients with stage I and II melanoma versus controls were found in two studies.[7,8] The greatest patient response was achieved in those patients with nodal disease. The overall 5-year survival in stage IIIb melanoma patients treated with IFN-α2b was 62 *vs* 36% non-treated patients.[9] In patients with disease limited to the skin and lymph nodes, the combination of isotretinoin and IFN-α has been useful (5 of 20 patients with a partial to complete response). The results of this study also supported the use of high dose IFN-α2b for patients at high risk of recurrence.[10] IFN-α2b therapy is appropriate for patients with regional nodal and/or in-transit metastasis and for node-negative patients with primary melanomas deeper than 4 mm.[11] Overall, the use of IFN as a single agent in metastatic malignant melanoma is useful in a minority of cases. In general, the combined use of IFN and chemotherapeutic agents such as dacarbazine and vindesine are the most effective regimens.[12]

Intralesional IFN-α has been used in the therapy of metastasis of advanced malignant melanoma. Fifty-one evaluable patients with histologically proven metastasic melanoma and at least one skin metastasis were treated intralesionally with IFN-α in two different protocols. Twenty-six of the patients were given highly purified natural IFN-α at 6 million international units (IU) three times per week. Twenty-five patients were given 10 million IU of recombinant IFN-α2b three times per week. Three of 51 patients showed a complete response (disappearance of all lesions of disease for at least 1 month) and six of 51 had a partial response (decrease for at least 1 month of more than 50% of the sum of diameters of all measurable lesions). In seven patients, tumor regression was apparent after 1 month of treatment. Partial remissions lasted between 2 and 6 months. The authors suggested that in order to take advantage of both the local and systemic effects of IFN-α therapy in melanoma, local therapy should be seriously considered

after resection of the primary tumor or regional lymph nodes.[13]

Eleven biopsy-proven cases of lentigo maligna (LM) in 10 patients were treated with perilesional and intralesional interferon α2b. Four cases had relapsed after surgery. The dose injected three times a week was 3 million IU for LM lesions that were 25 mm in diameter or smaller, and 6 million IU for LM lesions larger than 25 mm. The 11 LM lesions cleared after treatment without scarring. These results are satisfactory and warrant the need for controlled trials to establish efficacy and protocols for the use of IFN-α2b as a treatment for LM in selected cases when surgery is not an option.[14]

Kaposi's sarcoma

The use of IFN-α2a and IFN-α2b in the treatment of Kaposi's sarcoma (KS) in patients with acquired immune deficiency syndrome (KS/AIDS) due to human immunodeficiency virus is FDA approved.

The overall objective response rates with IFN-α2a and IFN-α2b equaled or surpassed those achieved with conventional cytotoxic chemotherapy. The recommended dosages of IFNs-α2a and 2b are 36 and 30 million IU subcutaneously respectively, three times a week. The average response rate of KS to high dose IFN-α therapy has been approximately 30%. In many cases, tumor recurrence occurs within 6 months in complete responders and the response to a second treatment is not reliable. These facts led to a current recommendation of maintenance treatment as long as adverse effects are tolerated.[15]

Basal cell carcinoma

Available recommended forms of treatment for basal cell carcinoma (BCC) include curettage and cautery, excision and cryosurgery. Buechner reported complete cure of nodular BCC when given at low doses (1.5 million IU IFN-α) three times weekly for 4 weeks in four patients.[16] The most recent results of a multicenter, placebo-controlled, randomized study of 172 patients with biopsy-proven BCC, confirmed the findings of earlier pilot studies that the optimal intralesional dose of IFN-α2b was 1.5 million IU, administered three times weekly for 3 weeks (Fig. 41.2). This IFN regimen resulted in an 86% complete response rate including no histologic evidence of residual BCC, compared with a 29% rate in the placebo group ($P<0.0001$). Nodular and superficial basal cell carcinomas were treated at the same dose, but for 3 weeks.[17] Similar doses, however, when used for aggressive (recurrent or morpheaform) BCC resulted in a complete cure in only 27% of patients.[18]

Intralesional IFN-α used over a 3-week period has had an overall success rate in most clinical trials between 70 and 100%, which is lower than the cure rate of primary surgical excision (95%) or cryosurgery (94 to 99%).[19] Based on these results, IFN treatment of BCCs can be regarded as an alternative to surgery in a number of selected cases of patients with nodular or superficial BCCs. Current guidelines for the management of basal cell carcinoma do not include interferon therapy, as this modality of treatment for BCC is considered expensive and time consuming. It would most likely constitute a non-surgical alternative in special individual low-risk cases.

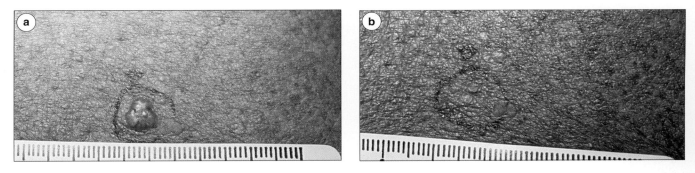

Figure 41.2 IL Interferon-α2b for BCC (1.5 × 10⁶ IU in 0.15 ml, 3 times/week for 3 weeks).

Squamous cell carcinoma

Squamous cell carcinoma (SCC) of skin constitutes 10–25% of non-melanoma skin cancers. The standard of treatment for this type of skin cancer is surgical excision or Mohs' surgery. IFN-α2b was used in the treatment of 34 biopsy proven SCC, localized in sun-exposed areas. The protocol used was 1.5 million IU of intralesional IFN-α2b three times weekly for 3 weeks. At the end of the study, 33 of 34 lesions revealed histologic absence of squamous cell carcinoma.[20] Another study evaluated the effectiveness and cosmetic results of intralesionally administered recombinant IFN-α2b in 27 invasive, and seven *in situ* SCCs (size from 0.5 to 2.0 cm in the longest dimension) at a dose of 1.5 million IU, three times a week for 3 weeks.[21] Over 97% of the SCCs were cured both clinically and histologically at 18 weeks, with a 96.2% cure rate of the 27 invasive lesions. The investigators and patients independently judged 93.9% of the cases to have a 'very good' or 'excellent' cosmetic result. IFN-α2b may be considered for special low risk cases of SCC in which surgery is not an option.

Keratoacanthoma

Keratoacanthomas are considered precancerous conditions and whether or not they are low grade SCCs is unclear. Grob and co-workers reported regression in five out of six large keratoacanthomas (greater than 2 cm in diameter) treated with intralesional IFN-α2a, 9–20 injections per patient with total resolution in 4–7 weeks.[22] Avoidance of scarring following surgery is a positive consequence from the use of IFN in this condition, but the number of injections and patient visits may discourage its use as an alternative treatment.

Cutaneous T-cell lymphoma

Cutaneous T-cell lymphoma (CTCL), including mycosis fungoides (MF) and Sézary syndrome, is a malignant proliferation of T cells, typically helper/inducer (CD4) lymphocytes with initial presentation in the skin. Most of the data on the use of IFN-α in CTCL therapy have come from studies using recombinant IFN-α2a.

A review of the literature by Bunn and co-authors,[23] revealed an overall response rate of 55% and a complete response of 17% among 207 patients with MF and the Sézary syndrome treated with IFN-α2a. As a monotherapy, recombinant IFN-α2a is an active agent with less toxicity when low doses are used, and with a greater activity in patients with early-stage disease. They believe

3 million units given three times each week subcutaneously is the optimal treatment based on their review. There was no apparent therapeutic difference between IFN-α2a and 2b.

IFN-α effectiveness depends upon the disease stage, being greater for skin-limited disease with higher remission rates shown in stage I patients (50–62% complete response), compared with stage IV patients (8–16% complete response).[24] Intralesional injection of plaques of mycosis fungoides with IFN-α2b, 1 million IU three times weekly for 4 weeks, produced substantial localized clinical and histological improvement with 10/12 plaques demonstrating complete regression localized to the IFN injected sites.[25]

The effect of combining psoralen ultraviolet A (PUVA) with subcutaneous injections of IFN-α2a in the treatment of 63 CTCL patients has also been studied.[26] The study subjects were 42 males and 21 women, with a median age of 62 and the following stages of disease distribution: stage IA, *n*=6; IB, *n*=37; IIA, *n*=3; IIB, *n*=3; III, *n*=12; and IVA, *n*=2. Subcutaneous IFN-α2a was administered at a maximum dose of 9 to 12 million IU three times a week, given simultaneously with PUVA up to the minimal erythema dose. The initial treatments were administered three times per week until complete skin clearing, then once a week for 4 weeks, followed by treatments once every 2–4 weeks for an indefinite period of time. Of the 63 patients, 47 (75%) obtained a complete response (CR), six obtained a partial response (PR), two were classified as non-responders and five had progressive disease. The median time to obtain remission was 7 months; the median duration of overall response was 32 months, with a range of 6–57 months. CRs were obtained in all stages of disease. These results confirm that CR rates obtained with the combination of IFN-α and PUVA are better than those reported for IFN-α or PUVA alone.

The responses of IFN-α plus retinoic acid receptor (RAR) retinoids with respect to all stages of cutaneous T-cell lymphoma have shown an overall response of 60% with a CR of 11%, similar to those of either modality when used alone.[27]

A prospective controlled study treated 14 patients with stage II CTCL with interferon-α2a and extracorporeal photochemotherapy (ECP).[28] ECP was performed twice a month on two consecutive days with oral 8-metoxy-psoralen, 0.5 mg/kg body-weight. IFN-α2a was injected SQ three times a week up to the maximal tolerated dose,

12 to 18 million units. Among stage IIa patients the response rate was 60%, in contrast to only 25% for those in stage IIb.

Actinic keratoses

A study comparing injections of intralesional IFN-α2b, 0.5 million IU three times weekly for 2–3 weeks, to injections with placebo, revealed up to 93% of actinic keratoses clearing completely following IFN-α2b injection, with no clearing occurring in the placebo injected group.[29] The clinical usefulness of this modality for treatment of actinic keratoses is quite limited because of the need for injections and multiple physician visits, which are not required by other treatments currently available.

Infantile hemangiomata

IFN-α2a and 2b have both been reported to induce involution of infantile hemangiomata. IFN-α2a at a dose of 3 million IU/m^2 for 4 months resulted in regression of at least 90% of the tumor in 42% of the patients. Because of reported neurologic abnormalities in infants treated with IFN, it should be reserved for life-threatening infantile hemangiomata, not amenable to other therapies.[30]

Contraindications

Relative contraindications are cardiac arrhythmias, depression or other psychiatric disorders, leukopenia, pregnancy and previous organ transplantation.

Adverse effects

The adverse effects of IFNs are dose-dependent and generally remit either during continued therapy or following dose reduction. In addition, the adverse effects are generally rapidly reversible upon cessation of therapy.

- *Influenza-like symptoms.* The most commonly associated adverse effects after IFN therapy are influenza-like symptoms such as fever, chills, myalgias, headache and arthralgia, and may be controlled with acetaminophen and tend to remit with continued administration of IFN (tachyphylaxis).

- *Cutaneous reactions.* Skin necrosis at the site of injection.

- *Rhabdomyolysis.* Fatal rhabdomyolysis and multiple organ failure occurred in a patient treated with high dose IFN-α2b (20 million IU i.v. twice daily).[31]

- *Cardiovascular effects.* Significant hypotension, arrhythmia or tachycardia (150 beats/min or greater) associated with IFN use can occur. Close monitoring of patients with a recent history of myocardial infarction or a history of an arrhythmic disorder is recommended.

- *Neurologic and psychiatric effects.* Spastic diplegia was reported in the treatment of infantile hemangiomata.[32] Depression and suicidal behavior (including suicidal ideation, attempts and completed

suicides) have been reported in association with IFN-α therapy.

- *Other adverse effects.*
  - Gastrointestinal disturbances
  - Neutralizing antibodies can develop in patients receiving IFN-α2a and 2b. They appear to be specific to the recombinant IFN and not neutralize natural IFN.
  - Immune-mediated complications are infrequent, with thyroid disorders being the most common ones. The clinical spectrum of IFN-induced connective tissue disorders ranges from typical lupus erythematosus to rheumatoid arthritis. Patients with previous autoimmune phenomena should be identified, and if possible, treated with alternative drugs.[33]

Pegylated IFN (PEG-IFN) is a chemically modified form of recombinant human IFN. Initial data obtained in animal and phase I studies suggest that PEG-IFN injected once a week may be superior to human IFN injected three times a week. The safety of this modified form of IFN appears to be comparable with human IFN.[34]

Use in pregnancy

Interferons belong to pregnancy category C and though it is unknown whether IFN is excreted into human milk, it has been shown to be excreted into mouse milk.

Drug interactions

Interferon may cause inhibition of the cytochrome P-450 enzyme system. Caution is advised when IFN is used in conjunction with potentially neurotoxic vinca alkaloids.

IMIQUIMOD

Introduction

Imiquimod is a potent stimulator of innate and cell mediated immune responses resulting in potent antiviral, antitumor and immunoregulatory properties. The rationale of using imiquimod in the treatment of skin cancer and other diseases was based on the efficacy of the interferons. Imiquimod 5% cream (Aldara®) is FDA approved for the treatment of external genital and perianal warts, but currently imiquimod is considered a therapeutic option for certain types of skin cancer, especially in those cases where surgery is not an option.

Mechanism of action

In vitro, imiquimod induces cytokine production, inducing IFN-α, tumor necrosis factor-α (TNF-α), IL-1, IL-6, IL-8, and IL-12 production by human peripheral blood mononuclear cells (Fig. 41.1). The cytokine producing cells are monocytes, macrophages and toll-like receptor 7 (TRL7)-bearing plasmacytoid dendritic cells. Cell mediated immunity is also stimulated by IFN-α, causing CD4 T-cells to produce the IL-12 β2 receptor. Imiquimod also causes responding cells to produce IL-12, which stimulates the production of IFN-γ by CD4 cells. IFN-γ stimulates cytotoxic T-lymphocytes responsible for killing virus-infected and tumor cells.

Recent evidence of the expression of FasR (CD95), a member of the tumor necrosis receptor family, on BCC cells after treatment with imiquimod was found (Fig. 41.3). Imiquimod induced FasR mediated apoptosis may contribute to the effectiveness of imiquimod 5% cream in the treatment of BCC.[35]

Percutaneous absorption of imiquimod from imiquimod 5% cream is minimal, with less than 0.9% of a radio-labeled 5 mg dose being recovered in urine and feces. The site of potential metabolism is unknown, as is the degree of protein binding, if any. The recommended frequencies of application for the non-FDA approved indications in the treatment of skin cancer are discussed below.

Indications

Actinic keratosis
Current treatment modalities for actinic keratosis (AK), which may be considered as SCC *in situ*, include local destruction, drug therapy, and photodynamic therapy. Stockfleth *et al.* described six case reports of men with AK, where imiquimod was applied three times a week for 6 to 8 weeks, with clearance of all treated AK lesions and no reports of recurrence (ranging from 2 to 12 months post-treatment).[36] In a randomized, double-blind study,[37] 36 patients with AK lesions applied imiquimod 5% or vehicle cream three times a week for 12 weeks or until clinical resolution of the lesions. Complete resolution occurred in 85% of the patients and partial resolution in 8%. Histological confirmation occurred 2 weeks after the last application of imiquimod. The clinical recurrence rate one year after treatment was 10% (2/25), compared with the recurrence present with other methods. Persaud

et al.[38] conducted a trial involving 22 patients with AKs, using imiquimod 5% cream against placebo applied three times per week for 8 weeks or until total clearance of lesions, with a statistically significant reduction in the average number of lesions on the imiquimod-treated side. Salache *et al.*[39] used imiquimod to treat 25 patients with AKs of the face and scalp. The medication was applied to the entire area once daily, three times a week for 4 weeks, followed by a rest period of 4 weeks. If any AKs were present at the end of a 4-week rest period, the entire area was re-treated for another cycle of 4 weeks, followed by another 4-week rest period. Each cycle then consisted of 8 weeks and a maximum of three cycles was permitted. If AKs were present after the third cycle (24 weeks), this was considered a treatment failure. For the intent-to-treat analysis, 82% of the sites were completely cleared. The authors noted that a cycled approach may lead to higher rates of patient acceptance, compliance, and satisfaction, and may benefit patients who would experience complete clearance with the first cycle, without having to re-treat the area or using the medication for longer periods of time. At the American Academy of Dermatology annual meeting in 2003, Dr Mark Lebwohl presented the results from four multi-center, double-blind, randomized, vehicle-controlled phase III safety and efficacy studies evaluating the treatment of AKs on the face or balding scalp with imiquimod 5% cream.[40] Two studies randomized the patients to imiquimod 5% cream (*n*=215) or vehicle (*n*=221), once daily, 2 days a week. The two other trials randomized the patients either to imiquimod cream (*n*=242) or vehicle (*n*=250) once daily three times a week for 16 weeks. Complete clearance rate was defined as subjects with zero clinical visible AK lesions in the treatment area at 8-week post-treatment visit. The conclusion of the studies was that imiquimod 5% cream, either once daily twice a week or once daily three times a week, was significantly better than the vehicle with respect to complete clearance rates (*P*<0.001). Patients achieved a complete clearance of 45% and 48% when treated twice a week and three times a week respectively, and the

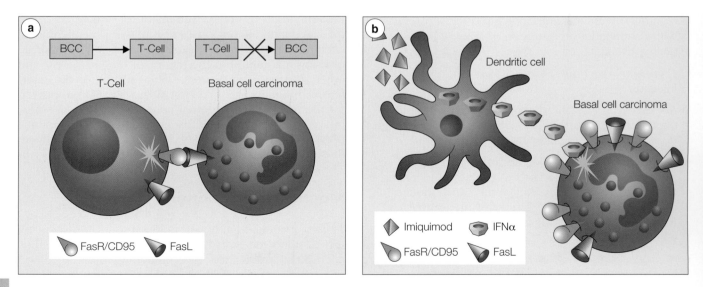

Figure 41.3 (a) Basal cell carcinoma cells are protected by failing to express the FasR/CD95 'Death receptor'; (b) imiquimod-induced BCC expression of FasR/CD95.

median clearance of AKs was 83.3% with the twice a week regimen. Imiquimod 5% cream was found to be safe to apply in the treatment of AKs. Figure 41.4 shows a case of a patient with actinic keratosis on the face, treated with imiquimod 5% cream following 5% 5-FU cream failure. Imiquimod 5% cream was recently approved by the FDA for the treatment of AKs.

Bowen's disease

In a phase II open-label study, 16 biopsy-proven plaques of Bowen's disease, with diameters ranging between 1 to 5.4 cm in diameter, were treated once-daily with imiquimod 5% cream for 16 weeks.[41] Of the 16 lesions treated, 15 were on the legs, and one was on the shoulder. Fourteen of the 15 patients (93% per protocol analysis) had no residual tumor present in their 6-week post-treatment biopsy specimens. One patient died of unrelated intercurrent illness before a biopsy specimen could be obtained. Ten patients completed 16 weeks of treatment, and 6 patients stopped treatment between 4 and 8 weeks because of local skin reactions that included superficial erosive changes associated with hemorrhagic crust. Patients were followed for 6 months without recurrences.

Several case reports have been published illustrating the efficacy of imiquimod in treating Bowen's disease of the penis. A 65-year circumcised white man presented with a squamous cell carcinoma in situ of the penis located on the dorsolateral penile shaft, extending to the corona and glans with approximately 45% of the penile shaft involved. Topical imiquimod 5% cream was applied nightly until intense erythema and superficial vesiculation developed at the application site. The patient received imiquimod cream during two cycles of 11 and 13 days, occurring one month apart. One month after discontinuation of the first cycle, there was clinical evidence of residual tumor. Re-evaluation 1 month after the second cycle, showed no clinical or histologic evidence of residual tumor.[42] Another case, a 41-year old uncircumcised man with a widespread *in situ* squamous cell carcinoma of the glans penis applied 5% imiquimod cream to the entire glans penis twice daily, three times a week for 12 weeks showing negative histological follow-up and remained disease free for 14 months after the treatment.[43] A 50-year-old HIV-1 positive man with perianal squamous cell carcinoma in situ received 16 weeks of 5% imiquimod cream, applied three nights a week to the external area of the involvement and within the anal canal. In the mornings and the remaining nights, the patient applied 5% fluorouracil to the same areas. The patient continued this therapy for 16 weeks, and at week 12 experienced a mixed bacterial infection that required oral and topical antibiotics. The erythema and residual superficial erosions healed after discontinuation of therapy. Three weeks later, four biopsy specimens taken from the area showed no evidence of residual dysplasia.[44] Another case involved a 52-year-old man with a diagnosis of Bowen's disease in a 2 cm plaque located mid shaft on the right side of the penis, the patient was treated with imiquimod 5% cream, three times weekly for 3 weeks, and experienced erythema, weeping and erosions at the site. One month after discontinuation of imiquimod, there was entire resolution of the lesion, with no residual or recurrent disease at 6 month follow-up.[45] Imiquimod has also been shown to be effective in combination with 5% fluorouracil (5-FU) therapy in immunosuppressed populations. Five cases of renal transplant patients treated with imiquimod and 5-FU for Bowen's disease in multiple areas following their transplants have been described.[46] Imiquimod 5% cream was applied to the plaques and to a 1 cm surrounding margin three nights a week. 5-FU was applied

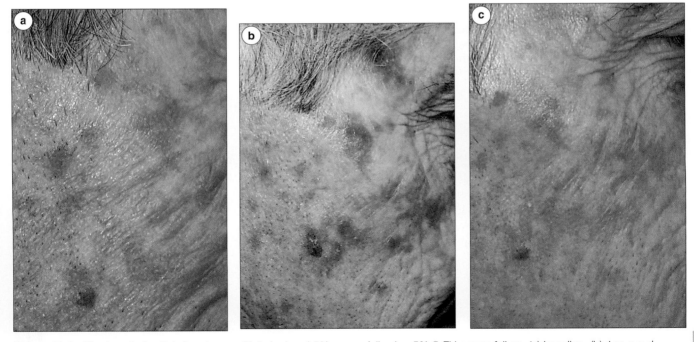

Figure 41.4 Treatment of actinic keratoses with imiquimod 5% cream following 5% 5-FU cream failure. (a) baseline, (b) 1 m q.o.d., (c) 1 m post Tx.

in the mornings and in the remaining four nights. Both medications were applied for 7 to 8 weeks in all patients, two weeks more than the time it took them to resolve clinically. Follow-up visits varied from 3 to 15 months with no evidence of residual lesions. Figure 41.5 shows a case of Bowen's disease of the face, which resolved after imiquimod once a day for 1 month.

Bowenoid papulosis

Bowenoid papulosis is histologically seen as a carcinoma *in situ*, despite the benign course of the condition. Treatments with excisional surgery, electrocoagulation, cryotherapy, and 5-FU have been attempted with variable success. A 38-year-old woman with bowenoid papulosis was treated with imiquimod 5% cream on alternating days for 10 days until the skin became visibly irritated. The cream was then applied once daily for another 10 days, but washed off after 2 hours. Complete clinical resolution was noted within 8 weeks and histology revealed no persisting or recurring disease. The patient remained clinically clear after more than 18 months after treatment.[47]

Vulvar intraepithelial neoplasias

A large percentage of vulvar intraepithelial carcinoma neoplasias (VIN) have been shown to harbor human papillomavirus (HPV). Vulvar intraepithelial squamous cell *in situ* is designated VIN 3. Imiquimod is thought to be a potentially beneficial treatment for patients with VIN of viral (HPV) etiology because of both its indirect antiviral and antineoplastic properties. Four cases of VIN 3 were treated with imiquimod 5% cream three times per week until lesions cleared, for a maximum of 16 weeks. The four patients had negative post-treatment biopsies, one patient recurred during the treatment and another patient recurred one year after imiquimod therapy.[48] A prospective study of 15 patients with high-grade VIN 3 examined the effects of imiquimod 5% cream self-applied three times weekly to vulvar lesions for 16 weeks. Local side effects were soreness, burning, erythema, ulceration and blisters. One patient required hospitalization, catheterization and analgesia because of the severity of the side-effects. From the 13 patients that were able to complete the study, four showed visible clinical improvement in the state of their condition, but only three had no evidence of VIN on a subsequent biopsy. The remaining patients showed no response to treatment. All four patients that responded clinically to the treatment relapsed 4 months after treatment. The authors feel that the side effects limited the frequency of cream application and therefore may have contributed to the patients' lack of response. An interesting finding was that patients who demonstrated a histological resolution of their VIN 3 continued showing koilocytosis as a sign of HPV infection, which may explain why patients relapsed so quickly after treatment.[49]

Melanoma

The recommended treatment for lentigo maligna (LM) is conventional surgery, using a 5–10 mm margin. Topical imiquimod 5% has also been of use in the treatment of LM. A case of a patient reluctant to have surgery for excision of a large LM of the scalp reported apparent complete resolution after 7 months of daily application of imiquimod 5% to an initial (the most pigmented) test area inside the lesion, followed by 3 months of application over the entire affected area. There was no evidence of LM in an incisional biopsy after stopping the treatment. No clinical recurrence was reported at 9-month follow-up.[50] A study involving 30 patients with histologic diagnosis of LM, *in situ* melanoma, treated with topical imiquimod was presented at the American Academy of Dermatology annual meeting in 2003.[51] Thirty patients older than 18 years with *in situ* melanomas were treated once daily for 3 months. One-month post treatment 4-quadrant biopsies were performed, as well as any other biopsies indicated by dermoscopic findings. One patient was re-classified as stage 1 and withdrawn from the study. One patient died from diabetic and lung disease not related to the study. Among the 28 evaluable subjects, 26 (93%) showed complete clinical and histological response. Ten patients required a rest period of more than 2 days, because of local severe reactions that occurred from week 2 to week 10, usually after 7–8 applications. Two of 28 patients experienced chills, malaise and headache; though both

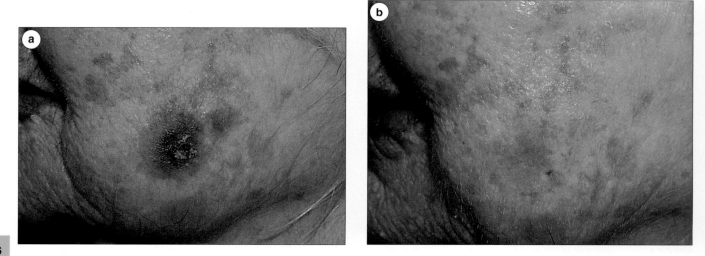

Figure 41.5 Bowen's disease treated with imiquimod 5% cream. (a) Once daily for 1 month, (b) 3 weeks after stopping treatment.

stopped early because they were considered to have local severe reactions, both were complete responders. The authors concluded that imiquimod 5% cream is a highly effective therapy for LM (*in situ* melanoma). A recent publication assessing the standard recommendation of 5-mm margins of resection of LM showed that it is adequate in less than 50% of cases.[52] If during long-term follow-up these patients remain free of recurrences and do not develop >stage 0 disease, we feel that imiquimod may represent a non-surgical alternative in treating LM beyond the 5-mm clinical margin, with excellent therapeutic and cosmetic results.

In a case of disseminated cutaneous metastatic melanoma lesion, with widespread lesions unsuitable for treatment with excision or radiotherapy and failing to improve after a cycle of dacarbazine alone, topical imiquimod 5% cream was used three times a week with continuance of dacarbazine. Twelve weeks after treatment with imiquimod was initiated, treated metastases were no longer detected on a second biopsy, which showed apoptotic melanoma cells.[53] A study of two patients with metastasic melanoma to the skin treated with imiquimod 5% cream was also reported recently.[54] The first, an 86-year-old woman with a history of melanoma on her right knee, presented with several skin melanoma metastases to her right lower leg, initially treated with carbon-dioxide laser ablation. No lymph nodes or visceral metastases were found. The other case, a 49-year-old man with a history of melanoma of the scalp treated with wide and deep resection, presented with multiple local recurrences around the surgical scar. These recurrences were initially treated with excision, carbon-dioxide laser vaporation and regional hyperthermia. The two patients received imiquimod 5% cream for application to the lesions three times per week in the evening, with a 1-cm surrounding margin. Patient 1 received the treatment for 4 months with complete clearing clinically and histologically. Patient 2 showed complete clearing of the skin after 8 months of treatment, and residual melanoma could not be detected.

Cutaneous T-cell lymphoma

In a case of stage IA cutaneous T-cell lymphoma (CTCL) refractory to topical steroid preparations and topical nitrogen mustard and carmustine, the patient was treated for 4 months with imiquimod 5% followed by complete clinical and histological clearance without recurrence at the treatment site at 10-month follow-up. The authors have initiated a double blind, placebo-controlled trial to better evaluate the efficacy of imiquimod in the treatment of CTCL.[55]

Cutaneous extramammary Paget's disease

Extramammary Paget's disease (EMPD) is an infrequent epidermal malignancy with a high rate of recurrences and associated with possible internal malignancies, occurring most commonly in the anogenital and vulvar regions. Two cases are reported of perineal and genital EMPD treated with imiquimod 5% cream, with clinical cure occurring after 7.5 to 12 weeks of application of imiquimod 5% on alternating days of the week.[56] Because many cases of EMPD occur in the anogenital region, this modality of treatment offers a convenient, non-invasive therapeutic option.

Actinic cheilitis

Actinic cheilitis can lead to invasive SCC and therapeutic alternatives used in the treatment of this entity include superficial destructive methods, topical fluorouracil and photodynamic therapy. A retrospective review of 15 patients with a biopsy-determined diagnosis, who received topical imiquimod as a single agent three times a week for the treatment of actinic cheilitis, showed clearance of the treated area in six patients after 4 weeks of treatment and in the remaining nine patients after week 6. All patients showed clinical resolution of their actinic cheilitis. Nine patients were followed up for at least 3 months without evidence of recurrence.[57]

Basal cell carcinoma

As discussed previously in this chapter, intralesional injections of IFN-α have been found to be effective in the treatment of basal cell carcinoma (BCC). The following clinical trials document the effectiveness of imiquimod 5% cream, an IFN-α inducer, in the treatment of superficial or nodular basal cell carcinomas (BCCs) at low-risk sites. The cosmetic outcome following topical treatment of BCC with imiquimod has been excellent. The initial study of topical imiquimod 5% cream for nodular and superficial BCC was a vehicle-controlled, 16-week, dose-ranging study.[58] The histologically confirmed cure rate varied depending upon the frequency of dosing, and the overall response rate was 83% (20/24) in the imiquimod-treated group and 9% (1/11) in the vehicle-treated group.

Superficial basal cell carcinoma

The first two phase II trials to examine the safety and efficacy of topically applied 5% imiquimod cream in the treatment of superficial BCC are summarized in Table 41.3.[58,59] These two randomized, multicenter studies reported that with a twice-daily application of imiquimod 5% cream, 100% efficacy is achieved. With the once daily dose, the response rate is around 88%, which is lower than the response rate seen in the commonly used modalities of treatment for primary BCC (92 to 96.8%).[19] In the 12-week, double-blind study the percentage of patients that experienced investigator-assessed severe reactions was higher in the once daily and twice daily regimens. In the twice-daily group, severe erythema and severe scabbing were recorded for 30% of the patients. Severe erosion and severe excoriation/ flaking, were each recorded for 10% of the patients. The authors considered that this regimen, twice-daily for 12 weeks, presented unacceptable safety profile because of severe local skin reactions at the treatment site. Similarly, in the 6-week, open-label study there was a clear dose-response gradient with the highest rate of severe local skin reactions, as assessed by the investigators, in the twice-daily regimen. From this regimen, 66.7% of the patients experienced severe local skin reactions.

With the data available from these two multicenter randomized studies, the once daily or five times a week dosage regimens had the highest efficacy results with acceptable safety profiles. The 6-week therapy appears

Table 41.3 Therapy of superficial BCC with 5% imiquimod cream

Type of study	Duration of therapy (weeks)	Total number enrolled	Schedule	n	Efficacy (intention to treat, %)
Phase II, randomized, double-blind, vehicle controlled, dose response[58] Distribution (%): trunk 56, limbs 38, face/neck 6.	12	128	Twice daily	10	100
			Once daily	31	87
			5 times a week	26	81
			3 times a week	29	52
			Vehicle	32	19
Multicenter, randomized open-label dose-response[59] Distribution (%): upper limbs 32, upper anterior trunk 14, upper posterior trunk 14.	6	99	Twice daily	3	100
			Once daily	33	88
			Twice daily, 3 times a week	30	73
			Daily, 3 times a week	33	67

to be as effective as the 12-week therapy for superficial BCC. At the American Academy of Dermatology annual meeting in 2003, Dr Marc Brown presented the results from four multicenter, double-blind, randomized, vehicle-controlled phase III safety and efficacy studies on the treatment of superficial basal cell carcinoma with imiquimod 5% cream for 6 weeks.[61] The patients had to have one primary (non-recurrent) sBCC, located on the limbs, trunk (non-anogenital), head, or neck, with diameters between 0.5 cm and 2.0 cm. Two studies randomized the patients to imiquimod 5% cream (n=185) or vehicle (n=179) once daily, 5 days a week. The two other trials randomized the patients either to imiquimod cream (n=179) or vehicle (n=181) once daily, 7 days a week for 16 weeks. The patients underwent tumor excision after a 12-week post-treatment period. A complete responder was defined as having no clinical (visual) evidence of BCC with no histological evidence of BCC at the target tumor site or having clinical evidence of BCC but no histological evidence at the target tumor site (and the histological findings when reviewed explained the incorrect clinical assessment). From these four studies, the authors concluded that imiquimod 5% cream is efficacious for the treatment of primary superficial BCC at the five times per week regimen, with a histological complete response rate of 82% (intent to treat). Imiquimod 5% cream is safely administered at both the seven times and five times per week regimen, the latter being the more efficacious and better tolerated of the two.

Nodular basal cell carcinoma

Two phase-II studies performed to determine the safety and efficacy of imiquimod 5% cream treatment of nodular BCC are described in Table 41.4.[61] The highest response rate that was achieved using this modality of treatment, in this particular clinical presentation of BCC, was 76% in the twice daily, 12-week group. The complete response rates in these two studies were not as high as the response seen in the 2 studies treating superficial BCC with imiquimod 5% cream (Table 41.3). The efficacy levels in the treatment of nodular basal cell carcinoma does not compare with the surgical excision success rate.[19] Therefore the candidates for this modality of treatment may be patients in which surgery, radiotherapy or cryotherapy is not an option.

Challenging cases with multiple or large BCCs

Examples of special cases of BCCs treated with imiquimod 5% cream include a case of a large (5 × 6 cm) superficial basal cell carcinoma,[63] a patient with basal cell nevus syndrome with multiple BCCs,[64] and the report of its use in two patients with xeroderma pigmentosum, in whom topical imiquimod decreased the rate of new tumor formation, permitting dermatologists to 'keep up' with the surgical treatment of these new lesions.[65] Further clinical trials are required to confirm imiquimod efficacy in larger BCCs and BCCs with aggressive growth patterns.

Infantile hemangiomata

A report on the efficacy of topical application of imiquimod in the treatment of two cases of postnatal-onset infantile hemangiomata in the proliferative state showed complete resolution of the lesions, which were located in the scalp, within 3 to 5 months. Though the development of erythema and crusting necessitated resting periods, both cases showed virtually complete clinical regression without scarring or neurologic abnormalities. Currently the authors have launched a larger clinical study with pathologic correlation and a mechanism-oriented investigation.[66] If treatment with imiquimod is not associated with spastic diplegia, which, albeit rare, limits the use of injected interferons, imiquimod 5% cream could be a valuable non-surgical treatment of infantile hemangiomata.

Major side-effects

The most common adverse reactions to imiquimod 5% cream are restricted to the site of application and include erythema (3%), ulceration (2%), edema (1%), excoriation (1%) and flaking (1%). Systemic adverse effects possibly or probably related to treatment include flu-like symp-

Table 41.4 Therapy of nodular BCC with 5% imiquimod cream

Type of study	Duration of therapy (weeks)	Total number enrolled	Schedule	n	Efficacy (intention to treat, %)
Randomized, double-blind, vehicle-controlled, dose-response[61] Distribution (%): face/neck 42, trunk 26, limbs 24.	12	92	Once daily	21	78
			Once daily, 5 days a week	23	70
			Once daily, 3 days a week	20	60
			Vehicle	24	13
Randomized, open-label dose-response[61] Distribution (%): face/neck 33, trunk 31, limbs	6		Once daily	35	71
			Twice daily, 3 days a week	31	42
			Once daily, 3 days a week	32	59

toms, fatigue, fever, headache, diarrhea and myalgia (in approximately 1–2% of patients).

Contraindications

None known.

Use in pregnancy

Imiquimod 5% cream belongs to pregnancy category B. It is not known whether topically-applied imiquimod 5% cream is excreted in breast milk.

Drug interactions

There are no known drug interactions with imiquimod 5% cream.

INTERLEUKIN-2

Key features

- Th1 type cytokine
- Used in clinical trials as an adjuvant therapy for metastatic melanoma and advanced CTCL
- Highly toxic at therapeutic doses

Introduction

Interleukin-2, secreted by CD4+ T lymphocytes after antigen recognition, has no direct effect on cancer cells. It is through stimulation of cytotoxic T lymphocytes, NK cells and macrophages that it exerts its antitumor activity (Fig. 41.1). Interleukin-2 also induces the synthesis of specific cytokines, including tumor necrosis factor, IL-1 IL-6 and IFN-γ.

Indications

Melanoma

Given its growth factor activity (promoting further T-cell activation and proliferation), IL-2 use has been investigated in the treatment of metastasic melanoma. The experience in the treatment of melanoma with IL-2 has suggested that maximum immunologic effect is achieved only in the context of high-dose therapy with, unfortunately, increased toxicity.[67] In clinical studies, high-dose intravenous (i.v.) IL-2 was administered at 600,000 to 720,000 IU/kg every 8 hrs on days 1 to 5 and 15 to 19 of the treatment course. Up to 20% of patients treated with this modality achieved objective responses.[68,69] When IL-2 was used in combination with available single, multi-agent chemotherapeutic regimens, the highest response rate achieved was 47%, in patients who received IL-2, IFN-α, cisplatin and dacarbazine, with a median survival duration of 10 months. It appears that this combination is statistically superior to either IL-2 alone or chemotherapy alone.[69] Results of ongoing trials may clarify the true value of the use of IL-2 in combination with chemotherapy, versus chemotherapy alone. The current use of histamine (see below) as an adjunct to IL-2 in metastasic melanoma and other malignant diseases may prolong the survival time of patients with metastasic melanoma to the liver.

Cutaneous T-cell lymphoma

Seven patients with advanced-stage (stage III–IVA) CTCL were treated with high dose recombinant IL-2, at a dose of 20 million IU/m^2/day by continuous infusion in a three-cycle, 30 day induction phase, and five-cycle monthly consolidation phase. IL-2 shows a CR in three patients (43%) and a PR in two patients (29%). Two of the remissions were durable (56–62 months).[70] An *in vitro* study evaluating the immunologic effects of adding IL-2 to IL-12 as a model to overcome refractoriness to recombinant human IL-12 for CTCL demonstrated synergism, enhancing the levels of IFN-γ and both the natural killer cell activity of 15 CTCL patients, as well as the T-cell surface IL-12 receptor expression in comparison with the effects of IL-12 or IL-2 alone.[71]

Contraindications

Patients with compromised general state, or specific cardiovascular pathology unable to tolerate the severity of IL-2 adverse effects.

Side-effects

Systemic high-dose IL-2 treatment is associated with severe toxic side effects such as cardiac toxicity, thrombocytopenia, hypotension, fever and vascular leak syndrome, resembling the clinical manifestation of septic shock, in addition to cardiovascular and respiratory toxicity.[72] The severity of the side-effects accompanying IL-2 systemic administration requires an ICU setting. Neurological and psychiatric disturbances may present as well.[73] Because of the notable disadvantages of its application, IL-2 has been used primarily in the treatment of metastatic melanoma, showing clinical benefit when used in high doses.

FUTURE OUTLOOK

Many of the future therapies are currently under investigation and for some, there is already promising data based on clinical experience. In this section, we will consider histamine, IL-12, granulocyte-macrophage and granulocyte colony stimulating factor (GM-CSF and G-CSF) and cyclooxygenase (COX) inhibitors as the agents that may become useful tools in immunotherapy against skin cancer.

Interleukin-12 (IL-12)

Interleukin-12 stimulates Th1 responses by direct effect on T cells, and also by induction of IFN-γ production by NK cells. IL-12 also augments the cytotoxic capacity of both NK and cytotoxic T cells. It seems to be essential for an optimal, early response against tumors.[74] IL-12 prevents the inhibitory effects of cis-urocanic acid (cis-UCA) on tumor antigen presentation by Langerhans cells (LCs). Cis-UCA may play an important role in photocarcinogenesis by inhibiting a tumor immune response.[75]

Cutaneous T-cell lymphoma
Based on the observations that CTCL presents with marked defects in IL-12 production, a phase I dose escalation trial with recombinant human IL-12 (rhIL-12) on patients with CTCL was conducted.[76] The study population consisted of 10 patients with the clinical and histological diagnosis of CTCL with plaques, tumors or erythrodermia (stage T1= two patients, stage T2= three patients, stage T3= two patients, stage T4= three patients). RhIL-12 was given at 50 ng/kg, 100 ng/kg, or 300 ng/kg 2 times a week subcutaneously. Treatment was performed for up to 24 weeks. A complete clinical response (CR) was defined as complete disappearance of all measurable and evaluable lesions for at least 1 month. Partial response (PR) was defined as at least 50%

disappearance of all CTCL skin lesions for at least 1 month. All patients with plaque disease had measurable clinical improvement while receiving rhIL-12. Two of these patients had a CR at week 7 and 8 respectively and both received a dose of 100 ng/kg. A previously detectable T-cell receptor rearrangement in the blood of a patient became undetectable at the time of the documented CR and remained undetectable at the conclusion of the treatment. Two other patients with plaque disease that received 100 ng/kg and 300 ng/kg, respectively, experienced a PR. Among the three patients with Sézary syndrome, only one completed the 24 weeks of treatment and had a documented PR. This patient started at 100 ng/kg, with dose escalation at week 4 to 300 ng/kg. Each of the two tumor-stage patients had rapidly progressive disease with numerous skin tumors at the time of the initiation of the rhIL-12. Direct intra-lesional therapy was given to the tumors. Both patients had progressive disease despite the treatment and both discontinued therapy. Adverse effects were short-lived (24 to 36 hrs) and consisted of fatigue, headache, or myalgias. Two patients had transient elevations of hepatic enzymes. One patient experienced severe depression that resolved within 1 week of discontinuation of the rhIL-12. The results of this trial suggests that rhIL-12, in the dose schedule used and administered subcutaneously, is both efficacious and without serious adverse effects. The authors announced the development of future phase II/III clinical trials based on the high response rate of patients with plaque stage CTCL.[76]

Histamine

Histamine protects NK cells and T cells against oxygen radical-induced dysfunction and apoptosis, and also maintains the activation of these cells by IL-2 and other lymphocyte activators.[77] Histamine, as an adjunct to IL-2, prolongs survival of patients with metastatic melanoma to the liver.[77] Histamine synergizes with IL-2 and IFN-α in vitro by protecting their target cells against oxidative inhibition (Fig. 41.1). Clinical trials with these regimens are underway in the treatment of metastasic malignant melanoma, acute myelogenous leukemia, and renal cell carcinoma.[78] There are expectations that the results of these ongoing studies will overcome the disappointing results of the clinical trials of immunotherapy with IL-2 and/or IFN-α in metastasic melanoma.

Cyclooxygenase inhibitors

Cyclooxygenase (COX)-2 levels are elevated in several types of human cancer tissues. Regular use of non-steroidal anti-inflammatory drugs (NSAIDs) significantly reduces the risk of spread of some cancers.[79] Epidemiological data and clinical studies were analyzed and compared with the results of studies of human tumor tissues, animal models, and cultured tumor cells. The results of these analyses were that COX-2 but not COX-1, is highly expressed in human colon carcinoma, squamous cell carcinoma of the esophagus, metastasic murine mammary tumor cells and skin cancer.[79,80] COX-

2 is inducible by the oncogenes ras and scr, as well as IL-1, hypoxia, benzo[a]pyrene, ultraviolet light, epidermal growth factor beta, and tumor necrosis factor alpha. COX-2 synthesizes prostaglandin E2 (PGE2), which stimulates bcl-2, inhibits apoptosis, and induces IL-6, which enhances haptoglobin synthesis. PEG2 is associated with tumor metastasis, IL-6 with cancer cell invasion and haptoglobin with implantation and angiogenesis. Evidence suggests that COX-2 expression may contribute to *in vivo* drug resistance in colorectal neoplasms.[81] Selective COX-2 inhibition is preferable to nonselective inhibition in reducing cancer cell proliferation, inducing apoptosis (Fig. 41.1), suppressing angiogenesis,[75] and sparing COX-1-induced cytoprotection of the gastro-intestinal tract.[79]

Granulocyte-macrophage and granulocyte colony-stimulating factor

Granulocyte-macrophage and granulocyte colony-stimulating factor (GM-CSF and G-CSF) have been used as rescue therapy on patients undergoing oncological therapy. There is recent evidence that their role in the treatment of cancer is not only supportive but that they may indeed have antitumor and immunomodulatory effects (Fig. 41.1).

A study of 17 patients with advanced solid tumors analyzed the mobilization of dendritic cells (DC) in cancer patients treated with granulocyte colony-stimulating factor and chemotherapy, and compared their baseline DC numbers with normal controls. The patients received intravenous chemotherapy with epirubicin and docetaxel on day 1, and agmen from day 2 until neutrophil recovery was achieved. Patient blood samples were collected at baseline and during the course of the therapy. Data from this study demonstrated after day 12 of treatment with G-CSF, patients with solid tumors increased the number of circulating DC 32-fold when compared with baseline. Isolation of DC from cancer patients is a critical aspect of many current immunotherapeutic strategies, therefore the possibility of a substantial increase in DC numbers during standard chemotherapy with G-CSF mobilization may be very useful.[82]

GM-CSF may provide an antitumor effect that prolongs survival in clinically disease-free patients with melanoma stage II and IV. Forty-eight patients with these characteristics were treated in a phase II trial with long term, chronic, intermittent GM-CSF after surgical resection of the disease.[83]

REFERENCES

1 Stockfleth E, Ulrich C, Meyer T, Christophers E. Epithelial malignancies in organ transplant patients: Clinical presentation and new methods of treatment. Recent Results Cancer Res 2002; 160:251–258.

2 Hellstrand C. Histamine in cancer immunotherapy: A preclinical background. Semin Oncol 2002; 29(3):35–40.

3 Dcnin N, Jurianz K, Ziporen L, et al. Complement resistance of human carcinoma cells depends on membrane regulatory proteins, protein kinases and sialic acid. Clin Exp Immunol 2003; 131:254–263.

4 Halliday GM, Le S. Transforming growth factor-beta produced by progressor tumor inhibits. while IL-10 produced by regressor tumor enhances, Langerhans cells migration from skin. Int Immunol 2001; 13:1147–1154.

5 Rabinowich H, Reichert TE, Kashii Y, et al. Lymphocyte apoptosis induced by Fas ligand-expressing ovarian carcinoma cells. Implications for altered expression of T cell receptor in tumor-associated lymphocytes. J Clin Invest 1998; 101:2579–2588.

6 Alamartine E, Berthoux P, Mariat C, Cambazard F, Berhoux F. Interleukin-10 promoter polymorphisms and susceptibility to skin squamous cell carcinoma after renal transplantation. J Invest Dermatol 2003; 120:99–103.

7 Rusciani L, Petraglia S, Alotto M, et al. Postsurgical adjuvant therapy for melanoma. Evaluation of a 3-year randomized trial with recombinant interferon-alpha after 3 and 5 years of follow-up. Cancer 1997; 79:2354–2360.

8 Creagan ET, Dalton RJ, Ahmann DL, et al. Randomized, surgical adjuvant clinical trial of recombinant interferon alfa-2a in selected patients with malignant melanoma. J Clin Onccl 1995; 13:2776–2783.

9 Doveil GC, Fierro MT, Novelli M, et al. Adjuvant therapy of stage IIIb melanoma with interferon alfa-2b: clinical and immunological relevance. Dermatology 1995; 191:234–239.

10 Kirkwood JM, Resnick GD, Cole BF. Efficacy, safety, and risk-benefit analysis of adjuvant interferon alfa-2b in melanoma. Semin Oncol 1997; 24:16S–23S.

11 Dubois RW, Swetter SM, Atkins M et al. Developing indications for the use of sentinel lymph node biopsy and adjuvant high-dose interferon alfa-2b in melanoma. Arch Derm 2001; 137:1217–1224.

12 Barth A, Morton DL. The role of adjuvant therapy in melanoma management. Cancer 1995; 75:726S–734S.

13 Wussow P Von, Block B, Hartmann F, Deicher H. Intralesional interferon-alpha therapy in advanced malignant melanoma. Cancer 1988; 61:1071–1074.

14 Cornejo P, Vanaclocha F, Polimon I Del, Rio R. Intralesional interferon treatment of lentigo maligna. Arch Dermatol 2000; 136(3):428–430.

15 Krown SE. Interferon and other biological agents for the treatment of Kaposi's sarcoma. Hem Oncol Clin N Am 1991; 5:311–322.

16 Buechner S. Intralesicnal interferon-alpha 2b in the treatment of basal cell carcinoma. J Am Acad Derm 1991; 24:731–734.

17 Greenway HT, Cornell RC, Tanner DJ, et al. Treatment of basal cell carcinoma with intralesional interferon. J Am Acad Derm 1986; 15:437–443.

18 Stenquist B, Wennberg AM, Gisslen H, et al. Treatment of aggressive basal cell carcinoma with intralesional interferon: evaluation of efficacy by Mohs surgery. J Am Acad Derm 1992; 27:65–69.

19 Telfer NR, Colver GB, Bowers PW. Guidelines for the management of basal cell carcinoma. British Association of Dermatologists. Br J Dermatol 1999; 141(3):415–423.

20 Ikic D, Padovan I, Pipic N, et al. Interferon therapy for basal cell carcinoma and squamous cell carcinoma. Int Jour Clin Pharm Ther Toxicol 1991; 29:342–346.

21 Edwards L, Berman B, Rapini RP, et al. Treatment of cutaneous squamous cell carcinoma by intralesional interferon-alpha 2b therapy. Arch Derm 1992; 128:1486–1489.

22 Grob JJ, Suzini F, Richard A, et al. Large keratoacanthomas treated with intralesional interferon-alpha 2a. J Am Acad Derm 1993; 29:237–241.

23 Bunn PA Jr, Hoffman SJ, Norris D, et al. Systemic therapy of cutaneous T-cell lymphomas (mycosis fungoides and the Sezary syndrome). Ann Intern Med 1994; 121:592–602.

24 Apisarnthanarax N, Talpur R, Duvic M. Treatment of cutaneous T-cell lymphoma: current status and future directions. Am J Clin Dermatol 2002; 3(3):193–215.

25 Vonderheid EC, Thompson R, Smiles KA, et al. Recombinant interferon-2b in plaque-phase mycosis fungoides-intralesional and low-dose intramuscular therapy. Arch Derm 1987; 123:757–763.

26 Chiarion-Silenu V, Bononi A, Veller Fornasa C, et al. Phase II trial of interferon-alpha 2a plus psoralen with ultraviolet light A in patients with cutaneous T-cell lymphoma. Cancer 2002; 95(3):596–604.

27 Apisarnthanarax N, Talpur R, Duvic M. Treatment of cutaneous T-cell lymphoma: current status and future directions. Am J Clin Dermatol 2002; 3(3):193–215.

28 Wollina U, Looks A, Meyer J, et al. Treatment of stage II cutaneous T-cell lymphoma with interferon alfa-2a and extracorporeal photochemotherapy: a prospective controlled trial. J Am Acad Dermatol 2001; 44(2):253–260.

29 Edwards L, Levine N, Weidner M, et al. Effect of intralesional interferon in actinic keratoses. Arch Derm 1986; 122:779–782.

30 Greinwald J, Burke D, Bonthius D, et al. An update on the treatment of hemangiomas in children with interferon alpha-2a. Arch Otolaryngol Head Neck Surg 1999; 125:21–27.

31 Reinhold U, Hartl C, Hering R, et al: Fatal rhabdomyolysis and multiple organ failure associated with adjuvant high dose interferon alpha in malignant melanoma. Lancet 1997; 349:540–541.

32 Barlow CF. Spastic diplegia as a complication of interferon alfa-2a treatment of hemangiomas of infancy. J Pediatr 1998; 132:527–530.

33 Pia R, Ben-Bassat I. Immune-mediated complications during interferon therapy in hematological patients. Acta Haematol 2002; 107:133–144.

34 Pehamberger H. Perspectives of pegylated interferon use in dermatological oncology. Recent Results Cancer Res 2002; 160:158–164.

35 Berman B, Sullivan T, de Araujo T, Nadji M. Expression of fas-receptor on basal cell carcinoma after treatment with Imiquimod 5% cream or vehicle. Br J Derm 2003; July.

36 Stockfleth E, Meyer T, Benninghoff B, Christophers E. Successful treatment of actinic keratosis with imiquimod cream 5%: a report of six cases. Br J Derm 2001; 144(5):1050–1053.

37 Stockfleth E, Meyer T, Benninghoff B, Salasche S, et al. A randomized, double-blind, vehicle-controlled study to assess 5% Imiquimod cream for the treatment of multiple actinic keratoses. Arch Derm 2002; 138:1498–1502.

38 Persaud AN, Shamuelova E, Sherer D, et al. Clinical effect of imiquimod 5% in the treatment of actinic keratoses. J Amer Acad Derm 2002; 47(4):553–556.

39 Salasche SJ, Levine N, Morrison L. Cycle therapy of actinic keratoses of the face and scalp with 5% topical imiquimod cream: An open label trial. J Amer Acad Derm 2002; 47(4):571–577.

40 Lebwohl M, Dinehart S, Whiting D, et al. Imiquimod 5% cream for the treatment of actinic keratosis: results from two phase III, randomized, double-blind, parallel group, vehicle-controlled trials. J Am Acad Derm 2003; in press.

41 Pehoushek J, Smith KJ. Imiquimod and 5% fluorouracil therapy for anal and perianal squamous cell carcinoma in situ in an HIV-1-positive man. Arch Derm 2001; 137(1):14–16.

42 MacKenzie Wood A, Kossard S, deLauney J, Wilkinson B, Owens M. Imiquimod 5% cream in the treatment of Bowen's disease. J Am Acad Derm 2001; 44:462–470.

43 Schroeder TL, Sengelmann RD. Squamous cell carcinoma in situ of the penis successfully treated with imiquimod 5% cream. J Amer Acad Derm 2002; 46(4):545–548.

44 Orengo I, Rosen T, Guill C. Treatment of squamous cell carcinoma in situ of the penis with 5% Imiquimod cream: A case report. J Am Acad Dermatol 2002; 47:S225–S228.

45 Thai K, Sinclair R. Treatment of Bowen's disease of the penis with imiquimod. J Am Acad Derm 2002; 46:470–471.

46 Smith KJ, Germain M, Skelton H. Squamous cell carcinoma in situ (Bowen's disease) in renal transplant patients treated with 5% imiquimod and 5% 5-fluorouracil therapy. Derm Surg 2001; 27(6):561–564.

47 Petrow W, Gerdsen R, Uerlich M, Richter O, Bieber T. Successful topical immunotherapy of bowenoid papulosis with imiquimod. Br J Derm 2001; 145(6):1022–1036.

48 Davis G, Wentworth J, Richard J. Self-administered topical imiquimod treatment of vulvar intraepithelial neoplasia: a report of four cases. J Reproduct Med 2000; 45(8):619–623.

49 Todd RW, Etherington IJ, Luesley DM. The effects of 5% imiquimod cream on high-grade vulvar intraepithelial neoplasia. Gynecol Oncol 2002; 85(1):67–70.

50 Ahmed I, Berth-Jones J. Imiquimod: a novel treatment for lentigo maligna. Br J Dermatol 2000; 143:843–845.

51 Naylor MF, Crowson N, Kuwahara R, et al. Treatment of lentigo maligna with topical imiquimod. Br J Dermatol 2003; 149:66–70.

52 Agarwal-Antal N, Bowen G, Gerwls J. Histologic evaluation of lentigo maligna with permanent sections: Implications regarding current guidelines. J Am Acad Derm 2002; 47:743–748.

53 Steinmann A, Funk JO, Schuler G, Driesch P von den. Topical imiquimod treatment of a cutaneous melanoma metastasis. J Amer Acad Derm 2000; 43(3):555–556.

54 Wolf H, Smolle J, Binder B, et al. Topical imiquimod in the treatment of metastasis melanoma to the skin. Arch Derm 2003; 139:273–276.

55 Suchin KR, Junkins-Hopkins JM, Rook AH. Treatment of stage Ia cutaneous T-cell lymphoma with topical application of the immune response modifier imiquimod. Arch Derm 2002; 138(9):1137–1139.

56 Zampogna JC, Flowers FP, Roth WI, Hassenein A. Treatment of primary limited cutaneous extramammary Paget's disease with topical imiquimod monotherapy. Two case reports. J Amer Acad Derm 2002; 47(4):S229–S235.

57 Smith KJ, Germain M, Yeager J, Skelton H. Topical 5% imiquimod for the therapy of actinic cheilitis. J Amer Acad Derm 2002; 47(4):497–501.

58 Beutner KR, Geisse JK, Helman D, et al. Therapeutic response of basal cell carcinoma to the immune response modifier imiquimod 5% cream. J Am Acad Derm 1999; 41:1002–1007.

59 Geisse J, Rich P, Pandya A, Gross K, et al. Imiquimod 5% cream for the treatment of superficial basal cell carcinoma: A double-blind, randomized, vehicle-controlled study. J Am Acad Derm 2002; 47:390–398.

60 Marks R, Gebauer K, Shumack S, et al. Imiquimod 5% cream in the treatment of superficial basal cell carcinoma: Results of a multicenter 6-week dose-response trial. J Amer Acad Derm 2001; 44(5):807–813.

61 Brown M. AAD meeting, San Francisco, 2003; in press.

62 Shumack S, Robinson J, Kossard S, et al. Efficacy of topical 5% imiquimod cream for the treatment of nodular basal cell carcinoma: comparison of dosing regimens. Arch Dermatol 2002; 138(9):1165–1171.

63 Chen TM, Rosen T, Orengo I. Treatment of a large superficial basal cell carcinoma with 5% Imiquimod: a case report and review of the literature. Dermatol Surg 2002; 28:344–346.

64 Kagy MK, Amonette R. The use of Imiquimod 5% cream for the treatment of superficial basal cell carcinomas in a basal cell nevus syndrome patient. Dermatol Surg 2000; 26:577–579.

65 Weisberg NK, Varghese M. Therapeutic response of a brother and sister with xerocerma pigmentosum to Imiquimod 5% cream. Dermatol Surg 2002; 28:518–523.

66 Martinez ML, Sanchez-Carpintero I, North PE, Mihm MC. Infantile hemangioma. Arch Dermatol 2002; 138:881–884.

67 Atkins M. Interleukin-2: clinical applications. Semin Oncol 29(7):12–17.

68 Allen I, Kupelnick ZB, Kumashiro M. Efficacy of IL-2 in the treatment of metastasic melanoma. Cancer Ther 1998; 1:168–173.

69 Allen I, Kupelnick B, Kumashiro M. Efficacy of interleukin-2 in the treatment of metastasic melanoma – systemic review and meta-analysis. Cancer Ther 1998; 1:168–173.

70 Baccard M, Marolleau JP, Rybojad M. Middle-term evolution of patients with advanced cutaneous T-cell lymphoma treated with high dose recombinant interleukin-2 [letter]. Arch Derm 1997; 133:656.

71 Zaki MH, Wysocka M, Everetts SE, et al. Synergistic enhancement of cell-mediated immunity by interleukin-12 plus interleukin-2: basis for therapy of cutaneous T-cell lymphoma. J Invest Dermatol 2002; 118(2):366–371.

72 Atkins MB. Interleukin-2: clinical applications. Semin Oncol 2002; 29(3):12–17.

73 Helgurea G, Morrison SL, Penichet ML. Antibody-cytokine fusion proteins: Harnessing the combined power of cytokines and antibodies for cancer therapy. Clin Immunology 2002; 105(3):233–246.

74 Grufman P, Karre K. Innate and adaptive immunity to tumors: IL-12 is required for optimal responses. Eur J Immunol 2000; 30(4):1088–1093.

75 Beissert S, Ruhlemann D, Mohammad T, et al. IL-12 prevents the inhibitory effects of cis-urocanic acid on tumor antigen presentation by Langerhans cells: implications for photocarcinogenesis. J Immunol 2001; 167(11):6232–6238.

76 Rook AH, Wood GS, Yoo EK, Elenitsas R, et al. Interleukin-12 therapy of cutaneous T-cell lymphoma induces lesion regression and cytotoxic T-cell responses. Blood 1999; 94(3):902–908.

77 Hellstrand K, Brune M, Naredi P, et al. Histamine: a novel approach to cancer immunotherapy. Cancer Invest 2000; 18(4):347–355.

78 Peter N. Histamine as an adjunct to immunotherapy. Semin Oncol 29(7):31–34.

79 Fosslien E. Molecular pathology of cyclooxygenase-2 in neoplasia. Ann Clin Lab Sci 2000; 30(1):3–21.

80 Kundu N, Smyth MJ, Samsel L, Fulton AM. Cyclooxygenase inhibitors block cell growth, increase ceramide and inhibit cell cycle. Breast Cancer Res Treat 2002; 76(1):57–64.

81 Keller JJ, Offerhaus GJ, Drillenburg P, et al. Molecular analysis of sulindac-resistant adenomas in familial adenomatous polyposis. Clin Cancer Res 2001; 7:4000–4007.

82 Radcliff F, Caruso D, Koina C, et al. Mobilization of dendritic cells in cancer patients treated with granulocyte colony-stimulating factor and chemotherapy. Br J Haematol 2002; 119:204–211.

83 Spitler L, Grossbard M, Ernstoff M, et al. Adjuvant therapy of stage III and IV malignant melanoma using granulocyte-macrophage colony-stimulating factor. J Clin Oncol 2000; 18:1614–1621.

Photodynamic Therapy in Skin Cancer

Colin A Morton

Key points

- Photodynamic therapy (PDT) is a selective non-invasive therapy.
- PDT is an approved therapy for non-hyperkeratotic actinic keratoses and basal cell carcinomas, and has several additional potential indications.
- PDT offers particular advantages for large and multiple lesions and those in sites where standard therapies have limitations.
- Superiority of cosmetic outcome following PDT is often observed over conventional therapies.
- PDT appears to be safe, with repeat treatments possible. Stinging/pain during treatment can be controlled, if required, by analgesia or local anesthesia.

INTRODUCTION

Photodynamic therapy (PDT) is a non-invasive therapy with proven efficacy in non-melanoma skin cancer. PDT involves the activation of a photosensitizing drug by visible light to produce activated oxygen species within target cells, resulting in their destruction.[1] Initially, systemic administration of photosensitizers was required, adding complexity to the procedure and resulting in the complication of generalized photosensitivity that could last several weeks. Subsequently, the use of the topically active agent, 5-aminolaevulinic acid (5-ALA), a precursor of the endogenous photosensitizer protoporphyrin IX (PpIX) was described, permitting simplification of the treatment process.[2]

PDT is emerging as an effective treatment for various cutaneous and non-cutaneous malignancies. Systemic photosensitization and endoscopic light delivery have permitted the treatment of many hollow organ tumors, including those in the esophagus, stomach, bronchus and bladder curing early superficial disease and palliating late disease. Evidence-based studies indicate that, in dermatology, topical PDT is effective in actinic keratoses on the face and scalp, Bowen's disease (squamous cell carcinoma *in situ*), superficial basal cell carcinomas (BCC) and has potential in nodular BCC (Table 42.1).[3] Case reports suggest it is also effective in treating localized plaques of cutaneous T-cell lymphoma. Topical PDT has moved from research to clinic with FDA approval of PDT using a 5-ALA preparation, Levulan (DUSA, USA), for actinic keratoses and European approval for PDT with the methyl ester of 5-ALA (MAL)

for actinic keratoses and basal cell carcinomas (PhotoCure, Oslo, Norway; Galderma, Paris, France). Topical PDT offers the potential of a practical non-surgical out-patient/office therapy in dermatology. Against the continued rise in incidence of cutaneous malignancy and aging population profiles in most parts of the world, developing safe, effective and patient-friendly therapies is of great importance (Table 42.2).

PDT may prove advantageous where size, site or numbers of lesions limit the efficacy and/or acceptability of conventional therapies.[4] Topical PDT studies consistently report a superiority of the cosmetic outcome with minimal or no scarring when compared to standard therapies: cryotherapy, topical 5-fluorouracil and surgery.

In addition to providing a novel therapy, fluorescence emitted by ALA-induced PpIX, can be utilized to provide a fluorescent diagnosis of cutaneous lesions. This permits the definition of surface tumor margins or recurrent disease where clinical delineation is difficult.[5] Refinement of this technique is still required, but offers an additional advantage of PDT. Surface tumor delineation can be visualized even using a simple Woods UV lamp prior to illuminating lesions with the PDT lamp.

Porfimer sodium (Photofrin, Axcan Pharma, Quebec, Canada) is the most widely used first generation systemic photosensitizer and has FDA approval in the US for esophageal and early lung cancer. It is also currently used off-label for treating non-melanoma skin cancers.

HISTORY

The term 'photodynamic therapy' was first used around 100 years ago by von Tappeiner following experiments using eosin and a combination of natural and artificial light in the treatment of skin cancer in 1903.[6] He realized the requirement for oxygen, describing the phenomenon as an oxygen-dependent photosensitization. The subsequent observation of selective localization of porphyrins to tumors and the demonstration of a photodynamic action involving hematoporphyrin in tumors raised interest in PDT. However, large doses of the crude photosensitizer were required and the consequent phototoxicity limited development. Partial purification produced hematoporphyrin derivative (HpD) re-ignited interest in this modality and PDT using HpD in human cancer was reported in 1967. The first trial was performed in 25 patients in 1978 in a variety of malignancies including squamous and basal cell carcinomas. Many studies have subsequently reported the successful use of PDT with the more purified form of HpD, porfimer sodium (Photofrin), in the treatment

Table 42.1   Advantages and disadvantages of topical photodynamic therapy

Advantages	Disadvantages
• Relatively selective treatment • Minimal or no scarring • Functional preservation of tissue • Treats field disease • Non-invasive • Multiple lesions may be treated simultaneously • Large lesions can be effectively treated • 'Difficult' anatomical sites for conventional therapy are usually suitable for PDT • Reduced adverse events compared with standard therapies • Safe 25 year experience suggests very low potential for carcinogenicity • Repeated treatments possible • Does not limit subsequent salvage therapies when used for palliation • No generalized photosensitivity • Supervised out-patient therapy ensures compliance • Good healing rate with ulceration very rare	• Prickling/burning/stinging sensations during and immediately following treatment are common • Local anesthesia/analgesia required for a minority of patients • Local erythema and edema following treatment • No histological confirmation of diagnosis nor of clearance • Treatment time-consuming and requires practice, space and staff • Initial high cost relative to certain standard therapies (offset by reduced adverse events) • Recurrence rates vary • Concern that deep disease may be left untreated rendering difficult salvage therapy at certain body sites • Hypo and hyper-pigmentation post therapy common, but temporary • Hair loss in hirsute sites observed, but much less than following radiotherapy.

of various malignancies. While HpD and porfimer sodium require systemic administration, Kennedy *et al.*[2] reported in 1990 the use of the topically active agent, 5-aminolaevulinic acid (5-ALA), which has been the focus of much research activity during the past decade.

HOW IT WORKS: THE PHOTOSENSITIZER

The photodynamic reaction concerns the activation of photosensitizers in target tissue following absorption of light of an appropriate wavelength. A poorly understood gradient of differential sensitizer concentration between tumor and surrounding tissue has been demonstrated following systemic delivery, but differs between sensitizer and tumor type. For skin tumors, the topical route of application of 5-ALA permits an additional method of tumor selectivity, with selective uptake through altered epidermis. 5-ALA is a precursor in the heme biosynthesis pathway of protoporphyrin IX (PpIX), an endogenous photosensitizer not normally present within tissue in therapeutically useful concentrations.[1,7] Exogenous administration of 5-ALA can increase the intracellular concentration of PpIX (Fig. 42.1), as 5-ALA is the first precursor of heme after the feedback control point and the conversion of PpIX to heme is relatively slow. Local application of 5-ALA is possible due to its increased passage, when in aqueous solution, through an abnormal epidermis thus restricting the photosensitization primarily to the tumor sites. Proliferating, relatively iron deficient tumor cells preferentially accumulate PpIX as iron is required for the final conversion of PpIX into haem. This tissue selectivity in 5-ALA photodynamic therapy can be demonstrated by the detection of PpIX-induced fluorescence. There is a relatively greater specificity with the methyl ester of 5-ALA (MAL) in comparison with 5-ALA due to increased lipophilicity, with a ratio of 9:1 compared with 2:1 for BCC compared with normal skin.

Szeimies *et al.* demonstrated a homogenous distribution of PpIX fluorescence of nodular and superficial (but not morpheic) BCC, including tumor lobules in deep dermis, 12 hrs after 10% ALA application.[8] Roberts *et al.* reported that PpIX distribution in BCC was most intense in those regions of tumor immediately adjacent to the dermis following application of 20% 5-ALA for 4 hrs to Bowen's disease and superficial BCC.[9]

For exogenous photosensitizers, including porfimer sodium, where systemic administration is required, there remains only a limited understanding of the mechanism of increased tumor accumulation/retention. Porous tumor vasculature, poor lymphatic drainage and increased low-density lipoprotein mediated endocytosis activity of tumor cells may each contribute.[1] Porfimer sodium is administered intravenously at a dose of 1 mg/kg, 48–72 hrs before therapy.

Several new agents are under evaluation for PDT. These include benzoporphyrin derivative monoacid, meso-tetra-(hydroxyphenyl)-chlorin (mTHPC), N-aspartyl chlorine, tin etiopurpurin, tetraphenylporphine sulfonate, zinc phthalocyanine and sulfonated aluminum phthalocyanines.[10] These new photosensitizers are more potent than porfimer sodium and are more rapidly cleared following systemic administration.

Meso-tetraphenylporphinesulfonate tetrasodium (mTPPS) and mTHPC have both been studied for topical use. mTPPS cleared 94% of 292 superficial BCC with a single treatment and a 10% recurrence rate. However, its development has been limited by prolonged photosensitivity and the potential for neurotoxicity.[11] In the only study of the topical use of mTHPC, a histological clearance of only 9/28 patches of Bowen's disease and 2/7 BCC was achieved and formulation was considered to be a problem.[12]

As 5-ALA is hydrophilic, to facilitate penetration most studies report the use of a 20% concentration in an oil-in-water emulsion. Enhancement of 5-ALA PDT has been attempted using the penetration enhancer dimethyl-

Table 42.2   Indications and contraindications to topical PDT for skin cancer

Indication with strong evidence-base of efficacy	Indication with anecdotal experience of efficacy	Insufficient current evidence of efficacy	Contraindication (evidence-based or due to PDT methodology)
• Actinic keratoses (non-hyperkeratotic, face and scalp)[a,t] • Bowen's disease • Superficial BCC[b] • Nodular BCC[b] (with debulking and repeat therapy)	• Actinic keratoses on acral sites • Erythroplasia of Queyrat • Localized cutaneous T-cell lymphoma	• Malignant melanoma • Squamous cell carcinoma • Cutaneous metastases • Kaposi's sarcoma • Extramammary Paget's • VIN	• Pigmented or hyperkeratotic actinic keratoses • Pigmented basal cell carcinomas • Morpheaform BCC • Xeroderma pigmentosum • Porphyria

Author's view of current status of topical PDT, based on the published literature. Indications with strong or anecdotal experience deserve consideration for PDT. Indications with insufficient evidence of efficacy are those where the strength of evidence currently should discourage the use of PDT.
[a]Licensed indication for ALA-PDT by FDA. [b]Licensed indication for MAL-PDT in Europe at 4/03.

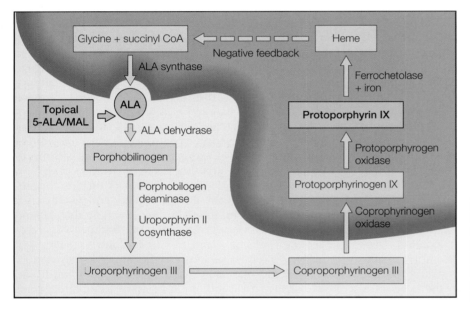

Figure 42.1   The heme cycle in ALA/MAL PDT. Regulation of heme synthesis – the accumulation within the mitochondria of protoporphyrin IX is central to ALA and MAL PDT. Cellular uptake mechanisms differ between ALA and MAL, but exogenous administration acts to temporarily promote the accumulation of PpIX.

sulfoxide, and the iron chelators desferrioxamine and ethylenediaminetetraacetic acid disodium. The latter agents have shown improved response rates with PDT in nodular BCC.[13]

Reported application intervals for 5-ALA are typically 3–8 hrs.[9] The optimal pre-illumination interval is probably disease dependent. 6 hrs application pre-treatment is possibly superior to 4 hrs for superficial BCC 1–2 mm thick.[14]

Mechanism of action of light

Light of appropriate wavelength for activation of the photosensitizer is required in the target tissue. While 635 nm light may penetrate up to 6 mm (compared with 1–2 mm for light at 400–500 nm), the therapeutically effective maximum depth of PDT will depend on sufficient light dose being delivered to tissue that also has sufficient photosensitizer to achieve a photodynamic reaction. The therapeutically effective depth of PDT in the skin is

therefore likely to be less, at 1–3 mm at 635 nm depending on the tissue.[1]

Most clinical applications of PDT have used red light around 630–635 nm to achieve adequate penetration. 5-ALA-induced photosensitivity has a porphyrin-like spectrum with maximum excitation at 410 nm and additional smaller peaks at 510, 545, 580 and 635 nm (Fig. 42.2).[15] Using shorter wavelength light could thus achieve more efficient activation of PpIX, but at the expense of depth of therapeutic effect.

Several light sources have been used in clinical PDT studies for cutaneous applications, including lasers, xenon arc/discharge lamps, incandescent filament lamps and solid-state light-emitting diodes (LEDs). Coherent light is not required for PDT. The development of energy-efficient LED sources has facilitated the development of large area, yet portable, red-light sources that are likely to become the most frequently used lights in clinical practice (Actilite, Galderma, Paris, France; Omlilux, Photo-therapeutics Ltd, Altringham, UK). Little comparison data exists between light sources with their different wavelength and intensity characteristics making simple dosage comparisons between studies extremely difficult for lesional tissue.

Actinic keratoses have been successfully treated using blue, green, red and broadband light sources. There is limited comparison evidence, in small numbers of patients and/or short follow-up periods, typically 3 months, making interpretation difficult. The FDA has approved a blue light source, the Blu-U (DUSA, USA), for use with the 5-ALA formulation Levulan for actinic keratoses. For superficial disease such as non-hyperkeratotic actinic keratoses, short wavelength blue light is a more efficient wavelength to use. This is near the maximum absorption wavelength of PpIX at 410 nm and may reduce the stinging/pain of PDT. In a randomized comparison of green with red light in Bowen's disease, however, green light was significantly inferior. This suggested deeper light penetration with longer wavelength red light is necessary to treat the entire thickness of disease (including skin appendages) in Bowen's disease.[16]

Dosimetry in PDT can presently be defined only in terms of explicit parameters, including the administered photosensitizer dose (and vehicle), the drug–light interval, and the wavelength/band, irradiance (mW cm^{-2}) and fluence (J cm^{-2}) of light. Total effective fluence, taking into account incident spectral irradiance, optical transmission through tissue, and absorption by photosensitizer, has been proposed as a method for more accurate dosimetry but light dosage can only be estimated from the energy fluence in practice.[17] Comparison of dosimetry between studies is thus prevented as a significant proportion of incident light may be of relatively ineffective wavelengths.

Fluence rates greater over 150 mW cm^{-2} may induce hyperthermic injury and should be avoided if the intention is to deliver a pure PDT effect. Fractionation (discontinuous illumination) may improve tumor responsiveness by permitting tissue re-oxygenation during 'dark' periods. MAL-PDT is approved on the basis of a double treatment one week apart, this 'long-interval' fractionation presumed to target residual disease before re-epithelialization and re-growth occur.

Choice of light source requires consideration of their relative efficiency for the photosensitizer used and for the indications proposed. One method of comparison is to map, for each lamp, the spectral output to PpIX absorption, total power, size of illumination field and ease and cost of use. Flexibility to adapt to the use of other photosensitizers should also be considered.

How the photodynamic effect is achieved

The rationale of the therapeutic efficacy of PDT is based on the cytotoxic action of products generated by excited photosensitizers.[1] When a photosensitizer absorbs light of the appropriate wavelength it is converted from a stable ground state to a short-lived singlet state that may undergo conversion to a longer-lived excited triplet state. This is the photo-active species responsible for the generation of cytotoxic products. This may either directly react with substrate by hydrogen atom or electron transfer to form radicals (type I reaction), or the triplet state can transfer its energy to oxygen directly to produce singlet oxygen. Singlet oxygen is highly reactive in biological systems (type II reaction), causing photo-oxidation and cell death (Fig. 42.3). The complete process, with excitation of photosensitizer, transfer of energy through intersystem crossings, to excitation of oxygen from its triplet state and the subsequent quenching of singlet oxygen through cytotoxic mechanisms, takes place in a time scale of microseconds.

The effect of PDT on cells depends on the concentration and localization of the sensitizer and its efficiency in that environment, the light dose reaching the cell and the oxygen supply. As the diffusion distance of singlet oxygen in cells is estimated to be only 0.1 µm, cell damage is likely to be close to the site of its generation. For lipophilic photosensitizers, including Photofrin and Protoporphyrin IX, inhibition of mitochondrial enzymes may be the key event in PDT cell death.

The predominant mechanism of action of PDT is presumed to be direct tumor cell kill. In PDT with

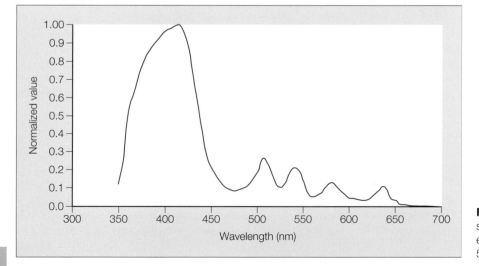

Figure 42.2 Protoporphyrin absorption spectrum – demonstrating maximum excitation at 410 nm, with further peaks at 510, 545, 580 and 635 nm.

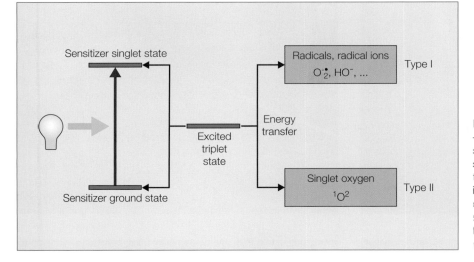

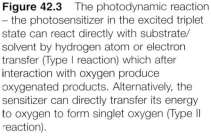

Figure 42.3 The photodynamic reaction – the photosensitizer in the excited triplet state can react directly with substrate/solvent by hydrogen atom or electron transfer (Type I reaction) which after interaction with oxygen produce oxygenated products. Alternatively, the sensitizer can directly transfer its energy to oxygen to form singlet oxygen (Type II reaction).

systemically administered photosensitizers, an important contribution to tumor destruction is also achieved via damage to the vascular supply. Topical ALA-PDT appears to rely on direct tumor cell destruction to achieve a therapeutic effect. Immunologic effects such as the elimination of small foci of cancer cells that have escaped PDT-induced cytotoxicity may also contribute to the success of PDT although its importance remains undetermined. Tumor-sensitized immune cells and the anti-tumor activity of inflammatory cells probably both contribute to this immune response.

TOPICAL PDT IN PRACTICE

Figure 42.4 demonstrates the sequence of preparation a patient would receive for MAL-PDT for extensive actinic keratoses. The extent of lesion preparation required remains unclear. Removal of overlying crust and scales with gauze soaked in saline, forceps, or by gentle curettage is probably helpful but no study has confirmed this. For nodular BCC treated by topical MAL-PDT, the need for lesion preparation is probably more critical. A debulking curettage, avoiding the edge of the lesion, facilitates effective therapy. This is unlike typical curettage as this gentle debulking is without the need for local anesthesia and by sparing the edges and base of the lesion, probably preserves the superior cosmesis that is consistently seen after PDT. A thin layer of photosensitizer is applied, typically of a thickness of only 1 mm, including a margin of 5–10 mm around the visible borders of lesions. An occlusive dressing to retain cream and to minimize ambient light exposure should then be applied. The patient is free to leave, returning 3 hrs later (4–6 hrs if standard ALA-PDT with red light), for removal of excess cream and optional check of surface fluorescence with an ultraviolet 'Woods' lamp (Fig. 42.5), (e.g. UVL-56, Upland CA, USA) – helpful in confirming PpIX generation at least in superficial part of the lesion. Levulan PDT for actinic keratoses involves mixing 5-ALA powder together with solution vehicle in the Levulan Kerastick, then dabbing gently the mixed solution onto lesions, allowed to dry, then re-applied. Patients leave the office, without the need for occlusion of lesions, but with advice to minimize light exposure and not to wash the treatment site. 14–18 hrs later, blue light is delivered via the Blu-U for 1000 seconds to provide a 10 J/cm^{-2} light dose.

There is the option for either pre-treatment application of a topical anesthetic, e.g. Ametop cream (Smith & Nephew, Cambridge, UK), applied following removal of excess 5-ALA 30–45 minutes prior to illumination, or provision during illumination of local injected anesthesia, e.g. 1–2% lidocaine. Analgesia prior to treatment is advocated by some practitioners while others recommend a fan or cool air system to minimize sensations of prickling/burning/stinging experienced during illumination with typical treatment times of 15 min.

It remains important to ensure that the entire lesion plus at least a 5 mm border is illuminated for the entire duration of treatment – and greater margins are important at mobile sites, e.g. the chest, where respiratory excursion necessitates a generous treatment field margin. The treatment site should then be protected from ambient light for up to 24–48 hrs. When MAL-PDT is used, the treatment is repeated after 1 week. For 5-ALA preparations, it is common to assess outcome after 6–8 weeks, before determining the need for repeat treatment. Comparison literature is currently lacking as to the optimal protocol.

INDICATIONS

Actinic keratoses

Topical ALA-PDT clears 71–100% of facial actinic keratoses in a single treatment (Fig. 42.6).[3] A single ALA-PDT treatment was as effective as 3 weeks of topical 5-fluorouracil in patients with extensive disease affecting both hands, a site where thick actinic keratoses may predominate.[18] Topical PDT with MAL and the 5-ALA formulation Levulan have been approved only for non-hyperkeratotic actinic keratoses of the face and scalp,

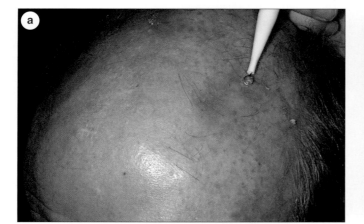

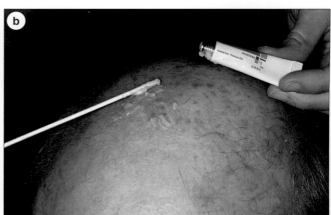

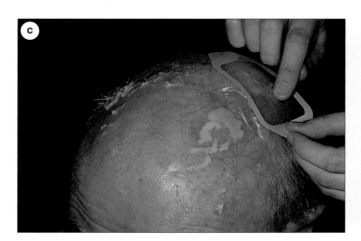

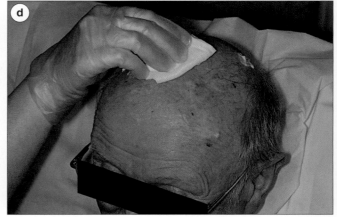

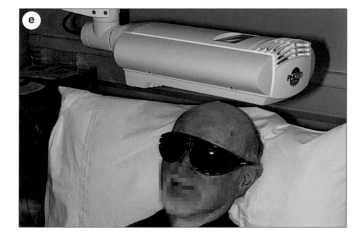

Figure 42.4 Preparation of a patient with widespread actinic keratoses on scalp for MAL-PDT: (a) Gentle crust removal. (b) Application of thin layer of ALA or MAL cream. (c) Occlusion of cream (followed by light occlusion). (d) Removal of excess cream. (e) Illumination, typical time, 15 min.

but thin/moderate thickness lesions can probably respond well at any site. The similarity of effect of single PDT with topical 5-fluorouracil still suggests potential benefit in patients with widespread acral disease. In these cases, scattered residual thick actinic keratoses could be treated by cryotherapy/curettage. This represents a practical combined therapy approach to a difficult management problem.

Most studies have assessed efficacy in Caucasian skin, but ALA-PDT for actinic keratoses in oriental patients achieved a clearance rate of 82% for facial lesions (although 3–6 treatments were required), suggesting pigmentation reduces response rate to individual treatments.[3]

Phase III trials using the 5-ALA formulation Levulan and blue light in 241 patients with non-hyperkeratotic lesions of the head, reported a 72% complete response at 12 weeks versus 20% for those treated by vehicle and light alone.[19] A randomized multi-center comparison of 699 actinic keratoses (thin or moderate thickness, 92% situated on the face or scalp) assesses MAL-PDT in comparison with cryotherapy.[20] Overall response rates, at 3 months, to a single treatment session were similar between the groups (69% for PDT, 75% for cryotherapy) but cosmetic outcome was superior in the PDT. In a second study of MAL-PDT compared with cryotherapy for AK (*n*=855), Foley *et al.*[21] demonstrated PDT to be

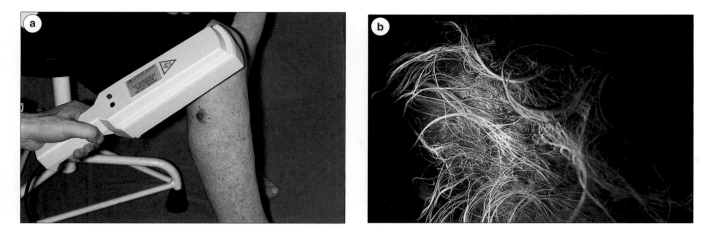

Figure 42.5 (a) Woods light illumination of lesion. (b) Intense surface fluorescence in BCCs on scalp that were difficult to delineate clinically, but clearly outlined using the Woods lamp.

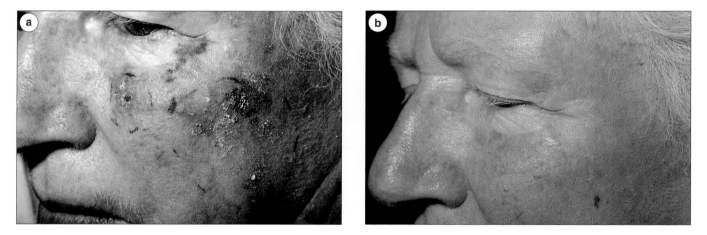

Figure 42.6 Extensive facial actinic keratoses before and following ALA-PDT. (a) Pre-PDT. (b) Following ALA-PDT.

more efficacious (91% for PDT, 68% for cryotherapy after 3 months), again with superior cosmesis with PDT. The latter study involved two treatments with PDT 7 days apart. In a recent North American trial of MAL-PDT for actinic keratoses, PDT demonstrated an 89% complete lesion response at three months versus 38% placebo treatment per protocol, with excellent or good cosmetic outcome reported in over 90% of PDT patients.[22]

Bowen's disease (squamous cell carcinoma *in situ*)

ALA-PDT is effective in the treatment of Bowen's disease with clearance rates of 90–100% and recurrence rates of 0–10% (Fig. 42.7).[3] Currently, there is no approved indication for topical PDT in Bowen's, but consistent high response rates between many studies will encourage off-label use.

A recent randomized trial has demonstrated that ALA-PDT is superior to topical 5-fluorouracil in Bowen's disease.[23] A total of 40 patients with 66 lesions received either 5% 5-fluorouracil, or ALA-PDT. PDT initially cleared 88% (29/33), compared with 67% (22/33) after 5-fluorouracil, with adverse events more frequent and

severe in the latter group. After 12 months, two recurrences in the PDT group and six in the 5-fluorouracil group reduced clearance to 82% and 48%, respectively with PDT significantly more effective. An earlier comparison of ALA-PDT with cryotherapy in Bowen's disease observed superior clearance with a single treatment (75 *vs* 50%) and fewer adverse events that included ulceration of 25% of the cryotherapy treatment sites.[4] The low incidence of ulceration following PDT is of particular importance in the elderly population developing Bowen's disease. Pain during cryotherapy was more severe than during PDT (*P*=0.01).

Topical ALA-PDT is probably as effective as current routine therapies in small, single patches of Bowen's disease, and may offer particular advantages for large and multiple lesions. In a study of 40 large (20–55 mm) lesions, an initial clearance rate after 1–3 treatments of 88% fell to 78% by 12 months. In the same study, 10 patients, each with three or more patches of Bowen's disease achieved an overall clearance rate with PDT of 89% after 12 months. The absence of serious adverse events and observed good cosmesis were again noted.[24] The treatment by PDT of digital and perianal lesions is also feasible with the advantages of tissue preservation and avoidance of loss of tissue function.

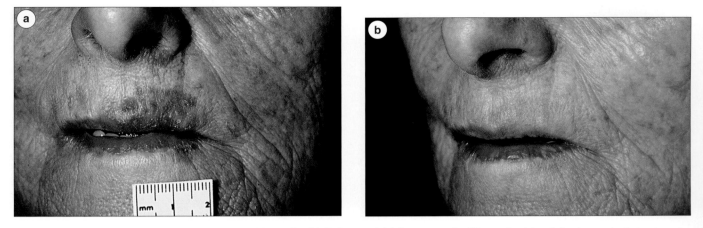

Figure 42.7 Bowen's disease on the upper and lower lip. (a) Before and (b) the same site 12 months later, following a single treatment with ALA-PDT.

Bowen's disease appears to respond well to PDT using systemic photosensitizers, but with the success of topical PDT, there would appear little need for this route of photosensitizer administration.

Open studies of ALA-PDT indicating a wide variance in initial response rates of 54–100% and in recurrence rates (0–69%) in the treatment of squamous cell carcinoma.[3] Until further studies with close follow-up are performed, it would appear advisable not to treat invasive squamous cell carcinomas by topical PDT. Experience of systemic photosensitizer use in squamous cell carcinoma also has demonstrated efficacy but with disappointingly high recurrence rates.

Basal cell carcinoma

Complete clearance rates, after follow-up periods of 3 to 36 months, were 87 and 53%, respectively in a review of 12 studies treating 826 superficial and 208 nodular BCC.[25] For tumors up to 1 mm thick, initial clearances of 81–100% are reported after 1–2 treatments (4–6 hrs 5-ALA application) (Fig. 42.8).[3] Limited data on depth of response is available for thicker superficial BCC although 6/6 up to 2 mm thick, treated at 6 hrs, cleared without recurrence over 6–16 months. Morpheic and pigmented lesions respond poorly to PDT.

Nodular BCC show improved response with ALA-PDT following the use of penetration enhancers. Prior debulking has increased rates to 90 and 92%, respectively. A randomized comparison study of ALA-PDT with cryotherapy for both superficial and nodular BCC observed no significant difference in response. However, fewer adverse events, shorter healing times and superior cosmesis followed PDT.[4]

The only current approved indication for topical PDT is in Europe for superficial and nodular BCC treated by MAL-PDT. Careful lesion preparation followed by a repeat treatment after 7 days appears important in achieving the high clearance rates reported. MAL-PDT has recently been reported to be as efficacious as cryotherapy for superficial BCC with 3 month clearance rates of 97% and

95% following 1–2 treatments of PDT or cryotherapy respectively.[26] PDT achieved superior cosmetic results. A comparison of MAL-PDT with surgery for nodular BCC reports similar 3-month clearance rates of 91 and 98%, with the number of recurrences at 12 months, 2 and 0, respectively. Cosmetic outcome was again superior with PDT.[27]

Systemic photosensitizer-derived PDT for BCC using hematoporphyrin derivative or Photofrin has achieved widely differing initial clearance rates of 52–100%. Topical PDT remains preferable to systemic PDT particularly for single lesions which provide similar high efficacy rates. Systemic PDT may, however, have a particular benefit for patients with basal cell nevus syndrome. The large number of lesions and apparent reduced efficacy with ALA-PDT, would favor treating large numbers of superficial lesions in a single hospital visit using Photofrin. The Roswell Park Group treated 588 superficial and nodular BCC in nine patients with PDT using Photofrin 1 mg/kg 48–96 hrs prior to illumination with an argon laser. Complete clinical response rates in the adults treated ranged from 82–98% after a follow-up of 28 months.[28]

However, long-term follow-up remains essential before a full comparison of topical PDT with standard therapies for BCC can be made. High recurrence rates are a particular early concern of a few studies of topical PDT. Long-term follow-up data indicates a 9% recurrence rate after 45 months (16–73 months) for ALA-PDT in superficial BCC (Fig. 42.9), that is comparable with the 7.5–10.1% 5-year recurrence rates reported for standard therapies in BCC (excluding Mohs).[29] A similar recurrence rate of 11% for superficial and nodular BCC is reported following MAL-PDT after a mean of 35 months.[4]

Cutaneous T-cell lymphoma

Selective uptake of photosensitizers into lymphocytes after topical PDT, with inhibition of T cells has been demonstrated in topical PDT of cutaneous T-cell lymphoma (CTCL). Several small case reports support the efficacy of repetitive treatments with 5-ALA PDT for

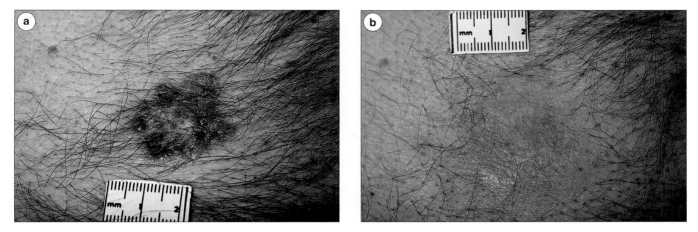

Figure 42.8 Superficial BCC on lower leg. (a) Pre- and (b) post ALA-PDT at 6 months after 2 treatments, 1 week apart.

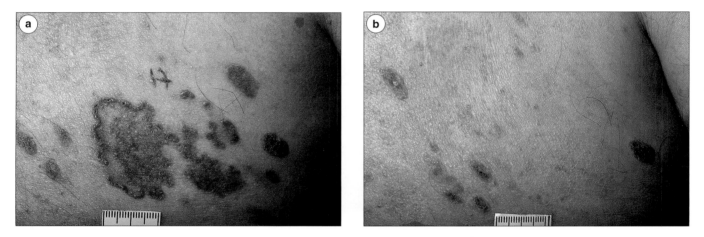

Figure 42.9 Large superficial BCC. (a) pre-PDT and (b) 36 months following ALA-PDT (2 cm ruler just visible).

localized plaque-stage CTCL, but single treatments appear less likely to be successful.[3] There is also one report of the successful clearance of a nodule of CTCL following ALA-PDT.

Non-NMSC cancer applications for topical PDT

The use of topical PDT in vulval intra-epithelial neoplasia (VIN) indicates benefit with multiple treatments, with histological grade of VIN as determinant of response. Topical PDT appears useful as an adjunctive therapy for extramammary Paget's disease. However, clearance of recurrent disease with intralesional 5-ALA and multiple treatments has been shown in one subject, suggesting its potential as monotherapy.[30]

Photofrin-mediated PDT has been studied in AIDS-related Kaposi's sarcoma with control of tumors up to 4 cm in diameter. Greatest effect was seen in studies where both superficial and interstitial laser light was used.

Overall response rates equivalent to other therapeutic modalities, have been achieved and merits further study.[7]

Topical ALA-PDT has not been reported in Kaposi's sarcoma with low efficacy anticipated.

The treatment of skin metastases by PDT has been widely studied. Photofrin-mediated PDT with and without interstitial light diffusing fibres has achieved some dramatic results, but with unpredictable overall response rates. Palliation is achievable for initial small metastases of breast cancer but appears unsuitable for advanced disease. Kennedy *et al.* used topical ALA-PDT to treat four patients with metastatic breast carcinoma.[2] Although strong protoporphyrin IX fluorescence was induced in percutaneous nodules, there was no effect of PDT, using surface illumination.

Experience of the successful treatment of cutaneous metastatic melanoma deposits by PDT is limited.[7] The reduced penetration of light into pigmented lesions reduces the potential for achieving a response with PDT with currently used photosensitizers. Systemic PDT has achieved initial response rates of up to 70% of treated lesions although recurrence rates are high, even if interstitial light fibres are used. Eight cutaneous metastases of melanoma failed to clear after topical ALA-PDT with only superficial tumor necrosis achieved in those amelanotic tumors and no response with melanotic metastases.

Adverse effects

Generalized photosensitivity up to 6–10 weeks following injection of porfimer sodium has been reported. However, no generalized photosensitivity reactions have been observed in clinical studies of topical PDT. ALA-induced PpIX appears to be almost completely cleared from the body within 24 hrs of its induction.

Pain or discomfort, often described as 'burning,' 'stinging' or 'prickling' restricted to the illuminated area, is commonly experienced during ALA-PDT.[3,7] It usually peaks within minutes of commencing light exposure and probably reflects nerve stimulation and/or tissue damage by reactive oxygen species. This discomfort can occasionally persist for hours, and rarely for a few days, at a reduced intensity. Most patients will tolerate ALA-PDT without anesthesia/analgesia. The face and scalp may be more susceptible to pain and large and/or ulcerated lesions are more likely to be painful. Strategies to reduce pain include prior topical/injected local anesthetic, premedication with benzodiazepine, cooling fans or spraying water on lesions during therapy. Since 5-ALA, but not 5-ALA methyl ester, is transported by GABA carriers, it is speculated that the ester might be less likely to provoke nerve fibre stimulation and hence pain.

Immediately following treatment, erythema and edema are common, with erosion, crust formation and healing over 2–6 weeks, but ulceration is very rare. A good cosmetic outcome following ALA-PDT is widely reported. Hyper- or hypo-pigmentation can occasionally be seen in treated areas and usually resolves within six months. Permanent hair loss has been observed following ALA-PDT, but is much less than that observed following radiotherapy.

PDT has the potential of promoting genotoxic effects including induction of DNA strand breaks, chromosomal aberrations and alkylation of DNA. However, porphyrin molecules also possess anti-mutagenic properties. ALA-PDT delays photocarcinogenesis in mice. Overall, evidence would indicate that the risk of cancer associated with PDT to be low, but in view of the latent period for carcinogenesis, careful reporting of malignancies in sites of prior PDT is advised.

FUTURE OUTLOOK

PDT is attractive because it permits repeat treatment on a tumor selective basis with minimal scarring and low systemic toxicity. The potential of this topical PDT is currently limited by the depth of therapeutic effect. The use of longer wavelength light with new photosensitizers and the advent of interstitial light delivery could further extend this depth.

Research is now underway to assess the potential of topical PDT as a cancer prevention therapy, through periodic treatments to high-risk patients, e.g. renal transplant recipients, to determine whether the treatment of sub-clinical disease can reduce the incidence of subsequent skin cancer development.

The potential to harness the clinical benefits of fluorescence diagnosis enhances the appeal of utilizing the photodynamic therapy process. Delineation of sub-clinical disease by fluorescence, followed by targeting of 'hot-spots', could offer substantial benefit to high-risk patients, currently enduring multiple surgical excisions, sometimes with grafting.

Emerging home topical therapies also offer many benefits, but the achievement of reported high efficacy depends on compliance with typically irritant medications. PDT offers the advantage of being a supervised outpatient therapy for the typically elderly patient population developing cutaneous malignancy, ensuring high compliance.

Treatment associated pain is widely discussed in connection with PDT. It is perhaps unfortunate that initial studies sought to minimize anesthesia in order to clearly study the PDT effect. Experience would suggest that some form of analgesia/local anesthesia is reasonable for multiple/large area disease, especially for facial sites. However, for single small lesion PDT treatments, experience from many studies (including the recent MAL-PDT studies) suggests that pain relief is rarely required. Refining pain/discomfort management in PDT is now the subject of close study.

Topical PDT has also been studied in many non-cancer indications. Experience of this modality in most applications remains limited but most attention has been towards studies supporting efficacy in viral warts, acne, and psoriasis.[30] The potential of PDT to become another tool of the dermatologist will encourage efforts to maximize the use of this therapy in oncologic-related skin disorders.

REFERENCES

1 Henderson BW, Dougherty TJ. How does photodynamic therapy work? Photochem Photobiol 1992; 55:145–157.

2 Kennedy JC, Pottier RH, Pross DC. Photodynamic therapy with endogenous protoporphyrin IX: Basic principles and present clinical experience. J Photochem Photobiol B Biol 1990; 6:143–148.

3 Morton CA, Brown SB, Collins C, et al. Guidelines for topical photodynamic therapy: report of a workshop of the British Photodermatology Group. Br J Derm 2002; 146:552–567.

4 Morton CA. The emerging role of 5-ALA-PDT in dermatology: is PDT superior to standard treatments? J Dermatol Treat 2002; 13(1):S25–S29.

5 Fritsch C, Lang K, Neuse W, Ruzicka T, Lehmann P. Photodynamic diagnosis and therapy in dermatology. Skin Pharmacol Appl Skin Physiol 1998; 11:358–373.

6 Daniell MD, Hill JS. A history of photodynamic therapy. Aust NZ J Surg 1991; 61:340–348.

7 Kalka K, Merk H, Mukhtar H. Photodynamic therapy in dermatology. J Am Acad Derm 2000; 42:389–413.

8 Szeimies RM, Sassy T, Landthaler M. Penetration potency of topical applied 5-aminolaevulinic acid for photodynamic therapy of basal cell carcinoma. Photochem Photobiol 1994; 59:73–76.

9 Roberts DJH, Cairnduff F. Photodynamic therapy of primary skin cancer: a review. Br J Plast Surg 1995; 48:360–370.

10 Sternberg ED, Dolphin D. Second generation photodynamic agents: a review. J Clin Laser Med Surg 1993; 11(5):233–241.

11 Santoro O, Banieramonte G, Melloni E, et al. Photodynamic therapy by topical meso-tetraphenylporphinesulfonate tetrasodium salt administration in superficial basal cell carcinomas. Cancer Res 1990; 50:4501–4503.

12 Gupta G, Morton CA, Whitehurst C, et al. Photodynamic therapy with meso-tetra(hydroxyphenyl)chlorin in the topical treatment of Bowen's disease and basal cell carcinoma. Br J Derm 1999; 141:385–386.

13 Warloe T, Heyerdahl H, Peng Q, Giercksky K-E. Photodynamic therapy with 5-aminolaevulinic acid induced porphyrins and skin penetration enhancer for basal cell carcinoma. SPIE 1994; 2371:226–235.

14 Morton CA, MacKie RM, Whitehurst C, et al. Photodynamic therapy for basal cell carcinoma: effect of tumor thickness and duration of photosensitizer application on response. Arch Derm 1998; 134:248–249.

15 Pottier RH, Chow YFA, LaPlante JP, et al. Non-invasive technique for obtaining fluorescence excitation and emission spectra in vivo. Photochem Photobiol 1986; 44:679–687.

16 Morton CA, Whitehurst C, Moore JV, MacKie RM. Comparison of red and green light in the treatment of Bowen's disease by photodynamic therapy. Br J Derm 2000; 143:767–772.

17 Moseley H. Total effective fluence: a useful concept in photodynamic therapy. Lasers Med Sci 1996; 11:139–143.

18 Kurwa HA, Yong-Gee SA, Seed PT, et al. A randomized paired comparison of photodynamic therapy and topical 5-fluorouracil in the treatment of actinic keratoses. J Am Acad Derm 1999; 41:414–418.

19 Ormrod D, Jarvis B. Topical aminolevulinic acid HCL photodynamic therapy. Am J Clin Derm 2000; 1(2):133–139.

20 Szeimies M, Karrer S, Radakovic-Fijan S, et al. Photodynamic therapy using topical methyl-5-aminolevulinate compared with cryotherapy for actinic keratosis: A prospective, randomized study. J Am Acad Derm 2002; 47:258–262.

21 Foley P, Freeman M, Vinciullo C, et al. A comparison of photodynamic therapy using Metvix with cryotherapy in actinic keratosis. J Eur Acad Derm Venereol 2001; 15(2):223.

22 Pariser DM, Lowe NJ, Stewart DM, et al. Photodynamic therapy with topical methyl aminolevulinate for actinic keratoses: results of a prospective randomized multicenter trial. J Am Acad Derm 2003; 48:227–232.

23 Salim A, Leman JA, McColl JH, et al. Randomized comparison trial of photodynamic therapy with topical 5-fluorouracil in Bowen's disease. Br J Derm 2003; 148:539–543.

24 Morton CA, Whitehurst C, McColl JH, et al. Photodynamic therapy for large or multiple patches of Bowen's disease and basal cell carcinoma. Arch Dermatol. 2001; 137:319–324.

25 Peng Q, Warloe T, Berg K, et al. 5-ALA based photodynamic therapy. Cancer 1997; 79(12):2282–2308.

26 Basset-Sequin N, Ibbotson S, Emtestam L, et al. Photodynamic therapy using Metvix is as efficacious as cryotherapy in BCC, with better cosmetic results. J Eur Acad Derm Venereol 2001; 15(2):226.

27 Rhodes LE, Rie M De, Enstrom Y, et al. A randomized comparison of excision surgery and PDT using methyl aminolevulinate in nodular basal cell carcinoma. Presented at the Annual Meeting of the American Academy of Dermatology, San Francisco, USA, 2003.

28 Buscaglia DA, Wilson BD, Shanler SD, et al. Photodynamic therapy with Photofrin successfully treats basal cell carcinomas in patients with basal cell nevus syndrome. Presented at the 5th International Photodynamic Association Meeting, Amelia Island, Florida, 1994.

29 Leman JA, Morton CA, MacKie RM. Treatment of superficial basal cell carcinomas with topical photodynamic therapy; recurrence rates and outcome. Br J Derm 2001; 145(59):17.

30 Ibbotson SH. Topical 5-aminolaevulinic acid photodynamic therapy for the treatment of skin conditions other than non-melanoma skin cancer. Br J Derm 2002; 146:178–188.

CHAPTER
43   Laser Surgery for Skin Cancer

Laurie Jacobson and Roy Geronemus

Key points

- Some premalignant and malignant cutaneous neoplasms can be treated effectively with laser surgery, photodynamic therapy, or laser-assisted photodynamic therapy.
- The lasers most commonly utilized to treat cutaneous neoplasms are the carbon dioxide and pulsed dye lasers.
- Patients who are poor surgical candidates (on a pacemaker, with a bleeding diathesis, etc.) can often be treated safely with laser surgery. In addition, for those patients who have multiple carcinomas (for example, those with basal cell nevus syndrome), laser therapy provides an excellent treatment option.
- Laser-assisted photodynamic therapy is a rapidly emerging tool used to treat actinic keratoses and actinic cheilitis without a lengthy recovery period or discomfort.
- In general, lasers should not be utilized to treat malignant melanoma unless surgery is not an option.

INTRODUCTION AND HISTORY

The term LASER was first presented by Maiman in 1960, and is an acronym for *l*ight *a*mplification by *s*timulated *e*mission of *r*adiation. Laser technology is particularly applicable to medicine due to its unique properties – monochromaticity, spacial coherence, and intense brightness. Monochromaticity refers to light emission at a single wavelength which translates therapeutically to selective absorption of its energy by a specific chromophore (light-absorbing compound). Spacial coherence allows for radiation to be focused onto a small spot facilitating high-energy delivery and the ability to target small cellular components. Due to the amplification process, lasers generate brightness that is greater than any natural light source.[1] Some of the first laser studies in medicine were performed on skin due to the accessibility of this organ. With the rapid evolution of laser technology, it is now possible to effectively eradicate most premalignant and malignant cutaneous neoplasms with laser surgery, photodynamic therapy, or laser-assisted photodynamic therapy.

The major components of every laser system include a power source, a gain medium and optical resonators. The power source pumps the randomly moving atoms to an excited state with use of electrical energy, effectively increasing the frequency of stimulated emission. Stimulated emission occurs when an electron in the excited state is stimulated by another photon of equivalent wavelength and frequency. Upon return to its resting state, this atom can now emit two photons of light energy of the same frequency and wavelength traveling the same direction in spacial and temporal phase. Optical resonators consist of a pair of mirrors at either end of the laser cavity, which amplify the stimulated emission. The energized photons travel back and forth, and at one end of the laser, one of the mirrors is partially reflective so that the laser light can be emitted. The most variable component of a laser is the gain medium, which refers to atoms or molecules that have been stimulated into an excited state. The medium can be gas (argon, carbon dioxide, or helium with neon), liquid (fluorescent dye dissolved in an organic solvent), solid (a simple crystal – ruby or alexandrite or an active element supported by crystal – Nd:Yag), or a semiconductor (diode). The gain medium determines the wavelength of light emitted.

According to the Grothus – Draper law of physics, a photochemical reaction in tissue can only occur provided light energy is absorbed. There are three chromophores (light absorbing compounds) that allow these reactions to occur in skin – hemoglobin, water, and melanin, each of which has its own specific peak absorption wavelengths. The wavelength of light emitted by a laser determines the biologic chromophore affected, and ultimately, its therapeutic potential. Laser light can be emitted in the ultraviolet range (100–400 nm), the visible range (400–720 nm), near infrared (720–1000 nm) and the mid- and far- infrared range (1000–10,000 nm). Yellow–orange laser energy (530–595 nm) has the ability to destroy vascular lesions because it closely matches oxyhemoglobin's peak absorption. Meanwhile, lasers that emit in the infrared range are primarily absorbed by water so that nonselective destruction of tissue occurs. Red and near-infrared laser energies (630–755 nm) are not strongly absorbed by blood and have the ability to destroy pigmented lesions due to melanin absorption.

Aside from the wavelength of light emitted from a laser, the other major parameter that determines its effect on tissue is the duration of exposure that the laser has upon the skin's surface. Laser light can be emitted in a continuous, pulsed, or q-switched mode. Continuous wave lasers deliver little to no variation in power output over time, but the emission can be shuttered to produce pulses that may vary from 0.01 to several seconds in duration. In general, these lasers produce less specifically localized injury than do pulsed lasers. A pulsed laser emits high energy, very brief pulses of light that are generally much shorter than those provided by shuttered continuous wave lasers. The energy delivered is not constant, but instead builds, peaks, and tapers off in less than one millisecond's time. Q-switched lasers deliver extremely high intensity pulses of nanosecond duration. An electromagnetic switch within the laser cavity allows for the accumulation of energy during the majority of the natural pulse time followed by its release in a powerful, brief pulse.

DESCRIPTION OF PROCEDURE/THERAPY

Lasers used for treatment of precancerous and cancerous skin lesions

Ruby
Although current use of the ruby laser for treatment of cutaneous cancers is limited, it was the first laser to be developed, and subsequently utilized, for that purpose. Ruby laser light, which emits energy at a wavelength of 694 nm, is primarily absorbed in skin by the chromophore melanin and slightly by hemoglobin. The active medium is ruby (aluminum oxide) crystal doped with chromium ions. Initial studies by Goldman using the ruby in the normal-mode (millisecond pulse duration) to treat basal cell carcinoma, squamous cell carcinoma, melanoma, Kaposi's sarcoma, mycosis fungoides, and breast cancer revealed the laser's ability to effect coagulation necrosis and its deeper reaction in pigmented lesions. Today's q-switched ruby laser emits higher energy in nanosecond pulse durations, allowing for selective melanosome destruction.

Argon
The argon laser has been used to treat lentigo maligna, Kaposi's sarcoma, Bowen's disease and bowenoid papulosis. Argon laser light emits energy at six different wavelengths, with peak emissions at 488 and 514 nm. Melanin and hemoglobin are its primary tissue chromophores and argon gas is its active medium. Treatment of cancer with this system is limited, due to its 1 mm maximal depth of coagulation.

Neodynium: yttrium-aluminum-garnet (Nd:Yag)
The Nd:Yag laser has been used to treat basal cell carcinoma, lentigo maligna, squamous cell carcinoma, bowenoid papulosis, actinic keratoses, leukoplakia, and Bowen's disease. The laser emits energy in the near infrared spectrum at 1064 nm, which does not have a specific skin chromophore and at 532 nm which is absorbed by both hemoglobin and melanin. Due to its lack of a chromophore at 1064 nm, treatment at this wavelength can penetrate the skin up to 6 mm.[2] This greater penetration gives it the ability to treat deeper, solid tumors, but it often does so with resultant atrophic and hypertrophic scarring.

Carbon dioxide
The carbon dioxide laser is unique in that it can be utilized in the focused mode to bloodlessly excise tissue or in the defocused mode to vaporize tissue. With emission of infrared light at 10,600 nm, it is strongly absorbed by tissue water and is perhaps the most widely used laser in the treatment of precancerous and cancerous lesions. Since 80% of skin is composed of water and vaporization is a rapid process, thermal damage to adjacent tissue is usually limited to 600 micrometers or less. Because infrared light is invisible, the aiming beam for the laser is a coaxially mounted helium-neon laser that emits low intensity red light at 632.8 nm.

The versatility this laser offers rests on its ability to change the focus of the beam. Maintaining the laser handpiece closer than 1 inch from the skin (focused mode) creates a small spot size, high-power density and high tissue temperature leading to tissue cutting. In contrast, by moving the handpiece away from the skin, the result is a larger spot size, lower-power density, and lower temperature generation leading to tissue vaporization. Benefits of the focused mode for excision include its ability to treat patients with highly vascular tumors, those taking anticoagulants, with a pacemaker, or with a bleeding diathesis. A major drawback with this mode involves the thermal damage to the margins of the excision, perhaps obscuring the histological analysis. This should be kept in mind if using the laser for Mohs micrographic surgery as sections will need to be cut more deeply into the block to obtain undamaged tissue, resulting in potential false positive analysis. Also regarding Mohs surgery, dehydrated sections obtained from laser excision may be difficult to adhere to glass slides. This can be alleviated with the use of albumin as a tissue adherent. The thermal damage and subsequent dehydration following laser excisions may compromise the viability of skin grafts or wound closures.

There are many advantages of this laser system over use of traditional scalpel surgery for excision of cancerous lesions. In the focused mode, it provides hemostasis by sealing off blood vessels that are 0.5 mm or less in diameter, and in the defocused mode large vessels can be sealed and coagulated, providing a bloodless surgical field. Carbon dioxide lasers are a viable treatment alternative for patients with a pacemaker since hemostasis is provided by the laser itself and there is no need for use of high frequency electric current (electrodessication). It also minimizes postoperative pain and edema by sealing off nerve endings and lymphatics, respectively. The laser does not come into contact with the surgical field, minimizing the risk of postoperative infection or transfer of malignant cells. Compared with techniques that rely on thermal destruction, carbon dioxide laser use results in minimal adjacent tissue injury and ultimately, decreased scarring.

A significant disadvantage of this treatment modality is the plume of smoke that is generated by vaporization of tissue. This can be ameliorated with attentive use of a smoke evacuator, protective masks, goggles and filters, but the risk of inhalation of aerosolized viral particles is real. This is especially concerning if the laser is used to treat bowenoid papulosis or verrucous carcinoma

(Buschke–Loewenstein) which harbor human papilloma virus particles.

Pulsed dye

Pulsed dye lasers emit light in the yellow portion of the visible spectrum and are used for the treatment of actinic keratoses via photodynamic therapy. The laser's active medium is rhodamine dye, an orange solid dissolved in a solvent, which is pumped by a flashlamp and delivered to tissue via fiber optics. Its primary tissue chromophore is oxyhemoglobin and, to a much lesser degree, melanin.

INDICATIONS AND CONTRAINDICATIONS

Precancerous and cancerous skin lesions treated with laser therapy

Actinic keratoses and actinic cheilitis

Actinic keratoses and actinic cheilitis are premalignant lesions, which are confined to the epidermis but may eventuate into invasive squamous cell carcinoma. A wide array of treatment modalities are available including cryotherapy, topical chemotherapy, electrodessication and curettage, chemical peels, and more recently available, photodynamic therapy and laser resurfacing. Potential risks and limitations of the ablative therapies (cryotherapy, electrodessication and curettage, medium depth chemical peels) include hypopigmentation, scarring, lengthy healing times, discomfort during treatment and inability to treat large body surface areas in a single session. Meanwhile, use of topical chemotherapy such as 5-fluorouracil leads to significant erythema and crusting, a lengthy recovery period, photosensitivity and discomfort. Patient compliance is often an issue with this modality due to the marked and unsightly inflammatory response elicited by the medication.

Photodynamic therapy (PDT) involves the application of photosensitizing drugs that are preferentially absorbed and concentrated in tumors and hyperproliferating tissues. A laser light source in the visible spectrum then activates the photosensitizer to create activated oxygen species. The topical photosensitizer most commonly utilized is 5-aminolevulinic acid (5-ALA), a precursor of the heme biosynthetic pathway, which generates the porphyrin metabolite protoporphyrin IX. Activation of photoreactive protoporphyrin IX by visible light produces singlet oxygen, which oxidizes tumors and hyperproliferative tissues leading to ultimate cell necrosis.

Historically, light sources that have been used for PDT include coherent light sources such as the argon dye laser (630 nm), gold vapor laser (628 nm), diode lasers, and Nd:Yag lasers and incoherent light sources such as a modified slide projector or high pressure lamps. Most commonly in practice, an incoherent blue light source has been utilized. Any light source can be used provided that it emits near the sensitizer's absorption peaks.[3] The hematoporphyrin derivatives such as protoporphyrin IX display peak absorption at 505, 540, 585, 630 nm.[3,4] Disadvantages of PDT include pain during the 15 min illumination period, post treatment

erythema and crusting that may last for weeks, photosensitivity, and 14–16 hr period between photosensitizer application and treatment time.

Foley et al.[4] assessed the efficacy and cosmetic outcome of actinic keratoses treated with cryotherapy against those treated with PDT. In their phase III trial, they used methyl 5-aminolevulinic acid followed by illumination with a red-light source. A total of 200 patients with 855 actinic keratoses were assessed at 3 months following treatment. They reported greater actinic keratosis clearance with PDT as well as superior cosmesis. While 83% of patients reported excellent cosmesis with PDT, that percentage fell to 51% with cryotherapy.

In 1999, Karrer et al.[5] demonstrated the efficacy of a pulsed laser light source for photodynamic therapy in the treatment of actinic keratoses. Prior to this study, continuous wave light sources had been primarily utilized for this purpose. Topical 5-aminolevulinic acid PDT was performed on actinic keratoses of the head for 24 patients. Patients were divided into two treatment groups irradiated with either an incoherent light source (160 mW/cm^2, 60–160 J/cm^2) or the long pulsed dye laser (585 nm, 18 J/cm^2). Those treated with the incoherent light source had 84% of lesions cleared while those treated with the LPDL had 79% clearance.

Importantly, the Karrer et al.[5] study not only demonstrated the long-pulse dye laser's efficacy, but also its decreased side effect profile when compared to use of an incoherent light source in the treatment of actinic keratoses. Instead of an average 15 min uncomfortable irradiation period with standard PDT, this time was decreased to 1.5 ms per spot (able to cover an entire face in less than 5 min). The downside of this treatment however, was a purpuric response that lasted for 2 weeks.

More recently, Alexiades et al.[6] demonstrated effective treatment of actinic keratoses without causing purpura using a 595 nm long-pulsed pulsed dye laser as the light source for photodynamic therapy (Figs 43.1–43.3). Topical 5-aminolevulinic acid was applied to over 3000 actinic keratoses for either three hours or overnight (14–16 hrs). Each lesion was subsequently irradiated with 1–4 non-overlapping pulses at 7.5 J/cm, pulse duration of 6–10 ms, 10 mm spot size and with a 30 ms cryogen spray followed by a 30 ms delay prior to each laser pulse.

Laser assisted photodynamic therapy for the treatment of actinic keratoses using a 595 nm laser appears to be a promising new option with fewer side effects and more pleasing aesthetic results than other treatment modalities. At 8 months follow-up, 90% of lesions treated on the head remained clear. In a subset of patients who did not respond to therapy, biopsies were performed. A total of 73% of these 30 lesions were neoplasms and not actinic keratoses, suggesting an even higher clearance rate than that reported. It is the variable pulse width option (1.5–40 ms) of the 595 nm laser that allows prevention of the unsightly purpura associated with other laser systems for PDT. Typically, purpura can be avoided with use of 6–40 ms pulse widths. Its dynamic cooling device provides a protective spray of liquid cryogen (tetrafluoroethane), which reduces the discomfort associated with pulsed dye laser treatments.[7] Additional

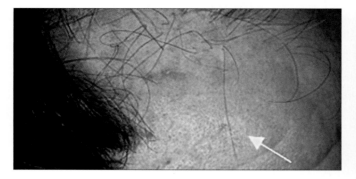

Figure 43.1 Right forehead with actinic keratoses prior to treatment.

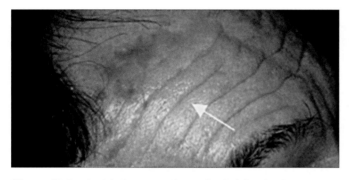

Figure 43.2 Actinic keratoses immediately following laser-assisted photodynamic therapy with increased erythema.

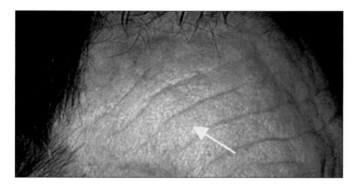

Figure 43.3 1-month following treatment, significant clearing of lesions.

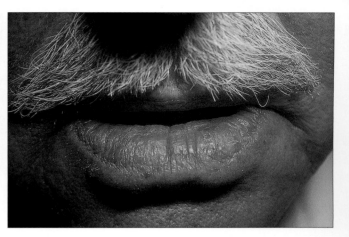

Figure 43.4 Diffuse actinic cheilitis of the lower lip prior to treatment. (From Geronemus, Dover, Arndt and Alora, Illustrated Cutaneous and Aesthetic Laser Surgery (2000); Appleton & Lange.)

benefits include the ability to treat large surface areas (60 lesions per min with 1 Hz and large spot size) and only slight to moderate erythema which resolved within 10 days. They were also able to demonstrate no difference in clearance of lesions whether the topical 5-ALA had been applied for 3 hrs or overnight, allowing patients to remain in the office between photosensitizer application and treatment.

The carbon dioxide laser is another light source that has been successfully utilized in the treatment of actinic keratoses and additionally, actinic cheilitis. In 1997, Trimas et al.[8] treated 14 patients with extensive actinic keratoses with carbon dioxide resurfacing and reported no recurrences at 6–24 months follow-up. In 1999, Massey and Eliezeri[9] treated two patients with extensive actinic

keratoses and history of cutaneous neoplasms who were also treated with resurfacing. Untreated or superficially treated areas did develop skin cancer while treated areas remained cancer and keratosis-free during the follow up period (33 and 52 months following therapy). It should be noted however, that Stratigos et al.[10] reported two patients who did not have evident actinic keratoses prior to resurfacing, but who ultimately developed non-melanomatous skin cancers within 6 months of the procedure. However, the authors conceded that these tumors likely existed even prior to the resurfacing procedure, but were not clinically evident. Since actinic keratoses are limited to the epidermis while neoplasms are thought to originate in follicular stem cells, this suggests that perhaps resurfacing can successfully treat actinic keratoses but not provide adequate prophylaxis for cancerous lesions.

Actinic cheilitis requires a rapid and effective treatment as it has the potential to eventuate into squamous cell carcinoma of the lip, a lesion with greater potential to metastasize than those occurring elsewhere on the face. Treatment options include surgical vermilionectomy, 5-fluorouracil, cryotherapy, electrocautery and carbon dioxide laser resurfacing. Studies have demonstrated successful treatment with carbon dioxide resurfacing for actinic cheilitis[11–13] (Figs 43.4–43.8). This treatment option is often associated with less scarring, superior cosmetic outcome, and decreased pain. Healing of resurfaced lips reportedly only takes 1–3 weeks.[11] A 1992 study assessed the number of passes required to effectively eradicate actinic cheilitis with the carbon dioxide laser.[14] Histological analysis of 23 biopsies from 14 patients showed that complete destruction of the epidermis was observed, irrespective of the number of carbon dioxide laser passes. PDT was performed successfully in three patients with cheilitis, using incoherent visible light and with no recurrence at one year follow up.[15] Early work with laser-assisted photodynamic therapy using a pulsed dye laser has also been promising for the treatment of these lesions (Alexiades-Armenakas et al., unpublished data) (Figs 43.9 and 43.10).

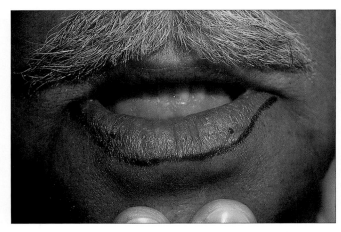

Figure 43.5 The vermilion border has been outlined with a purple marking pen. (From Geronemus, Dover, Arndt and Alora, Illustrated Cutaneous and Aesthetic Laser Surgery (2000); Appleton & Lange.)

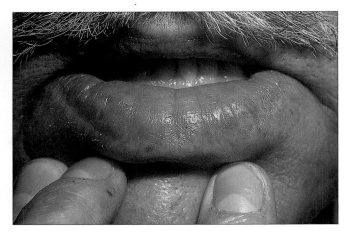

Figure 43.8 Six weeks after treatment, the lower lip is completely healed. (From Geronemus, Dover, Arndt and Alora, Illustrated Cutaneous and Aesthetic Laser Surgery (2000); Appleton & Lange.)

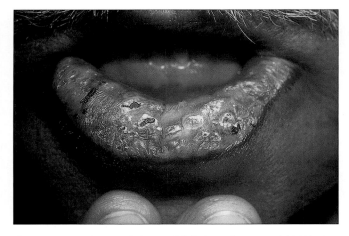

Figure 43.6 Using a defocused CO_2 laser beam and 10 W of power, the lip has been diffusely coagulated. Several charred areas represent focal vaporization. (From Geronemus, Dover, Arndt and Alora, Illustrated Cutaneous and Aesthetic Laser Surgery (2000); Appleton & Lange.)

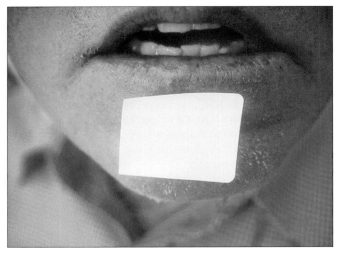

Figure 43.9 Pre-treatment: scaly, erythematous confluent patch of actinic cheilitis on the lower lip.

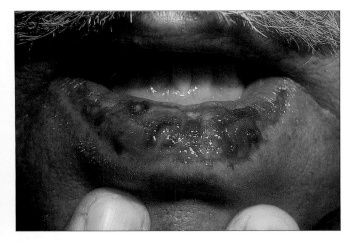

Figure 43.7 One week after treatment, there is hemorrhagic crusting of the lower lip without residual edema. (From Geronemus, Dover, Arndt and Alora, Illustrated Cutaneous and Aesthetic Laser Surgery (2000); Appleton & Lange.)

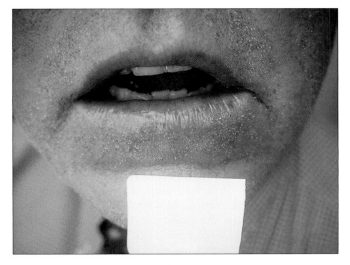

Figure 43.10 Post-treatment: 1 month following laser-assisted photodynamic therapy, significant clearance of lesions.

Basal cell carcinomas

Basal cell carcinomas are the most common type of tumor found in humans, with an incidence of approximately 900,000 cases annually in the US. While the vast majority of BCC are treated with excision, Mohs micrographic surgery, or electrodessication and curettage, effective eradication can also be achieved using the CO_2 laser as well as with photodynamic therapy. Use of laser therapy or PDT may be most helpful for patients with multiple superficial BCC, such as those with basal cell nevus syndrome, or for those who are not good surgical candidates.

The carbon dioxide laser can cause superficial tissue damage over a large area by moving the handpiece away from the skin, in its defocused, or vaporization mode. While early studies in the late 1970s demonstrated BCC clearance rates as low as 50% with the CO_2 laser,[16] recent publications have been far more promising. Wheeland et al.[17] combined traditional curettage with carbon dioxide vaporization of 370 superficial BCC and did not find any recurrences with a follow up ranging from 6–65 months. Iyer et al.[18] treated 61 superficial and nodular BCC with a 4–6 mm margin of healthy tissue with the CO_2 ultrapulse laser with two to eight passes. The number of passes performed was dictated by elimination of the clinical appearance of the tumor. Three cases recurred with an average follow up period of forty months.

Campolmi et al.[19] demonstrated successful CO_2 vaporization of small BCC via intraoperative examination of tissue and clinical follow-up. A total of 140 patients with superficial or nodular BCC less than 1.5 cm were treated with superpulsed CO_2 (1–3 mm spot size, 2–3 ms pulse duration). Skin scraping samples for cytology or biopsies were taken at three points during therapy – prior to treatment, when the papillary dermis was visible and following vaporization of the lesion. The skin samples demonstrated BCC in the specimens obtained prior to and during therapy, but all were clear of tumor following treatment. In addition, there were no recurrences at three-year follow up. In a similar study, Horlock et al.[20] examined 35 patients with 51 BCC treated with the carbon dioxide laser followed by excision and histological analysis of the tumor bed following treatment. Superficial BCC were successfully ablated provided they were lasered to a depth of at least the middle dermis. In contrast, nodular BCC were only eradicated provided they were less than 10 mm in diameter and depth of treatment to the lower dermis was achieved. Humphreys et al.[21] found that superficial BCCs could be successfully treated provided use of three passes and a 4 mm margin of normal tissue were removed.

Benefits of treatment of BCC with the carbon dioxide laser include fast treatment, rapid recovery (7–10 days), minimal scarring, bloodless surgical field, minimal postoperative pain and acceptable cosmetic outcomes. While it is clearly not the treatment of choice for infiltrative, morpheaform, and large nodular BCC, CO_2 vaporization is a viable option for those with multiple superficial BCC or those who simply cannot tolerate surgery (wear a pacemaker, are allergic to lidocaine, etc.).

Carbon dioxide vaporization may be the best treatment option for patients with basal cell nevus syndrome as patients often have multiple BCC that require treatment in a single session. Basal cell nevus syndrome (Gorlin's syndrome) is an autosomal dominant inherited condition, which is associated with abnormalities of the central nervous and skeletal systems in addition to multiple basal cell carcinomas. Simultaneous treatment of numerous cutaneous cancers poses a difficult problem in these patients. Cryosurgery and electrodessication and curettage often leave patients with slowly healing wounds and extensive scarring and hypopigmentation. Studies performed by Nouri et al.,[22] Grobbelaar et al.,[23] and Krunic et al.[24] demonstrated successful eradication of multiple BCC in a single session as well as minimal postoperative scarring, preservation of adjacent normal tissue, rapid treatment, and low postoperative pain.

Photodynamic therapy is another treatment option for basal cell carcinoma. Marmur et al.[25] performed a literature review and found few studies with more than ten patients investigating the use of PDT in the treatment of basal cell carcinomas. These studies had follow up periods ranging from 6 to 35 months, demonstrating recurrence rates ranging from 10–30%. They suggested that currently PDT should only be reserved for those patients who cannot undergo surgical therapy. Fritsh et al.[26] followed 35 patients with 100 superficial BCC. Those BCC greater than 4 cm responded poorly despite three treatment sessions with ALA-PDT. Meanwhile, Morton et al.[27] suggest that PDT should be used as a first line treatment modality for patients who have either large or multiple BCC. With one to three treatment sessions utilizing delta-ALA PDT, 40 patients with large BCC and three patients with multiple BCC showed 88 and 90% clearance of lesions, respectively.

Wang et al.[28] compared the efficacy of superficial and nodular BCC treated with cryotherapy versus PDT. With 1-year follow-up, of the 44 patients treated with ALA-PDT, 25% had a histologically proven recurrence. Meanwhile, of the 39 patients treated with cryotherapy, 15% had a recurrence. In addition, 30% of the lesions in the PDT treated group required an additional treatment. They reported decreased healing time as well as superior cosmesis in the PDT-treated group while pain associated with both procedures was comparable. Clearly, while PDT is not the current treatment of choice for BCC, it is a rapidly evolving research area, which holds great promise.

Squamous cell carcinoma/Bowen's disease/erythroplasia of Queyrat

Squamous cell carcinomas are the second most common tumor found in humans. Due to their potential to metastasize, invasive SCCs should be treated definitively via excision or Mohs micrographic surgery, modalities in which marginal control can be adequately assessed. Conversely, SCC in situ, also known as Bowen's disease, is a superficial lesion that is confined to the epidermal portion of skin and can be treated effectively via non-surgical means such as with cryotherapy, electrodessication and curettage, radiotherapy, lasers or with photodynamic therapy. These non-surgical treatment modalities are especially helpful for those lesions in which surgical removal would result in loss of function, severe disfigurement, or scarring.

Bowenoid papulosis is an eruption of papules or plaques on the genitalia that does not have full thickness atypia but has scattered dysplastic keratinocytes within the epidermis.[29] It is caused by human papillomavirus infection and in some cases, can eventuate into Bowen's disease or invasive SCC. In 1986, Landthaler *et al.*[30] reported successful treatment of six patients with bowenoid papulosis and two with vulvar Bowen's disease in the genital region treated with the argon, Nd:Yag, and carbon dioxide lasers (Figs 43.11 and 43.12). Due to the limited depth of coagulation of the argon laser to only 1 mm and primary chromophores of hemoglobin and melanin, they

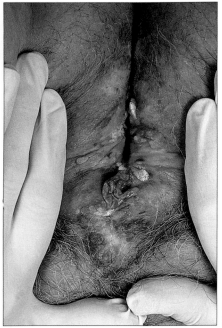

Figure 43.11
Bowenoid papulosis prior to treatment.

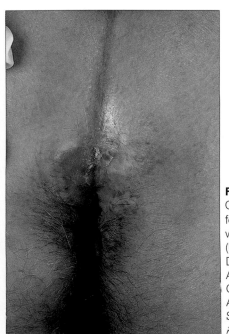

Figure 43.12
Clearance of lesions following treatment with the CO$_2$ laser. (From Geronemus, Dover, Arndt and Alora, Illustrated Cutaneous and Aesthetic Laser Surgery (2000); Appleton & Lange.)

suggested that it be used only for lesions that are erythematous macules or pigmented flat topped papules. It was not suited for treatment of leukoplakia-like whitish lesions or for thicker lesions. Those lesions which were thicker or leukoplakia-like were successfully treated with Nd:Yag or carbon dioxide laser therapy.

Nonsurgical treatment, including laser therapy, for treatment of erythroplasia of Queyrat, or SCC *in situ* of the penis, is worthy of serious consideration since partial and complete penectomies are the standard surgical treatment options available (with a recurrence rate of 19% with amputation). Preservation of sexual function and excellent cosmesis are benefits provided by laser surgery. Van Bezooijen *et al.*[31] reported treatment of 19 cases with a margin of 2 mm or less using the carbon dioxide or Nd:Yag lasers (Figs 43.13–43.15). Retreatment was required in three cases due to incomplete lesion removal at 2-month follow-up. In addition, five patients presented with a true relapse at an average of 25 months following treatment, all of whom were subsequently treated with the carbon dioxide laser and have remained disease free at 5-year follow-up. A single patient who had been clear at 5-year follow-up presented at 6-year follow-up, with an invasive penile SCC. They conclude that use of larger margins (5–8 mm) may be indicated in light of the observed recurrence rate in addition to close follow-up. They also conclude that the carbon dioxide laser should be the laser of choice for these lesions as the Nd:Yag causes deep tissue coagulation, does not cut well and larger defects are created.

In a similar study, Tietjen and Malek[32] reported treatment of 52 men with lesions ranging from PENIN (dysplastic premalignant penile intraepithelial neoplasia) to SCC *in situ* to invasive disease who were treated with carbon dioxide, Nd:Yag, or KTP (potassium-titanyl-phosphate) lasers. Not only were grossly visible lesions treated but also those which displayed aceto-whitening. Postoperative sites were painless despite their appearance otherwise and the cosmetic results were excellent. Complications included pain secondary to infection in one patient with diabetes and lymphedema in another. A total of five patients had a recurrence including one with PENIN, one with SCC *in situ*, two with T1 invasive SCC, and one with T2 invasive SCC. They suggest laser treatment for all such lesions except those patients who have deeply invasive (T2 stage), a history of diabetes, immunosuppression or are on anticoagulation therapy.

Laser therapy has also been successful for treatment of Bowen's disease of the finger. Again, preservation of function and cosmesis is vital in this location, and attempts to avoid surgery and its associated risks of contracture should be considered. In 1996 Gordon and Robinson[33,34] reported five cases of Bowen's disease of the finger of which four were successfully treated with carbon dioxide vaporization using 2 mm margins. None of their patients developed problematic scarring or contracture. They did note that treatment down to the level of the hair follicles would likely require deeper vaporization with increased risk of scar tissue, but since the fingers have few hair follicles, treatment to that level may not be a necessity. They also suggest that any area of nail fold involvement have avulsion of the nail to expose the affected area for sufficient treatment.

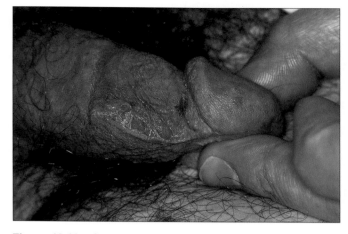

Figure 43.13 Squamous cell carcinoma of the distal shaft and glans of the penis prior to treatment. (From Geronemus, Dover, Arndt and Alora, Illustrated Cutaneous and Aesthetic Laser Surgery (2000); Appleton & Lange.)

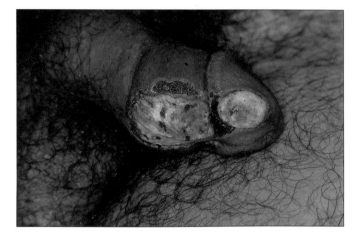

Figure 43.14 Visible abnormal tissue as well as margins of normal skin were vaporized using a defocused CO_2 laser beam and 20 W of power. (From Geronemus, Dover, Arndt and Alora, Illustrated Cutaneous and Aesthetic Laser Surgery (2000); Appleton & Lange.)

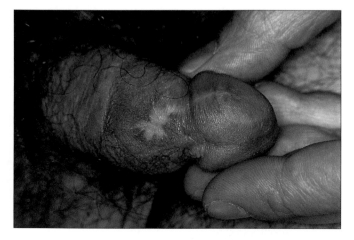

Figure 43.15 Some 6 weeks after treatment, the tumor is completely clear and there is residual pliable scarring with focal depigmentation.

Lentigo maligna

Lentigo maligna, or melanoma *in situ*, generally occurs on the chronically sun-exposed regions of the head and neck of elderly patients. The traditional treatment has been local surgical excision with 5- to 10-mm margins of normal skin. This definitive treatment is currently the gold standard of treatment due to the risk for progression to invasive melanoma. Limitations of this modality include removal of functionally vital tissue that may not have had disease involvement and a delay in margin assessment with the potential requirement for further resection. Though controversial, many cases are currently treated using Mohs micrographic surgery. Detractors believe that assessment of hematoxylin-eosin stained frozen sections of melanocytic lesions is particularly difficult. Alternative non-surgical approaches to treatment include cryosurgery, irradiation and laser therapy. While treatment of lentigo maligna via non-surgical modalities is enticing, there is lack of convincing evidence that laser therapy of such lesions is appropriate unless surgery is not an option.

Treatment of lentigo maligna has been performed in isolated cases using the argon, Q-switched ruby, carbon dioxide and Nd:Yag lasers with mixed results. In a 1984 case report, Arndt reported successful treatment of a nasal lentigo maligna treated with the argon laser[35] (14.5 J/cm², 50 ms). At 8-month follow-up, not only was there a reported excellent cosmetic result, but the lesion was clear both on clinical exam and on histological examination. Notably, however, Arndt reported at 4-year follow-up a histologically proven lentigo maligna contiguous with the previously treated site (Figs 43.16–43.19).[36] He also reported successful treatment of two other lentigo malignas utilizing the argon laser. Successful reports utilizing the Q-switched ruby laser include those by Thissen[37] and Geronemus[38] in which a single patient who was followed for 1 year and three of four patients who were followed for 6–24 months, respectively, were clear of tumor. Conversely, Lee *et al.*[39] describe treatment of two atypical appearing solar lentigines treated with the ruby laser that recurred as lentigo maligna at 1 and 2 years follow-up.

CO_2 laser treatment was performed successfully in four patients with lentigo maligna.[40] Kopera *et al.* treated patients with two passes in the defocused mode with excellent cosmetic results as well as no evidence of recurrence at 11–20 months follow-up. Meanwhile, mixed results were noted when LM was treated with the Q-switched Nd:Yag by Orten *et al.*[41] Two of five patients were successfully treated at 3.5 year follow-up, both of whom received treatment with 532 nm and 1064 nm wavelengths. Those patients who were treated with either 532 nm or 1064 nm had recurrences or did not clear at the time of treatment.

Malignant melanoma

Wide surgical excision remains the standard of care for removal of cutaneous malignant melanoma. Laser procedures are not recommended therapy for these neoplasms as histological analysis of the excised tissue is often difficult due to thermal damage of the tissue margins. Grob[42] reported a case in which an erythematous lesion had been removed with a carbon dioxide laser, only to recur 1 year later as an amelanotic melanoma.

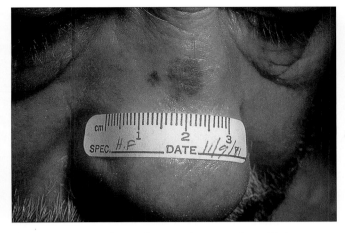

Figure 43.16 Lentigo maligna on the nose of an elderly gentleman prior to treatment. (From Geronemus, Dover, Arndt and Alora, Illustrated Cutaneous and Aesthetic Laser Surgery (2000); Appleton & Lange.)

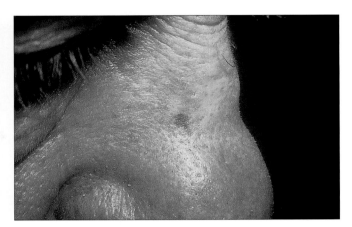

Figure 43.19 Lentigo maligna has reappeared, 4 years later, near the inferior margin of the previous lesion. (Reprinted with permission from Arndt KA. New pigmented macules appearing 4 years after visible light CW and quasi-CW laser treatment of lentigo maligna. J Am Acad Dermatol 1986; 14:1092.)

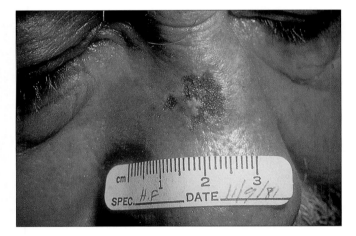

Figure 43.17 Immediately after treatment using the argon laser, a continuous beam, a 1.0 mm spot, and 10 W of power. (From Geronemus, Dover, Arndt and Alora, Illustrated Cutaneous and Aesthetic Laser Surgery (2000); Appleton & Lange.)

On the other hand, metastatic lesions of melanoma have been palliatively treated with the carbon dioxide laser.[43–46] Strobbe *et al.*[43] reported having treated 469 in-transit or satellite lesions in 15 patients. While treatment was easily performed and wound healing was rapid, there was a high incidence of recurrence. They suggest that if lesions are few, excision may be the preferred option, however for those with a large number of lesions, carbon dioxide therapy is advised. Lingam[44] reported successful eradication of metastatic lesions in eight of 14 patients in whom isolated limb perfusion had failed.

FUTURE OUTLOOK

Although lasers are generally not the treatment of choice for most cutaneous neoplasms, they are an effective modality for precancerous lesions such as actinic keratoses and actinic cheilitis and provide an alternative for those patients who are not good surgical candidates. They are especially suited to cases in which both the retention of cosmetic and functional aspects of tissue are vital. Due to the rapid evolution of laser technology, it is likely that new lasers and techniques will be developed which will improve our ability to treat skin cancer in the future.

REFERENCES

1 Freedberg IM, Eisen AZ, Wolff K, et al. Fitzpatrick's dermatology in general medicine. New York, NY: McGraw-Hill; 1999:2901–2921.

2 Anderson RR, Margolis RJ, Watanabe S, et al. Selective photothermolysis of cutaneous pigmentation by Q-switched Nd:Yag laser pulses at 1064, 532, and 355 nm. J Invest Derm 1989; 93:28–32.

3 Fritsch C, Goerz G, Ruzicka T. Photodynamic therapy in dermatology. Arch Derm 1998; 134:207–214.

4 Foley P, Freeman M, Vinciullo C, et al. A comparison of photodynamic therapy with Metvix and cryotherapy in actinic keratosis. Eur Acad Dermatol Venerol 2001; 15(2):223.

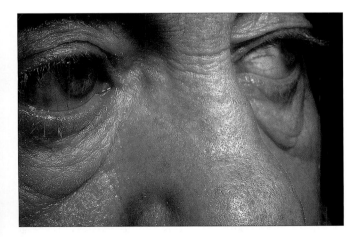

Figure 43.18 Some 6 weeks after treatment, there is complete healing with total clearing of the lesion. (From Geronemus, Dover, Arndt and Alora, Illustrated Cutaneous and Aesthetic Laser Surgery (2000); Appleton & Lange.)

5 Karrer S, Baumler W, Abels C, et al. Long-pulse dye laser for photodynamic therapy: investigations in vitro and in vivo. Surg Med 1999; 25:51–59.

6 Alexiades-Armenakas M, Bernstein L, Mafong E, Geronemus R. Laser-assisted photodynamic therapy of actinic keratoses. Arch Dermatol 2003; 139:1313–1320.

7 Waldorf HA, Alster TS, McMillan K, et al. Effect of dynamic cooling on 585-nm pulsed dye treatment of port-wine stain birthmarks. Derm Surg 1997; 23:657–662.

8 Trimas SJ, Ellis DA, Metz RD. The carbon dioxide laser. An alternative for the treatment of actinically damaged skin. Derm Surg 1997; 23(10):885–889.

9 Massey RA, Eliezri YD. A case report of laser resurfacing as a skin cancer prophylaxis. Derm Surg 1999; 25(6):513–516.

10 Stratigos AJ, Tahan S, Dover JS. Rapid development of nonmelanoma skin cancer after CO_2 laser resurfacing. Arch Derm 2002; 138(5):696–697.

11 David LM. Laser vermilion ablation for actinic cheilitis. J Derm Surg Oncol 1985; 11(6):605–608.

12 Dufresne RG Jr, Garrett AB, Bailin PL, Ratz JL. Carbon dioxide laser treatment of chronic actinic cheilitis. J Am Acad Derm 1988; 19:876–878.

13 Zelickson BD, Roenigk RK. Actinic cheilitis. Treatment with the carbon dioxide laser. Cancer 1990; 65(6):1307–1311.

14 Johnson TM, Sebastien TS, Lowe L, Nelson BR. Carbon dioxide laser treatment of actinic cheilitis. Clinicohistopathologic correlation to determine the optimal depth of destruction. J Am Acad Derm 1992; 27:737–740.

15 Stender IM, Wulf HC. Photodynamic therapy with 5-aminolevulinic acid in the treatment of actinic cheilitis. Br J Derm 1996; 135:454–456.

16 Adams EL, Price NM. Treatment of basal cell carcinomas with a carbon-dioxide laser. J Derm Surg Onc 1979; 5(10):803–806.

17 Wheeland RG, Bailin PL, Ratz JL, Roenigk RK. Carbon dioxide laser vaporization and curettage in the treatment of large or multiple superficial basal cell carcinomas. J Derm Surg Onc 1987; 13(2):119–125.

18 Iyer S, Bowes L, Kricorian G, Friedli A, Fitzpatrick R. Treatment of basal cell carcinoma with the pulsed carbon dioxide laser. Dermatol Surg, in press.

19 Campolmi P, Brazzini B, Urso C, et al. Superpulsed CO_2 laser treatment of basal cell carcinoma with intraoperatory histopathologic and cytologic examination. Derm Surg 2002; 28(10):909–911.

20 Horlock N, Grobbelaar AO, Gault DT. Can the carbon dioxide laser completely ablate basal cell carcinomas? A histologic study. Br J Plast Surg 2000; 53:286–293.

21 Humphreys TR, Malhotra R, Scharf MJ, et al. Treatment of superficial basal cell carcinoma and squamous cell carcinoma in situ with a high-energy pulsed carbon dioxide laser. Arch Derm 1998; 134(10):1247–1252.

22 Nouri K, Chang A, Trent JT, Jimenez GP. Ultrapulse CO_2 used for the successful treatment of basal cell carcinomas found in patients with basal cell nevus syndrome. Derm Surg 2002; 28(3):287–290.

23 Grobbelaar AO, Horlock N, Gault DT. Gorlin's syndrome: the role of the carbon dioxide laser in patient management. Ann Plast Surg 1997; 39(4):366–373.

24 Krunic AL, Viehman GE, Madani S, Clark RE. Microscopically controlled surgical excision combined with ultrapulse CO_2 vaporization in the management of a patient with the nevoid basal cell carcinoma syndrome. J Derm 1998; 25(1):10–12.

25 Marmur E, Schmults CD, Goldberg DJ. Photodynamic therapy for non-melanoma skin cancer. Surg Med 2003; 47:S15.

26 Fritsch C, Goerz G, Ruzicka T. Photodynamic therapy in dermatology. Arch Derm 1998; 134:207–214.

27 Morton CA, Whitehurst C, McColl JH, Moore JV, MacKie RM. Photodynamic therapy for large or multiple patches of Bowen's disease and basal cell carcinoma. Arch Derm 2001; 137(3):319–324.

28 Wang I, Bendsoe N, Klinteberg CA, et al. Photodynamic therapy vs. cryosurgery of basal cell carcinoma results of a phase III clinical trial. Br J Derm 2001; 144(4):832–840.

29 Freedberg IM, Eisen AZ, Wolff K, et al. Fitzpatrick's dermatology in general medicine. New York, NY: McGraw-Hill; 1999:823–839.

30 Landthaler M, Haina D, Brunner R, Waidelich W, Braun-Falco O. Laser therapy of bowenoid papulosis and Bowen's disease. J Derm Surg Oncol 1986; 12(12):1253–1257.

31 Bezooijen BPJ van, Horenblas S, Meinhardt W, Newling DWW. Laser therapy for carcinoma in situ of the penis. J Urol 2001; 166(5):1670–1671.

32 Tietjen DN, Malek RS. Laser therapy of squamous cell dysplasia and carcinoma of the penis. Urology 1998; 52(4):559–565.

33 Gordon KB, Robinson J. Carbon dioxide laser vaporization for Bowen's disease of the finger. Arch Derm 1994; 130(10):1250–1252.

34 Gordon KB, Garden JM, Robinson JK. Bowen's disease of the distal digit. Outcome of treatment with carbon dioxide laser vaporization. Derm Surg 1996; 22(8):723–728.

35 Arndt KA. Argon laser treatment of lentigo maligna. J Am Acad Derm 1984; 10:953–957.

36 Arndt KA. New pigmented macule appearing 4 years after argon laser treatment of lentigo maligna. J Am Acad Derm 1986; 14(6):1092.

37 Thissen M, Westerhof W. Lentigo maligna treated with ruby laser. Acta Derm Venereol 1997; 77(2):163.

38 Kauvar ANB, Geronemus RB. Treatment of lentigo maligna with the Q-switched ruby laser. Lasers Surg Med 1995; Suppl 7:48.

39 Lee PK, Rosenberg CN, Tsao H, Sober AJ. Failure of Q-switched ruby laser to eradicate atypical-appearing solar lentigo: report of two cases 1998; 38:314–317.

40 Kopera D. Treatment of lentigo maligna with the carbon dioxide laser. Arch Derm 1995; 131(6):735–736.

41 Orten SS, Waner M, Dinehart SM, Bardales RH, Flock ST. Q-switched neodymium:yttrium-aluminum-garnet laser treatment of lentigo maligna. Otolaryngol Head Neck Surg 1999; 120(3):296–302.

42 Grob M, Senti G, Dummer R. Delay of the diagnosis of an amelanotic melanoma due to CO_2 laser treatment–case report and discussion. Schweiz Rundsch Med Prax 1999; 88(37):1491–1494.

43 Strobbe LJ, Nieweg OE, Kroon BB. Carbon dioxide laser for cutaneous melanoma metastases: indications and limitations. Eur J Surg Oncol 1997; 23(5):435–438.

44 Lingam MK, McKay AJ. Carbon dioxide laser ablation as an alternative treatment for cutaneous metastases from malignant melanoma. Br J Surg 1995; 82(10):1346–1348.

45 Hill S, Thomas JM. Use of the carbon dioxide laser to manage cutaneous metastases from malignant melanoma. Br J Surg 1996; 83(4):509–512.

46 Waters RA, Clement RM, Thomas JM. Carbon dioxide laser ablation of cutaneous metastases from malignant melanoma. Br J Surg 1991; 78(4):493–494.

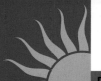

CHAPTER
44

Mohs Surgery: The Full Spectrum of Application

Gregory M Bricca and David Brodland

Key points

- Mohs micrographic surgery (MMS) is the best solution to the dichotomy of complete removal of the skin cancer and tissue conservation.
- Excision is effective for removal of the primary, non-metastatic skin cancer but not metastatic disease. Therefore, excisional margins, whether microscopically controlled or not, should be designed for the primary malignancy, not metastasis.
- MMS has been shown to be highly effective in basal cell and squamous cell carcinomas and a growing body of knowledge is validating its effectiveness in many other types of cutaneous malignancies as well.
- Refinement of the MMS technique has resulted in improvement of its effectiveness and convenience for both the patient and surgeon.
- The indications for MMS are best determined on a patient-to-patient basis and upon the premise that MMS provides the highest cure rates combined with maximal tissue conservation.

INTRODUCTION

There are two seemingly dichotomous precepts that every surgeon faces when treating skin cancer. First and foremost is the complete removal of the skin cancer. All forms of excisional and destructive therapy improve the chance of achieving this goal by widening and deepening the tissue removed.

The other precept, tissue conservation, moderates the temptation to widen and deepen the excision or destruction more than necessary. Why is the goal of complete cancer removal at odds with tissue conservation? The answer is that even the most skilled eye in identifying tumor margins is unacceptably inaccurate. Each millimeter of clinically tumor free skin margin that the surgeon removes increases the statistical probability that subtle or clinically occult tumor extensions will be entirely removed. Unfortunately, each millimeter increase in the tumor free margin enlarges the area of skin removed by the increase squared. Naturally, this becomes a very important consideration in tissue sensitive areas of the body.

Dr Frederick Mohs recognized in 1936 when he began performing chemosurgery for skin tumors that microscopic confirmation of tumor free margins was more accurate than by visual means.[1] He was convinced that

microscopically controlled margins would therefore improve the cancer clearance rate over the standard practice of visualizing tumor margins followed by the excision of the tumor plus a margin of clinically tumor free skin. Through meticulous records, Dr Mohs was able to confirm improved cure rates even in the most difficult of skin cancers.[2] The incorporation of the fresh tissue technique into Mohs surgery made it increasingly feasible to focus on removing smaller margins of normal skin while maintaining the high cure rates.[3]

Today, Mohs micrographic surgery (MMS) virtually eliminates the old dichotomy between complete cancer removal and tissue conservation. The technique has continued to evolve making its use more practical, less time consuming and more convenient for both the patient and physician. Vast numbers of studies have confirmed and reconfirmed cure rates never before achieved for basal cell carcinoma (BCC) and squamous cell carcinoma (SCC). Cure rates are routinely as high as 98 or 99%.[4-8]

Recent studies have begun to validate MMS's effectiveness with other tumor types as well. Mohs surgeons were initially hesitant to utilize their technique in the removal of tumors other than BCC and SCC either because of the unfamiliarity of rarer tumors or due to concern about its efficacy in tumor systems which have the potential for metastasis. These concerns were not prohibitive to Dr Mohs. Throughout his career, he treated what would still be considered very unconventional malignancies such as breast and thyroid cancer, malignancies of the floor of the mouth in addition to cutaneous malignancies such as melanoma, dermatofibrosarcoma protuberance, soft tissue sarcomas, etc.[9]

DESCRIPTION OF PROCEDURE

The original Mohs fixed tissue technique involved the application of zinc chloride paste fixative directly to the skin. The paste is allowed to fixate the tissue for a variable period of time, usually over night. The patient returns in the morning and the fixated tissue is removed and processed for mounting on a slide. Chemosurgery is still used by some Mohs surgeons, however, the prolongation of the process makes it significantly less convenient for the patient and physician.

The most commonly practiced form of MMS today is the fresh tissue technique. This involves snap-freezing the excisional specimen, flattening the leading edge of the specimen into a flat, two-dimensional plane and cutting sections in a cryostat to be placed on a glass slide and stained. This entire process can be performed in 15 to 30 min depending on the complexity of the tissue and the Mohs histotechnician's skill.

MMS entails four important steps (Fig. 44.1). The first step is the identification and delineation of the tumor margins. Often, the only margins that can be assessed are the lateral margins. However, occasionally deep dermal or subcutaneous extensions can be palpated better than seen. The clinically identifiable margins are then marked.

The second step is the excision of the tumor. The tumor is typically debulked either by scalpel excision of the obvious tumor or by curettement. Although this is a very crude method of determining the extent of the tumor, it occasionally helps to characterize a tumor as either superficial or deep. The first tissue specimen is then excised with a margin of skin beyond the clinically obvious lateral margins. This margin varies from less than 1 mm in small, well-defined BCC and SCC to 6–10 mm for larger, more aggressive or ill-defined tumors such as melanoma, Merkel cell, DFSP, MFH, etc. Incisional angles range from 15 to 30 degrees to the skin to perpendicular depending on the desired depth of the excision. In the process of tissue excision, nicks are made in the skin that are perpendicular to and cross the

incision line. Typically, they are placed at 3, 6, 9 and 12-o'clock positions on a circular incision. Larger, more complex shaped tumors may require more than four nicks.

Next, the tissue is carefully divided into pieces small enough to be easily flattened and to fit on a glass slide. The divided wound edges and/or nicks are inked with tissue dyes that can be seen microscopically and help accurately identify and orient the tissue. A map of the tissue depicting the divisions and the color coding of the tissue is made and the specimen is then taken to the Mohs laboratory. The sections are flattened and mounted with tissue mounting medium on a microtome platform or chuck. They are then sectioned into 2–6 μm thick sections and placed on a slide. The slides are then stained; typically with hematoxylin and eosin or toluidine blue.

Once the slides are stained and cover slipped, they can be viewed under the microscope. The Mohs surgeon evaluates the microscopic slide and looks for residual tumor. First, the sections are checked by the surgeon for quality and completeness. If portions of the tissue sections are incomplete or unreadable due to sectioning technique, the physician requests a re-cut in order to be able to evaluate 100% of the margin. The tissue is then examined and any residual tumor is identified and indicated on the map.

If margins remain positive, the map is taken back to the bedside and used to precisely identify the location of the persistent tumor. Another specimen is excised being sure to remove the entire tissue margin that would contain the residual tumor. Tissue uninvolved by the residual tumor, however, is left untouched. A map of the second stage tissue is then made after it has been dyed and is taken back to the Mohs lab again to be processed and evaluated microscopically.

This process is repeated until a tumor free plane is confirmed microscopically. Once complete removal of the tumor is assured, the wound can be evaluated for its suitability for second intention wound healing, reconstruction or referral to a colleague in another subspecialty for reconstruction.

INDICATIONS AND CONTRAINDICATIONS

MMS is the most meticulous technique in evaluating all excision margins and confirming complete tumor extirpation. Traditionally, it has been taught that MMS is indicated in cases of recurrent cancer, cancer located in high risk areas such as the periocular, nasal, perioral and auricular skin, in tumors greater than 2 cm in size and those that have histologic features associated with aggressive behavior.[10] Relative indications would include any cancer where it is felt important to achieve a high cure rate or conserve the maximum of normal tissue.

Some debate has arisen as to whether it is appropriate to perform MMS on certain types of skin cancers, most notably small and/or very superficial skin cancers. The issue of whether it is appropriate to use MMS begs the question of when it is ever inappropriate to meticulously and thoroughly check the entire excisional margin. On the contrary, when is it appropriate to excise

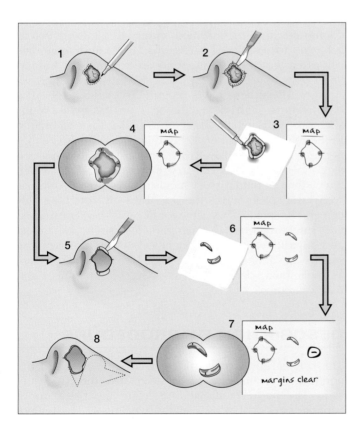

Figure 44.1 MMS technique. (1) First step. Careful physical examination under bright lighting with delineation and marking of tumor margins. (2) Second step. Excision of tumor. (3) Third step. Inking of tissue with tissue dye. A map of the tissue with color coding is made. (4) Fourth step. Microscopic examination of prepared slides and identification of residual tumor. Corresponding marks are made on the map. (5–7) Repeat steps 2, 3 and 4 until histologically tumor free margins are obtained. (8) Reconstruction of defect.

a malignancy but elect to not confirm complete tumor removal histologically or to use a less thorough microscopic method? All tumors, even small ones, can have ill-defined margins. Therefore, what appears to be a small lesion may in fact be substantially larger (Fig. 44.2). For this reason, when the practitioner elects to perform standard excisional surgery on a tumor, it is prudent to excise a margin of normal appearing skin beyond the clinically identifiable tumor. There are studies which have attempted to establish guidelines for margins of excision of tumors without micrographic control.[11–14] When it is practical to elect to excise the clinical tumor plus the safety margins which would statistically give at least a 95% chance of histologically tumor free margins, then standard excision is very reasonable. However, given the availability of micrographically controlled excision, a 95% cure rate should be considered the standard of care for most tumors, especially for common tumors such as BCC and SCC.

Another frequently raised question is whether or not MMS is appropriate to use in tumors that are potentially metastatic. In short, any time it is considered reasonable to attempt to cure a tumor that has metastatic potential by means of excision, the Mohs surgical technique of excision is certainly a reasonable treatment option. Simplistically stated, if excision with clinically tumor free margins augmented by partial microscopic examination of the margins is an acceptable treatment, then how could an argument be made that excision with a more thorough microscopic confirmation of tumor free margins not be considered rational therapy?

Two arguments have been made against the use of MMS for potentially metastatic tumors. The first is that the use of frozen section pathology is inadequate in identifying positive margins. The second is that when the Mohs technique is used and narrower clinically tumor free margins are taken than are routinely recommended for wide excision of these tumors, the patients are put at greater risk for recurrence or metastasis.

Studies have confirmed that the frozen section technique is accurate in identifying positive margins.[15] Furthermore, studies done comparing the cure rates of MMS with standard wide excision of potentially metastatic tumors have shown at least equivalent efficacy. Having said that, not all physicians practicing MMS feel confident enough in their ability to histologically identify some of the less common tumors to perform micrographic surgery on them. This underscores the extreme importance of high quality training when treating tumors that have potential for metastasis. It is doubly important that the treating physician is competent to perform micrographic surgery through extensive training that provides a high volume of cases of every tumor type.

Another concern raised about MMS and potentially metastatic tumors is whether or not 'local recurrence' is more likely with margins taken using micrographic surgery versus wide margins of 1–3 cm. It must be remembered that the key therapeutic principle in malignancies where there is no evidence of metastasis is to remove the primary tumor with the hope that metastasis has not yet occurred. No study has ever shown that the chance of metastasis is less when wider excisions of the primary tumor are undertaken. In this situation, the basic tenet and the most important duty of the surgeon in treatment of a primary tumor is to be sure that it is extirpated in its entirety. Failure to do so results in persistent disease and the ongoing risk of metastasis from the residual primary tumor. On the other hand, increasing the width of the surgical margin in an attempt to treat occult tumor that is discontiguous (metastatic to nearby tissue) has never been convincingly shown to provide a survival benefit. Therefore, the surgeon's attention should not be focused on how many centimeters of tumor free margin is wide enough, but rather on how wide the subclinical contiguous extension of the patient's primary tumor is.

Since many studies of the efficacy of margin width consider 'local recurrence' to be any tumor that arises within a certain distance of the incision line (e.g. 2 cm for melanoma) a distinction between residual, unexcised primary tumor and satellite or in transit metastatic tumor is impossible. When one does distinguish between residual primary tumor versus satellite or in transit metastasis, persistence within the margins of excision can be expected to be low, in both micrographically controlled

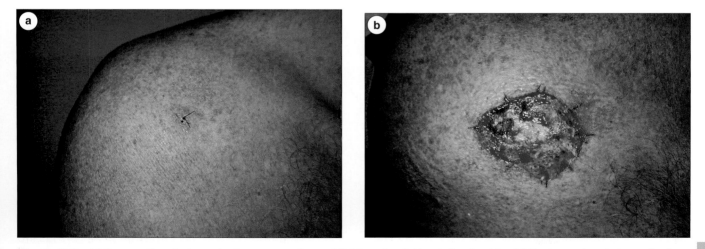

Figure 44.2 (a) Preoperative photograph of an apparently small BCC on the right anterior shoulder. (b) Postoperative photograph after three stages of MMS. Clinically occult tumor resulted in a larger than expected defect.

excisions and excisions performed with wide margins of normal appearing tissue. The reasons for low marginal persistence are different, however. In the case of wide excisions without complete histologic confirmation of tumor free margins, the wide margins of normal tissue increases the likelihood of complete tumor removal. On the other hand, the MMS technique confirms complete extirpation of the primary tumor by careful and meticulous histologic examination of all tissue margins. In the case of incomplete excision, this technique enables precise localization of residual tumor through the mapping procedure.

Currently, there are no side-by-side, randomized, controlled studies comparing the efficacy of excision with predetermined clinically tumor free margins and MMS excision in tumors with metastatic potential. Studies of the cure rates of both forms of excision in many potentially metastatic tumors have been performed independent of each other. Comparison of cure rates of these studies would likely indicate that the cure rates with MMS are no worse than those of the standard wide excision technique.

The role of MMS as the 'gold standard' of excision for BCC and SCC has been well established.[5,6] Its efficacy in terms of cure rates, tissue conservation and practicality in even difficult tumors is well documented. The remainder of the chapter will be dedicated to reviewing the literature pertinent to the use of MMS in a wide spectrum of cutaneous malignancies.

MELANOMA

MMS of melanoma has been extensively studied. It would seem that as with all forms of excision, treatment of melanoma with MMS prior to metastasis is highly effective. There are other issues, however, which have caused some to doubt whether the patient is as well treated with MMS as wide excision.

Melanoma exhibits a wide variety of clinical presentations. In general, melanoma in situ tends to be macular or patch-like, whereas invasive melanomas are generally nodular or plaque-like. Melanoma can present in a wide variety of colors and although surface changes are not always present they may include erosion, ulceration, crusting, or appendage loss. Melanoma is potentially very aggressive and often exhibits early regional nodal or distant metastasis. Survival rates plummet once metastasis occurs regardless of subsequent therapy.

Melanoma is a tumor of melanocytic origin and may be divided into two groups: in situ and invasive. Melanoma in situ (MIS) is characterized by a proliferation of atypical melanocytes either singly or in nests distributed throughout all levels of the epidermis. MIS may involve adnexal structures, but individual cells do not penetrate the dermo-epidermal junction. Invasive melanoma exhibits atypical dermal melanocytes that may be epithelioid, spindle-shaped, or nevus cell-like. There is no maturation with descent into the dermis. These cells may be arranged in a fascicular fashion or may be in solid sheets. Individual cells often have hyperchromatic nuclei, prominent nucleoli and mitoses are common.

Given melanoma's propensity for histologic invasion and metastasis, early diagnosis and complete excision provides the greatest chance for cure. Adaptation of MMS for the treatment of melanoma was first proposed by Frederic Mohs. He supported his reasoning in a 1950 review which included his first 20 patients.[16] In 1989, 200 melanomas treated with Mohs' fixed tissue technique were summarized and after stratification by Clark's level, it was found that MMS provided comparable cure rates to wide local excision (WLE) with the added benefit of tissue conservation.[17] A later study using the fresh tissue technique on 103 consecutive melanoma patients (n=77, follow-up 2.5 years and n=26, follow-up 5 years) demonstrated survival rates and recurrence rates at least as good as those found after WLE.[17] The most definitive study to date (n=535, follow-up at least 5 years in 99.5% of patients) compared MMS with WLE in the treatment of melanoma.[14] After stratification by Breslow depth, it showed local recurrence rates, metastasis rates and five year Kaplan–Meier survival rates comparable with or better for patients in the MMS treatment group. This same study reported 83% of melanomas completely excised with 6 mm margins, 95% with 9 mm margins and 99% clear in 15 mm. Larger tumors and those located on the head, neck, hands and feet required larger margins as a group.

The initial margin of normal skin removed in the aforementioned study was 6 millimeters. Positive margins identified by microscopic viewing are mapped and precisely identified for further excision, in effect tailoring the surgical defect to involve only the affected skin. The relatively small margins used to clear melanoma in MMS are in contrast to the historical belief that wider margins result in higher cure rates. More recent data shows similar patient outcomes with more narrow margins.[18] These results lend credence to the MMS technique of analyzing the entire tissue rather than depending on excising widely into clinically normal skin.

Melanoma patients often present for MMS with significant anxiety over their diagnosis and prognosis. Prior to performing the procedure, it is important to discuss the details of each patient's specific tumor in regards to prognosis and treatment options. Often patients appreciate physicians who spend time to answer these questions with specific data and statistics. Pertinent personal and family historical details and a review of systems geared towards revealing symptoms of metastatic disease should be obtained. A full skin and lymph node examination should be performed on the day of MMS and education about self skin and lymph node examination should be provided. A discussion about the degree of risk for family members in developing melanoma may be appropriate at some point during care.

MMS excision of melanoma is performed by first assessing the viewable tumor borders. Some surgeons opt to use a Wood's lamp to aid in identifying the perimeter. A skin marker is used to delineate the area and it is then anesthetized. It is prudent to inject beyond the perimeter of obvious tumor. Excision is then performed with predetermined margins of clinically normal skin and into the deep subcutaneous tissue. Excision through fascia has not proven to be beneficial.[19] Excised tissue is then marked, mapped and submitted for histologic preparation.

Significant debate still occurs regarding the best method of tissue processing in melanoma. Whether fresh frozen or paraffin-embedded tissue is used, it is absolutely imperative for the histotechnician to produce thin (2–4 μm), evenly stained sections without artifact. Although some authors find frozen sections unreliable in the evaluation of melanoma, one study found frozen sections to be 100% sensitive and 90% specific (n=221 specimens).[15] The addition of immunostains makes melanoma more obvious on both paraffin-embedded and frozen sections. When compared to S-100 and HMB-45, MART-1 is rapidly becoming the immunohistochemical marker of choice for increasing sensitivity for melanoma on frozen sections. Its high sensitivity for all melanocytes aids in abetting one of the primary challenges of reading all melanocytic lesions, namely the distinction between normal melanocyte density, melanocytic hyperplasia in sun damaged skin, isolated atypical melanocytes and melanoma.

Lymph node dissection, chemotherapy, radiation therapy and immunotherapy are under study as treatment modalities for melanoma, but have as yet not shown reproducible disease specific survival benefit. Their use is debatable. In many treatment centers, sentinel lymph node biopsy (SLNB) has become the standard of care. Although SLNB offers no reproducible survival benefit, it does provide prognostic information and may be a requirement for entry into adjuvant therapy trials. On the other hand, patients noted to have palpable lymphadenopathy after MMS may achieve improved disease free survival and quality of life if therapeutic lymph node dissection is performed.[20]

SPINDLE CELL TUMORS

Dermatofibrosarcoma protuberans

Dermatofibrosarcoma protuberans (DFSP) presents as one or multiple erythematous, firm nodules or plaques. Most occur on the trunk, but the head and neck are also common locations. DFSP is a rare, dermal tumor with a propensity for deep invasion and extensive sub-clinical spread. Longstanding lesions can invade subcutaneous tissue, muscle, fascia and bone, but metastasis is rare. The subtle and insidious growth characteristics combined with their dermal/subcutaneous location often leads to delayed diagnosis and presentation of very large tumors. MMS is an ideal treatment for DFSP because microscopic tracking of the tumor results in removal of tumor even when sub-clinical spread is extensive.

DFSP is a contiguous tumor that is thought to arise from fibroblasts. It is readily viewable on frozen section and paraffin embedded permanent section tissues. Meticulous preparation of subcutaneous fat, muscle, cartilage, or bone may be necessary for examination of deep DFSPs. CD34 immunostaining is used with both frozen section and paraffin-embedded permanent section tissues to differentiate DFSP from other spindle cell tumors and benign fibroblasts. Immunohistochemical staining is often useful at the periphery of DFSPs, where cellularity may decrease.

Recurrence rates for DFSP after treatment with MMS are reported at 1.6% (n=64, follow-up 5–96 months),

whereas recurrence rates after treatment of DFSP by WLE are reported at 20% (n=489, follow-up 1–360 months).[21] Predilection for extensive sub-clinical spread makes pre-determination of excision margins difficult. Parker and Zitelli[13] reviewed 20 patients who all were microscopically free of tumor with 2.5 cm peripheral margins, while Ratner et al.[22] presented a patient not microscopically free of tumor with excision margins as large as 12.0 cm. The wide variation between the clinical and microscopic margins necessary to completely excise a DFSP illustrates the great potential not only for tissue preservation in asymmetrical tumors, but also for an overall reduction in treatment failures. Even though the tumor free margin taken with MMS is significantly less than what has been recommended for standard WLE, most Mohs surgeons' first stage of excision is often with 5–10 mm margins. Subsequent stages of excision are with 3–5 mm margins. Preoperative palpation of the tumor can occasionally identify subtle dermal or subcutaneous tumor extensions and is therefore a critical aspect of the examination.

Most DFSP recurrences occur within three years after primary surgical excision,[23] and some surgeons opt for delayed closure of surgical defects after a period of observation. Although many patients have a heightened awareness of any changes in their skin after diagnosis of DFSP, routine and thorough skin examination should be undertaken semi-annually for the first five years. Lymph node examination should be performed in patients with longstanding or deeply invasive tumors since rare lymph node metastases may occur. Distant or visceral metastases are exceedingly rare and routine screening with CAT/MRI scans is not warranted.

Atypical fibroxanthoma

Atypical fibroxanthoma (AFX) is an intradermal, spindle cell tumor of mesenchymal origin occurring most commonly on the head and neck. They most often present as small, firm nodules with eroded or crusted surfaces. AFX typically exhibits low to moderate malignant potential and recurrences are most commonly due to incomplete excision.

Atypical fibroxanthoma is easily identifiable on frozen section tissue. Polymorphic and pleomorphic spindle cells with occasional mitotic figures are most often confined to the dermis, but occasionally extend into the subcutis. AFX tumor cells tend to become sparser near the tumor periphery necessitating close examination of high quality frozen sections. Special stains are rarely, if ever required to clear an AFX microscopically.

Davis et al.[24] showed no recurrences (n=19, mean follow-up 29.6 months) in patients treated with MMS, while Fretzin and Helwig[25] reported a 9% recurrence rate (n=101, mean follow-up 4.1 years) in patients treated with WLE. The difference in recurrence rates is not likely due to unequal follow-up durations since the vast majority of AFX recurrences are within 24 months.[24] The meticulous examination of excision margins inherent in MMS is the most rational explanation for the difference in recurrence rates and the available data suggests that MMS is at least equivalent to WLE in the treatment of AFX.

541

Follow-up should include thorough skin examination. Regional metastases are rare, but tend to occur in large, ulcerated lesions, in previously irradiated sites or in immunocompromised patients.[24] These high risk patients should have regular, regional lymph node examination, but screening examination with MRI or CAT scans has not been confirmed as being helpful.

Malignant fibrous histiocytoma

Malignant fibrous histiocytoma (MFH) is the most common soft tissue sarcoma of late adulthood and is an aggressive spindle cell tumor of deep tissue.[26] These lesions most often present as an expanding, painless mass of several months duration. Common sites of involvement include the extremities and retroperitoneum. MFH exhibits spread along fascial planes, often extending for considerable distances between muscle fibers.[27] Treatment is primarily surgical, but specific guidelines outlining optimal peripheral excision margins have not been firmly established. The role of adjuvant therapy is also uncertain, mainly because of tumor rarity. High recurrence rates and the potential for local invasiveness and metastatic spread make complete removal of the primary tumor critical once evaluation for metastasis is negative.

MFH is commonly divided into four histologic subtypes, with the storiform-pleomorphic variant being the most common. Mesenchymal cells or fibroblasts are favored over histiocytes as the cell of origin in MFH.[27] MFH is often considered a deeper version of AFX, but at the time of diagnosis, it may also be confused with other spindle cell tumors such as DFSP or pleomorphic variants of liposarcoma and rhabdomyosarcoma. After diagnosis is made, either frozen or paraffin section slide preparation can be used for histologic evaluation of surgical margins. MFH is easily identifiable microscopically and special stains are rarely required to clear the surgical margins.

MMS was reported effective in treating MFH by Brown and Swanson[28] who showed a 9% recurrence rate (n=22, mean follow-up 3 years). Their study included five AFX cases as well, but they did not specify in which tumor type the recurrences occurred. Heuther et al.[29] reported recurrence in 43% of patients (n=7, mean follow-up 3.8 years) after MMS and Weiss and Enzinger[26] reported recurrence in 44% of patients (n=196, follow-up 2–15 years) after WLE. Proposed peripheral excision margins may be quite large in WLE and amputation is occasionally deemed necessary in advanced extremity tumors. Initial excision margins with MMS are narrower but are typically at least 5–10 mm, which is more generous than is typical with more common tumors such as BCC and SCC. MMS offers comparable recurrence rates to conventional wide local excision.

Metastasis rates are approximately 40–50%, with the lungs and lymph nodes being the two most common sites. Risk of metastasis appears to correlate with size and depth of the primary tumor.[26] In advanced cases, radiation therapy plays an important role. It may be used in combination with surgery for better local control, particularly in high-grade lesions and in cases with positive surgical margins after attempted wide local excision. In unresectable tumors, MMS allows for determination of margins that remain microscopically positive. This may be useful in directing adjunctive radiotherapy to residual tumor after surgical excision. The role of adjuvant chemotherapy remains investigational.

Complete surgical resection at the time of diagnosis is most likely to afford the best chance for recurrence free survival. MMS offers careful and complete margin evaluation in tumors such as MFH, which have a tendency for extensive subclinical spread. Given the aggressive nature of MFH, the optimal surgical treatment is still uncertain, but MMS demonstrates comparable recurrence rates to traditional WLE with the possible added benefit of tissue conservation.

Leiomyosarcoma

Superficial leiomyosarcoma (LMS) is subdivided into tumors arising from the arrector pili smooth muscle in the dermis (primary cutaneous LMS) or from the smooth muscular perimeter of subcutaneous vasculature. Tumors arising from the arrector pili muscles have a better prognosis than subcutaneous tumors, but distinguishing between the two is not always possible as tumor cells may infiltrate both the dermis and subcutis.

Diagnosis of LMS on permanent section tissue may require special stains to distinguish it from other spindle cell tumors such as fibrosarcoma, MFH, AFX and DFSP. Desmin, vimentin, muscle specific actin and S100 may all be helpful for this purpose.[30] Biopsy proven LMS is not difficult to identify on frozen sections and special stains are not often used during MMS.

Cutaneous LMS is locally invasive and surgical excision is the treatment of choice. Its rarity has prevented development of widely accepted treatment guidelines. Wide local excision is the traditional treatment and is associated with recurrence rates of 14% (n=21, follow-up 1–10+ years)[31] to 40% (n=65, follow-up 2–360 months).[32] Primary cutaneous LMS has been successfully treated with MMS. Huether, Zitelli and Brodland[29] reported recurrence in 14% (n=7, mean follow-up 4.3 years). The patient that had the recurrence had a recurrent tumor at the time of initial MMS.

The rarity of this tumor precludes specific follow-up protocols. Examination of patients should be long term as recurrences have occurred as long as 5 years postoperatively.[32] LMS is regarded as relatively resistant to radiotherapy and chemotherapy. Therefore, it is imperative to optimize chances for complete resection at the time of diagnosis. Despite the small numbers of patients studied, MMS appears comparable to wide local excision in the treatment of primary cutaneous LMS.

SPINDLE CELL TUMOR – NOT OTHERWISE SPECIFIED

Spindle cell tumor, not otherwise specified (SCT–NOS) was introduced by Heuther et al.[29] and is a dermal spindle cell tumor for which no definitive diagnosis may be assigned. The spindle cells in SCT–NOS assume patterns and architecture often mimicking DFSP, MFH, melanoma, SCC, or AFX, but immunophenotyping is indeterminate or incomplete. In a series of 15 patients[29] treated with MMS, there was no recurrence after a mean follow-up of 4.6 years.

INFANTILE DIGITAL FIBROMATOSIS

Infantile digital fibroma (IDF) is a rare tumor often occurring on the digits in young children. IDFs may grow rapidly and invasively, remain unchanged for extended periods of time, or spontaneously resolve. IDF is an unencapsulated dermal tumor composed largely of myofibroblasts with cytoplasmic inclusion bodies which stain positively for actin filaments. IDF is identifiable on frozen section tissue using hematoxylin and eosin, Masson's trichrome and actin immunostain.[30]

A case of IDF treated with MMS was halted prior to obtaining tumor free margins. The rationale for stopping before complete clearance was to avoid damage to the underlying joint space. Despite the positive margins after MMS in this case, no tumor was evident at 2 years of follow-up.[32] Deep tumor margins often invade fascia, making tumor clearance challenging without causing structural or functional damage.

The treatment of choice for IDF is still debated, but surgery is often used in aggressive cases and in cases where parental anxiety is high. In these cases, further study into the treatment of IDF with MMS to determine recurrence rates is warranted.

MICROCYSTIC ADNEXAL CARCINOMA

Microcystic adnexal carcinoma (MAC) usually presents as deeply invasive, poorly marginated plaques frequently arising periorally, perinasally, periocularly, or on the scalp. MAC exhibits a contiguous growth pattern and often invades nerves, with persistent or longstanding tumors also invading underlying subcutaneous fat, muscle, cartilage, bone, salivary glands and lymph nodes.[34,35] It often blends into surrounding normal skin, making clinical identification of tumor borders difficult. It is clinically misdiagnosed approximately 30% of the time,[36] and even though it is slowly growing, MAC is often sizable at the time of diagnosis. MAC often arises in previously irradiated sites. Acne treatment with X-ray,[35] and therapeutic radiation for treatment of a periocular rhabdomyosarcoma,[37] are two cited examples. There is evidence that more aggressive growth patterns and increased morbidity may occur in immunocompromised patients.[38] The combination of involvement of structurally sensitive area, potential for deep invasion and clinically indistinct tumor borders make MMS the ideal treatment for MAC.

Microcystic adnexal carcinoma is thought to arise from pluripotent keratinocytes capable of differentiation toward hair follicles or sweat ducts. It is identifiable on frozen section tissue with hematoxylin and eosin or toluidine blue stains showing the typical small nests and strands of cells exhibiting variable ductal differentiation. MAC is easily confused with syringoma, desmoplastic trichoepithelioma and sclerosing BCC. The presence of perineural invasion supports the diagnosis of MAC. It is primarily a dermal tumor, but may invade the subcutaneous tissue, especially when there is perineural involvement. The quality of the histologic sections in MMS must be excellent, as small nests of subcutaneous MAC may be the only clue that wider excision is necessary for complete tumor clearance. When excellent frozen sections are unattainable, some surgeons utilize paraffin-embedded, permanent sectioning after excision.

Excision of MAC with the MMS technique often surprises even the most experienced surgeon, as tumors often exhibit significant sub-clinical extension, resulting in sizable defects. One study showed that the average defect after microscopically controlled excision was four times that of the clinically apparent size at presentation.[36] MAC treated with MMS recurs in less than 5% of cases (n=25, follow-up 2–67 months) and MAC treated with traditional excision recurs in approximately 41% of cases (n=29, follow-up 6–360 months).[38] The higher recurrence rates with WLE undoubtedly result from difficulty in visualization of peripheral tumor margins and inability to microscopically view 100% of the excision margin. In contrast, the higher cure rates with MMS translate into fewer office visits and improved cost effectiveness.

Tumor recurrence has been reported to occur up to 30 years after initial excision[34] and careful follow-up after MMS treatment of MAC over many years is important, especially in high-risk patients. MAC is not prone to metastatic spread and adjuvant radiation therapy and lymph node dissection have been used in only a limited number of cases. Use of adjuvant therapy after MMS excision of MAC is justifiably rare.

MERKEL CELL CARCINOMA

Merkel cell carcinoma (MCC) is an aggressive tumor with a propensity for early in-transit, regional nodal and distant metastasis.[39] Two year survival rates have been reported as low as 30%.[40] It occurs with equal distribution in Caucasian men and women. Tumors are usually reddish nodules and arise most often on the sun-exposed areas of the head and neck, but also may occur on the extremities or trunk. These tumors are frequently non-tender and their rapid growth often leads to large size prior to biopsy and treatment.

Merkel cells are neuroendocrine cells that reside in the basal layer of the epidermis and are presumably the cell of origin for this tumor. MCC appears as sheets or solid nests of small, uniform, oval cells. Tumor cells are readily identifiable in frozen section tissue. Meticulous preparation of thin, evenly stained sections are essential for accurate microscopic examination. Staining specificity for Merkel cells can be increased with various immuno-histochemical antibodies, including those directed against chromogranin, neuron specific enolase and cytokeratin.

MCC has a propensity to metastasize, raising the issue of how to best treat primary tumors that are clinically stage I. Studies comparing MMS to conventional wide local excision in regards to tumor persistence and regional lymph node recurrence after surgery, suggest comparable cure rates between MMS and conventional surgery. In a retrospective patient review, O'Connor et al.[41] reported an 8.3% marginal persistence rate (*n*=12, mean follow-up 36 months) after MMS and a 31.7% marginal persistence rate (*n*=41, mean follow-up 60 months) after conventional WLE. Boyer et al.[42] reported regional lymph node metastases in 15.6% (*n*=45, mean follow-up 27.8 months) after MMS, while Allen et al.[43] reported regional lymph node metastases in 39.2% (*n*=102, median follow-up 35 months) after WLE. Distant metastasis rates occurring after MMS remain low (1–2%)[46] while they are reported to be 25.4%[43] after WLE.

WLE is dependent upon the ability of the surgeon to accurately identify the tumor margin on physical examination prior to excision. A recent study involving 18 patients was unable to show statistical differences in disease specific survival or recurrence rates with increasing clinically tumor free margin widths.[44] This outcome not only exemplifies the inherent inaccuracy in identifying clinical tumor borders, but also shows that widening excision margins is not the critical factor in survival. The decreased persistence and local recurrence rates associated with MMS undoubtedly hinge upon the ability to view 100% of the excised margin microscopically.

MCC is distinctly sensitive to radiation, but utilization of adjuvant radiation after excision is still debated. When used in conjunction with MMS, postoperative radiation may enhance local control.[39,41,42] This is especially true in cases where primary tumors are large and/or recurrent and in cases where clearance of tumor margins microscopically is not possible. Despite short-term improvement in tumor size and regional nodal spread, there is no evidence supporting increased long-term survival rates with postoperative radiation.

There is a paucity of data published on complete lymph node dissection after MMS. When used after WLE, there is improvement in disease free survival, but no overall survival benefit.[43] Sentinel lymph node biopsy is less invasive than complete dissection of an entire nodal basin and is associated with lower morbidity. Zeitouni et al.[45] described two cases where SLNB was utilized in conjunction with and prior to MMS. Positive SLNs were demonstrated in one of these patients and complete lymph node dissection followed. SLNB may provide valuable prognostic information and may make dissection of entire nodal basins more selective. There is no reported consistently reproducible survival benefit with either SNLB or CLND.[43,46,47]

Data detailing the use of chemotherapy in conjunction with MMS is sparse as well. In a review of patients with advanced MCC treated with conventional excision, Voog et al.[48] found 60% response rates (69% for locoregional disease and 57% for distant metastases). Median overall survival after starting chemotherapy was nine months. This supports the current theory that response rates are relatively high, but not durable. The role of chemotherapy in treatment of advanced MCC is debatable, but the available data suggests that it should not have a primary role in non-disseminated cases.

Disease persistence, recurrence, or metastasis occurs within 24 months in the large majority of patients.[43] Since MCC is prone to aggressive growth and potential metastasis, it is prudent to perform careful skin and lymph node examinations for years after the primary

excision. MMS tailors treatment of individual tumors to provide comparable cure rates while potentially sparing normal tissue in cosmetically and structurally sensitive areas. MCC has been compared with malignant melanoma in invasiveness and its ability to metastasize early. As in malignant melanoma, local persistence, regional spread and distant metastases are predictors of poor outcome. Early diagnosis and complete excision of the primary tumor using MMS is an effective treatment option for MCC.

SEBACEOUS CARCINOMA

Sebaceous carcinoma (SC) is a rare, invasive tumor most often appearing on the upper eyelids. It presents most often as a painless, yellowish nodule or plaque and is frequently mistaken for chronic inflammatory processes such as chalazion or blepharoconjunctivitis. BCC also can mimic SC, but BCC more commonly occurs on the lower eyelid. SC is also commonly misdiagnosed as SCC. SC is aggressive, with invasion often into orbital structures or regional lymph nodes. Regional lymph node metastasis is estimated at 17–28%.[49] Metastasis has also been reported to tissues such as muscle, liver, spleen, viscera and brain.

Meibomian glands are ocular adnexal structures considered to be in higher concentration on the upper eyelid and are the site of SC origin in most cases. Other potential sites of origin include other sebaceous glands common to the region: the Zeis glands of the cilia, sebaceous glands of the eyebrows, sebaceous glands of the caruncle and sebaceous glands of eyelid surface hair follicles.[3] SC occurs in extraocular sites as well, but regardless of location has been treated successfully with MMS.

One review estimated that correct initial permanent section histopathologic diagnosis was made in only 22.5% of cases of SC.[50] Pathologic misdiagnosis of SC may be a function of its rarity and its microscopic similarity to BCC with sebaceous differentiation. Separating SC from BCC with sebaceous differentiation can be challenging and microscopic characteristics favoring SC include: vacuolated cell cytoplasm, high mitotic index, strong staining with Oil Red O and on occasion the presence of diffuse, pagetoid spread. Other prominent features include basophilic cells, vesicular nuclei, prominent nucleoli and vacuolated cytoplasm. The presence of pagetoid spread, poor differentiation and invasive growth pattern were microscopic features noted to be harbingers of poor prognosis in a review of 104 SC cases.[51] SC is identifiable on meticulously prepared frozen sections and Doxanas et al.[50] suggest that frozen section control in the presence of pagetoid spread may allow for preservation of conjunctiva and lid margin. Others find that overnight paraffin-embedded sectioning provides clearer slides for more accurate viewing and therefore, better control.[52] Aggressive growth pattern and non-specific clinical and histologic diagnosis often result in advanced disease at presentation for primary treatment.

Despite these reported difficulties in accurate diagnosis of SC, MMS has been used very effectively in treatment of primary tumors. Spencer et al.[53] reported

11.1% recurrence (n=18, mean follow-up 37 months) after MMS treatment of SC, whereas 5-year recurrence rates with traditional excision are approximately 32%.[49,54] In addition to comparable recurrence rates, MMS may also preserve normal tissue in this structurally sensitive area when compared with traditional excisional techniques.

Postsurgical management of SC patients should consist of meticulous skin examination. Ratz *et al.*[49] suggest postsurgical follow-up at 1, 3 and 6 months, then every 3 months for the next year, every 6 months for the following year and once yearly thereafter. Adjunctive radiotherapy, chemotherapy and lymph node dissection are not frequently used in conjunction with MMS. Radiation therapy should be reserved for recurrent, metastatic, or non-resectable tumors. No reproducible benefit in disease free survival has been demonstrated with chemotherapy or lymph node dissection after Mohs surgical treatment of SC.

ANGIOSARCOMA

Angiosarcoma (AS) is a very aggressive tumor with 5-year survival rates estimated to be as low as 12%.[55] These tumors have a wide array of clinical appearances, from ill-defined, dusky patches or plaques to ulcerated tumors. The patch/plaque-like lesions often blend imperceptibly into surrounding normal skin and they tend to be larger at the time of diagnosis. The higher recurrence and lower survival rates suggested for this subtype may be due to a longer delay in diagnosis or to difficulty in microscopic identification.

AS is an endothelial cell derived dermal tumor that often infiltrates subcutaneous tissues. Microscopic features may include various levels of differentiation, multicentricity and subtle tumor extension. Poorly differentiated tumors are generally more challenging to view microscopically as they stain less intensely than well-differentiated tumors. When present, multicentricity and subtle tumor extension can cause inaccuracy in the microscopic evaluation of clinically ill-defined tumors. Frozen section and paraffin-embedded permanent section tissues have both been used in conjunction with MMS in the treatment of AS.

The medical literature contains small case series and anecdotal case reports of MMS being used for excision of primary cutaneous AS of the head and neck[56–58] and recurrence/survival rates appear comparable to conventional excision. Definitive comparisons between the two methods of surgical treatment are unavailable however, because the rarity of this tumor has limited trial sizes. Treatment guidelines are based on small case series. Some surgeons opt to sample a tumor's perimeter with preoperative punch biopsies. Performing these in a grid-like pattern aids in determining tumor borders. Bullen and colleagues[56] suggest the following treatment algorithm for AS: for tumors less than 5 cm in size – consider MMS plus radiation and for tumors larger than 5 cm in size – consider peripheral margin assessment followed by radiation or electron beam therapy. When compared with conventional excision, MMS offers the potential advantage of accurately identifying peripheral margins without requiring the extra step of performing punch biopsies. In unresectable tumors, MMS also allows for determination of margins that remain microscopically positive. This may be useful in directing adjunctive radiotherapy to residual tumor after surgical excision.

AS is highly aggressive and the large majority of cases that go on to exhibit tumor persistence, regional nodal, or distant metastasis declare themselves within 2 years after primary surgical excision. Frequent follow-up is prudent in all AS patients. When surgery fails to control AS, radiation therapy may be used in conjunction with IL-2 or as a solo treatment for palliation. On the other hand, chemotherapy has not been shown to be effective and is not routinely used in conjunction with MMS. The role of MMS in the treatment of AS is still evolving.

EXTRAMAMMARY PAGET'S DISEASE

Extramammary Paget's disease (EMPD) usually presents as a persistent, reddish plaque occurring in areas with high concentrations of apocrine glands. These areas include the vulva in females, the scrotum in males and the perianal area in both sexes. EMPD is frequently clinically misdiagnosed as chronic dermatides such as inverse psoriasis, lichen simplex chronicus, or dermatophytosis. EMPD notoriously contains cells that imperceptibly extend peripherally and unpredictably for long distances beyond the borders of clinically involved skin. Therefore, MMS is a logical treatment choice for this potentially invasive skin cancer in these structurally sensitive areas.

EMPD is identifiable on frozen section tissue. Paget's cells contain abundant, pale cytoplasm and large pleomorphic nuclei. They are arranged either singly or in small groups in the basal or parabasal regions with mitoses often present. Subtle tumor extensions may be identified using CEA immunostaining. Other protocols for use with frozen section tissue include mucicarmine and PAS.[30] Some groups suggests using Mohs surgical excision in conjunction with horizontal paraffin-embedded sections.

EMPD can be divided into epidermal disease and invasive disease. Epidermal disease is contained by the basement membrane while invasive disease occurs either through direct extension or through association with subjacent internal malignancy. It is widely accepted that disease associated with internal malignancy rapidly disseminates and has poor prognosis. Invasive disease occurs in a minority of cases with estimates ranging from 0–45%.[59–62] In a review of 73 cases, the overall recurrence rate after excision was 44%. More specifically, EMPD in this study limited to the epidermis only had recurrence of 36%, whereas EMPD associated with invasive disease had recurrence of 67%.[63]

Since clinical borders are difficult to ascertain, application of 5-FU for 10 days prior to excision, or performing punch biopsies of the surrounding area have been suggested to estimate tumor perimeter.[64] Poorly delineated tumor borders make complete resection of EMPD in a single layer a rare occurrence. Coldiron *et al.*[65] reported recurrence rates of 23% (n=48, mean follow-up 39 months) in EMPD cases treated with MMS and recurrence rates of 33% (*n*=112, mean follow-up 54 months) in EMPD cases treated with conventional surgical excision. Fanning et al.[66] reported recurrences in 31% (*n*=58) of EMPD patients treated with radical vulvectomy and in 43% (*n*=32) of EMPD patients treated with wide excision after median follow-up of 7 years.

MMS recurrence rates in EMPD approach those of conventional excision and this may be due to challenging histology, subtle adnexal spread, large area and therefore higher risk of physician error. A potential advantage of MMS in the treatment of EMPD over conventional excision is cost savings. MMS uses local anesthesia in the outpatient setting, whereas conventional excision usually uses general anesthesia in the operating room.

CASE REPORTS OF RARE TUMORS

Hidradenomas are rare and may occur at any site on the body. They occasionally become large and it may be difficult to histologically differentiate benign lesions from those with malignant transformation. One group treated a large, longstanding hidradenoma with MMS and obtained 1.5 years of disease free follow-up.[67] Another group suggests MMS as the treatment of choice for large or recurrent hidradenomas.[68]

Separation of malignant from benign granular cell tumors is occasionally difficult as well. Malignant cases are often noted only after metastasis. Therefore, Dzubow and Kramer[69] recommend MMS for treatment of clinically malignant behaving granular cell tumors. Others have used MMS for its tissue conserving properties in treating granular cell tumors in structurally sensitive areas such as the corona of the penis.[70]

Eccrine porocarcinoma is an aggressive tumor with an estimated 20% recurrence rate and MMS has been reported successful in a single case report.[71] In this report, the authors suggest that CEA, EMA, cytokeratin and S100 immunostains may be helpful in identifying tumor cells on frozen section tissue.

Most mucinous carcinomas of the skin are metastatic from other sites, but when this is ruled out, primary mucinous carcinoma may be treated with MMS. Two cases of primary mucinous carcinoma were treated with MMS without recurrence in 4 and 5 years.[72]

The majority of cylindromas are benign, but rare transformation into a malignant form may occur. Malignant forms are more likely to exhibit increased mitotic figures, anaplasia, stromal invasion and focal necrosis. A case of malignant cylindroma required two MMS treatments prior to obtaining 4 years of recurrence free survival.[73]

Malignant schwannoma, also called malignant peripheral nerve sheath tumor, is a rare entity occurring most often on the proximal extremities in young and middle-aged adults. Padilla and Shimazu[74] present a case of malignant schwannoma treated with MMS without recurrence after 5 years follow-up.

Papillary eccrine adenomas are often ill-defined and recurrences have been reported after incomplete excision. Jackson and Cook[75] reported a case of persistent papillary eccrine adenoma excised using the Mohs fresh tissue technique.

Apocrine adenocarcinoma is an aggressive primary cutaneous tumor with a propensity to recur locally after attempted surgical excision. There have not been reports of multi-focality, skip areas, or direct blood vessel invasion by this tumor. Dhawan et al.[76] recommend excision of apocrine adenocarcinoma with MMS.

Eccrine adenocarcinoma is difficult clinically to distinguish from eccrine adenoma. Histologic features suggesting malignancy are: increased number of mitoses, atypical cellular forms, perineural or lymphatic or vascular invasion, extension into deep tissues. Since eccrine adenocarcinoma does not grow in a contiguous pattern, Dzubow et al.[77] favor the MMS technique used in a debulking fashion followed by conservative marginal re-excision and lymph node dissection in clinically warranted cases.

Primary cutaneous adenoid cystic carcinoma is characterized by frequent local recurrences and infrequent metastasis after excision attempts. The cribriform islands of tumor produce abundant mucin and Chesser et al.[78] recommend treatment of cutaneous adenoid cystic carcinoma with MMS. Toluidine blue staining may be superior to hematoxylin and eosin staining because the mucin stains metachromatically with the former.

Further study is needed to assess the efficacy of MMS for the treatment of tumors with contiguous growth patterns. Any lesion that requires excision with clear surgical margins is a potential candidate. Certainly not all tumors excised with the MMS technique have appeared as case reports in the literature. In addition to the tumors described above (excluding case reports of rare tumors), the authors have treated the following tumors with the MMS technique: desmoplastic trichoepithelioma, trichoepithelioma, trichofolliculoma, trichoadenoma, Spitz nevus, deep penetrating nevus, cylindroma, eccrine spiradenoma, eccrine poroma, eccrine acrospiroma, pilomatricoma, chondroid syringoma, cystadenoma, sebaceous adenoma, myoepithelial carcinoma of the parotid gland metastatic to the skin, clear cell acanthoma, granular cell tumor and glomus tumor.

FUTURE OUTLOOK

In theory, MMS should enable the physician to successfully excise all cutaneous tumors that are contiguous. The limitations of the procedure revolve around the ability of the surgeon to accurately identify neoplastic cells by frozen section and the difficulty of the Mohs technician to consistently prepare sections that are histologically complete without distracting artifact. In some instances, inflammatory reactions mask underlying tumor. Small clusters or single elements of tumors such as melanoma, Merkel cell or DFSP may be extremely difficult to recognize.

In order for the cure rate for MMS to improve, accepted criteria must be established to aid recognition of dysplastic cells viewed by frozen sections. Histologic features that distinguish normal from dysplastic cells, whether aided by special stains or viewed with standard preparations, need to be developed. Attention should be paid to refining the technique of frozen section preparation so that even technicians with less experience might attain reliable, complete sections.

If the ability to recognize even minimal dysplasia is improved and the quality of specimen preparation approaches the ideal, the Mohs procedure will even more closely approach the theoretical cure rate of 100% for tumors with contiguous spread. Only then will the practical application of the procedure reach the level of accuracy embedded within the concepts developed long ago by Dr Mohs.

REFERENCES

1 Brodland DG, Amonette R, Hanke CW, Robbins P. The history and evolution of Mohs micrographic surgery. Derm Surg 2000; 26(4):303–307.

2 Chemosurgery MFE. A microscopically controlled method of cancer excision. Arch Surg 1941; 42:279.

3 Tromovitch TA, Stegeman SJ. Microscopically controlled excision of skin tumors: chemosurgery (Mohs): fresh tissue technique. Arch Derm 1974; 110:231–232.

4 Swanson NA, Taylor WB, Tromovitch TA. The evolution of Mohs surgery. J Derm Surg Oncol 1982; 8:650–654.

5 Rowe DE, Carroll RJ, Day CL Jr. Prognostic factors for local recurrence, metastasis and survival rates in squamous cell carcinoma of the skin, ear and lip: implications for treatment modality selection. J Am Acad Derm 1992; 26:976–990.

6 Rowe DE, Carroll RJ, Day CL Jr. Long term recurrence rates in previously untreated (primary) basal cell carcinoma: implications for patient follow-up. J Derm Surg Oncol 1989; 15:315–328.

7 Robins P. Chemosurgery: My 15 years of experience. J Derm Surg Oncol 1981; 7(10):779–789.

8 Miller PK, Roenigk RK, Brodland DG, Randle HW. Cutaneous micrographic surgery: Mohs procedure. Mayo Clin Proc 1992; 67:971–980.

9 Mohs FE. Chemosurgery in Skin Cancer, Gangrene and Infections. Springfield, Ill: Charles C. Thomas; 1956.

10 Roenigk RK, Roenigk HH Jr. Dermatologic Surgery: Principles & Practice. New York, NY: Marcel Dekker; 1996.

11 Wolf DJ, Zitelli JA. Surgical margins for basal cell carcinoma. Arch Derm 1987; 123:213–215.

12 Brodland DG, Zitelli JA. Surgical margins for excision of primary cutaneous squamous cell carcinoma. J Am Acad Derm 1992; 27:2241–2248.

13 Parker TL, Zitelli JA. Surgical margins for excision of dermatofibrosarcoma protuberans. J Am Acad Derm 1995; 32:233–236.

14 Zitelli JA, Brown CD, Hanusa BH. Surgical margins for the excision of primary cutaneous melanoma. J Am Acad Derm 1997; 37:422–429.

15 Zitelli JA, Moy RL, Abell EA. The reliability of frozen sections for evaluation of surgical margins of melanoma. J Am Acad Derm 1991; 24:102–106.

16 Mohs FE. Chemosurgical treatment of melanoma: a microscopically controlled method of excision. Arch Derm 1950; 62:269–279.

17 Zitelli JA, Mohs FE, Larson P, et al. Mohs micrographic surgery for melanoma. Derm Clin 1989; 7:833–843.

18 Balch C, Soong S-J, Smith T. Long-term results of a prospective surgical trial comparing 2 cm vs. 4 cm excision margins for 740 patients with 1–4 mm melanomas. Ann Surg Oncol 2001; 8:101–108.

19 Kenady DE, Brown BW, McBride CM. Excision of underlying fascia with a primary malignant melanoma: effect on recurrence and survival rates. Surgery 1982; 92(4):615–618.

20 Karakousis CP. Therapeutic node dissections in malignant melanoma. Ann Surg Oncol 1998; 5:473–482.

21 Gloster HM, Harris KR, Roenigk RK. A comparison between Mohs micrographic surgery and wide surgical excision for the treatment of dermatofibrosarcoma protuberans. J Am Acad Derm 1996; 35:82–87.

22 Ratner D, Thomas CO, Johnson TM, et al. Mohs micrographic surgery for the treatment of dermatofibrosarcoma protuberans. J Am Acad Derm 1997; 37:600–613.

23 Pack GT, Tabah EF. Dermatofibrosarcoma protuberans: a report of thirty-nine cases. Arch Surg 1951; 62:391–411.

24 Davis JL, Randle HW, Zalla MJ, et al. A comparison of Mohs micrographic surgery and wide excision for the treatment of atypical fibroxanthoma. Derm Surg 1997; 23:105–110.

25 Fretzin DF, Helwig EB. Atypical fibroxanthoma of the skin. A clinicopathologic study of 140 cases. Cancer 1973; 31:1541–1552.

26 Weiss SW, Enzinger FM. Malignant fibrous histiocytoma – an analysis of 200 cases. Cancer 1978; 41:2250–2266.

27 Enzinger FM. Weiss SM. Soft Tissue Tumors: Malignant Fibrohistiocytic Tumors. St Louis, MO: Mosby; 1988:273.

28 Brown MC, Swanson NA. Treatment of malignant fibrous histiocytoma and atypical fibrous xanthomas with micrographic surgery. J Derm Surg Oncol 1989; 15:1287–1292.

29 Huether MJ, Zitelli JA, Brodland DG. Mohs micrographic surgery for the treatment of spindle cell tumors of the skin. J Am Acad Derm 2001; 44:656–659.

30 Weedon D. Skin Pathology. San Francisco: Harcourt Publishers Limited; 1998.

31 Bernstein SC, Roenigk RK. Leiomyosarcoma of the skin: treatment of 34 cases. Derm Surg 1996; 22:631–635.

32 Fields JP, Helwig EB. Leiomyosarcoma of the skin and subcutis. Cancer 1981; 47:156–159.

33 Albertini JG, Welsch MJ, Conger LA, et al. Infantile digital fibroma treated with Mohs micrographic surgery. Derm Surg 2002; 28:959–961.

34 Burns MK, Chen SP, Goldberg LH. Microcystic adnexal carcinoma: ten cases treated by Mohs micrographic surgery. J Derm Surg Oncol 1994; 20:429–434.

35 Cooper PH, Mills SE. Microcystic adnexal carcinoma. J Am Acad Derm 1984; 10:908–914.

36 Chiller K, Passaro D, Scheuller M, et al. Microcystic adnexal carcinoma: forty-eight cases, their treatment and their outcome. Arch Derm 2000; 136:1355–1359.

37 Antley CA, Carney M, Smoller BR. Microcystic adnexal carcinoma arising in the setting of previous radiation therapy. J Cutan Pathol 1999; 26:48–50.

38 Carroll P, Goldstein GD, Brown CW. Metastatic microcystic adnexal carcinoma in an immunocompromised patient. Derm Surg 2000; 26:531–534.

39 Gollard R, Weber R, Kosty MP, et al. Merkel cell carcinoma: review of 22 cases with surgical, pathologic and therapeutic considerations. Cancer 2000; 88:1842–1851.

40 Linjawi A, Jamison WB, Meterissian S. Merkel cell carcinoma: important aspects of diagnosis and management. Am Surg 2001; 67:943–947.

41 O'Connor WJ, Roenigk RK, Brodland DG. Merkel cell carcinoma: comparison of Mohs micrographic surgery and wide local excision in eighty-six patients. Derm Surg 1997; 23:929–933.

42 Boyer JD, Zitelli JA, Brodland D, et al. Local control of primary Merkel cell carcinoma: review of 45 cases treated with Mohs micrographic surgery with and without adjuvant radiation. J Am Acad Derm 2002; 47:885–892.

43 Allen PJ, Zhang ZF, Coit DG. Surgical management of Merkel cell carcinoma. Ann Surg 1999; 229:97–105.

44 Gillenwater AM, Hessel AC, Morrison WH, et al. Merkel cell carcinoma of the head and neck: effect of surgical excision and radiation of recurrence and survival. Arch Otolaryngol Head Neck Surg 2001; 127:149–154.

45 Zeitouni NC, Cheney RT, Delacure MD. Lymphoscintigraphy, sentinel lymph node biopsy and Mohs micrographic surgery in the treatment of Merkel cell carcinoma. Derm Surg 2000; 26:12–18.

46 Wasserberg N, Schachter J, Fenig E, et al. Applicability of the sentinel node technique to Merkel cell carcinoma. Derm Surg 2000; 26:138–141.

47 Hill ADK, Brady MS, Coit DG. Intraoperative lymphatic mapping and sentinel lymph node biopsy for Merkel cell carcinoma. Br J Surg 1999; 86:518–521.

48 Voog E, Biron P, Martin J-P. Chemotherapy for patients with locally advanced or metastatic Merkel cell carcinoma. Cancer 1999; 85:2589–2595.

49 Ratz JL, Luu-Duong S, Kulwin DR. Sebaceous carcinoma of the eyelid treated with Mohs' surgery. J Am Acad Derm 1986; 14:668–673.

50 Doxanas MT, Green R. Sebaceous gland carcinoma: review of 40 cases. Arch Ophthalmol 1984; 102:245–249.

51 Rao NA, Jidoyat AA, McLean IW, et al. Sebaceous carcinoma of the ocular adnexa: a clinicopathologic study of 104 patients with 5-year follow-up data. Hum Path 1982; 13:113–122.

52 Yount AB, Bylund D, Pratt SG, et al. Mohs micrographic excision of sebaceous carcinoma of the eyelids. J Derm Surg Oncol 1994; 20:523–529.

53 Spencer JM, Nossa R, Tse DT, et al. Sebaceous carcinoma of the eyelid treated with Mohs micrographic surgery. J Am Acad Derm 2001; 44:1004–1009.

54 Dixon RS, Mikhail GR, Slater HC. Sebaceous carcinoma of the eyelid. J Am Acad Dermatol 1980; 3:241–243.

55 Holden C, Spittle M, Jones E. Angiosarcoma of the face and scalp, prognosis and treatment. Cancer 1987; 59:1046–1057.

56 Bullen R, Larson PO, Landeck TE, et al. Angiosarcoma of the head and neck managed by a combination of multiple biopsies to determine tumor margin and radiation therapy: report of three cases and review of the literature. Derm Surg 1998; 24:1105–1110.

57 Clayton BD, Leshin B, Hitchcock MG, et al. Utility of rush paraffin-embedded tangential sections in the management of cutaneous neoplasms. Derm Surg 2000; 26:671–678.

58 Goldberg DJ, Kim YA. Angiosarcoma of the scalp treated with Mohs micrographic surgery. J Derm Surg Oncol 1993; 19:156–158.

59 Helwig EB. Graham JH. Anogenital (extramammary) Paget's disease: a clinicopathologic study. Cancer 1963; 16:387–403.

60 Fenn ME, Morley GW, Abell MR. Paget's disease of the vulva. Obstet Gynecol 1971; 38:660–670.

61 Chanda J. Extramammary Paget's disease: prognosis and relationship to internal malignancy. J Am Acad Derm 1985; 13:1009–1014.

62 Jones RE, Austin C, Ackerman AB. Extramammary Paget's disease. A critical reexamination. Am J Derm 1979; 1:101–132.

63 Mohs FE, Blanchard L. Microscopically controlled surgery for extramammary Paget's disease. Arch Derm 1979; 115:706–708.

64 Eliezri YD, Silvers DN, Horan DB. Role of preoperative topical 5-fluorouracil in preparation for Mohs micrographic surgery of extramammary Paget's disease. J Am Acad Derm 1987; 17:497–505.

65 Coldiron BM, Goldsmith BA, Robinson JK. Surgical treatment of extramammary Paget's disease: a report of six cases and a reexamination of Mohs micrographic surgery compared with conventional surgical excision. Cancer 1991; 67:933–938.

66 Fanning J, Lambert HCL, Hale TM, et al. Paget's disease of the vulva: prevalence of associated vulvar adenocarcinoma, invasive Paget's disease and recurrence after surgical excision. Am J Obstet Gynecol 1999; 180:24–27.

67 House NS, Helm KF, Maloney ME. Management of a hidradenoma with Mohs micrographic surgery. J Derm Surg Oncol 1994; 20:619–622.

68 Will R, Coldiron B. Recurrent clear cell hidradenoma of the foot. Derm Surg 2000; 26:685–686.

69 Dzubow LM, Kramer EM. Treatment of a large, ulcerating, granular-cell tumor by microscopically controlled excision. J Derm Surg Oncol 1985; 11:392–395.

70 Gardner ES, Goldberg LH. Granular cell tumor treated with Mohs micrographic surgery: report of a case and review of the literature. Derm Surg 2001; 27:772–774.

71 Snow SN, Reizner GT. Eccrine porocarcinoma of the face. J Am Acad Derm 1992; 27:306–311.

72 Weber PJ, Hevia O, Gretzula JC, et al. Primary mucinous carcinoma. J Dermatol Surg Oncol 1988; 14:170–172.

73 Lo JS, Peschen M, Snow SN, et al. Malignant cylindroma of the scalp. J Derm Surg Oncol 1991; 17:897–901.

74 Padilla RS, Shimazu C. Malignant schwannoma treated by Mohs surgical excision. J Derm Surg Oncol 1991; 17:793–796.

75 Jackson EM, Cook J. Mohs micrographic surgery of a papillary eccrine adenoma. Derm Surg 2002; 28:1168–1172.

76 Dhawan SS, Nanda VS, Grekin S, et al. Apocrine adenocarcinoma: case report and review of the literature. J Derm Surg Oncol 1990; 16:468–470.

77 Dzubow LM, Grossman DJ, Johnson B. Chemosurgical report: eccrine adenocarcinoma – report of a case, treatment with Mohs surgery. J Derm Surg Oncol 1986; 12:1049–1053.

78 Chesser RS, Bertler DE, Fitzpatrick JE, et al. Primary cutaneous adenoid cystic carcinoma treated with Mohs micrographic surgery toluidine blue technique. J Derm Surg Oncol 1992; 18:175–176.

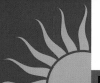

CHAPTER
45

Surgical Excision for Skin Cancer

Daihung V Do, Niels Krejci-Papa and Gary S Rogers

Key points

- Surgical excision is the cornerstone for the surgical management of most cutaneous neoplasms.
- All excision specimens should be sent for histologic analysis and margin assessment which may be of diagnostic and prognostic significance.
- In the absence of high risk features, non-melanoma skin cancers of the head and neck under 2 cm in diameter may be conservatively excised with little risk for recurrence.
- When possible, lesions suspicious for melanoma should be biopsied *in toto* by excisional technique with the long-axis paralleling lines of lymphatic drainage.
- The initial treatment for melanoma should include resection with 5 mm margins (for *in situ* lesions), 1 cm margins (for tumors 0.01–2.00 mm of invasion), 1–2 cm margins (for tumors greater than 2.00 mm invasion) and depth to fascia with consideration for sentinel lymph node biopsy if appropriate criteria are met.

INTRODUCTION

Surgical excision is the primary approach in the treatment of cutaneous neoplasms. In general, the objective is to completely remove the tumor and enable histological examination for diagnostic and/or prognostic information. Detailed knowledge of the underlying anatomy, surgical complications, local recurrence rates, and appropriate resection margins are integral in providing optimal treatment, maximizing tumor removal and producing a good cosmetic outcome.

HISTORY

The surgical management of melanoma and other cutaneous neoplasms has advanced considerably since Laennec first described the disease 'melanoma' in 1806.[1] William Norris was the first to advocate surgical excision with margins to reduce the rate of local recurrence in 1857. Based on his post mortem examination of a single patient with advanced melanoma, William Sampson Handley recommended wide local excision, regional lymph node dissection, and even amputation in 1907. For the next 50 years, his recommendation served as the basis for the treatment of melanoma. Advances in our knowledge of tumor prognostication, tumor biology and

surgical technology helped to eliminate radical surgery for melanoma and other skin cancers. Today, the surgical management of both melanoma and non-melanoma skin cancers can, in the vast majority of cases, be performed under local anesthesia in an office setting. The trend is towards more conservative resection margins and less aggressive surgical techniques.

PREOPERATIVE CONSIDERATIONS

Antibiotics

Antibiotic prophylaxis is often considered to reduce the risk of post-surgical complications such as wound infections or endocarditis. Antibiotics should not be used to compensate for poor sterile technique. Transient bacteremia occurs frequently with common activities such as tooth brushing or chewing. Only bacteremias with pathogenic organisms are likely to cause complications. Bacteremia occurs in 0.7% of immunocompetent patients undergoing cutaneous surgery[2] which is equivalent to the rate of bacteremia found in normal healthy adults without evidence of focal infection.[3]

Postoperative wound infections may have a range of consequences from life-threatening to a detrimental effect on the cosmesis of the resultant scar. For most routine dermatologic surgeries that involve clean or clean-contaminated wounds and have a low risk for wound infection, antibiotic prophylaxis is not necessary.[4] For procedures in which there is an increased risk for wound infection (location near nose, mouth, external ear canal, perineum, groin, etc.), administration of prophylactic antibiotics may be considered. Cephalexin, dicloxacillin, clindamycin, or ciprofloxacin may be given orally one hour prior to the start of the procedure depending on the anticipated pathogenic bacteria. Others have recommended either dicloxacillin or clindamycin to be added to the lidocaine anesthetic solution used for local anesthesia.[5]

Infective endocarditis is caused by bacterial invasion of the endocardium of the heart and may be life-threatening. Patients with underlying structural heart defects are at risk for developing endocarditis secondary to surgical intervention. Antibiotics are commonly given for endocarditis prophylaxis even though there are no randomized controlled trials that show antibiotics reduce the rate of endocarditis in patients at risk. Use of antibiotics should be weighed against their adverse effects, which include allergic drug reactions, interactions with other medications (e.g. coumadin), emergence of bacterial resistance, and medication cost. The indications for endocarditis prophylaxis in patients undergoing cutaneous surgery are not well-defined. The American Heart Association (AHA) guidelines (Table 45.1) for endocarditis prophylaxis[6] did not directly address prophylaxis in patients undergoing dermatologic surgery. The guidelines suggest that clinically significant bacteremia was unlikely to occur after procedures performed on 'surgically scrubbed skin'. However, the definition of what constitutes surgically scrubbed skin and what skin preparation methods qualify as such was not elaborated.

Factors influencing the decision on whether to provide antibiotic prophylaxis can be broken down into site-specific factors and host-specific factors. Site-specific factors include the location of the site as well as its potential for bacterial contamination and the intactness of the skin at the surgical site. Wounds near the nose, mouth, external auditory canal, genitalia, and anus are more likely to have high bacterial loads prior to surgery and are difficult to decontaminate. Furthermore, during the postoperative period, they are more likely to become contaminated due to high levels of endogenous bacterial flora. Skin that is not intact permits preoperative entry of pathogenic organisms that may pervade the peri-operative site beneath the skin surface. Surgical scrubbing would not be expected to clear the operative site of such organisms. Host-specific factors include history of valvular heart disease, prosthetic valves and joints, and prior history of endocarditis. In general, patients can be stratified into high, moderate, and low risk groups as defined by the American Heart Association (Table 45.2).

Given the low incidence of bacteremia in patients undergoing cutaneous surgery in sites, which can be reasonably prepped with betadine or chlorhexidine, routine endocarditis prophylaxis for patients with no risk factors is not necessary.

The prophylactic regimens recommended by the American Heart Association (AHA) are shown in Table 45.1. In general, patients should receive amoxicillin unless they have an allergy to penicillins. In that case, clindamycin, cephalosporins, or azithromycin/clarithromycin should be given. Cephalosporins should be avoided in penicillin-allergic patients with a history of immediate hypersensitivity reactions. In patients unable to take oral medications, ampicillin should be given intramuscularly or intravenously. For patients with penicillin allergies who are unable to take oral medications, clindamycin or cefazolin should be administered intravenously. Ideally, patients who require antibiotic prophylaxis will be identified at the initial consultation and given a prescription for the appropriate antibiotic. They should be instructed to take the prescribed antibiotic one hour prior to surgery.

Table 45.1 Antibiotic regimens for cutaneous surgery for endocarditis prophylaxis[6]

Situation	Regimen
Standard	Amoxicillin Adults: 2 g PO × 1 Children: 50 mg/kg PO × 1
Penicillin allergic	Clindamycin Adults: 600 mg PO × 1 Children: 20 mg/kg PO × 1 Cephalexin/Cefadroxil Adults: 2 g PO × 1 Children: 50 mg/kg PO × 1 Azithromycin/Clarithromycin Adults: 500 mg PO × 1 Children: 15 mg/kg PO × 1
Unable to take oral medications	Ampicillin Adults: 2 g IM/IV × 1 Children: 50 mg/kg IM/IV × 1
Unable to take oral medications and penicillin allergic	Clindamycin Adults: 600 mg IV × 1 Children: 20 mg/kg IV × 1 Cefazolin Adults: 1 g IM/IV × 1 Children: 25 mg/kg IM/IV × 1

All oral antibiotics should be administered 1 hour prior to the beginning of the procedure. All intravenous antibiotics should be administered within 30 min of the start of the procedure. Cephalosporins should not be used in individuals with a history of immediate-type hypersensitivity reaction such as urticaria, angioedema, or anaphylaxis to penicillins.

Table 45.2 Endocarditis risk groups as defined by the American Heart Association[6]

Risk category	Host-specific factors
High	• Prosthetic cardiac valves • Previous history of bacterial endocarditis • Complex cyanotic congenital heart diseases (single ventricle states, transposition of the great arteries, tetralogy of Fallot) • Surgically constructed systemic pulmonary shunts or conduits
Moderate	• Most other congenital cardiac malformations (other than those listed above and below) • Acquired valvular dysfunction (e.g. rheumatic heart disease) • Hypertrophic cardiomyopathy • Mitral valve prolapse with valvular regurgitation and/or thickened leaflets
Low	• Isolated secundum atrial septal defect • Surgical repair of atrial septal defect, ventricular septal defect, or patent ductus arteriosus (without residua beyond 6 months) • Previous coronary artery bypass graft surgery • Mitral valve prolapse without valvular regurgitation • Physiologic, functional, or innocent heart murmurs • Previous Kawasaki disease or rheumatic fever without valvular dysfunction • Cardiac pacemakers (intravascular and epicardial) and implanted defibrillators

Anticoagulants

Anticoagulants are taken by a small, but ever growing number of patients undergoing cutaneous surgery. Because of the theoretical risk of increased hemorrhagic complications in these patients, antithrombotic agents have traditionally been withheld perioperatively. Aspirin is usually withheld 5–10 days prior to surgery. Coumadin is most commonly discontinued 3–7 days prior to surgery. The indication for anticoagulation is an important factor in determining whether it should be discontinued. Aspirin has been found to significantly reduce the risk of myocardial infarction[7] and is regarded by some as a measure of the quality of care of a healthcare system. Discontinuing coumadin therapy in the setting of mechanical heart valves is dangerous since discontinuation would present an unacceptably high risk for thrombotic complications.

Although few studies have examined the role of anticoagulation in cutaneous surgery, at the current time, the weight of evidence is against brief discontinuation of anticoagulation prior to surgery. The risk of developing serious hemorrhagic complications in patients taking anticoagulants is low (0–1.6%)[8–10] and is similar to patients not on anticoagulant therapy. Furthermore, the risk of serious bleeding perioperatively is not decreased with brief periods of anticoagulant discontinuation.[8] In agreement with these findings, cutaneous surgeons have been shown to be unable to predict a patient's anticoagulation status based on intraoperative visual inspection.[11]

Thrombotic complications have been estimated to occur in 1 in 13,000 surgeries[12] in which anticoagulation was discontinued perioperatively. Comparison of thrombotic complications in patients remaining on anticoagulation therapy was not addressed. Although they occur much less frequently than hemorrhagic events, thrombotic complications are more likely to be life-threatening and lead to significant morbidity and mortality. Therefore, current recommendations suggest anticoagulation with either aspirin or coumadin should not be discontinued perioperatively unless surgery involves the orbital fat pad where retrobulbar hemorrhage may result in blindness. For patients on coumadin, it may be prudent to check their INR prior to surgery to confirm that it is not beyond the therapeutic range as supratherapeutic INRs may be more likely to result in hemorrhagic complications. Other anticoagulants such as clopidogrel (Plavix) and enoxaparin (Lovenox) have not been extensively studied and recommendations concerning their use in patients undergoing cutaneous surgery cannot be made at this time.

Pacemakers

Electrosurgical instruments are often used during surgical excisions for hemostasis and may interfere with the function of pacemakers and implantable cardiovertor-defibrillators (ICDs). Interference with the sensing circuitry of demand pacemakers may lead to improper triggering of pulses or reprogramming of the device.[13] Electrosurgical interference with ICDs may lead to inappropriate delivery of intracardiac shocks. For patients undergoing excisions at sites distant from the implanted device, bipolar electrosurgical instruments such as coagulation forceps should be used because current flows between the two electrode tips and is less likely to interfere with remotely located sensing electrodes. When operating near cardiac devices, electrocautery should be used since no current is introduced into the patient. Consultation with the primary cardiologist, temporary reversion to fixed-rate pacing, and deactivation of ICDs devices prior to surgery are additional options that should be considered.[13]

Allergies

Patients should be queried about their allergies at initial consultation and certainly prior to the start of the procedure. Every effort should be made to avoid using medications or substances in patients with a known allergy to these allergens. Lidocaine is an amide anesthetic, and true lidocaine allergy is rare. More commonly, adverse reactions are either due to a direct effect of the lidocaine or due to an added preservative. Larger bottles of lidocaine with epinephrine contain methylparabens as a preservative. Cutaneous reactions may occur if patients sensitized to parabens are anesthetized with lidocaine with epinephrine. Two percent lidocaine without epinephrine does not contain any parabens and may be used safely in these patients. Patients with allergies to iodine should be prepped with chlorhexidine or 70% alcohol rather than betadine. Non-latex gloves should be worn by care providers for patients with latex allergies.

Medical considerations

A thorough history and physical examination should be performed prior to undertaking a surgical excision. Factors that may adversely affect patient outcome should be anticipated and appropriate circumventions pursued so that the operation may proceed smoothly. Requirements for general anesthesia either due to patient anxiety (young age, psychiatric history) should be determined. Oxygen dependence during surgery should be assessed, particularly for procedures located near the mouth or nose in which electrosurgical instruments are necessary for hemostasis.

EXCISIONAL PROCEDURES

The treatment of skin cancer by surgical means generally entails (1) obtaining a tissue diagnosis to guide management and (2) complete removal of the tumor. Generally, histologic diagnosis should be established prior to the definitive surgical therapy for a tumor. Biopsies to confirm the diagnosis can either be excisional or incisional.

In an excisional biopsy, the whole lesion is removed (Fig. 45.1a) and submitted for pathologic analysis. It is the method of choice for melanocytic lesions suspicious for malignant melanoma. Because the whole lesion is available for histologic examination, sampling error is avoided. Furthermore, the depth of the lesion and other pertinent factors may be assessed. These factors are vitally important for the subsequent management of the patient with respect to sentinel lymph node biopsy, interferon therapy, wide local excision, and overall prognosis. Finally, excisional biopsies have the advantage of removing the entire primary tumor, which may be of diagnostic significance in neoplasms challenging the dermatopathologist's diagnostic skills.

In some circumstances, the size or anatomic location of a lesion may make complete removal with primary closure impractical or impossible. In these instances, an incisional biopsy in which a portion of the lesion is removed may be preferable (Fig. 45.1b). With melanocytic neoplasms, care should be taken to include the part of the lesion most likely to be diagnostic (e.g. the darkest or raised part of a lesion) in the sample removed. The topic of biopsy procedures is covered in greater depth elsewhere in this volume.

Once the tissue diagnosis is obtained, consideration must be given to the most appropriate management of the patient's cancer. Under rare circumstances, no treatment is the 'best' option; often the most difficult decision the physician must make with their patient and reserved for extreme circumstances. For many skin cancers, in particular basal cell carcinoma (BCC) and squamous cell carcinoma (SCC), the dermatologist has a broad armamentarium of treatment choices. Treatment options are based on patient factors, e.g. anatomic site, age, co-morbid conditions, etc. and tumor characteristics, e.g. primary versus recurrent tumor, histopathologic features among other criteria. The best therapeutic option considers not only long-term recurrence risk, but treatment risks, co-morbidity, patient convenience and full understanding of the patient's needs and expectations.

For some diseases, such as malignant melanoma, surgical resection is the primary therapeutic option. There must be clear and convincing reasons to chose another treatment modality. The issue of how wide and deep a resection is necessary to treat primary melanoma has been long debated and is reviewed later in this chapter.

Shape/orientation of excision

The shape of the planned excision will be influenced by the tumor's location and the direction of relaxed skin tension lines in the area (Fig. 45.2). Most commonly, lesions are excised in a fusiform ellipse, which is formed by two arcs (Fig. 45.3a). Although not technically an ellipse which has two different radii and no sharp angles, the fusiform shape has been referred to as an ellipse in the surgical literature based on its resemblance to an ellipse. Excisions with this shape are most often used in areas in which the relaxed skin tension lines are straight (Fig. 45.3) and in situations in which primary closure is most appropriate. The length to width ratio should be about 3–4:1 and the angles formed at the ends should approximate a 30° angle to avoid producing standing cones of tissue, so-called 'dog-ears', at the ends.

Once the tumor has been excised, the wound edges are undermined to reduce the tension across the wound and to enable eversion of the edges. The defect is then closed primarily meaning that the edges of the defect are

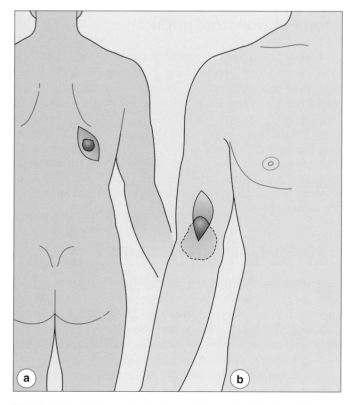

Figure 45.1 Excisional vs incisional biopsy. (a) Excisional biopsy of a lesion suspected to be malignant melanoma. The ellipse drawn contains the lesion in toto. (b) Incisional biopsy of a lesion suspected to be a malignant melanoma. Since complete excision would be difficult, only a portion of the lesion is removed.

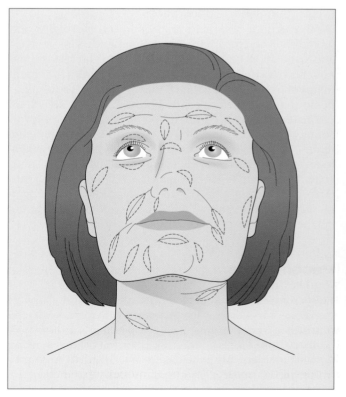

Figure 45.2 Excision orientation incorporating relaxed skin tension lines (lines of Langer).

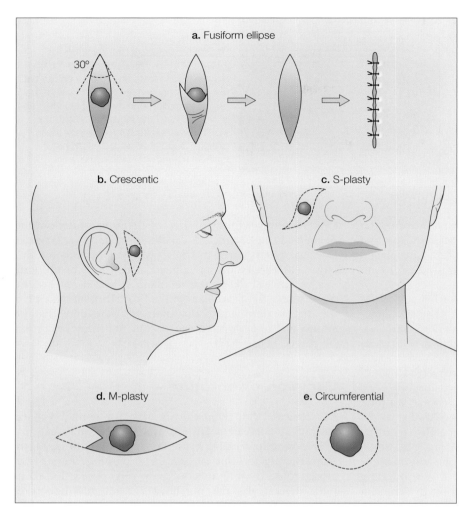

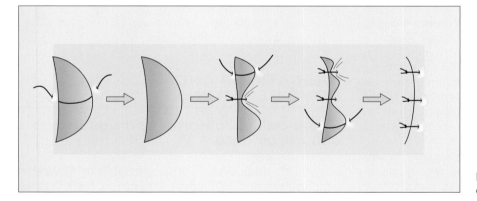

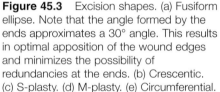

Figure 45.3 Excision shapes. (a) Fusiform ellipse. Note that the angle formed by the ends approximates a 30° angle. This results in optimal apposition of the wound edges and minimizes the possibility of redundancies at the ends. (b) Crescentic. (c) S-plasty. (d) M-plasty. (e) Circumferential.

Figure 45.4 Closing by following the rule of halves.

sutured together to form a line. Generally, dissolvable deep sutures are placed to remove dead space, stabilize wound edges and offload tension from the wound to the suture. Cutaneous sutures are then placed to finely appose wound edges and provide slight eversion to aid wound healing and scar cosmesis. Primary closures are the simplest to perform and often yield the smallest scar. In older patients, the scar may often be hidden within rhytides if the excision has been properly planned.

An alternative approach uses crescent shapes or 'C' shapes that are either formed by a line and an arc or two arcs in the same direction with one having a greater degree of curvature than the other (Fig. 45.3b). In anatomic areas in which the relaxed skin tension lines are curved such as the preauricular area or the area of the cheek lateral to the nasolabial fold, crescentic excisions may result in a better cosmetic outcome than an excision with a fusiform ellipse because the resultant scar would better follow these lines.

When closing a crescentic excision, the side with greater curvature will always have tissue redundancies due to its greater length. These defects are best closed following the rule of halves to equally distribute the excess tissue along the length of the defect (Fig. 45.4).

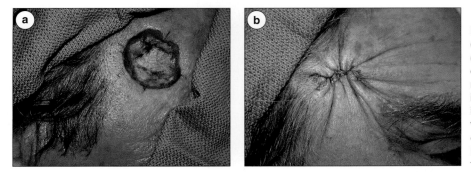

Figure 45.5 Purse string closure. (a) Circular defect on the right temple. (b) Defect closed with a purse string closure. Skin pleats are introduced but will resolve after several months. The final scar is much smaller than the original defect and is preferable to the large linear scar that would have resulted from primary linear closure. Superficial simple interrupted Prolene sutures are visible and were used to finely oppose the skin edges.

This is performed by first placing a deep suture in the center. Then, another suture is placed between the first suture and one of the tips. Additional sutures are placed to bisect the remaining defect until the wound edges are adequately apposed.

An S-shaped or double convex excision (Fig. 45.3c) is used when the skin tension lines vary in opposite directions at the edges of the ellipse or on convex surfaces. The resultant scar may attract less attention due to its curviness than a linear scar.

M-shaped excisions are used to decrease the overall length of a scar or to avoid an important anatomic landmark. They are based on a fusiform ellipse with the middle of the 'M' resting on the edge of the circular defect (Fig. 45.3d). The resultant scar will form a Y-shape.

Circumferential excisions (Fig 45.3e) are performed around the circumference of the lesion plus any margins desired and result in the least sacrifice of surrounding normal skin. They are used in situations in which a purse-string closure (see below) or healing by secondary intention is planned. Alternatively, circumferential excisions can be used in situations in which the axis of relaxed skin tension lines cannot reliably be determined prior to excision. When circular lesions are excised, the long axis of the resultant oval-shaped defect will lie parallel to the relaxed skin tension lines. Once this oval is closed along its long axis, tissue redundancies at the ends may be corrected. Circumferential excisions have the added benefit of minimally disrupting lymphatic drainage, which is of importance if subsequent sentinel lymph node biopsy is being considered.

Purse string closures may be used to close circumferential defects (Fig. 45.5). Absorbable monofilament sutures such as Vicryl or PDS are placed intradermally around the perimeter of the defect, the ends of the suture are drawn tight, and then tied with a surgeon's knot. The resultant closed wound demonstrates multiple pleats due to tissue redundancy along the shorter circumference of the defect once the purse string is tied. These pleats will even out over 1–3 months. Superficial sutures to further reduce the defect size may be placed taking shallow bites to avoid inadvertently lacerating the previously placed intracuticular suture. The superficial sutures may be removed in 2–4 weeks. Purse string closures have a number of advantages. They result in a much smaller scar than would result from a fusiform excision. The quality of the scar is often good with close matching of skin texture and color compared to grafts. It is rapidly performed and may be used to temporarily

close wounds while margins on permanent sections are being evaluated. Variations on the purse string are possible. Because pleats form in the skip area between bites, if larger skip areas are introduced at the ends of the long axis of an oval defect the resultant closed defect will be more linear than circular (Fig. 45.6a). In patients with a thin friable dermis in which there is a possibility that the suture will tear through the dermis, cuticular bites may be placed (Fig. 45.6b).

Excision orientation

For tumors with a significant risk for spread via the lymphatics such as melanoma and Merkel cell carcinoma, it is desirable to orient the long axis of the fusiform ellipse along the line of lymphatic drainage rather than along relaxed skin tension lines (Fig. 45.7). Excisions performed in this manner have the potential benefit of removing microsatellite metastasis en route to the draining lymph node basin. If the tissue margins are involved, re-excision will result in a smaller scar than if the primary tumor had been removed with an ellipse following the relaxed skin tension lines.

INDICATIONS AND CONSIDERATIONS

Basal cell carcinoma and squamous cell carcinoma

In general, surgical excision is an excellent method of treating BCC and SCC when borders are well defined, adequate margins can be taken, the defect can be closed primarily without significant anatomic distortion, and the rate of recurrence is low. In choosing a treatment modality for these tumors, considerations of local recurrence are paramount. The primary advantage of excision over destructive modalities such as cryotherapy or curettage and electrodesiccation is that margins can be assessed histologically.

The National Comprehensive Cancer Network has established guidelines for excision of BCC and SCC based on a review of the available literature by a panel of experts.[14] Tumors are classified by their likely rate of recurrence. Low risk tumors are those located on the trunk or extremities with diameter less than 2 cm; and tumors located on the head and neck outside of the

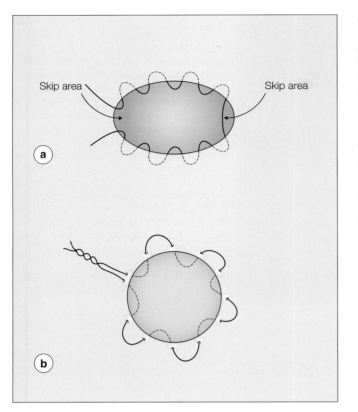

Figure 45.6 Variations on the purse string. (a) Skip areas at the ends of the ellipse are introduced to result in a more linear closure. The skin in the skip area forms a larger pleat when the suture is tied. (b) Cuticular variation. This variation of the purse is useful in locations in which the dermis is thin or fragile. The sutures have a cutaneous component, which prevents the suture from tearing through the weak dermis.

H-zone of the face (Fig. 45.8) such as the cheeks, forehead, neck, and scalp.

The H-zone or mask-areas of the face denotes anatomic areas in which there is a high rate of recurrence.[15] Tumors within these areas tend to be near free margins where considerations of tissue conservation are paramount. Cancers within these areas should be referred for Mohs micrographic surgery or radiation, which have a track record for lower rates of recurrence and better cosmetic outcome.

If the clinical border is poorly defined, then there is a greater likelihood of either excising too little tissue around the cancer, which will result in incomplete removal and a high rate of recurrence, or excising too much tissue with unnecessarily large margins. These tumors may be best treated with Mohs surgery in which intraoperative histologic margin assessment can be undertaken to properly define tumor borders.

Both BCC and SCC may in some settings spread along nerves (neurotropism). Once the tumor invades the nerve, spread along the perineurium may result in relatively distant tumor recurrences. Such spread may be unpredictable because as the tumor tracks proximally and invades a ganglion, it may subsequently spread along the course of another nerve or enter the cranial cavity. Patients may be asymptomatic for years before developing dysesthesia, pain, numbness, or motor

deficits depending upon the nerve involved.[16] The incidence of neurotropism is approximately 4% for SCCs.[17] Factors associated with neurotropism include tumor size greater than two centimeters, location of the forehead, and prior therapy.[18] The local recurrence rate after surgical excision of SCCs that demonstrate neurotropism is 47.2% in contrast to less than 1% for Mohs micrographic surgery.[17] Often, neurotropism is discovered upon histologic examination of an excision specimen. These tumors should subsequently be considered for management by Mohs micrographic surgery for maximum local control. Approximately 50% of patients symptomatic for neurotropic spread of their cancer exhibit evidence of perineural disease when imaged with CT or MRI.[16] Perhaps due to larger tumor burden, radiologic evidence of perineural spread is associated with a worse prognosis.[16]

Margins

Because tumors often extend beyond their clinical borders, it is necessary to excise a small margin of normal-appearing skin around tumors to ensure complete resection. The current recommendation is that tumors located on the trunk and extremities measuring less than 2 cm in diameter should be excised with 4 mm margins for BCCs[19] and 4–6 mm margins for SCCs.[20] Well differentiated SCCs should be excised with 4 mm margins. Moderately to poorly differentiated SCCs should be excised with 6 mm margins.[20] Tumors measuring more than 2 cm in diameter should be excised with at least 10 mm margins.[19]

Curettage is often used prior to excision to help establish the margins of the tumor. Better assessments of tumor border enable subsequent excision with appropriate margins to be more effective. Indeed, for BCC, curettage prior to excision has been shown to result in a 24% decrease in surgical failure rate (incomplete resection) compared with excision without prior curettage.[21] However, a similar benefit for curettage prior to excision for SCC was not seen, possibly due to firmer consistency of the tumor, or tumor tissue mechanics (higher keratin content) similar to normal skin resulting in less suitability for curettage.

Management of incomplete excisions

For BCCs with well-defined borders that are surgically excised with 3 mm margins, the rate of incomplete excisions (i.e. tumor extends to margin of surgical resection specimen) is 4%.[22] At least 30–50% of incompletely excised BCCs recur clinically.[23–25] Recurrence may be manifested by a sensation of pruritus or tingling, ulceration/crusting, papule near incision scar, oozing or bleeding, or firm swelling in the surgical area.[26] When BCCs recur, they are usually deeper and more aggressive and necessitate more extensive surgery, especially if flaps were used to repair the original defect.[25]

Because recurrent BCCs may be difficult to recognize clinically and tend to act more aggressively in terms of tissue infiltration, it is recommended that patients with

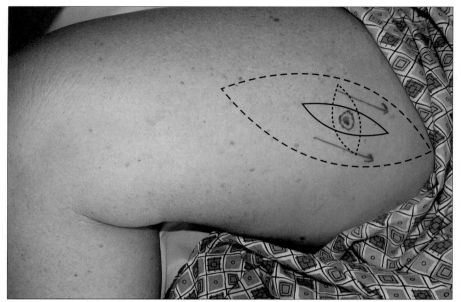

Figure 45.7 Excision oriented along the path of draining lymphatics as determined by lymphoscintigraphy or Sappy's lines of lymphatic drainage. Lymphatics in this patient drain in the direction of the arrows drawn. A fusiform ellipse with narrowest margin 1 cm around tumor and with the long axis oriented parallel to these arrows was drawn around the lesion (solid line). An excision oriented in this manner will resect the draining lymphatic ducts, which travel in the superficial fat. A fusiform ellipse oriented along the relaxed skin tension lines (dotted line) will transect the draining lymphatic ducts and alter lymphatic flow. If the margins of the excision specimen are involved, re-excision will result in a considerably larger defect since the entire scar must be removed with an additional margin (dashed line).

incomplete excisions undergo immediate surgical resection of remaining tumor rather than waiting for clinical signs and symptoms of recurrence.[26] However, in certain settings such as elderly or debilitated patients with tumors in non-critical sites, watchful waiting with close clinical follow up may be justifiable. In patients with multiple medical problems and competing co-morbidities, it may be acceptable to delay surgical resection. In patients with superficial BCCs that are located anywhere except the central face or ears measuring less than 1 cm in diameter with incompletely resected tumor involving less than 4% of the margin, the risk of clinically occult recurrence is low. These patients may safely be followed clinically until signs of recurrence manifest.[27]

Recurrence

Recurrence rates may be reported as raw, strict, or modified life-table rates.[28] Because BCC and SCC are slow growing, 5-year recurrence rates are usually used to judge the effectiveness of this treatment modality. The 2- and 5-year recurrence rates for surgical excision are 2.8 and 10.1%, respectively.[29] These rates are approximately the same as those for curettage and electrodesiccation (4.7% and 7.7%), radiation therapy (5.3% and 8.7%) and cryotherapy (3.7% and 7.5%).

BCCs on the neck, trunk, and extremities have a low 5-year recurrence rate of 0.7%.[15] For BCCs on the head, there is a correlation of recurrence rates with size. Small BCCs on the head measuring less than 6 mm in diameter have a 5-year recurrence rate after surgical excision of 3.2% compared with larger basal cells measuring more than 6 mm that have a recurrence rate of 8–9%.[15]

After surgical excision, SCCs have a 5-year recurrence rate of 8.1%.[17] Recurrent SCCs that undergo surgical excision have a much greater 5-year recurrence rate of 23.3%.[17]

The histologic type of a tumor can also influence post-excision recurrence rates. Superficial and nodular BCCs have a low risk of recurrence. Morpheaform, sclerosing, infiltrative, and micronodular types of BCC often have poorly defined clinical margins and are, in many cases, best treated by Mohs micrographic surgery or radiation if wide surgical margins are inappropriate.[14,15]

Well-differentiated SCCs have a low rate of local recurrence and may be excised surgically if the clinical margins are distinct. Moderately or poorly differentiated SCCs may necessitate wider surgical margins or Mohs micrographic surgery.[17] Tumors that recur after destructive modalities such as curettage and electrodesiccation or cryotherapy may be safely excised if they meet the above criteria for size and location.[14,15,17]

Recurrent BCCs that undergo *subsequent* surgical resection have a 5-year rate of recurrence of 17.4%.[30] When recurrent BCCs undergo Mohs micrographic surgery, the 5-year recurrence rate is 5.6%.[30] Thus, Mohs micrographic surgery should be considered for recurrent BCCs.

Melanoma

Surgical removal is the mainstay of therapy for malignant melanoma. Excision alone will provide long-term disease-free survival of the majority of these patients with stage I and II disease. Patients who are at risk for nodal involvement (thick tumor or presence of ulceration) should undergo sentinel node biopsy and, if necessary, lymph node dissection. Patients with advanced melanoma should be managed with a multidisciplinary approach.

Excision technique

In practical terms, it is advisable to first outline the biopsy scar or, if a pigmented lesion is still present, the outlines of the pigment using a Woods lamp. The

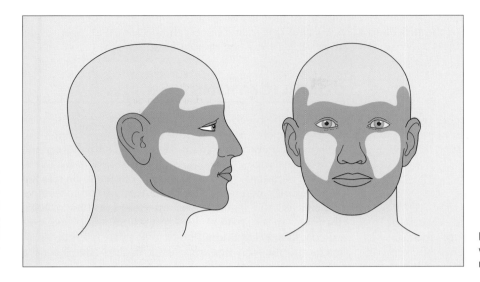

Figure 45.8 H-zone of the face (purple) which denotes areas of higher risk for recurrence of BCC and SCC.

appropriate margin is then drawn around the previous outline. This should all be performed before the administration of local anesthesia, which may distort tissues and obscure subtle tissue margins. Prior to excision, consideration should be given to the melanoma thickness, and whether a sentinel node biopsy is indicated which could be performed simultaneously with the melanoma excision, thus reducing the number of surgical visits for the patient. There is no clear evidence regarding the depth of melanoma excision, however excision to the mid-fat for melanoma *in situ* and excision to the muscle fascia for invasive melanoma is conventionally performed.

Excision margins for primary melanoma have been the source of considerable controversy. The first published recommendations come from William Sampson Handley who recommended large lateral and deep excision margins based on the autopsy of a single patient with melanoma metastatic to the lymph nodes.[31] Petersen[32] advocated the need for 5 cm lateral excision margins in their paper in 1962. In their opinion, an aggressive incision was needed to prevent local and in transit recurrence, which is an ominous prognostic sign and is associated with poor survival. Finally in 1977, Breslow and Macht[33] demonstrated that prognosis was more closely related to tumor thickness than the width of the excision margins.

More recently, several prospective studies have demonstrated that narrow surgical margins of 1–2 cm provided the same outcome as wider margins of 3–4 cm with respect to patient survival and local control.[34–37] A randomized prospective study from Milan[38] compared excision margins of 1 cm and of 3 cm from 612 patients with thin stage I melanoma and found similar rates for subsequent development of metastatic disease and disease-free survival. Currently the American Academy of Dermatology recommends excision margins or 0.5 cm for melanoma *in situ*, 1 cm margins for melanomas thinner than 2 mm, and 2 cm margins for melanomas thicker than 2 mm.[39]

Ackerman argues that a tumor that is excised with even the thinnest microscopic margins of healthy tissue surrounding it is in essence removed and no additional healthy tissue should be sacrificed.[40] Kelly *et al.*, in a prospective study, found that recurrences of *in situ* superficial spreading melanoma occurred more frequently when margins of 0.5 cm or less were used.[41]

One reason that controversy still persists is the fact that the nomenclature surrounding a local recurrence is imprecise. The cardinal difference is that of 'tumor persistence' at the margin of resection and local metastasis, or 'satellitosis' within 5 cm of the surgical scar. Both are called 'recurrent melanoma'. Tumor persistence is most frequently encountered in patients with poorly defined lentigo maligna melanomas where cosmetic considerations dictate narrow margins. Recurrences in this setting represent incomplete removal of the original tumor, i.e. *in situ* disease present at the margin, and as such carry a prognosis identical to that of the primary tumor.[42,43] In contrast, recurrences that are adjacent to the scar, and usually appear as dermal (or subcutaneous) papules, represent satellite metastases. Epidermotropic metastases can 'home' to scars. The pathologist can usually differentiate this form of satellitosis from incomplete resection. Satellitosis is a metastatic event, which has a prognostic impact equivalent to lymph node or visceral metastasis.[43] Because of the stark contrast in prognosis, every effort should be made to ascertain into which of these categories a local recurrence falls.

Lentigo maligna

Lentigo maligna deserves special consideration. If left untreated, it will invade the dermis and is then thought to behave as aggressively as any other melanoma. In a study by Zitelli[42] the majority of patients would appear to have inadequate resection margins if treated by standard surgery guidelines for patients with *in situ* melanomas on the head and neck. This percentage falls within the reported range of local recurrence for head and neck melanoma.[43] In addition, the face is the cosmetically most sensitive area of the body, and a difference in excision margins of a few millimeters can require a dramatically different defect closure with distinct cosmetic results. It is for this reason that there is intense interest in the use of Mohs micrographic surgery for lentigo maligna and lentigo maligna melanoma of the head and neck.[44]

Other cutaneous neoplasms

Other cutaneous tumors may be managed by surgical excision but lower rates of local recurrence are often achieved with Mohs micrographic surgery.

Merkel cell carcinoma

For patients with Stage I disease (local disease with no evidence of lymph node involvement or metastasis), wide local excision is acceptable. Margins of 3 cm or greater are associated with better local control but there is no difference in survival compared with excision with narrower margins.[45] Mohs surgery has been shown to result in better local control (8.3% local recurrence rate) compared with standard surgical excision (31.7%).[46]

Sebaceous carcinoma

Surgical excision with frozen section control in the absence of orbital involvement results in a 5-year recurrence rate of 9–36%[47] and a 5-year mortality rate of 18–30%.[48] If there is orbital involvement, exenteration is recommended. A small number of patients with this rare tumor have been treated with Mohs surgery with a 3-year local recurrence rate of 11.1%,[49] which appears promising. Because sebaceous carcinoma sometimes exhibits discontinuous spread, some authors have advocated an additional 4–5 mm Mohs 'assurance layer' to remove small discontinuous tumor foci beyond the edge of the Mohs defect in addition to peripheral biopsies.[50]

Microcystic adnexal carcinoma

Simple excision of microcystic adnexal carcinoma results in a high rate of recurrence of 47%.[51] Multiple excisions with postoperative margin assessment until margins are clear results in a 1.5% per person-year recurrence rate.[52] Mohs surgery offers a similarly low local recurrence rate but requires fewer procedures for patients.[51,52]

Soft-tissue sarcomas

The local recurrence rate after surgical excision of cutaneous leiomyosarcomas is 32%.[53] Because of their potential for recurrence, these tumors should be widely excised with a 3–5 cm margin down to and including the fascia.[54] Small numbers of patients have been treated with Mohs surgery with promising results.[55]

Wide local excision of dermatofibrosarcoma protuberans with at least a 3 cm margin results in a local recurrence rate of 20–54%.[54] Because of the frequency of local recurrence at the deep margin, excision down to

and including fascia is recommended. Mohs surgery is becoming the treatment of choice for DFSP and results in a 0–2.3% local recurrence rate.[56]

COMPLICATIONS

Postoperative bleeding can be a significant complication of surgical excision. It typically manifests by oozing from the surgical incision, ecchymoses, or hematoma formation. In most instances, bleeding may be stopped with firm pressure applied for at least 15 minutes. Significant bleeding may occur if there is inadequate intraoperative hemostasis, the patient has an inherent hematologic disorder, or the patient has supratherapeutic levels of anticoagulants. Expanding hematomas may exert pressure across the incision line and result in flap edge necrosis or dehiscence of the wound.

Wound infections may result from intraoperative lapses in sterility, from the introduction of bacteria intraoperatively from the nose or mouth or post-operatively from urine or feces for operative sites in the perineum. Importantly, hematomas and tissue necrosis at wound edges may predispose to wound infections by providing a rich medium for bacterial growth.

Dehiscence may result from factors related to the surgery such as poor choice of suture material, wound closure under excessive tension, premature suture removal, or postoperative trauma. Patient-specific factors such as poor nutrition, chronic debility, and advanced age may also predispose to dehiscence.

Scars typically contract with time. If the excision is not properly planned, scar contracture may result in functional defects such as decreased range of motion if the site is located over or near a joint, or ectropion if the axis of contracture is perpendicular to the free margin of the eyelid. Cosmetic defects may occur if scar contracture leads to asymmetry or if a keloid develops. The key to avoiding these complications is appropriate preoperative planning and proper postoperative follow up so that scar revision may be undertaken if necessary as early as possible.

CONCLUSION

Surgical excision is the mainstay of therapy for most skin cancers. Over the past several decades, surgical margins have been reduced from radical resection to conservative removal of the cancer. In planning surgery to treat a patient's cancer, the physician must have a thorough knowledge of the patient's medical history as well as the tumor's characteristics. Surgical risks and alternatives must be reviewed prior to any procedure. As much as possible, the resection margins should be based on acknowledged guidelines, and wound closure technique should be determined prior to commencing the surgery. All tissue resected should be submitted for histologic examination. Careful planning, early management of complications and review of wound care with the patient are essential to obtaining good outcomes.

FUTURE OUTLOOK

The use of immune response modifiers as an adjunct for surgical treatment is being evaluated both preoperatively and postoperatively. Topical imiquimod has been used to treat small superficial and nodular BCC. Theoretically, larger tumors may not respond as well to topical treatment, due to limited penetration. However, topical use may result in a reduction in the size of large tumors, which may require a less extensive surgical operation, which may be of value for tumors located in cosmetically sensitive areas.

Imiquimod has been used in treating lentigo maligna in a limited number of patients who were not candidates for surgery. However, the use of imiquimod following resection of lentigo maligna may be of benefit as an adjunctive treatment. First, imiquimod may induce the destruction of any residual melanoma cells that were not resected. Second, imiquimod may induce the destruction of the atypical melanocytic hyperplasia that typically surrounds lentigo maligna and may be present around the operative site. Such melanocytic hyperplasia may represent premalignant precursors that have developed many, but not all the somatic mutations necessary for a neoplastic phenotype. Destruction of this melanocytic hyperplasia may reduce the incidence of a second primary melanoma due to a field effect.

The development of instrumentation to non-invasively visualize tumor margins will lead to more narrow surgical margins being taken for cancer removal. *In vivo* confocal microscopy enables the real-time high resolution imaging of live tissue without the need for tissue fixation and processing. With near-infrared instruments, subcellular detail down to 200–350 μm may be visualized. A number of diagnostic features with this type of imaging have been elucidated for BCCs[57] and melanoma[58] to assess margins. Although the sensitivity and specificity of these criteria have not been determined, confocal microscopy may enable cutaneous surgeons to preoperatively define tumor borders with greater accuracy and consequently enable the further reduction of surgical margins and local recurrence rates.

REFERENCES

1 Balch CM, Milton GW, Shaw HM, Soong SJ. Cutaneous melanoma: Clinical management and treatment results worldwide. Philadelphia, PA: JB Lippincott; 1985.

2 Carmichael AJ, Flanagan PG, Holt PJ, Duerden BI. The occurrence of bacteraemia with skin surgery. Br J Derm 1996; 134:120–122.

3 Wilson WR, Scoy RE Van, Washington JA 2nd. Incidence of bacteremia in adults without infection. J Clin Microbiol 1976; 2:94–95.

4 Haas AF, Grekin RC. Antibiotic prophylaxis in dermatologic surgery. J Am Acad Derm 1995; 32:155–180.

5 Huether MJ, Griego RD, Brodland DG, Zitelli JA. Clindamycin for intraincisional antibiotic prophylaxis in dermatologic surgery. Arch Derm 2002; 138:1145–1148.

6 Dajani AS, Taubert KA, Wilson W, et al. Prevention of bacterial endocarditis. Recommendations by the American Heart Association [comment]. JAMA 1997; 277:1794–1801.

7 Roncaglioni MC. Low-dose aspirin and vitamin E in people at cardiovascular risk: a randomised trial in general practice. Lancet 2001; 357:89–95.

8 Otley CC, Fewkes JL, Frank W, Olbricht SM. Complications of cutaneous surgery in patients who are taking warfarin, aspirin, or nonsteroidal anti-inflammatory drugs. Arch Derm 1996; 132:161–166.

9 Alcalay J. Cutaneous surgery in patients receiving warfarin therapy. Derm Surg 2001; 27:756–758.

10 Bartlett GR. Does aspirin affect the outcome of minor cutaneous surgery? Br J Plast Surg 1999; 52:214–216.

11 West SW, Otley CC, Nguyen TH, et al. Cutaneous surgeons cannot predict blood-thinner status by intraoperative visual inspection. Plast Reconstr Surg 2002; 110:98–103.

12 Kovich O, Otley CC. Thrombotic complications related to discontinuation of warfarin and aspirin therapy perioperatively for cutaneous operation. J Am Acad Derm 2003; 48:233–237.

13 LeVasseur JG, Kennard CD, Finley EM, Muse RK. Dermatologic electrosurgery in patients with implantable cardioverter-defibrillators and pacemakers. Derm Surg 1998; 24:233–240.

14 Network NCCN. NCCN Practice Guidelines for Nonmelanoma Skin Cancer. NC: NCNN; 2002.

15 Silverman MK, Kopf AW, Bart RS, Grin CM, Levenstein MS. Recurrence rates of treated basal cell carcinomas. Part 3: Surgical excision. J Derm Surg Oncol 1992; 18:471–476.

16 Williams LS, Mancuso AA, Mendenhall WM. Perineural spread of cutaneous squamous and basal cell carcinoma: CT and MR detection and its impact on patient management and prognosis. Int J Radiat Oncol Biol Phys 2001; 49:1061–1069.

17 Rowe DE, Carroll RJ, Day CL Jr. Prognostic factors for local recurrence, metastasis, and survival rates in squamous cell carcinoma of the skin, ear, and lip. Implications for treatment modality selection. J Am Acad Derm 1992; 26:976–990.

18 Lawrence N, Cottel WI. Squamous cell carcinoma of skin with perineural invasion. J Am Acad Derm 1994; 31:30–33.

19 Wolf DJ, Zitelli JA. Surgical margins for basal cell carcinoma. Arch Derm 1987; 123:340–344.

20 Brodland DG, Zitelli JA. Surgical margins for excision of primary cutaneous squamous cell carcinoma. J Am Acad Derm 1992; 27:241–248.

21 Chiller K, Passaro D, McCalmont T, Vin-Christian K. Efficacy of curettage before excision in clearing surgical margins of nonmelanoma skin cancer. Arch Dermatol 2000; 136:1327–1332.

22 Bisson MA, Dunkin CS, Suvarna SK, Griffiths RW. Do plastic surgeons resect basal cell carcinomas too widely? A prospective study comparing surgical and histological margins. Br J Plast Surg 2002; 55:293–297.

23 Gooding CA, White G, Yatsuhashi M. Significance of marginal extension in excised basal-cell carcinoma. N Engl J Med 1965; 273:923–924.

24 Silva SP De, Dellon AL. Recurrence rate of positive margin basal cell carcinoma: results of a five-year prospective study. J Surg Oncol 1985; 28:72–74.

25 Richmond JD, Davie RM. The significance of incomplete excision in patients with basal cell carcinoma. Br J Plast Surg 1987; 40:63–67.

26 Robinson JK, Fisher SG. Recurrent basal cell carcinoma after incomplete resection. Arch Dermatol 2000; 136:1318–1324.

27 Berlin J, Katz KH, Helm KF, Maloney ME. The significance of tumor persistence after incomplete excision of basal cell carcinoma [comment]. J Am Acad Dermatol 2002; 46:549–553.

28 Silverman MK, Kopf AW, Grin CM, Bart RS, Levenstein MJ. Recurrence rates of treated basal cell carcinomas. Part 1: Overview. J Derm Surg Oncol 1991; 17:713–718.

29 Rowe DE, Carroll RJ, Day CL, Jr. Long-term recurrence rates in previously untreated (primary) basal cell carcinoma: implications for patient follow-up. J Derm Surg Oncol 1989; 15:315–328.

30 Rowe DE, Carroll RJ, Day CL, Jr. Mohs surgery is the treatment of choice for recurrent (previously treated) basal cell carcinoma. J Derm Surg Oncol 1989; 15:424–431.

31 Handley WW. The pathology of melanotic growths in relation to their operative treatment. Lancet 1907; 1:996–1003.

32 Petersen NC, Bodenham DD, Lloyd OC. Malignant melanomas of the skin. Br J Plast Surg 1962; 15:49–92.

33 Breslow A, Macht SD. Optimal size of resection margin for thin cutaneous melanoma. Surg Gynecol Obstet 1977; 145:691–692.

34 Balch CM, Urist MM, Karakousis CP, et al. Efficacy of 2-cm surgical margins for intermediate-thickness melanomas (1 to 4 mm). Results of a multi-institutional randomized surgical trial. Ann Surg 1993; 218:262–269.

35 Karakousis CP, Balch CM, Urist MM, et al. Local recurrence in malignant melanoma: long-term results of the multi-institutional randomized surgical trial. Ann Surg Oncol 1996; 3:446–452.

36 Bono A, Bartoli C, Clemente C, et al. Ambulatory narrow excision for thin melanoma (< or = 2 mm): results of a prospective study. Eur J Cancer 1997; 33:1330–1332.

37 Heaton KM, Sussman JJ, Gershenwald JE, et al. Surgical margins and prognostic factors in patients with thick (>4 mm) primary melanoma. Ann Surg Oncol 1998; 5:322–328.

38 Veronesi U, Cascinelli N, Adamus J, et al. Thin stage I primary cutaneous malignant melanoma. Comparison of excision with margins of 1 or 3 cm. N Engl J Med 1988; 318:1159–1162.

39 Sober AJ, Chuang TY, Duvic M, et al. Guidelines of care for primary cutaneous melanoma. J Am Acad Derm 2001; 45:579–586.

40 Ackerman AB, Sheiner AM. How wide and deep is wide and deep enough? A critique of surgical practice in excisions of primary cutaneous malignant melanoma. Hum Pathol 1983; 14:743–744.

41 Kelly JW, Sagebiel RW, Calderon W, et al. The frequency of local recurrence and microsatellites as a guide to reexcision margins for cutaneous malignant melanoma. Ann Surg 1984; 200:759–763.

42 Zitelli JA, Brown CD, Hanusa BH. Surgical margins for excision of primary cutaneous melanoma. J Am Acad Derm 1997; 37:422–429.

43 Brown CD. Surgical guidelines for malignant melanoma. Curr Probl Dermatol 2001; 13:114–118.

44 Kaufmann R. Surgical management of primary melanoma. Clin Exp Derm 2000; 25:476–481.

45 Goessling W, McKee PH, Mayer RJ. Merkel cell carcinoma. J Clin Oncol 2002; 20:588–598.

46 O'Connor WJ, Roenigk RK, Brodland DG. Merkel cell carcinoma. Comparison of Mohs micrographic surgery and wide excision in eighty-six patients. Derm Surg 1997; 23:929–933.

47 Nelson BR, Hamlet KR, Gillard M, Railan D, Johnson TM. Sebaceous carcinoma. J Am Acad Derm 1995; 33:1–18.

48 Doxanas MT, Green WR. Sebaceous gland carcinoma. Review of 40 cases. Arch Ophthalmol 1984; 102:245–249.

49 Spencer JM, Nossa R, Tse DT, Sequeira M. Sebaceous carcinoma of the eyelid treated with Mohs micrographic surgery. J Am Acad Derm 2001; 44:1004–1009.

50 Snow SN, Larson PO, Lucarelli MJ, Lemke BN, Madjar DD. Sebaceous carcinoma of the eyelids treated by Mohs micrographic surgery: report of nine cases with review of the literature. Derm Surg 2002; 28:623–631.

51 Friedman PM, Friedman RH, Jiang SB, et al. Microcystic adnexal carcinoma: collaborative series review and update. J Am Acad Derm 1999; 41:225–231.

52 Chiller K, Passaro D, Scheuller M, et al. Microcystic adnexal carcinoma: forty-eight cases, their treatment, and their outcome. Arch Derm 2000; 136:1355–1359.

53 Fields JP, Helwig EB. Leiomyosarcoma of the skin and subcutaneous tissue. Cancer 1981; 47:156–169.

54 Fish FS. Soft tissue sarcomas in dermatology. Derm Surg 1996; 22:268–273.

55 Holst VA, Junkins-Hopkins JM, Elenitsas R. Cutaneous smooth muscle neoplasms: clinical features, histologic findings, and treatment options. J Am Acad Derm 2002; 46:474–491.

56 Nouri K, Lodha R, Jimenez G, Robins P. Mohs micrographic surgery for dermatofibrosarcoma protuberans: University of Miami and NYU experience. Derm Surg 2002; 28:1060–1064.

57 Gonzalez S, Tannous Z. Real-time, in vivo confocal reflectance microscopy of basal cell carcinoma. J Am Acad Derm 2002; 47:869–874.

58 Langley RG, Rajadhyaksha M, Dwyer PJ, et al. Confocal scanning laser microscopy of benign and malignant melanocytic skin lesions in vivo. J Am Acad Derm 2001; 45:365–376.

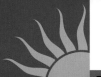

CHAPTER

46

Regional Lymph Node Surgery for Patients with Malignant Melanoma

James Jakub, Solange Pendas and Douglas S Reintgen

Key points

- Lymphatic mapping and sentinel lymph node biopsy has become the standard of care for the nodal staging of patients with malignant melanoma.
- The American Joint Committee on Cancer Melanoma Staging Committee states that in order to determine pathological stage of the patient with melanoma, both the microstaging of the primary tumor and nodal staging is necessary.
- The information gained from the lymphatic mapping procedure identifies patients who are candidates for complete node dissection and adjuvant Interferon alfa therapy.
- Lymphatic mapping and sentinel lymph node biopsy require a multi-disciplinary approach with collaboration from nuclear medicine, surgery and pathology to perform the technique and provide accurate nodal staging.
- Clinical trials are addressing whether this surgical strategy for the regional basin contributes to a survival benefit for the patient with melanoma.

INTRODUCTION

Melanoma incidence is rising.[1] This tumor affects young persons who are in the most productive years of their lives. Accordingly, melanoma constitutes a major public health problem. Since the early 1990s, the care of patients with melanoma has changed dramatically with the development of new lymphatic mapping techniques that reduce the cost and morbidity of nodal staging, the emergence of more sensitive assays for occult melanoma metastases, and the identification of interferon alfa-2b as an effective adjuvant therapy for melanoma patients who are at high risk for recurrence.

The development of intraoperative lymphatic mapping and selective lymphadenectomy has made it possible to map the lymphatic flow from a primary tumor and to identify its so-called sentinel lymph node (SLN) or nodes (SLNs) in the regional basin. Integration of this technique, in association with detailed pathologic examination of the SLN, into the surgical treatment of melanoma offers the potential for more conservative operations that not only result in lower morbidity but also permit more accurate staging.

RATIONALE

Many factors are known to predict the risk for metastatic disease in melanoma patients. In evaluating treatments for melanoma, it is crucial to take into account prognostic factors that can accurately categorize patients into different risk groups for metastasis. If this is not done, it is difficult to determine whether differences between treatment regimens are due to the treatments themselves or merely reflect imbalances of prognostic factors.

The presence or absence of lymph node metastases is the single most powerful predictor of recurrence and survival in melanoma patients: the 5-year survival rate is approximately 40% lower in patients who have lymph node metastases. A great deal of time and effort has been expended on identifying prognostic factors based on primary tumor variables (e.g. Breslow's tumor thickness, ulceration, primary site, and sex). However, multiple regression analyses performed on many collected populations in the literature indicate that once melanoma metastasizes to the regional nodes, primary site prognostic factors contribute relatively little to the prognostic model compared with the patient's lymph node status. This finding suggests that many melanoma patients might benefit from an accurate nodal staging procedure.

NODAL STAGING

Elective lymph node dissection

Elective lymph node dissection (ELND) has been the mainstay of the surgeon's armamentarium for nodal staging of melanoma patients. ELND removes clinically negative nodes, as opposed to therapeutic dissection, which removes nodes with gross, palpable tumor involvement. Opinions are divided as to whether ELND actually extends survival or whether it is solely a staging procedure. Two prospective, randomized trials failed to demonstrate improved survival in melanoma patients treated with ELND in comparison with patients who underwent wide local excision (WLE) alone as primary surgical therapy.[2,3] Retrospective studies using large databases suggested that there were subpopulations of melanoma patients who did benefit from ELND.[4]

The controversy may have been laid to rest by the results of the Intergroup Melanoma Trial, which is the first randomized study to prove enhanced survival after surgical treatment of clinically occult metastatic melanoma. Only patients with intermediate-thickness melanoma (tumor thickness, 1.0 to 4.0 mm) were eligible. In addition, the Intergroup Melanoma Trial was the first prospective study to require preoperative lymphoscintigraphy to identify and remove all basins at risk for metastasis. Without preoperative lymphoscintigraphy to provide a map for the surgeon, ELND may be misdirected in more than 50% of head and neck dissections and trunk dissections[5]. Moreover, so-called in transit nodes (defined as nodes outside the classic anatomic basin between the primary site and the regional nodes), which are equally at risk for metastasis, may be missed in 5% of patients.[6]

In the Intergroup Melanoma Trial, overall survival was not significantly longer in patients who underwent WLE and ELND than in those who underwent WLE of the primary site coupled with observation of the regional basins. There were, however, two well-defined subsets of the ELND group that exhibited a significant increase in overall survival: patients with melanomas 1.1 to 2.0 mm thick and patients younger than 60 years.[7] Stratification by tumor thickness was part of the original design of the trial, but the age-related benefit only became apparent with retrospective subgroup analysis. Now with follow-up that extends to 10 years, Balch has shown in this trial that the survival curves of the two groups have continued to separate secondary to late recurrences and deaths in the group treated with just a WLE. In addition, the P value for differences in survival for the entire study has decreased from 0.25 to 0.09 with the longer follow-up, suggesting that there may be a survival benefit associated with surgery in and of itself to the regional nodal basin.[8]

Given these results and those of three national prospective randomized trials investigating adjuvant Interferon alfa-2b, including the initial Eastern Cooperative Oncology Group (ECOG) 1684, which was the impetus for FDA approval of interferon alfa-2b as the first effective adjuvant therapy[9] for high risk recurrence melanoma, a strong argument can be made that when the risk of nodal metastasis reaches a certain defined level, a nodal staging procedure should be done. At the Lakeland Regional Cancer Center (Lakeland, FL), the level of primary melanoma thickness to consider nodal staging is 0.76 mm or greater. The nodal staging procedure recommended and performed is lymphatic mapping and SLN biopsy.

INTRAOPERATIVE LYMPHATIC MAPPING AND SELECTIVE LYMPHADENECTOMY

Intraoperative lymphatic mapping and selective lymph-adenectomy was developed as a method of assessing regional lymph node status more accurately than ELND could while reducing both morbidity and expense. This technique relies on two concepts: first, that different regions of the skin have specific patterns of lymphatic drainage to the regional lymphatic basin; and second, that for a given skin region, there is a specific lymph node (i.e. a sentinel lymph node) or nodes in the basin to which the cutaneous lymphatic vessels drain first. These concepts were borne out by initial animal studies

using either vital blue dye[10] or radiocolloid[11] (which has been shown to map the same lymphatic pathways and label the same nodes as vital blue dye). Lymphatic mapping and selective lymphadenectomy was initially proposed by Morton and associates,[12,13] who used a vital blue dye method. These investigators showed that the SLN is the first node or nodes in the lymphatic basin into which the primary melanoma consistently drains (though not necessarily the closest to the primary). They also hypothesized that the status of the SLN, if it was negative for metastases, would reflect the status of higher nodes (i.e. nodes farther down the lymphatic drainage pathway, second tier nodes). Subsequent work on intraoperative mapping and selective lymphadenectomy confirmed that the SLN is the first site of metastatic disease and demonstrated that if the SLN or nodes are histologically negative, then the remainder of the lymph nodes in the basin are histologically negative as well.[14,15] These findings suggest that melanoma patients can be accurately staged with procedures that are less extensive than complete dissection.

SLNs can be mapped from different primary site locations, and more than one node in the same basin can be an SLN, depending on the primary site. Fine dermal lymphatic vessels coalesce to form several major lymphatic trunks that eventually drain to the regional lymphatic basin. Because cutaneous lymphatic vessels converge rather than diverge, one can perform intraoperative mapping from various skin sites and still harvest only one or two SLNs from the basin. The small number of specimens facilitates detailed pathologic examination: the pathologist can readily perform serial sections of the nodes and use immunohistochemical methods to look for micrometastatic disease. More intensive pathologic examination of one or two SLNs appears to identify patients with micrometastatic lymph node metastases more accurately than routine examination of all the regional lymph nodes.

Unusual or ambiguous drainage patterns. Lympho-scintigraphy has been used in patients to map patterns of lymphatic drainage from various primary skin sites. Early assessments of lymphatic flow patterns, such as those of the nineteenth century anatomist, Sappey,[16] were based on anatomic dissections of cadavers and do not accurately reflect lymphatic flow patterns in living humans. The watershed areas of the body are much larger than originally described by Sappey, and there is no clinically predictable lymphatic flow from a melanoma until it is located 10 cm off the midline or 10 cm off Sappey's line (a line running between the umbilicus and L2 in the back). In addition, the entire head and neck region is a watershed area. Cutaneous lymphatic flow frequently cannot be predicted on the basis of anatomic site, and areas of ambiguous or multidirectional flow are significantly more extensive than classical descriptions predicted.[17]

A number of unusual cutaneous drainage patterns and pathways have been noted from work from the Sydney Melanoma Unit in Australia:[17] 26% of melanomas on the back drained to an in transit node near the scapula in the intermuscular space, 20% of melanomas near the umbilicus drained to an internal mammary node, some posterior scalp melanomas drained to lymph nodes at the base of the neck, and at least one forearm melanoma drained directly to a lymph node in the ipsilateral neck. Krag and coworkers[18,19] have also noted some unusual lymphatic drainage patterns: one melanoma on the right upper back drained directly to a node in the right midclavicular space, almost at the apex of the right lung, another melanoma on the lower back drained to an SLN along the neurovascular bundle under the 12th rib, and two lower extremity melanomas drained to SLNs in the popliteal fossa.

PATIENT SELECTION

Selective lymphadenectomy and SLN biopsy are currently being evaluated in a randomized trial sponsored by the National Cancer Institute, the goal of which is to determine whether this surgical strategy by itself extends the survival of the melanoma patient. Even if this trial demonstrates no inherent survival benefit, there are additional considerations that support use of the procedure in certain populations. Data from the interferon alfa-2b trials cited earlier[9] suggest that all patients whose melanoma is more than 0.75 mm thick should undergo a nodal staging procedure so that adjuvant therapy can be administered in a selective fashion. If T4N0 patients are removed from the analysis of this trial and only patients with lymph node metastases are considered, disease-free survival (DFS) increases by 82% ($P = 0.0006$) with adjuvant therapy and overall survival increases by 24% ($P = 0.006$). Given such a difference in both DFS and overall survival, one would naturally want to offer these patients interferon alfa-2b therapy. Accordingly, one would need to identify patients with nodal metastases who might benefit from such therapy. Lymphatic mapping and SLN biopsy is the least morbid and most cost-effective way of determining which melanoma patients have lymph node metastases.

In female patients with melanomas less than 0.76 mm thick, the risk of nodal metastasis is less than 1%. Therefore, SLN biopsy is not indicated in this population. However, in male patients whose primary site is on the trunk, the incidence of occult nodal metastases may be as high as 9%. For this reason, even if the primary lesion is less than 0.76 mm thick, lymphatic mapping may be considered in this population.

In patients whose tumors are 0.76 to 1.0 mm thick, the risk of nodal metastasis is less than 6%. The procedure can be offered as an option in this population. In our experience, these patients usually elect to undergo SLN biopsy despite the low risk of occult nodal metastasis. The morbidity of the procedure is low, and the finding of a positive SLN can radically affect subsequent treatment decisions. If the patients have a positive SLN, the standard recommendation is to take that patient back to the operating room for a complete lymph node dissection (CLND) and offer adjuvant interferon alfa-2b. Several prognostic factors have been shown to identify patients with thin melanomas who are at higher risk (approximately 10%) for metastatic disease and death at 5 years: tumors at Clark level III or greater, ulcerated primaries, regressed lesions, male gender, and axial melanomas.[20] Patients with 4 or 5 of these prognostic factors should be treated as if they have thicker lesions,

and their SLNs should be harvested even if the primary lesions are less than 0.76 mm thick.

Melanoma patients with intermediate thickness lesions (between 1–4 mm) probably have the most to benefit from lymphatic mapping and SLN biopsy. The procedure can be used to stage patients in order to offer adjuvant therapy in a selective fashion and it may contribute to a survival benefit as shown with the long term follow-up of the Intergroup study.[8]

In patients with thick (>4.0 mm) melanomas, the rate of occult systemic metastasis is 70%, and that of occult nodal metastasis is 60% to 70%. Consequently, in the past, procedures involving the regional nodes (i.e. ELND) were not recommended, because there was no survival benefit. However, now that effective adjuvant therapy is available, lymphatic mapping and SLN biopsy should be offered to these patients as a staging procedure. Survival is decreased in patients with thick melanomas and documented nodal microscopic disease compared with patients with thick melanomas and no sign of nodal spread.[21] Accordingly, some medical oncologists observe T4 patients unless nodal metastasis is documented.

A crucial question to be answered is, what is the standard of surgical care for melanoma patients with tumors thicker than 0.75 mm? Given that over 25 reports in the literature have shown how the histology of the SLN is indicative of the histology of the rest of the nodes in the basin, one can conclude that if the surgeon has adequate support from nuclear medicine and pathology services, there is no need to perform ELND. If such support is unavailable, if intraoperative mapping cannot be done (as, perhaps, when WLE of the primary melanoma has already been performed), or if the results of mapping are equivocal, then the ELND guidelines from the Intergroup Melanoma Surgical Trial[7] should be followed. If this approach is taken, ELND should be guided by preoperative lymphoscintigraphy for identification and dissection of all basins at risk for metastasis.

Finally, previous extensive primary site surgery constitutes a general technical contraindication to lymphatic mapping. Patients who have undergone rotational flap closure or Z-plasty reconstruction are considered ineligible for this procedure.

DEFINITION OF AN SLN

A node is considered to be the SLN if it meets one of three criteria:

- The node is blue.

- The node has a blue-stained afferent lymphatic leading to it. Occasionally, a node is full of tumor and has a dilated blue-stained lymphatic vessel leading to it, but it does not take up the dye or the radiocolloid readily. This scenario is realized intraoperatively because the node is hard to direct palpation. Despite the lack of uptake of the mapping reagent, such nodes must be considered SLNs.

- The node has an *in vivo* activity ratio (radioactivity in the SLN/neighboring non-SLN) of 3:1 or an *ex vivo* activity ratio of 10:1.

This definition is a purely anatomical definition in that any node that is connected to the primary site with an afferent lymphatic has to be considered an SLN. Thus, the SLNs are not the nearest nodes to the primary site in the regional basin, are not just the hottest nodes in the basin, are not only the blue nodes. SLNs are nodes in the regional basin that meet the above criteria. A node will not accumulate enough blue dye in order for the surgeon to see it, or will not accumulate enough radiocolloid with the appropriate activity ratios unless it has this direct connection to the primary site. And if the node in the regional basin has this direct connection, then it is equally at risk for harboring metastatic disease and has to be identified and harvested.

TECHNIQUE

The technique of intraoperative mapping varies considerably from center to center. We will describe the nuances of the technique as it is performed at Lakeland Regional Cancer Center (LRCC), detailing the steps that are important for successful mapping. It cannot be emphasized enough that successful intraoperative SLN mapping requires close collaboration between the surgeon, the nuclear radiologist, and the pathologist, with each member of the team playing a critical role.

An initial caveat regarding the timing of the procedure in relation to WLE is in order. Data from LRCC indicate that when lymphatic mapping is done after WLE, the dissection tends to be more extensive than it needed to be. More SLNs are removed and more regional basins dissected than when lymphatic mapping is done before WLE. Moreover, the rate at which so-called skip metastases are detected appears to be increased. With lymphatic mapping and SLN biopsy becoming the standard of care in the US for nodal staging to identify melanoma patients who are candidates for adjuvant therapy and a possible survival benefit, it is essential that patient care not be compromised by extensive primary site surgery before lymphatic mapping.

Step 1: Preoperative lymphoscintigraphy

Patients come to the nuclear medicine suite early on the day of operation or the afternoon before the procedure and undergo preoperative lymphoscintigraphy with the injection of 450 µCi in 1 ml of filtered technetium-99-labeled sulfur colloid (^{99m}Tc-SC). Dynamic scans are performed 5 to 10 minutes after injection of the radiocolloid, and the location of the SLN in the basin is marked with an intradermal tattoo. All regional lymphatic basins at risk for metastatic spread, along with in transit nodes and SLNs, are identified and marked for harvesting. A typical case of a patient with a right foot intermediate thickness primary melanoma will be illustrated.

Pre-operative lymphoscintigraphy is used to provide a 'road map' to the surgeon of cutaneous lymphatic flow patterns from the primary melanoma. The following information is provided by this study:

- Identifies all nodal basins at risk for metastatic disease. This is especially important with melanomas of the trunk or the head and neck, whose lymphatic drainage patterns cannot be reliably predicted by clinical judgment or classic anatomic guidelines.

- Identifies any in transit nodes that can be tattooed by the nuclear radiologist for later harvesting. An in-transit node is defined as a node somewhere between the primary site and the regional basin but located outside any classic anatomical landmarks of a regional basin.

- Identifies the location of the SLN in relation to the rest of the nodes in the basin.[22] Because the location of the SLN may vary within a basin, it is important to mark the position of the SLN in reference to other nodes so that harvesting may be done with local anesthesia through a minimal incision. Preoperative lymphoscintigraphy can accomplish this task quite well, especially in the groin and the head and neck area, where the lymph nodes are more superficial. The axilla is the most difficult area to map: here, the best preoperative lymphoscintigraphy can do is to determine whether the node is located anteriorly, posteriorly, superiorly, or inferiorly in the basin. Use of hand-held gamma probes during SLN mapping has reduced the need to mark SLN locations during preoperative lymphoscintigraphy. However, intradermal tattooing to mark the location of the SLN can confirm the site and thereby make the surgical procedure more efficient.

- Estimates the number of SLNs in the regional basin that will have to be harvested.

The timing of the injection of the mapping reagent has an impact on the success of the procedure. Whereas vital

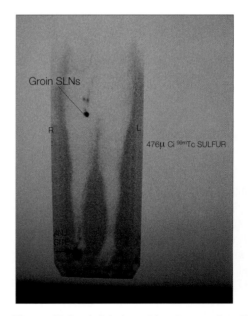

Groin SLNs

R L

476µ Ci ^{99m}Tc SULFUR

Figure 46.1 A right lateral foot intermediate thickness melanoma is injected peri-tumor with approximately 450 µCi of technetium sulfur colloid. After 10 min, images are obtained to visualize migration of the injected radiocolloid to the right groin where a number of sentinel lymph nodes (SLN) are visualized.

blue dyes typically travel to the regional basin within a matter of minutes, most radiocolloids are concentrated in the SLN over a period of hours. Activity ratios (ratio of radioactivity in the SLN vs surrounding tissue or non-SLNs) for ^{99m}Tc-SC are highest 2 to 6 hours after injection, which is helpful to the surgeon in three respects. First, the higher ratios make the SLN easier to locate. Second, the radiocolloid can be injected by the nuclear radiologist hours before the actual operation, and the surgeon does not need a special license for radioactivity handling. Third, cases are easier to schedule because there is a 2- to 24-hr window during which the intraoperative mapping can be easily accomplished. Other groups have shown that one can perform effective lymphatic mapping for melanoma the next day (16–24 hrs) after the injection of the radiocolloid. Counts are decreased because of the short half-life of technetium (6 hrs), but 'hot-spots' of radiocolloid concentration in the SLN are still recognizable due to the fact that once the radiocolloid enters the first node it is trapped there by the dendritic cells of the node and very little passes through to second tier nodes.[23]

In the illustrative case, the right foot melanoma is seen to drain into the right groin (Fig. 46.1 – arrows mark the primary site and the SLN). There is no in-transit activity noted in the popliteal space.

Step 2: Intraoperative lymphatic mapping and identification of SLN

The patient is taken to the OR 2 to 24 hrs later, and 1 ml/direction of drainage of 1% isosulfan blue dye (Lymphazurin) is injected around the primary site. If the patient has thin skin, the afferent lymphatics can be visualized emanating from the primary site (Fig. 46.2). The primary site and the regional basin are prepared and draped, and 10 minutes is allowed for the vital blue dye to travel to the SLN. Attention is then directed initially to the regional basin. The radioactive hot spot in the regional basin is identified with the hand-held gamma probe, and the *in vivo* activity ratio is noted. If shine-through from the injected radioactivity at the primary site is a problem, WLE of the primary may be performed first. An incision is made over the hot spot, and small flaps are created in all directions to allow identification of the blue-stained afferent lymphatic vessels. Surgical dissection is aided by visualization of the stained afferent lymphatic vessel leading down to the blue-stained node and by the use of the hand-held gamma probe to direct dissection down to the SLN. If, as is sometimes the case, one becomes confused as to what is proximal and what is distal on the afferent lymphatic vessel, the probe can be used to identify the direction of dissection. In the illustrated case, since a skin graft was needed to close the anticipated defect at the primary site, a full thickness skin graft is harvested from the area of the SLN biopsy. In this way, patients are saved an extra wound to heal that would have been necessary if the graft was not harvested from this site (Fig. 46.3). In Figure 46.4, the right groin is opened over the 'hot spot' identified with the hand-held gamma probe and the afferent lymphatics leading to the SLNs are visualized as wisps of blue-stained channels.

Radiocolloid and vital blue dye mapping techniques are complementary, and there is no reason why the two approaches should not be used simultaneously to improve the chances of locating the SLN successfully. Either may be crucial in a given instance, depending on the location of the primary in relation to the regional basin. If the

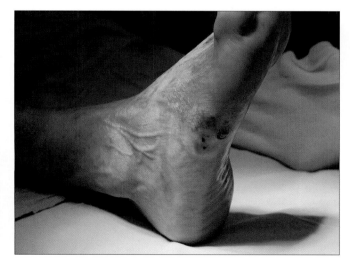

Figure 46.2 The patient is then brought to the operating room and given general anesthesia. The right foot primary site is injected with the vital blue dye-mapping agent. If the patient has 'thin' skin, the blue dye can be seen being taken up by the lymphatics that stream up the leg. This blue dye migrates to the regional basin (right groin) to stain the SLN and gives the surgeon a visual clue as to the location of the SLN.

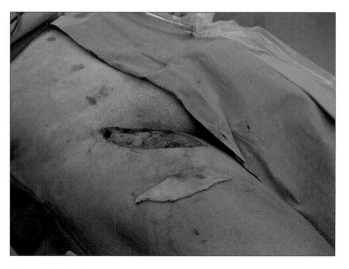

Figure 46.3 After allowing the blue dye and radiocolloid to migrate to the regional basin (right groin), an ellipse of skin is taken over the SLN area to later be used as a full-thickness skin graft to cover the skin defect from the primary site wide local excision on the right foot. This saves the patient a third incision and a third wound to heal.

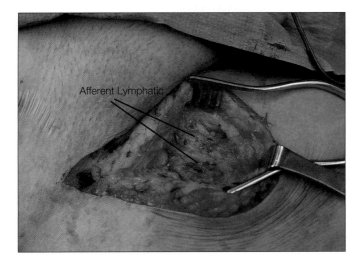

Figure 46.4 Upon opening the skin over the 'hot-spot' in the groin detected by the hand-held probe, wisps of blue-stained afferent lymphatics are seen entering the SLNs.

primary site is close to, overlying, or in a direct line to the basin, so that the gamma probe is likely to encounter shine-through, use of vital blue dye may be the only technique that permits successful mapping. Only 1 to 5% of the injected radiocolloid dose is delivered to the regional basin. Therefore, even if the radioactivity from the primary site is reduced by performing WLE first, there is enough diffusion of the injectate that enough radioactivity may remain at that site to increase the background level in the basin to the point where mapping with the radiocolloid alone is impossible. Alternatively, when one is mapping a fatty axilla or the head and neck region, it may be impossible to follow a wisp of blue-stained afferent lymphatic vessel to the SLN. Large flaps are especially to be avoided in the head and neck area because of the surrounding vital structures. In this setting, the ability of the gamma probe to locate the hot spot through the skin before the incision is made is a tremendous advantage.

A key issue with intraoperative radiocolloid mapping is how to define an SLN in terms of accumulated radio-activity. To do this, clinicians must use so-called activity (or localization) ratios. Measurement of the absolute level of radioactivity in a node is not sufficient, because in each harvest, there are a number of crucial variables: different radiocolloid doses are injected at the primary site, the injection is sometimes unevenly distributed around the primary site, the time interval between injection and harvest is not constant, the distance between the primary site and the regional basin is not always the same, and varying degrees of shine-through may be present. The effects of these variables can be eliminated by determining the *in vivo* activity ratio (i.e. the ratio of the radioactivity in the SLN to the background radioactivity). *In vivo* radioactivity is measured in counts/10 s with the SLN fully exposed. Background activity is estimated by counting four areas in the basin equidistant from the injection site and away from the SLN. Perhaps most helpful is the *ex vivo* activity

ratio (i.e. the ratio of the radioactivity in an excised SLN to that in an excised neighboring non-SLN), which has the virtue of eliminating all shine-through. At LRCC, we define an SLN as a node with an activity ratio of 3:1 or higher *in vivo* or 10:1 or higher *ex vivo*. In our experience, 98% of SLNs exhibit these ratios.

Occasionally, pass-through of the blue dye or the radiocolloid occurs but rarely, if ever, to the point where it results in mistaken identification of a higher node as an SLN. That is, one typically does not see non-SLNs that are stained blue or that have activity ratios of 3:1 *in vivo* or 10:1 *ex vivo*. When the radiocolloid does pass through the SLN, it is distributed to multiple higher nodes, thereby helping to raise the background radiation level. However, it is not concentrated to any large extent in any one higher node.

Step 3: Removal of SLN

Once the SLN is identified, the entire node is removed by means of sharp dissection or the electrocautery. Afferent and efferent lymphatic vessels entering or exiting the SLN, some of which (afferent) are stained blue, are controlled with hemostatic clips because the electrocautery will not seal these vessels. This measure decreases the risk of postoperative wound seroma. If the opportunity presents itself without the risk of increased morbidity, a neighboring non-SLN may be removed to provide an internal control, and the *ex vivo* activity ratio may be calculated. In the illustrated case, two blue-stained SLNs have been dissected so that they are only

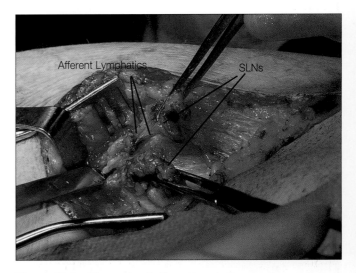

Figure 46.5 Blue-stained afferent lymphatic vessels are seen entering two blue-stain nodes. These nodes are also 'hot' compared with surrounding nodes and tissue due to the migration of the radiocolloid into the SLN. A combination (blue-dye and radiocolloid) mapping technique is used to ensure that all the SLNs are removed with the initial operation, since they are all equally at risk for metastatic disease. The mean number of SLNs removed for melanoma cases is two per basin. Many times melanomas located on the trunk or head and neck area drain in multiple directions to multiple lymphatic basins. If this is the case, then all basins identified to be at risk for the spread of the melanoma have to be dissected and the SLNs harvested.

connected to the underlying tissue by their afferent lymphatic from the lower leg (Fig. 46.5).

The radioactivity level in the excised SLN is checked with the hand-held gamma probe to confirm that the node has been correctly identified as the SLN (Fig. 46.6). The residual radioactivity in the basin is then checked with the probe to verify that all SLNs have been removed. If radioactivity has not fallen to the background level, the probe should be used to direct additional dissection to remove more SLN(s). A secondary benefit of radio-colloid mapping is its ability to provide immediate verification that all SLNs have been removed from the lymphatic basin: if all of the radiolabeled SLNs have in fact been excised, the radioactivity in the basin must return to its background level. When only vital blue dye is used for mapping, it often proves necessary to perform further dissection (and create more flaps) to locate additional blue-stained lymphatics and verify that all SLNs have been excised.

In addition, as noted (see Step 1: Preoperative Lymphoscintigraphy, above), the radiocolloid has a much longer retention time than the dye and tends to be concentrated in the SLN. When harvest occurs 2–24 hrs after injection of the radiocolloid, activity ratios are double what they are when mapping is done immediately after injection.[24] What works against the surgeon if there is a long interval between the injection of the radiocolloid and the harvest is the fact that the half-life of technetium is only 6 hrs. With a next day harvest, the radioactivity counts may have been cut in half 2–3 times.

Step 4: Pathologic examination of SLN

Once the SLN has been harvested, it is submitted for detailed pathologic examination. The examination may include serial sectioning, immunohistochemical staining with S-100, Melanin A and/or HMB-45 monoclonal anti-

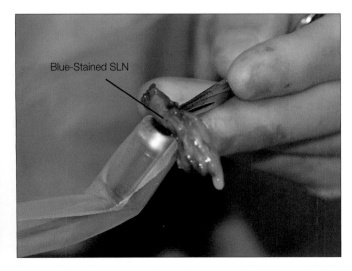

Blue-Stained SLN

Figure 46.6 Once removed, the blue-stained SLN is counted to ensure that it is also 'hot' and has an appropriate ratio of radioactivity (10:1 ratio of activity in the SLN vs surrounding non-SLNs or surrounding tissue).

bodies, and perhaps reverse transcriptase-polymerase chain reaction (RT-PCR) analysis.

COMPLICATIONS

Complications of lymphatic mapping are rare. All SLN harvests are performed without any postoperative drainage, and this contributes to the low morbidity of the procedure. A seroma develops in about 10% of patients, but it is easily handled with percutaneous aspiration. Surgical site infections are rare, and wound healing is better than with ELND because large flaps are not needed for the dissection. Investigators from the SunBelt Melanoma Trial recently reported the complication rate of lymphatic mapping in over 1202 patients on the trial and compared this to 277 patients who required a CLND as part of the trial. The incidence of seroma, lymph-edema and wound problems was 3% *vs* 7.9%, 0.7% *vs* 9.8% and 1.7% *vs* 11.9%, respectively. Each significant difference favored the SLN dissection alone arm.[24]

REPORTED RESULTS

In the initial report by Morton and associates,[12] in which mapping was done with vital blue dye alone, SLNs were successfully identified in 194 of 237 lymphatic basins, and 40 (21%) of the 194 specimens contained metastatic melanoma detected either by routine histologic examination with hematoxylin-eosin staining (12%) or by immunohistochemical staining exclusively (9%). Metastases were present in 47 (18%) of 259 SLNs, whereas non-SLNs were the exclusive site of metastasis in only two of 3079 nodes from 194 dissections, for a false negative rate of 1% (with nodes rather than patients as the unit of analysis).

Given that lymphatic mapping can be evaluated only in patients with metastatic disease, because these are the only patients in whom a skip metastasis (i.e. the SLN is histologically negative but nodes farther down the drainage pathway are histologically positive) could be documented, the investigators' findings in these patients are of considerable interest. Of 40 patients with histologically positive nodes, SLN mapping identified 38, for a 5% false negative rate. In 72% of basins, a particular primary site drained to a single SLN; in 20%, to two SLNs; and in 8%, to three or more SLNs. Surgeons successfully identified SLNs in 72 to 96% of attempts, depending on where the surgeons were on the learning curve. Overall, groin mappings were the most successful (89% success rate). Axillary mapping was generally successful as well (78% successful SLN identification). The investigators concluded that a learning curve of 60 cases would be necessary, which meant that the procedure would have to be restricted to major medical centers that treat large numbers of melanoma patients. This caveat notwithstanding, the new technique clearly was capable of accurately identifying patients with occult lymph node metastases who might benefit from radical lymphadenectomy.[12,13]

Surgical trials at several other institutions[11,14,15,18,19] confirmed two essential points. First, nodal metastasis from cutaneous primary sites follows an orderly, nonrandom, progressive pattern. Second, SLNs in the lymphatic basins can be individually identified, and their status reflects the presence or absence of melanoma metastases in the remaining nodes in the basins. In an initial study of 42 patients with intermediate-thickness melanomas from Moffitt Cancer Center (MCC, Tampa, FL),[14] SLN harvesting was followed by complete node dissection to confirm the low incidence of skip metastases in this population. None of the patients in this study had skip metastases: eight had a positive SLN, with the SLN as the only site of disease in seven of the eight, and 34 had a histologically negative SLN, with the rest of the nodes in the basin also histologically negative. Analysis of the results proved that the SLN was the first and favored site of metastatic disease. Preoperative lymphoscintigraphy was performed in this trial to define all basins at risk for metastatic disease, and intraoperative mapping was performed with isosulfan blue dye alone. The rate of technical failure was 10%.

A trial at the University of Vermont employed radiocolloid for intraoperative mapping after it was determined that in some cases, use of the vital blue dye was difficult if not impossible.[11,18] The investigators studied 100 patients with melanoma arising at a wide variety of primary sites. All of the patients underwent lymphoscintigraphy 1 to 24 hours before intraoperative mapping and SLN excision. A hand-held gamma probe was used to facilitate accurate identification and removal of the SLNs. Incisions were made directly over the hot spot to minimize dissection. Further dissection, if needed, was guided by the probe. The SLNs were successfully located in 98% of the patients, a markedly better result than was obtained in previous reports.

Subsequently, this same melanoma consortium published updated findings.[19] Between February 1993 and October 1994, 121 patients with invasive melanomas and clinically negative nodes were enrolled in a study comparing two different approaches to intraoperative mapping. In one group (64% of patients), mapping involved only injection of a radiocolloid (unfiltered ^{99m}Tc-SC, ^{99m}Tc-human serum albumin (^{99m}Tc-HSA), or Microlite (Dupont, Billerica, MA)) around the primary site and use of a hand-held gamma probe. The SLN was successfully identified in 97.6% of the patients in this group. In the other group (36% of patients), both vital blue dye and radiocolloid were used. All of the blue-stained SLNs also yielded radioactive hot spots, and in four patients the blue dye was not identified in any of the lymph nodes, which meant that mapping would have been unsuccessful if blue-staining had been the only mapping technique applied. Preoperative lymphoscintigraphy was used in 93% of the patients, with a technical failure rate of 10%. The radiolabeled SLNs could not be successfully imaged in these 12 patients preoperatively, but with the help of the hand-held gamma probe, the SLNs could be identified intraoperatively. This result suggests that a hand-held gamma probe is more sensitive at identifying SLNs than a scintillation camera. The reason may be that the probe accumulates data for scanning the basin in seconds, compared with the 5 to 10 min needed for the camera to produce images. This difference probably also explains why multiple nodes are sometimes imaged on preoperative lymphoscintigraphy when 1 to 2 hrs have elapsed between radiocolloid injection and imaging. Intraoperative mapping, on the other hand, readily identifies the SLN or nodes and does not identify second tier nodes as SLNs simply because they do not accumulate enough radiocolloid to make them 'hot' with the appropriate activity ratios. This finding is true if technetium sulfur colloid and not human serum albumin is used as the mapping agent.[25] Micrometastatic disease was present in 15 (12.4%) of the 121 patients studied, and the SLN was the only metastatic site in 10 of the 15. After a minimum follow-up of 220 days, one regional nodal recurrence was observed in an SLN-negative patient.

The addition of intraoperative radiolymphoscintigraphy to vital blue dye lymphatic mapping made SLN localization easier and more widely applicable.[26] The first study in the literature that employed a combination mapping technique was from the MCC. In this study 106 consecutive patients with cutaneous melanoma thicker than 0.75 mm at all primary site locations underwent lymphatic mapping using a vital blue dye and radiocolloid.[26] A total of 200 SLNs and 142 neighboring non-SLNs were harvested from 129 basins. 70% of the SLNs demonstrated blue staining, and 84% were identified as radioactive hot spots. When the two intraoperative mapping techniques were used in conjunction, the SLN could be identified in 96% of the nodal basins sampled. Routine histology identified SLN micrometastases in 15% of patients, and two patients had micrometastatic disease in nodes that were hot but not blue-stained. These data suggest that radiocolloid localization identifies more SLNs, some of which are clinically important in that they contain micrometastatic disease.

Another study used a combination of vital blue dye and radiocolloid (^{99m}Tc-HSA) mapping in a series of 30 patients with melanoma from all primary sites.[27] The SLN stained blue and was the most radioactive site in 27 patients (90%). In five of 13 patients undergoing groin dissection, radiolymphoscintigraphy identified two SLNs in the drainage basin. In each case, the presence of the second inguinal SLN was suggested by the high residual radioactivity after removal of the first node, not by the blue dye. Radioactivity decreased to background levels after excision of the second node. The investigators concluded that radiolymphoscintigraphy can be used not only to confirm blue-dye identification of an initial SLN but also to detect additional SLNs that are not easily identified with the dye technique alone.

In a subsequent MCC trial that used isosulfan blue dye and ^{99m}Tc-SC as mapping agents,[26] only patients with a positive SLN underwent complete node dissection. After 3 years of follow-up, two recurrences in regional basins were observed in patients whose previous SLN biopsy was negative. Serial sectioning and immunohistochemical staining of the SLN block found no abnormal cells. However, both patients' SLNs were RT-PCR-positive for messenger RNA (mRNA) for the tyrosinase gene,[28] which suggests the presence of micrometastatic disease that was missed by more conventional tests.

In another study, the Sydney Melanoma Unit reported an 87% success rate in identifying SLNs.[29] There was a pronounced learning curve, in that the success rate for the last 100 patients was 97%. Cutaneous lymphoscintigraphy was performed in 800 melanoma patients and was used to guide subsequent SLN harvesting. 23% of patients were found to have micrometastatic disease. Initially, the SLNs underwent frozen sectioning for occult metastases, but the 9% false negative rate led the investigators to switch to permanent sections, an approach that allowed the pathologist 2 to 5 days to perform a detailed examination. Patients found to have a positive SLN were returned to the OR for complete node dissection. When preoperative lymphoscintigraphy was followed by intraoperative mapping using vital blue-dye staining in conjunction with radiocolloid (^{99m}Tc-ATS) injection and a hand-held gamma probe, a 1.9% false negative rate was reported.

Finally, valuable findings are anticipated from the NCI-sponsored prospective trial now under way (see National Protocols, below). Survival data from this trial are unlikely to be available before 2005.

Recent reports would suggest that the lymphatic mapping procedure is applicable to all primary sites of the body, including the head and neck area, probably the most technically demanding area.[30,31] These reports illustrate that a combination mapping technique employing both vital blue dye and colloid is essential. False negative SLN biopsy rates are slightly higher (10% vs 1–2%) when compared with performing lymphatic mapping in extremity and trunk melanoma. But these rates are low enough to offer the procedure to patients with head and neck melanoma considering that the only alternative to obtain the nodal staging information is with the more radical and morbid CLND.

PATTERNS OF FAILURE AFTER A NEGATIVE SLN BIOPSY

Several of the earlier studies found that SLN mapping had a false negative rate, defined as a negative SLN with positive higher nodes, of less than 4%, as determined by concomitant formal lymph node dissection.[12–15] However, they did not clearly establish the long-term risk of failure within the mapped nodal basin after a negative SLN alone. This issue was addressed by a joint study from MCC and the M. D. Anderson Cancer Center (Houston, TX).[32] In this study, patients with cutaneous melanoma whose tumor was at least 1.0 mm thick or was categorized as Clark level IV or higher were eligible for mapping and SLN biopsy. All patients underwent preoperative lymphoscintigraphy, and only those with a histologically positive SLN underwent complete lymphadenectomy. A total of 618 patients underwent mapping with successful identification of at least one SLN; of these, 518 had histologically negative SLNs. After a minimum follow-up of 3 months and a median follow-up of 18 months, 32 (6%) of the 518 patients had recurrent disease and nine (1.7%) of the 518 had their first recurrence in a basin where the SLN was negative at the previous mapping. Patients with a histologically negative SLN had significantly better DFS (P<0.001) and

distant disease-free survival (P<0.001) than those with a histologically positive SLN. When SLNs from the nine patients whose SLNs were determined to be free of metastatic disease on initial review were retrospectively reexamined by serial sectioning or immunohistochemistry, occult nodal metastases were present in seven (77%) of the nine. These data established the durable long-term accuracy of lymphatic mapping and SLN biopsy.

Optimal nodal staging requires not only accurate identification of the SLN but also careful examination of the SLN with special pathologic techniques. It is likely that many false negative SLN biopsies do not actually reflect true skip metastases but are the result of micrometastases missed on routine pathologic examination. In the study cited, it is clear, given the subsequent recurrences, that the missed micrometastases represented clinically relevant disease. The recurrences could have been prevented if the SLNs had undergone detailed histologic examination initially, the micrometastases had been found, and complete node dissection had been performed.

Other explanations of false positive SLN biopsies have been proposed. One is that after a negative SLN biopsy, some regional basins are seeded with metastatic cells from in transit metastases or local recurrences. In transit metastasis occurs in 2 to 3% of patients and could be a source of skip metastases.

CLINICAL IMPLICATIONS

The information generated by this experience has been used to change the standards for surgical management of melanoma so that only patients with evidence of nodal metastatic disease are subjected to the morbidity and expense of complete node dissection.[24,33] Initial studies showed the usefulness of lymphatic mapping with either vital blue dye or radiocolloid in obtaining such evidence. However, it is now clear that the success rate of SLN identification increases markedly when the two mapping approaches are combined as described. A combined mapping approach identifies SLNs both more accurately and more completely: it removes more SLNs and results in a lower incidence of positive nodes on subsequent complete lymph node dissection (CLND).

In 85–94% of melanoma patients, the SLN is the only site of metastasis. At MCC and LRCC, we have seen no patients with melanomas less than 2.8 mm thick in whom nodes other than SLNs harbored metastases. It has been hypothesized that a melanoma must reach a certain thickness before it sheds enough cells to involve higher nodes beyond the SLN, and this hypothesis is supported by data from the M. D. Anderson Cancer Center showing no positive higher nodes after a positive SLN biopsy in patients with melanomas less than 2.5 mm thick. It appears that metastatic cells are concentrated in SLNs in much the same way that vital blue dyes and radiocolloids are. Thus, for many melanoma patients (in particular, those whose tumors have not reached the critical thickness just specified), to locate the SLN is essentially to define the limit of metastatic spread. Accordingly, lymphatic mapping, by identifying SLNs (and thus defining the extent of disease) with a high degree of accuracy, can be extremely useful in helping clinicians make more informed therapeutic decisions – for example, regarding eligibility for adjuvant therapy or the possibility of forgoing CLND. Based on this data, a multi-center regional trial (Florida Melanoma Trial II) has been instituted that will randomize patients with a microscopic positive SLN into either adjuvant therapy alone vs a CLND and adjuvant therapy. This trial will attempt to answer the question of the role of CLND in patients with low volume metastatic disease in their regional basin. It will also be the first trial to use molecular staging procedures (RT-PCR analysis) to define SLN positive disease and make a treatment decision based on molecular staging.

The findings of the studies cited demonstrate that intraoperative lymphatic mapping and SLN biopsy yields accurate pathologic staging, does not lower care standards, decreases morbidity (e.g., lymphedema is virtually absent, and early return to work or normal activity is facilitated), makes possible rational yet less aggressive surgical and adjuvant medical approaches, and reduces costs.[33] A report from a comprehensive database assembled from the major melanoma centers throughout the world by the AJCC melanoma staging committee illustrates the power of this new technique to stage patients with melanoma. With over 25,000 patients with melanoma in the database, the study showed that if melanoma patients with tumor thickness 1.0 mm or greater were staged to be node negative with a clinical exam, they had a 5-year survival of 65%. If patients with melanoma and a tumor thickness greater than or equal to 1 mm were staged to be node negative with an ELND, the 5-year survival was 75%. However, the 5-year survival of a similar population of patients with melanoma who were staged to be node negative with lymphatic mapping and SLN biopsy was 90%.[34] These differences in survival among the three groups were significant and underscores the fact that micrometastatic disease is missed less often with the lymphatic mapping technique than with a clinical exam of the nodal basin or an ELND. It is apparent from this report that the lymphatic mapping procedure is the preferred method to stage the patient with melanoma, since it identifies a more uniform population of truly node negative patients. Clinical exam of the regional basin and even an ELND to stage the regional nodes will miss micrometastatic disease. Lymphatic mapping and SLN biopsy is the most accurate method for staging melanoma patients to be either node negative or node positive.

NATIONAL PROTOCOLS

The first national multicenter study addressing lymphatic mapping for melanoma was the Multicenter Selective Lymphadenectomy Trial (Donald Morton, principal investigator), which started in 1993 and is funded by the NCI (Grant No. PO1 CA29605-12). This trial focuses on the effect of lymphatic mapping and SLN biopsy on survival. Melanoma patients with intermediate or thick tumors (1.0 mm) are randomly selected to receive either WLE plus observation of the nodal basins or WLE plus SLN harvesting. The study differs from previous studies

of ELND in that only some of the patients (i.e. those with a positive SLN) undergo CLND. If this study demonstrates a survival benefit, then there will be two good reasons to perform SLN: (1) to remove the node at highest risk for metastatic disease so that a CLND can be performed to contribute to a survival benefit and (2) to identify patients who are candidates for adjuvant therapy.

The second national trial examining the role of this new procedure in treating melanoma is the industry-sponsored Sunbelt Melanoma Trial, in which 60 institutions across the country, equally divided between university centers and community hospitals, are participating. In this study, melanoma patients whose tumors are at least 1.0 mm thick are undergoing lymphatic mapping and SLN harvesting. SLNs are examined with routine histology, serial sectioning, and immunohistochemical staining. If an SLN is negative on the initial screen, an RT-PCR assay based on a panel of four melanoma-specific markers (at least two of which must be positive for a positive result) is performed. Patients whose SLNs are negative on histology and RT-PCR assay are observed. Patients whose SLNs are histologically negative but positive on RT-PCR assay are randomly selected to undergo either observation, CLND or CLND plus adjuvant interferon alfa-2b. It is conceivable that patients in the second category might have a very small volume of tumor that is confined to the SLN and thus might be cured with SLN harvesting alone, thereby avoiding the side effects attendant on CLND or adjuvant interferon therapy. Another arm of this trial is designed to focus on the role of adjuvant interferon alfa-2b in patients with microscopic nodal disease. In the cooperative group study that found interferon alfa-2b to be effective adjuvant therapy,[9] 85% of the patient population had gross nodal disease. It remains to be determined whether patients with minimal disease in the regional basin (i.e. those with only one positive microscopic SLN) benefit from this adjuvant therapy. As of early 2003, the study had enrolled over 2500 patients.

A regional trial has been instituted (Florida Melanoma Trial II, 7/2001, Principal Investigator, Douglas Reintgen, MD) that involves the random selection of SLN-positive melanoma patients to undergo either observation of the remaining nodes in the basin plus adjuvant therapy with high dose Interferon alfa-2b or CLND plus adjuvant therapy. The data suggest that the SLN is the only site of disease in 80 to 94% of cases (depending on whether the initial SLN harvested used single agent or combination mapping techniques). Thus, the focus of this study would be on defining the role of CLND in patients with microscopic stage III disease documented by SLN biopsy. This will also be the first national study that will use molecular staging (RT-PCR assays) to determine the status of the SLN.

FUTURE OUTLOOK

Lymphatic mapping and SLN biopsy has changed the standard of care for the patient with melanoma. The technique has proven to have less morbidity than the old methods of nodal staging, such as the elective lymph node dissection. In addition, the ability to perform a more detailed examination of the SLN allows for a more accurate staging. This nodal staging will continue to be improved upon with the introduction of molecular assays for metastatic disease.

Largely based on the reverse transcriptase polymerase chain reaction, tests are being developed that have the sensitivity of identifying one abnormal melanoma cell in a background of a million normal lymphocytes, two orders of magnitude greater in sensitivity than what the naked eye can find under the microscope. In the future, the possibility of 'ultra-staging' exists in that the SLN, peripheral blood and bone marrow will be examined to come closer to identify patients who are surgically cured of their disease. In this way patients with the appropriate nodal characteristics can be spared the side effects of more radical surgery or the toxicities of adjuvant therapy.

REFERENCES

1 Jemal A, Murray T, Samuels A, Ghafoor A, Ward E, Thun M. Cancer statistics, 2004. CA Cancer J Clin 2004, January; 54:8–29.

2 Veronesi U, Adamus J, Bandiera DC, et al. Inefficacy of immediate node dissection in stage I melanoma of the limbs. N Engl J Med 1977; 297:627–630.

3 Sim FH, Taylor WF, Pritchard DJ, et al. Lymphadenectomy in the management of stage I malignant melanoma: a prospective randomized study. Mayo Clin Proc 1986; 61:697–705.

4 Reintgen DS, Cox EB, McCarthy KS, et al. Efficacy of elective lymph node dissection in patients with intermediate thickness primary melanoma. Ann Surg 1983; 198:379–385.

5 Norman J, Cruse CW, Wells K, et al. A redefinition of skin lymphatic drainage by lymphoscintigraphy for malignant melanoma. Am J Surg 1991; 162:432–437.

6 Tanabe KK. Lymphatic mapping and epitrochlear node dissection for melanoma. Surgery 1997; 121:102–104.

7 Balch CM, Soong SJ, Bartolucci AA, et al. Efficacy of an elective regional lymph node dissection of 1–4 mm thick melanoma for patients 60 years of age or younger. Ann Surg 1996; 224:255–268.

8 Balch C, Soong S-J, Ross MI, et al. Long-term results of a multi-institutional randomized trial comparing prognostic factors and surgical results for intermediate thickness melanomas (0.0 to 4.0 mm). Ann Surg Oncol 2000; 7:87–97.

9 Kirkwood JM, Strawderman MH, Ernstoff MS, et al. Adjuvant therapy of high-risk resected cutaneous melanoma: the Eastern Cooperative Oncology Group Trial EST 1684. J Clin Oncol 1996; 14:7–17.

10 Wong JH, Cagle LA, Morton D. Lymphatic drainage of skin to a sentinel lymph node in a feline model. Ann Surg 1991; 214:637–641.

11 Alex JC, Krag DN. Gamma-probe-guided localization of lymph nodes. Surg Oncol 1993; 2:137–143.

12 Morton DL, Wen DR, Wong JH, et al. Technical details of intraoperative lymphatic mapping for early stage melanoma. Arch Surg 1992; 127:392–399.

13 Morton DL, Wen DR, Cochran AJ. Management of early-stage melanoma by intraoperative lymphatic mapping and selective lymphadenectomy or 'watch and wait'. Surg Oncol Clin North Am 1992; 1:247.

14 Reintgen DS, Cruse CW, Berman C, et al. An orderly progression of melanoma nodal metastases. Ann Surg 1994; 220:759–767.

15 Ross M, Reintgen DS, Balch C. Selective lymphadenectomy: emerging role of lymphatic mapping and sentinel node biopsy in the management of early stage melanoma. Semin Surg Oncol 1993; 9:219–223.

16 Sappey MPC. Injection, preparation et conservation des vaisseaux lymphatiques. Thèse pour le doctorat en médecine, No. 241. Paris, Rignoux Imprimeur de la Faculté de Médecine, 1843.

17 Uren RF, Hoffman-Giles RB, Shaw HM, et al. Lymphoscintigraphy in high-risk melanoma of the trunk: predicting draining node groups, defining lymphatic channels and locating the sentinel node. J Nucl Med 1993; 34:1435–1440.

18 Krag DN, Meijer SJ, Weaver DL, et al. Minimal-access surgery for staging of melanoma. Arch Surg 1995; 130:654–658.

19 Krag D, Meijer S, Weaver D, et al. Minimal access surgery for staging regional nodes in malignant melanoma (abstract). The 48th Cancer Symposium, Society of Surgical Oncology, Boston, 1995.

20 Slingluff C, Vollmer R, Reintgen D, et al. Lethal thin malignant melanoma. Ann Surg 1988; 208:150–161.

21 Ross M, Reintgen DS, Gershenwald J, et al. The margin of resection for deep (> 4.0 mm) primary melanoma. J Clin Oncol, in press.

22 Reintgen DS, Albertini J, Berman C, et al. Accurate nodal staging of malignant melanoma. Cancer Control. J Moffitt Cancer Center 1995; 2:405.

23 Hung JC, Wiseman GA, Wahner HW, et al. Filtered technetium-99m-sulfur colloid evaluated for lymphoscintigraphy. J Nucl Med 1995; 36:1895–1901.

24 Wrightson WR, Reintgen DS, Edwards M, et al. Morbidity of sentinel lymph node biopsy (Abstract). 54th Annual Cancer Symposium, Society of Surgical Oncology, Washington, DC, 15–18 March 2001.

25 Meyer CM, Lecklitner ML, Logie JR, et al. Technetium-99m sulfur-colloid cutaneous lymphoscintigraphy in the management of truncal melanoma. Radiology 1979; 131:205–209.

26 Albertini J, Cruse CW, Rapaport D, et al. Intraoperative radiolymphoscintigraphy improves sentinel lymph node identification in melanoma patients. Ann Surg 1996; 223:217–224.

27 Essner R, Foshag L, Morton D. Intraoperative radiolymphoscintigraphy: a useful adjunct to intraoperative lymphatic mapping and selective lymph-adenectomy in patients with clinical stage 1 melanoma (abstract). The 47th Cancer Symposium, Society of Surgical Oncology, Houston, Texas, 1994.

28 Wang X, Heller R, VanVoorhis N, et al. Detection of submicroscopic metastases with polymerase chain reaction in patients with malignant melanoma. Ann Surg 1994; 220:768–774.

29 Thompson JF, McCarthy WH, Robinson E, et al. Sentinel lymph node biopsy in 102 patients with clinical stage 1 melanoma undergoing elective lymph node dissection (abstract). The 47th Cancer Symposium, Society of Surgical Oncology, Houston, Texas, 1994.

30 Byrd D, Nason K, Eary J, Young R. Utility of sentinel lymph node dissection in patients with head and neck melanoma (Abstract). The 54th Annual Cancer Symposium, Society of Surgical Oncology, Washington, DC, 15–18 March 2001.

31 Medina-Franco H, Beenken S, Heslin M, Urist M. Sentinel lymph node biopsy for cutaneous melanoma of the head and neck (Abstract). The 54th Annual Cancer Symposium, Society of Surgical Oncology, Washington, DC, 15–18 March 2001.

32 Gershenwald J, Thompson W, Mansfield P, et al. Patterns of failure in melanoma patients after successful lymphatic mapping and negative sentinel node biopsy (abstract). The 49th Cancer Symposium, Society of Surgical Oncology, Atlanta, Georgia, 1996.

33 Reintgen DS, Einstein A. The role of research in cost containment. Cancer Control: J Moffitt Cancer Center 1995; 2:429.

34 Dessureault S, Soong S, Ross M, et al. Improved survival for node-negative patients with intermediate-to-thick melanomas (>1.0 mm) staged with sentinel lymph node (SLN) biopsy. 54th Annual Cancer Symposium, Society of Surgical Oncology, Washington, DC, 15–18 March 2001.

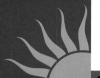
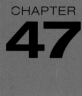
CHAPTER
47

Reconstructive Surgery for Skin Cancer

Shan R Baker

Key points

- Flaps are best classified by their method of transfer. The most common modes of movement are referred to as advancement, pivotal and hinged.
- Pivotal flaps may involve rotation, transposition or interpolation.
- Advancement flaps require stretching of the skin and are best suited for areas of reasonable skin elasticity.
- Attention should be directed to cosmetic units and boundaries. Ideally scars are placed within cosmetic junctions and flaps will not cross cosmetic boundaries.

INTRODUCTION

Skin cancer is the most common malignancy affecting man, with the majority of these occurring on the face. Important risk factors associated with the development of cutaneous malignancy include: fair complexion, light hair, blue or green eyes, Fitzpatrick Type I skin (propensity to burn and never tan), outdoor occupation, and Celtic ancestry. Many of these factors are colinear variables.

The incidence of cutaneous malignancies is sharply increasing and the greater number of persons developing skin cancer translates into an increasing demand for facial, plastic and dermatologic surgeons skilled in the repair of facial defects. This chapter will confine its discussion to reconstruction after removal of skin cancer using grafts and local flaps. A comprehensive discussion of local flaps cannot be achieved in a single chapter. However, given that most skin cancers occur in the face, an attempt is made to answer the most important question: what is the preferred local flap for a defect at a given location on the face?

LOCAL FLAP CLASSIFICATION

The author defines a local cutaneous flap as a skin flap designed immediately adjacent to or near the location of the defect for which the flap is designed to repair. There are a number of methods of classifying local flaps. Flaps may be classified by the nature of their blood supply (random *vs* arterial), by configuration (rhomboid, bilobe, etc.), by location (forehead, cheek, lip) and by the method of transferring the flap. Classifying flaps by method of transfer which is to say method of tissue movement is usually the most convenient way of discussing them relative to their use in repairing facial cutaneous defects (Table 47.1).[1-3] This classification divides local flaps into pivotal, advancement and hinged. Hinge flaps have specific and limited indications and will not be discussed in this chapter. Advancement in the majority of situations depends on stretching the flap skin in the direction of flap movement. Such flaps are subjected to an increase in wound closure tension. In contrast pivotal flaps rotate about a point at their base and in their purest form are not stretched. Thus, they are not subjected to an increase in wound closure tension. However, in the vast majority of circumstances when using pivotal flaps, tissue movement is achieved through a combination of pivoting and advancement. That is, movement of most pivotal flaps is aided by stretching (advancement) of the flap skin. Surgeons often speak of combined mechanisms of tissue movement such as 'advancement rotation flap'. For clarity, the major mechanism of tissue transfer should dictate the term given to describe a particular flap, unless both mechanisms are of approximately equal importance.

Pivotal flaps

There are three types of pivotal flaps: rotation, transposition and interpolated. All pivotal flaps are moved toward the defect by rotating the base of the flap around a pivotal point. Except for island flaps, which have been skeletonized to the level of their nutrient vessels, the greater the pivot, the shorter is the effective length of the flap. This reduction in effective length must be accounted for when designing pivotal flaps (Fig. 47.1). As the flap pivots in an arc around its relatively fixed pivotal point, redundant tissue, known as a standing cutaneous deformity (dog ear), develops at the base.

Rotation flaps

Rotation flaps are pivotal flaps with a curvilinear configuration. They are designed immediately adjacent to the defect and are best used to close triangular defects. In such instances, the triangular-shaped defect is covered by a portion of the standing cutaneous deformity, thus facilitating the pivotal movement of the flap (Fig. 47.2). This flap usually makes use of some advancement, and when it does, the vector of greatest wound closure tension is along a line from the base of the flap to a distal point of the curvilinear border (Fig. 47.3). A back cut at the base of the flap shifts the position of the pivotal point,

Table 47.1   Classification of local cutaneous flaps by method of transfer
Pivotal:
Rotation
Transposition
Interpolated
Advancement:
Unipedicle
Bipedicle
V-Y
Hinged

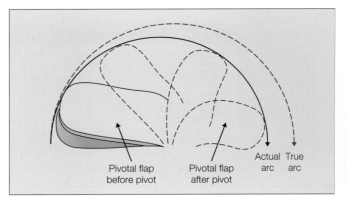

Figure 47.1   Pivotal flaps move about a pivotal point. Their effective length decreases as flap pivots.

and thus changes the wound closure tension vector as well as the location of the standing cutaneous deformity.

A primary defect is the skin defect that the surgeon wishes to repair. A secondary defect is created at the donor site of the flap used to repair the primary defect. Inherent with rotation flaps is the unequal lengths of the flap's border compared to the width of the primary and secondary defect. To equalize this discrepancy, it may be necessary to excise an equalizing Bürow's triangle at some point along the curvilinear periphery of the incision. This triangle should have the same width as the width of the primary defect. Excision of a Bürow's triangle has the effect of equalizing the lengths of the two sides of the incision. Another solution that avoids the need for an equalizing triangle is to change the movement of the flap from one that is purely pivotal to one that is both pivotal and advancement. Stretching the flap in essence lengthens the peripheral border of the flap so that it approaches the sum width of the primary and secondary defect. As a general rule, when designing rotation flaps on the face, the length of the incision should be four times the width of the defect. With this 4:1 ratio, excision of a Bürow's triangle is usually not necessary. To avoid a standing cutaneous deformity at the base of the flap, the defect's shape ideally should have a triangular configuration with a height-to-width ratio of 2:1. In addition, if the arc of the flap's incision is to be a completely symmetrical curve, the height of the triangular defect should be 0.5 to 1 times the radius of the curve of the flap.

There are several advantages of the rotation flap. The flap has only two sides; thus it lends itself to placing one side in a border between aesthetic regions of the face. The flap is broad based, and therefore its vascularity tends to be reliable. There is great flexibility in the design and positioning of the flap. When possible, the flap should be designed so that it is inferiorly based, which promotes lymphatic drainage and minimizes flap edema.

Disadvantages of rotation flaps are relatively few. The defect itself must be somewhat triangular or must be modified by removing normal tissue to create a triangular defect. The configuration of the flap includes a right angle at the distal tip and the surgeon must take care in positioning the tip so that it is not subjected to excessive wound closure tension and vascular compromise. The curvilinear incision necessary to create the flap does not easily lie in relaxed skin tension lines (RSTLs). As with all pivotal flaps, rotation flaps develop standing cutaneous deformities at their base, which may not be easily removed without compromising the vascularity of

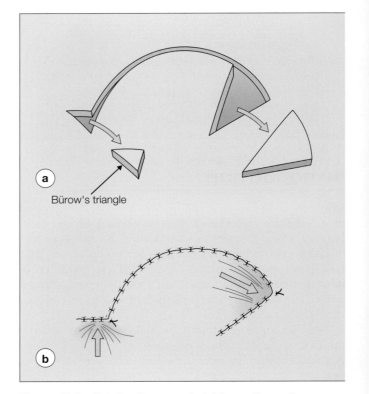

Figure 47.2   Rotation flaps are pivotal flaps with curvilinear configuration. They are useful for closure of (a) triangular-shaped defects. (b) Excision of Bürow's triangle facilitates flap transfer.

the flap. Second stage revision in which the standing cutaneous deformity is removed may be necessary.

Transposition flaps

In contrast to rotation flaps, which have a curvilinear configuration, transposition flaps have a linear configuration. Both are pivotal flaps moving about a pivotal point, and their effective length decreases as they pivot (Fig. 47.1). This reduction in effective length must be considered when designing such flaps. Rotation flaps must be designed in such a way that one border of the flap is also a border of the defect for which it is intended for repair. Like rotation flaps, transposition flaps may be designed so that one border of the flap is also a border

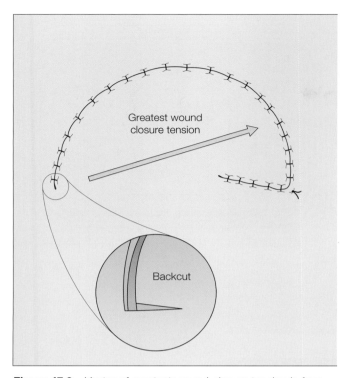

Figure 47.3 Vector of greatest wound-closure tension is from pivotal point, to point on peripheral border. Back cut shifts position of pivotal point, reduces wound-closure tension and alters location of standing cutaneous deformity.

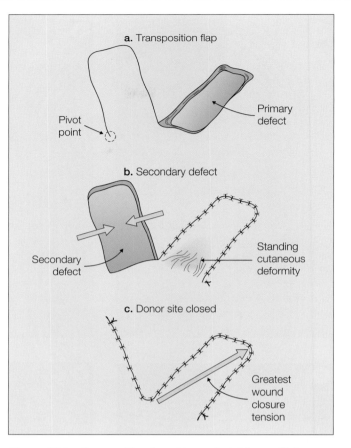

Figure 47.4 Transposition flaps (a) are pivotal flaps with linear configuration. Flap may be constructed at some distance from defect (b) with its axis independent from axis of defect. Base of flap must be contiguous with defect (c).

of the defect. However, it may also be designed with borders that are removed from the defect (Fig. 47.4). In this circumstance only the base of the flap is contiguous with the defect. If the flap is stretched as it pivots, the greatest wound closure tension is along a vector from the pivotal point to the most peripheral border of the flap.

The ability to construct a flap some distance from the defect with its axis independent from the linear axis of the defect is one of the greatest advantages of transposition flaps. This fact enables the surgeon to recruit skin at variable distances from the defect, selecting areas of greatest skin elasticity or redundancy for donor sites. In addition, the ability to select a variable site for harvesting a flap may allow the selection of a donor site that will provide the best possible donor scar.

Transposition is the most common method of transferring local flaps to skin defects of the head and neck. A transposition flap is a reconstructive option for small-to-medium sized defects of almost any conceivable configuration or location, thus making it the most useful of local flaps in head and neck reconstruction. Two types of transposition flaps frequently used are rhombic flaps and bilobe flaps. Rhombic flaps depend upon advancement for part of their tissue movement, but the majority of movement is pivotal (Fig. 47.5). A rhombus is an equilateral parallelogram. A rhombus defect consists of two equilateral triangles placed base to base to form a rhombus with adjacent angles of 60° and 120°. All sides and the short diagonal of the defect must be equal in a 60° to 120° rhombus defect and flap. Once the 60° to 120° rhombus defect has been created with all sides equal, the flap is designed by directly extending

the short diagonal. This creates the first side of the flap and should be extended a distance equal to all other sides. The second side of the flap, again equal to all other sides, is drawn parallel to one of the adjacent borders of the defect.[4]

The greatest wound closure tension when using a rhombus flap is at the donor site and has been calculated to be 20° from the short diagonal line across the base of the flap.[4] Wide undermining of the surrounding tissue has minimal effect on the wound closure tension. Thus, when designing the flap, skin mobility and extensibility are important. Understanding the vector of the resultant wound closure tension is critical to avoid distortion of surrounding structures. For every rhombus defect, four potential flaps may be designed. The surgeon can quickly visualize the resulting scar and approximate vector of maximum wound closure tension by drawing the flap and then covering the two parallel sides of the flap with his or her fingers.

The design of the rhombus flap is more complex than most other facial skin flaps because of the geometry and option of placing the flap in four separate locations about a rhombus defect. The author does not use the rhombus flap or its variations frequently, primarily because approximately half of the entire length of the scar that results from such repair is not parallel or does not lie within RSTLs. This disadvantage is most important in the area of the forehead and temple, where skin creases are

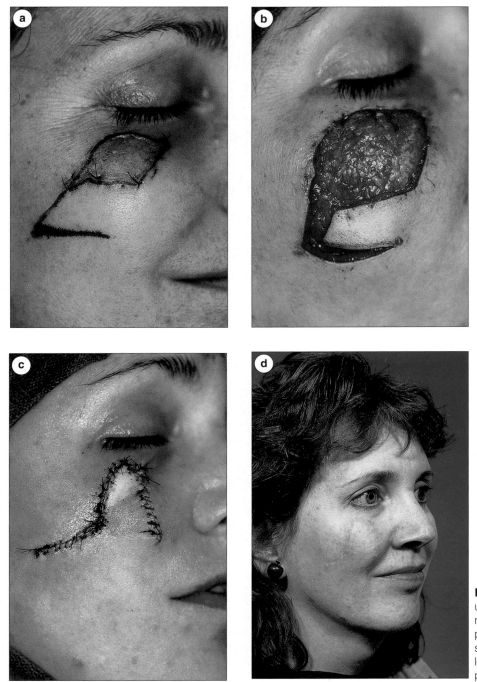

Figure 47.5 Rhombic flaps depend upon advancement for part of their tissue movement, but majority of movement is pivotal. (a) Lentigo maligna outlined by sutures. Rhombic flap designed. (b) Skin lesion excised, flap incised. (c) Flap in place. (d) 7 months postoperative.

more prominent. RSTLs are less important in the cheek, where creases are not as prominent, the skin is thinner and the resulting scar from the use of a rhombus flap tends to blend better with adjacent skin.

The bilobe flap is a double transposition flap that shares a single base. Each lobe of the flap has a separate pivotal point and thus each has a standing cutaneous deformity.[5] It was originally designed for repair of nasal defects, but has frequently been used to reconstruct cheek defects as well. In the classic design of the bilobe flap, the axis of the primary and secondary lobes as well

as the defect, were all separated by an angle of 90° (180° total). This design transferred the tension of the wound closure through a 90° arc, which is more than the usual 45° to 60° pivot of a single transposition flap. This greater movement about a pivotal point assists to minimize wound closure tension of the primary and secondary defects.

The major disadvantage of the bilobe flap is that the majority of the incision necessary to create the two lobes of the flap produce scars that do not parallel RSTLs. The resulting scar is also lengthy due to the requirement of elevating two lobes.

Interpolated flap

The interpolated flap, like the transposition flap, is a pivotal flap that has a linear configuration, but differs from transposition flaps in that its base is not contiguous with the defect. Thus, the pedicle must cross over or under intervening tissue (Fig. 47.6). If the pedicle passes over intervening tissue, the flap must subsequently be detached in a second surgical procedure. This is the greatest disadvantage of such flaps. On occasion, the pedicle can be de-epithelialized or reduced to subcutaneous tissue only and brought under the intervening skin to allow a single-stage reconstruction. Passing flaps through a subcutaneous tunnel may either compromise the vascularity of the pedicle or create a contour deformity along its path.

The paramedian forehead flap used to repair large defects of the nose is the arched type of interpolated flap. This flap is exceedingly reliable because of its axial design based on the supratrochlear artery and vein. An axial flap is one which has a named artery and vein incorporated into the base of the flap. The flap is designed so that the vessels extend along the axis of the flap providing an ample blood supply to the skin. When such vessels are not part of the local flap, the flap is said to have a random blood supply. The base of the paramedian forehead flap is placed in the glabellar region and is centered over the supratrochlear artery and vein on the same side as the majority of the nasal defect. The origin of the supratrochlear artery is consistently found to be 1.7–2.2 cm lateral to the midline[6] and usually corresponds to a line that represents the vertical tangent of the medial border of the eyebrow. The vessels exit the orbit by piercing the orbital septum and passing under the orbicularis oculi and over the corrugator supercilii muscle. At the level of the brow, the artery passes through the orbicularis and frontalis muscle and continues upward vertically in a subcutaneous plane. Because of this, the portion of the flap cephalic to the level of the eyebrow and extending up to the level of the anterior hairline can be trimmed of its frontalis muscle and most of the subcutaneous fat without harming the blood supply to the skin of the flap.[7]

Similar to the interpolated paramedian forehead flap used for nasal reconstruction, the melolabial interpolated flap transferred from the cheek to the nose is a reliable flap for resurfacing alar defects. Unlike the forehead flap, the cheek flap has a random blood supply and cannot safely be thinned of as much of its subcutaneous fat as the forehead flap. Interpolated flaps have the advantage of crossing over rather than through the intervening tissue between flap donor site and the defect, so they do not distort boundaries between aesthetic regions of the face. This insures a completely natural appearing border between the cheek or forehead and the nose. Another advantage of an interpolated flap is that it can be harvested in regions of redundant tissue, at sites removed from the immediate area of the defect.

Advancement flaps

Advancement flaps have a linear configuration and are moved by sliding toward the defect. This involves stretching the skin of the flap. Thus advancement flaps work best in areas of greater skin elasticity. The most basic advancement flap is the simple linear layered closure, which involves undermining and direct advancement of tissue side-to-side to close the defect primarily. This closure does not create a secondary defect and additional incisions are made only for the removal of standing cutaneous deformities. However, the term advancement flap usually refers to a flap created by incisions, which allow for a 'sliding' movement of tissue. This transfer is achieved by moving the flap and its pedicle in a single vector. Advancement flaps may be categorized as single pedicle, bipedicle or V-Y.

Single pedicle advancement flap

A single pedicle advancement flap is created by parallel incisions, which allow a 'sliding' movement of tissue in a single vector toward a defect. The movement is in one direction and the flap advances directly over the defect. As a consequence, the flap must be developed adjacent to the defect, and one border of the defect becomes the leading border of the flap. Repair with an advancement flap involves both primary and secondary tissue movement (Fig. 47.7). In primary movement, the incised flap

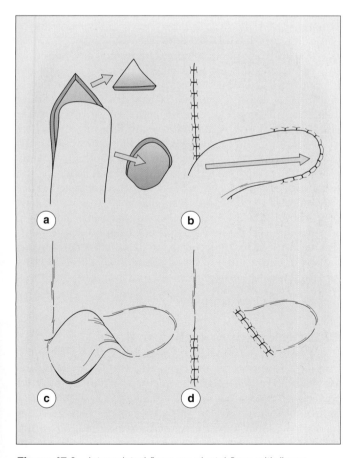

Figure 47.6 Interpolated flaps are pivotal flaps with linear configuration. (a,b) Pedicle passes over intervening tissue. (c,d) Such flaps require subsequent pedicle division and flap inset.

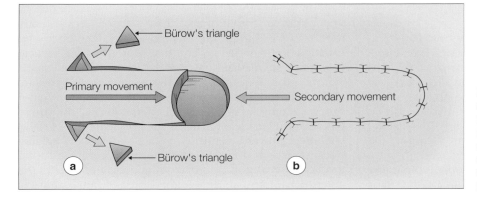

Figure 47.7 A single pedicle advancement flap is created by parallel incisions which enable 'sliding'. (a) Primary movement of tissue in single vector toward defect. (b) Secondary movement of surrounding skin immediately adjacent to defect occurs in direction opposite of primary movement.

is slid toward the defect by stretching the flap skin. Secondary movement of surrounding skin and soft tissue immediately adjacent to the defect occurs in a direction opposite the direction of the movement of the advancing border of the flap. This secondary movement may either help in repair, by providing less wound closure tension, or may be detrimental, by displacing free margins of facial structures. Complete undermining of the advancement flap as well as the skin and soft tissue around the pedicle is important to enhance tissue movement. In contrast to pivotal flaps, which form a single standing cutaneous deformity, two deformities are created with all single pedicle advancement flaps. These may require excision. Excision of standing cutaneous deformities (Bürow's triangles) may also facilitate movement of the flap (Fig. 47.7).

Unlike the pivotal flap, in which the standing cutaneous deformity must be dealt with at the base of the flap, the deformities that develop from advancement can be excised anywhere along the length of the flap and not necessarily adjacent to the base. This is because of the mechanism of tissue movement. Excision of standing cutaneous deformities of advancement flaps is predicated on the most optimal site for excision. Typical excisions are placed in RSTLs or in borders between aesthetic regions of the face. When the flap is sufficiently long, standing cutaneous deformities can be subdivided into multiple small puckers of tissue that need not be excised but can merely be 'sewn out'.

In certain locations on the face, single pedicle advancement flaps work particularly well: the forehead (particularly in the vicinity of the eyebrow), helical rim, upper and lower eyelids and medial cheek. Mucosal advancement flaps are useful for vermilion reconstruction.

Bilateral advancement flaps are commonly combined to close various defects, resulting in H or T-shaped repairs depending on the configuration of the defect. Repair in this manner is often referred to as an H-plasty or T-plasty (Figs 47.8 and 47.9). In both cases, advancement flaps are designed on opposite sides of the defect and advance toward each other. Each flap is responsible for covering a portion of the defect. The resulting standing cutaneous deformities are often excised partly in the area of the defect and partly along the linear axes of the flaps. The two flaps do not necessarily have to be of the same length. The length of the flap is determined primarily by the elasticity and redundancy of tissue at the donor site.

V-Y advancement flap

The V-Y advancement flap is unique in that the V-shaped flap is not stretched or pulled toward the recipient site, but rather achieves its advancement by recoil or by being pushed forward. Thus, the flap is allowed to move into the recipient site in a nearly tension-free fashion. The secondary triangular donor defect is then repaired with wound closure tension by advancing the two borders of the remaining wound toward each other. In so doing, the wound closure suture line assumes a Y configuration, with the common limb of the Y representing the suture line resulting from closure of the secondary defect (Fig. 47.10). The flap is optimally designed so that the common limb of the Y falls in the boundary of neighboring aesthetic regions or within a natural crease, fold or wrinkle.

V-Y advancement is particularly useful when a structure or region requires lengthening or release from a contracted state. For instance, V-Y advancement is helpful in releasing contracted scars that are distorting adjacent structures such as the vermilion or eyelids. The affected area of distorted vermilion or eyelid is incorporated into the V-shaped flap and advanced toward the lip or eye to restore natural topography (Fig. 47.11). The skin borders adjacent to both sides of the secondary defect are then advanced toward each other and sutured. The suture line becomes the vertical or common limb of the Y configuration. The V-Y advancement flap may also be designed on a subcutaneous pedicle. In this case the flap is stretched toward the defect rather than allowed to recoil (Fig. 47.12). This type of flap is discussed in detail in a later portion of this chapter.

Bipedicle advancement flaps

Bipedicle advancement flaps are used primarily for repair of large defects of the scalp. The flap is designed adjacent to the defect and is advanced into the defect at right angle to the linear axis of the flap. This leaves a secondary defect, which usually must be repaired with a split-thickness skin graft. As a consequence, bipedicle flaps are rarely used for reconstruction of the face and neck. The exception to this is the use of bipedicle advancement flaps for relining limited full-thickness nasal defects of the hemi-tip or ala, which have a vertical

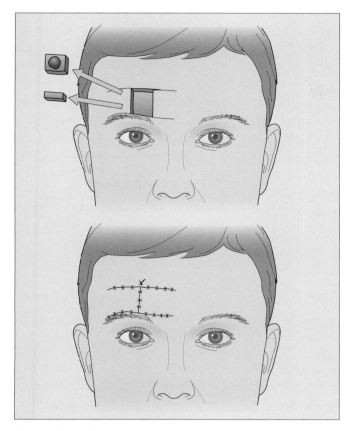

Figure 47.8 Bilateral advancement flaps may be combined to repair defect resulting in H-shaped repair. Removal of skin adjacent to defect may facilitate positioning scars along aesthetic borders (i.e. eyebrow).

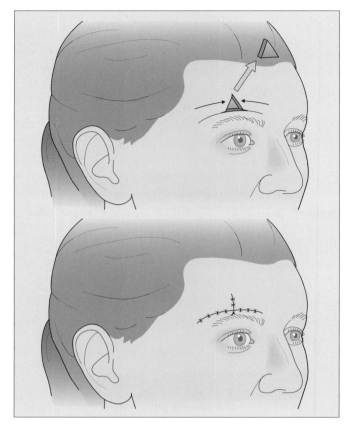

Figure 47.9 T-plasty occurs when opposing advancement flaps are created by making a single incision for each flap. Standing cutaneous deformities from advancement are removed at defect site and wound repair assumes a T-shaped closure.

height of no more than 1.0 cm. The flap consists of vestibular skin and mucosa based medially on the septum and laterally on the floor of the nasal vestibule. An extended intercartilaginous incision is made and the flap is elevated off the under surface of the alar cartilage and mobilized inferiorly to re-line the ala or hemi-tip. The donor site on the inner aspect of the cartilage is covered with a thin full-thickness skin graft. The bipedicle flap is thin and provides natural physiological material for the interior of the nasal passage with sufficient vascularity to support the concomitant use of free cartilage grafts placed over the lining flap for structural support of the construction.[8]

DEFECT ANALYSIS

The face is divided into aesthetic facial regions, which include the principle masses of the face: forehead, eyelids, cheeks, nose, lips, mentum, and auricles (Fig. 47.13). Additionally, these aesthetic regions may be subdivided into an abundance of anatomical components separated by boundaries. Most notably are the following: frontal, supraorbital, orbital, infraorbital, zygomatic, buccal, parotid, masseteric, mental, labial, nasal, temporal and auricular.[9] The nose may further be divided into aesthetic units including the dorsum, sidewalls, tip, facets, columella, and alae.[10] Aesthetic regions and units of the face and nose are outlined by anatomical boundaries and have topographic variations and regional differences in skin color, thickness and texture. Whenever possible it is important to position incisions in borders of the regions (aesthetic borders) or units. This will better camouflage scars. In addition, when possible, it is advantageous to use a local flap harvested from the same facial region where the defect is located. This will insure tissue replacement with skin that has similar hair growth patterns, texture and color as that of the resected skin. When a defect occupies two adjacent facial regions, it is preferred to develop individual flaps for repair of the portion of the defect occupying a given facial region. This will ensure better preservation of the topography between the regions and will position the majority of the scars in aesthetic borders.

In assessing a facial defect, the surgeon must determine the most appropriate method of reconstruction.[1] Several issues enter the decision-making process. First the closure must not conceal residual tumor so the reconstructive surgeon must be comfortable with the fidelity of the extirpative method. Second, the risk of tumor recurrence must be assessed; the reconstructive method of choice may be altered by this consideration. Finally, given these factors, the surgeon should select the technique that will render the best possible aesthetic and functional result.

In assessing a given defect, the surgeon should evaluate its complexity in terms of missing tissue layers,

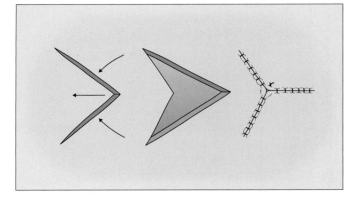

Figure 47.10   V-Y advancement flap is not stretched or pulled toward recipient site, but rather achieves movement by recoil or by being pushed forward. Donor site is repaired by advancement of opposing borders of secondary defect creating a Y-shaped wound repair.

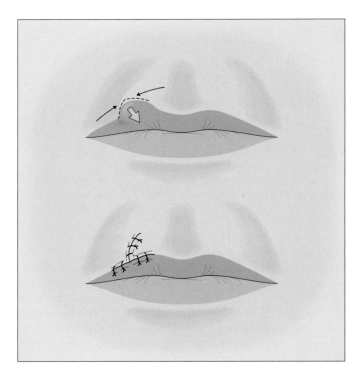

Figure 47.11   V-Y advancement flap is useful when a structure (vermilion) requires release from contracted state.

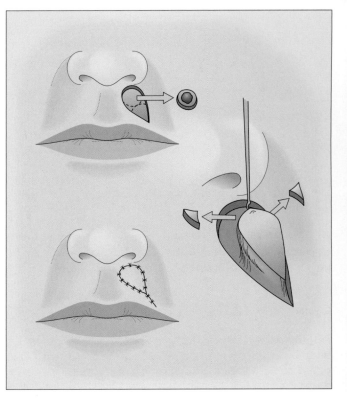

Figure 47.12   V-Y advancement flap may be harvested on subcutaneous pedicle. In such circumstances, flap is stretched toward defect rather than allowed to recoil.

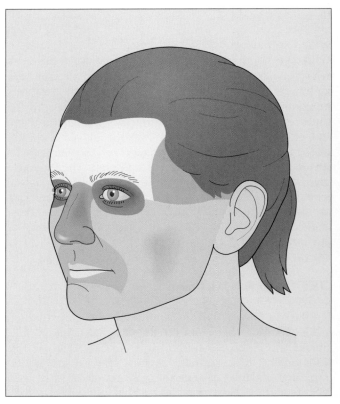

Figure 47.13   Aesthetic facial regions.

topography, and aesthetic region/unit involvement. On initial consideration, the surgeon should evaluate the applicability of immediate vs. delayed reconstruction.[11] Options for cutaneous repair include healing by second intention (granulation), primary wound closure with or without M-plasty, skin graft, and local or distant flap repair (Table 47.2). Optimally, each layer of absent tissue should be repaired with like tissue. When possible, the cutaneous defect should be closed with skin of similar thickness, color, and texture as that of the missing skin. Missing cartilage should be replaced by appropriately positioned, contoured and sculptured cartilage. Mucosa should generally be repaired with neighboring mucosal tissue. Surgical judgment is critical in the decision-making

Table 47.2   Options in repair of facial cutaneous defects
Healing by granulation
Primary wound closure
Local flaps
Regional and distant flaps
Microvascular flaps
Composite grafts
Full thickness skin grafts
Split-thickness skin grafts

process. The scope of this chapter is limited to a discussion of local flaps and grafts for repair of facial cutaneous defects.

Skin grafts

Split-thickness skin grafts generally are not used for facial reconstruction except as a temporary cover because of the marked contraction that occurs and the stark color, thickness and texture mismatch with neighboring tissue. Exceptions would include repair of extensive scalp defects and repair of defects resulting from excision of deeply invasive tumors or those with unreliable surgical margins where close postoperative surveillance of the area of resection is especially important. In contrast to split-thickness skin grafts, full thickness skin grafts (FTSG) enjoy widespread use in the repair of well-circumscribed, relatively superficial wounds of the face, especially the nose. Appropriate inconspicuous sites from which to harvest these grafts include the pre or post-auricular regions, supraclavicular skin, and occasionally, the melolabial fold (Fig. 47.14). With FTSG, the full thickness of the epidermis and dermis is harvested and subsequently transplanted. Subcutaneous tissue is appropriately removed from the graft. Dermal appendages are typically preserved, thus any hair on the graft is likely to grow. Because FTSG are thicker than split-thickness skin grafts, there is less contraction and the grafts are less atrophic in appearance. FTSG are also more resistant to trauma than their split-thickness counterpart. FTSG are particularly useful in the closure of defects affecting the nasal tip unit, lateral surface of the auricle, and the eyelids (Fig. 47.15). The appearance of skin grafts may often be improved by dermabrasion of the graft and adjacent skin 6–8 weeks following successful grafting.

PREFERRED FLAPS

Typically a number of different flap designs can be considered for any given facial cutaneous defect. However, in the majority of cases, one or two flap designs are usually preferred and this is determined by a host of factors. Location and size of the facial defect are the two most important factors governing the selection of a specific local flap. The region of the face where the defect is located is important because the skin of each region

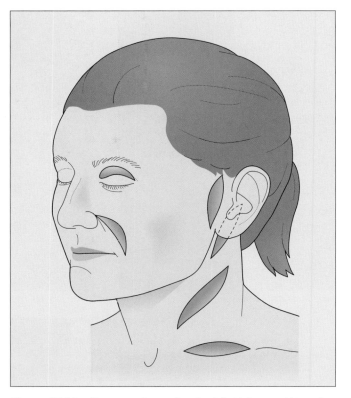

Figure 47.14   Common donor sites for full-thickness skin grafts.

has certain intrinsic properties. The most important of these properties is elasticity and redundancy; each of which may influence the method of repair. The facial region also determines the adjacent facial structures that may be distorted or in other ways suffer impairment of function following repair of a defect.

The size of the defect is the other important factor affecting the selection of the preferred local flap. For instance, potential donor sites for a flap must provide sufficient skin to close the defect and still achieve secondary closure of the donor site. Larger defects of the face and neck may be difficult to resurface with local flaps without considerable impairment in form or function. In such circumstances, the surgeon must select a regional flap or skin graft that may be aesthetically less pleasing but perhaps will provide a more functional repair. These decisions are determined by clinical judgment. The defect size will also influence the degree of secondary tissue movement that may result and this in turn may affect free margins of adjacent facial structures.

Scalp

Large (≥6 cm) partial thickness scalp defects are best repaired with a full-thickness skin graft. The galea aponeurosis severely limits tissue movements causing flap repair of even small defects to be difficult. The preferred method of reconstruction of the majority of small-to-intermediate size defects (defined as those that can be repaired with the remaining scalp tissue) is the utilization of two or more rotation flaps. Rotation flaps have curvilinear configurations and as such they are

581

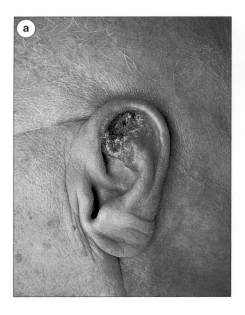

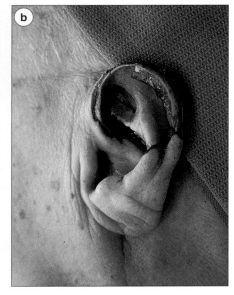

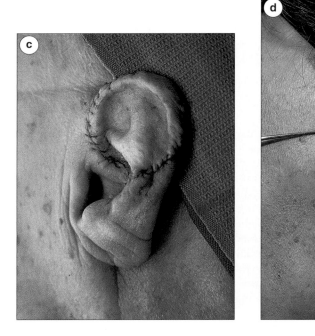

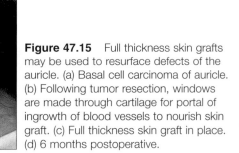

Figure 47.15 Full thickness skin grafts may be used to resurface defects of the auricle. (a) Basal cell carcinoma of auricle. (b) Following tumor resection, windows are made through cartilage for portal of ingrowth of blood vessels to nourish skin graft. (c) Full thickness skin graft in place. (d) 6 months postoperative.

ideally suited for spherical-shaped contours such as the scalp. Rotation flaps are transferred by a pivoting movement rather than depending on stretching of the flap for movement as required by advancement flaps. Because of the inelasticity of scalp tissue, advancement flaps are poorly suited for scalp reconstruction.

In general, multiple rotation flaps are preferred to the use of a single flap for scalp reconstruction. Each flap is designed to pivot on an independent pivotal point. When using two rotation flaps, the flaps may be designed to pivot in opposite directions creating an O-T configuration of the wound repair, or in the same direction, as an O-Z repair (Fig. 47.16).[12] Using more than one rotation flap is advantageous because it recruits tissue for reconstruction from different locations on the scalp. Within limits, the greater the number of flaps used, the more diffuse is the tissue recruitment. Likewise, the burden of the repair of the secondary defect is shared by

the number of flaps utilized. Two or three rotation flaps work best for reconstructing most scalp defects. When utilizing three flaps, each flap is responsible for repairing one-third of the surface area of the defect. Wound closure is accomplished by pivoting all three flaps in the same direction. Repair of the defect has an appearance of a pinwheel, and wound closure configuration resembles the closing of a camera lens.[12]

When using a single rotation flap, the parameter of the arc of the flap should be at least four times the diameter of the scalp defect. Sometimes one or two back cuts at the base of the flap are necessary to reduce wound closure tension. On rare occasions, the secondary defect must be skin-grafted or left to heal by secondary intention. Standing cutaneous deformities are not resected at the base of scalp flaps at the time of transfer because resection has the effect of reducing the width of the base of the flap and may impair vascularity. In addition, deformities tend to flatten over a 4–6 week interval. Usually after 6 weeks, any remaining deformity may be removed safely because recipient site vascularity is sufficient to maintain flap viability.

Forehead

The most effective technique for reconstruction of the forehead usually involves one or more advancement flaps. In spite of the relative inelasticity of forehead skin, the use of advancement flaps *vs* pivotal flaps is preferred because they typically produce the best cosmetic results. This is because incisions necessary for advancement flaps may be placed in the horizontal furrows of the forehead or along the border of the eyebrow depending on the location of the defect. Transposition flaps do work well in the region of the temple, but more medially

on the forehead it becomes difficult to close the donor site when such flaps are used.

Dividing the forehead into three zones (median, paramedian, lateral) assists in planning reconstruction. In spite of a wound closure scar that is perpendicular to relaxed skin tension lines, defects of the central one-third of the forehead may be repaired in a vertical orientation with a predictably good aesthetic result (Fig. 47.17). This is probably due to the natural dehiscence or attenuation of the frontalis muscle in this portion of the forehead. In contrast, defects located solely within the paramedian and lateral zones of the forehead are best repaired with closure oriented in a horizontal axis.

Advancement flaps should be designed with horizontal orientations that facilitate scar camouflage and that minimizes any vertical component to the repair. Vertical scars in the paramedian and lateral zones of the forehead are perpendicular to forehead furrows and their appearances are accentuated by contraction of the frontalis muscle.

Because of the inelasticity of forehead skin, bilateral advancement flaps are typically designed on opposite sides of the defect. This arrangement reduces the degree of tissue movement required compared to using a single flap. Two opposing advancement flaps recruit tissue from two separate areas of the forehead and this has the

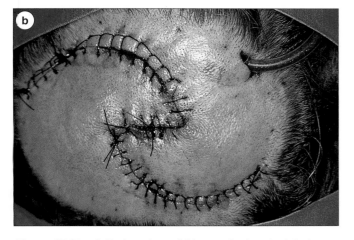

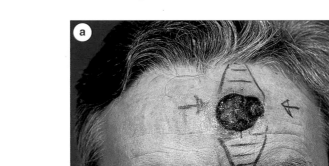

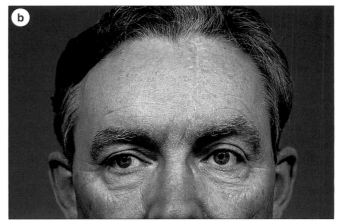

Figure 47.16 O-Z plasty is useful for repair of scalp defects. (a) 4 cm full thickness vertex scalp defect. Rotation flaps designed to pivot in same (clockwise) direction. (b) Wound repair assumes Z-shaped closure.

Figure 47.17 Defects of central forehead may be repaired with vertical orientation with predictably good aesthetic results. (a) 3.5 × 3.0 cm skin defect of central forehead repaired by primary closure. Areas marked for excision represent standing cutaneous deformities. (b) 10 months postoperative.

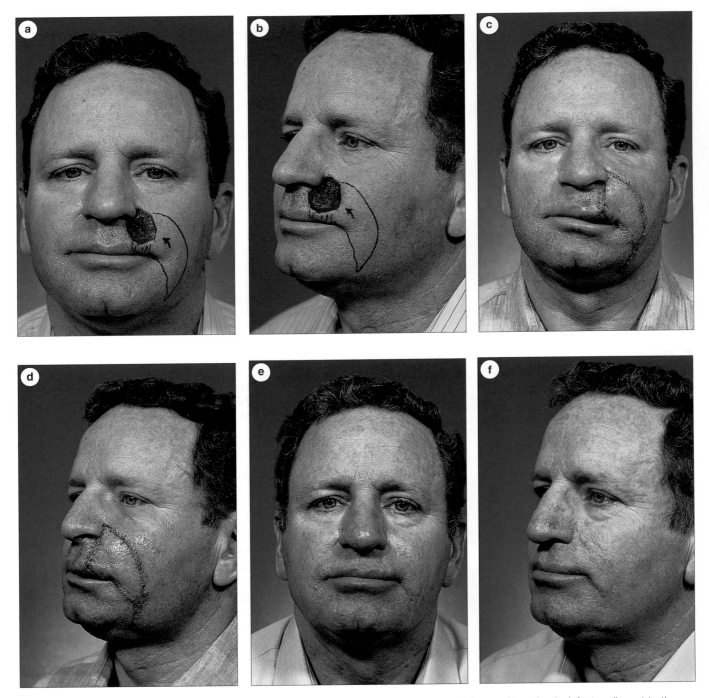

Figure 47.20 V-Y Subcutaneous pedicle island advancement flaps are particularly useful for repairing cheek defects adjacent to the ala. (a,b) 4 × 3.5 cm cutaneous defect of lip and cheek. V-Y subcutaneous pedicle island flap is designed for repair. Remaining skin of lateral upper lip marked for excision. (c,d) Flap in place. (e,f) 2 years, 8 months postoperative.

accommodate the thickness of the advancement flap. The leading border of the skin island is fixed in place and the wound surrounding the remaining perimeter subsequently closed, such that wound closure tension is equally distributed over the entire length of the flap. The donor site is closed in a V-Y fashion, taking care to compensate for any differences in the length of the opposing margins of the donor site.

Cutaneous pedicled advancement flaps are probably the least useful of the three types of flap designs preferred for repairing medial cheek defects. When tissue advancement is used for repair of the medial cheek, it often takes

the form of primary wound closure. Standing cutaneous deformities are removed in aesthetic boundaries when possible (Fig. 47.21). If incisions are necessary to create a flap, they are designed so they are placed in the natural lines of the face. Two parallel or slightly divergent incisions are made adjacent to the defect and the flap is elevated in the subcutaneous plane and advanced over the defect. If the flap does not stretch sufficiently, it may be necessary to excise Burow's triangles on either side of the flap's base. These triangular excisions help equalize the distance between the sides of the flap and the wound margins.

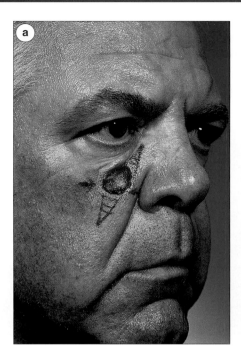

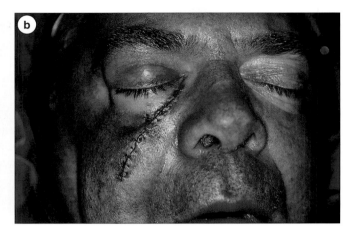

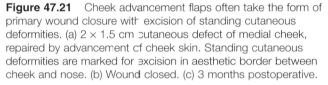

Figure 47.21 Cheek advancement flaps often take the form of primary wound closure with excision of standing cutaneous deformities. (a) 2 × 1.5 cm cutaneous defect of medial cheek, repaired by advancement of cheek skin. Standing cutaneous deformities are marked for excision in aesthetic border between cheek and nose. (b) Wound closed. (c) 3 months postoperative.

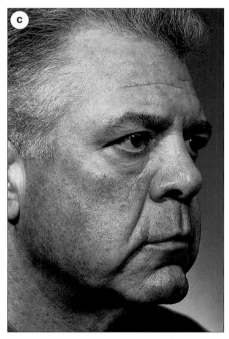

Lateral cheek

Lateral cheek skin has less subcutaneous fat and is more adherent to the underlying fascia than is medial cheek skin. For this reason, subcutaneous pedicle island advancement flaps work less well here since such flaps depend on ample subcutaneous tissue for movement. The preferred flap for smaller defects of the lateral cheek are transposition flaps. Larger defects are best repaired with rotation advancement flaps designed to recruit upper cervical skin into the flap (Fig. 47.22). Transposition flaps are usually superiorly based and the skin immediately above the angle of the mandible serves as the donor tissue for the flap. This is because skin of the inferior posterior cheek is more redundant and mobile

compared to skin located in the posterior superior cheek near the temple. The increased mobility is attributed to the presence of the platysmal muscle covering the mandible.

Large defects (>3–4 cm) located in the lateral cheek are most easily reconstructed with rotation advancement flaps. From the lateral inferior border of the defect a curvilinear incision extends downward and posteriorly below the earlobe and then backward to the posterior hairline. From there, the incision extends inferiorly along the posterior border of the sternocleidomastoid muscle. Flaps are based medially and inferiorly and can provide a flexible means of transferring large areas of skin from the remaining cheek and upper cervical regions.

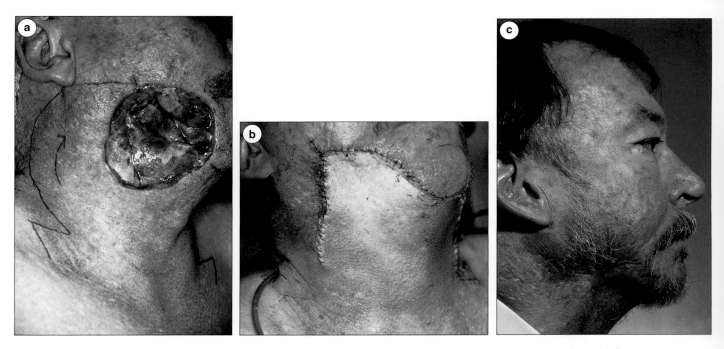

Figure 47.22 Large lower cheek and upper neck defects can be repaired with cervical rotation advancement flaps. (a) Cutaneous defect following removal of squamous cell carcinoma. Bilateral cervical rotation advancement flaps are designed to recruit upper cervical skin for purpose of repair. (b) Wound closed. (c) 3 months postoperative.

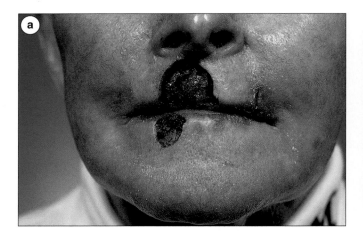

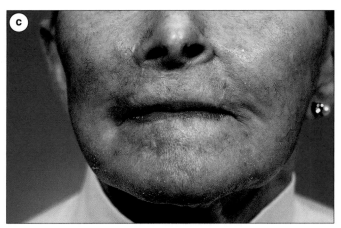

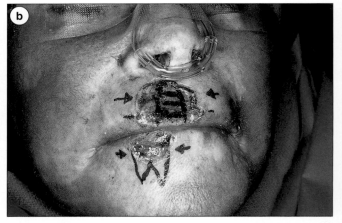

Figure 47.23 Cutaneous defects of the lips can often be repaired by performing full thickness excisions of the lip in the area of the defect followed by primary closure. (a) Skin and soft tissue defects of upper and lower lip. (b) Both defects converted to full thickness by excising muscle and mucosa. Lower lip defect repaired in W-plasty fashion. Upper lip defect repair with primary closure. (c) 7 months postoperative.

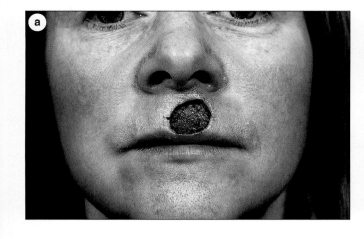

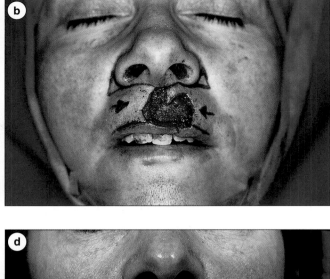

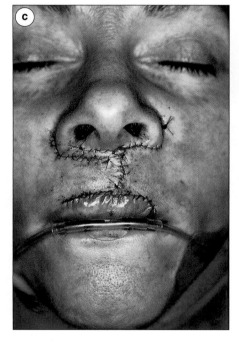

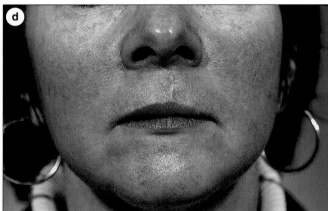

Figure 47.24 Cutaneous defects of the central upper and lower lips that cannot be closed primarily can be repaired most favorably using bilateral advancement flaps. (a) 3 × 2.5 cm upper lip cutaneous defect. (b) Bilateral advancement flaps are designed so incisions are in vermiliocutaneous border and adjacent to nasal sil. Bürow's triangles are marked in alar facial sulcus bilaterally. Wound closed. (c) Bilateral standing cutaneous deformities have been removed from vermilion below and alar facial sulcus above. (d) 8 months postoperative.

Central lip

Depending on the laxity of the lips, cutaneous defects approaching one half of the width of the lip may be converted to full-thickness excisions of the lip followed by primary closure (Fig. 47.23). The majority of skin defects of the central upper and lower lips that cannot be closed primarily can be repaired most favorably using bilateral advancement flaps. For the upper lip, incisions for opposing advancement flaps are made along the vermiliocutaneous border and immediately below the nasal sil (Fig. 47.24). For the lower lip incisions are placed in the vermiliocutaneous border and the mental crease. Although the skin of the lips is elastic it is tightly adherent to the underlying muscle and must be dissected sharply from the orbicularis oris as there is little subcutaneous fat present. It is usually necessary to remove a Bürow's triangle from the vermilion to prevent excessive bunching when the opposing borders of the two advancement flaps are approximated.

Lateral lip

Cutaneous defects of the lateral aspect of the upper and lower lips are best repaired using rotation flaps or subcutaneous island pedicled advancement flaps (Fig. 47.25). Skin is recruited from the adjacent perioral area. In general, flaps from the medial cheek should not be used because by necessity they traverse the melolabial crease and obliterate this important aesthetic boundary. Rotation flaps should be designed so that the incision for the flap lies in or parallel to the melolabial crease. The skin flap is elevated from the orbicularis oris and is based on the ample subcutaneous fat located immediately lateral to the commissure. In the case of upper lip defects, a back cut below the level of the commissure may be necessary to facilitate sufficient tissue movement. A standing cutaneous deformity develops as the flap pivots and should be excised along the vermilion border to prevent the flap from distorting the vermilion.

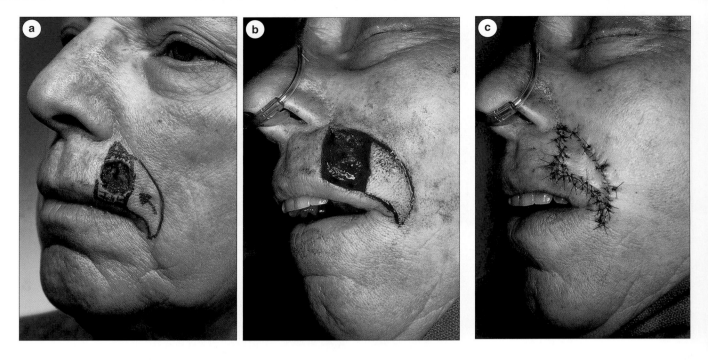

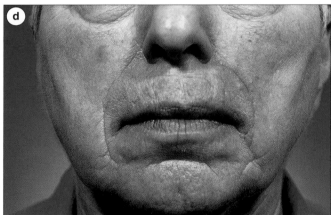

Figure 47.25   Cutaneous defects of the lateral upper lip can be repaired with V-Y subcutaneous pedicle island advancement flap. (a) Cutaneous defect of upper lateral lip. V-Y subcutaneous pedicle island advancement flap designed for repair. Skin of lip is marked for removal to place scar at vermiliocutaneous border. (b) Flap recruits skin from perioral area. (c) Wound closed. (d) 3 months postoperative.

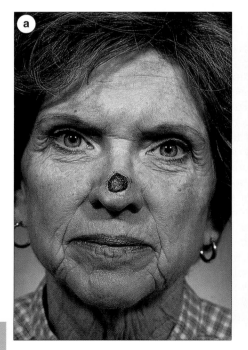

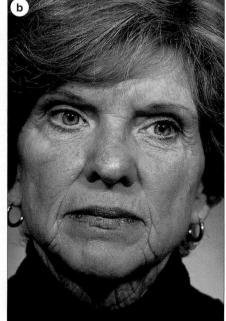

Figure 47.26   A bilobe nasal flap is the preferred method of repairing cutaneous defects that are 1.5 cm or less on the central nasal tip. (a) Cutaneous defect of nasal tip. (b) 2 months following repair of defect with bilobe nasal flap.

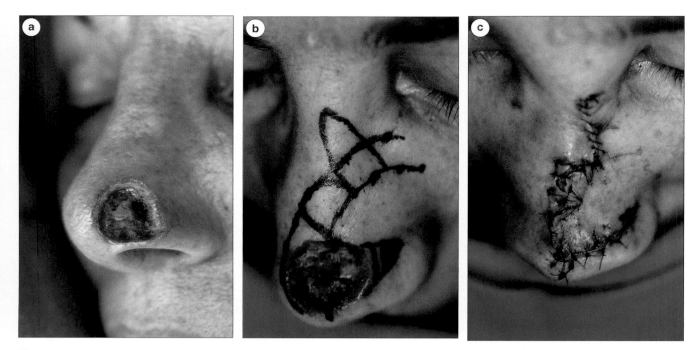

Figure 47.27 Although bilobe nasal flaps work best for repair of defects of the central tip, they may be used to repair the lateral tip. (a) 2 × 2 cm cutaneous defect of lateral nasal tip. (b) Bilobe nasal flap designed for repair. (c) Flap in place. Standing cutaneous deformity removed from left alar groove.

Subcutaneous pedicle island advancement flaps are ideally suited for repair of lateral skin defects of the upper lip. They do not work as well for defects of the lower lip. As discussed earlier, this flap design is also ideal for medial cheek defects adjacent to the nasal alae. The flap is dissected in a similar fashion to the method discussed for its use in repairing medial cheek defects.

Nose

The two most commonly used local flaps for repair of cutaneous defects of the nose and in which the donor site is confined to the nose are the subcutaneous pedicle island advancement flap and the bilobe flap.[14] The island flap is used for repair of defects located at the anterior aspect of the alar groove. The bilobe flap is used to repair small cutaneous defects of the nasal tip and caudal dorsum.

Small defects (1.5 cm or less in size) located in the region of the anterior alar groove between the ala and tip can be effectively repaired with a subcutaneous pedicle island advancement flap. It is based on subcutaneous tissue and portions of the transverse nasalis muscle. A triangular-shaped flap with its base making up the cephalic border of the defect is designed with the apex of the flap positioned laterally. The posterior border of the flap rests in the alar groove. The anterior border extends cephalically and slightly medially from the defect and is designed to recruit skin of the nasal sidewall. The anterior border then arcs laterally to meet the posterior border in the alar facial sulcus. The flap is incised to the level of the perichondrium of the nasal cartilages. The adjacent nasal skin is undermined widely and the proximal and distal one-third of the flap is undermined in the subcutaneous plane. The central third of the flap remains pedicled on the subcutaneous tissue. The flap is advanced and secured at the recipient site first and then the donor site is closed creating a V-Y configuration to the repair.

Bilobe nasal flaps are the preferred flap to repair 1–1.5 cm cutaneous defects of the central tip or caudal dorsum (Fig. 47.26).[14] They may also be used to repair skin defects of the lateral nasal tip (Fig. 47.27). However, when the defect encroaches on the nostril margin, there is a greater likelihood of elevation of the nostril as the wound heals. A distance equal to the radius of the defect is measured from the lateral border of the defect to the pivotal point of the two lobes of the bilobe flap (Fig. 47.28). Two arcs are drawn with their centers at the pivotal point. One arc passes through the center of and the other tangential to the distal border of the defect. The base of both lobes of the flap arise from the first arc. The height of the first lobe extends to the second arc. The height of the second lobe is twice the height of the first lobe and tapers to a point. The width of the first lobe equals the width of the defect. The width of the second lobe may be 25% less than the first lobe. The axis of the defect and the two lobes of the flap are approximately 45° apart for a total of 90 to 110°. The donor site of the second lobe is closed first. The first lobe is transposed and the standing cutaneous deformity removed. The second lobe is then transposed and trimmed to fit precisely without wound closure tension.

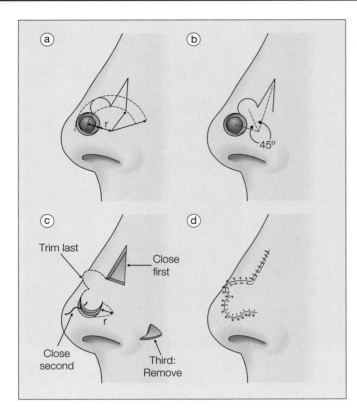

Figure 47.28 Design of bilobe nasal flap. (a) Two arcs are drawn with their centers at pivotal point one radius length from lateral border of defect. Base of both lobes rest on smaller arc. Height of first lobe extends to second arc. Height of second lobe is twice that of first lobe and is triangulated. (b) Axis of defect and two lobes of flap are approximately 45° apart for a total tissue pivotal movement of 90° to 110°. (c,d) Donor site of second lobe closed first. First lobe is transposed and standing cutaneous deformity removed in alar groove. Second lobe is then trimmed to fit precisely donor site of first lobe.

FUTURE OUTLOOK

The mission of reconstruction is a reparative attempt to restore 'normalcy' following a damaging surgical effort. We have progressed significantly beyond simply 'filling the hole' or 'patching the wound.' Future efforts will be directed at further understanding of the subtle aesthetic components of what visually determines a 'normal' face as well as what detracts from that impression. As creativity evolves, new flap designs will emerge. Better

methods of wound and scar management will also aid in achieving more 'natural' results. Methods to encourage flap survival are actively being investigated.

Reconstruction is a blend of artistry, technical skill and science. The integration of these areas will guarantee satisfaction for both patient and physician.

REFERENCES

1 Clevens RA, Baker SR. Defect analysis and options for reconstruction. Otolaryngol Clin N Amer 1997; 30(4):495–517.

2 Baker SR. Reconstruction of facial defects. In: Krause CJ, ed. Otolaryngol Head Neck Surg, 3rd edn., Philadelphia, PA: Mosby; 1998:527–559.

3 Baker SR. Local cutaneous flaps in soft tissue augmentation and reconstruction in the head and neck. Otolaryngol Clin North Am 1994; 27:139–159.

4 Bray DA. Rhombic flaps. In: Baker SR, Swanson NA eds. Local Flaps in Facial Reconstruction. St. Louis, MO: Mosby; 1995:151–163.

5 Zitelli JA. Bilobe flaps. In: Baker SR, Swanson NA eds. Local Flaps in Facial Reconstruction. St. Louis, MO: Mosby; 1995:165–180.

6 Baker SR, Alford EL. Mid-forehead flaps. Oper Tech Otolaryngol Head Neck Surg 1993; 4:24–30.

7 Menick FJ. Aesthetic refinements in use of the forehead flap for nasal reconstruction: the paramedian forehead flap. Clin Plast Surg 1990; 17:607–622.

8 Baker SR. Internal lining flaps. In: Baker SR, ed. Principles of Nasal Reconstruction. St. Louis, MO: Mosby; 2002:31–47.

9 Cook TA, Guida RA. Soft tissue technique. In: Papel ID, Nachlas NE, eds. Facial Plastic and Reconstructive Surgery. St. Louis, MO: Mosby; 1992:2.

10 Burget GC, Menick FJ. Subunit principle in nasal reconstruction. Plast Reconstr Surg 1985; 76:239–247.

11 Thomas JR, Frost TW. Immediate versus delayed repair of skin defects following resection of carcinoma. Otolaryngol Clin North Am 1993; 26:203.

12 Baker SR. Options for reconstruction in head and neck surgery. In: Cummings CW, Fredrickson JM, eds. Otolaryngology Head and Neck Surgery, Update 1. St. Louis, MO: Mosby; 1989:192–248.

13 Rustad TJ, Hartshorn DO, Cleven RA, et al. The subcutaneous pedicle in melolabial reconstruction. Arch Otolaryngol Head Neck Surg 1998; 124:1163–1166.

14 Baker SR. Nasal cutaneous flap. In: Baker SR ed. Principles of Nasal Reconstruction. St. Louis, MO: Mosby; 2002:103–121.

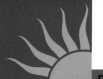

CHAPTER
48

Radiation Therapy in the Treatment of Skin Cancers

Jay S Cooper

Key points

- Radiation therapy should exploit both physical and radiobiologic factors to treat tumors optimally.
- Radiation therapy is curative for >90% of primarily treated basal and squamous cell carcinomas of the skin; the cosmetic appearance years later is a function of the manner in which the treatment course is fractionated.
- Malignant melanomas are the least sensitive type of skin tumor; however, 25% of metastatic malignant melanomas completely regress following radiation therapy. Elective irradiation of high-risk tumor beds substantially improves local-regional control of disease.
- Kaposi's sarcomas are universally responsive to radiation therapy in all clinical settings. The role and nature of radiation therapy depends on the overall health status of the patient.
- The role of and response to radiation therapy for mycosis fungoides depends upon the stage of the disease. Both 'spot radiation' and total skin electron beam radiation therapy have roles and offer benefits.

INTRODUCTION

Promiscuous exposure to the newly discovered X-ray first produced irritative and blistering effects in the skin of investigators approximately 100 years ago. Soon, physicians began to exploit these effects to kill tumors. Many decades of successful use of radiation therapy for cutaneous tumors followed. Yet, radiation therapy currently is being selected for the treatment of skin cancers less often than in prior years. In part this *appropriately* reflects the increasing variety of effective alternative therapies for skin cancer. But, has the pendulum swung too far? A recent survey[1] revealed that radiation therapy was used as first-line treatment for just 8% of the basal cell carcinomas treated in the UK and only 2% in The Netherlands. Certainly, radiation therapy is not the best treatment for all skin cancers, but it does represent an effective alternative for many. Hopefully, this chapter will provide sufficient information to (1) familiarize the reader with concepts of modern radiation therapy, (2) explain why two different radiation regimens can produce exactly the same short term effects (such as tumor control), but vastly different long-term effects (such as cosmetic appearance), and (3) suggest radiation therapy

as a possible treatment in situations where it offers a better alternative than other forms of management.

PRINCIPLES OF RADIATION THERAPY

Biologic factors

Cellular changes in response to radiation therapy reflect both biologic processes and physical processes that determine the outcome of treatment. All tissues are less likely to be damaged or killed by the same dose of radiation when their cells are in specific phases of the cell cycle (cells in S, G1 and early G2 are less sensitive), when oxygen is less plentiful, when they have a relatively long time to repair radiation-induced damage before being damaged again, and when they have sufficient time to grow and divide between fractions of treatment. The '4Rs' of radiobiology (Reassortment, Reoxygenation, Repair and Repopulation) help explain why radiation therapy generally is most effective when a fractionated regimen is used. Regaud and Ferroux[2] long ago performed a series of experiments in radiation fractionation, examining the effect of radiation on scrotal skin and testicular function. When radiation was administered in a single fraction there was no dose that could be delivered to a rabbit's testes that would be sufficient to cause sterility without producing unacceptable reactions in the scrotal skin as well. In contrast, when the radiation was given in a fractionated manner, it was possible to sterilize the animals without producing complications in the irradiated skin. Thus, to understand the literature the reader must understand the precise implications of the dose-fractionation pattern employed.

For most human neoplasms, curative-intent external beam radiation therapy is delivered in one fraction per day, 180–200 cGy per fraction, 5 days per week to total doses of 5000–7000 cGy. (Radiation is currently measured in 'Gray' or in units 1/100 as large, centiGray (cGy). One cGy numerically equals one rad, the previous standard of dose.) However, skin tumors are among the smallest neoplasms at the time of discovery and are so superficial that it is relatively easy to protect nearby normal tissues. Consequently, one can 'get away' with a wide variety of regimens that would not be tolerated in other anatomic sites and more variations have been used for the radiotherapeutic management of cutaneous tumors than could be used for tumors arising in other tissues in the body. Each of these variations has a predictable influence on the outcome of treatment (both in the short term and in the long term).

The concept of equivalent dose

Because the total dose is not independent of the manner in which it is administered, it would be useful to have a biologic-dose-equivalent number that compared different fractionation patterns, if it could be defined accurately. It is possible to expose patches of skin to differing courses of radiation and define 'equivalent doses' by scoring the degree of *acute* (short-term) damage produced shortly after treatment. From such experiments, it became clear that as the total length of a treatment course increased, the greater the numerical total dose had to be, to produce an equivalent reaction.

Ellis took this concept one step further by describing a mathematical formula that related the total numerical dose, the number of fractions, and the total time of a course of treatment to a single number termed the nominal standard dose (NSD). (In the NSD equation, the influence of the number of fractions exceeds the influence of the total time. The generally cited form of the equation is $D = NSD \times N^{.24} \times T^{.11}$ where D represents the total numerical dose, N represents the number of fractions and T represents the total time in days of the course of radiation.) Orton and Ellis[3] subsequently simplified matters by publishing a set of derivative tables, written in TDF (time-dose-fractionation) units, that allow physicians to look up the equivalent acute responses based on the daily dose, number of fractions per week and total number of fractions. Unfortunately, it is now clear that the amount of damage that is evident in the acute phase of a reaction does not accurately predict what will happen in the long term.

Although the radiobiologic laws that govern the production of damage are not yet understood completely, it is now becoming apparent that damage has at least two components, termed alpha (α) and beta (β). Some cells are killed by a single interaction (α killing). The number of cells killed in this manner is directly proportional to the dose-per-fraction. However, other cells merely are damaged. Such cells appear to have more than one target that needs to be destroyed for the radiation to be lethal (β killing); the killing of such cells by radiation is proportional to the square of the dose-per-fraction.

This concept has many implications for the clinical application of radiation therapy. (The ratio of α to β killing appears to be an intrinsic property of individual tissues. For many rapidly dividing tissues, including tumors, the α/β ratio appears to be about 10. For slowly growing tissues, such as normal connective tissues, the α/β ratio is closer to three. Because late complications are believed to occur in slowly proliferating normal tissues, late complications are made worse by larger doses per fraction. One commonly expressed form of the alpha-beta model is $E = n(\alpha d + \beta d^2)$ where E is the cell kill (measured in logs), n is the number of fractions and d is the dose in Gray of a single fraction of radiation.) For the current discussion, the concept predicts that for an equivalent amount of short-term damage, larger daily fractions will produce greater long-term damage, because the cells involved in long-term damage are disproportionately affected by beta killing.

In practice, this concept implies that two different radiation regimens may be equally effective in controlling cutaneous carcinomas (and may produce similar short-term cosmetic changes), but the one that uses the higher-dose-per-fraction to reach the same total dose will inevitably lead to a poorer long-term cosmetic appearance.

Physical factors

Superficial quality X-ray radiation

X-rays are massless, chargeless, electromagnetic packages (photons) of energy that are generated when electrons, produced from an electrically excited filament and accelerated across an electric potential, interact with a heavy metal target. Because some of the resulting X-rays are of relatively low energy, a filter typically is placed in the beam to absorb the less penetrating rays preferentially; 2 mm of aluminum filtration is common for the approximately 100 kV peak (kVp) energy 'superficial quality' X-ray machine. The amount of filtration chosen represents a balance between the need to 'harden' (i.e. increase the average energy of) the beam without decreasing intolerably its intensity (dose rate). Therefore, the precise amount of penetration of a superficial quality beam depends both on the energy of the progenitor electrons (kVp of the tube) and the subsequent filtration of the beam.

Superficial quality X-rays, no matter how highly filtered, cannot penetrate very far into tissue because they are attenuated rapidly by interactions with atoms in the tissues traversed. Under typical circumstances the intensity of a 100 kVp superficial quality X-ray beam decreases to 90% (i.e. loses 10%) of its maximum deposited energy (surface dose) after traversing only 0.5 cm of tissue. (Superficial X-rays interact maximally with tissues as soon as they encounter them and therefore are well-suited for treatment of relatively thin lesions close to or involving a tissue surface.) It drops to 50% of its maximum intensity by 2 cm. Because most cutaneous tumors lie within a few mm of the skin surface, superficial quality X-rays more than adequately penetrate such neoplasms. However, some tumors are too thick to be irradiated this way.

Electron beam radiation

Electron beam producing linear accelerators are now far more common than superficial quality X-ray producing units. To some degree a relatively low energy electron beam (e.g. 6 MeV (million electron volt)) and a superficial quality X-ray (e.g. 100 kVp) are similar. Because of their mass and charge, electrons can penetrate only limited distances through tissue before interacting and expending all of their energy. The greater the initial energy of the electron, the further it will travel through tissue. But, it will always dissipate its energy over a far shorter track then would a photon of the same energy. For example, a 6 million volt electron beam will homogeneously irradiate (< 10% variance) the first 2 cm it encounters. Yet it effectively will not penetrate more than 3 cm. Because it may be advantageous, particularly in the treatment of cutaneous neoplasms, to have a beam that penetrates a fixed, limited distance into tissue, linear accelerators often are designed to allow electrons to be used directly for treatment. In fact, most accelerators have the ability to produce electrons at several different energies allowing the physician to select the energy (and depth of penetration) that most closely matches the patient's needs. However, dermatologically relevant electron beams are sufficiently energetic that, if unmodified, relatively spare the first few millimeters of tissue they traverse. Consequently, tissue equivalent material (bolus) generally is placed on the skin over the lesion during treatment to ensure 'full dose' to the surface of the tumor and simultaneously decrease the penetration of the beam into deeper tissues.

Field size

Radiation therapy sometimes is denigrated because it does not permit histologic examination of the margins of the treated area as does surgery. Consequently, normal appearing tissue margins need to be slightly greater than is absolutely required for surgery. Fortunately, this typically can be done with little consequence to the patient. However, margins must be selected with the knowledge that the biologic effect of a dose is influenced by the volume of tissue irradiated; the greater the volume of tissue irradiated, the greater will be the biologic effect of physically identical doses of radiation. Experience and judgment are therefore required to select the optimum 'normal tissue' margin to be irradiated. For the typical, well-demarcated lesion a margin of 0.5 to 1.0 cm is adequate. Large tumors and those with less well-defined edges may require up to 2 cm margins. Poorly-demarcated tumors are usually better treated by Mohs' surgery; in the odd circumstance when radiation therapy is chosen, small circumferential punch biopsies can be used to map the tumor edge, beyond which a generous margin should be applied.

Anatomic site

The nature of the normal tissues in various anatomic sites also influences the response to radiation. Skin that is subjected to physical trauma tends to blister and/or ulcerate following radiotherapy. Consequently, there are relatively few situations in which a small basal cell carcinoma of the arms, legs or trunk would not be better treated by an alternative modality. In contrast, mucosal surfaces tolerate radiation therapy well. Squamous cell carcinomas of the lip are often good candidates for treatment by radiation therapy.

Some sites are ideally suited for treatment by radiation therapy. Tumors of the eyelids or at the tip of the nose tend to have a better cosmetic result when treated by a well-fractionated course of radiotherapy, as compared with surgery. However, when tumors are treated on the eyelids, the eye needs to be anesthetized and an appropriate shield placed directly on the globe, underneath the lid, to protect the lens from unnecessary radiation. Doses of only a few hundred cGy, even when given in many fractions, may be sufficient to cause a cataract.

Beam shape and profile

The simplest technique for irradiation of a small cutaneous lesion uses nothing more than a single *en face* beam and a custom-fabricated lead cut-out to demarcate a single field. For superficial X-rays, the cut-out (approximately 1 mm of lead or equivalent depending upon the energy and filtration of the superficial beam used) is placed directly on the skin, under the end of the cone of the X-ray unit to produce an irregularly shaped field of radiation that coincides with the shape of the tumor plus a uniform normal tissue margin. In contrast, the cut-out for an electron beam typically is placed in a holder within the 'electron cone' of the accelerator, approximately 50 cm from the patient's skin, and tends to be fabricated from a lead-equivalent alloy (that can be melted and poured to fit any shape), which needs to be approximately 1 cm thick.

One other difference between superficial X-rays and electrons is pertinent to the current discussion. The cross-sectional areas that electron beams effectively irradiate do not diverge with penetration into tissues in the same manner as occurs with X-ray beams. In essence, for an identical area of skin treated, the area treated by a dermatologically relevant electron beam is constricted (*vs* an X-ray beam) as the electron beam approaches its maximum depth. Consequently, a slightly larger area of skin needs to be irradiated by an electron beam to have equivalent coverage at the base of some tumors.

Although most tumors that arise from the integument are relatively thin, flat and of limited size, techniques more complex than a single irregularly shaped, *en face* X-ray or electron beam field may be required for lesions that are extensive, thick, on a curved surface or adjacent to critical anatomic sites. For example, complex techniques are mandatory for total skin electron beam therapy for cutaneous lymphoma.

In some circumstances, it may be preferable to irradiate tumors by placing radioactive materials either in them (implant brachytherapy) or adjacent to them (surface mold brachytherapy), thereby relatively sparing the surrounding normal tissues from damage. These techniques require the tumor to be relatively small and accessible. Tumors irradiated in this fashion are exposed to continuous treatment; at least in theory, this eliminates concern about regrowth in between fractions. Because the pattern of dose deposition from brachytherapy differs so greatly from external beam therapy, it is even more difficult to equate such treatments than it is to compare two different external beam regimens.

TREATMENT OF BASAL AND SQUAMOUS CELL CARCINOMAS

Basal cell and squamous cell carcinomas can be treated effectively by several different modalities and the selection of radiotherapy for a particular basal or squamous cell carcinoma depends less on the likelihood of tumor control than on the anticipated cosmetic and functional results. These considerations tend to favor radiation therapy for lesions arising on or near the eyelids, nose, ears and lips. There is rarely reason to favor radiation therapy elsewhere in the body if the lesion can readily be excised without substantial cosmetic and/or functional consequence.

Opinion versus evidence-based medicine

In recent years, some dermatologists have abandoned radiation therapy as 'an older treatment modality'. Kuijpers *et al*'s 2002 review entitled 'Basal Cell Carcinoma: Treatment Options and Prognosis, a Scientific Approach to a Common Malignancy'[4] is illustrative of this bias. The authors performed an 'extensive review of the literature' seeking to find 'evidence-based' justification for selection of treatment of tumors in follow-up to their 1999 work entitled 'A Systemic Review of Treatment Modalities for Primary Basal Cell Carcinomas'.[5] In both analyses, they relied nearly exclusively on one manuscript (by Silverman *et al*.[6]) as the basis of their analysis of radiation therapy and compared different modalities essentially by recurrence rates. Despite quoting a 7% recurrence rate after radiation therapy of basal cell carcinomas, well within the range of other treatments, radiation therapy was deemed a secondary choice for treatment after concluding, 'evidence-based guidelines could not be developed'. The reader is therefore urged to read the literature carefully and come to his/her own conclusions.

Do basal cell and squamous cell carcinomas react similarly to irradiation?

Basal cell and squamous cell carcinomas arising in the skin respond similarly to radiotherapy and logically are discussed together. This does not imply that they are identical and several series suggest a higher recurrence rate for squamous cell carcinomas than basal cell carcinomas treated identically (see later). However, basal cell and squamous cell carcinomas arising in the skin are relatively radioresponsive lesions and both types can be eradicated with unremarkable doses of radiotherapy. In part this truth reflects their inherent responsiveness and in part reflects the superficial nature of skin tumors and the small field sizes needed to encompass them, allowing physicians to inflict skin reactions, in small areas of skin, that would be intolerable over large volumes or deep within the body, to heal with relatively little problem. This may explain the current tendency for basal cell and squamous cell carcinoma of the skin to be treated with dose fractions that are considerably larger than are the fractions typically used for other types of neoplasms. Numerous such dose-fractionation schemes have proven effective in controlling such lesions and there is no universal standard. Some physicians modify their treatment based on the size of the lesion, while others modify based on its histology. There is no compelling evidence to demonstrate that any of these time-tested regimens is significantly more likely to eradicate a cutaneous basal or squamous cell carcinoma than is an alternative regimen. Perhaps, all of these accepted regimens are so good at eradicating these tumors that one should wonder if they are too aggressive. Of course, there is no concern about eradicating too many tumors, unless the treatment also leads to unnecessary side-effects.

Dose, time, fractionation

The New York University Skin and Cancer Unit long ago opted to adopt standardized dose fractionation schemes based on histology and the desire to find schemes that could be applied to the majority of lesions treated by dermatologists. All basal cell carcinomas received 680 cGy twice per week for a total of 2½ weeks; squamous cell carcinomas received 680 cGy twice per week for 4 weeks.

More often, basal and squamous cell carcinomas are treated according to a size-graduated scale, with larger lesions receiving larger numerical total doses delivered in smaller daily fractions. For example, Solan *et al*.[7] recommend 4000 cGy in 10 to 16 fractions for small lesions and 4500 cGy in 15 to 18 fractions to 6000 cGy in 20 to 30 fractions for larger lesions.

Tumor control: rates and modifiers

Silverman *et al*.[6] reviewed the outcome of 862 primary basal cell carcinomas uniformly treated with 680 cGy for 5 fractions over 2.5 weeks between 1955 and 1982. The 5-year recurrence rate was 7.4% and larger tumor size was the only independent factor that correlated with local recurrence. Petrovich *et al*.[8] reported the outcome of radiotherapy in 646 patients who had carcinomas of the eyelids, pinna, or nose (72% basal cell, 18% squamous cell carcinoma and 10% mixed). Using a size-graduated philosophy, they observed 5, 10, and 20-year control rates of 99%, 98%, and 98%, respectively, for 502 tumors less than 2 cm in diameter. For larger tumors between 2 and 5 cm in diameter the 5 and 10 year control rates dropped to 92% and 79%, respectively and for still larger tumors 60% at 5 years and 53% at 8 years.

There appears to be a slightly higher local recurrence rate for squamous cell carcinoma as compared with basal cell carcinoma. Solon *et al*.[7] reported that 96% (426/444) of basal cell carcinomas and 92% (144/156) of squamous cell carcinomas were controlled for at least 4 years after radiation therapy. Lovett *et al*.[9] observed that size-for-size basal cell carcinomas exhibited better control following radiotherapy: for lesions less than 1 cm control was 97% (86/89) *vs* 91% (21/23); for tumors 1–5 cm control was 87% (116/133) vs 76% (39/51) and for lesions greater than 5 cm control was 87% (13 of 15) *vs* 56% (9/16), for basal cell and squamous cell carcinoma, respectively.

The influence of specific anatomic sites relates more to the difficulty of applying other forms of treatment and/or the cosmetic implications of any form of treatment than to the radiocurability of tumors that just happen to arise at these sites. Size for size, there appears to be no difference in response of lesions situated at different anatomic sites. Lesions near embryologic fusion planes tend to extend relatively deeply and require more penetrating therapy (radiation or other). Lesions of the eyelids often can be cured without needing to resort to complex plastic repairs. Lesions of the medial orbit can be irradiated with preservation of the functioning tear duct. Lesions adjacent to cartilage, once thought to be inappropriate for treatment by radiation because of the fear of subsequent chondronecrosis, are now known to be suitable for fractionated radiotherapy.

The success rate of radiotherapy also depends upon knowing when to treat a patient by alternative means. Lesions arising on skin subjected to continual trauma tend not to be treated ideally by radiotherapy. For this reason, lesions on the extremities (particularly the hands, legs and feet) usually are better treated surgically. Lesions of the trunk typically can be excised and the defect closed primarily in one session. For such patients it is unnecessarily inconvenient to attend for repetitive fractions of radiation. In addition, cosmetic considerations will not likely be as important for lesions on the trunk as on the face. This is not to say that such lesions cannot be treated by radiotherapy, merely that radiotherapy usually is not the treatment of choice.

Technical aspects of treatment

Although it is beyond the scope of this chapter to discuss technical details of radiotherapy for all lesions, some comments about general principles, for typical lesions, should be helpful. The treatment portal for well-defined lesions should include radial margins of 0.5–1 cm of normal appearing tissue. For poorly defined lesions, an additional 0.5 cm margin seems prudent.

Margins must be applied to the depth of the tumor as well. Because of the continued penetration of a superficial X-ray beam beyond the depth of a tumor, some apparently 'normal tissue' deep to the tumor always is irradiated to nearly the same dose as the base of the tumor. To provide the desired dose at the base of a tumor, some authors[10] advocate selecting a treatment beam that has a half-value depth (D½) equal to the depth of the tumor. (For superficial X-rays, the maximum dose occurs at the surface of the skin. The 'half-value depth', also known as the 'half-dose depth', represents the depth in tissue that receives a dose that is numerically equal to ½ of the surface dose). In clinical practice, various half-value depths can be obtained from machines of different energy (as the kilovoltage increases the half-value depth increases) and/or filtration (as the filtration increases the intensity of the beam decreases, but the X-rays that pass through the filter are of higher average energy yielding a greater half-value depth). Three other factors affect depth dose to a lesser degree: (1) field size (increasing field size increases scatter and increases depth dose), (2) tissue type (dense tissues decrease depth), (3) source to skin distance (increasing source skin distance increases depth dose).

Properly administered radiotherapy always aims to deliver the required dose to a lesion with as little dose as possible to surrounding and underlying tissues. Matching the half-value depth to the thickness of the lesion represents a strategy that intentionally delivers only 50% of the surface dose to the base of a lesion to spare still deeper tissues. Alternatively, one can view this as delivering twice the needed dose to the surface of the tumor, as well as adjacent normal tissues.

An alternative approach attempts to treat the entire tumor to approximately the same dose. For this philosophy, the base of the tumor should receive no less than 90% of the surface dose and the entire tumor receives a dose with less than 10% variation. In practical terms, for thin tumors, a superficial X-ray beam of approximately 100 kV often will accomplish this objective. X-ray treatment of tumors by this philosophy unavoidably delivers more radiation to the underlying normal tissues as compared with D½ techniques. Provided that all tumor cells receive sufficient dose, the difference between treating with a D½ philosophy and a 90% isodose philosophy therefore reflects the choice between placing the 'extra' normal tissue radiation at the surface (D½ philosophy) or in underlying tissues (90% isodose philosophy).

For the vast majority of cutaneous carcinomas elective irradiation of regional lymph node beds is unnecessary; however, such treatment should be considered for very large, ulcerated or recurrent squamous cell carcinomas.

Cosmetic considerations

The preceding comments about efficacy of radiotherapy would be unimportant (in light of the alternatives of treatment) unless the cosmetic appearance of at least some irradiated lesions was comparable with those treated by surgery. The abundance of alternative effective forms of therapy for basal and squamous cell carcinoma allows physicians to compare them both for efficacy and cosmetic effects.

As previously discussed, large-dose-per-fraction radiation therapy is not likely to result in an optimal cosmetic appearance years later. This should not be interpreted as saying that large-dose-per-fraction therapy is inherently bad; for the elderly outdoorsman who is not at all concerned about the appearance of his skin, it may be ideal! However, for the cosmetically sensitive younger patient it is ill-advised.

It is generally acknowledged that the cosmetic appearance of irradiated lesions shortly after treatment is excellent. Particularly for lesions of the eyelids, nose, and ears, the short-term cosmetic appearance of lesions treated by irradiation generally exceeds that attainable by surgery (Figs 48.1–48.3). More problematic is the cosmetic appearance years after treatment. There is little doubt that changes in coloration and thinning of the skin can become evident over the long term. In some patients, this change can be pronounced and associated telangiectasia can render the cosmetic appearance unsightly. Precisely how frequently the results become cosmetically unacceptable is less clear.

Bart et al.[11] reported a general tendency for cosmetic results to deteriorate over time. Within one year of therapy, 74% of their patients had good or excellent cosmetic results (following the use of their standardized high-dose-per-fraction scheme) whereas between 3 and 5 years, the corresponding percentage was 68% and between 9 and 12 years, 49%. This prompted the authors to recommend that radiotherapy not be advised for patients who are less than 40 years old.

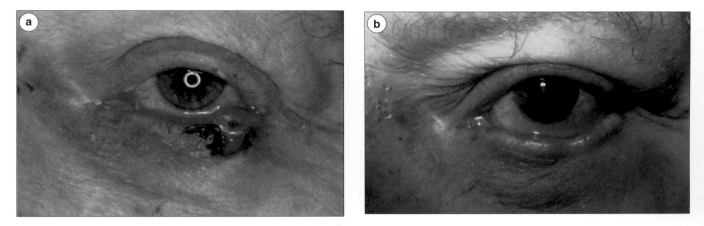

Figure 48.1   (a) Basal cell carcinoma of lower eyelid prior to treatment. (b) Same patient, 2 months following completion of radiotherapy. Patient was treated with superficial quality X-rays, a custom cut-out and an eye shield.

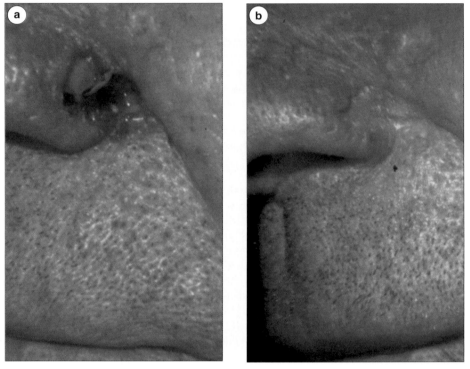

Figure 48.2   (a) Terebrant-type, infiltrating basal cell carcinoma prior to treatment. (b) Same patient, 3 months following radiotherapy. Because of the deeply infiltrative nature of this tumor, the patient was treated with cobalt therapy and bolus.

Oddly, there are very few reports describing differences in cosmetic outcome based on dose-fractionation. Brennan *et al.*[12] attempted to do precisely that by investigating the cosmetic appearance of tissues following three different dose fractionation schemes. Patients were randomly assigned to receive three fractions of 987 cGy each (total dose 2961 cGy), seven fractions of 513 cGy each (total dose 3591 cGy), or ten fractions of 380 cGy each (total dose 3870 cGy). All three schemes produce an equivalent NSD dose. When measured 2 years later, there was no difference in the cure rate or cosmetic result obtained by any of these dose-fractionation schemes. Whether longer follow-up or smaller fractions of 180–200 cGy, for example, as is customary for non-cutaneous lesions would have produced different results remains to be proven.

A recent randomized trial reported by Avril *et al.*[13] and Petit *et al.*[14] has been viewed by some as proof that radiotherapy leads to a poorer cosmetic outcome than does surgery. However, I believe this complex trial cannot be interpreted so simply. Although 93% of lesions were 2 cm or less, surgery was not as simple as might be assumed: frozen section assessment of the tumor margins was obtained for 91% of patients and 39% required additional resection. Following histologic examination of the permanent tumor specimen 3% patients required additional resection of residual disease, 3% required additional surgery to improve the appearance of the scar or correct an ectropion and 1% needed radiation therapy. The radiation therapy also differs substantially from the approximately 100 kV superficial X-rays or equivalent electrons discussed throughout this chapter: 55% of tumors were treated by implantation of interstitial radioactive sources (brachytherapy); 33% were treated by 50 kV contact X-ray therapy delivered in two *large* fractions of 1800 to 2000 cGy *each* spaced 2 weeks apart

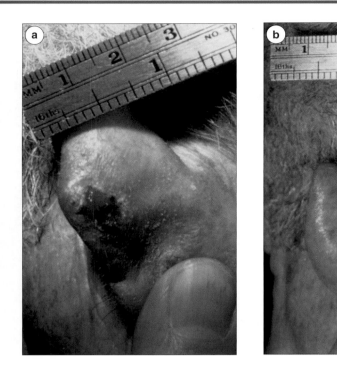

Figure 48.3 (a) Centrally ulcerated basal cell carcinoma on posterior helix of ear. (b) Same patient, 2 months following superficial X-ray radiotherapy. The lesion healed over completely and chondritis did not develop.

(treatment that predictably will give poorer cosmetic results than a more fractionated, smaller individual-size fraction regimen) and only 12% were treated with more conventional 85 to 250 kV therapy of 200–400 cGy per fraction, 3–4 times per week, up to 6000 cGy. Results of the trial were described as 'surgery' or 'radiotherapy' independent of the specific treatment delivered. Despite this, after 24 months and 36 months, the observed differences were relatively small. However, after 48 months, 69% of patients considered their cosmetic appearance 'good' following radiotherapy *vs* 87% after surgery; 8% of patients deemed their result poor after radiotherapy *vs* 2% after surgery. Surgery was not better in every anatomic location: the percentage of good cosmetic results was equal for tumors arising on the nose. This study demonstrates better cosmetic outcome for surgery only when compared to radiotherapy done in the same manner as was used in the trial … a manner I would not recommend if optimal cosmetic outcome is important!

A poll of our patients[15] irradiated 10 or more years previously according to a graduated treatment scale based on the size of their lesions, found them to be very satisfied with their cosmetic result. Fifty percent rated the appearance of the irradiated region 'excellent'. The data recently reported by Locke *et al.*[16] yielded a similar conclusion. The most common fractionation scheme they used (in 68% of their patients) delivered daily doses of no more than 300 cGy and total doses of 4001 to 6000 cGy. With these regimens 53% of their patients had excellent cosmetic results and 94% had good or excellent results.

Salvage by radiation therapy

Radiation therapy sometimes can be used to eradicate basal or squamous cell carcinomas that have recurred after surgical therapy. Caccialanza *et al.*[17] retrospectively reviewed the outcome of salvage radiotherapy for 249 lesions that had recurred after a variety of non-radiologic treatments. The 5-year cure rate was 83.6% and 'good or acceptable' cosmetic results were observed in 92.6% of the lesions that were controlled.

Non-melanoma summary and perspective

Numerous time-tested, dose-fractionation schemes are capable of curing cutaneous basal and squamous cell carcinomas in a high percentage of cases, similar to other methods of treatment. Whether size or histology should be used to select the proper dose for an individual patient is an archaic question; they both should influence the choice. The selection of radiotherapy as the treatment of choice should be based on the needs and desires of the individual patient. Patients who are poor candidates for surgical therapy (based on their overall health status) may remain good candidates for radiation therapy. For patients who can tolerate surgery, optimum treatment reflects the balance between patient-appropriate cosmetic results, lack of toxicity and convenience of the patient. If cosmetic appearance is important and if radiation therapy is chosen, a regimen that relies on relatively small doses-per-fraction and minimizes the dose delivered to adjacent skin surface is preferable.

TREATMENT OF MALIGNANT MELANOMA

Unlike the other tumors included in this chapter, malignant melanoma is not very radioresponsive. In fact, for many years malignant melanoma was believed to be impervious to radiation until data demonstrated that radiotherapy palliated distressing signs and symptoms of metastatic disease in more than 50% of patients. However, there does appear to be a basic biologic difference in the way some melanomas respond to radiotherapy, when compared with other types of neoplasms.

High-dose-per-fraction radiotherapy

At least some melanomas appear to have a greater than average ability to tolerate damage inflicted in a single dose and subsequently recover from some or all of it. Several groups published data that correlated better response with larger individual size fractions and not with total dose. For example, Habermalz and Fisher[18] observed no responses in 11 lesions treated with individual dose fractions of 200–500 cCy, while 29 of 33 lesions treated with 600 cGy or more per fraction regressed. However, others published response rates for malignant melanomas treated with conventionally fractionated techniques that appeared to be as good, while others claimed that high-dose per fraction techniques are more likely to induce short-term tumor regression, but are inferior to conventional techniques when measured by their ability to produce long-term local control.

To clarify the situation, the Radiation Therapy Oncology Group (RTOG) conducted a prospective randomized trial[19] for metastatic malignant melanomas comparing 800 cGy delivered four times at weekly intervals ('high-dose-per-fraction therapy') vs 250 cGy daily for 20 fractions over 26–28 days ('conventional-dose-per-fraction therapy'). (By NSD calculations, these regimens should produce approximately equivalent acute response.) The results showed no difference in response rates between the techniques. There was a 24.2% complete response rate (plus a 35.5% partial response rate) for lesions treated with high-dose-per-fraction radiation vs a 23.4% complete response (plus a 34.4% partial response rate) following conventional radiation. Thus, for the typical malignant melanoma, there does not appear to be a substantial difference in response to the two regimens. On the other hand, this trial clearly demonstrates that metastatic malignant melanomas do respond to radiation therapy and that complete response can be expected approximately 25% of the time.

Potentially curative radiotherapy

Although surgery generally is considered the treatment of choice for lentigo maligna and lentigo maligna melanoma, radiation has been used for these lesions, particularly in Europe. Typically, doses of 8000–10,000 cGy are delivered over the course of four or five fractions from a very low energy (10–20 kV) X-ray apparatus (the Miescher technique). Such beams are attenuated to 50% of their initial intensity by only 1 mm of tissue. Consequently, the Miescher technique can be viewed as superficial radiocautery rather than radiotherapy. There is no question, however, that it controls lentigo maligna in at least 95% of cases.

The main and formidable limitation of the Miescher technique relates to its inability to treat lesions of any substantial thickness. To overcome this problem, Harwood and Cummings[20] used more penetrating radiation, ranging from 100 kV to 280 kV, and scaled down their doses to the radiotherapy (not radiocautery) range. In general, they treated lentigo malignas and lentigo maligna melanomas with doses similar to those used for basal cell carcinomas. Lesions smaller than 2 cm generally received a dose of 3250 cGy in 5 fractions over one week while lesions 2–5 cm received 4500 cGy in ten fractions over 2 weeks. With follow-up ranging from 1½ to 13 years, 15 of 17 lentigo malignas and 21 of 23 lentigo maligna melanomas were controlled by initial radiotherapy. Similarly, Panizzon[21] used superficial X-ray therapy and reported a 100% cure rate for lentigo maligna and an 89% cure rate for lentigo maligna melanoma after 7.5 years of follow-up.

Even thicker disease sometimes can be effectively treated. Harwood et al.[22] irradiated 37 superficial spreading or nodular melanomas of the head and neck region. Six of these patients had undergone only incisional biopsy and had gross residual disease; 15 had undergone gross surgical removal, but in 11 histologic examination showed tumor to be present at the margin of the excision and 16 had gross local or regional recurrent disease following surgery. Four of the six lesions treated following biopsy were locally controlled and 14 of the 15 lesions treated for presumed microscopic size residual disease were similarly locally controlled. In contrast, only two of the 16 recurrent melanomas were controlled locally. However, radiation therapy has not gained wide acceptance as a curative treatment of macroscopic-size disease and questions remain about the potential role of radiation therapy in this setting.

Elective treatment of high-risk melanomas

Most recently, radiation therapy has been electively applied in situations where a high-risk for recurrence remains despite expertly done surgery (e.g. following resection of aggressive primary tumors, resection of locally recurrent disease or resection of metastases in regional lymph nodes). For example, Lee et al.[23] reported a 30% nodal basin recurrence rate following resection of histologically involved lymph nodes and correlated some pretreatment factors with even greater risks: extracapsular extension of disease (63%), multiple nodes invaded by tumor (46% for 4–10 nodes and 63% for >10 nodes), and cervical lymph node involvement (43%).

The risk of local-regional recurrence in these high-risk situations can be substantially reduced by elective radiation therapy. Following surgery, Ang et al.[24] electively irradiated 174 patients who had high-risk malignant melanomas. Of these, 79 patients had malignant melanomas at least 1.5 mm thick, 32 patients had clinically detectable regional nodal disease and 63 patients had recurrent previously resected disease. Treatment consisted of a total of 3000 cGy delivered in five fractions over two-and-one-half weeks. After a median follow-up of 35 months only six patients experienced isolated local-regional recurrence, nine patients experienced both local-regional and distant recurrence and 58 patients developed solely distant metastatic disease. Overall, the

5-year actuarial local-regional control rate was 88%, which far exceeded the historical experience at the same institution.

O'Brien et al.[25] similarly reported a non-randomized comparison of patients who had high-risk malignant melanomas treated with or without elective radiation. Forty-five patients (65% having at least two involved lymph nodes and 48% having extracapsular extension (ECE) of disease) received six fractions of 5.5 Gy each and only 6.5% experienced local-regional failure. A total of 107 other patients (40% having 2+ involved nodes and 19% having ECE) received no RT and experienced an 18.7% local-regional failure rate. The respective 5-year survival rates were 40% and 35%.

Corry et al.[26] used conventionally fractionated elective radiation therapy (typically 5000–6000 cGy delivered at 200 cGy per day) for 42 high-risk malignant melanomas. After 5 years follow-up, the first site of treatment failure was nodal alone in 20%; an additional 2% experienced simultaneous nodal and distant recurrence of disease. In this series the overall 5-year survival rate was 33%; 52% developed distant metastases, despite remaining loco-regionally free of disease.

We[27] also have used high-dose-per-fraction elective radiation therapy for high-risk malignant melanomas. Our patients had multiple involved lymph nodes (21 patients), close or microscopically involved surgical margins (nine patients), extracapsular extension of disease (six patients), previously resected, recurrent disease (three patients), and/or primary tumors more than 4 mm thick (four patients). In general, if the melanoma was considered high-risk because of a characteristic of the primary tumor or local recurrence, the primary tumor bed, the regional nodal bed and the in-transit pathways were included in the treatment portal, assuming that the resulting treatment portals were not excessively large. If the high-risk feature related to the nodal bed and the primary tumor was not considered high-risk or was excised years ago and the bed was subsequently free of recurrence, the primary tumor bed was not irradiated. Our patients experienced an 84% local-regional control rate at five

years. Unfortunately, the high-risk nature of the tumors that identified our patients for elective irradiation appear to have made them prone to develop distant metastases that presumably disseminated from the primary tumor sites before they were irradiated. Consequently, our patients had a 5-year survival rate of only 39%.

Thus the emerging literature suggests that elective irradiation of high-risk malignant melanomas improves the local-regional control rate, unfortunately without improving overall survival.

Elective irradiation should also be considered in the postoperative management of desmoplastic melanomas. This uncommon variant has a propensity for infiltrative growth, perineural spread and local recurrence with a relatively diminished likelihood of regional or distant metastases. These features suggest that elective irradiation should be helpful in their management and some groups advocate routine postoperative irradiation of desmoplastic melanomas. However, there currently is no prospective controlled trial data to support or refute this practice.

TREATMENT OF KAPOSI'S SARCOMA

Kaposi's sarcoma (KS) occurs in four different clinical settings ('classic' KS, 'epidemic' African KS, transplant-related KS and AIDS-related, 'epidemic' KS), but is highly radiosensitive in all four (Figs 48.4 and 48.5). In fact, there likely is no substantial difference in the radio-sensitivity of the disease between the variants and the results of treatment are remarkably consistent world-wide. For example, Stein et al.[28] writing from Johannesburg General Hospital in South Africa, compared response to irradiation in all four groups and concluded 'Kaposi's sarcoma showed a very high response rate to radiation therapy, regardless of variant, radiation modality or schedule.' However, the benefit of radiation therapy varies; the more localized the disease the greater the potential contribution of radiation therapy.

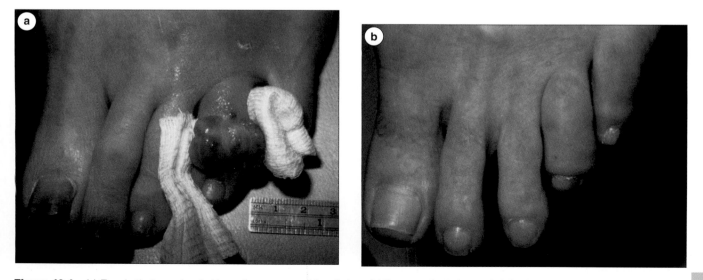

Figure 48.4 (a) Exophytic-type classic Kaposi's sarcoma of fourth toe. (b) Same patient, 1 month following treatment. Because of the bulky nature of his tumor, the patient received cobalt therapy with bolus.

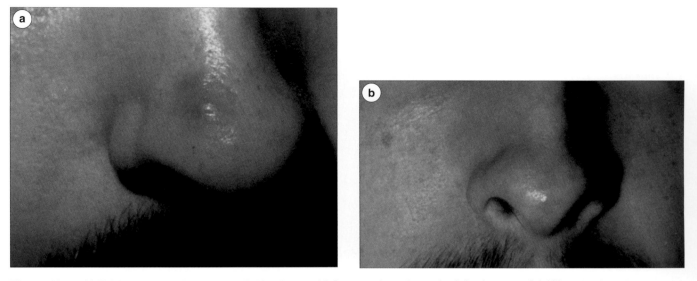

Figure 48.5 (a) Epidemic Kaposi's sarcoma of skin of nose. (b) Same patient, 4 months following superficial X-ray treatment.

'Classic' Kaposi's sarcoma

Because classic Kaposi's sarcoma tends to be a slowly progressive disease that remains confined to the legs for many years, the highly radioresponsive nature of the lesions often renders radiation therapy the treatment of choice. Radiotherapy generally is delivered solely to involved areas of skin plus a small normal appearing tissue border, although elective irradiation of adjacent clinically uninvolved areas has been advocated.

Fenig et al.[29] reviewed the outcome of radiation therapy in 123 Israeli patients who had classic KS. Radiotherapy produced an 88% objective (complete (CR) plus partial (PR)) response rate and symptomatic relief in 95% of patients. Similarly, Tombolini et al.[30] using doses ranging from 800 cGy in 1 fraction to 3000 cGy in 10 fractions observed a 92% objective response rate (54% complete response, 38% partial response) and complete remission of symptoms in all patients. Our own experience[31,32] treating 82 classic Kaposi's sarcomas in New York with doses ranging from 650 cGy in 1 fraction to 3500 cGy in 10 fractions demonstrated that more than 50% of classic KS lesions regressed completely and did not recur during a minimum follow-up of 10 years. We were also able to correlate the intensity of the treatment and the likelihood of long-term response. Doses of 2750 cGy or more delivered in ten fractions over 2 weeks, or their equivalent, were associated with significantly better long-term local control. A dose of 3000 cGy in ten fractions over 2 weeks appeared to provide an optimal balance between tumor control and rapidity of treatment.

Because of the potential for multicentric involvement by classic Kaposi's sarcoma, Holecek and Harwood[33] explored an alternative approach utilizing extended field radiotherapy, encompassing at least half a limb and including at least 15 cm of clinically normal skin proximal to the nearest clinically apparent lesion. They reported 10 of 12 patients so treated experienced complete response that persisted from 1 to 10 years. They compared this with patients treated to involved fields only in earlier years at the same institution. A total of 337 lesions were treated in 16 patients. (Two patients developed KS while on immunosuppressive therapy following renal transplant.) Twenty-four of the lesions were 'not assessable,' 249 regressed completely and 64 regressed partially. Although 800 cGy in a single fraction was used routinely for extended field therapy, varying doses were used for local radiotherapy. In that some of the lesions treated by local radiotherapy (which attained only partial response) were treated with doses as low as 300 cGy in a single fraction, it is difficult to separate the roles of field size vs dose in assessing the effectiveness of the method.

Harwood[34] subsequently reported the results of extended field radiotherapy for Kaposi's sarcoma in a total of 30 patients (including the 12 previously described) who were not getting immunosuppressive therapy. Twenty-three of these patients received only a single fraction of 800 cGy; 19 of them were reported to be in complete clinical remission from three months to five years after radiotherapy. Seven patients were given fractionated extended field radiotherapy; five of them were reported to be in complete remission between 2 and 14 years following treatment.

AIDS-related KS

After the initial 'epidemic' explosion, the incidence of AIDS-related Kaposi's sarcoma has dramatically declined in response to highly active anti-retroviral therapy (HAART). Moreover, the typically disseminated nature of epidemic KS not infrequently requires a more widespread systemic approach to the palliation of distressing lesions than radiation therapy can provide. Thus the current role for radiation therapy is considerably diminished compared with a decade ago.

Yet, there remain selected patients who can benefit from radiation therapy and the individual lesions remain as highly radiosensitive as those in classic Kaposi's sarcoma. Objective response rates to radiation therapy (complete and partial response) often exceed 90% although residual benign pigmentation remains in 20–40%, the rate varying inversely with the dose delivered.

As in classic KS, there appears to be a dose–response relationship for AIDS-related KS. Stelzer and Griffin[35] conducted a landmark prospective randomized trial testing three different dose regimens in epidemic Kaposi's sarcomas: 800 cGy in one fraction, 2000 cGy in ten fractions, or 4000 cGy in 20 fractions. Complete response occurred in 50% of tumors treated with 800 cGy, 79% of tumors treated with 2000 cGy and 83% of tumors treated with 4000 cGy. In addition, in the 4000 cGy group recurrence was less frequent, the median time to recurrence was longer and residual purple pigmentation was less likely to be evident.

Saran and colleagues[36] also suggest that the likelihood of complete response is approximately 40% lower when comparing total doses below 2000 cGy to larger doses. However, the ideal dose for any lesion represents the likely effects of that dose viewed in terms of the patient's needs. every patient does not need the maximum tolerated dose. Harrison et al.[37] conclude 'a single fraction of 8 Gy is an appropriate treatment for acceptable response and normal skin pigmentation within a group of patients in whom the median life expectancy is limited'. Similarly, de Wit et al.[38] state 'a single dose of 800 cGy is an effective treatment for patients with a predicted survival of only a few months'.

Selection of dose should also reflect the likelihood of inducing toxicity at a given anatomic site. Belembaogo et al. and Kirova et al.[39,40] irradiated 643 patients with doses ranging from 1000 to 3000 cGy and observed objective responses in 92% of cutaneous lesions with 'acceptable' (7% grade I, 70% grade II, and 23% grade III) toxicity. Oral mucosal reactions were frequent after relatively low doses, prompting the authors to recommend 3000 cGy in fractionated doses for cutaneous EKS (to small local fields), 2000 cGy for lesions involving eyelids, conjunctiva, and genitals and 1500 cGy for oral lesions.

Conill et al.[41] treated 251 cutaneous lesions with doses ranging from 800 cGy in one fraction (68% of irradiated tumors) to 3000 cGy in ten fractions (27% of irradiated tumors) and concluded that radiation therapy provides 'excellent local control with minimal toxicity'. Based on their experience, Stein et al.[42] conclude 'radiation therapy can provide good to excellent palliation with only minimal side-effects, producing a lesser impact on the hematological and immunological system than chemotherapy'.

TREATMENT OF MYCOSIS FUNGOIDES (CTCL)

Mycosis fungoides, like most lymphomatous tumors, is very sensitive to ionizing radiation. Both plaques and tumor nodules typically regress completely following modest doses of radiation. Because of the relatively large number of treatments that can induce regression of mycosis fungoides, radiation therapy can be used as an adjunct to other therapies ('spot' radiation therapy) or as the principal therapy (total skin electron beam therapy, TSEB) with or without other treatments (Fig. 48.6).

Dose and response

Single fraction doses of only a few hundred cGy may be sufficient to control individual lesions; however, fractionated radiotherapy is usually chosen because of its vastly superior cosmetic result. Cotter et al.[43] reviewed the response of 191 lesions in 20 patients who received fractionated irradiation for mycosis fungoides. Complete response to treatment was noted in all lesions that received more than a numerical total of 2000 cGy. Unfortunately, local recurrence was noted, despite initial

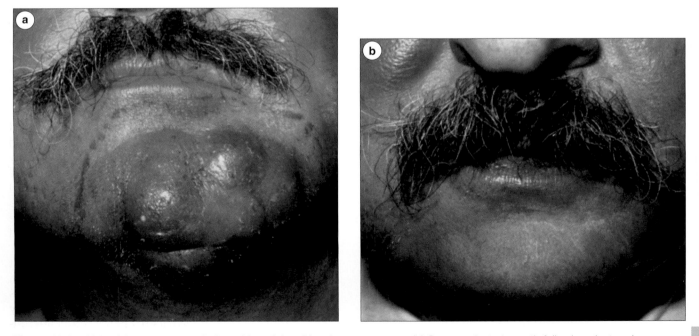

Figure 48.6 (a) Nodular stage mycosis fungoides of the chin prior to treatment. (b) Same patient, 1 month following electron beam treatment. Note new lesions on right cheek.

complete response, when relatively small doses were used. The in-field recurrence rate was 42% in patients receiving 1000 cGy or less, 32% in patients receiving 1001–2000 cGy, 21% in patients receiving 2001–3000 cGy and 0% in patients receiving more than 3000 cGy. This prompted the authors to recommend tumor doses equivalent to at least 3000 cGy delivered at 200 cGy per fraction, five fractions per week for long-term local control. And the intention of obtaining long-term control appears to be appropriate; in contrast to the relatively long survival times associated with mycosis fungoides, the authors observed that 83% of local recurrences became evident within 1 year of treatment and all were evident within 2 years.

Technical aspects

The optimal technique for irradiation of mycosis fungoides is highly dependent upon the presentation of disease. Isolated plaques and nodules can be treated with 'spot-therapy,' delivered for its palliative potential. Thin plaques are treated suitably either by superficial X-rays or relatively low energy electron beams and bolus. As plaques get thicker, electron beams become preferable. Tumor nodules usually require moderate energy electron beams (8 or 10 MeV beams will effectively irradiate 2.5–3.5 cm into tissue). Large nodules that wrap around a curved surface, such as the lateral aspect of the chest wall or an extremity, sometimes are best treated by tangentially directed X-ray beams with tissue compensation techniques and/or bolus.

The technical development of the linear accelerator has provided a means of delivering superficial radiation to very large segments of skin. By delivering treatment at relatively great distances from the source, the entire body can be encompassed. Each accelerator has its own unique characteristics requiring detailed individual dosimetric measurements, but in general electron beams of approximately 4 MeV are used. (It is possible to degrade a higher energy electron beam by interposing a plastic 'spoiler' in the beam.) This effectively irradiates an approximately 1 cm rind of tissue. Because of the relatively great intensity of the beams that can be produced by modern linear accelerators, the dose rate at the skin surface is acceptable despite the fall off of dose secondary to distance. However, photon contamination of the beam must be carefully measured; the bone marrow should not receive more than 70 cGy for the entire course of treatment to avoid hematologic toxicity.

There appears to be a small subset of patients (approximately 5%) who have very limited disease ('minimal' stage IA) at presentation who are effectively treated with localized superficial radiation therapy.[44,45] Relapse of treated disease appears to be very rare, progression of disease in other anatomic sites uncommon (and when it occurs amenable to further therapy) and 10-year survival assured.

Unfortunately, most patients have much wider involvement of the skin at presentation and when radiation therapy is chosen as the primary treatment modality all skin surfaces need to be relatively homogeneously irradiated. Recently, the European Organization for Research and Treatment of Cancer (EORTC) has published consensus guidelines for total skin electron beam radiation of mycosis fungoides.[46] For patients who have previously untreated limited patches and/or plaques (more than 'minimal' disease but less than 10% of their skin surface involved, with or without clinically enlarged, but histologically uninvolved lymph nodes) TSEB offers the prospect of long-term progression-free survival. Approximately 95% of patients will experience complete response of disease and 50% will survive for at least 10 years free of progression of disease. If patches and/or plaques affect more than 10% of the skin, TSEB plus an adjuvant therapy, such as PUVA, should be considered. Approximately 90% of patients will have a complete response to TSEB, but 10-year progression-free survival is likely to be less than 20%. Once tumor nodules have formed (with or without clinically enlarged, but histologically uninvolved lymph nodes), TSEB can offer 'effective palliation' and combinations of therapies are generally required. Patients who have their tumors confined to a relatively limited area have a 5-year progression-free survival rate of approximately 45%, but with more extensive disease uncommonly survive for 5 years without experiencing progression of disease. Generalized erythroderma generally (approximately 75%) can be controlled by TSEB. Histologically involved lymph nodes generally require photon beam radiation therapy for control.

Radiation therapy may also be useful after recurrence of disease. Following other therapies, recurrent limited patches and/or plaques remain suitable for TSEB with the potential for long-term progression-free survival. More advanced recurrent disease generally is better treated by combined modality therapy. Recurrent disease following TSEB that produced a complete or substantial partial response appears to be potentially suitable for a repeat course of TSEB with somewhat attenuated doses. The second course of TSEB appears to be tolerable and capable of producing substantial responses again.[47]

The recent reviews of the outcome of TSEB (with or without PUVA or nitrogen mustard) from Creteil, France,[48] Dijon, France,[49] New Haven, Connecticut[50] and Stanford, California[51] demonstrate the universal consistency of results despite the differences in the precise manner in which TSEB is delivered.

FUTURE OUTLOOK

Radiation therapy already provides highly effective, relatively non-toxic therapy for a variety of tumors and recent years have witnessed a move away from ablative surgery to radiation therapy (with or without chemotherapy) for tumors of the head and neck, breast, esophagus, prostate and anus. Why should cancers arising in the skin be different? Moreover, a number of radiosensitizing and radioprotective drugs, that change the relative sensitivity of tumors to the adjacent normal tissues (either by making the tumors more sensitive or the normal tissues more resistant to damage), are in development or clinical trial and offer the potential of even more effective treatment. In addition, when more effective systemic therapies are developed for malignant melanomas, the value of elective irradiation of high-risk tumors beds will increase. Physicians who ignore the long proud history of dermatologic radiation therapy and think that radiation therapy is passé may be very surprised by the future.

REFERENCES

1 Thissen MR, Neumann HAM, Berretty PJM, et al. De behandeling van patienten met basalecelcarcinomen door dermatologen in Nederland. Ned Tijdschr Geneeskd 1998; 142:1563–1567.

2 Regaud C, Ferroux R. Discordance des effets des rayons X, d'une part dans la peau, d'autre part dans les testicule par he fractionement de la dose: diminution de l'efficacite dans le peau, maintien de h'efficacite dans le testicule. Compt Rend Soc Biol 1927; 97:431–434.

3 Orton CG, Ellis F. A simplification in the use of the NSD concept in practical radiotherapy. Br J Radiol 1973; 46:529–537.

4 Kuijpers D, Thissen M. Neumann M. Basal cell carcinoma: treatment options and prognosis: a scientific approach to a common malignancy. Am J Clin Derm 2002; 3(4):247–259.

5 Thissen M, Neumann M, Schouten L. A systemic review of treatment modalities for primary basal cell carcinomas. Arch Derm 1999; 135:1177–1183.

6 Silverman MK, Kopf AW, Grin CM, et al. Recurrence rates of treated basal cell carcinomas, Part 4: X-ray therapy. J Derm Surg Oncol 1992; 18(7):549–554.

7 Solan MJ, Brady LW, Binnick SA, et al. Skin. In: Perez CA, Brady LW, eds. Principles and Practice of Radiation Oncology, 3rd edn. Philadelphia, PA: Lippincott-Raven; 1997:723–744.

8 Petrovich Z, Kuisk H, Langholz B, et al. Treatment results and patterns of failure in 646 patients with carcinoma of the eyelids, pinna, and nose. Am J Surg 1987; 154(4):447–450.

9 Lovett RD, Perez CA, Shapiro SJ, et al. External irradiation of epithelial skin cancer. Int J Radiat Oncol Biol Phys 1990; 19(2):235–242.

10 Goldschmidt H., ed. Treatment planning. In: Goldschmidt, H., ed. Physical Modalities in Dermatologic Therapy. New York, NY: Springer; 1978:68.

11 Bart PS, Kopf AW, Petratos MA. X-ray Therapy of Skin Cancer: Evaluation of a 'Standardized' Method for Treating Basal-Cell Epitheliomas. The 6th National Cancer Conference Proceedings, 1970.

12 Brennan D, Young CM, Hopewell JW, et al. The effects of varied numbers of dose fractions on the tolerance of normal human skin. Clin Radiol 1976; 27(1):27–32.

13 Avril MF, Auperin A, Margulis A, et al. Basal cell carcinoma of the face: surgery or radiotherapy? Results of a randomized study. Br J Cancer 1997; 76:100–106.

14 Petit JY, Avril MF, Margulis A, et al. Evaluation of cosmetic results of a randomized trial comparing surgery and radiotherapy in the treatment of basal cell carcinoma of the face. Plast Reconstr Surg 2000; 105:2544–2551.

15 Cooper JS. Patients' perceptions of their cosmetic appearance more than ten years after radiotherapy for basal cell carcinoma. Radiat Med 1988; 6:285–288.

16 Locke J, Karimpour S, Young G, et al. Radiotherapy for epithelial skin cancer. Int J Radiat Oncol Biol Phys 2001; 51(3):748–755.

17 Caccialanza M, Piccinno R, Grammatica A. Radiotherapy of recurrent basal and squamous cell skin carcinomas: a study of 249 re-treated carcinomas in 229 patients. Eur J Derm 2001; 11(1):25–28.

18 Habermalz HI, Fischer JJ. Radiation therapy of malignant melanoma. Cancer 1976; 38:2258–2262.

19 Sause WT, Cooper JS, Rush S, et al. Fraction size in external beam radiation therapy in the treatment of melanoma. Int J Radiat Oncol Biol Phys 1991; 20:429–432.

20 Harwood AR, Cummings B. Radiotherapy for malignant melanoma: A re-appraisal. Cancer Treat Rev 1981; 8:271–282.

21 Panizzon RG. Die roentgenweichstrahlentherapie als alternative bei alteren patienten. In: Burg G, Hartmann AA, Konz B, eds. Onkologische Dermatologie. Fortschritte der dermatologischen und onkologischen dermatologie, BAND 7. Heidelberg: Springer; 1992:263–267.

22 Harwood AR, Dancuart F, Fitzpatrick P, et al. Radiotherapy in nonlentiginous melanoma of the head and neck. Cancer 1981; 48:2599–2605.

23 Lee RJ, Gibbs JF, Proulx GM, et al. Nodal basin recurrence following lymph node dissection for melanoma: implications for adjuvant radiotherapy. Int J Radiat Oncol Biol Phys 2000; 46(2):467–474.

24 Ang KK, Peters LJ, Weber RS, et al. Postoperative radiotherapy for cutaneous melanoma of the head and neck region. Int J Radiat Oncol Biol Phys 1994; 30(4):795–798.

25 O'Brien CJ, Petersen-Schaefer K, Stevens GN, et al. Adjuvant radiotherapy following neck dissection and parotidectomy for metastatic malignant melanoma. Head Neck 1997; 19(7):589–594.

26 Corry J, Smith JG, Bishop M, et al. Nodal radiation therapy for metastatic melanoma. Int J Radiat Oncol Biol Phys 1999; 44(5):1065–1069.

27 Cooper JS, Chang WS, Oratz R, et al. Elective radiation therapy for local-regional control of resected high-risk malignant melanomas. Cancer J 2001; 7:498–502.

28 Stein ME, Lachter J, Spencer D, et al. Variants of Kaposi's sarcoma in Southern Africa. A retrospective analysis (1980–1992). Acta Oncol 1996; 35(2):193–199.

29 Fenig E, Brenner B, Rakowsky E, et al. Classic Kaposi sarcoma: experience at Rabin Medical Center in Israel. Am J Clin Oncol 1998; 21(5):498–500.

30 Tombolini V, Osti MF, Bonanni A, et al. Radiotherapy in classic Kaposi's sarcoma (CKS): experience of the Institute of Radiology of University 'La Sapienza' of Rome. Anticancer Res 1999; 19:4539–4544.

31 Cooper JS. The influence of dose on the long-term control of classic (non-AIDS associated) Kaposi's sarcoma by radiotherapy. Int J Radiat Oncol Biol Phys 1988; 15(5):1141–1146.

32 Cooper JS, Sacco J, Newall J. The duration of local control of classic (non-AIDS-associated) Kaposi's sarcoma by radiotherapy. J Am Acad Derm 1988; 19:59–66.

33 Holecek MI, Harwood AR. Radiotherapy of Kaposi's sarcoma. Cancer 1978; 41:1733–1738.

34 Harwood AR. Kaposi's sarcoma. Arch Derm 1981; 117:775–778.

35 Stelzer KJ, Griffin TW. A randomized prospective trial of radiation therapy for AIDS-associated Kaposi's sarcoma. Int J Radiat Oncol Biol Phys 1993; 27(5):1057–1061.

36 Saran F, Adamietz IA, Mose S, et al. The value of conventionally fractionated radiotherapy in the local treatment of HIV-related Kaposi's sarcoma. Strahlenther Onkol 1995; 171(10):594–599.

37 Harrison M, Harrington KJ, Tomlinson DR, et al. Response and cosmetic outcome of two fractionation regimens for AIDS-related Kaposi's sarcoma. Radiother Oncol 1998; 46(1):23–28.

38 Wit R de, Smit WG, Veenhof KH, et al. Palliative radiation therapy for AIDS-associated Kaposi's sarcoma by using a single fraction of 800 cGy. Radiother Oncol 1990; 19(2):131–136.

39 Belembaogo E, Kirova Y, Frikha H, et al. Radiotherapy of epidemic Kaposi's sarcoma: the experience of the Henri-Mondor Hospital. Cancer Radiother 1998; 2(1):49–52.

40 Kirova YM, Belembaogo E, Frikha H, et al. Radiotherapy in the management of epidemic Kaposi's sarcoma: a retrospective study of 643 cases. Radiother Oncol 1998; 46(1):19–22.

41 Conill C, Alsina M, Verger E, et al. Radiation therapy in AIDS-related cutaneous Kaposi's sarcoma. Dermatology 1997; 195(1):40–42.

42 Stein ME, Spencer D, Kantor A, et al. Epidemic AIDS-related Kaposi's sarcoma in southern Africa: experience at the Johannesburg General Hospital (1980–1990). Trans R Soc Trop Med Hyg 1994; 88(4):434–436.

43 Cotter GW, Baglan RJ, Wasserman TH, et al. Palliative radiation treatment of cutaneous mycosis fungoides – a dose response. Int J Rad Oncol Biol Phys 1983; 9:1477–1480.

44 Micaily B, Miyamoto C, Kantor G, et al. Radiotherapy for unilesional mycosis fungoides. Int J Radiat Oncol Biol Phys 1998; 42(2):361–364.

45 Wilson LD, Kacinski BM, Jones GW. Local superficial radiotherapy in the management of minimal stage IA cutaneous T-cell lymphoma (mycosis fungoides). Int J Radiat Oncol Biol Phys 1998; 40(1):109–115.

46 Jones GW, Kacinski BM, Wilson LD, et al. Total skin electron radiation in the management of mycosis fungoides: Consensus of the European Organization for Research and Treatment of Cancer (EORTC) Cutaneous Lymphoma Project Group. J Am Acad Derm 2002; 47(3):364–370.

47 Becker M, Hoppe RT, Knox SJ. Multiple courses of high-dose total skin electron beam therapy in the management of mycosis fungoides. Int J Radiat Oncol Biol Phys 1995; 32(5):1445–1449.

48 Kirova YM, Piedbois Y, Haddad E, et al. Radiotherapy in the management of mycosis fungoides: indications, results, prognosis. Twenty years experience. Radiother Oncol 1999; 51(2):147–151.

49 Maingon P, Truc G, Dalac S, et al. Radiotherapy of advanced mycosis fungoides: indications and results of total skin electron beam and photon beam irradiation. Radiother Oncol 2000; 54(1):73–78.

50 Quiros PA, Jones GW, Kacinski BM, et al. Total skin electron beam therapy followed by adjuvant psoralen/ultraviolet-A light in the management of patients with T1 and T2 cutaneous T-cell lymphoma (mycosis fungoides). Int J Radiat Oncol Biol Phys 1997; 38(5):1027–1035.

51 Chinn DM, Chow S, Kim YH, et al. Total skin electron beam therapy with or without adjuvant topical nitrogen mustard or nitrogen mustard alone as initial treatment of T2 and T3 mycosis fungoides. Int J Radiat Oncol Biol Phys 1999; 43(5):951–958.

CHAPTER
49 Vaccine Therapy for Melanoma

Jean-Claude Bystryn and Sandra R Reynolds

Key points

- Vaccines are a promising, but still experimental treatment for melanoma.
- Vaccines stimulate immune responses against melanoma and by so doing, increase resistance against this cancer.
- Numerous melanoma vaccines against melanoma are being developed. The most effective is not known.
- The more melanoma antigens in a vaccine, the more likely it is to be effective.
- All vaccines are given with an adjuvant, to increase the potency of the vaccine.
- Vaccines are usually used to treat resected stage IIb and III melanoma. Some studies suggest they are also effective in limited stage IV disease.
- Melanoma vaccines have been clinically effective in two randomized trials, one of which was double-blind.
- Vaccines have much less toxicity than many other therapies for melanoma.

INTRODUCTION

There is a critical need for improved treatments for melanoma that is at high risk of recurrence following surgical excision. The only one currently available and approved by the FDA, interferon alfa 2b (IFNα2b), has limited effectiveness and frequent side-effects. Vaccines are a novel, but still experimental, treatment for melanoma. They are attractive because they may permit the safe and selective destruction of melanoma cells. Thus, development of such vaccines is currently the focus of a major effort by the scientific community and the pharmaceutical industry. The rationale for believing that melanoma vaccines may be effective, the relative advantages and disadvantages of the different approaches used to construct such vaccines and the results obtained to date are summarized below.

THE RATIONALE FOR VACCINES AGAINST MELANOMA

There are multiple reasons for believing that the progression of melanoma in humans is influenced by immunological factors,[1] and that stimulation of these factors with vaccines can markedly increase resistance to this cancer. The two most compelling observations that support this rationale are these:

- There are defense mechanisms in humans that can kill melanoma cells and do so selectively, without harming normal melanocytes. They are evidenced by partial tumor regression in 15–20% of primary melanomas,[2,3] and by the rare, but dramatic, spontaneous and complete regression of advanced melanoma.[4] The partial regression that occurs in primary melanoma is actually visible to the naked eye as areas of white depigmentation within the tumor (an example of which is illustrated in Figure 49.1). It accounts for the white in the red, white and blue color description of melanoma. The white areas are due to the destruction of melanoma cells. As these regression events occur spontaneously without any treatment, they clearly indicate that humans possess protective mechanisms with the ability to destroy melanoma cells. These defense mechanisms are very selective, as they destroy melanoma cells without harming adjacent normal melanocytes. This is evident from the skin adjacent to areas of regression in primary melanomas, it remains normally pigmented (Fig. 49.1), i.e. non-malignant melanocytes are not harmed by the process destroying the malignant cells. The selectivity of this process indicates it is immunological, because only the immune system has the exquisite ability to recognize the difference between malignant and normal cells. Stimulating these immune defenses is the purpose of vaccines.

- In mice, moreover, vaccines can markedly increase resistance to melanoma. Murine B16 melanoma is invariably and rapidly fatal when injected into mice. Yet, most mice pre-immunized to vaccines against melanoma can survive injection of a lethal dose of melanoma cells that invariably kills all non-immunized animals,[5] as illustrated in Figure 49.2. The protection is specific for melanoma. Melanoma vaccine-immunized mice are not protected against an unrelated tumor. This fact indicates that the protective mechanisms are immunologic in nature.

A number of additional observations support that immune mechanisms play an important role in slowing the progression of melanoma. These include the presence on melanoma cells of antigens that are either unique or present in larger amount than on normal melanocytes, the ability of these antigens to stimulate antibody and/or

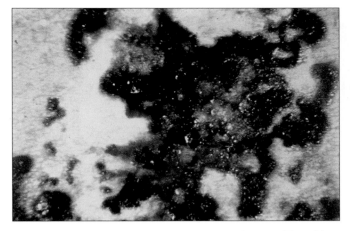

Figure 49.1 Partial regression of primary melanoma. The white areas within this primary cutaneous melanoma are areas of tumor regression, indicating that there are defense mechanisms in humans that kill melanoma cells. Note that the skin immediately adjacent to regressing areas remains normally pigmented, indicating that the defense mechanism selectively attacks malignant cells. (Image courtesy of New York University Department of Dermatology.)

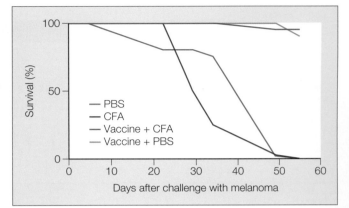

Figure 49.2 Prevention of melanoma in mice by vaccine immunization. Groups of 10 syngeneic C57BL/6J mice were immunized to an irradiated whole B16 melanoma cell vaccine admixed with saline (PBS) or with Freund's adjuvant (CFA) or to saline or the adjuvant alone. One week following 5-weekly immunizations, all mice were challenged with a lethal dose of B16 melanoma cells. Note that 1 month later, 90% of vaccine immunized mice are alive whereas all control mice are dead.

T cell responses in patients with melanoma, and the infiltration of lymphocytes into melanoma nodules of vaccine-treated patients.[6] There are correlations between the presence of these immune responses and an improved clinical outcome, indicating that these responses can play an active role in controlling the progression of melanoma.[7–11]

Thus, there are theoretical reasons for believing that vaccines can increase resistance to melanoma in animals and humans and practical observations that they actually do so in animals. Our challenge is to develop vaccines that will be as effective in humans.

REQUIREMENTS FOR A VACCINE TO BE EFFECTIVE

Melanoma vaccines are intended to stimulate patients' immune system to react more strongly and effectively against their own melanoma, and by so doing destroy the tumor or slow its progression. To do so, the vaccines must satisfy a number of requirements; the two most important are these:

- The vaccine must contain antigen(s) that can stimulate tumor-protective immune responses.

- Some of these antigens must be present on a patient's own tumor, otherwise the vaccine-induced immune responses will be unable to recognize and attack the tumor.

A number of other requirements must be satisfied for a vaccine to be clinically effective and practical to use, as discussed below. In addition, vaccines must be safe to use, their composition well characterized, and their manufacture reproducible. To retain their potential to provide cost-effective therapy, the vaccines should be relatively simple to prepare and administer.

To be effective, immune responses induced by vaccines must also be strong. For that reason, all melanoma vaccines are actually composed of two distinct components: (1)

Tumor antigen(s), which stimulate anti-tumor immune responses and (2) *an adjuvant*, which is intended to enhance the potency of these responses. An adjuvant is necessary, and used with all vaccines, because the immune responses induced by tumor antigens alone are weak. Each of these two components is discussed separately.

CHALLENGES IN THE DESIGN OF MELANOMA VACCINES

There are, however, problems satisfying each of the requirements described.

Selection of antigens used to prepare the vaccine

This is the most important issue in constructing cancer vaccines because the vaccine must contain antigens that can stimulate tumor-protective immunity or it will not work. Unfortunately, these antigens are unknown. Many antigens associated with melanoma have been identified and in some cases purified (Table 49.1).[12–31] However, whether any of these are the ones that stimulate tumor-protective immunity, is not known. Establishing this ability is arduous. It requires that a large-scale phase III randomized trial be conducted with each antigen, to demonstrate objectively whether it can slow the progression of melanoma. Taking into account the number of candidate antigens, the size and expense of phase III trials and the limited number of melanoma patients available, the process of analysis for every currently known antigen and for new ones that will be discovered is not practical.

Antigenic heterogeneity of tumors

Another complication in selecting vaccines is the requirement that some of the antigen(s) that stimulate

Table 49.1   Melanoma vaccines in clinical trials

Vaccine	Adjuvant	Investigator/company	Phase trial
Non-purified			
Whole cells (Canvaxin)[a]	BCG	CancerVax[12]	III
Whole cells (M-Vax)[b]	DNP / BCG	Avax[14]	III
Whole cells[a]	IL-2 Viral-transduced	Belli[17]	I
Whole cells[b]	IFN-γ Viral-transduced	Chiron[18]	I
Whole cells[b]	GM-CSF Viral-transduced	Parmiani[19]	I
Whole cells[b]	IL-7 Viral-transduced	Schadendorf[20]	I
Whole cells[a]	IL-4 Viral-transduced	Sanatonio[21]	I
Cell lysate (Melacine)[a]	Detox	Sondak[13]	III
Cell lysate[a]	Vaccinia oncolysate	Wallack[15]	III
Cell lysate[a]	Vaccinia oncolysate	Hurley[16]	III
Cell lysate[b]	Dendritic cells	Chang[31]	I
Semi-pure			
Shed antigens[a]	Alum, IL-2-liposomes	Bystryn[29]	II/III
Oncophage[b]	Heat-shock protein complexes	Antigenics[30]	III
Pure or defined			
GM2 ganglioside	KLH + QS21	Progenics[26]	III
GD3 anti-idiotype	BCG, QS-21	Chapman[27]	I
GD2 anti-idiotope (TriGem)	QS-21	Titan[28]	I/II
gp100, tyrosinase[c]	IFA,GM-CSF	Weber[22]	I/II
gp100[c]	QS-21, Montanide ISA-51	Slingluff[23]	I
MART-1, MAGE-3, gp100[c]	Dendritic cells	Banchereau[24]	I
Tyrosinase, gp100[c]	Dendritic cells	Weber[25]	I

[a]Allogeneic
[b]Autologous
[c]Peptide

protective immunity be expressed by the tumor intended for treatment. Unfortunately, the expression of tumor antigens by melanoma cells is heterogeneous. The pattern of antigens expressed by melanomas in different individuals, between different tumor nodules in the same individual, and even between different melanoma cells within the same tumor nodule is variable.[32–34] This problem is particularly acute, because the actual antigens expressed by residual melanoma cells in a patient is unknown at the time treatment is instituted. A solution suggested to circumvent this problem is to prepare autologous vaccines from a patient's own tumor. However, this does not satisfactorily resolve the problem because there is no assurance that the antigens present in the tumor tissue used to prepare the vaccine will be the same as those present in the residual tumor(s) that need treatment.

Antigen modulation

The pattern of antigens expressed by tumor cells changes during tumor progression.[35] In part, this reflects the morphological and functional changes which occur in tumors as they metastasize; and it results also in part, from immunological pressures acting in a manner analogous to the development of drug-resistance in bacteria. Vaccine-induced immune responses destroy tumor cells bearing the targeted antigen(s), which results in the selection and expansion of surviving cells that lack these targets and are now resistant to the action of the vaccine.

Thus, one does not know which antigens should be used to construct melanoma vaccines, whether these antigens are expressed by the tumor to be treated, or whether they will still be there once treatment begins.

HLA restriction of vaccine-induced immune responses

Some immune responses, which play a critical role in tumor-protective immunity, such as CD8+ and CD4+ T cell responses, are HLA restricted. An antigen will induce these responses only in patients who have a specific HLA antigen. This is because of two requirements which must be fulfilled to activate T cells: (1) the antigen must be bound or presented as a peptide by an HLA molecule on the surface of antigen-presenting cells and (2) the T cells must be capable of recognizing the bound peptide. Each peptide normally binds with only one type of HLA molecule. As there are a large number of HLA molecules and as the expression of each varies from individual to individual, only a minority of patients will express the HLA molecule required to bind a particular peptide. Even the most common HLA molecule (HLA-A*O2) is expressed by only 40% of Caucasians, the population most at risk for melanoma. Many HLA molecules are expressed by only a few percent of patients to be treated.

As a result of HLA restrictions on the ability of tumor antigens to stimulate immune responses, and the variable expression of antigens on melanoma cells, the proportion of patients who can theoretically benefit from vaccines prepared from any one antigen is small. Even if the antigen is universally expressed on all melanoma cells, and is presented by the most common HLA phenotype, no more than 40% of the population at risk would be a candidate for treatment with that antigen. As the frequency of expression of the antigen in tumors, and as the frequency of an HLA molecule expression (in the population), decreases, the proportion of patients that can actually benefit from the treatment will also decrease.

HLA-unrelated heterogeneity in patient's ability to develop immune responses to the same antigen

In addition, there is also heterogeneity which is independent of HLA restriction in the ability of different patients to develop antibody and cellular immune responses to antigens.[36] Different patients who express the same HLA phenotype and who are immunized identically to the same antigen can vary in their ability to develop a cellular immune response to that antigen. This is not due to lack of immune competence on the part of the patients, since patients who do not respond to one antigen will respond well to another antigen presented by the same HLA molecule, whereas patients who responded to the first antigen may not respond to the second. There is similar heterogeneity in the ability of individuals to develop antibody responses,[37] as illustrated in Figure 49.3. This further limits the proportion of patients that can develop effective anti-tumor immune responses to any single antigen.

Number of antigens required to induce effective protective immunity

It is unknown whether clinically effective tumor-protective immunity can be induced by immunization to a single antigen or whether responses against multiple antigens are required for cancer cells to be killed or prevented from replicating. Even if immune responses to a single antigen can kill melanoma cells, it seems logical that stimulating responses to multiple antigens should do so even more effectively. Thus, the larger the number of antigens in a vaccine the better it should work. However, there is a price to be paid for increasing the number of antigens in a vaccine.

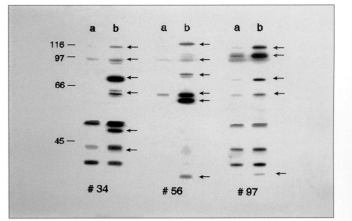

Figure 49.3 Patient-to-patient heterogeneity in antibody response to vaccine immunization. The figure illustrates antibody responses against antigens in fresh melanoma tumor tissue measured by immunoblotting before (lanes a) and after (lanes b) treatment with a polyvalent melanoma vaccine. Note that the antibodies induced by vaccination in the three patients are directed against different pattern of antigens. (Image courtesy of New York University Department of Dermatology.)

THE RATIONALE FOR POLYVALENT VACCINES

One strategy that can minimize the problems listed above is to construct polyvalent vaccines containing a large number of different tumor-associated antigens. It is evident that the greater the number of antigens in a vaccine, the greater the chances it will contain the unknown antigens that stimulate tumor-protective immunity. There will be greater chances, too, that at least some of these antigens will be expressed by the patient's own tumor and that the antigen(s) will be able to stimulate desired immune responses. Furthermore, stimulation of immune responses against multiple targets on the melanoma cells should increase the chances of killing these cells. Reflecting this evolving strategy, the field of melanoma vaccines has moved sharply in the direction of creating polyvalent vaccines during the past year, as opposed to vaccines made from a single purified antigen, which was the prior trend.

STRATEGIES TO CONSTRUCT POLYVALENT VACCINES AND THEIR RELATIVE ADVANTAGES AND DISADVANTAGES

One of three strategies can be used to construct polyvalent cancer vaccines that contain many tumor antigens. The strategies differ in the purity and number of tumor antigen(s) used to prepare the vaccine. The antigens can be: (1) non-purified, (b) partially purified or (c) pure. None of the strategies are completely satisfactory; each has certain advantages and disadvantages listed in Table 49.2 and discussed below. There is currently no ideal way of constructing cancer vaccines and the decision as to which of these strategies appears most advantageous is somewhat subjective.

Table 49.2 Cancer vaccine design strategies

Purity of antigen(s) used to construct vaccines	Advantages and disadvantages
Non-purified	Includes all relevant antigens; bulk of vaccine is irrelevant material
Partially-pure	Includes most relevant antigens; excludes most irrelevant antigens
Pure	Includes only pure antigen(s); Clinical relevance of antigen uncertain.

The essential difference between these three different vaccine-design strategies is in the number and concentration of tumor antigens in the vaccine. The dilemma is that while non-purified vaccines contain multiple tumor antigens and thus are more likely to contain relevant antigens, these account for only a small fraction of the material in the vaccine and the bulk of the material in the vaccine is irrelevant. Conversely, vaccines prepared from pure antigens contain a high concentration of antigen, but because the number of antigens available to construct such vaccines is sharply limited, it is uncertain whether the ones selected are the 'correct' antigens to stimulate protective immunity. Partially purified vaccines strike a middle course between these two polar approaches.

Non-purified or cellular vaccines

The traditional method to construct cancer vaccines is to prepare them from whole tumor cells or non-purified extract of these cells. The tumor cells are often pooled from different donors to increase the number of tumor antigens in the vaccine. Examples of such vaccines, which are currently in advanced clinical trials, include Canvaxin, a polyvalent vaccine prepared from three lines of intact, irradiated, melanoma cells combined with BCG as an adjuvant[12]; Melacine, which is a mechanical lysate of two melanoma cell lines admixed with Detox as an adjuvant[13]; whole, autologous melanoma cells conjugated to a hapten[14]; and lysates of cells infected with vaccinia or other non-pathogenic viruses.[15–16] The tumor cells can also be genetically engineered to express certain cytokines such as GM-CSF or other molecules or antigens that hopefully will increase their ability to stimulate desired immune responses.[17–21] Genetic vaccines made from DNA or RNA extracted from tumor cells also fall in the category of non-purified vaccines as the DNA that is administered as the vaccine will code for many molecules other than the one of interest.

Cellular vaccines can be made either from the patient's own tumor cells (autologous vaccines) or from other patients' cells (allogenic vaccines). Autologous vaccines are claimed to have an antigenic profile that will more closely resemble that present on a patient's remaining tumor tissue. However, this claim is uncertain because of the heterogeneity in the profile of antigens expressed by melanoma cells between and within different tumor nodules in the same individual. Furthermore, such vaccines are limited to patients with advanced disease who have sufficient tumor tissue for vaccine preparation. They are costly, requiring that a custom vaccine be made for each individual patient.

What is the major advantage of non-purified vaccines? They contain the widest variety of tumor antigens. Thus, they are more likely to contain the as yet unidentified antigen(s) essential for vaccine activity, and they obviate the need to identify and purify each individual such antigens. Because the vaccines contain a broad range of tumor antigens, particularly if prepared from a pool of tumor cells, they have an increased chance of containing relevant antigens expressed by the individual tumor to be treated. For the same reason, the vaccines are more likely to contain antigens that are recognized in the context of the patient's own HLA haplotype and ones that can trigger immune responses in a particular patient. Vaccines prepared from whole tumor cells may be inherently more immunogenic, because antigens tend to lose potency as they are purified. Furthermore, the multiple antigens in non-purified vaccines have the potential to stimulate immune responses to multiple targets on tumor cells, which is more likely to result in cell kill and clinical effectiveness.

The major drawback to this approach is that the active antigens constitute only a small fraction of the material in the vaccine. The overwhelming bulk of the material in the vaccine is irrelevant and dilutes the concentration of the relevant antigens increasing the technical difficulty of preparing reproducible and well-characterized vaccine formulations. In addition, the non-antigenic material in the vaccine may potentially decrease its effectiveness due to the presence of suppressive or immuno-inhibitory factors[38] or the stimulation of competitive immune responses to unrelated antigens, and may potentially increase toxicity. The concern that the immune responses that are induced are difficult to measure has been resolved by the development of assays permitting the measurement of antibody[37] and T cell responses[36] to individual antigens in such vaccines.

Vaccines prepared from pure, defined antigens

The polar approach is to prepare polyvalent vaccines from cocktails of purified antigens.[22–28] It has become feasible as a result of the identification and purification of melanoma-associated antigens recognized by antibodies or T cells.[39] Use of peptides that are recognized by T cells and derived from melanoma-associated antigens is particularly favored because these can be identified and readily manufactured. Their amino acids can be substituted to increase their binding affinity to HLA and hence boost their immunogenicity.[40,41]

The major advantages of this approach are: pure antigen vaccines are more easily characterized and prepared in a reproducible manner, and the concentration of antigen(s) in the vaccine is high. It is believed that the immune responses they induce can be measured more easily, although assays are now available to measure responses to individual antigens induced by vaccines containing multiple antigens. The approach is elegant, taking advantage of recent major advances in our understanding of melanoma immunology; and for these reasons it is attractive to scientists. However, the approach has a number of drawbacks. The major one is that the antigens that stimulate tumor-protective immunity and thus should be used to make the vaccine, remain unknown. The vaccines are made from available antigens and not necessarily from those that should be used. Many of the antigens used for such vaccines are intended to stimulate CD8+ T-cell responses and hence are HLA-restricted. That fact, together with the less-than-universal expression of these antigens in different melanomas, means that such vaccines cannot be used in many patients. The number of antigens in such vaccines is also strictly limited to the small number that have been identified and sequenced. This number is further constricted by intellectual property rights issues which make it difficult to obtain permission to use many of these antigens.

The purified vaccine in the most advanced stage of clinical testing is a ganglioside vaccine constructed from GM2 conjugated to KLH and administered with the adjuvant QS-21.[26] Other purified antigen vaccines are still in early phases of clinical trials. Most of these are prepared from peptides derived from the melanoma-associated antigens MAGE-1, MAGE-3, Melan A/Mart-1, tyrosinase or gp100 that are recognized by CD8+ T cells.[22–25] Some vaccines are prepared from the antibodies to gangliosides GD2 and GD3. The use of these anti-idiotype monoclonal antibodies is an alternate approach to stimulate responses to tumors using a purified protein.[27,28,42]

Vaccines prepared from partially purified antigens

The third design strategy attempts to balance the advantages and disadvantages of the two approaches described above. It does so by preparing vaccines from tumor cell extracts, which are enriched in the cellular elements most likely to contain tumor antigens relevant for vaccine therapy and depleted of material likely to be irrelevant.

The advantages of this approach are: (1) it retains the most critical element required for vaccine effectiveness (i.e. the vaccines contain a broad cocktail of tumor antigens), while (b) being much purer than vaccines prepared from whole tumors or their extracts. Partially purified vaccines contain fewer antigens than cellular vaccines but many more than vaccines prepared from cocktails of purified antigens. While not as pure as the latter vaccines, they contain much less irrelevant material than cellular vaccines.

Two examples of this approach are in clinical trial. One is a polyvalent vaccine made from antigens shed by melanoma cells into culture medium.[29] It exploits the natural phenomenon of the rapid release or shedding of surface material by cells in culture. Because cell-surface material is released much more rapidly than the bulk of unrelated cellular material, which is in the cytoplasm and the nucleus, it is partially purified and enriched in surface antigens. To increase the representation of melanoma antigens in the vaccine, the cell lines used for vaccine production were selected based on each expressing different and complementary patterns of melanoma-associated antigens. This vaccine contains multiple melanoma antigens, including MAGE-1, MAGE-3, MelanA/Mart-1, tyrosinase, gp100, S100, TRP-1 and numerous immunogenic antigens ranging in MW from 30 to 150 kD, which are expressed by melanoma *in vivo*.[36,43] The vaccine is made from allogenic melanoma cell lines maintained in master and working cell banks to produce a generic vaccine that can be administered to all patients.

The other approach to partially purified vaccines is to prepare them from autologous heat shock proteins (HSP).[30,44] HSP are a family of proteins made in response to stress. The ones most commonly used for vaccine production are HSP70 and gp96. They function as chaperones that transport peptides within cells. Purified HSP provides a source of multiple processed peptides that include both normal self-peptides and tumor antigen-derived peptides.[30,44] These peptides may be enriched for those able to bind to HLA class I. The HSP vaccine furthest in development is Oncophage, which is based on purified gp96 HSP.[30] Comparative information on the spectrum of melanoma antigens present in HSP versus shed antigen vaccines is lacking. HSP vaccines must be made from the patient's own tumor cells, which like all autologous vaccines, restricts their use to patients with sufficiently bulky melanomas to provide the material required for vaccine preparation. HSP vaccines must be individualized for each patient.[30]

ADJUVANTS

The immune responses induced by tumor antigens are weak, often of short duration. Hence, a critical element of all cancer vaccines is an adjuvant, which is used to enhance their ability to stimulate strong immune responses. A large number of adjuvants are available and more are being developed. A discussion of adjuvant strategies is beyond the scope of this review. Briefly, these include:

- modifications of the physical or biochemical properties of the antigens[45]
- various types of emulsions or bacterial extracts such as alum
- incomplete Freund's adjuvant, BCG, QS21, or Detox
- slow release vehicles such as liposomes
- immunomodulators such as IL-2, IL-4, IL-7, IFN-8, GMCSF
- T-helper cell epitopes[23]
- the use of antigen-presenting cells such as dendritic cells.[24,25,31]
- coupling the antigen to strongly immunogenic molecules such as KLH[46] or to a hapten[14]
- binding the antigen to the surface of inert beads or other structures such as ISCOMs

- using recombinant techniques to express the antigen of interest on viruses such as vaccinia or adenoviruses[47]
- transfecting tumor cells to express molecules that hopefully will increase their immunogenicity.[17–21]

The selection of an appropriate adjuvant is complicated because, while all of these approaches can enhance vaccine immunogenicity, little is known about their relative effectiveness. Another complication to adjuvant selection is that different adjuvants potentiate humoral and cellular immune responses differently and their effect will vary depending on the antigen with which the adjuvant is coupled. Thus, results obtained with one vaccine-adjuvant combination will not necessarily translate to another vaccine coupled with the same adjuvant.

One of the more effective adjuvant strategies is to present the antigen on dendritic cells (DC). These are professional antigen-presenting cells that are most potent for initiation of T cell immunity.[24,25,31,48] A variety of approaches are available to load the antigen(s) onto the DC, but it is not clear which results in the most effective vaccine. Early clinical trials with DC pulsed with melanoma peptides have shown immune responses and some clinical responses.[49] This approach is limited by the need to obtain DC from the patient to be treated so that a custom vaccine must be prepared for each person. This increases the cost and the time required to prepare the vaccine.

Another promising approach is to encapsulate the vaccine into liposomes together with a small amount of a cytokine such as IL-2 or GM-CSF that can upregulate immune responses. This has the advantage of greatly prolonging the half-life of the cytokine and delivering it together with the vaccine antigen(s) to draining lymph nodes where stimulation of immune cells occurs. This approach has been shown to markedly increase melanoma vaccine-induced cellular immune responses in humans.[50]

In summary, adjuvants are required to improve the effectiveness of vaccines for melanoma. Although a large choice is available, it is unclear which is best. These choices, however, further complicate the selection of the vaccine to be considered in treating of patients.

RESULTS OF CLINICAL TRIALS

Because a wide variety of approaches are available to prepare the antigenic component of vaccines and an equally expansive range of adjuvants is available to enhance the activity of these antigens, a large number of melanoma vaccines are currently in clinical trial. A partial listing of them is provided in Table 49.1. However, little solid information is available on the clinical effectiveness of most of these vaccines as the bulk are still in early phase I or II clinical trials.

Three criteria are used to evaluate the clinical activity of tumor vaccines: safety, immunological activity (ability to stimulate immune responses against melanoma), and clinical effectiveness (ability to slow the progression of melanoma).

IMMUNOLOGICAL ACTIVITY

Immunological activity is the most common end-point currently used to judge the activity of cancer vaccines. It is an important parameter as vaccines will not be effective unless they can stimulate potent and clinically effective anti-tumor immune responses. Unfortunately, it is difficult to use this end-point to compare the activity of different vaccines. Results depend on the type of immune responses that are measured, how they are measured, and when they are measured. Complicating this problem is that the assay procedures used to measure these responses are not standardized. In addition, the clinical relevance of the different types of vaccine-induced immune response remains unclear.

The frequency with which vaccines induce anti-tumor immune responses and the type of response they stimulate is related to the nature of the vaccine and the manner in which it is administered. For example, it is difficult to demonstrate antibody responses to peptide-based vaccines by contrast. Ganglioside vaccines stimulate antibody but not cellular responses, and cellular and protein-based vaccines can stimulate both type of responses. Potent adjuvants can markedly increase the frequency with which the same vaccine stimulates antibody and/or cellular responses.

Clinical relevance of different types of vaccine-induced immune responses

Both antibody and cellular immune responses against melanoma can be induced by vaccine-treatment.[7–11,51–54] Which is the more important mediator of protective immunity and which should be used as the end-point is unclear. The dogma, based mostly on animal studies, is that cellular responses are more important. In humans, however, as many studies show a good correlation between vaccine-induced antibody responses and improved clinical outcome[7–9,51] as with T-cell responses.[10,11,52–54] Probably both types of responses are important, and their relative importance may depend on the actual nature of the response, the antigens against which they are directed, and possibly the stage of the disease. Critical evaluation of this issue is difficult, as few trials evaluate both types of responses concurrently, and the remaining correlations are based on analysis of only small numbers of patients.

Effect of assay procedure on the analysis of vaccine-induced immune responses

A variety of assays are used to measure antibody and cellular responses to vaccine-treatment. These differ not only in the type of response that they measure but also on the specificity of the response which is measured and include:

- the antigen(s) against which the response is directed

Table 49.3   Methods for measuring vaccine-induced, antigen-specific, CD8+ T-cell responses

Method	Difficulty	Sensitivity (%)	Reproducibility
Limiting dilution analysis	++++	+++	+
ELISPOT	++	0.001–0.01	+++
Tetramer assay	++	0.01–0.0125	++
Cytokine flow cytometry	++	0.01–0.1	++

- the functional significance of the response, i.e. can it kill tumor cells or conversely block the killing

- the sensitivity of the assay (for example pre-incubation of T cells with antigen prior to assay greatly increases the sensitivity of the assay but at the price of decreasing the ability to quantify the magnitude of the response). Currently, there are efforts to develop a battery of standard immune tests that would simplify comparing the results of different trials.[55] This effort has progressed furthest for assay of CD8+ T-cell responses, where there is emerging agreement that the best tests are ELISPOT, cytokine flow cytometry and tetramer assays (Table 49.3).

Impact of assay timing on the detection of vaccine-induced immune responses

The frequency and magnitude of vaccine-induced immune responses are also influenced by the time elapsed from onset of immunization and by the number of immunizations. The responses increase with time to an optimum level and with the number of immunizations. However, too intensive immunizations can sometimes lead to tolerance.

CLINICAL EFFECTIVENESS

There is increasing evidence that melanoma vaccines can be clinically effective, based on 4 different sets of observations: (1) correlations between vaccine-induced immune responses and improved clinical outcome, (2) the effect of vaccine treatment on intermediate markers of clinical outcome, (3) comparisons of survival with that of historical controls, and most convincingly (4) the results of randomized trials.

Correlations between vaccine-induced immune responses and improved clinical outcome have been observed in multiple studies. Improved outcome was seen in patients with antibody[7–9,51,56] or with T-cell responses[10,11,52–54] so that both types of responses appear to be important. Whether or not a correlation is present appears to depend on the antigen against which the responses are directed. Thus, in one recent study a correlation was found between vaccine-induced CD8+

T-cell responses to MAGE-3 and improved outcome, but none with responses to tyrosinase.[10] Caution must be used when interpreting correlations in studies involving small number of patients, as the power and hence the confidence of such analysis is limited.

It has recently been found that molecular markers of melanoma can be present in the blood of melanoma patients, even those with resected disease. The markers include melanoma cells in the blood,[57] and individual proteins and antigens such as LDH, S100, melanoma-inhibitory activity,[58] and total serum ganglioside levels. What is interesting is that the presence of these markers can decrease in patients treated with melanoma vaccines, and that there can be a correlation between the decrease in marker and improved clinical outcome. For example, in a recent study[57] the proportion of patients with circulating melanoma cells decreased by over 55% following treatment with a polyvalent vaccine and the recurrence-free survival of those patients in whom melanoma cells disappeared during vaccine treatment was significantly longer than that of patients in whom circulating melanoma cells appeared, as illustrated in Figure 49.4.[57] The treatment-associated clearance of these markers from blood suggests the vaccines are clinically effective and that they may also be clearing tumor deposits elsewhere in the body, possibilities supported by the improved clinical outcome of patients whose marker level decreases compared with those whose level increases or remains stable.[57]

Vaccine treatment also appears effective in prolonging survival in historically controlled studies. Most convincing are those involving large numbers of patients. Two are particularly compelling. Morton's group reported that in

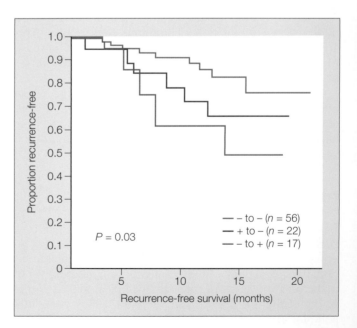

Figure 49.4 Kaplan–Meier analysis of recurrence-free survival as a function of vaccine-associated changes in circulating melanoma cells. Patients negative for circulating melanoma cells at the beginning and the end of vaccine treatment (green line), positive for melanoma cells at baseline but negative after vaccine treatment (red line), who became positive for circulating melanoma cells while on vaccine treatment (blue line).

a matched-pair analysis the 5-year overall survival rate of 107 patients with resected stage IV melanoma treated with a whole-cell vaccine was 39% compared to 19% for the control group.[12] Bystryn et al.[59] reported that the overall survival of 94 vaccine-treated patients with stage IV disease was two to four times longer than that of similar historical controls matched for site of metastatic disease and presence of measurable disease, the two most powerful risk factors in stage IV melanoma. Particularly striking was that 35% of patients with resected, non-visceral, disease survived 5 years, compared with 13% for historical controls. Morton's group reported similar results in stage IV disease.[12]

A number of vaccines have been reported to induce occasional partial or complete regression of established tumors. As similar remission rate occurs with almost all other modalities used to treat melanoma, the significance of this observation is unclear.

There are now two randomized, concurrently controlled trials, in which melanoma vaccine-treated patients had a higher survival than the control group. One is a double-blind and placebo controlled trial of a polyvalent, shed antigen, melanoma vaccine developed by Bystryn. The vaccine contains multiple melanoma-associated antigens including MAGE-1, MAGE-3, MelanA/MART-1, gp100, S100, tyrosinase, TRP-1, TRP-2 and a number of other antigens with MW ranging from 30 to 150 kDs. It stimulates antibody responses to multiple melanoma associated antigens which are expressed in vivo by melanoma,[43] cellular responses to a patient's own melanoma in vivo,[6] and CD8+ T cell responses to multiple peptides derived from MAGE-1, MAGE-3, MART-1, tyrosinase and TRP-1, which are presented by the class I HLA phenotypes most common among melanoma patients.[36] The recurrence-free and overall survival of patients with stage III disease treated

with this vaccine was approximately 50% longer[60] and that of patients with early stage IV disease two to four times longer than that of similar historical controls.[59] In a double-blind and placebo-controlled trial in ASCC stage IIIb disease, the recurrence-free survival of the melanoma vaccine treated patients was over twice as long as that of patients treated with placebo vaccine,[39] see Figure 49.5. This difference was statistically significant after Cox multivariate analysis ($P=0.03$). However, the results must be interpreted cautiously, as they are based on a small number of patients.

The other promising randomized trial is that of Melacine, a vaccine prepared from the lysate of two melanoma cells line adjuvanted with Detox. The vaccine was developed by Mitchell and is commercialized by Corixa. The response rate and median survival of patients with stage IV melanoma treated with the vaccine or with standard chemotherapy using the Dartmouth regimen were similar, but toxicity of the vaccine treatment was less; resulting in improved quality of life.[61] A randomized trial of this vaccine in resected stage II melanoma has been conducted in 689 patients by SWOG.[13] Overall there was no difference in recurrence-free survival between the vaccine-treated and an observation only control group. However, in a pre-planned subset analysis the relapse-free survival was significantly prolonged in patients that were HLA-A2 or C3 positive.[13] These results suggest that the HLA type of patients can influence the results of vaccine therapy. This vaccine has been approved for sale in Canada, but not by the FDA in the US.

Another vaccine in advanced clinical trials is Canvaxin, an irradiated, whole melanoma cell, polyvalent, vaccine developed by Morton and associates at the John Wayne Cancer Center (Santa Monica, CA) and currently commercialized by CancerVax. In a case-controlled study, the recurrence-free and overall survival of stage III and IV patients treated with this vaccine was longer than that of similar historical patients treated by the same investigator.[12] This vaccine is currently in two large scale phase III trials with results that are still pending.

A vaccine prepared from the purified ganglioside GM-2 has also been in a large scale randomized trial. An initial randomized trial was conducted in 122 patients with resected AJCC stage III melanoma immunized to the vaccine + BCG or to BCG alone.[62] There was no significant difference in recurrence-free survival between the two groups. However, the outcome was significantly better in patients with an antibody response to the vaccine.[62] An improved GM2 vaccine was constructed by conjugating GM2 to KLH and using QS-21 as an adjuvant, which significantly augmented antibody responses. But in a multicenter trial, the GM2 vaccine was less effective than interferon-alfa.[26] However, the trial may have been interrupted early, before the full benefits of vaccine treatment became evident. Two other large randomized trials of melanoma vaccines have been conducted in resected melanoma at high risk of recurrence. In both, the vaccine consisted of vaccinia viral lysates of melanoma cells.[15,16] In neither trial was there a difference in outcome between the vaccine treated and control groups.

Numerous other melanoma vaccines are in clinical trials in the US and in Europe (see Table 49.1 for a partial list). A listing of melanoma vaccines in active clinical

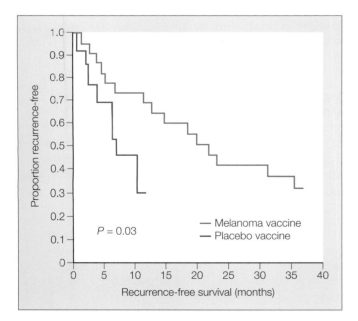

Figure 49.5 Recurrence-free survival of patients with resected stage IIIB melanoma immunized to a polyvalent melanoma vaccine or to a placebo vaccine in a double-blind trial (n=38). The difference in outcome between the two groups was significant.[29]

trial, and a description of the entry requirements, can be obtained from the National Cancer Institute at 301-496-4000 or at www.nci.nih.gov.

INDICATIONS AND CONTRAINDICATIONS

Indications

Vaccines are still experimental. However, taking into account the limited effectiveness of standard therapy for melanoma and the major toxicity it causes, experimental therapy is considered a standard of care for patients with resected melanoma at high risk of recurrence.[63,64] Thus melanoma vaccines can be offered to patients who are candidates for this treatment. Because vaccines are experimental, they can only be administered in the context of a clinical trial.

There is no standard criteria for determining whether or not a patient is a candidate for vaccine treatment. The eligibility and exclusion criteria are set by the investigator(s) conducting a particular trial, so that it is necessary to contact each trial to determine what these are. Generally, the type of patient most often treated with vaccines are those with resected melanoma that has a high chance of recurrence, i.e. AJCC stage IIB (primary lesions 4 mm or thicker) or with stage III (metastatic to regional nodes) disease. A few trials are being conducted in patients with thinner primary melanoma (primary lesions 1.5 to 4 mm in thickness) and with disseminated stage IV disease, either resected or with limited tumor load. While it is often believed that vaccines will not be effective in patients with advanced disease, two historically controlled large studies suggest they can be effective in that setting.[12,59]

Contraindications

There are few contraindications to vaccine treatment. They include widely disseminated disease, known allergies to any of the components used to construct the vaccine, concurrent administration of immunosuppressive agents or underlying medical conditions that would contraindicate the use of the particular adjuvant used with a vaccine.

Potential risks

Melanoma vaccines have proven very safe to use. There has been little toxicity in the several thousand patients who have been treated to date. The toxicity that has occurred was usually due to the adjuvant rather than to the vaccine.

The most common side-effects are local reactions at the site of injection such as induration, swelling, or pain. Ulcerations can occur if an irritating adjuvant such as BCG or Detox is used. Other potential toxicities include swelling of nodes, chills, fever and infections. The more serious side-effects are usually due to the adjuvant and

depend on the adjuvant used. They can range from self-limited transfusion type of reactions to dendritic cell vaccines to very severe systemic toxicity in patients receiving high doses of cytokines such as IL-2.

There are two potentially severe, but theoretical, side-effects. One is enhancement of tumor growth, which could occur if vaccine induces the wrong type of immune response. This can occur in animals. It has been reported in a few vaccine-treated patients with advanced disease where it is not possible to determine whether the rapid tumor growth resulted from the vaccine or from the natural behavior of advanced melanoma. In the vast majority of melanoma vaccine trials no adverse impact on tumor progression has been reported. As discussed above, the evidence is that vaccines work, not that they make things worse. The other concern is that of inducing autoimmunity, particularly against normal melanocytes, as evidenced by vitiligo or uveitis. These changes have not been associated with functional disturbances or induction of autoimmunity to other organs. However, autoimmunity may become a larger problem as stronger adjuvants are used to enhance the immunogenicity of the vaccines.

Lastly, the FDA now requires that patients be informed about the highly unlikely possibility of contracting bovine spongiform encephalopathy or Creutzfeld–Jakob disease if any of the reagents used to prepare the vaccine (such as the fetal calf serum or trypsin used in the preparation of whole cell vaccines or the amino acids used to prepare peptide vaccines) are of ruminant or human origin.

As all cancer therapy has toxicity, the real issue is not whether vaccines have toxicity or not, but whether it is more common or severe than alternate treatments. Vaccines are clearly less toxic than current FDA approved therapy for resected melanoma at high risk of recurrence. This is interferon alfa-2b, which causes major toxicity (grade 3 or 4) in two-thirds of patients.[65] By contrast, for example, less than 1% grade 3 toxicity and no grade 4 toxicity was observed in a group of over 200 patients treated with a shed antigen vaccine. Thus, vaccine treatment, whatever its merit, provides a quality of life advantage.

PREVENTION OF CANCER WITH VACCINES

No discussion of cancer vaccines should end without mention of their unique and potentially most significant application: use in preventing cancer in normal individuals. Several observations suggest that this may ultimately be feasible. It is well-established that cancer vaccines can prevent tumors in animals.[5,66] It is also clear, in animals, that vaccines are more effective in preventing cancer than in treating the disease once it is established. As noted above, cancer vaccines appear to be clinically effective in some patients. Consequently, the logic of the animal studies suggests that it should be feasible for vaccines to prevent cancer in man and that, in fact, this might prove to be easier than treating patients who already have the disease.

FUTURE OUTLOOK

Two basic issues need to be addressed in the future to advance the vaccine treatment of melanoma. Large scale, randomized, clinical trials need to be conducted to determine objectively whether any of the promising vaccines currently in phase I or II clinical trials can actually slow the progression of melanoma. There must be a continued effort to develop improved vaccine formulations that can more effectively stimulate strong and protective anti-tumor immune responses. Here two primary problems must be addressed. The major one is to develop a mix of melanoma-associated antigens that can stimulate clinically beneficial anti-tumor immune responses. The other is to develop potent adjuvants that can safely, easily and powerfully boost the frequency and magnitude of these responses. More strategies are available to reach both goals that can possibly be evaluated in clinical trials. Selecting among these will be a challenging task.

ACKNOWLEDGMENTS

Supported in part by NIH grant No. 1 R01 CA89270 and by grants from the Rose M Badgeley Residual Trust and the Catherine and Henry Gaisman Foundation.

REFERENCES

1 Bystryn J-C, Shapiro RL, Oratz R. Cancer vaccines: Clinical applications: Partially purified tumor antigen vaccines. In: V DeVita, S Hellman, and SA Rosenberg, eds. Biologic Therapy of Cancer, 2nd Edition. Philadelphia, PA: JB Lippincott; 1995:668–679.

2 Gromet MA, Epstein WL, Blois MS. The regressing thin melanoma. A distinctive lesson with metastatic potential. Cancer 1978; 42:2282–2292.

3 Balso M, Schiavon M, Cicogna PA, et al. Spontaneous regression of subcutaneous metastasis of cutaneous melanoma. Plast Reconstr Surg 1992; 90:1073–1076.

4 Kopf AW. Host defense against melanoma. Hosp Pr 1971; 6:116.

5 Bystryn J-C. Antibody response and tumor growth in syngeneic mice immunized to partially purified B16 melanoma associated antigens. J Immunol 1978; 120:96–101.

6 Oratz R, Cockerall C, Speyer JL, et al. Induction of tumor-infiltrating lymphocytes in human malignant melanoma metastases by immunization to melanoma antigen vaccine. J Biol Response Modif 1989; 8:355–358.

7 Hsueh EC, Gupta RK, Qi K, et al. Correlation of specific immune responses with survival in melanoma patients with distant metastases receiving polyvalent melanoma cell vaccine. J Clin Oncol 1998; 16:2913–2920.

8 Livingston PO, Wong GY, Adluri S, et al. Improved survival in stage III melanoma patients with GM2 antibodies: a randomized trial of adjuvant vaccination with GM2 ganglioside. J Clin Oncol 1994; 12:1036–1044.

9 Miller K, Abeless G, Oratz R, et al. Improved survival of patients with melanoma with an antibody response to immunization to a polyvalent melanoma vaccine. Cancer 1995; 75:495–502.

10 Reynolds SR, Zeleniuch-Jacquotte A, Shapiro RL, et al. Vaccine-induced CD8+ T cell responses to MAGE-3 correlate with clinical outcome in patients with melanoma. Clin Can Res 2003; 9:657–662.

11 Jäger E, Gnjatic S, Nagata Y, et al. Induction of primary NY-ESO-1 immunity: CD8+ T lymphocyte and antibody responses in peptide-vaccinated patients with NY-ESO-1+ cancers. Proc Natl Acad Sci 2000; 97:12198–12203.

12 Hsueh EC, Essner R, Foshag LJ, et al. Prolonged survival after complete resection of disseminated melanoma and active immunotherapy with a therapeutic cancer vaccine J Clin Oncol 2002; 20:4549–4554.

13 Sosman JA, Unger JM, Liu PY, et al. Adjuvant immunotherapy of resected, intermediate-thickness, node-negative melanoma with an allogeneic tumor vaccine: impact of HLA class I antigen expression on outcome. J Clin Oncol 2002; 20:2067–2075.

14 Berd D. M-Vax: an autologous, hapten-modified vaccine for human cancer. Expert Opin Biol Ther 2002; 2:335–342.

15 Wallack MK, Sivanandham M, Blach CM, et al. Surgical adjuvant active specific immunotherapy for patients with stage III melanoma: The final analysis of data from a phase III, randomized, double-blind, multicenter vaccinia melanoma oncolysate trial. J Am Coll Surg 1998; 187:69–79.

16 Hersey P, Coates AS, McCarthy WH, et al. Adjuvant immunotherapy of patients with high-risk melanoma using vaccinia viral lysates of melanoma: results of a randomized trial. J Clin Oncol 2002; 20:4181–4190.

17 Belli F, Arienti F, Sule-Soso J, et al. Active immunization of metastatic melanoma patients with interleukin-2 transduced allogeneic melanoma cells: evaluation of efficacy and tolerability. Cancer Immunol Immunother 1997; 44:197–203.

18 Abdel-Wahab Z, Weltz C, Hester D, et al. A phase I clinical trial of immunotherapy with interferon-γ gene-modified autologous melanoma cells. Cancer 1997; 80:401–412.

19 Soiffer R, Lynch T, Mihm M, et al. Vaccination with irradiated autologous melanoma cells engineered to secrete human granulocyte-macrophage colony stimulating factor generates potent anti-tumor immunity in patients with metastatic melanoma. Proc Natl Acad Sci USA 1998; 95:13141–13146.

20 Moller P, Sun Y, Dorbic T, et al. Vaccine with IL-7 gene-modified autologous melanoma cells can enhance the anti-melanoma lytic activity in peripheral blood of patients with a good clinical performance status: a clinical phase I study. Brit J Can 1998; 77:1907–1916.

21 Arienti F, Belli F, Napolitano F, et al. Vaccination of melanoma patients with interleukin 4 gene-transduced allogeneic melanoma cells. Hum Gene Ther 1999; 10:2907–2916.

22 Weber J, Sondak VK, Scotland R, et al. Granulocyte-macrophage-colony-stimulating factor added to a multipeptide vaccine for resected stage II melanoma. Cancer 2003; 97:186–200.

23 Slingluff CL Jr, Yamshchikov G, Neese P, et al. Phase I trial of a melanoma vaccine with gp100(280–288) peptide and tetanus helper peptide in adjuvant: immunologic and clinical outcomes. Clin Can Res 2001; 7:3012–3024.

24 Banchereau J, Palucka AK, Dhodapkar M, et al. Immune and clinical response in patients with metastatic melanoma to CD34+ progenitor derived dendritic cell vaccine. Can Res 2001; 61:6451–6458.

25 Lau R, Wang F, Jeffery G, et al. Phase I trial of intravenous peptide-pulsed dendritic cells in patients with metastatic melanoma. J Immunotherapy 2001; 24:66–78.

26 Kirkwood JM, Ibrahim JG, Sosman JA, et al. High-dose interferon alfa-2b significantly prolongs relapse-free and overall survival compared with GM2-KLH/QS-21 vaccine in patients with resected stage IIB-III melanoma: results of intergroup trial E1694/S9512/C509801. J Clin Oncol 2001; 19:2370–2380.

27 McCaffery M, Yao TJ, Williams L, et al. Immunization of melanoma patients with BEC2 anti-idiotypic monoclonal antibody that mimics GD3 ganglioside: enhanced immunogenicity when combined with adjuvant. Clin Can Res 1996; 2:679–686.

28 Foon KA, Lutzky J, Baral RN, et al. Clinical and immune responses in advanced melanoma patients immunized with an anti-idiotype antibody mimicking disialoganglioside GD2. J Clin Oncol 2000; 18:376–384.

29 Bystryn J-C, Zeleniuch-Jacquotte A, Oratz R, et al. Double-blind trial of

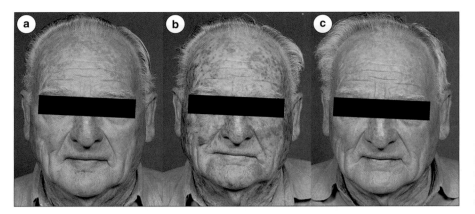

Figure 50.1 Male with multiple actinic keratoses and treated with 5% 5-FU (Efudex®) b.i.d. (a) Pre-treatment. (b) After 2 weeks. (c) Post-treatment after 1 month course of treatment.

topical 5-FU formulation experience some degree of facial irritation (Fig. 50.2).

The maximum severity rating of facial irritation in patients treated with topical 5-FU 0.5% microsphere-based cream once daily was moderate or severe in 80.5% of patients after 2 weeks and 90% of patients after 4 weeks (n= 40).[3,4]

To avoid the undesirable effects of treatment, some investigators and many practitioners have tried 'pulse therapy' to help decrease associated irritation.[5] Unfortunately, pulse therapy does not appear to be reliably effective for treatment of AKs (Epstein).[6] As described by Jeffes et al.,[7] the maxim of 'no pain no gain' appears to be true with topical 5-FU therapy.

Regardless of the proprietary formulation and concentration of topical 5-FU that is applied, the patient needs to be forewarned that erythema, inflammation and erosions are anticipated and expected throughout the course of therapy. Because of the protracted inflammatory reaction, it is important that treatment be planned around important social or work related activities. Upon completion of the course of topical 5-FU therapy, resolution of the associated inflammatory reaction and symptoms of local irritation can be hastened by the use of a mid-potency topical corticosteroid applied to the zone of inflammation twice daily over a period of 1–2 weeks. Specific patient instructions during use of topical 5-FU include avoidance of the ocular and periocular regions, uninvolved peri-orbital areas and mucous membranes. Inadvertent application to the intertriginous areas, penis or scrotum can result in significant irritation with local intolerability. Patients with marked seborrheic dermatitis should be treated prior to beginning topical 5-FU.

As stated above, for thick lesions and for areas other than the head and neck, topical 5-FU is not as effective. Longer therapy or combining 5-FU with other treatments may be beneficial. Robinson and Kligman[8] reported that combining tretinoin 0.1% with 5% 5-FU applied to the extremities for 2 weeks followed by 3 weeks of 5-FU 5% cream was more effective than 5 weeks of 5-FU 5% therapy alone. Bercovich[9] reported that tretinoin 0.05% at bedtime and 5-FU 5% cream twice daily for 12–28 days was significantly more effective than the 5-FU 5% cream alone.

For hyperkeratotic AKs of the extremities, the authors have found the combination therapy approach of spot treatment with liquid nitrogen cryotherapy or application of trichloroacetic acid (TCA) 35% solution, prior to initiating or after completing a course of topical 5-FU therapy, produces optimal results.

Less than 10% of a dose of 5-FU 5% cream applied topically to intact skin is reported to be absorbed systemically.[10] However, application to diseased skin may enhance absorption of 5-FU by up to 75 times greater than absorption from healthy skin.[11] Fortunately, systemic reactions related to topical application of 5-FU appear to be extremely rare. Systemic absorption of 5-FU may be significantly increased in patients with DPD (dihydropyrimidine dehydrogenase) deficiency, resulting in a potential risk of severe toxicity[12] although this has not been a clinical problem in our experience. A comparison of systemic absorption after application of 5-FU based on urinary excretion parameters evaluated 5-FU 5% cream applied twice daily and 5-FU 0.5% microsponge cream applied daily up to 28 days.[13] Urinary excretion after application of 5-FU 0.5% microsponge cream was 1/40th of what was observed with 5-FU 5% cream despite only a 1/10th difference in drug concentration. The clinical significance of this systemic absorption differential is not clear.

For basal cell carcinoma (superficial), only the 5-FU 5% is recommended at this time, although data is limited. Application should be twice daily to cover the lesion plus a few mm margin. Treatment should last for at least 3–6 weeks. Treatment may be needed for 10–12 weeks to completely clear lesions. Careful follow-up is needed to be certain of a cure. Inadequate treatment may resolve only the superficial component and make the diagnosis of recurrence difficult. The authors prefer to use this only for multiple (or in difficult treatment areas) superficial basal cell carcinoma. It may be useful for palliation in patients unable to tolerate other forms of treatment.

Topical 5-FU has been used for the treatment of squamous cell carcinoma *in situ* (Bowen's disease, erythroplasia de Queyrat), with variable and unpredictable results. Data regarding efficacy is very limited. Results are variable and unpredictable and the formulations used are not routinely available.[14–17] Bergman,[18] however, recently reported treating 26 patients with Bowen's disease noting only two recurrences with follow-up periods of up to 10 years.

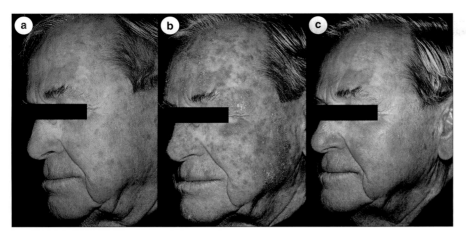

Figure 50.2 Male with multiple actinic keratoses treated with 0.5% 5-FU (Carac®) q.d. (a) Pre-treatment. (b) After 2 weeks. (c) Post-treatment.

Topical imidazoquinolines

Recent studies have demonstrated the effectiveness of the imidazoquinolines as immune response modifiers for the treatment of skin cancer. Topical imiquimod 5% cream is FDA-approved in the US for the treatment of external genital warts and non-hypertrophic AKs. Effective treatment has been correlated with enhanced innate and acquired immune responses facilitated by imiquimod application.[19,20] Topical imiquimod is devoid of direct antiviral and antineoplastic properties. It is currently believed that imiquimod facilitates immunologic recognition of disease and augments natural immune response, at least partially through increased synthesis and/or release of multiple cytokines (i.e. interferon-alpha, tumor necrosis factor-alpha), chemokines, several interleukins, indirect stimulation of interferon-gamma, enhancement of Langerhans cell migration to regional lymph nodes, promoting the activation and recruitment of targeted T-lymphocytes and augmentation of apoptosis.[21]

Topical imiquimod 5% cream has been reported to be effective for the treatment of AKs, superficial and nodular basal cell carcinoma and squamous cell carcinoma in situ.[21–23] Specific cytokines and activated T-lymphocytes infiltrating tumor islands have been demonstrated in both naturally regressing and interferon-treated basal cell carcinoma and squamous cell carcinoma *in situ*, findings that are believed to correlate at least partially with the mechanism of action of imiquimod, which is described in depth elsewhere in this volume.[22,23]

Several investigations, including case report collections and controlled studies, have established that imiquimod 5% cream is effective for the treatment of AKs.[24–26] In some patients, treated AKs were described as recurrent after prior treatment with other modalities (i.e. cryotherapy, 5-FU). For treatment of AKs, topical imiquimod is applied at bedtime two to three applications per week. The usual duration of therapy is 6–8 weeks. However, longer durations (up to 12 weeks) or repeated courses of therapy may be used based on clinical response. Individual case reports of patients treated with topical imiquimod twice weekly for AKs involving the forehead and dorsum of the hands demonstrated significant clearance of lesions and maintenance of remission over a period of 9 months.[26]

Suggested protocols for the use of topical imiquimod in the treatment of AKs allow for reduction in application frequency and the use of short rest periods off of therapy (1–4 weeks) upon the development of a brisk local cutaneous inflammatory response.[26] The use of rest periods allows for reduction in the intensity of inflammation without sacrificing efficacy. If AK lesions persist after completion of the rest period, therapy may be restarted with reduction in dosing frequency by one less application per week. Unlike topical 5-FU, where the inflammatory reaction is a 'by-product' of direct cytotoxic activity, the erythema associated with topical imiquimod use reflects the induction of a directed therapeutic inflammatory response.

A preliminary, open-label investigation using topical imiquimod 'cycle therapy' for treatment of AKs included patients presenting with five to twenty lesions involving multiple 'cosmetic units' (scalp, cheeks, temples, forehead).[27] A treatment 'cycle' was defined as application of imiquimod 5% cream three times per week for 4 weeks followed by a 4-week 'rest period' off therapy; a maximum of three treatment cycles were utilized if clinical examination demonstrated persistent AK lesions. Imiquimod was applied to the entire 'cosmetic unit' under treatment. A single cycle of therapy produced a complete clearance rate of 46% of treated cosmetic units. A second treatment cycle provided an additional complete clearance rate of 36%; the complete clearance after two cycles totaled 82%. The use of a 4-week rest period allowed for resolution of erythema and optimal assessment of lesion clearance (Fig. 50.3).

Several studies have evaluated the efficacy of topical imiquimod in the treatment of basal cell carcinoma, primarily for superficial and small, low-risk nodular subtypes.[22,28–30] The mechanism of action is believed to relate at least partially to induction of local release of interferons; cytokines are induced which enhance expression of BCC surface receptors that allow for binding of activated T-lymphocytes.[22,31] A variety of dosing regimens have been assessed with studies utilizing similar protocols.

Eradication of tumor after treatment with topical imiquimod was confirmed by histologic evaluation of excised treatment sites, completed at 6 weeks post-therapy.[21,22,28,29]

with scalp lesions and for thinner AKs. Hyperkeratotic AKs are less responsive to ALA/PDT, likely reflecting incomplete penetration of 5-ALA solution into AK lesions (Fig. 50.6).

ALA 30% applied to AKs under occlusive dressing for three hours followed by red laser light exposure (630 nm) has demonstrated comparable efficacy to the blue light regimen using ALA 20% described above.[7] The blue light photoactivation regimen requires a longer time delay. From a practical perspective, the patient must visit the physician in the late afternoon for application of the ALA 20% solution to the individual AK lesions and return the next morning for controlled blue light exposure.

Local inflammatory reactions are commonly observed with ALA-PDT.[44] Some degree of burning and/or stinging has been observed in essentially all patients during active treatment and within the 24 hr period after ALA-PDT therapy. Erythema, scaling and focal areas of crusting are observed in the majority of treated patients with approximately one-third demonstrating perilesional edema. Disadvantages of ALA/PDT include marked discomfort in some patients, inconvenience related to timed patient visits and costs related to drug acquisition, equipment (light source), space and personnel time.

ALA/PDT appears to be as efficacious as 5% 5-FU and cryosurgery in the treatment of actinic keratoses.[45–47]

ALA/PDT has also shown promising results for mycosis fungoides (MF). Although data is preliminary the efficacy appears promising. Edstrom et al.[48] reported 10 patients having 10 plaque stage lesions and two tumors. A good clinical response was reported in seven of nine MF plaques and complete clearance with follow up of 4–19 months. The two tumors did not respond to treatment.

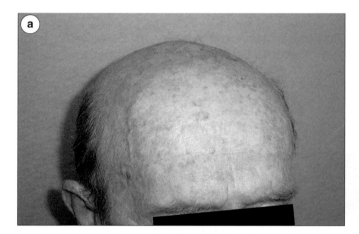
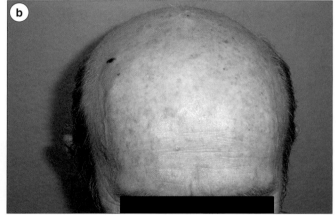
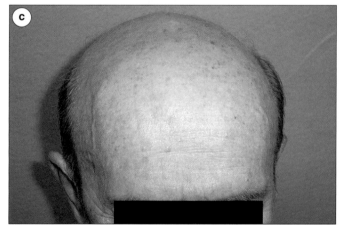

Figure 50.5 Male with multiple actinic keratoses on the scalp treated with topical diclofenac 3% gel b.i.d. (a) Pre-treatment. (b) After 30 days. (c) Post-treatment of a 90-day course. (Images courtesy of Dr Christopher Nelson.)

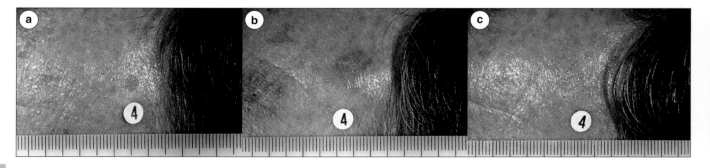

Figure 50.6 Treatment of actinic keratoses on forehead with topical ALA-PDT. (a) Pre-treatment. (b) 1 week post-treatment. (c) 6 weeks post-treatment.

ALA/PDT shows promise for the treatment of superficial or nodular basal cell carcinoma.[49,50] Preliminary results show that ALA/PDT and cryosurgery were compatible in terms of efficacy, but the healing time and cosmetic outcome were better with ALA/PDT.[51] ALA/PDT may be advantageous for large superficial lesions especially in areas where function and healing are at risk or if good cosmetic results are especially important. As with topical 5-FU and cryosurgery, close follow-up is needed to be certain that not only the superficial component is destroyed leaving behind the deep component of the tumor. Detection of recurrence (persistence) may be difficult at times.

ALA/PDT has also been reported to be effective for squamous cell carcinoma *in situ* (Bowen's disease) with response rates from 88–100% with a low recurrence rate and good cosmetic results.[52,53] ALA/PDT does not appear to be an effective treatment for invasive squamous cell carcinoma based on current data.

Metvix (methyl aminolevulinic, an ester of 5-ALA (M-ALA), Photocure ASA, Oslo) is a new form of photosensitizer which has been shown to be effective for both actinic keratoses[54] and basal cell carcinoma when activated by light. It appears to have somewhat better selectivity for actinic keratoses and cancer cells. Also, it is more convenient since it is applied 3 hrs before treatment rather than 14–18 hrs for ALA. It appears to be as good as or better than cryosurgery for both actinic keratoses and basal cell carcinomas with shorter healing time, better cosmetic results and much lower incidence of hypopigmentation.

As expected, M-ALA PDT is associated with local skin reactions such as pain, crusting and erythema. For basal cell carcinomas the surface is lightly curetted prior to application of M-ALA cream. The lesions are retreated in 1 week.

PDT with M-ALA is becoming popular in Europe and in Australia. Studies involving over 25,000 patients with basal cell carcinoma or actinic keratoses in 14 countries around the world have been conducted. Overall, this therapy appears to be as effective as cryotherapy for actinic keratoses[54] and superficial basal cell carcinoma, but with the added advantage of a superior cosmetic result. It also appears to be effective for nodular basal cell carcinoma[55] and 'difficult to treat' and recurrent basal cell carcinoma.[56] M-ALA PDT is not yet approved for use in the US.

OTHER TOPICAL CHEMOTHERAPY AGENTS

Retinoids

Vitamin A (retinol) plays an important role in normal epithelial growth and differentiation. Retinoids have been shown to normalize differentiation in photoaged skin. Recent studies suggest a relative deficiency of retinol in epithelial cancers.[57,58] Correction of this retinol deficiency may be of therapeutic value for cutaneous malignancies and pre-malignancy.

The potential benefit of topical retinoids for the treatment of AKs has been suggested by studies demonstrating partial or complete clearance of AKs in many patients treated with oral etretinate[59] and a potential synergistic effect against AKs when low-dose oral isotretinoin therapy is used in combination with topical 5-FU. The limitations of systemic toxicity and tetrogenicity obviate the widespread use of systemic retinoids for treatment of AKs, however, their use may be beneficial in selected cases in patients with immunosuppression associated with multiple AKs and frequent development of squamous cell carcinomas.

Prolonged use of topical retinoids has been shown to decrease the number and size of AKs. Prolonged application of tretinoin 0.1% cream applied once or twice daily for facial AKs produced a gradual and significant decrease in the size and number of lesions over a period of six to fifteen months.[30] Similar results were reported with the use of topical isotretinoin.[60] Based on currently available data, topical retinoid therapy for AKs is not comparable to available therapies that are proven to be consistently effective such as 5-FU. As discussed above in the section on topical 5-FU, topical retinoids may be combined with topical 5-FU treatment for AKs involving the extremities. Although topical retinoids are not recommended as monotherapy for AK, their adjunctive use may be chemopreventative with potential for reduction of AKs on a long-term basis and they have been shown to reduce photoaging. In addition to FDA approval for treatment of acne vulgaris, both topical tretinoin and topical tazarotene are FDA approved for the treatment of photoaging.[61,62] Although a preliminary observation in a small collection of patients suggested that basal cell carcinoma may respond to treatment with topical tazarotene, additional study is needed.[63]

Colchicine

Colchicine is an alkaloid obtained by the corm and seeds of the meadow saffron *Colchicum autumnale* (Liliaceae)[64] and known since antiquity as a poison. It has potent antimitotic activity through its interaction with tubulin protein hindering the assembly of microtubules with selective destruction of tumor cells. An 8% solution has been reported to be effective in penile condylomata acuminata.[65] A 0.5% colchicine ointment has been reported to be effective for psoriasis.[66]

The beneficial effects of topical colchicine were first reported by Marshal in 1968.[67] More recently Grimaitre *et al.* confirmed that a topical application of a 1% colchicine gel is safe and effective for the treatment of actinic keratoses.[64] In a double blind placebo controlled study they reported complete clearing of solar keratoses in 7 of 10 patients treated twice daily to the forehead for 2 months. Treatment was interrupted when a strong inflammatory response developed usually by 10 days. No recurrences were noted after 2 months of follow-up and no systemic absorption was noted.

Only those lesions with a strong inflammatory reaction showed a very good cosmetic result. The reaction appeared to be selective for the actinic keratoses and sparing the surrounding normal skin. Further studies on this approach and comparison to other treatments are needed.

Table 52.1 AJCC Melanoma Classification System

T classification	Thickness	Ulceration status
T1	≤1.0 mm	a: Without ulceration and level IV/V b: With ulceration or level IV/V
T2	1.01–2.0 mm	a: Without ulceration b: With ulceration
T3	2.01–4.0 mm	a: Without ulceration b: With ulceration
T4	>4.0 mm	a: Without ulceration b: With ulceration
N classification	**No of metastatic nodes**	**Nodal metastatic mass**
N1	1 node	a: Micrometastasis b: Macrometastasis
N2	2–3 nodes	a: Micrometastasis b: Macrometastasis
N3	4 or more metastatic nodes Matted nodes Intransit metastasis(s)/satellite(s) with metastatic node(s)	
M classification	**Site Serum**	**LDH**
M1a	Distant skin, subcutaneous, or nodal metastases	Normal
M1b	Lung metastases	Normal
M1c	All other visceral metastases	Normal
	Any distant metastasis	Elevated

T, tumor; N, node; M, metastasis; LDH, lactate dehydrogenase

Table 52.2 Staging groups for cutaneous melanoma

	Clinical staging			Pathologic staging		
	T	N	M	T	N	M
O	Tis	No	Mo	Tis	No	Mo
IA	T1a	No	Mo	T1a	No	Mo
IB	T1b	No	Mo	T1b	No	Mo
	T2a	No	Mo	T2a	No	Mo
IIA	T2b	No	Mo	T2b	No	Mo
	T3a	No	Mo	T3a	No	Mo
IIB	T3b	No	Mo	T3b	No	Mo
	T4a	No	Mo	T4a	No	Mo
IIC	T4b	No	Mo	T4b	No	Mo
III	Any T	N1	Mo			
		N2				
		N3				
IIIA				T1-4a	N1a	Mo
				T1-4a	N2a	Mo
IIIB				T1-4b	N1a	Mo
				T1-4b	N2a	Mo
				T1-4a	N1b	Mo
				T1-4a	N2b	Mo
				T1-4a/b	N2c	Mo
IIIC				T1-4b	N1b	Mo
				T1-4b	N2b	Mo
				Any T	N3	Mo
IV	Any T	Any N	Any M1	Any T	Any N	Any M1

is, in situ

high risk for developing advanced disease who would best benefit from adjuvant therapy. It will be of interest whether future revision of the staging system will incorporate preliminary data correlating the molecular detection of melanoma cells by means of reverse-transcriptase polymerase chain reaction (RT-PCR) in regional lymph nodes[2] or peripheral blood[3] with clinical outcome.

The AJCC staging system divides patients into four stages depending on whether tumors are only localized to the skin (stage I and II), have regional metastases (to lymph nodes or satellite or in-transit intralymphatic sites, stage III), or have distant metastatic disease (stage IV). Subgroups are based on the interplay of the above-described prognostic factors and reflect the prognostic heterogeneity of patients with the same tumor. Traditionally, the high-risk group is described as subjects with primary deep melanomas (T4N0M0) or stage III disease, whereas intermediate risk group includes patients with melanoma thickness ≥1.0 mm. We summarize the data on adjuvant therapy for melanoma of intermediate and high-risk patients.

The past of adjuvant therapy

Non-interferon (IFN) based adjuvant treatments have been largely ineffective

Table 52.3 summarizes the most important randomized controlled trials (RCT) for intermediate and high-risk cutaneous melanoma that have tested non IFN-based regimens in an adjuvant setting.[4–23] Chemotherapy as a single agent, in combination with other chemotherapeutic agents, hormones, or biologics, except under special settings (isolated limb perfusion), have not improved DFS and OS in any reported prospective randomized multicenter studies to date. Single-center studies that have not utilized the current accepted rigorous standards of concurrent randomized comparators have suggested that adjuvant therapy with vindesine has benefit in stage III melanoma.[24] However, these results have not been reproduced in RCTs. Following early suggestion of benefit from small single-institution non-randomized trials, negative results were also obtained using megestrol acetate, vitamin A, and non-specific immunostimulants such as BCG, *Corynebacterium parvum*, or transfer factor.

Melanoma vaccines have been extensively investigated for more than three decades and are presented with greater detail elsewhere in this textbook

Table 52.3   Most important randomized controlled trials of adjuvant non IFN-based therapy of cutaneous melanoma

Study reference	Enrolled patients (n)	Stage	Treatment arms	Average follow-up (years)	Comments
1. Chemotherapy					
Veronesi 1982[4]	931	II III	DTIC BCG DTIC + BCG Observation	5	NS
Lejeune, 1988[5]	325	I IIA IIB	DTIC Levamisole Placebo	4	NS
Fisher 1981[6]	181	II III	CCNU Observation	3	NS
Koops 1998[7]	832	II III	Isolated limb perfusion + hyperthermia Observation	6.4	BS
Meisenberg 1993[8]	39	III	Autologous bone marrow transplant Observation	NA	NS
2. Vitamins, Hormones					
Meyskens 1994[9]	248	II III	Vitamin A Observation	8	NS
Markovic 2002[10]	262	IIB III	Megestrol Observation	4.5 min	NS
3. Non specific immunostimulants					
Czarnetzki 1993[11]	353	II	BCG (RIV) BCG (Pasteur) Observation	6	NS
Paterson 1984[12]	199	I II	BCG Observation	4	NS
Balch 1982[13]	260	I II	Corynebacterium parvum Observation	2	NS
Lipton 1991[14]	262	III	Corynebacterium parvum BCG	4–9	BS
Quirt 1991[15]	577	I IIA IIB III	Levamisole BCG BCG + levamisole Observation	8	NS
Spitler 1991[16]	216	I IIA IIB III IV	Levamisole Placebo	10	NS
Miller 1988[17]	168	II III	Transfer factor Observation	2	NS
4. Vaccines					
Sondak 2002[18]	689	IIA	Melacine with DETOX Observation	5.6	NS
Hershey 2002[19]	700	IIB	Vaccinia melanoma cell lysate Placebo	8	Trend on RFS/OS
Wallack 1998[20]	250	III	Vaccinia melanoma oncolysate Placebo	3	NS
Wallack 1995[21]	250	II	Virus allogeneic polyvalent melanoma cell lysate	2.5min	NS
Livingston 1994[22]	123	III	GM2-BCG-Cytoxan BCG alone-Cytoxan	5	NS
Bystryn 2001[23]	38	III	Polyvalent shed antigen Placebo	2.5	S

DITC, dacarbazine; BCG, Bacille Calmette-Guerin; min, minimal duration of follow up; NS, non statistically significant; S, statistically significant; NA, non available; BS, borderline significance; RFS, relapse free survival; OS, overall survival; GM2, ganglioside GM2.

Table 52.5   Phase II clinical trials evaluating treatment schedules for metastatic melanoma

Study reference	Enrolled no patients	IFN-α subspecies	Dose range (MU/m^2)	Schedule	Route	Overall response rate	CR	PR
Ernstoff 1983[37]	17	2b	10–100	qd (5 d/week, × 4 weeks)	i.v.			2
Creagan 1984[38]	23	2a	50	q2d (3 ×/week, × 3 months)	i.m.	20	1	5
Creagan 1985[39]	35	2a + cimetidine	50	q2d (3 ×/week, × 12 weeks)	i.m.	23	0	8
Creagan 1984[40]	31	2a	12	t.i.w. × 3 months	i.m.	23	3	4
Legha 1987[41]	a. 35	2a	(a) Escalating 3→36, q3d	(a) Induction × 70 d, then maintenance	i.m.	1	0	3
	b. 31		(b) Fixed 18	(b) t.i.w.		6	0	2
Hersey 1985[42]	20	2a	Escalating 15→50	t.i.w.	i.m.	10	2	0
Neefe 1990[43]	97	2a	Escalating 3→36	3 MU for 10 d then escalate over 10 d	s.c.	8	6	2
Dorval 1986[44]	22	2b	10	t.i.w.		24	2	4
Coates 1986[45]	15	2a	20	5 d/week, every 2 weeks	i.v.	0	0	0

CR, complete remission; PR, partial remission; i.v., intravenously; i.m., intramuscularly; s.c., subcutaneously; d, day; q.d., every day; t.i.w., three times a week; MU, mega units.

dosing, route of administration, and duration of therapy. The trials are summarized based on high-, intermediate-, and low-dose regimens.

High dose IFN-α regimens are of two types: one evaluated by the Eastern Cooperative Group (ECOG) and US Intergroup, is comprised of an induction phase consisting of one month of daily i.v. bolus IFN-α2b, followed by a prolonged (11 month) maintenance with lower doses that approach the maximum tolerable dosage given s.c.[46–48] The other is a regimen evaluated in a single trial conducted by the North Central Cancer Treatment Group (NCCTG) utilizing a high dose of IFN-α2a administered i.m. thrice weekly for 12 weeks.[49]

The *E1684* trial was the first randomized controlled trial that showed a significant prolongation in DFS and OS in patients with deep primary tumor (>4 mm, T4N0M0), or the presence of regional lymph node metastases (TxN1–3M0, AJCC stage III).[46] In transit, satellite, or extracapsular spread of disease was excluded and all patients had pathologic staging of regional lymph nodes before enrollment. Patients were assigned either to the treatment arm group which received IFN-α2b i.v. at 20 MU/m^2 per day, 5 days per week for 4 weeks followed by three times weekly s.c. injections at 10 MU/m^2 per day for 48 weeks or to the observation group. After a median follow-up time of more than 6.9 years, the estimated 5-year RFS rate in the IFN-α2b treated group was 37% (30–46%, 95% confidence interval, 95 CI) versus 26% in the observation group (19–34%, 95 CI) whereas the 5-year overall OS in the IFN-α2b treated group was 46% (39–55%, 95 CI) versus 37% in the observation arm (30–46%, 95 CI). Although the patients with deep primary, node-negative melanoma were underrepresented (11% of the overall

accrual of patients) it appeared that the node-positive patients benefited the most from IFN-α2b therapy, the impact of which was manifested early in the first year of treatment. The results of this pivotal trial led the United States Food and Drug Administration (FDA) to approve the above regimen as the standard of care for adjuvant therapy of high-risk melanoma patients.

The substantial toxicities associated with high-dose i.v. IFN-α2b and the joint discussion of alternatives with the World Health Organization (WHO) led to the parallel evaluation of low-dose IFN-α2a and IFN-α2b (3 MU s.c. three times a week). The WHO trial 16 of low dose IFN-α2a versus observation was initially reported as effective[50] that was later at maturity, dismissed.[51] ECOG intergroup trial E1690 compared the benefit of the E1684 high-dose, one-year regimen as well as the low-dose regimen of IFN-α2b at 3 megaunits s.c. three times a week for 2-years *vs* observation.[47] High risk for relapse was defined in the WHO as nodal disease whereas in the E1690 it was defined as lymph node involvement, detected clinically or pathologically at elective lymph node dissection, or deep (>4 mm) primary lesions without clinically or pathologically defined nodal disease. In E1690, patients were spared the need for pathologic staging of regional nodes if there was no clinical evidence of node metastasis and the primary tumor was at least 4 mm deep (T4, stage IIB). Also in E1690, 75% of patients had stage III disease, and 25% had deep primary disease without pathologically staged regional lymph node involvement – more than double the fraction of patients with this stage of disease that entered the E1684 trial. E1690 was unblinded by the external data monitoring committee before reaching the planned number of events because of the improved OS of groups in this

Table 52.6 Phase III trials of adjuvant IFN-α therapy in patients with melanoma at intermediate and high risk for relapse

Study reference	Enrolled patients (n)	Stage	Treatment arm[a]	Outcome	DFS	OS
High dose						
Eastern COG-E1684	287	IIB III	IFN-α2b 20 MU/m^2 i.v. q.d. 5 d/week × 4 weeks then 10 MU/m^2 s.c. t.i.w. × 48 weeks		S^b	S
Eastern COG-E1690	642	IIB III	IFN-α2b 20 MU/m^2 i.v. q.d. 5 d/week × 4 weeks then 10 MU/m^2 s.c. t.i.w. × 48 weeks vs 3 MU t.i.w. × 2 years	S NS	NS	NS
Eastern COG-E1694	774	IIB III	IFN-α2b 20 MU/m^2 i.v. q.d. 5 d/week × 4 weeks then 10 MU/m^2 s.c. t.i.w. × 48 weeks vs GMK vaccine 1 cc s.c. on d1, 8, 15, 22 q12 weeks (weeks 12 to 96)	S S	NS	NS
NCCTG 83-7052	262	IIB III	IFN-α2a 20 MU/m^2 i.m. q.d. × 3 months		NS	NS
Intermediate dose						
EORTC 18952	1418	IIB III	IFN-α2b 10 MU s.c. 5 d/week × 4 weeks then 10 MU s.c. t.i.w. × 1 year vs IFN-α2b 10 MU s.c. 5 d/week × 4 weeks then 5 MU s.c. t.i.w. × 2 years	NS ?	S	?
Low dose						
WHO-16	444	IIB III	IFN-α2a 3 MU s.c. t.i.w. × 3 years		NS	NS
AIM HIGH (UKCCCR)	654	IIB III	IFN-α2a 3 MU s.c. t.i.w. × 2 years		NS	NS
ECRTC 18871/DKG-80	830	IIB III	IFN-α2b 1 MU s.c. alternate days, × 1 year vs IFN-γ 0.2 mg s.c. alternate days × 1 year vs Iscador M®	NS NS	NS NS	NS NS NS
Scottish Melanoma COG	96	II III	IFN-α2b 3 MU s.c. t.i.w. × 6 months		NS	NS
Austrian Melanoma COG	311	II	IFN-α2a 3 MU s.c. q.d. × 3 weeks then 3 MU s.c. t.i.w. × 1 year		NS	NS
French Melanoma COG	499	II	IFN-α2a 3 MU s.c. t.i.w. × 18 months		NS	NS

[a]All clinical trials also include an observation arm, except the ECOG trial E1694.
[b]Statistical comparisons with the observation group.
COG, cooperative group; WHO, World Health Organization; EORTC, European Organization for Research and Treatment of Cancer; UKCCCR, United Kingdom Committee for Cancer Research; NCCTG, North Central Cancer Treatment Group; DKG, German Cancer Society; Iscador M®, popular mistletoe extract (placebo); MU, mega units; i.v., intravenously; s.c., subcutaneously; d, day; q.d., every day; t.i.w., three times a week; DFS, disease free survival; OS, overall survival; S, statistically significant; NS, non-significant; GMK, ganglioside GM2 coupled to keyhole limpet hemocyanin (KLH). ?, data have not yet reached maturation.

study and the low projected likelihood that the survival results would differ to the extent that had originally been stipulated for either treatment. Thus, at a median follow-up of 4.3 years, and in an intention to treat analysis, 5-year relapse-free survival of those treated with high-dose IFN was significantly better than that of the observation group (44 vs 35%, P 2=0.05 log-rank test) but the 5-year OS estimates were similar for all three groups (52% high dose vs 53% low dose, vs 55% observation). Subset analysis reached statistical significance for relapse-free benefit patients with 2–3 positive lymph nodes, but not in other groups. The low-dose arm had no significant relapse interval or survival benefit.

The unexpected results of high dose IFN-α2b in the E1690 trial were explained in part on the basis of the overall improvements observed between E1684 and E1690 for RFS and OS outcomes – where the patients on the observation arms of the E1690 and E1684 clinical trials differed at a significance level of P=0.001. When evaluated in terms of RFS, the improvement in 5-year RFS was 35% vs 26, and 5-year OS 54 vs 37%, respectively for observation (Fig. 52.3). As already noted, the

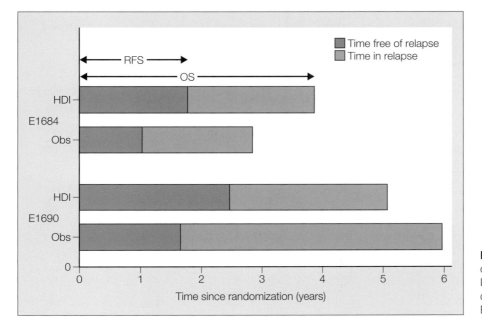

Figure 52.3 Relapse-free (RFS) and overall survival (OS) benefits of high-dose IFN-α2b (HDI) vs observation (Obs) demonstrated in each of the ECOG trials E1684 and E1690.

demographic analysis reveals that the E1690 trial recruited more patients with T4N0 disease (25%) and a smaller proportion of relapsed patients than the prior E1684 trial. Of potentially greater significance, as the US FDA approved high-dose IFN for the treatment of high-risk melanoma in 1995, many of the patients assigned to the observation arm of E1690 to 'cross over' to receive IFN-α2b high-dose therapy as a 'salvage' regimen were outside the trial when relapse occurred. This opportunity did not exist for patients in the earlier E1684 trial. Finally, the large fraction of patients who entered E1690 with deep T4 primary tumors and were not surgically staged with lymphadenectomy, presented the frequent scenario of nodal relapse in previously undissected regional nodes, coupled with the advent of a therapy for this (IFN-α2b) that was the tested agent in the E1690 trial. *Post hoc* analysis of the actual crossover frequency in fact demonstrated a significant and asymmetrical delivery of IFN-α2b therapy for patients who were assigned to observation in E1690, at relapse. Thus, the use of IFN in post-protocol therapy for patients who entered the study in high numbers with deep primary melanoma and relapsed thereafter may have confounded the detection of an OS benefit without significantly affecting the DFS impact in this trial.

The subsequent *E1694* trial[48] tested a vaccine that had shown a trend toward relapse interval benefit in a single institution phase III study at Memorial Sloan Kettering Cancer Center (MSKCC). It was undertaken to develop a therapy that would be superior to high-dose IFNα2b treatment. This study was the first in which high-dose IFNα2b treatment was taken as the standard of adjuvant therapy against which new options were tested. Thus, this trial also had the capacity to resolve the controversy regarding the benefit of high-dose IFN-α2b on OS which arose following the E1690.[48]

The GMK vaccine consists of the purified ganglioside GM2 coupled to keyhole limpet hemocyanin (KLH) and combined with the new and more potent QS-21 adjuvant, piloted at MSKCC by Livingston.[52] This modified GM2 regimen induced more consistent high-titered IgM and IgG antibodies than the original GM2-BCG vaccine that had previously improved RFS in stage III melanoma at MSKCC. An important observation in the first trial was that patients who produced IgM anti-GM2 antibodies benefited most from the vaccine, affording an intermediate endpoint for the E1694 phase III multicenter trial.[53] It was felt to be ethically difficult to continue with an observation arm, given the well-publicized E1684 data and despite the question interjected by the subsequent E1690 results. Eligible patients for E1694 had either deep primary tumors (>4.0 mm) without clinical evidence of lymph node metastasis (T4N × M0, AJCC stage IIB), based on clinical or pathologic grounds, or nodal metastatic disease, after completion of lymphadenectomy (T × N1–2M0, AJCC stage III).

This trial was unblinded after a median follow-up of 1.3 years by the external data safety and monitoring committee when the interim analysis revealed the superiority of high dose IFN-α2b in terms of both RFS (hazard ratios (HR), 1.47 (1.14–1.90, 95% CI)) and OS (HR 1.52 (95% CI 1.07–2.15)). These results demonstrated a 33% lower relapse and death rate for IFN-α2b, compared with the GMK vaccine. Despite the absence of an observation arm, E1694 has served as powerful confirmation of the original E1684 results. This trial is the largest adjuvant trial ever conducted in the US for resected high-risk melanoma patients of the GMK arm developed antibody IgM and IgG responses to GM2 more often than patients in the original MSKCC trial.

One of the concerns in this trial is whether the GMK vaccine adversely influenced outcome, making high-dose IFN-α2b appear effective artefactually. The antibody responses induced by the GMK have been analyzed to address this question, as all vaccine recipients were serially monitored for the induction of anti-GM2 antibody responses. The results dispelled worries that the vaccine adversely influenced outcome – patients who developed antibody response by day 29 demonstrated a trend to OS benefit (*P*=0.06). The vaccine arm outcome for E1694 was similar to, or slightly better than, the observation arm of the immediate preceding Intergroup trial with identical entry criteria, E1690.

Why GMK did not better influence outcome is unanswered. However, the GMK arm provided a reasonable comparator for IFN, confirming the benefit of this therapy as it was independently tested against observation in the original trial E1684. Together, these results make high dose IFN-α2b the logical standard of care for adjuvant therapy of resected high risk melanoma patients.

INDICATIONS AND CONTRAINDICATIONS

Eligibility and toxicity profile of the high dose IFN-α2b regimen

High dose IFN-α2b therapy is currently the standard of care for patients with high risk for relapse. Table 52.7 demonstrates indications, contraindications and cautions in use of high dose IFN-α2b therapy. Eligible patients are not restricted for age but should maintain a performance status of ECOG 0 or 1 (i.e. have normal activity, or have some symptoms but otherwise be nearly fully ambulatory) and have no significant hematologic, cardiac, hepatic or psychiatric co-morbidities. Appropriate dosage adjustments need to be done for any hepatic, renal, or hematologic impairment.

High-dose IFN-α2b is associated with a number of potential adverse events ranging from flu-like symptoms that may interfere with daily activities and pose a threat to patients' compliance to severe (life-threatening) toxicities that mandate dose interruption, or modification as well as aggressive supportive care.[54] Table 52.8 summarizes the most common grade III/IV toxicities and the frequency with which they have been observed in the three Cooperative Group phase III studies of this

modality, the proposed mechanisms of each toxicity and potential strategies for management of each toxicity. Up to 78% of patients receiving high-dose IFN-α2b experience at least one event of ≥ grade III toxicity, 50% required dose reduction for grade 2–4 toxicities and 23% could not complete the 1-year regimen in the original E1684 trial. The incidence and severity of these symptoms is primarily dose-related (Table 52.6). Most toxicities observed with high-dose IFN-α2b are fully reversible with dose interruption, often allowing resumption of therapy at a dose reduction of 33%. Some toxicities are more frequent than others (i.e. constitutional 48% *vs* hepatic 15%).

It is important to distinguish toxicities associated with peak dose exposure (i.e. the induction component of the E1684 regimen) from those that are associated with cumulative and continuous exposure (i.e. the maintenance phase of E1684 and the other alternate-daily regimens). In fact, many patients tolerate the induction i.v. therapy phase with little difficulty, only to develop insidiously progressive toxicity during the maintenance phase. However, others tolerate maintenance with little difficulty but experience acute effects of the induction regimen that require dose interruption and reduction.

The maintenance phase requires attention to the patient's complaints; some noting difficulty with the treatment at the start of each week while others have problems that mount over the week (signifying cumulative effects). Some acute effects demonstrate tachyphylaxis, and dissipate over time (fever, chills, malaise), whereas others are chronic and cumulative (anorexia, fatigue). Patients need to understand the scope and likely intensity of toxicity, and that persisting functional decrements of more than 25–33% will result in dose or dose reduction until day-to-day functions have resumed a level that is at least 60% of normal. Careful follow-up of laboratory and clinical findings is critical to the successful safe delivery of this therapy. Follow-up is recommended weekly, during induction therapy and monthly, during maintenance (for at least 3 months) and at 3-monthly intervals to the conclusion of the year of therapy, once the patient has achieved a stable and acceptable profile.

Despite concerns regarding the toxicity of high dose IFN-α2b, experience gained in a succession of nationwide Intergroup studies has demonstrated that this regimen can be safely administered and is tolerable for the majority of patients. While 23% of patients enrolled in E1684 did not complete a year of therapy due to toxicity, only 13% of patients in the Intergroup E1690 study discontinued treatment for toxicity, and in the largest and most recent Intergroup trial E1694, only 1% of patients who were assigned to high-dose IFN-α2b were withdrawn from treatment before the close of the year for toxicity. Close follow-up for early detection of side effects, especially the potentially life-threatening hepatic, hematologic and neurological toxicities, is mandatory.

Quality of life analyses have been performed. Using the quality-adjusted Time Without Symptoms or Toxicity (Q-TWiST) methodology, Cole *et al.* have shown that treatment with high-dose IFN-α2b results in a significant improvement in quality-adjusted time once the time with

---

Table 52.7 Indications, contraindications, cautions for high dose IFN-α2b therapy

Indications
- ECOG performance status 0 or 1

Contraindications
- Pregnancy, lactation
- Infancy
- Autoimmune diseases
- Immunosuppression (i.e. organ transplantation)
- Decompensated liver disease
- Severe neuropsychiatric diseases (i.e. depression)
- Myelosuppression
- Life threatening infection

Cautions
- Diabetes mellitus
- Cardiovascular disease
- Pulmonary disease
- Renal disease

Table 52.8 Toxicity and its management in patients with melanoma undergoing high dose IFN-α2b therapy

Adverse event	All grades (%) E1684 (n=143)	Grade 3/4 (%)	E1690 (n=216) E1694 (n=394)	Proposed mechanism	Management
Myelosuppression	64	57	59	IP-10, IL-1 release	Dose reduction
Liver toxicity	44	28	27	Suppress activity of certain cytochrome P450 isoenzymes	Dose reduction
Fatigue	67	23	21	Acts as ACTH-like, DA-agonist (acute), or DA-antagonist (chronic) Via IL-1, -2, -6, and TNF-α affects HPA axis Thyroid dysfunction	Behavioral[†] Pharmacologic[‡] SSRIs Megestrol Stimulants
Myalgia	52	17	4	IL-1, IL-6, TNF-α	Tylenol[†] Demerol[‡]
Nausea	46	8	4	IFN-α, IL-1, 5-HT3	Chlorpromazine[†]
Vomiting	28	9	10		Metoclopramide[†] Ondasetron[‡] Graniserton[‡]
Neuropsychiatric	46	5	5	Disturbance of HPA/HPG axis (IL-6 and glucocorticoids) Dysregulation of NE-/5HT3-ergic neurotransmitters	

IP-10, IFN-inducible protein; IL, interleukin; ACTH, adrenocorticotropic hormone; DA, dopamine; HPA, hypothalamus–pituitary–adrenal axis; HPG, hypothalamus–pituitary–gonadal axis; TNF-α, tumor necrosis factor-alpha; NE, norepinephrine; 5-HT3, serotonin; SSRI, serotonin selective reuptake inhibitors.

toxicity is factored out, even presuming the worst valuations of time with toxicity.[55] Kilbridge has reported strikingly poorer valuations of time with asymptomatic relapse than might generally be presumed and rather better valuations of time with toxicity.[56] These, together, provide useful tools to portray the utility of treatment for individual patients, using indices that are specific for each individual patient.

Alternatives to high dose IFN-α2b therapy

Low-dose IFN-α therapy may have a better toxicity profile, but does not improve OS significantly or RFS durably in high- or intermediate-risk melanoma.

Several European studies including those of the World Health Organization (WHO) and the European Organization for Research and Treatment of Cancer (EORTC), as well as the American E1690 study have asked whether lower doses of IFN-α2 administered over a longer period of time may improve upon DFS and OS without the toxicities of the high-dose regimen. In patients with *high-risk* melanoma, the results have been disappointing. The preliminary favorable results in 2-year RFS of the WHO Melanoma Program Trial 16, published after a 3-year median follow-up of patients randomized to receive low dose IFN-α2a (3 MU s.c. t.i.w. for 3 years) *vs* observation (46%, [36–54% 95CI], *vs* 27%, [18–35% 95CI])[50] dissipated completely after longer follow-up of 7.3 years.[51] Similarly, the recently published United Kingdom Coordinating Committee for Cancer Research (UKCCCR) AIM-HIGH (adjuvant IFN in mela-

noma high risk) trial on patients randomized to receive either low dose IFN-α2a (3 MU s.c. t.i.w., for 2 years), observation showed no significant difference in OS or DFS between the two arms after only 3.1 years median follow-up.[43,57] Even lower doses of IFN-α2b (1 MU) or IFN-γ (0.2 mg), administered s.c. every other day for 12 months showed no benefit in comparison with an untreated control group or with a fourth arm treated with Iscador M®, a popular extract of mistletoe, the latter added to the EORTC design by the German Cancer Society (DKG) after median follow-up of 5.5 years.[58] Similarly, a small underpowered Scottish study comparing treatment with low dose IFN-α2b (3 MU s.c. t.i.w. for 6 months) *vs* observation in intermediate and high risk melanoma patients, has shown no improvement in RFS and OS with low doses of IFN.[59]

Low-dose IFN-α2 has not shown any evidence of significant OS benefit in melanoma patients with intermediate risk for relapse, defined as primary tumors of ≥1.5 mm without regional lymph node metastasis based on clinical (but not pathological) grounds. Improvement in RFS has been shown in two randomized controlled clinical trials.[46,47,60,61] The Austrian Melanoma Cooperative Group compared low dose IFN-α2a (3 MU s.c. every day for 3 weeks, followed by 3 MU s.c. three times a week, for 1 year) with observation. After a median follow-up of 3.4 years, there was an improvement in DFS (*P*=0.02) in an intention-to-treat analysis without any noted improvement in OS. Similarly, improvement in RFS was shown in the subsequent French Melanoma Cooperative Group trial comparing low dose IFN-α2a (3 MU s.c. three times a week, for 18 months) with observation. A trend (*P*=0.059) towards improved OS of the IFN-treated *vs* the observation group was noted as well, although both RFS and OS differences appeared to erode within several years of treatment in this experience. The role of intermediate dose IFN-α2b in high-risk melanoma patients remains to be defined.

It is important to evaluate preliminary reports of any current trial with caution and to avoid interim reports of trials before they reach maturity, save where trials require interruption for outcome differences that an external data safety monitoring committee regards as compelling. There is a tendency to report trials at premature and interim assessments that ought to be eschewed in favor of definitive mature assessments.

FUTURE OUTLOOK

Pegylated IFNs

In an attempt to improve quality of life, optimize patient compliance and improve the integrated 'area under the concentration-time curve' (AUC) of therapy with IFN, longer-acting forms of IFN have been developed through attachment to larger molecules that may serve as a reservoir. Pegylation is the attachment of polyethylene glycol, a linear, hydrophilic, uncharged polymer, to a molecule in order to prolong its pharmacokinetic profile and reduce renal clearance without significant alteration of the volume of distribution. This results in many-fold increase in half life. Two forms of pegylated IFN are commercially available: Pegylated IFN-α2a (Pegasus; Hoffman-La Roche, Nutley, NJ) and pegylated IFN-α2b (PEG-Intron; Schering Plough Corporation, Kenilworth, NJ) that retain antiviral activity at variably diminished levels. A preliminary phase I/II study in a variety of metastatic solid tumors, especially renal cell carcinoma and melanoma, suggests that pegylated IFNs are safe and well-tolerated in advanced solid tumors.[62,63] It remains to be seen whether these forms of IFN-α2 will reach or exceed the antitumor or other effects of recombinant IFN-α2 in randomized controlled studies for melanoma. In the adjuvant setting of node positive melanoma patients the EORTC 18991 trial is currently evaluating the impact of long-term maintenance therapy of 5 years with pegylated-IFNa (PEG-Intron) compared with observation.

Open questions in the adjuvant therapy of melanoma with IFN-α2b

Previous clinical studies raised several interesting questions:

- What is the contribution of the induction phase of the high dose E1684 IFN-α2b regimen to the overall benefit?

Since there was no significant benefit in OS with high dose i.m. IFN-α2a in the NCCTG 83-7052 clinical trial, in which no i.v. induction phase was included, the initial 4-week i.v. phase that has been a cornerstone of E1684, E1690 and E1694 is perhaps not necessary for the benefit observed in E1684. This hypothesis is being tested in two phase III trials, Intergroup E1697 comparing

4 weeks high dose i.v. IFN-α2b in stage T3–T4 or N1 (microscopic) melanoma versus observation and the Sunbelt melanoma trial, where patients are offered 1 month of induction therapy or observation if the sentinel node demonstrates only molecular evidence of tumor involvement by RT-PCR evaluation.

- Is there any additional benefit from combining chemotherapy and other biologicals with IFN?

Studies of metastatic melanoma using combination chemotherapy (cisplatin, vinblastine and dacarbazine, CVD) with biotherapy (IFN-α and interleukin-2) have shown higher response rates (44.8%, $P=0.001$) than IL-2 therapy alone, IL-2 plus IFNa and IL-2 plus chemotherapy in phase II trial.[64] Therefore, biochemotherapy has been tested both in the neoadjuvant setting in node-positive disease in small phase II studies[65,66] and in the adjuvant setting in high risk melanoma. The current Intergroup phase III trial by SWOG (S0008) and joined by ECOG and CALGB tests this regimen for three months *vs* high dose IFN-α2b. Although the results of the latter trial are awaited with interest, initial enthusiasm has been moderated by the results of an Intergroup study in metastatic disease that has shown no survival benefit of biochemotherapy *vs* biotherapy alone.[67]

- Will any subgroups with completely resected melanoma benefit from IFN-α2b more than others?

Sentinel lymph node biopsy, the results of which correlates with DFS and OS, and the preliminary data correlating the molecular detection of melanoma cells by RT-PCR with clinical outcome, challenge the homogeneity of the patient population in ECOG studies 1684, 1690, 1694 and raise the question of whether only some patient subgroups benefit from the relatively toxic regimen. The Sunbelt Melanoma Trial, by using the above described 'ultra-staging', will attempt to identify those patients who may benefit most from adjuvant therapy.[68]

- Is there any additional benefit to be obtained by combining melanoma vaccines with IFN-α2b?

More specific and less toxic than high dose IFN-α2b vaccines have improved DFS or OS. More specifically, stage III melanoma patients with circulating antibodies to GM2 gangliosides, have shown improved RFS.[53] Also, Melacine®, an allogeneic melanoma cell lysate combined with the DETOX adjuvant, has been used in the adjuvant setting with encouraging results.[69] These two vaccines are being tested in a phase III randomized controlled trial setting along with IFN-α2b. Preliminary results from the phase II ECOG trial E2696 show that patients treated with the GMK vaccine (ganglioside GM2 given with bacillus Calmette–Guerin vaccine) combined with IFN-α2b had longer RFS than patients who received the GMK vaccine alone.[70]

Defining subgroups of patients who will most likely respond to IFNs

The obstacle of high dose IFN-α2b toxicity may be overcome by defining patient subgroups that are likely to respond to IFN-α2b. So far, neither disease stage, nor any clinical or demographic feature of melanoma patients has been correlated with favorable response to IFN-α2b. Results from the E2690 laboratory corollary of Intergroup adjuvant trial E1690 show that (a) in the pretreatment tumor biopsies IFN-α2b treatment *in vitro* resulted in upregulation of HLA-DR and downregulation of molecule ICAM, and (b) at 1 month in patients receiving the high dose regimen there was significant elevation of the percentage of CD4+CD3+ (T helper cells).[62,71]

More precise knowledge of the IFN's molecular mechanism of action and novel molecular research tools, such as microarray assays[63,64,72,73] and proteomic spectra in serum generated by mass spectroscopy will hopefully define patient subpopulations with different patterns of natural history and patients in whom therapy is more predictable.[74,75]

REFERENCES

1 Balch CM, Buzaid AC, Soong SJ, et al. Final version of the American Joint Committee on Cancer staging system for cutaneous melanoma. J Clin Oncol 2001; 19(16):3635–3648.

2 Shivers SC, Wang X, Li W, et al. Molecular staging of malignant melanoma: correlation with clinical outcome. JAMA 1998; 280(16):1410–1413.

3 Mellado B, Colomer D, Castel T, et al. Detection of circulating neoplastic cells by reverse-transcriptase polymerase chain reaction in malignant melanoma: association with clinical stage and prognosis. J Clin Oncol 1996; 14(7):2091–2097.

4 Veronesi U, Adamus J, Aubert C, et al. A randomized trial of adjuvant chemotherapy and immunotherapy in cutaneous melanoma. N Engl J Med 1982; 307(15):913–916.

5 Lejeune FJ, Macher E, Kleeberg U, et al. An assessment of DTIC versus levamisole or placebo in the treatment of high risk stage I patients after surgical removal of a primary melanoma of the skin. A phase III adjuvant study. EORTC protocol 18761. Eur J Cancer Clin Oncol 1988; 24(suppl. 2):S81–S90.

6 Fisher RI, Terry WD, Hodes RJ, et al. Adjuvant immunotherapy or chemotherapy for malignant melanoma. Preliminary report of the National Cancer Institute randomised clinical trial. Surg Clin North Am 1981; 61(6):1267–1277.

7 Koops HS, Vaglini M, Suciu S, et al. Prophylactic isolated limb perfusion for localized, high-risk limb melanoma: results of a multicenter randomized phase III trial. European Organization for Research and Treatment of Cancer Malignant Melanoma Cooperative Group Protocol 18832, the World Health Organization Melanoma Program Trial 15, and the North American Perfusion Group Southwest Oncology Group-8593. J Clin Oncol 1998; 16(9):2906–2912.

8 Meisenberg BR, Ross M, Vredenburgh JJ, et al. Randomized trial of high-dose chemotherapy with autologous bone marrow support as adjuvant therapy for high-risk, multi-node-positive malignant melanoma. J Natl Cancer Inst 1993; 85(13):1080–1085.

9 Meyskens FL Jr, Liu PY, Tuthill RJ, et al. Randomized trial of vitamin A versus observation as adjuvant therapy in high-risk primary malignant melanoma: a Southwest Oncology Group study. J Clin Oncol 1994; 12 (10):2060–2065.

10 Markovic S, Suman VJ, Dalton RJ, et al. Randomized, placebo-controlled, phase III surgical adjuvant clinical trial of megestrol acetate (Megace) in selected patients with malignant melanoma. Am J Clin Oncol 2002; 25(6):552–556.

11 Carnetzki BM, Macher E, Suciu S, Thomas D, Steerenberg PA, Rumke P. Long-term adjuvant immunotherapy in stage I high risk malignant melanoma, comparing two BCG preparations versus non-treatment in a randomized multicentre study (EORTC Protocol 18781). Eur J Cancer 1993; 29A(9):1237–1242.

12 Paterson AH, Willans DJ, Jerry LM, Hanson J, McPherson TA. Adjuvant BCG immunotherapy for malignant melanoma. Can Med Assoc J 1984; 131(7):744–748.

13 Balch CM, Smalley RV, Bartolucci AA, Burns D, Presant CA, Durant JR. A randomized prospective clinical trial of adjuvant *C. parvum* immunotherapy in 260 patients with clinically localized melanoma (Stage I): prognostic factors analysis and preliminary results of immunotherapy. Cancer 1982; 49(6):1079–1084.

14 Lipton A, Harvey HA, Balch CM, Antle CE, Heckerd R, Bartolucci AA. *Corynebacterium parvum* versus bacille Calmette–Guerin adjuvant immunotherapy of stage II malignant melanoma. J Clin Oncol 1991; 9(7):1151–1156.

15 Quirt IC, Shelley WE, Pater JL, et al. Improved survival in patients with poor-prognosis malignant melanoma treated with adjuvant levamisole: a phase III study by the National Cancer Institute of Canada Clinical Trials Group. J Clin Oncol 1991; 9(5):729–735.

16 Spitler LE. A randomized trial of levamisole versus placebo as adjuvant therapy in malignant melanoma. J Clin Oncol 1991; 9(5):735–740.

17 Miller LL, Spitler LE, Allen RE, Minor DR. A randomized, double-blind, placebo-controlled trial of transfer factor as adjuvant therapy for malignant melanoma. J Clin Oncol 1991; 9(5):735–740.

18 Sondak VK, Liu PY, Tuthill RJ, et al. Adjuvant immunotherapy of resected, intermediate-thickness, node-negative melanoma with an allogeneic tumor vaccine: overall results of a randomized trial of the Southwest Oncology Group. J Clin Oncol 2002; 20(8):2058–2066.

19 Hersey P, Coates AS, McCarthy WH, et al. Adjuvant immunotherapy of patients with high-risk melanoma using vaccinia viral lysates of melanoma: results of a randomized trial. J Clin Oncol 2002; 20(20):4181–4190.

20 Wallack MK, Sivanandham M, Balch CM, et al. Surgical adjuvant active specific immunotherapy for patients with stage III melanoma: the final analysis of data from a phase III, randomized, double-blind, multicenter vaccinia melanoma oncolysate trial. J Am Coll Surg 1998; 187(1):69–77.

21 Wallack MK, Sivanandham M, Balch CM, et al. A phase III randomized, double-blind multi-institutional trial of vaccinia melanoma oncolysate-active specific immunotherapy for patients with stage II melanoma. Cancer 1995; 75(1):34–42.

22 Livingston PO, Wong GY, Adhuri S, et al. Improved survival in stage III melanoma patients with GM2 antibodies: a randomized trial of adjuvant vaccination with GM2 ganglioside. J Clin Oncol 1994; 12(5):1036–1044.

23 Bystryn JC, Zeleniuch-Jacquotte A, Oratz R, Shapiro RL, Harris MN, Roses DF. Double-blind trial of a polyvalent, shed-antigen, melanoma vaccine. Clin Cancer Res 2001; 7(7):1882–1887.

24 Retsas S, Quigley M, Pectasides D, Macrae K, Henry K. Clinical and histologic involvement of regional lymph nodes in malignant melanoma. Adjuvant vindesine improves survival. Cancer 1994; 73(8):2119–2130.

25 Minev BR. Melanoma vaccines. Semin Oncol 2002; 29(5):479–493.

26 Morton DL, Hsueh EC, Essner R, et al. Prolonged survival of patients receiving active immunotherapy with Canvaxin therapeutic polyvalent vaccine after complete resection of melanoma metastatic to regional lymph nodes. Ann Surg 2002; 48(9):438–448.

27 Hall S. A commotion in the blood. Life, death, and the immune system. New York, NY: Henry Holt; 1997.

28 Stark GR, Kerr IM, Williams BR, Silverman RH, Schreiber RD. How cells respond to interferons. Annu Rev Biochem 1998; 67:227–264.

29 Veer MJ de, Holko M, Frevel M, et al. Functional classification of interferon-stimulated genes identified using microarrays. J Leukoc Biol 2001; 69(6):912–920.

30 Belardelli F, Ferrantini M. Cytokines as a link between innate and adaptive antitumor immunity. Trends Immunol 2002; 23(4):201–208.

31 Zou W, Machelon V, Coulomb-L Hermin A, et al. Stromal-derived factor-1 in human tumors recruits and alters the function of plasmacytoid precursor dendritic cells. Nat Med 2001; 7(12):1339–1346.

32 Gresser I, Belardelli F. Endogenous type I interferons as a defense against tumors. Cytokine Growth Factor Rev 2002; 13(2):111–118.

33 McCarty MF, Bielenberg D, Donawho C, Bucana CD, Fidler IJ. Evidence for the causal role of endogenous interferon-alpha/beta in the regulation of angiogenesis, tumorigenicity, and metastasis of cutaneous neoplasms. Clin Exp Metastasis 2002; 19(7):609–615.

34 Grander D, Sangfelt O, Erickson S. How does interferon exert its cell growth inhibitory effect? Eur J Haematol 1997; 59(3):129–135.

35 Thyrell L, Erickson S, Zhivotovsky B, et al. Mechanisms of Interferon-alpha induced apoptosis in malignant cells. Oncogene 2002; 21(8):1251–1262.

36 Kirkwood JM, Ernstoff MS, Davis CA, et al. Comparison of intramuscular and intravenous recombinant alpha-2 interferon in melanoma and other cancers. Ann Intern Med 1985; 103(1):32–36.

37 Ernstoff MS, Reiss M, Davis CA, Rudnick SA, Kirkwood JM. Intravenous (IV) recombinant alpha-2 interferon (IFNα-2) in metastatic melanoma (abstr C-222). Proc Am Soc Clin Oncol 1983; 2:57.

38 Creagan ET, Ahmann DL, Green SJ, et al. Phase II study of recombinant leukocyte A interferon (r-IFN-A) in disseminated malignant melanoma. Cancer 1984; 54:2844–2849.

39 Creagan ET, Ahmann DL, Green SJ, Long HJ, Frytak S, Itri LM. Phase II study of recombinant leukocyte A interferon (IFN-rA) plus cimetidine in disseminated malignant melanoma. J Clin Oncol 1985; 3(7):977–981.

40 Creagan ET, Ahmann DL, Green SJ, et al. Phase II study of low-dose recombinant leukocyte A interferon in disseminated malignant melanoma. J Clin Oncol 1984; 2(9):1002–1005.

41 Legha SS, Papadopoulos NE, Plager C, et al. Clinical evaluation of recombinant interferon alfa-2a (Roferon-A) in metastatic melanoma using two different schedules. J Clin Oncol 1987; 5(8):1240–1246.

42 Hersey P, Hasic E, MacDonald M, et al. Effects of recombinant leukocyte interferon (rIFN-alpha A) on tumour growth and immune responses in patients with metastatic melanoma. Br J Cancer 1985; 51(6):815–826.

43 Neefe JR, Legha SS, Markowitz A, et al. Phase II study of recombinant alpha-interferon in malignant melanoma. Am J Clin Oncol 1990; 13(6):472–476.

44 Dorval T, Palangie T, Jouve M, et al. Clinical phase II trial of recombinant DNA interferon (Interferon alpha 2b) in patients with metastatic malignant melanoma. Cancer 1986; 58(2):215–218.

45 Coates A, Rallings M, Hersey P, Swanson C. Phase-II study of recombinant alpha 2-interferon in advanced malignant melanoma. J Interferon Res 1986; 6(1):1–4.

46 Kirkwood JM, Strawderman MH, Ernstoff MS, et al. Interferon alfa-2b adjuvant therapy of high-risk resected cutaneous melanoma: the Eastern Cooperative Oncology Group Trial EST 1684. J Clin Oncol 1996; 14(1):7–17.

47 Kirkwood JM, Ibrahim JG, Sondak VK, et al. High- and low-dose interferon alfa-2b in high-risk melanoma: first analysis of intergroup trial E1690/S9111/C9190. J Clin Oncol 2000; 18(12):2444–2458.

48 Kirkwood JM, Ibrahim JG, Sosman JA, et al. High-dose interferon alfa-2b significantly prolongs relapse-free and overall survival compared with the GM2-KLH/QS-21 vaccine in patients with resected stage IIB–III melanoma: results of intergroup trial E1694/S9512/C509801. J Clin Oncol 2001; 19(9):2370–2380.

49 Creagan ET, Dalton RJ, Ahmann DL, et al. Randomized, surgical adjuvant clinical trial of recombinant interferon alfa-2a in selected patients with malignant melanoma. J Clin Oncol 1995; 13(11):2776–2783.

50 Cascinelli N, Bufalino R, Morabito A, Mackie R. Results of adjuvant interferon study in WHO melanoma programme. Lancet 1994; 343(8902):913–914.

51 Cascinelli N, Belli F, MacKie RM, et al. Effect of long-term adjuvant therapy with interferon alpha-2a in patients with regional node metastases from cutaneous melanoma: a randomised trial. Lancet 2001; 358(9285):866–869.

52 Helling F, Zhang S, Shang A, et al. GM2-KLH conjugate vaccine: increased immunogenicity in melanoma patients after administration with immunological adjuvant QS-21. Cancer Res 1995; 55(13):2783–2788.

53 Livingston PO, Wong GY, Adluri S, et al. Improved survival in stage III melanoma patients with GM2 antibodies: a randomized trial of adjuvant vaccination with GM2 ganglioside. J Clin Oncol 1994; 12(5):1036–1044.

54 Kirkwood JM, Bender C, Agarwala S, et al. Mechanisms and management of toxicities associated with high-dose interferon alfa-2b therapy. J Clin Oncol 2002; 20(17):3703–3718.

55 Cole BF, Gelber RD, Kirkwood JM, et al. Quality-of-life-adjusted survival analysis of interferon alfa-2b adjuvant treatment of high-risk resected cutaneous melanoma: an Eastern Cooperative Oncology Group study. J Clin Oncol 1996; 14(10):2666–2673.

56 Kilbridge KL, Cole BF, Kirkwood JM, et al. Quality-of-life-adjusted survival analysis of high-dose adjuvant interferon alpha-2b for high-risk melanoma patients using intergroup clinical trial data. J Clin Oncol 2002; 20(5):1311–1318.

57 Hancock BW, Wheatley K, Harris S, et al. AIM HIGH: Adjuvant interferon in Melanoma (HIGH risk) – United Kingdom Coordinating Committee on Cancer Research randomized study of adjuvant low dose extended duration interferon alfa 2a in high risk resected malignant melanoma. J Clin Oncol 2003; 22(1): 53–61.

58 Eggermont AMM, Kleeberg UR, Ruiter DJ, Suciu S. The European Organization for research and Treatment of Cancer Melanoma Group Trial Experience with more than 2000 patients evaluating adjuvant therapy treatment with low or intermediate doses of interferon Alpha-2b. Alexandria, VA: ASCO; 2001.

59 Cameron DA, Cornbleet MC, Mackie RM, et al. Adjuvant interferon alpha 2b in high risk melanoma – the Scottish study. Br J Cancer 2001; 84(9):1146–1149.

60 Pehamberger H, Soyer HP, Steiner A, et al. Adjuvant interferon alfa-2a treatment in resected primary stage II cutaneous melanoma. Austrian Malignant Melanoma Coop Group. J Clin Oncol 1998; 16(4):1425–1429.

61 Grob JJ, Dreno B, Salmoniere P de la, et al. Randomised trial of interferon alpha-2a as adjuvant therapy in resected primary melanoma thicker than 1.5 mm without clinically detectable node metastases. French Cooperative Group on Melanoma. Lancet 1998; 351(9120):1905–1910.

62 Motzer RJ, Rakhit A, Ginsberg M, et al. Phase I trial of 40-kD branched pegylated interferon alfa-2a for patients with advanced renal cell carcinoma. J Clin Oncol 2001; 19(5):1312–1319.

63 Bukowski R, Ernstoff MS, Gore ME, et al. Pegylated interferon alfa-2b treatment for patients with solid tumors: a phase I/II study. J Clin Oncol 2002; 20(18):3841–3849.

64 Legha SS, Ring S, Eton O, et al. Development of a biochemotherapy regimen with concurrent administration of cisplatin, vinblastine, dacarbazine, interferon alfa, and interleukin-2 for patients with metastatic melanoma. J Clin Oncol 1998; 16(5):1752–1759.

65 Buzaid AC, Colome M, Bedikian A, et al. Phase II study of neoadjuvant concurrent biochemotherapy in melanoma patients with local-regional metastases. Melanoma Res 1998; 8(6):549–556.

66 Gibbs P, Anderson C, Pearlman N, et al. A phase II study of neoadjuvant biochemotherapy for stage III melanoma. Cancer 2002; 94(2):470–476.

67 Keilholz U, Gore ME. Biochemotherapy for advanced melanoma. Semin Oncol 2002; 29(5):456–461.

68 McMasters KM. The Sunbelt Melanoma Trial. Ann Surg Oncol 2001; 8(9):41S–43S.

69 Mitchell MS, Darrah D, Stevenson L. Therapy of melanoma with allogeneic melanoma lysates alone or with interferon-alfa. Cancer Invest 2002; 20(5/6):759–768.

70 Kirkwood JM, Ibrahim J, Lawson DH, et al. High-dose interferon alfa-2b does not diminish antibody response to GM2 vaccination in patients with resected melanoma: results of the Multicenter Eastern Cooperative Oncology Group Phase II Trial E2696. J Clin Oncol 2001; 19(5):1430–1436.

71 Kirkwood JM, Richards T, Zarour HM, et al. Immunomodulatory effects of high-dose and low-dose interferon alpha2b in patients with high-risk resected melanoma: the E2690 laboratory corollary of intergroup adjuvant trial E1690. Cancer 2002; 95(5):1101–1112.

72 Certa U, Seiler M, Padovan E, Spagnoli GC. High density oligonucleotide array analysis of interferon-alpha2a sensitivity and transcriptional response in melanoma cells. Br J Cancer 2001; 85(1):107–114.

73 Veer MJ de, Holko M, Frevel M, et al. Functional classification of interferon-stimulated genes identified using microarrays. J Leukoc Biol 2001; 69(6):912–920.

74 Barthe C, Mahon FX, Gharbi MJ, et al. Expression of interferon-alpha (IFN-alpha) receptor 2c at diagnosis is associated with cytogenetic response in IFN-alpha-treated chronic myeloid leukemia. Blood 2001; 97(11):3568–3573.

75 Petricoin EF, Ardekani AM, Hitt BA, et al. Use of proteomic patterns in serum to identify ovarian cancer. Lancet 2002; 359(9306):572–577.

CHAPTER
53

The Treatment of Disseminated Melanoma

Andrew Pippas and Douglas S Reintgen

Key points

- Chemotherapy has not been very effective for the treatment of disseminated melanoma.
- Multi-agent chemotherapy protocols when compared with single agent studies for Stage IV melanoma have generally given better response rates but similar survival.
- Surgical resection of isolated Stage IV melanoma is a reasonable alternative to consider, particularly if the patient can be rendered free of disease.
- Immunotherapy agents have shown activity in metastatic melanoma. Interferon alfa-2b is an approved adjuvant therapy for resected Stage III melanoma and high dose interleukin-2 therapy for Stage IV disease can give response rates of 16% with durable complete response rates of 6%.

INTRODUCTION

Melanoma spreads both through the lymphatic system and the bloodstream and this feature explains the distinction between melanoma and other skin cancers. In fact, it is rare for squamous cell carcinomas and basal cell carcinomas of the skin to metastasize. Treatment for the primary melanoma is directed both at providing local control and preventing distant, systemized progression. Although surgery can cure 90% of patients with superficial lesions, the prognosis remains very poor in patients with locally advanced, disseminated or recurrent systemic disease.

EPIDEMIOLOGY

In the US and Canada, the incidence of melanoma has increased at a rate greater than all other malignancies, except lung cancer in women. In 2002, approximately 5% of patients were diagnosed with Stage IV (systemic metastases) melanoma at diagnosis and another 15–20% of all melanoma patients will eventually experience Stage IV disease. Systemic spread is felt by many oncologists to be incurable and the 5-year survival supports this supposition and is currently a poor 3%. The second significant feature of melanoma is the relatively young age of onset. The median age of patients entering clinical trials is 45–55 years. Advanced melanoma rates second

to leukemia in terms of years of lost life[1] and is a significant public health problem for the US, even more so than some of the more common cancers that physicians deal with such as breast and colon cancer.

PROGNOSTIC FACTORS IN THE METASTATIC (STAGE IV) SETTING

The 2002 revised version of the AJCC staging system for Stage IV melanoma incorporates two prognostic factors: site(s) of metastasis and elevated LDH.[2] Patients with distant metastasis to skin, non-regional lymph nodes or subcutaneous tissue, have a better prognosis than patients with metastasis at *any* other sites. The serum LDH has been identified recently as the most predictive independent factor for reduced survival in multivariate analysis for this stage of melanoma. Patients with an elevated LDH and Stage IV disease have a very poor prognosis (Fig. 53.1).

Additional favorable factors identified by the Eastern Cooperative Oncology Group (ECOG) in reviewing patients entering their clinical trials was normal appetite, absence of nausea, vomiting or fever, and normal performance status at the time of diagnosis of Stage IV disease.[3]

TREATMENT OPTIONS

Surgery

Surgical removal of Stage IV metastatic deposits should be considered in all patients with limited metastatic disease. Several series have shown 5-year survival rates of approximately 20% in patients taken to surgery with the intent of achieving a complete resection (Table 53.1). This is comparable with the benefit achieved in patients who have an isolated, palpable regional nodal reoccurrence who undergo a complete lymphadenectomy. The complete response rate achieved with surgical resection is better than anything that can be achieved with a systemic therapy.

Patients with pulmonary lesions are often asymptomatic and clinicians must remember that a third of patients with a history of melanoma and lung nodules have other reasons for their lung findings (either benign disease or new lung primary cancers). In a large series of patients from a single institution, 2% (34/1750) of patients were able to undergo surgery for apparent liver

655

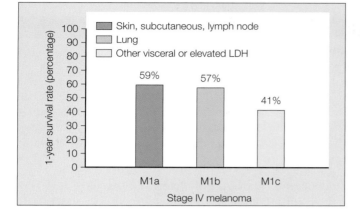

Figure 53.1 Comparison of 1-year survival rates in patients with advanced melanoma.

Table 53.2 Common chemotherapy agents used in advanced melanoma and their effectiveness[23]

Agent	Response (%)	Comment
Dacarbazine	20 (5% complete response)	Inexpensive
BCNU	18	Lipophilic
Fotemustine	10–20	High hepatic extraction rate
Cisplatin	15–23	No difference between 100 vs 200 mg/m²
Vinblastine	12	

Table 53.1 Survival in melanoma patients with resected metastatic disease by anatomic site[20–22]

Site of metastasis	5-year survival (%)
Non-visceral	10–61
Pulmonary	21
Gastrointestinal	26
Hepatic	29
Pancreas	24

only metastasis. Of the 18 patients with a complete resection, 29% were alive at 5 years representing only 0.5% of the initial cohort. In addition, the majority of these patients received post-surgical vaccines or chemotherapy. This analysis reveals the limitation of surgery for most patients with Stage IV disease. Only a tiny minority of Stage IV patients present with resectable disease and only 20–30% of these patients will be alive at 5 years.

Cytotoxic therapy

Single agent chemotherapy

Multiple agents have been used in metastatic melanoma. Many of these drugs have been available for over 20 years and have modest activity. Table 53.2 outlines the most common agents, their efficacy and unique features.

Unlike other malignancies such as breast or lung cancer where newer agents such as the taxanes have demonstrated an improvement in efficacy as third generation drugs, the treatment of melanoma has not seen an analogous advancement in effective drug development. Temozolomide is a pro-drug that converts rapidly at physiologic pH to form MTIC, the active moiety of dacarbazine (DTIC). Unlike DTIC, temozolomide crosses the blood–brain barrier and is converted to MTIC. Although temozolomide has activity against a wide variety of CNS tumors, including gliomas, its activity in Phase I–III studies of melanoma has been equal to DTIC.

Cytotoxic chemotherapy

Combination therapy

Several combinations of agents with non-overlapping toxicities have been designed for treatment of Stage IV metastatic melanoma. Most regimens have DTIC as the principle agent with the addition of one to three other drugs. Examples as shown in Table 53.3.[4]

Initial reports from single institutions have usually demonstrated encouraging high response rates with these multiple agent combinations. The BOLD (bleomycin, oncovin, lomustine, dacarbazine or DTIC) chemotherapy regimen was initially described at Duke University and gave response rates of 25–30%. Subsequently the Dartmouth protocol was described (cisplatin, DTIC, bleomycin, tamoxifen) and had a 55% response rate in initial reports from single institutions and was considered in the 1980s to be a standard regimen. Unfortunately when studied in multi-institutional settings, response rates were lower.

An analysis of the addition of various chemotherapy agents with activity against melanoma to DTIC has failed to demonstrate a synergistic benefit (Table 53.4).[5]

Randomized trials of DTIC vs poly-chemotherapy have been conducted in community and cooperative group settings, demonstrating slightly higher response rates for multi-agent treatment. Nonetheless, the largest trial randomized 240 patients to either the Dartmouth regimen or DTIC and demonstrated no survival advantage (7 month median survival).[6] Furthermore, a higher response rate (18.5% vs 10.2%) did not achieve statistical significance for the Dartmouth combination. As a result of this trial, most medical oncologists have accepted that combination chemotherapy has yet to be proven superior to DTIC.

Immunotherapy

Interferon and interleukin-2

The suggestion that melanoma may respond to immunotherapy protocols stems from several observations. Up to 5% of patients with metastatic melanoma have no identifiable cutaneous primary. This suggests that the primary site has regressed by inherent immune activity but the metastatic cells change in a way to evade the

Table 53.3 Response rates with combination chemotherapeutic agents[4,24]

Regimen	Response (%)
BOLD (1980)	22–44
CDBT (1984, Dartmouth)	15–55
CVD (1989)	20–40

Table 53.4 Response rates for DTIC in combination with other chemotherapeutic agents[5]

Regimen	Response (%)	No.
DTIC + VA/CDDP/Nu/Nu	19	1147
DTIC + two agents	25	1662
DTIC + three agents	30	440

Table 53.5 Randomized trials comparing either chemotherapy (DTIC or combination treatment) or chemotherapy with IFN have not demonstrated an improvement in response rate or survival[8]

Regimen	No.	DTIC response (%)	Survival (months)
DTIC	69	15	10
DTIC + IFN	68	21	9.3
DTIC + tamoxifen	66	18	8.0
DTIC + IFN + tamoxifen	68	19	9.1
		P=NS	P=NS

immune system, grow, and cause a clinical recurrence. Also, up to 20% of biopsies from melanoma lesions demonstrate areas of spontaneous regression.[7]

The two most studied immune modulating agents are the interferons and interleukin-2. The efficacy of IFN in the treatment of melanoma is reviewed in greater detail in Chapter 52. High dose interferon α (IFN) has anti-proliferative effects and low dose IFN has anti-angiogenic properties. IFN also has immune modulating effects by causing an increase in natural killer cell activity suggesting that its mechanism of action is multi-modal.

Investigators have had difficulty in establishing a clear dose–response relationship between IFN and melanoma. IFN has not been consistently shown to manifest clinical efficacy as a single agent in Stage IV disease. This is in contradistinction to national multi-center studies through the ECOG cooperative group that have shown efficacy for high dose interferon alfa-2b used as an adjuvant in resected Stage III melanoma (regional nodal disease). Response rates in Phase I–II studies vary between 5–15% in patients treated with widely varying doses (3 million units/day to 15 million units/m² per day). With the exception of a single clinical trial reported in 1991, multiple randomized trials of either chemotherapy (DTIC or combination treatment) or chemotherapy with IFN have not demonstrated an improvement in response rate or survival.[8]

A large Phase III trial (ECOG 3698) has been recently reported (Table 53.5).[8] This study confirmed the absence of benefit for IFN when added to DTIC.

Interleukin 2 (IL-2), a T cell growth factor, was identified in 1976. It has no direct cytotoxic effects on melanoma cells. The therapeutic effects of IL-2 are mediated by activating natural killer (NK) cells to form lymphokine activated killer (LAK) cells which have been shown to lyse melanoma cells *in vitro* and *in vivo*. In addition, IL-2 generates nitric oxide, which is felt to augment anti-tumor efficiency.

The multi-factorial effects of high dose IL-2 contribute to its toxicity which limits its use in community settings.

More recently, however, these effects have significantly diminished by screening patients for adequate cardiac and pulmonary function. Also, increased experience with the agent and reducing the mean number of doses (from 13 to 8) given during the first cycle have had favorable effects in this area (Table 53.6).[9]

The response to high dose IL-2 has been updated based on multi-institutional experience in 270 patients with long follow-up.[9] The complete response rate in patients with disseminated disease is 6% with a partial response of 10%. More importantly, the median duration of response has not been reached in CR patients; disease progression was not observed in any patient who had responded for longer than 30 months. Response rates have been associated with site of Stage IV disease (subcutaneous only – 53%, distant lymph node only – 22%, visceral – 16%), the amount of lymphocytosis generated post-treatment and the development of vitiligo in the patient.[10]

Bio-chemotherapy

Pre-clinical rationale

Given the modest efficacy of either single or combination chemotherapy or immunotherapy alone, bio-chemotherapy has been pursued in an attempt to enhance tumor response by combining classes of agents with different mechanisms and non-overlapping toxicities. *In vitro* and early clinical data demonstrated that treatment with cisplatin did not compromise the ability to generate NK and LAK cell responses to IL-2. Clinical trials have shown treatment with IL-2 and IFNα did not have a negative impact in the likelihood of responding to chemotherapy.[11] Multiple IL-2 based regimens have been published using a variety of chemotherapeutic agents in combination.[12] Multiple regimens using IL-2 given subcutaneously or via a continuous infusion have also been published.

The largest experience with bio-chemotherapy comes from the MD Anderson Phase II trials.[13] Toxicities were substantial with a 64% incidence of neutropenic fever, 54% incidence of bacteremia and a 50% incidence of thrombocytopenia requiring transfusions. A modified (cisplatin, velban, dacabazine) CVD-BIO regimen reduced the dose of velban to a total of 4.8 mg/u² per cycle, added

657

Table 53.6 Decrease in significant side effect of IL-2 therapy in advanced melanoma patients over time[9]

Event	1985 Incidence (%)	1997 Incidence (%)
Hypotension	81	31
Neuro-psychiatric changes	19	8
Line sepsis	16	4
Pulmonary edema	12	3
Death	1–3	<0.1

Table 53.8 Response rates and survival using bio-chemotherapy[11]

	No.	Objective response (%)	Survival (months)
IL-2	710	15	8.0
IL-2/IFN	911	17	11.0
IL-2/CT	523	22	9.4
CT	4426	29	8.6
IL-2/IFN/CT	1141	41	9.8
		$P<0.0001$	NS

Note no difference in survival among the evaluated protocols.

Table 53.7 Response rates for bio-chemotherapy protocols[12]

Regimen	Patients	Complete	Partial	Overall
CVD/IL-2 CIV/IFN	53	21	43	64
CVD/IL-2 CIV/IFN	40	20	28	48
CVD/Tamoxifen/IL-2/IFN	45	23	34	52
CBDT/IL-2 Subcut/IFN	53	19	23	42

C, Cisplatin; V, Velban; D, DTIC; B, BCNU.

Table 53.9 NIH study showing improved survival using bio-chemotherapy[13]

Regimen	No.	Complete response (%)	RR (%)	Survival (weeks)
CVD	92	2	25	9.2
CVD-BIO	91	7	48	11.9
		$P=0.001$		$P=0.06$

prophylactic GCSF support and reduced the number of cycles from six to four in the hope of improving tolerance and preserving response. Unfortunately, as had been seen in other Phase II trials, this regimen had a high incidence (11/19 responding patients) of CNS metastasis as the first site of relapse (Table 53.7).[12,14]

The initial assessment of bio-chemotherapy was a significant improvement in response rates compared with either chemotherapy or immunotherapy alone in patients with advanced melanoma. A meta-analysis of 7711 patients found the highest response rate for bio-chemotherapy. Unfortunately, overall survival did not improve using these therapeutic approaches (Table 53.8).[11]

Several large randomized trials of bio-chemotherapy compared with chemotherapy alone have been conducted. The National Institutes of Health (NIH) reported on 102 patients randomized to cisplatin, dacarbazine and tamoxifen or the same chemotherapy with high-dose IL-2 and interferon added. Neither response rates nor survival differed significantly.[15] More recently, the MD Anderson Cancer Center experience using sequential CVD-BIO (a regimen in a phase 2 setting) has shown significantly improved overall response rates compared with CVD alone (Table 53.9).[13]

Although response rates nearly doubled in the CVD-BIO arm, survival in the combination arm did not quite achieve statistical significance. By comparison with earlier phase 2 studies, the CR rates were also dramatically lower reflecting the inclusion of patients treated adjuvantly with interferon who had failed this systemic therapy. An additional disturbing finding was the development of brain metastasis in 40% of these patients.

The modified CVD-BIO regimen developed by Atkins et al. had demonstrated similar response rates to 'standard'

CDV-BIO with less neutropenia, hypotension, and gastrointestinal toxicity.[16] These improvements made it possible to test bio-chemotherapy in a multi-institutional, cooperative group setting (Intergroup trial E3695). The final results of this important study are pending at the time of this writing. Preliminary results, however, indicate no improvement in overall survival or time to progression in favor of the CVD-BIO regimen.

CURRENT STANDARDS OF THERAPY FOR DISSEMINATED MELANOMA

The absence of active chemotherapy or immunotherapy for metastatic melanoma makes selecting a course of therapy for an individual patient difficult. Nonetheless, several guidelines can be established:

- All patients should be considered for metastasectomy since patients who are able to undergo a complete resection may have a 20–25% 5-year survival.
- Single agent chemotherapy with DTIC/temozolomide confers the same survival benefit as multi-agent chemotherapy and is appropriate for poor performance patients.
- Multi-agent chemotherapy or bio-chemotherapy has higher response rates than single-agent treatment. This approach is useful in patients with symptomatic metastatic disease.
- High dose IL-2 should be considered for all patients with a good performance status.

FUTURE OUTLOOK

Future research will hopefully unlock some of the mysteries of advanced melanoma and lead to more effective therapies than are currently available today. Several experimental approaches for patients with disseminated disease are currently being investigated.

Vaccines in Stage IV melanoma have shown in phase II studies response rates of 10–15%. Two recent studies have used an autologously derived tumor-heat shock protein (HSP96) peptide vaccine producing 2 CR and 3 stable disease in 28 patients with very long response durations.[17] Canvaxin (Cancer-Vax), an irradiated preparation of whole melanoma cell from three allogenic cell lines, has shown 5-year survival rates of 39% compared with 19% for closely matched historical controls.[18] Both vaccines are undergoing phase III evaluation in national multi-center studies.

Novel chemotherapeutic approaches include the combination of docetaxel and temozolomide as first line therapy, showing 27% overall response with only 8% of patients developing CNS metastasis. This is far fewer than the 40–60% of patients with CNS relapse in other clinical trials of Stage IV therapy.[19]

In melanoma cells, BCL2, a proto-oncogene which can block apoptosis, is expressed in up to 100% of cases. Over-expression of BCL2 has been associated with chemo-resistance. A phase I-II using an anti-sense oligonucleotide against BCL-2 mRNA showed a 40% decline in BCL-2 protein expressed in melanoma cells with increased tumor-cell apoptosis, further augmented by dacarbazine treatment. A phase III trial of front line therapy with either DTIC vs DTIC and anti-sense BCL2 oligonucleotide is ongoing.

Thalidomide, an inhibitor of TNF-α, has been studied in varying doses with limited benefit. Nonetheless, the combination of thalidomide and temozolomide given in a prolonged schedule has shown response rates of 20–30% in patients with both visceral and CNS metastasis. Revimid, a more potent analog of thalidomide, has shown activity in phase I studies. Both agents are being studied in ongoing phase III studies.

REFERENCES

1 Flaherty L. Rationale for Intergroup Trial E3695. Comparing concurrent biochemotherapy with Cisplatin, Vinblastine and DTIC alone in patients with metastatic melanoma. Cancer J Sci Am 2000; 6(Suppl 11):515–520.

2 Balch CM, Buzard AL, Soong SJ, et al. Final version of the American Joint Committee on cancer staging system for cutaneous melanoma. J Clin Oncol 2001; 19:3635–3648.

3 Ryan L, Kramer A, Border E. Prognostic factors in metastatic melanoma. Cancer 1993; 71:2995.

4 Philip A, Flaherty L. Biochemotherapy for melanoma. Cur Onc Rep 2000; 2:314–321.

5 Nathan FE, Benet D, Mastrangeto MJ. Chemotherapy of melanoma. In: Perry MC, ed. Chemotherapy Source Book. Philadelphia, PA: Williams and Williams; 1997:1043–1069.

6 Atkins MB, Gollob JA. Chemotherapy and cytokine-based immunotherapy for high risk and metastatic melanoma. Advances in Oncology 2001; 15:22–29.

7 Crowson AN, Magro CM, Barnhill RL, Mihm MC. Pathology. In: Balch CM, Houghton AN, Sober AJ, Soong SJ (eds). Cutaneous Melanoma. 4th edition. St Louis, MO: Quality Medical Publishing; 2003: 171–206.

8 Falkson CI, Ibrahim J, Kirkwood JM, et al. Phase III trial of Dacarbazine versus Dacarbazine with interferon α-2b and Tamoxifen in patients with metastatic malignant melanoma. An Eastern Cooperative Oncology Group Study. J Clin Oncol 1998; 16:1743–1751.

9 Atkins MB, Lotze MT, Dutcher JP, et al. High-dose recombinant interleukin 2 therapy for patients with metastatic melanoma analysis of 270 patients treated between 1985 and 1993. J Clin Oncol 1999; 17:2105–2116.

10 Schwartzentruber DJ, Rosenberg SA. Interleukins. In: Balch CM, Houghton AN, Sober AJ, Soong SJ. Cutaneous Melanoma. 4th edition. St Louis, MO: Quality Medical Publishing; 2003: 623–643.

11 Allen LE, Kupelnick B, Kumashiro M. Efficiency of Interleukin-2 in the treatment of metastatic melanoma; systematic review and meta-analysis. Cancer 1998; 1:168–173.

12 Lotze MT, Dallal RM, Kirkwood JM, et al. Cutaneous melanoma. In: Devita VT, Hellman S, Rosenberg SA, eds. Cancer Principles and Practice of Oncology, 6th edn. Philadelphia, PA: JB Lippincott; 2001:2012–2069.

13 Eton O, Legha SS, Bedikian AY, et al. Sequential bio-chemotherapy versus chemotherapy for metastatic melanoma; results from a phase III randomized trial. J Clin Oncol 2002; 20:2045–2052.

14 McDermott DF, Mier JW, Lawrence DP, et al. A phase II pilot trial of concurrent bio-chemotherapy with Cisplatin, Vinblastine, Dacarbazine, interleukin-2 and interferon α-2b in patient with metastatic melanoma. Clin Cancer Res 2000; 6:2201–2208.

15 Rosenberg SA, Yang JC, Schwartzentuber DJ, et al. Prospective randomized trial of patients with metastatic melanoma using chemotherapy with Cisplatin, Dacarbazine and Tamoxifen alone or in combination with Interleukin-2 and Interferon alfa-2b. J Clin Oncol 1999; 17:968–975.

16 Atkins MB. The treatment of metastatic melanoma with chemotherapy and biologics. Curr Opin Oncol 1997; 9:205–213.

17 Belli F, Testori A, Rivoltini L, et al. Vaccination of metastatic melanoma patients with autologous tumor derived heat shock protein gp96-peptide complexes: clinical and immunologic findings. J Clin Oncol 2002; 20:4169–4180.

18 Hsueh EC, Essner R, Foshag LJ, et al. Prolonged survival after complete resection of disseminated melanoma and active immunotherapy with a therapeutic cancer vaccine. J Clin Oncol 2002; 20:4549–4554.

19 Bafaloukos D, Gogas H, Georgoulias V, et al. Temozolomide in combination with docetaxel in patients with advanced melanoma: a phase II study of the Hellenic Cooperative Oncology Group. J Clin Oncol 2002; 20(2): 420–425.

20 Rose DM, Essner R, Hughes MD, et al. Surgical resection for metastatic melanoma to the liver. Arch Surg 2001; 136: 950–955.

21 de Wilt JHW, McCarthy WH, Thompson JF. Surgical treatment of splenic metastases in patients with melanoma. J Am Coll Surg 2003; 197: 38–43.

22 Reintgen DS, Thompson W, Garbutt J, Seigler HF. Radiologic, endoscopic and surgical considerations of melanoma metastatic to the gastrointestinal tract. Surgery 1984; 95: 635–639.

23 Atkins MB, Buzaid AC, Houghton AN. Chemotherapy and biochemotherapy. In: Balch CM, Houghton AN, Sober AJ, Soong SJ (eds). Cutaneous Melanoma. 4th edition. St Louis, MO: Quality Medical Publishing; 2003: 589–604.

24 Thompson JA, Gold PJ, Markowitz DR, et al. Updated analysis of an outpatient chemoimmunotherapy regimen for treating metastatic melanoma. The Cancer Journal from Scientific America 1997; 3: S29–S34.

CHAPTER 54

Indoor Tanning

James M Spencer

Key points

- Indoor tanning is a US$5 billion a year industry, utilized daily by millions of Americans.
- Increasing in popularity.
- Utilizes bulbs that contain UVB amounts similar to the sun and UVA content several multiples higher.
- Convincingly linked to the development of photoaging and squamous cell carcinoma and is highly likely to be linked to the development of melanoma and basal cell carcinoma.

INTRODUCTION

All life on earth depends on energy from the sun. Without the sun, the earth would be dark, cold and lifeless. The sun emits a broad spectrum of electromagnetic radiation, a very small portion of which is the ultraviolet range. This small portion has a number of effects on the skin, including stimulating the production of vitamin D, producing a sunburn, producing a tan and most importantly, causing photoaging and skin cancer. The development of indoor tanning over the last 20 years has allowed the public to receive ever greater doses of ultraviolet (UV) radiation, all with the sole purpose of cosmetic tanning. By every indication, the use of indoor tanning is increasing. At the same time, the incidence of skin cancer has reached epidemic proportions. It is quite likely that the popularity of indoor tanning plays a role in this epidemic and will continue to do so in the future.

HISTORY OF TANNING

Attitudes about UV exposure and tanning have changed dramatically over the last 100 years and the popularity of indoor tanning must be seen in this context. During the nineteenth century, fair skinned populations (particularly those of upper socioeconomic classes) avoided excessive sun exposure.[1] The link between sun exposure and skin cancer was not yet appreciated but the cosmetic results of UV exposure were. Sunburn, suntan, and photoaging were to be avoided. The poor cosmetic outcome of excessive UV exposure was appreciated and acted upon. Sun-protective clothing with broad brimmed hats and parasols were the norm. By the end of the nineteenth century, a change in attitudes about tanning began to emerge. This change was driven by the changing status of women and emerging medical information about UV light. First, the status of women improved and offered greater choices in life, including being able to engage in a number of activities that resulted in greater UV exposure. More importantly, medical information was being disseminated that supported the idea of the health benefits of UV radiation. At the beginning of the twentieth century, Neils Finsen received the Nobel prize for reporting the successful use of UV radiation for the treatment of cutaneous tuberculosis.[2] This led to the notion that UV light could treat or even prevent infectious disease as well as be helpful for a host of medical conditions as diverse as rheumatic diseases, gout, renal disease, diabetes, obesity and respiratory afflictions.[1] By the 1920s, it was appreciated UV light stimulated vitamin D production in the skin and thus was both therapeutic and preventative for rickets.[3] These observations led to the widely held view that a tan was healthy and to be encouraged. This feeling that a tan 'looks healthy' persists to this day and is often sited by indoor tanners as a reason for attending indoor tanning salons.[4] By the 1930s, the manufacture and sale of UV lamps for health purposes became big business.[5] These were typically carbon arc or quartz mercury vapor lamps with significant UVC emission (Fig. 54.1). They were available for office and home use with purported systemic health benefits. Ocular damage from shorter wavelength emission was appreciated so simple glass filters to block wavelengths below 280 nm were advocated by groups such as the AMA.[6]

By the 1940s, the development of antibiotics and other advances in medicine made the use of UV radiation for systemic disease obsolete. Except for dermatologic conditions such as psoriasis, there is little use for UV light in medicine today. However, the idea that a tan is 'healthy' has clearly persisted even if the public is not sure why UV exposure would be healthy. At the same time the medical use of UV light was declining, the period following the Second World War saw a dramatic increase in the popularity of tanning for cosmetic purposes. Tanned skin was seen not only as 'healthy' but also as attractive and beautiful. The cosmetic desirability of a tan has been reinforced by the entertainment and advertising industries where tanned models and actors are both beautiful and desirable.

Since the 1970s, a growing industry has emerged to fill the public's desire for a tan: the indoor tanning salon. UV emitting lamps are manufactured and sold to salons, spas and health clubs for the purpose of producing a cosmetically desirable tan. The indoor tanning industry estimates that there are currently over 60,000 indoor

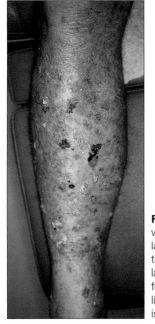

Figure 54.1 The leg of a patient who built his own carbon arc UV lamp for indoor tanning as a teenager in the 1940s. He used the lamp to tan himself and charged his friends for the same use. He is now literally covered with skin cancers, as is shown on his leg.

tanning facilities and 180,000 indoor tanning units in the US. Almost 30 million North Americans go to an indoor tanning facility each year.[7] As the industry developed and enlarged in the 1980s, it was fueled by the claim that indoor tanning bulbs used 'safe' UVA radiation and thus one could tan without any danger. The bulbs used at that time were never 100% UVA but always contained some amount of UVB. Since that time, bulbs in current use contain ever greater amounts of UVB. The industry is aggressively promoting indoor tanning as not only safe but actually healthy in a systemic way, much like the claims from 100 years ago. An understanding of the scientific evidence on artificial UV radiation and its effects on humans may allow these claims to be rationally evaluated.

MECHANISMS OF INDOOR TANNING

The ultraviolet spectrum is defined as electromagnetic radiation with a wavelength from 100 to 400 nm. Although there is some variability in the literature, the most commonly used division of the UV spectrum is that of the International Commission of Illumination (IARC, 1992), which divides the UV spectrum into UVC, UVB and UVA. UVC is defined as 100–290 nm. These wavelengths from the sun are filtered by the ozone layer and do not reach the earth's surface. UVC is still used in germicidal lamps to kill bacteria, and presumably is the portion responsible for the effects reported by Finsen on cutaneous tuberculosis.[2] The shorter the wavelength the more energetic the radiation. Therefore, UVC is the most energetic portion of the UV spectrum. It is highly mutagenic and carcinogenic and has not been used in medical or cosmetic UV lamps in decades. UVB is 290–320 nm, while UVA is 320–400 nm. Natural sunlight reaching the earth's surface contains both UVB and UVA, with the amount of UVA far in excess of UVB. The amount of UVA that reaches the earth's surface is fairly constant, while the amount of UVB is quite variable, depending on such factors as the latitude, the season of the year, the time of day, air pollution, and cloud cover. Nonetheless, natural sunlight most often contains 95% UVA and 5% UVB. Despite being only around 5% of UV radiation, UVB is of shorter wavelength and thus more energetic. For many biologic phenomena, UVB plays a greater role than 5% would suggest.

Indoor tanning bulbs utilized in the 1980s were often advertised as 'UVA only' and thus safer. During that time, no bulb was 100% UVA and therefore there was always some amount of UVB.[8] However, UVB is more efficient at inducing a tan so the current trend is to use bulbs with UVB content approximating that of natural sunlight. While many models are on the market for commercial use, measurements conducted in tanning salons suggest bulbs in current use have UVB emittance similar to the sun, while UVA emittance can be several times higher. For example, in Quebec the Joint Committee of the Ministère de la Sante[9] measured UVA and UVB output from various tanning beds used in tanning salons. UVB output was found to be in the range of 1.1–5.0 W/m^2, while the sun at its zenith gives off 1.0–2.2 W/m^2. In contrast, the UVA output from the various models ranged from 150–200 W/m^2 while natural sunlight in Quebec ranged from 46–68 W/m^2. Thus indoor tanners were receiving UVB doses equivalent to the sun and UVA doses about four times higher than the sun. Similarly, it was found that the most popular indoor tanning bulbs in Switzerland emitted UVB in amounts similar to the sun there, while UVA emission is 10 to 15 times higher than the sun.[10] The 'UVA only' marketing technique is no longer used, but rather most bulbs seem to emit UVB ranges similar to natural sunlight with greatly enhanced emissions of UVA.

The goal of indoor tanning is to produce a tan and this has pushed the addition of UVB back into these bulbs. Two types of tanning are seen in human skin in response to UV radiation: immediate pigment darkening and delayed tanning. Immediate pigment darkening occurs in response to UVA, develops within minutes of exposure and is short lived. It is thought to result from the oxidation of preexisting melanin in the skin and is seen more prominently in darker-skinned individuals. Delayed tanning is the cosmetic goal of indoor tanners. Delayed tan develops 48 to 72 hrs after UV exposure and is persistent. It is induced primarily by UVB and, to a much lesser extent, by UVA. The exact mechanism of delayed tan formation is unclear. An intriguing series of experiments have shown that addition of thymidine dinucleotides to cell culture and guinea pig skin can induce melanin production.[11,12] Thymidine dinucleotides mimic UV induced DNA damage and thus the signal to produce a tan may be DNA damage and the ensuing repair process.

UVB is primarily responsible for a delayed tan. An action spectrum for delayed tanning has essentially the same shape as the action spectrum for erythema (sunburn) and to the development of squamous cell carcinoma in animals: very high in the UVC range then falling through the UVB range to reach a low level in the UVA range (Fig. 54.2). Thus the wavelengths that most efficiently induce a tan also induce a burn and, in animals, also induce squamous cell carcinoma. That is not to say that UVA alone cannot induce a burn or a skin cancer in animals, only that much higher doses are required to do so. Since UVB is so much more effective at inducing a burn than UVA, tanning bed manufacturers promoted the idea of a 'safe' UVA tan by removing the 'burning' UVB radiation. However, since tanning salon customers want to develop a tan, it is more efficient to add increasing amounts of UVB to the bulbs to do so. Today, we are left with bulbs containing the same amount of UVB as natural sunlight, and with a UVA content 4–15 times higher. Therefore, tanning salon customers can receive the amount of UVB they would have gotten at the beach and several multiples more UVA.

ACUTE AND CHRONIC EFFECTS OF INDOOR TANNING

The effects of indoor tanning can be divided into acute and chronic. The first and foremost acute effect is that customers want to develop a tan. It can be safely assumed they are in fact developing a tan or the marketplace would quickly drive tanning salons out of business. The tanning industry mentions a sense of well being indoor tanners develop as a benefit of indoor tanning. Seasonal affective disorder (SAD) is a recognized emotional state thought to result from prolonged lack of visible light. However, there is no evidence UV light is effective for SAD. A postulated mechanism for the effect of light is an elevation in circulating endogenous opioid peptides, which may produce pleasure. In a recent study, six sessions in a tanning bed over 3 weeks produced no increase in either β-endorphin immunoreactive material or met-enkephalin.[13]

Acute adverse events include erythema (sunburn), phototoxic reactions, photoallergic reactions, photosensitive disease exacerbation, and corneal burns. The avoidance of these acute complications is something everyone can agree on. It is equally clear acute adverse events occur with some regularity. A survey of 203 indoor tanners in Quebec showed 26.1% experienced one or more acute adverse events.[9] The survey showed 17.7% had a sunburn, 14.8% reported skin dryness, 3% reported ocular burning or itching and 1.5% reported nausea. Similarly, Rivers[14] reported 22% of experimental volunteers receiving indoor tanning developed a sunburn, 27% had itching, 15% had dry skin and 4% had nausea.

There is very little regulation of indoor tanning salons, so there is great variability in operator safety. The manufacturers of indoor tanning equipment are regulated at the federal level by the FDA while operators of tanning salons are regulated at the state level. Some states have stringent safety regulations while others have minimal to no requirements. Furthermore, in those states that have regulations, it is not at all clear how these regulations are enforced or who would do so. At a minimum, a history for photosensitivity or photo-sensitizing medications should be taken. Diseases known to be exacerbated by UV radiation, such as dermatomyositis, lupus erythematosus, pellagra, and porphyria, should be identified. Children should not be allowed equipment use unescorted by a parent, if at all. Eye protection should be mandatory for all users and exposure times should be carefully monitored by the salon operators. Bulb fluence and equipment hygiene should be regularly checked. These safety standards are often minimally applied or ignored altogether.

Despite the fact that it is in the tanning industry's interest to avoid unwanted acute adverse events, the industry has lobbied vigorously to avoid legislation at

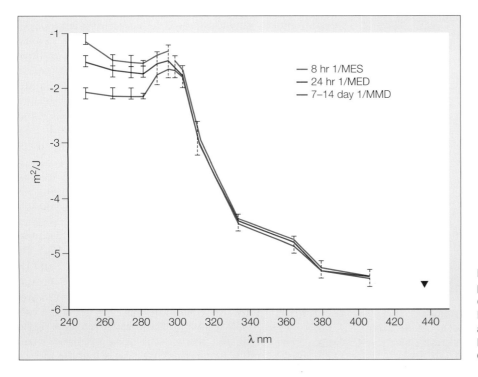

Figure 54.2 The action spectrum for the production of erythema (sunburn) and delayed pigmentation (tanning). (From Parrish JA. Erythema and melanogenesis action spectra of normal human skin. Photochem Photobiol 1982; 36:187–191. © Allen Press, Inc.)

the state and federal level. For example, eye protection is recommended by all parties (including FDA regulations), yet corneal burns from indoor tanning devices show this recommendation is often ignored. A survey of ophthalmologists in Wisconsin showed that over a 1-year period, 152 patients were seen for eye burns caused by indoor tanning equipment.[15]

The chronic effects of indoor tanning are of much greater concern and the source of much tension between the indoor tanning industry and the medical profession. A tan will fade in a few weeks, so there is no long-term cosmetic benefit. Since the point of indoor tanning is cosmetic enhancement, it is ironic that the long-term effect may be photoaging, which leads to wrinkled, leathery, discolored skin. Aging of the skin is divided into intrinsic aging, which is those changes that occur from the passage of time, and photoaging, which are changes induced by ultraviolet radiation.[16]

The changes of intrinsic aging are relatively minor from a cosmetic point of view. Photoprotected skin in elderly people is somewhat dry with mild flaking and has a slight increase in laxity. Histologically, there is flattening of the rete ridges with little change in overall epidermal thickness. In the dermis, there is a loss of dermal thickness in the range of about 20%. The dermis

itself is relatively avascular and acellular. There is a decrease in both collagen and elastin content but the changes are not dramatic. In contrast, the changes of photoaging can be quite dramatic. Clinically, photoaged skin is wrinkled, leathery, sallow and characterized by discolorations such as lentigos, actinic keratoses, and telangiectasias (Fig. 54.3). Histologically, there is an increase in dermal cellularity resembling an inflammatory response. There is loss of blood vessels, with remaining vessels becoming dilated and tortuous. There is extensive loss of collagen and elastin, with thickened tangles of elastotic material termed solar elastosis.

The precise action spectrum of photoaging in human skin has not been determined, but it seems both UVA and UVB play a role. In mice, an elastotic reaction similar to human photoaging can be produced by prolonged exposure to UVB.[17] On the other hand, human skin exposed to subMED doses of UVA daily for only 1 month demonstrated many of the histologic changes characteristic of photoaging.[18] This last finding is particularly important because it developed without a sunburn. The indoor tanning industry often argues no deleterious effects of UV light seen in the absence of a sunburn. However, chronic exposure to subMED doses of ultraviolet light leads to the undesirable appearance of photoaging.

INDOOR TANNING AND SKIN CANCER

The development of skin cancer represents the greatest potential danger of indoor tanning. Ultraviolet exposure causes skin cancer. Short-term recreational tanning salon exposure causes molecular alterations believed essential in the development of skin cancer similar to outdoor sun exposure.[19] Cyclobutane pyrimidine dimers in DNA and *p53* protein expression have been detected in epidermal keratinocytes even after a single UV exposure from a tanning bed.

However, the pattern of exposure and its relationship to skin cancer development is less well understood. All three common types of skin cancer, basal cell carcinoma (BCC), squamous cell carcinoma (SCC), and melanoma, are caused by ultraviolet light, but the exposure pattern responsible for the three appears to differ. Animal models of SCC are available and allow detailed studies. Since no such animal models exist for BCC and melanoma, we must rely on epidemiologic studies of human populations which are much more difficult to perform.

In experimental animals, both UVB and UVA can induce SCC but UVB is much more efficient at doing so. The action spectra for SCC follows that of tanning and burning: high in the UVB range, and falling at higher wavelengths (Fig. 54.4). While UVB is more efficient at inducing skin cancer, it must be emphasized UVA by itself can induce SCC in experimental animals.[20] Animal studies allow the examination of the pattern of exposure that induces skin cancer. The important question to ask is: for a given total dose of UV radiation, what is the carcinogenic potential of giving all the radiation as a single large dose versus the same total dose in many small fractions? The relevance to this question is that the indoor

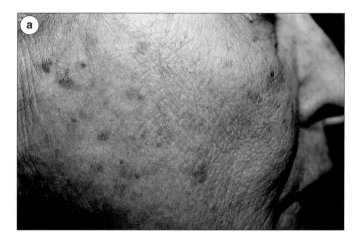

Figure 54.3 (a) The cheek of an 83-year-old woman showing the changes of photoaging. (b) The photoprotected buttock cheek of the same woman, showing only the mild changes of intrinsic aging.

tanning industry argues that single large doses that result in sunburns are carcinogenic, while many small doses such as tanners could receive is not. This question can be answered for SCC in experimental animals. Under conditions meant to simulate what indoor tanners receive, many small doses are more carcinogenic than the same total dose given in a few large doses.[21] The important point is that subMED doses of UV light can and do cause squamous cell carcinoma. Many small doses such as those that an indoor tanner might receive is more carcinogenic than the sunburn a vacationer might experience.

This pattern of exposure in experimental animals for the development of SCC is supported by epidemiologic evidence in humans. There is roughly a linear relationship between UV exposure and SCC development throughout life.[22] The development of SCC correlates with outdoor occupation[23] and is more likely in chronically exposed areas such as the face and hands, again suggesting chronic low dose exposure leads to the development of SCC.

The action spectrum and pattern of exposure for BCC is not clear because there is no animal model for this tumor. Human epidemiologic studies suggest recreational exposure before the age of 20 is most correlated with the development of BCC.[24] This suggests that 'large doses', such as one might receive on a day at the beach, are more carcinogenic than chronic low dose exposure, such as one might get with an outdoor occupation. However, the question is still open, as it may be that an individual's carcinogenic potential is 'saturated' after a certain level of UV exposure, which explains why adult UV exposure does not seem to play a role in BCC development. Furthermore, BCC is typically seen on the head and neck which are areas subject to chronic exposure.

The action spectrum and pattern of exposure for melanoma also is unknown as there is no good animal model to study the UV–melanoma relationship. The fish *Platyfish xiphophorus* develops melanocytic tumors in response to UV radiation but may not be the best representative of human skin. Nonetheless, studies using this fish model suggest UVA may be the most efficient at melanoma induction.[25] The pattern of exposure has not been addressed in experimental animals. Human epidemiologic studies suggest melanoma is associated with high dose intermittent sun exposure, especially childhood sunburns.[26] Melanoma does not correlate with outdoor occupation but rather correlates with higher income levels and indoor occupation.[27] The implication is that these individuals would be more likely to develop a severe sunburn on vacation, putting them at higher risk for melanoma later in life. In men, the most common site to develop a melanoma is on the back. This is a location not chronically exposed but rather a location likely to receive a sunburn on vacation. These epidemiologic observations have led indoor tanning advocates to argue that sunburns cause melanoma but that chronic low dose exposure does not. This argument is then taken a step further: if only people were tan, then they would not get a sunburn and the incidence of melanoma would go down.

The 'tans' *vs* 'burns' debate provides no real rationale for indoor tanning for several reasons. First and foremost, it is clear that the development of photoaging and SCC is favored by chronic low dose UV exposure such as might be received by an indoor tanner. These observations alone make a compelling case for avoiding indoor tanning. Second, even if it is true that only sunburns cause melanoma while tanning does not, people can and do frequently burn in indoor tanning devices. Third, the most high-risk individuals do not tan very well and these individuals are the most likely to go to a tanning salon. Fair skinned people are those most likely to seek indoor tanning and are the least likely to successfully develop a tan without burning. This is the group most likely to develop melanoma, so for the highest risk individuals the tan *vs* burn debate is irrelevant. Lastly, many people think if they get a 'base tan' at a tanning salon before their beach vacation they would be less likely to develop a harmful sunburn. However, studies suggest that the tan received from indoor tanning provides an SPF of about 4, which is hardly adequate protection for a day at the beach.

Although melanoma is the least common of the three types of skin cancer, it has received the greatest research interest in terms of its relationship to indoor tanning because it accounts for the greatest number of deaths from skin cancer. More than 20 case control studies have investigated a possible link between indoor tanning and melanoma.[28] The majority found no relationship, while seven showed a significant positive association between indoor tanning and melanoma. Most of the studies are flawed by methodological problems but the most recent, more rigorously designed studies have found a positive correlation. A recent study of 571 first time melanoma patients compared with 913 healthy controls found a significantly elevated odds ratio of 1.8 between indoor tanning and melanoma.[29] No study has ever suggested

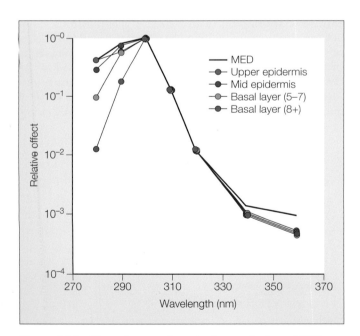

Figure 54.4 The action spectrum for the production of DNA photoproducts in human epidermis has the same shape as the erythema action spectrum. The action spectrum for the development of SCC in experimental animals follows the same shape.

that indoor tanning decreases the risk of melanoma as has been proposed by the indoor tanning industry.

Fewer epidemiologic studies of the relationship of BCC and SCC and indoor tanning have been performed. However, the most recent raise the possibility of an association between indoor tanning and non-melanoma skin cancer. Karagas et al.[30] compared 603 patients with BCC, 293 patients with SCC, to 540 matched controls. A positive correlation with indoor tanning and the development of non-melanoma skin cancer was noted, with an odds ratio of 2.5 for SCC and 1.5 for BCC. In addition, a recent population-based study of 10.2 million persons in Sweden noted an increase in the rate of SCC with the greatest increase occurring in in-situ lesions on normally covered sites.[31] The strong cohort effect suggests a contribution by intentional tanning. Combined with the animal studies on the development of SCC, it would seem indoor tanning is a significant risk factor for the development of non-melanoma skin cancer.

TANNING AND VITAMIN D

Recently, the indoor tanning industry has begun to promote the health benefits of vitamin D synthesis in the skin in response to UV radiation. Vitamin D_3 is synthesized in the skin in response to UVB. It is then converted in the liver to 25-OH-D_3, and finally to 1,25-OH-D_3 in the kidneys. It is estimated that 10–15 min of noon-time sun on the cheeks is more than adequate for Vitamin D production. However, in the complete absence of sun exposure, dietary sources are completely adequate. In a study of children with xeroderma pigmentosum who practice rigorous and complete sun avoidance, vitamin D levels were normal.[32] In another study of patients in Australia given sunscreen to use consistently for 1 year, vitamin D levels remained within the normal range.[33] Dietary sources include fortified milk, margarine and eggs. Vitamin D has properties of a vitamin, but also those of a hormone. It is important for regulating calcium and phosphorus that is important for mineralization of the bones, neuromuscular function and various cellular activities.

It has been hypothesized, with little experimental support, that vitamin D may provide chemoprevention for a variety of cancers. This was first suggested for colon cancer more than 20 years ago[34] and then for breast cancer.[35] The proposed role for vitamin D was suggested principally on the geographic distribution of these cancers in the US. The incidence of many cancers varies geographically but not in any obvious pattern. An exception is breast cancer, which was noted many years ago to have a higher mortality in northern latitudes in the US and lower in southern. The pattern is not absolute: while the mortality rate of breast cancer is higher as one moves north along the east coast of the US, it is not higher as one moves north along the west coast. There are many possible explanations for this observation, and the significance of this pattern is not clear. One explanation proposed is that sun exposure is the variable that explains this pattern. It has also been hypothesized that increased serum vitamin D levels in response to greater UVB exposure must be the explanation. The

implication is the vitamin D provides chemoprevention for breast cancer and colon cancer.

Over the last 20 years, little experimental evidence has supported this idea. However, the indoor tanning issue has seized upon this rather obscure argument to promote a radical idea: that indoor tanning is healthy and prevents cancer. The indoor tanning industry is prevented by the FDA from advertising this 'health benefit', but would very much like to do so. They have vigorously lobbied the government to be allowed to but have been unsuccessful to date. Given the fact that adequate levels of vitamin D are obtained through the diet and one could take additional oral supplementation if so desired, there is little reason to believe there is any 'health benefit' to indoor tanning. The link of indoor tanning to the development of photoaging and SCC is clear, and the link to BCC and melanoma is highly probable, while any chemopreventative effect has no experimental or epidemiologic support. Furthermore, even if there is a chemopreventative effect of vitamin D, it could be obtained through diet.

FUTURE OUTLOOK

The indoor tanning industry is prohibited by the federal government from marketing their devices for any purpose other than cosmetic tanning. The industry has lobbied the government for permission to advertise the 'health benefits' of indoor tanning (Table 54.1). The industry itself currently estimates they are a US$5 billion a year business, so the potential for effective lobbying is quite real. However, given current market trends, the industry may not need this marketing tool. In a recent survey of undergraduate and graduate students at a major midwestern university, 47% of students had used indoor tanning equipment in the last 12 months.[36] An extraordinary finding of this survey was that more than 90% of these students were aware that premature aging of the skin and skin cancer were possible complications of indoor tanning. Young people value a tanned look as desirable and this desire seems to outweigh dangers to their health. As long as tanned skin is seen as healthy and beautiful, we can expect to see an increase, rather

Table 54.1 Suggested 'benefits' of indoor tanning
Lowers your heart rate
Reduces your risk for health disease
Stimulates your body's natural SAFE production of Vitamin D
Reduces your risk for many types of cancer
Increases bone density
Increases metabolism, burns fat
Increases sex drive
Makes you feel happy
And, makes you more attractive
Source: Indoor Tanning Association President, Dan Humiston's speech, 2002; available from: www.indoor-tanning.org

than a decrease, in indoor tanning and an increase in the development of resultant skin cancer.

REFERENCES

1 Albert MR, Ostheimer KG. The evolution of current medical and popular attitudes toward ultraviolet light exposure: part I. J Am Acad Derm 2002; 47:930–937.

2 Finsen NR. Phototherapy. London: Edward Arnold; 1901.

3 Hess AF, Weinstock M. A study of light waves in their relation to rickets. JAMA 1923; 80:687–690.

4 Mawn VB, Fleischer AB Jr. A survey of attitudes, beliefs, and behavior regarding tanning bed use, sunbathing, and sunscreen use. J Am Acad Derm 1993; 29:959–962.

5 Albert MR, Ostheimer KG. The evolution of current medical and popular attitudes toward ultraviolet light exposure: part II. J Am Acad Derm 2003; 48(6):909–918.

6 Acceptance of sunlamps. JAMA 1933; 100:1863–1864.

7 Humiston D. Speech. Indoor Tanning Association President, 2002. Online. Available from: www.tanningtruth.com.

8 Spencer JM, Amonette RA. Indoor tanning: risks, benefits, and future trends. J Am Acad Derm 1995; 33(2):288–298.

9 Joint Committee on Exposure to Ultraviolet Rays. Artificial tanning in Quebec, Government du Quebec, Ministère de la Sante et des Services Sociaux. Joint Committee on Exposure to Ultraviolet Rays; 1999.

10 Gerber B, Mathys P, Moser M, et al. Ultraviolet emission spectra of sunbeds. Photochem Photobiol 2002; 76:664–668.

11 Gilchrest BA, Zhai S, Eller MS, Yarosh DB, Yaar M. Treatment of human melanocytes and S91 melanoma cells with the DNA repair enzyme TV endonuclease enhances melanogenesis after UV irradiation. J Invest Derm 1993; 101:666–700.

12 Eller MS, Yaar M, Gilchrest BA. DNA damage and melanogenesis. Nature 1994; 372:413–416.

13 Gambichler T, Bader A, Vojvodic M, Avermaete A, Schenk M, Altmeyer P, Hoffmann K. Plasma levels of opioid peptides after sunbed exposure. Br J Derm 2002; 147:1207–1211.

14 Rivers JK, Norris PG, Murphy GM, et al. UVA sunbeds: tanning, photoprotection, acute adverse effects, and immunologic changes. Br J Derm 1989; 120:767–777.

15 MMWR. Injuries associated with ultraviolet tanning devices. JAMA 1989; 261:3519–3520.

16 Yaar M, Gilchrest B. Aging of the skin. In: Fitzpatrick TB, Eisen AZ, Wolff K, et al., eds. Dermatology in General Medicine, 6th edn. New York, NY: McGraw Hill.

17 Kligman LH, Sayre RM. An action spectrum for ultraviolet induced elastosis in hairless mice: Quantification of elastosis by image analysis. Photochem Photobiol 1991; 53:237–240.

18 Lavker RM, Veres DA, Irwin CJ, Kaidbey KH. Quantitative assessment of cumulative damage from repetitive exposures to suberythmogenic doses of UVA in human skin. Photochem Photobiol 1995; 62:338.

19 Whitmore SE. Morison WL, Potten CS, Chadwick C. Tanning salon exposure and molecular alterations. J Am Acad Derm 2001; 44(5):775–780.

20 Weelden H Van, Gruijl FR de, Putte SCJ van der, et al. The carcinogenic risk of modern tanning equipment: is UVA safer than UVB? Arch Derm Res 1988; 280:300–307.

21 Forbes PD, Davies DE, Urbach F. Experimental ultraviolet carcinogenesis: wavelength interactions and time–dose relationships. Natl Cancer 1st Monogr 1978; 50:31–38.

22 Armstrong BK, Kricker A. Epidemiology of sun exposure and skin cancer. Cancer Surv 1996; 26:133–153.

23 Gallagher RP, Hill GB, Bajdik CD, et al. Sunlight exposure pigmentation factors, and risks of nonmelanocytic skin cancers. Arch Derm 1995; 131:164–169.

24 Kricker A, Armstrong BK, English DR. Does intermittent sun exposure cause basal cell carcinoma? A case–control study in Western Australia. Int J Cancer 1995; 60:489–494.

25 Setlow RB, Grist E, Thompson K, et al. Wavelengths effective in induction of malignant melanoma. Proc Natl Acad Sci USA 1993; 90:6666–6670.

26 Ellwood JM, Gallagher RP, Hill GB, et al. Cutaneous melanoma in relation to intermittent and constant sun exposure: the Western Canada Melanoma Study. Int J Cancer 1985; 35:427–433.

27 Gallagher RP, Ellwood JM, Threlfall WJ, et al. Socioeconomic status, sunlight exposure and risk of malignant melanoma: the Western Canada Melanoma Study. J Natl Cancer Inst 1987; 79:647–652.

28 Swerdlow AJ, Weinstock MA. Do tanning lamps cause melanoma? An epidemiologic assessment. J Am Acad Derm 1998; 38(1):89–98.

29 Westerdahl J, Ingvar C, Masback A, et al. Risk of cutaneous melanoma in relation to use of sunbeds: further evidence for UV-A carcinogenicity. Br J Cancer 2000; 82(9):1593–1599.

30 Karagas MR, Stannard VA, Mott LA, et al. Use of tanning devices and risk of basal cell and squamous cell skin cancers. J Natl Cancer Inst 2002; 94(3):224–226.

31 Hemminki K, Zhang H, Czene K. Time trends and familial risks in squamous cell carcinoma of the skin. Arch Derm 2003; 139:885–889.

32 Sollitto RB, Kraemer KH, DiGiovanna JJ. Normal vitamin D Levels can be maintained despite rigorous photoprotection: six years' experience with xeroderma pigmentosum. J Am Acad Derm 1997; 37(6):942–947.

33 Marks R, Foley PA, Jolley D, et al. The effects of regular sunscreen use on vitamin D levels in an Australian population. Results of a randomized controlled trial. Arch Derm 1995; 131(4):415–421.

34 Garland FC, Garland CF. Do sunlight and vitamin D reduce the likelihood of colon cancer? Int J Epidemiol 1980; 9(3):227–231.

35 Garland FC, Garland CF, Gorham CD, et al. Geographic variation in breast cancer mortality in the United States: a hypothesis involving exposure to solar radiation. Prev Med 1990; 19(6):614–622.

36 Knight JM, Kirincich AN, Farmer ER, et al. Awareness of the risks of tanning lamps does not influence behavior among college students. Arch Derm 2002; 138(10):1311–1315.

CHAPTER
55

Photo Documentation for Skin Cancer

William Slue Jr

Key points

- Digital imaging is replacing film for documenting lesions suspicious for skin cancer.
- Understanding how to take effective digital images is critical.
- Maintaining and storing digital image archives for accurate and efficient access important.
- Baseline photography useful in following patients at high risk for skin cancer.

INTRODUCTION

Photography plays a very important role in the recording of skin cancers. Images are extremely useful tools for teaching, identification of location and morphology and patient follow-up. The ability to properly document suspicious and/or high-risk skin lesions often plays a critical role in the management of skin cancer patients.

A BASIC APPROACH TO SKIN CANCER PHOTOGRAPHY

For dermatologic purposes, there are three basic views of the patient that are photographed.[1-4] These views are: scan, location and detail. A scan is taken a distance from the patient and shows approximately half of the body (Fig. 55.1). This is very useful in showing the distribution of lesions. A location shot is closer and shows where on the body the lesion is located (Fig. 55.2). Detail photographs are close-ups that show the morphology of the lesion (Fig. 55.3).[5]

On a normal lens (50–60 mm) there are numerical markings that will identify how far the camera is from the lesions being photographed.[6] These markings will also allow the determination of the image size in relation to life size (i.e. 1:2 means that the image size is one half of life size; 1:4 means that the image size is one quarter of life size). This system holds true in the 35 mm film setting; in the digital setting the computer chip creates a larger image than seen in a film camera. As a result, you may need to make your own markings on the lens to achieve the desired setting. For most skin cancers the detail setting (1:2 or 1:4) can be used. For other views, the photographer can make a measurement such as 1:8 for the location and 1:12 for the scan. Consistently using these settings will result in an easy and consistent way to standardize skin cancer images and have reproducible conditions for before and after pictures.

Another technique to keep in mind for creating consistent before and after pictures is body focusing. Body focusing is a technique that can be used to insure the same camera distance to the patient in the after picture as was used in the before. It is most easily done when using the same setting each time your patients are being photographed. Using the 'three views' method insures that body focusing can be easily employed since the camera setting will remain constant.[2] Instead of rotating the lens to focus, move your body back and forth slightly to bring the image into focus. The best way to do this is to stand with one leg in front of the other and shift forward and back. Once the focus has been achieved, the picture is taken. The lens also should be set at the same setting when taking the 'after' picture. Since the lens setting has not changed from the before to the after, you know that the clinical information will be exactly the same size in both images.

When photographing skin cancer or other dermatological lesions a few rules will help. It is often hard to determine the size of lesions in a detail view photograph. A ruler will help provide information on size. Take care to avoid using a ruler with a commercial advertisement. Printed ads on the rulers distract from the clinical information being presented. Plain rulers well suited to dermatological photography can be obtained through Shamrock Scientific Specialty Systems (http://www.shamrocklabels.com/sssim011.htm) and other similar suppliers (Fig. 55.4). Additionally, clothing, jewelry and glasses should not be seen in the photographs; they are distracting and irrelevant.

The goal of skin cancer photography is to maximize clinical information while minimizing irrelevant data. Items such as underwear, objects in the exam room, doorknobs and other irrelevant information should not be included. When you look through the camera's viewfinder, ask yourself 'what am I photographing?' If elements are seen in the viewfinder that are distracting or irrelevant try to avoid them. Consider changing the angle of the photograph, move closer to the patient, or switch the camera from a horizontal view to a vertical one in order to crop these things out of the picture. Another distracting element may be a recent biopsy site. It is always better to photograph the patient before the biopsy is performed rather than to have a healing wound as a distraction.

The most important image in photographing skin cancer is typically the detail view. Image sharpness

669

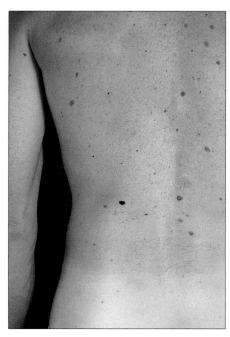

Figure 55.1 Scan view showing distribution of lesions.

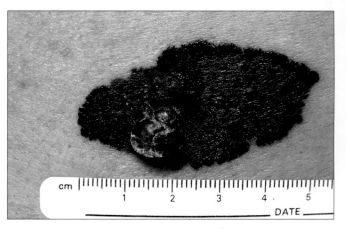

Figure 55.3 Detail view showing lesion morphology.

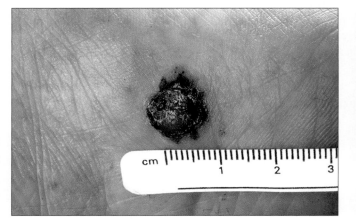

Figure 55.4 Ruler in image helping to document size.

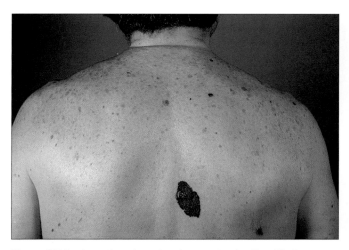

Figure 55.2 Location view showing anatomic site of lesion.

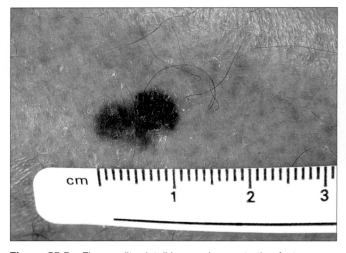

Figure 55.5 Fine quality detail image demonstrating features that help make the diagnosis of melanoma in this pigmented lesion.

is critical. Photographic professionals often hear 'the image is good enough' but this may not be true. Is the image good enough because you have a low standard of image sharpness? Is it good enough for the colleagues you are sharing this image with? The standard of image sharpness should be that the skin markings and the hair leaving the follicle can be clearly seen. Such standards will allow you to see skin morphology to be seen and also will assist in arriving at a correct diagnosis. A good detail or close-up image will show translucency of skin, dryness, follicular involvement and telangiectasia. With pigmented lesions, a close-up photo will allow viewers to note subtle changes that will often enhance the ability to recognize early melanoma (Fig. 55.5).

To optimize lesional photography it is also important to understand the concept of depth of field. Depth of field refers to the area of the photograph that is in sharp focus. Since the size of the lens opening (also called f-stop or aperture) is inversely proportional to the amount of depth of field, a simple rule to remember is that the smaller the lens opening, the greater the depth of field. This means that a lens opening of f22 or f16 is required instead of f5.6 or f4. Having a smaller aperture setting will require a flash output to be strong enough to give adequate light; the shutter speed never changes during flash photography. Figure 55.6a, b illustrates this concept.

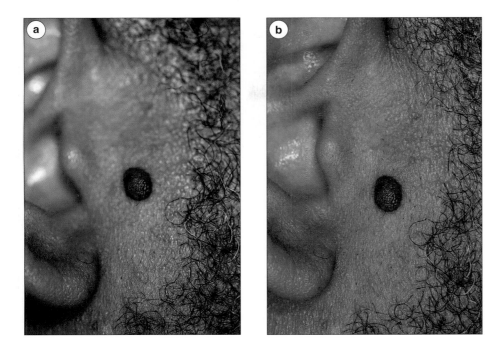

Figure 55.6 (a) Image with large lens opening and small depth of field. (b) Image with small lens opening and greater depth of field. Compare (a) with all areas of the image in focus versus (b) where only the lesion is in focus.

The image with good depth of field (Fig. 55.6b) has the entire image in sharp focus; however the image with the small depth of field (Fig. 55.6a) has only some of the hairs in focus with the majority of the background soft.

THE EVOLUTION OF PHOTO DOCUMENTATION

Since 1998, when a chapter on dermatologic photography in a surgery textbook was published, so much has changed.[6] At that time, film cameras were the standard and the complexities of achieving proper exposures the focus of photographic efforts. Today, we are fully in the digital age and film is steadily being replaced by digital imaging.

At the time of the writing of this chapter, there are over 65,000 new digital cameras on the market[7] and it is not a simple task to determine the appropriate choice in a given setting. Most dermatologic photographic professionals had finally found film systems that worked quite well and have now been forced to become fully digital. Some of this pressure has been related to the diminished availability of standard films (our department has been forced to switch films three times in the last couple of years as each previous film was discontinued). Many processing labs are closing or phasing out their film services and replacing them with digital options. Scientific meetings now typically occur where the only projector available is an LCD (digital) projector and those in need of a slide projector are left unable to display their presentations.

In this evolutionary era, some controversies are present. In the ever evolving digital imaging arena, there is a constant influx of smaller, faster, better cameras. Each new model, while usually an improvement over the last, often comes with a heftier price tag and the previous less expensive models are unavailable. Others believe that digital images are not as good as 35 mm film images.

While this was certainly true several years ago, the current higher end digital cameras are more than capable of producing images that rival and/or even exceed film. The question remains: what will happen if film becomes as difficult to find as Betamax tapes or vinyl records? The bottom line is that we cannot continue to hold on to the past or ignore the future.

What factors influence a physician in making the switch from film to digital documentation? One of the key factors is that with a digital approach you can instantly view images and store them on very compact and portable media. The ability to find images quickly can also easily be achieved using applicable software. Images can be sent to colleagues with a click of a button, whether for a consultation or a patient referral.

SELECTING THE APPROPRIATE DIGITAL CAMERA FOR A CLINICAL SETTING

The selection of a digital camera for an office setting can be reduced to two choices: A point-and-shoot (or consumer) camera or an SLR (single lens reflex) camera. Price is often the most important consideration. At this time, the approximate cost of a digital point-and-shoot camera is between US$200 and US$800, while the SLR varies between US$1800 and US$5000. It is very important to understand the applications of both cameras in skin cancer photography before making a decision of which to purchase.

The point-and-shoot is a smaller, lighter camera that often appeals to potential buyers because of its portability and ease of use. Several point-and-shoot cameras can take clear and crisp close-up photographs and this function can be enhanced by attaching a device called a close-up attachment scale manufactured by Canfield Scientific (Fig. 55.7). Although several point-and-shoot cameras can give very good close-up photographs of clinical lesions

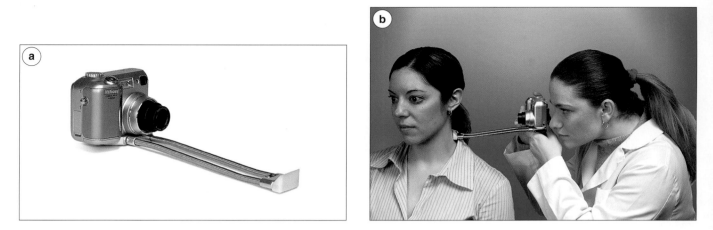

Figure 55.7 (a) Point and shoot digital camera with close-up attachment scale. (b) Correct use of a point and shoot digital camera at a fixed distance and constant lighting. (Images courtesy of Canfield Scientific.)

it is important to keep in mind that many do not have this ability. Therefore, when shopping for a point-and-shoot camera, make sure the model you are considering has a macro setting for close-up imaging or the camera will be useless for detailed pictures when photographing skin cancer. Another consideration for point-and-shoot cameras is that the attached flash is often too strong for macro use so close-up pictures tend to be over-exposed and all details washed out. It is recommend that these cameras be tested in a clinical setting before making a decision.

A point-and-shoot camera can also fall short when used for location and scan photographs. Because many of these cameras have relatively low resolution, pictures taken at a distance contain little clear detail. For this reason, point-and-shoot cameras often cannot be reliably used for before-and-after photography. In before and after pictures it is imperative that every set of photographs be taken under the same lighting, with the same exposure and distance from subject[1] (Fig. 55.7b). If this is not done, before-and-after pictures will be open to major criticism. Also, because point-and-shoot cameras often have automatic zoom lenses and do not allow you to have control over exposure, the results may not be consistent enough to be trusted.

For those who have been using an SLR film camera, the switch to a digital SLR camera is virtually a natural one (Fig. 55.8). The same technique that has been used to achieve good clinical images is simply brought over to the new digital camera system. One can easily begin by using the 'three views' method described previously in this chapter.

There are several other technical considerations that must be taken into account when selecting a digital camera for skin cancer photography. The camera you choose must have a resolution that is sufficient for capturing all the detail necessary; whether for patient follow-up, publication or another use. Camera resolution is most commonly expressed in pixel (short for 'picture element') count. The sensor in a digital camera is composed of pixels, which are tiny light-sensitive squares. The number of pixels in the image is approximately equal to the number of pixels on the camera sensor. This

number is referred to as the image's resolution. The term 'megapixel', which is found on most digital cameras, simply means one million pixels. The greater the number of pixels in an image, the higher the resolution will be. And the higher the resolution, the better and larger the print that can be made and the more clearly zoomed in on details can be displayed on a screen.

It is important that the digital camera chosen should have a minimum available resolution of 3 megapixels. This will ensure that images will be crisp and contain all necessary data required for making a high-quality print or magnified on-screen viewing. If a photograph is taken of an important case and a lower resolution camera is used, the result will typically be unacceptable in terms of sharpness and resolution. That is because the low resolution image lacks detail and may also appear jagged. The higher the photograph's resolution, the more printing and viewing options exist. If images are only used for patient charts and will only be viewed on computer monitors, using the camera's middle-quality (normal) setting should provide sufficient quality. However, if pictures are being taken for a study or to be submitted for publication, the highest quality setting your camera offers should be employed. The resolution can easily be adjusted downward on a computer later but there is a limit to how effectively photo resolution can be adjusted upward. This means sharp, clear, small prints can be made from high-resolution photos, but a rich, detailed, large print cannot be made from a low-resolution one.

The most commonly used file formats in digital photography are TIFF (short for 'tagged image file format') and JPEG (short for 'joint photographic experts group') and are defined as:

TIFF: This file format is uncompressed. Choosing TIFF means that you are always assured of getting all the image quality captured and processed by the camera. But TIFF files can be quite large, so only a few will fit onto a memory card. Because the files are larger, they can take a while to be written to the card making it necessary to wait a few seconds before you can take another picture.

JPEG: This file format is compressed, which means that the picture information is squeezed to a smaller size before it is stored on the memory card. Though this

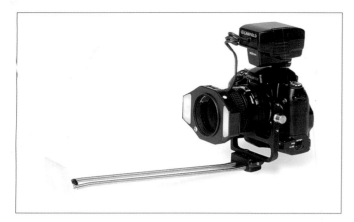

Figure 55.8 Single lens reflex digital camera also utilizing close-up attachment scale. (Image courtesy of Canfield Scientific.)

compression does not alter the photo's resolution, it does come at the expense of varying loss of detail and clarity in the photo. Typically, a camera will offer several JPEG settings, each offering progressively more compression (which translates into being able to store more photos on the memory card), with a commensurate drop in image quality. JPEG compression is often measured on a scale of 0–12. The lower numbers represent higher compression. Heavily compressed JPEGs give much smaller files sizes and greatly reduce sharpness and image quality. A higher number such as 11 or 12 will result in a much higher quality image and a larger file.

The differences in these two formats are important to be aware of, not only because several digital cameras offer both TIFF and JPEG settings, but because most publications prefer TIFFs to be submitted and JPEG files are almost exclusively preferred as e-mail attachments. The file format does not affect the resolution of the photo, but if a JPEG setting is chosen that compresses the photo heavily, the detail in the photo will be irretrievably damaged. The resulting visual damage of compression is called JPEG artifacting and often appears as a pattern of large, square blocks sprinkled through the picture (Fig 55.9a, b). JPEG artifacting limits the ability to make a quality print from the photo, even

though the resolution of the photo was not changed by the JPEG compression. It can also make images appear blurry and low in contrast when viewed on screen. Important details crucial in tracking skin lesions may be lost.

Although it would seem that choosing TIFFs as a format (if the camera has this option) would be the best solution, this is usually not the case. Since TIFF files are uncompressed, they take up much more space on a memory card. They also can take some time to save onto the card while using the camera and so there may be a wait of several seconds in between shots. Also, once downloaded on a computer, larger files take much longer to open and take up much more space on the hard drive or server. For this reason, it is recommended to photograph at the highest JPEG setting (often called 'fine' or 'best'). This will maximize both the resolution and clarity of photos and also prevent having excessively large files that can take too much time to download and open on a computer.

The highest-quality, lowest-compression JPEG setting on most cameras offers marginally less quality than TIFF, but without the difficulties associated with very large image sizes. The difference in quality between a best-quality JPEG and a TIFF is barely noticeable, even though the JPEG will be six to eight times smaller when stored on the card. The same cannot be said of the lower-quality JPEG settings since clarity and detail diminish quickly with compression.

It helps to be familiar with appropriate resolutions for photographic files. For most printers, a resolution for 300 dpi (dots per inch) is sufficient. Also, remember that when the size of an image on your computer is increased, the effective resolution is lessened. However, the amount of information contained in a photographic file remains the same. Therefore, if the size of an image on a page is doubled, the print resolution is halved. For instance, with a 3 × 3 inch 300 dpi image enlarged to 6 × 6 inches in a page layout or word processing program before printing, the effective resolution is only 150 dpi.

When using images only for screen viewing, they can be saved at 96 dpi. This resolution is appropriate for most monitors that are not capable of displaying finer reso-

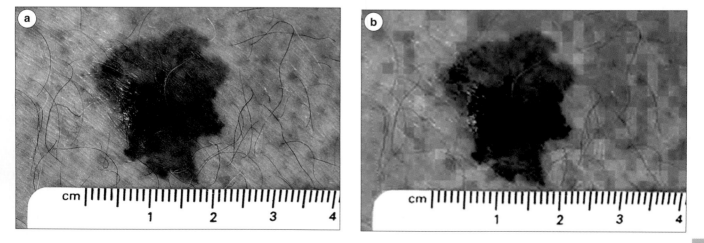

Figure 55.9 (a) Comparison of an uncompressed digital photograph of a melanoma versus (b) one with significant compression. Note the loss of crispness of the lesion and hairs in (b) along with 'pixelation'.

lutions. Therefore, if images of a higher resolution will never need to be printed, it is a good idea to save them at the lower resolution so they take up less storage space on a hard drive or server.

OPTIMIZING STORAGE OF DIGITAL IMAGES

Since many are now switching from 35 mm photos to digital, it is also important to consider what computer hardware should be used for archiving and retrieval. There are many forms of storage available, including Zip disks, tape, CDs and DVDs. Some storage media have a longer lifespan than others. A Zip disk, for example, if used over and over again, can malfunction causing all the data on the disk to be lost. Backing up image data on CDs is a fairly inexpensive solution, but finding the particular image you are searching for can be complicated if all you have is a pile of unlabeled disks for storage. To combat this problem, CD jukeboxes are a possible solution for high-volume data management. These storage systems support retrieval, archiving and backup applications. While DVD is a relatively new technology, it is a convenient backup medium, due to the large amount of information a single disk can hold (more than six times that of a CD).

Keeping everything on a computer hard drive is very risky; it can crash, erasing all data stored on it. For that reason, it is best to have everything backed up in an alternative place. Servers are often available for just this purpose; they can be within the building, or space can be rented on an external server. It is suggested that an information technology expert be contacted to discuss backup needs. Regardless of the storage media and software chosen, it is necessary to back *everything* up.

Storage and retrieval software is another important issue to consider. Good database software will assist in image capture and make it possible to store images so that they can be easily retrieved. Many database programs will allow searching for images using the patient's name, date photographs were taken, the diagnosis, procedure performed, the physician's name, or by a patient number (Fig. 55.10). Many different database software packages are on the market, although very few are specifically geared toward skin cancer photography. One such system is Canfield Scientifics' Photo File and Mirror software (www.canfieldsci.com). These two particular packages were designed specifically for medical photography. Using this software, images can be transferred directly into the database from the camera without the use of cards or disks. Another imaging database system specific to medical photography is iBase (*www.ibase.com*) which exhibits many of the same features. When making your software decision, always keep in mind which functions are most important for your practice.

Search and query functions usually rank as one of the most important tools a database can provide. Unless the images stored in the database are easily retrievable, they are nearly useless. For example, if dysplastic nevi are being followed, it is important that a patient's previous photographs be accessible when they arrive for their current appointment for photographic comparison (Fig. 55.11). Also, if there are several physicians using the same database, it is important that each patient's images be tagged with the attending physician's name so that each of the doctors can pull up a list of their particular patients. It can also be very important to be able to use diagnoses, patient names or assigned patient numbers as search criteria. Another helpful feature to look for is software that will store the dates all photographs were taken so that an accurate timeline can be established.

USE OF PHOTOGRAPHY FOR BASELINE COMPARISON EXAMINATION OF PATIENTS AT HIGH RISK FOR SKIN CANCER

Total-body photography has been found useful in the identification of thin melanomas in patients who have dysplastic nevi when used in conjunction with regular cutaneous examinations by the physician and patient education in the art of self-examination of the skin.

There are many ways that such documentation can be accomplished. For the patient with a few lesions a simple Polaroid (Macro 5) can be used to capture the clinical information. For a patient with many pigmented lesions, a more extensive approach is necessary. A 35 mm camera with a normal macro lens and on camera flash or a studio lighting set-up by a professional medical photographer has served this purpose for many years. The body is divided into 25 sections (Table 55.1), an adhesive ruler is placed on the back and the camera lens is focused at 3 ft from the patient (the front on the lens usually has this information). The photographs are taken using the body focusing technique previously described in this chapter. The photographer stands 3 ft from the patient, with one foot in front of the other and shifts slightly back and forth until the image is in sharp focus. This will create sharp images that consistently have the same image size in each exposure. With the ruler in place, it becomes an easy task to know the size of all lesions. A quick test in the manual mode of a camera will determine the correct f-stop for usage. Simply using the automatic mode may seem easier, but it often does not provide a reliable result and consistent image quality.

For those that have made the transition to digital, an SLR digital camera is best suited for total-body photography. Point and shoot digital cameras demonstrate a real weakness capturing pigmented lesions from a distance. Professional photographers use a digital back to capture their images as it is superior to film and provides excellent images of skin markings in pigmented lesions and use a controlled studio environment to maximize results. The data can be collected and stored in a digital archive (Fig. 55.12). It should be noted that such a setup can be quite expensive (US$20,000 and above) and typically is not practical for the average physician environment.

Other wavelengths beyond visible light are being employed to enhance clinical photography. Long wave UVA (360 nm) lighting can be used to accentuate pigmentary changes associated with dermatoheliosis (Fig.

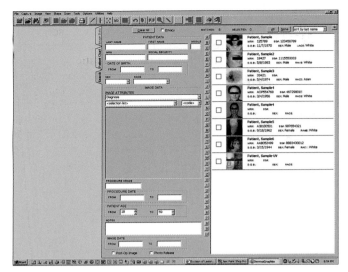

Figure 55.10 Screen from software package that allows for storage and retrieval of patient and lesion images.

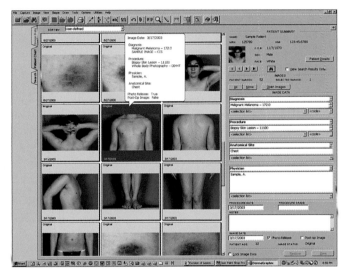

Figure 55.11 Lesion image search screen.

	Table 55.1 Anatomic sites for photographs in whole-body series
1.	Posterior upper aspect of the thorax
2.	Posterior left lower aspect of the thorax
3.	Posterior right lower aspect of the thorax
4.	Posterior aspect of the thigh
5.	Posterior aspect of the leg
6.	Lateral aspect of the right leg having the left leg in front
7.	Lateral aspect of the right thigh
8.	Lateral right aspect of the thorax, arm raised
9.	Lateral right aspect of the face and neck (including the top of the shoulder)
10.	Posterior aspect of the right arm
11.	Posterior aspect of the right forearm and the hand
12.	Lateral left aspect of the face and neck (including the top of the left shoulder)
13.	Posterior aspect of the left arm
14.	Posterior aspect of the left forearm and the hand
15	Lateral left aspect of the thorax, arm raised
16.	Lateral aspect of the left thigh
17.	Lateral aspect of the left leg having the right leg in front.
18.	Anterior aspect of the legs
19.	Anterior aspect of the thighs
20.	Anterior aspect of left inner thigh
21.	Anterior aspect of right inner thigh
22.	Anterior right lower aspect of the thorax
23.	Anterior left lower aspect of the thorax
24.	Anterior upper aspect of the thorax
25.	Anterior aspect of the face and inner aspect of right and left arm

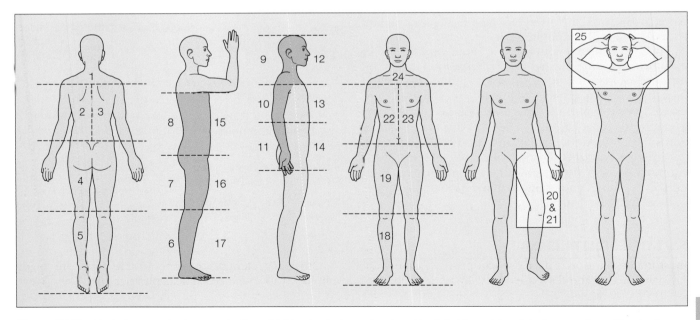

Figure 55.12 Typical anatomic site organization of full body photography stored in digital format for clinical comparison. (Numbering as per Table 55.1.)

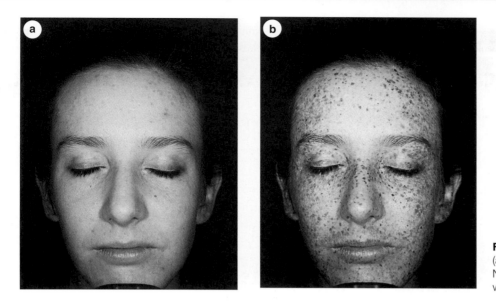

Figure 55.13 Photo of face taken in (a) visible light versus (b) long-wave UV. Note accentuation of photo-damage when viewed under UV lighting.

55.13a, b). Infrared bands (700–1000 nm) are also being used to display newer features that can be helpful in differential diagnosis of pigmented lesions. This approach is more fully described in Chapter 36.

OTHER CONSIDERATIONS IN SKIN CANCER PHOTOGRAPHY

Although a database is an invaluable tool to keep images catalogued and accessible, some images may eventually be used for more than patient follow-up. A patient may request copies of their images to be sent to another consulting physician, prints might need to be made for a chart, or you may wish to use some images for lectures or publication. For these reasons, images should also be exportable from the software in TIFF or JPEG format. These files can then be printed (although most image cataloging applications have a built-in printing function), e-mailed to other physicians involved directly in the patient's care, used in PowerPoint presentations, or burned to a CD and sent for publication.

Finally, a patient should sign a photography consent form before having pictures taken. Permission should be obtained at that time for all possible future uses of the images including patient follow-up, teaching, lecture usage, publication and clinical pathology correlations. Recently in the US, the HIPAA (Health Insurance Portability and Accountability Act of 1996) regulations governing medical records have made obtaining patient consent necessary. It was always good practice, but now it is even more important to have written, informed consent from the patient.

FUTURE OUTLOOK

The change from film to digital photography will be complete within the next few years. Major advances in both hardware and software for photo documentation have been occurring and will continue to do so. Better and faster methods of image capture and more efficient methods of data storage will continue to evolve. No matter what methods are employed, photo documentation will continue to play a critical role in the management of patients with or at high risk of the development of skin cancer.

ACKNOWLEDGMENT

I would like to thank Anne Stoecker and Canfield Scientific for their contribution to this chapter.

REFERENCES

1 Slue WE. Photographic cures for dermatologic disorders. Arch Derm 1989; 125:160–162.

2 Slue WE. Snapshot versus medical photographs. Cutis 1993; 51:345.

3 Slue WE. Better dermatologic office photography: getting started. Cutis 1994; 54:177–178.

4 Slue WE. Better dermatologic office photography: taking the photograph. Cutis 1994; 54:271–272.

5 Kopf AW, Slue W, Rivers JK. Photographs are useful for detection of malignant melanoma in patients who have dysplastic nevi. J Am Acad Derm 1988; 19:1132–1134.

6 Slue WE. Photography. In: Ratz JL, ed. Textbook of Dermatologic Surgery. Philadelphia, PA: Lippincott-Raven; 1998:75–94.

7 Progue D. State of the art; photography is easy; it's the shopping that's hard. The New York Times 2003; 3 April (Section G):1.

CHAPTER
56

Medical and Legal Aspects of Skin Cancer Patients

Abel Torres

Key points

- A common reason for a malpractice action is a failure in communication between the physician and patient.
- When a complication occurs during skin cancer treatment, maintaining the patient's trust is key to successful patient care and is helped by availability and close communication between the physician, the patient and significant others.
- Avoid discussing and making premature conclusions regarding an adverse event/complication in skin cancer care until all the facts are clear.
- Informed consent/refusal is based on the principle of autonomy and requires a meeting of the minds between the physician and patient which is more of a process than an act.
- When practicing innovative therapy for skin cancer treatment consider which reputable similarly situated skin cancer specialists would support that kind of treatment as expert witnesses.

INTRODUCTION

The treatment of skin cancer involves the art and science of medicine. In addition, physicians and patients have legal rights and responsibilities as it relates to medical treatment. For the most part those rights and responsibilities parallel good patient care. Thus, it is incumbent upon physicians treating skin cancer to balance the art and science with those legal rights and responsibilities. Yet, the current medico-legal environment in the US has created a malpractice climate that is causing doctors to limit the care they provide to patients and sometimes leave the practice of medicine altogether.[1] The result is that patient care is currently being adversely impacted.[1] Politics will determine part of the outcome of the current malpractice crisis, but physicians can also play a role directly by understanding the legal issues involved and managing them appropriately to effect good patient care, minimize malpractice exposure and avoid having to limit care. This is the reason for this chapter on the medico-legal aspects of skin cancer.

The legal responsibilities of patients and physicians are governed by Federal and State Legislative Statutes, Administrative rules, Regulations and Common Law promulgated by the Courts. Therefore, the legal rights and responsibilities of physicians and patients may vary from state to state. Although this chapter should serve as a useful educational tool for the physician, it is not a substitute for the advice of an attorney when potential or actual medico-legal issues arise.

MEDICAL MALPRACTICE

The most common legal risk for physicians caring for skin cancer patients is medical malpractice. One in five dermatologists may face a medical liability claim, but 35% of the claims are either dropped or dismissed in favor of the physician.[2,3] According to an analysis conducted on 78,712 malpractice cases, improper medical performance accounted for one-third of all claims and the second most common medical misadventure claim was for 'Errors in Diagnosis'.[2,3] A significant number of claims against dermatologists are related to conditions and procedures dealing with skin cancer management and surgical procedures.[3]

Medical Malpractice Law is based on a number of different theories (causes of action) which the accuser (plaintiff) can use to bring an action against the doctor (defendant). This section discusses medical malpractice as it relates to the Tort Law of Negligence (which compensates individuals for the losses they suffer due to the unreasonable acts of another person).

Negligence is the result of conduct which involves the breach of a duty to conform to a standard which in turn results in a foreseeable harm to another.[4] Medical negligence requires: the establishment of a duty by the physician, the breach of that duty by the physician, a reasonably close causal connection between the conduct and the resulting injury (Actual and Proximate Cause) and an actual injury (Damages).[4]

A duty to a given patient will generally exist when the physician–patient relationship is established. This usually requires some form of contact with the patient which can even consist of gratuitous advice or service and can even lack physical contact.[5,6] The courts will usually imply the duty to have been present, if the physician undertook to treat the patient or if his/her actions created a reasonable expectation of treatment by the patient.[7] If the physician does not want to establish a relationship by telephone or other contacts with individuals, the physician or staff should be careful about giving advice or directions upon which the person may rely for treatment. In fact, in certain circumstances it would probably be prudent to assert this to the individual and remind the individual to seek further advise or evaluation from another physician or remind the individual that they may need future assessment in a setting where they can be properly evaluated.

A patient appointment is usually considered to be an agreement to see a patient and not sufficient to establish a relationship. Some courts have ruled that if the appointment is for treatment of a specific problem, in certain circumstances, this may constitute an agreement to treat a specific illness and thus imply a relationship.[8] Thus, it would be prudent for a dermatologist to follow-up on appointments missed by patients, especially where the physician is the only one capable of providing the service.

If a physician owes a duty to his patients, what is the scope of that duty? A physician owes a duty to his patients to act with the knowledge, care and skill exercised by reasonable and prudent practitioners under similar circumstances.[9] Although the standard that a physician is held to is usually the standard in the community in which doctors practice, increasingly as a result of modern tools of communication such as the internet, that standard is held to be to, conform to the knowledge, care and skill practiced by physicians nationally.[10] If a physician performs a procedure traditionally performed by a specialist, the physician will likely be held to the standard of that specialty.[11]

The breach of a duty by a physician requires a showing that the physician deviated from the standard of care.[4,9,10] Unless the act is within the common knowledge of a non-medical person or covered by the doctrine of *Res Ipsa Loquitur*, expert testimony by another physician is required to show what that standard was and that a breach of duty occurred. The reason there is a need for expert testimony is that lay people cannot be expected to fully understand the nuances of medical decision making without the proper training.

For the skin cancer specialist, a standard of care issue that can arise is, how much of a skin exam is enough? Should the exam focus only on the lesion in question, or should a complete skin exam be performed? Some physicians advocate that a complete exam is essential since a physician is better situated to advise the patient of an important versus unimportant lesion. If this is held to be the standard of care, then physicians that do not offer to perform a complete exam on their patients may fail to meet the standard of care if they only examine the mole on the face and fail to find the melanoma on the back.

Other skin cancer specialists counter that such an approach puts a tremendous economic strain on an already broken health care system for an unproven benefit. They argue that education of patients would have a more effective and wider impact than random complete skin exams and preserve funds for actual treatment of skin cancer. For these physicians, the standard of care can be met with a focused exam.

Unfortunately, establishing the standard of care has essentially become a battle of opposing experts for the hearts and minds of judges or juries with the most persuasive expert usually prevailing. Thus, the reality for a dermatologist wishing to practice within the standard of care is that a dermatologist should choose what is in the patient's best interest. However, one must keep in mind that if the dermatologist follows the path of the majority, it will make it easier to find supportive expert witnesses should a malpractice suit ensue. Other important issues arise in this area. For example, if the dermatologist is practicing a form of innovative therapy followed by few, if any practitioners, this will make it that much harder to find supportive expert witnesses. The latter, unfortunately, is a disincentive to promoting innovation in health care and promotes more of a herd mentality. Yet, should we not encourage innovation in health care? For many years, according to the majority, the standard of care in the treatment of melanoma, was that the wider and deeper the excision, the better it was for the patient. Today, thanks to a courageous few, we realize what a disservice was done by adhering to this majority standard of care. So what is the standard of care when the Mohs Micrographic Surgery Technique is used to treat melanoma and the randomized prospective studies have addressed instead 1.0, 2.0, and 4.0 cm wide local excisions? Is the fact that this is not the majority practice or the focus of the major prospective studies, put this out of the standard of care? What is the lesson to be gleamed from prior unproductive majority practices for melanoma? Does the evidence-based medicine seal of approval need to be present for a practice to be within the standard? These issues can be argued in an endless cycle of point *vs* counterpoint, without a clear answer. Aggravating this problem further is that since the future role of practice guidelines in establishing the standard of care is unclear, physicians would be well advised to be familiar with practice guidelines as they relate to their area of practice. A dermatologist should select what is in the patient's best interests, but in today's legal climate, would be wise to inquire if the innovative skin cancer care he chooses to use is supported by at least some other reputable practitioners in the community.

As previously mentioned, an exception to the need for expert testimony is the doctrine of *Res Ipsa Loquitur*, 'The Thing Speaks for Itself'. Under this doctrine, a plaintiff does not need to prove a breach of the standard of care if the injury is of the type that could not occur absent negligence, the defendant was in control of the situation or instrumentality that caused the injury and the plaintiff did not cause the injury.[12] Although *Res Ipsa Loquitur* is not accepted in all of the US, dermatologists need to be aware of its acceptance in their state and its implication that negligence can be presumed in certain situations without the benefit of having a live expert whose credibility can be tested.

Even if there is a breach of duty by the physician, it is not necessarily medical negligence, unless the patient-plaintiff can establish that he/she was actually damaged (injured) and there was a foreseeable and actual causal link between the breach of the standard of care and the injury to the patient.[13,14] This damage can be physical, such as a scar, or it can be psychological, such as anxiety, depression and even 'fear of' contracting a disease. Skin cancer is a condition often fraught with many anxieties, fears and misunderstandings. Physicians should communicate carefully with their patients and look to address their anxieties and fears regarding skin cancer, therefore promoting good patient care while at the same time pre-empting possible legal damages.

Even if a physician is found to be negligent, a court judgment may be reduced or nullified if the patient-plaintiff was also negligent by helping to cause the injury or did not take steps to mitigate the damage. If patients do not advise the physician that there is a problem, or fail to follow instructions, the patients may be held accountable for their non-compliance. Thus, it is prudent for physicians to follow-up on their care of patients, or provide readily available access for patient questions or concerns. This is true not only because this approach promotes good skin cancer care but also so that patients are held accountable for their actions. This is also important since problems with proper timing of care and monitoring of patients appear to be at the top of the list when malpractice claims are ranked according to the size of the payout.[15]

CONSENT/REFUSAL FOR TREATMENT

In the treatment of skin cancer, obtaining consent for treatment would appear to be an oxymoron. Yet, physician failure to obtain informed consent or informed refusal could potentially result in legal allegations of an intentional tort (assault or battery), breach of contract, or negligence. For instance, how much consent does a skin cancer specialist need to obtain for a skin exam or refusal of an offered exam? Negligence appears to be the most frequently employed allegation in instances where informed consent or informed refusal was not obtained or was defective.[16] It is of paramount importance that physicians understand the nuances involved in obtaining proper consent for the treatment of skin cancer.

Simple consent

Consent by a patient permits the physician to provide treatment (touch the patient). It consists of the right by an individual to agree to treatment, based in the law of battery and the underlying concept that a person should be free from harmful or offensive touchings.[17] Rendering treatment to (touching) an individual without consent can result in a claim of a battery or a claim of assault (a fear of a harmful or offensive touching) and can subject the physician to a claim not covered by malpractice insurance.[18] A battery may also occur if the physician exceeds the scope of the patient's consent in providing the wrong treatment or performing the wrong procedure.[19] Absent, a misrepresentation by the physician, patient consent to the treatment (touching), constitutes a complete defense to an action for battery.[20]

Consent can be implied or expressed, oral or written. The courts have found implied consent to be present when the conduct of the patient indicates awareness and understanding of the planned treatment with the patient having an opportunity to withdraw.[21] Express consent can be in writing or orally. Relying on implied consent is risky since the burden will generally rest on the physician to prove that the patient's conduct implied

consent. Oral consent poses the problem of proving that consent was given while express written consent provides better evidence, should the veracity of consent be at issue.

Informed consent

Obtaining consent to treatment may avoid an action for battery but the physician still needs to obtain informed consent to treatment.[22] Generally, treatments involving medicines or medical and surgical procedures or devices are subject to informed consent requirements. To educate patients and protect patient autonomy in medical decision making, states require physicians to obtain informed consent which constitutes an affirmative decision by a competent individual to permit the physician to treat the patient in an agreed manner. Informed consent carries the obligations of obtaining patient consent prior to treatment, and disclosure of sufficient information so that patients can decide what treatment is in their best interest.[23] In contrast, an informed refusal situation is a special type of informed consent usually encountered when a competent individual decides to forego a recommended test or treatment. Both informed consent and refusal generally require disclosure of: uncommon but material (serious) risks, and common (likely) risks even if not (material) serious.[24]

In judging whether disclosure is adequate, a physician can use the two standards that the courts use as a guide. One standard is the Professional Standard, which promotes that a physician reveal the same information that other physicians would disclose in the same or similar circumstances.[25] The other standard, named the Legal Standard, is that a physician reveal the information that a reasonable person would consider material in deciding whether to undergo treatment.[26] The standard used by the courts varies according to the laws of each state.[27,28] Dermatologists should acquaint themselves with the standard used in their jurisdiction to ensure that their disclosure is both medically and legally adequate.

Informed consent and refusal takes on special importance in the treatment of skin cancer since there are so many modalities for treating these neoplasms. In addition, some skin cancer specialists may offer a complete skin exam which a patient may refuse. The best way for physicians to avoid problems with informed consent and informed refusal issues is to fully communicate. Patients need to be informed of the diagnosis or potential diagnosis, its natural course if untreated, the recommended treatment along with its potential benefits and risks, and the alternative viable treatments including their potential benefits and risks.[29] During the process of obtaining informed consent and/or informed refusal, the patient's questions can be answered and concerns addressed.

In general, courts have rejected a general duty to disclose a treatment or procedure a physician does not recommend.[30] This type of reasoning has been validated in an appeals court case from California (*Parris v Sands*).[31] But, the *Parris v Sands* court case implied that in a case involving surgery, cancer diagnosis, cancer treatment or other serious life-threatening procedures, there may need to be a different scope of discussion for alternative treatments depending on the situation. The Connecticut Supreme Court case of *Logan v Greenwich Hospital Association* also articulated that a patient might reasonably rely upon a specialist to provide further information. Thus, dermatologists should be careful when choosing not to discuss alternative treatments and should keep reasonably abreast with medical advances. Courts generally place the responsibility for obtaining informed consent on the physician, although nurses and other non-physicians can help inform the patient (Table 56.1).

MEDICAL RECORDS

A patient's medical records serve as a tool for planning patient care and as a chronological record. In addition, the contents of a medical record many times will be the only credible evidence available in a legal situation.[32] Thus, the completeness and accuracy of medical records is important for patient care and for malpractice defense.

The record should include positive or negative findings which are essential or customarily recorded for patient care.[33] All sources of information including discussions with the patient or related third parties in or out of the office should be documented whenever possible.[33] The record should reflect pertinent informed consent discussions, diagnostic considerations, treatment plans, as well as any instructions or warnings given to the patient and related third parties.[33]

A medical record should mainly include information for the patient's care and avoid self serving entries such as risk prevention activity by the physician or economic issues (failure of the patient to pay) unless they have a bearing on patient care.[33] Adverse events or complications are best documented in the records using terms that describe the event and avoid premature conclusions.[33] Threats and complaints by the patient or others are best recorded as to how they may impact patient care.[33] Statements must be accurate and not deliberately misleading.[33]

Altering a medical record can affect the record's credibility and the credibility of the physician, as well as create legal liability.[33] A record should not be altered unless it will benefit the patient (e.g. to note an error regarding an allergy).[33] Some attorneys recommend that any corrections should be initialed and dated and the erroneous entry lined out unless an error is recognized while making a new entry in a page with no other entries where it may be appropriate to rewrite the page.

Any alteration attributable to the physician may undermine the usefulness of the record for patient care or for the defense of the physician even if the alteration is insignificant or the facts of the case do not support a finding of malpractice (Table 56.2).[33]

Many in the field of risk management believe that a written, as opposed to oral informed consent or informed refusal that is signed by the patient and incorporated into the medical record before treatment is given or withheld, constitutes good documentation and may diminish a patient's perception of the chance for successful litigation. Some risk managers advocate that if oral informed consent is obtained, a note be recorded in the patient's medical record by the physician regarding the informed consent or refusal. Others further advocate that the patient signs or initials that note and/or also have the patient sign a written consent document. When documenting that informed consent has been obtained, the physician is often faced with the issue that writing voluminous amounts is not very efficient for patient care and carries the risk of the physician inadvertently not documenting a disclosed risk or alternative. On the other hand a skimpy note in the chart may be argued to be perfunctory and not indicative of the interactive process required of informed consent.

The preferred approach by this author is to maximize the patient's chart use for patient care purposes by recording a brief note in the patient's chart that reflects a broad description stating that the risks(R), benefits(B) and alternatives(A) of a particular diagnosis and or treatment plan were discussed with the patient and that consent or refusal to treatment was obtained. To avoid the implication that this is a perfunctory note, the author generally advocates that the brief note indicate that an issue or issues particularly relevant to the patient in question was discussed. For example, 'R,B,A, of surgical excision was discussed with the patient with emphasis

Table 56.1 Checklist for informed consent/refusal requirements

- Competent adult or authorized decision maker
- Common (likely) even if not serious (material) risks
- Uncommon but serious (material) risks
- Less need to discuss common knowledge or unlikely non-material risks

Table 56.2 Checklist for medical record keeping

- Should be complete but concise
- Avoid self serving or disapproving comments
- Should be consistent (avoid long notes in response to risk management which in a sea of brief notes may herald unwanted suspicion)
- Describe the facts and make conclusions when essential for patient care (e.g. wound dehisced, but avoid premature conclusion as to why unless pertinent)
- Alter only if essential for patient care and show no intent to mislead by, lining out items, initialing and dating the change or when possible entering a new note that refers to the correction without altering the initial entry.
- Only release copy of records after receiving proper authorization and according to HIPAA guidelines.
- Consider keeping billing records separate from patient care records.
- Always document from a patient care perspective (e.g. if documenting a threat explain the potential effect on physician–patient relationship, etc.)

on this patients high risk of scarring or pigmentary changes'. When feasible, the author also has the patient read, discuss and sign a written informed consent form that is placed in the chart, but this should be decided by the circumstances involved.

The patient's record is subject to an ethical and legal duty of confidentiality and under the US Federal Health Insurance Portability and Accountability Act (HIPAA) as well as State laws unauthorized release of that information can have serious civil and or criminal consequences for a physician. Physicians should be well aware of HIPAA and corresponding state laws, which in some cases may be even stricter than HIPAA. A physician's medical records are his/her private property, but HIPAA and most states allow the patient access to the records either directly, or through an authorized representative such as a physician, a lawyer, insurance company or other statutory exceptions.[34] Any release of records should be authorized in writing by the patient and carefully documented. A copy of the record should be released since the record could get lost and it is the physician's responsibility to keep those records safe.

ADVERSE EVENTS AND COMPLICATIONS IN SKIN CANCER TREATMENT

Macmillan's dictionary defines a complication as a difficulty, hurdle or obstacle and an adverse event as: 'not helpful to what is wanted, unfavorable, bad, poor or harmful'.[35] Not every complication is an adverse event, but since an adverse event is likely to lead to patient dissatisfaction and can activate the legal process, we will discuss complications as if they are adverse events.[36] The management of a clinical/surgical complication requires that the clinician approach the event in a manner that minimizes the impact to the desired clinical outcome and the activation of the legal process. A crucial element needed in dealing with adverse clinical/surgical events is one that emphasizes strengthening the trust between the patient and the clinician, since this erosion in trust can impede patient care and result in litigation.[37]

Honesty is the cornerstone of trust

Few would disagree with honesty being the cornerstone of trust, but dishonesty is not always so clear. Some physicians advocate that if a mistake is intercepted before it harms the patient, it should be disclosed internally to correct a system weakness but not disclosed to the patient and risk needless damage to patient trust. Is not disclosing this type of mistake, dishonesty?[36] Similarly, medical care and medical decision making can be simple or complex and the end result of a medical intervention is unpredictable.[38] What may be considered the correct approach for one person may in fact be the wrong approach for another and whether an intervening act or omission is a mistake may be better judged by the final outcome. Do these intervening acts or omissions need disclosure to assure honesty or would this needlessly erode patient trust and ultimately patient care?

In 1996, a survey of patients' attitudes towards doctors' mistakes was published in the *Archives of Internal Medicine*. The survey interviewed 149 responding patients, randomly chosen from among 10,000 patients seen at Loma Linda University Medical Center, a Health Sciences University Medical Center located in Loma Linda, California, which includes a medical school. The patients were presented with three hypothetical scenarios of a minor, moderate and severe mistake made by a doctor. The survey revealed that patients want physicians to acknowledge their mistakes no matter how minor, but would lose some measure of trust with a disclosure by the physician. Yet, it was even more damaging to the physician–patient trust if the physician failed to disclose a mistake and it was later discovered by the patient. The latter circumstance was more likely to lead the patient to sue or report the doctor.[39] Thus, it is clear that patients value honesty in their interactions with doctors and physicians would do well to keep honesty foremost as a guide to their actions when dealing with adverse events. The physician needs to honestly communicate with the patient, but should not engage in a premature rush to honesty without a full reconciliation of the facts since this may in fact be dishonest communication and lead to needless erosion of patient trust, impede corrective action and possibly result in premature litigation.

Remedying an adverse event

It goes without saying that when an adverse event occurs, the clinician needs to take positive measures to minimize the impact of that adverse event on the desired clinical outcome.

Positive measures
Positive measures refers to dealing with the situation in a manner that is productive. Empathy or sympathy with the patient's distress is productive in that it communicates that you are concerned about their well-being. On the other hand, expressing premature remorse when the facts have not been fully sorted out may lead to distrust and hinder patient care. Expressing self criticism or thinking out loud may stimulate the physician to be creative in remedying the situation since physicians are trained to consider differential diagnoses no matter how unlikely and ultimately discard those that are not plausible. However, a non-medically trained individual can misconstrue a differential diagnosis as a list of mistakes or omissions that occurred or incompetence by the physician. This is similar to a pilot discussing her options over the loudspeaker when the airplane is having difficulties. The latter would not be appreciated or inspire confidence with the passengers. Thus, physicians should problem solve but be careful about thinking out loud in the presence of the patient.

Another positive measure is to acknowledge any complaint by a patient as an opportunity to gather more data and investigate a situation. Physicians would do well not to dismiss a patient's complaint, no matter how trivial. One of the most important productive positive measures is to make sure that the patient's medical needs are appropriately addressed including referral for consultations, as needed. Procrastinating a referral is a negative measure that could force the patient to shop around for help and risks treatment by clinicians that may not be properly trained for the problem or who may make comments to hide their own inadequacies. Comments by other healthcare providers have been documented to be a frequent source for undermining the physician–patient trust and initiating litigation.[36]

Communication

People are social beings that seek comfort from others such as family and friends (support group). When an adverse event occurs it is to those same individuals that the patient will look to for comfort and advice. If the support group understands what is happening they can assist the patient, provide reassurance and avoid making inflammatory remarks. Aside from the inflammatory remarks of other healthcare practitioners precipitating litigation, so too do the remarks of friends and family.

In communicating with an angry patient and their support group, a physician should empathize and accept responsibility for the care of the patient but not accept blame prematurely. The discussion should center around factual issues, clearing up misperceptions and clarifying the course of action that will be taken. Premature opinions by the physician should be avoided and any theories by the patient and support group should be acknowledged with the clarification that further data will be gathered and all possibilities explored. Premature finger pointing without all the facts should be avoided since the pointer may be mistaken and human nature is such that it only makes others defensive and wanting to point back, initiating an endless cycle of blame.

Access must be present at all times. Physicians should make sure that they or a designated member of their staff are readily available or reachable by the patient or support group to answer questions and assist as needed. If the physician is not available to the patient to discuss their concerns, they will look for someone who will listen.

In our haste to communicate honestly with the patient, we must not forget that patients have a right to privacy.[40] HIPAA rules underscore the need to protect confidentiality.[41] Thus, prior to initiating any communication with a patient's support group, a physician should procure the patient's consent for this action, preferably with documentation in writing and depending on the jurisdiction, HIPAA regulations or more stringent local laws may mandate the process to be followed. Physicians should keep abreast of these rules and regulations.

Facts vs assumptions (opinions)

When an adverse event occurs, nothing should be assumed and the situation should be investigated fully. The facts as understood by the patient, physician and the healthcare team need to be understood and reconciled. When an adverse event occurs, the comments that take place in and out of the office as well as perceptions of the facts by the patient, physician and staff can vary widely. It is not uncommon for a patient or staff member to be aware of a fact that the physician has not been

made privy to. It is also common knowledge that if you whisper a comment in a person's ear and wait to hear the comment as it travels around a circle of people, the comment you hear at the end will often be very different from what you initially said. It is only reasonable to expect that such a distortion of the facts can occur in a clinical setting that involves the patient, their support group, physicians and the clinical staff. Becoming aware of and understanding all the facts allows us to clear up misperceptions by the patient, physician and/or the staff.

The physician should address all inquiries from the patient and support group himself or, alternatively, designate a staff member for that task in order to assure consistency for the patient, accuracy of communications and ease anxieties. It can be confusing for a patient to hear different explanations to their questions and any differences can be interpreted by the patient as inconsistencies or hint at subterfuge.

It is important to avoid voicing premature opinions without weighing all the facts. Unfortunately, the legal process can misinterpret any comment or opinion by a physician or staff member as an admission of guilt.[42] Yet, the sharing of opinions helps to stimulate discussion, learning, and quality assurance and physicians are often trained to discuss differential diagnoses with the health care team.

Thus, it is only natural that physicians would carry on these same type of exercises in their offices and discuss opinions with their staff as to what occurred during an adverse event. However, it is not uncommon for a physician or staff member to be asked during a deposition about what comments or opinions have been voiced out of the courtroom in an effort to ferret out these so called admissions. Therefore, it is wiser for physicians to discuss only facts with their staff or others until they have sufficient facts to arrive at a valid opinion and conclusion. Nevertheless, the need to speak out loud or express an opinion is often a way for a physician to release anxiety. Fortunately, the legal process allows us the privilege of communicating with our spouse, attorney and sometimes clergy to express our frustrations and opinions without fear of repercussion.

Documentation

A well-documented patient chart will assure that the information needed to take care of a patient is available. The physician should factually record the adverse event and response and unless it adds to the care of the patient, premature opinions and conclusions should be avoided. The key consideration should be how any entry will help the patient's care. Thus, the record should only be altered when essential for patient care.

Preserving the medical record and evidence

The patient's medical record is important for patient care and as evidence, and should be carefully handled to preserve its accuracy and confidentiality.[32–34] As such, the original records should never be released unless mandated by legal proceedings.[32–34] This protects the accuracy and reliability of the records. Commonly, a medical device may be used in providing patient care and an adverse event can be the result of a defective device. Therefore, advice from a manufacturer or vendor regarding the device should be sought if needed, but the device used should not be returned until its defect or lack of defect has been properly documented. A manufacturer may be subject to strict product liability for its devices, which can ease the litigation burden for the physician.[43]

Legal advice

If a physician receives requests for patient records, summons, legal complaint, or a threat or demand for compensation, they should immediately inform their attorney and/or medical malpractice carrier since failure to do so can result in non-coverage by the carrier. The advisability of writing off a bill should be discussed with and coordinated with an attorney or malpractice carrier. Some patients will see this as a gesture of goodwill, while others will see it as an admission of guilt and sue regardless of the adjustment. The courts and the National Practitioner Data Bank have not considered writing off a bill as either an admission of guilt or a reportable incident.[36] Patients may have paid for a service with specific expectations. Just as we would not want to pay in full for a service that was only partially performed, a patient may not want to pay in full for a procedure that only partially met their expectations. It behooves the physician to understand the motives behind his patient's request to accurately assess whether writing off a bill can help defuse a potentially inflammatory situation after an adverse event. The author disagrees with nay-sayers that insist writing off a bill is never an option. Table 56.3 summarizes the physician's approach to dealing with medico-legal complications.

SUMMARY

When dealing with an adverse event, treating physicians should take positive and not negative measures. They should be honest with the patient and the family as

appropriate. All facts should be reconciled with the health care team (office staff). Assessments and interventions should be well documented in the medical record with special care not to alter or give the appearance of altering the medical record. Any type of evidence involved in the occurrence should be preserved. Contacting the physician's liability carrier, risk management service or attorney should also be foremost in the mindset of the physician since risk of litigation is part of the definition of an adverse event.

FUTURE OUTLOOK

The US legal system is geared towards maintaining the standard of care for all patients. We are more likely to become aware of its presence when a complication/adverse event occurs. Complications are to be expected in the care of skin cancer patients. Most complications will not necessarily result in adverse events and even when an adverse event occurs, maintaining patient trust is important for good patient care. Unfortunately, the current legal climate does not promote a climate of maintaining the trust between the physician and patient, which is essential for good patient care. Tort reform would be welcome in the future but does not seem imminent. Until then, the approach described in this chapter can help keep the lines of communication between the physician and patient open.

REFERENCES

1 Eisenberg D, Siegger M. The doctor won't see you now. Time Magazine, 9 June, 2003:46–62.

2 Altman, J. The National Association of Insurance Commissioner's (NIAC) Medical malpractice closed claim study, 1975–1978. J Am Acad Dermatol 1981; 5:721.

3 Physicians Insurers Association of America: PIAA Data Sharing Reports. 1 January, 1985–31 December, 1987. Lawrenceville, NJ: Copyright Physicians Insurers Association of America; 1988.

4 Prosser L, Owen DG, Keeton RE. Prosser and Keeton on the Law on Torts, 5th edn. St Paul: West Publishing Co; 1984: Section 30, 41:187.

5 *Hiser v Randolph*, 617 P.2d 774 (Ariz 1980)

6 *Hamil v Bashline*, 305 A2d 57 (1973)

7 *Betesh v United States*, 400 F Supp. 238 (DC1974)

8 *Lyons v Grether*, 239 SE 2d 103 (1977)

9 Fiscina FS. Medical Law for the Attending Physician. Carbondale, IL: Southern Illinois Press; 1982.

10 Sills, H. What is the Law? Dental Clin North Am 1982; 26:256.

11 Rapp JA, Rapp RT. Medical Malpractice: A Guide for the Health Sciences. St. Louis MO: CV Mosby Co.; 1988.

12 Prosser L, Owen DG, Keeton RE. Prosser and Keeton on the Law on Torts, 5th edn. St Paul: West Publishing Co; 1984; Ch. 6, Section 39:252–260.

13 Flamm MB. Medical malpractice: physician as defendant. In: Falk KH and ACLM, eds. Legal Medicine: Legal Dynamics of Medical Encounters, 2nd edn., Ch. 41. St Louis, MO: CV Mosby; 1991: 525–534.

Table 56.3	Complications – mnemonic
'COMPLICATIONS'	
C	Be candid, commiserate, acknowledge the complaint
O	Discuss facts, not opinion
M	Mitigate, address medical needs
P	Take positive, not negative measures
L	Accept responsibility, not liability
I	Investigate fully
C	Clarify, not criticize, and consult
A	Accessibility is important
T	Truth leads to trust
I	Inform carrier
O	Organize meeting to outline risks, benefits and alternatives
N	Note and document, not alter
S	Save evidence, sincerity above all

14 Prosser L, Owen DG, Keeton RE. Prosser and Keeton on the Law on Torts, 5th edn. St Paul: West Publishing Co; 1984, Ch. 7, Section 44:263–309.

15 Balsamo RR, Brown MD. Risk Management. In: American College of Legal Medicine, eds. Legal Medicine: Legal Dynamics of Medical Encounters, 3rd edn., Ch. 20. St Louis, MO: CV Mosby; 1995:237–259.

16 Meisel A, Kabnick L. Informed consent to medical treatment: an analysis of recent legislation. U Pitt Law Review 1980; 407:410.

17 *Schoendorff v New York Hospital*, 211 NY 215 (1914).

18 *Bommareddy v Superior Court*, 222 Cal.App. 3d 1017 (1990).

19 *Ashcraft v King*, 228 Cal.App.3d 604 (1991).

20 Prosser L, Owen DG, Keeton RE. Prosser and Keeton on the Law on Torts, 5th edn. St Paul: West Publishing Co; 1984:113.

21 Frank, T. Flannery, et al., Consent to Treatment, Legal Medicine: Legal Dynamics of Medical Encounters. St. Louis, MO: CV Mosby Company, 1988.

22 Waltz & Sheuneman, Informed consent to therapy. Nw.U L Rev 1970; 64(5):628.

23 *Cobbs v Grant*, 8 Cal 3d.229, 502 P.2d 1, (1972)

24 *Canterbury v Spence*, 150 US App. DC 263, 464 F2d 772 (1972)

25 Redden EM, Baker, BC. Medicolegal problems in the management of patients with skin cancer. In: Friedman RJ, Rigel DS, Kopf AW, et al. eds. Cancer of the Skin, Ch. 41. Philadelphia, PA: WB Saunders; 1991:603–610.

26 *Natanson v Kline*, 350 P2d 1093 (1960).

27 Altman, J. One in five hit with malpractice claims in past ten years. Dermatology Marketing and Practice Management 1988; 2:2.

28 *Sard v Hardy*, 281 Md. 432 (1977).

29 *Logan v Greenwich Hosp. Ass'n,* 191 Conn. 282 (1983).

30 *Cobbs v Grant*, 8 Cal.3d 229 (1972).

31 *Parris v Sands*, 93 Daily Journal DAR 16233.

32 Holder AR. The importance of medical records. JAMA 1974; 228:118–119.

33 Tennenhouse J., Kasher MP. Risk Prevention Skills. San Rafael: Tennenhouse Professional Publications 1988:69.

34 Moorman CT, Armitage DT, Griggs EF, Hirsh HL. Medical records. In: Falk KH and ACLM, eds. Legal Medicine: Legal Dynamics of Medical Encounters, 2nd edn., Ch. 23. St Louis, MO: CV Mosby; 1991:237–253.

35 Levey JS. Macmillan Dictionary for Children, 2nd edn. New York: Simon and Schuster; 1989:12.

36 Keyes C., ed. Responding to Adverse Events. Forum: Risk Management Foundation of the Harvard Medical Institutions Inc., Adverse Events, 1997; 18(1):2–5.

37 Localio AR, Lawthers AG, Brennan TA, et al. Relationship between malpractice claims and adverse events due to negligence. N Engl J Med 1991; 325(4):245–251.

38 Anderson CA, ed. Evaluation and Management (F/U) Services Guidelines. Current Procedural Terminology. Chicago: AMA Press; 2001:1–7.

39 Witman A., Park D, Hardin S. How do patients want physicians to handle mistakes? A survey of internal medicine patients in an academic setting. Arch Int Med 1996; 156:2565–2569.

40 National Commission for the Protection of Human Subjects of Biomedical and Behavioral Research. The Belmont Report: Ethical Principles and Guidelines for the Protection of Human Subjects in Research, DHEW Pub No. (05) 78-0012. Washington DC: US Govt. Printing Office; 1979.

41 Health Insurance Portability and Accountability Act of 1996, Pub. L No.104–191 (Codified at 42 USC Section 1320d (1996).

42 California Jury Instructions 2.25: Extrajudicial Admissions, Cautionary Instructions. BAJI, 9th edn. 2000; 1:27.

43 California Jury Instructions 9.003: Products Liability – Strict Liability in Tort – Defect in Manufacture. BAJI, 9th edn. 2000; 5:324.

Index